D0667623

ANNUAL REVIEW OF
PHARMACOLOGY
AND TOXICOLOGY

EDITORIAL COMMITTEE (1985)

ANNUAL REVIEW OF PHARMACOLOGY AND TOXICOLOGY

VOLUME 25, 1985

ROBERT GEORGE, *Co-editor*

University of California School of Medicine, Los Angeles

RONALD OKUN, *Co-editor*

University of California School of Medicine, Los Angeles

ARTHUR K. CHO, *Associate Editor*

University of California School of Medicine, Los Angeles

ANNUAL REVIEWS INC.   4139 EL CAMINO WAY   PALO ALTO, CALIFORNIA 94306 USA

ANNUAL REVIEWS INC.
Palo Alto, California, USA

International Standard Serial Number: 0362–1642
International Standard Book Number: 0–8243–0425-X
Library of Congress Catalog Card Number: 61–5649

Annual Reviews Inc. and the Editors of its publications assume no responsibility for the statements expressed by the contributors to this *Review*.

Typesetting by Kachina Typesetting Inc., Tempe, Arizona; John Olson, President
Typesetting coordinator, Jeannie Kaarle

PRINTED AND BOUND IN THE UNITED STATES OF AMERICA

Annual Review of Pharmacology and Toxicology
Volume 25 (1985)

CONTENTS

(Continued)   v

viii

SOME RELATED ARTICLES IN OTHER *ANNUAL REVIEWS*

From the *Annual Review of Immunology*, Volume 3 (1985):

The Atomic Mobility Component of Protein Antigenicity, John A. Tainer, Elizabeth D. Getzoff, Yvonne Paterson, Arthur J. Olson, and Richard A. Lerner

Immunobiology of Myasthenia Gravis, Experimental Autoimmune Myasthenia Gravis, and Lambert-Eaton Syndrome, Jon Lindstrom

From the *Annual Review of Medicine*, Volume 36 (1985):

Beta-Adrenergic Blocking Drugs, John G. Gerber and Alan S. Nies

Elimination Half-Life of Drugs: Value and Limitations, David J. Greenblatt

Alzheimer's Disease, Donald L. Price, Peter J. Whitehouse, and Robert G. Struble

From the *Annual Review of Neuroscience*, Volume 8 (1985):

The GABA-ergic System: A Locus of Benzodiazepine Action, John F. Tallman and Dorothy W. Gallager

Adenosine as a Neuromodulator, Solomon H. Snyder

Neuropeptide Function: The Invertebrate Contribution, Michael O'Shea and Martin Schaffer

Applications of Monoclonal Antibodies to Neuroscience Research, Karen L. Valentino, Janet Winter, and Louis F. Reichardt

Neuropeptides in Identified Aplysia *Neurons*, Rashad-Rudolf J. Kaldany, John R. Nambu, and Richard H. Scheller

From the *Annual Review of Physiology*, Volume 47 (1985):

Physiology and Pharmacology of Gap Junctions, David C. Spray and M. V. L. Bennett

High-Energy Phosphate Metabolism in Vascular Smooth Muscle, Thomas M. Butler and Marion J. Siegman

Nucleotide Metabolism by Endothelium, Jeremy D. Pearson and John L. Gordon

Extracellular Functions of Nucleotides in Heart and Blood Vessels, Che Su

The Nature and Regulation of the Receptors for Pituitary Growth Hormone, J. P. Hughes and Henry G. Friesen

Mode of Action of Pituitary Growth Hormone on Target Cells, Olle G. P. Isaksson, Staffan Edén, and John-Olov Jansson

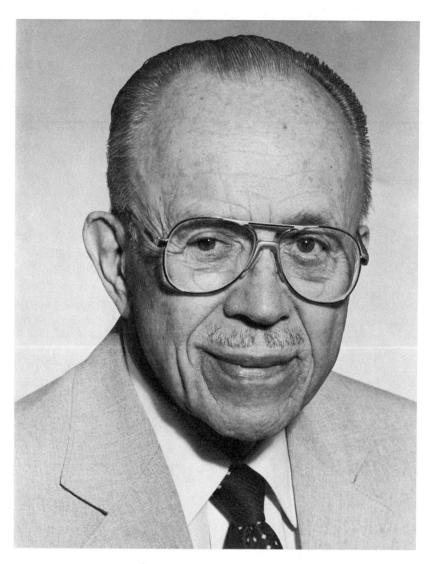

Arnold D. Welch

Ann. Rev. Pharmacol. Toxicol. 1985. 25:1–26

REMINISCENCES IN PHARMACOLOGY: AULD ACQUAINTANCE NE'ER FORGOT[1]

Arnold D. Welch

Division of Cancer Treatment, National Cancer Institute, National Institutes of Health, Bethesda, Maryland 20205

INTRODUCTION

Avoidance of personal pronouns in reminiscences is difficult; nevertheless, the main theme of this memoir will relate insofar as possible to its subtitle (with apologies to Robert Burns). Of necessity, this peripatetic writer has interacted with a great many colleagues during a period of over half a century. Marcia Davenport, in her autobiography (1), wrote beautifully, "I look back across the years and know of course that the real substance of my life, as of all lives, is the men and women with and through whom I have lived." And so it has been with me.

ORIGINS

My life began (7 November 1908) in a small New Hampshire town to which my parents had moved, after illnesses and business reverses, from Lynn, Massachusetts (where we were to return when I was eight). Of my ancestors, many of whom had settled in these areas in the seventeenth century, only the Reverend Stephen Bachiler seems particularly memorable (he even possessed a coat of arms!): he founded the first church in Lynn and then left hurriedly to

---

[1]The US Government has the right to retain a nonexclusive royalty-free license in and to any copyright covering this paper.

launch the town of Hampton, New Hampshire. The Reverend Stephen left a great many descendants, both in the colonies and in England (where he returned in his nineties); one of these, my maternal grandfather, was Colonel Joseph DeMerritt Batchelder (a colonel of what I have not discovered). Although at least doubly descended from Stephen, I had from 500 to 2000 lineal ancestors in the seventeenth century, of whom he was one; of the other 99.9% but little is known: par for the course in the USA. The original Welch in the colonies also derived from England, but the term *Welch* originally meant foreigner (a term appropriately applied to the vexatious Celts of Wales); hence, the surname Welch does not certify a Welshman. I especially regret that I cannot safely claim descent from the illustrious William Henry (Popsy) Welch, one of the founding fathers of The Johns Hopkins Medical School: Popsy died a bachelor. My sometimes mildly annoying middle name, DeMerritt, presumably was once de Mérite; this name, shared with my grandfather, was derived from his mother's family and now belongs to one of my grandsons (he is not yet old enough to regret its other connotations).

EDUCATION (THROUGH 1931)

My education began in the home, where my stern father's demands engendered little mutual affection. When I was seven he began, rather unsuccessfully, to expose me to French and Spanish; nevertheless, I am now grateful for his teaching, because my interests in linguistics, etymology, and grammar resulted (which perhaps contributed to my alleged editorial talents and to my being dubbed a *which*-hunter). The death of my mother when I was thirteen devastated me and adversely affected my scholastic performance. Fortunately, two years later my father retired to Florida, where I had a wonderful science teacher who encouraged my scholarship and devotion to chemistry. [This led to my eventual membership in the *23 Club* (in the Federated Societies *2* stands for biochemistry and *3* for pharmacology); for the older pharmacologists, however, such membership was a kiss of death. Times indeed have changed; otherwise, an invitation to write this prefatory chapter surely could not have been extended.]

My entrance into the University of Florida was helped by my successful competition for a scholarship, which so surprised my father and a bachelor uncle that I received more financial and moral support than I had expected; nevertheless, I always had at least one job while at the university. In spite of such distractions, I attained certain honors, such as Phi Beta Kappa, Phi Kappa Phi, and even Blue Key. In my fifth year, I began my studies in pharmacology; my first paper, with B. V. Christensen, appeared in 1932 in the *Journal of Pharmacology and Experimental Therapeutics*. My initial textbooks were those of Sollmann (whom I was to succeed at Western Reserve University in 1944) and of Meyer & Gottlieb as translated by Velyien E. Henderson (who was to guide my research to a PhD in 1934 at the University of Toronto). I was pleased in 1973 to receive the DSc (hc) from Florida thanks to my good friend Tom Maren.

Before moving to Toronto, I spent a pre-fellowship summer session in physiological chemistry at the University of Minnesota. The then chairman was not inspiring, but the professor of pharmacology at Minnesota, Arthur Hirsch-felder, gave me friendship, lab space, and an introduction to toxicology. A belated offer from Toronto's Henderson afforded me, then a lowly MS, the monetary equivalent of a post-doctoral teaching fellowship (then $1500). In those terrible depression years, such a fellowship was manna from heaven. My release from the anticipated fellowship in P-chem made it available to a friend from the University of Florida, Earle Arnow. A few years after finishing his PhD and MD, Arnow joined Sharp & Dohme as director of biochemical research. He succeeded me as director of research in 1944 and went on to an outstanding career at Merck, Sharp & Dohme and later at Warner-Lambert.

Here I must note the almost incredible effects on human lives that the apparently inconsequential act of a single individual can have. Henderson's belated offer to me, which had resulted only from the last-moment defection of a young MD unknown to me, had great impact on my life, on that of Arnow, on those of several thousand of our medical and graduate students, post-docs, and almost innumerable colleagues.

TORONTO YEARS (1931–1935)

The years in Toronto were eventful and sometimes chilling, both literally and figuratively. My initial course in physiology, presented by Best & Taylor before their classic textbook was first published, was stimulating. In Toronto I formed a deep and lifelong friendship with Tom Jukes (we even shared digs[1] for two years before he went off, as Dr. T. H. Jukes, to Berkeley as a post-doc). Both Charlie Best and Fred Banting befriended us; from them I learned a bit about the real story of insulin. I learned much more from Brock, the chief "diener" in pharmacology, a good friend of mine as well as of Sir Frederick-to-be. How Banting handled another of the four main scientific participants at Toronto when Collip refused to disclose his method for partial purification of the pancreatic principle is not to be found in most sources, but perhaps can be surmised. Henderson supported Banting when McLeod, with whom Banting was forced to share the Nobel Award, was unable to find funds for him. Although Best, a medical student, did not share the honor of the prize, Banting

---

[1]My first experiment in clinical pharmacology resulted from Tom's and my discovery that our lonely bottle of medicinal Scotch was being mysteriously emptied. Suspecting the nephew of our motherly landlady, I carefully calculated the necessary (but non-lethal) amount of emetine and added it to the residual spirit. The culprit identified himself very audibly and further problems were avoided without retaliation.

promptly gave him half of his share of the money, which shamed McLeod into doing likewise for Collip, while McLeod was offered a Scottish chair. Best had earned his MD by 1925; then, shortly after a few years with Dale in London (under whom he earned a DSc), he was appointed chairman of physiology at Toronto at the age of thirty. Thus, when I first met Best in 1931 he was only ten years older than I.

I grew very intolerant of the apparent complacency of many pharmacologists, who had neither the training for nor any interest in probing molecularly into drug actions. Certainly the idea that new drugs would some day be designed was yet to come (2). Classical pharmacologists regarded biochemistry with anathema rather than anticipation. Henderson, although he sometimes took a rather dim view of my biochemical leanings, was very tolerant, all things considered. It was Best, however, who encouraged my initial delvings into structure-activity relationships, especially among analogs of choline (later I continued these studies with Tom Jukes). Best and others had already shown choline to be required by depancreatized dogs maintained with insulin, and he encouraged my further studies of mechanisms with Huntsman.

New approaches to mechanistic studies of drug action had been initiated by the splendid book by A. J. Clark, poorly titled *Applied Pharmacology,* which introduced much biophysical analysis, but it was the work of Otto Loewi in Graz in 1920 that began the biochemical revolution. Vagal neurotransmission was shown to involve a biochemically labile entity [later identified as acetylcholine (ACh)] that was enzymically inactivated. Indeed, Loewi demonstrated that one of the most classical of drugs, eserine or physostigmine, exerts its powerful actions by inhibiting the inactivating enzyme. (Henderson moved promptly into this area and carried out his important studies on the chorda tympani nerve, ACh, and the submaxillary gland; however, it was his paper on the mechanism of erection that prompted many requests for reprints!) Loewi also probed the sympathetic neurotransmitters, which had been anticipated by Elliott and by Langley, although their studies had had little impact. The structure-activity studies of congeners of adrenaline by Dale and his associates Barger and Dudley offered clues not fully recognized at first. Nevertheless, the work of the brilliant Dale, by then Sir Henry (who had noted in 1914 that synthetic ACh mimicked the effects of parasympathetic nerve stimulation and that ACh was quickly inactivated by a tissue extract), led to the Nobel Prize for him and Loewi in 1936.[2]

---

[2]Had I had the courage of my convictions (a dated notebook outlines my reasoning), as well as the necessary experience and encouragement, I might have identified L-noradrenaline (the synthetic DL-form was then termed arterenol) as the sympathin E postulated by Cannon. Indeed, I obtained arterenol as well as D- and L-acids for its possible resolution, but other pressures prevailed. Hence, it remained for U. S. von Euler over ten years later to establish that L-noradrenaline is indeed the excitatory sympathetic neurotransmitter. As one wag recently stated, "You lose some and you lose some."

During my graduate years the adrenal medulla fascinated me, especially the claim by Kendall (of later cortisone fame) that the remarkable stability of adrenaline in the gland, compared with that of the pure compound, was attributable to its conjugation with lactic acid. With post-doc Don Heard, I perfused fresh bovine glands; we reported that gland-derived ascorbate in the perfusate prevented the oxidative inactivation of the catecholamines. This and another report on the mechanisms of oxidation and stabilization of adrenaline caught the attention of the Coris, who then used ascorbate to protect minute amounts of adrenaline during their studies on glycogenolysis. This fortunate circumstance led to correspondence, a meeting, a job and an MD degree for me.

Martin Roepke and I studied ACh as a cation and showed, with a model system, that it possibly was attached to an anionic receptor in or on cells. This led to my conviction that the quaternary N of ACh might be replaceable (so to speak) by quaternary P or As and that such synthetic compounds might behave qualitatively like ACh. Indeed they did, perfectly, although the P-analog exhibited 10–20% of the activity of ACh, while the As-analog had 1–2% of its activity. We also prepared the planar molecule: $(CH_3)_2S^+$-CH_2-CH_2-O-CO-CH_3 (Cl^-). This too was highly active and, like the other analogs, was inactivated by choline esterases, potentiated by eserine, and blocked by the classical drug atropine.[3]

Despite (or because of) these often exciting days, the Chief finally put his foot down and gave me some new alkaloids to study, saying that it would be good for me to learn some neuropharmacology. Perhaps the *real* reason was that these compounds had come from the Canadian National Research Council and had to be studied and I was the rather unwilling victim. The most interesting of these hydrastine-like alkaloids, bicuculline, was a powerful convulsant. Who could have guessed that nearly forty years later, when bicuculline had become a valuable tool in the study of GABA, I would be introduced by Professor Curtis in Canberra as the father of bicuculline? Indeed, Henderson was the father and I only an illegitimate son. The visit in Australia gave me then, as has occurred many times later, an opportunity to renew my warm friendship with Adrien Albert, the author of a real classic, *Selective Toxicity,* new editions of which continue to be in demand.

Henderson lectured to medical students cloaked in a decrepit baccalaureate gown. He always began by peering over his pince-nez with a somewhat

---

[3]In the synthesis of the S-analog of ACh, we were too impatient to wait for $(CH_3)_2S$ to be delivered and chose to synthesize it; fortunately, this was on a Saturday, because our attention wandered for a few moments and exothermia took over. Stinking $(CH_3)_2S$ shot out of the reflux condenser; the mess was cleaned up and the stench, to our relief, was abated by Monday. Had the disaster occurred on a weekday, the medical building would have been evacuated and our own evacuation could well have been permanent.

sardonic grin. After saying, in a very British manner, "In my laẃwst lect-chaw," he would continue in the speech of Upper Canada. The students loved it, although as individuals they were terrified of him, not without reason. The only other staff member, George Lucas, PhD, who was perhaps appropriately listed on the departmental letterhead as Ass. Prof., did not lecture. Henderson regularly took Tom Jukes, the post-docs, and me for an hour or two on Saturday mornings to drill us in scientific German. He even certified (doubtless with his fingers crossed) that Tom and I were qualified for our language requirements in French and German. May this very kindly scholar, who hid behind a mask of acerbity, rest in peace, as I wrote most sincerely in an obituary after his sudden death.

ST. LOUIS YEARS (1935–1940)

Under Carl Cori in St. Louis I became for a second time a scientific great-grandson of the reputed father of pharmacology, Schmiedeberg (actually a pupil of Bucheim in Dorpat). One of Schmiedeberg's pupils was H. H. Meyer; Henderson, in turn, had worked with Meyer in Marburg, and Cori also had worked with Meyer in Vienna and with Loewi in Graz. Cori's pharmacological credentials were as good as or better than those of certain classical pharmacologists who regarded Cori as an unsuitable occupant of the chair of pharmacology at Washington University, where the Coris had moved from Buffalo; their MD degrees had been earned in 1920 from the German University of Prague. Observed in Vienna by a Dr. Gaylord of the New York State Institute for the Study of Malignant Diseases (later to become the Roswell Park Memorial Institute), Carl and Gerty Cori were recruited in 1922; they were world-famous for their work in carbohydrate metabolism by 1931 (hence, a disgrace to pharmacology!). Carl Cori's thoughtful kindness to me was displayed immediately upon my arrival in St. Louis, albeit he mandated that I must obtain medical qualifications. This he made possible by wangling free tuition (as well as advanced standing) and by raising (somehow) my initial stipend from $600 to $800 (per year, not per month!). My wife, Mary, became an assistant mainly to the Coris; however, we also published two choline papers together. I published only once with Cori, a review on adrenaline; all other Cori-Welch papers are by Mary Welch. Initially, I had expected to be an assistant to the Coris, but Carl suggested that I prepare three research proposals; of these, he might approve one for my independent investigation (one was found approvable); otherwise, I would be his assistant. How many times have I wondered what would have have happened had I worked with the Coris rather than independently? Note what happened to Earl Sutherland, who later worked with Cori and then independently on what proved to be cyclic AMP; he succeeded me at Western Reserve in 1953 and won the Nobel Prize, as the Coris had in 1947.[4]

Cori approved my proposal to study arsenocholine as a labeled form of choline (in those days carbon-14 was not yet available, and the mass spectrometer for work with nitrogen-15 was not dreamed of). I hoped that arsenocholine not only would be nontoxic, but also would serve as a metabolic mimic of choline. The resynthesis of arsenocholine (not a job for one man) was made possible with the help of Sidney Colowick, then a new technician Cori loaned me.[5]

Arsenocholine worked like a charm as a lipotropic agent. It was converted to some extent by the liver to the arsenic analog of betaine $[(CH_3)_3As^+\text{-}CH_2COO^-]$. Clearly, the analog had to be synthesized, because betaine $[(CH_3)_3N^+\text{-}CH_2COO^-]$ had been found to be lipotropically active (transmethylation not yet having been discovered, it was thought that betaine might be reduced to choline); however, synthetic arsenobetaine proved not to be lipotropically active. Surprisingly, my S-analog of choline was too toxic to detect lipotropic activity (instability?); sulfobetaine $[(CH_3)_2S^+\text{-}CH_2\text{-}COO^-]$, however, was very effective as a lipotropic agent. It was likely, therefore, that sulfobetaine and betaine were donating one or more of their methyl groups for the biosynthesis of choline. Before this hypothesis could be tested and transmethylation established, duVigneaud, who knew of my work, renamed sulfobetaine dimethylthetine and hastened to publish without appropriate reference to my studies. Even some gods have feet of clay!

During my first post-MD year (1939–1940), Richard Landau, then a fourth-year medical student, did his BSc (Med) with me (Landau for many years has been a professor of medicine at Chicago and the distinguished editor of *Perspectives in Biology and Medicine*). We found great pleasure in working together then and in the friendship that has continued. The gold salts of choline-fractions derived from lecithin isolated from rats fed arsenocholine analyzed correctly with respect to the ratios of N:As:Au; thus, these fractions

[4]In competition for my attention with heavy teaching and research was an uninspiring course in anatomy. The professor (Terry) cared little for function and even less for holders of the PhD. When the female pelvis was dissected, I was attending the Federation meetings; hence, I was given an incomplete and told to report in June. I did, albeit reluctantly, as the speed and poor quality of my dissection displayed. Terry descended upon Cori (who also disliked anatomy and, I suspect, Terry as well) to complain about my performance. In no uncertain terms, Cori told me to get with it and do a perfect dissection. I did one so well that Terry found no hiatuses in my knowledge, but he barely passed me. I take some pride in the fact that, in spite of the magnanimous Terry, I graduated three years later (cum laude) with membership in Alpha Omega Alpha.

[5]Shortly after he had returned to Cori, Colowick, a chemical engineer then without experience with the tools of biochemistry, allowed the ungreased top of a desiccator to crash on the concrete floor directly in front of Cori's office. Cori emerged in horror (how short funds were in those days!) and said in essence, "This guy has gotta go." I like to believe that without my pleading this first of Cori's PhD students might have been lost to science and to his great career in biochemistry.

represented a mixture of choline and arsenocholine, the latter having functionally replaced much of the choline (3).

The days in St. Louis were exciting: the discovery and synthesis of the "Cori-ester" (glucose-1-phosphate); my close friendships with Carl and Gerty, Helen Graham, Gerhard Schmidt, F. O. Schmitt, my late brother-in-law Gordon H. Scott, Evarts Graham, the great surgeon, who offered me a career in anesthesiology, and many others of my colleagues; even those in my own medical class (dear friends still) who had to suffer my lectures and my grading of their papers. The offer to head a new research department of pharmacology at Sharp & Dohme (before its merger with Merck) came in 1940, at a time when I had no intention of ever leaving Cori. One sour note had been heard, however; the dean, despite Cori's urging, refused to promote me unless I did some "proper pharmacology," i.e. work on new sulfonamides. In my "spare time" I had already written (1937) the very first review of the "sulfa" drugs at the request of the *Journal of Pediatrics* (as I recall, it contained less than 40 references!). The mandate of the dean I found intolerable; thus, despite the belated offer of a promotion, an increase in salary from $2500 to $3500 per year, and a technician, I reluctantly parted from my dear friends, although I almost returned as Cori's successor in pharmacology only six years later. I had been elected to membership in ASPET in 1937 at age 28; however, when I became director of pharmacological research at Sharp & Dohme my membership was canceled, as the bylaws then required. Accordingly, the directory indicates that my membership dates from 1942, when, bylaw reform having occurred, I was reelected.

SHARP & DOHME (S & D) YEARS (1940–1944)

William A. Feirer (MD and DSc from The Johns Hopkins University), who had recruited me as director of pharmacological research, had just become director of research of S & D. We remained very close friends until he died only a few years ago. In view of my rejection of the sulfa drugs at Washington University, it was ironical, to say the least, that important discoveries of new sulfonamides by Jim Sprague and M. L. (Mel) Moore made study in this area mandatory for me while I was building a new department of pharmacology at S & D, the first of four. The small initial group included Paul A. Mattis, DSc, a most helpful colleague who later joined me in Cleveland, Albert Latven, a super technician, the animal man, and myself; however, the group grew rapidly to some twenty-five or thirty. The first of the new sulfonamides to show promise was a sulfamethylpyrimidine, which appeared superior to sulfapyrimidine, i.e. sulfadiazine; indeed, equal dosages gave much higher blood levels of the new drug, termed sulfamerazine. The latter was much better absorbed than sulfadiazine after oral administration, while renal clearance took twice as long; hence, equal blood levels of the chemotherapeutically equivalent drugs could be maintained by half as much sulfamerazine given at eight-hour, rather than four-hour, intervals. It seemed that we had a winner.

Feirer proposed that our findings be reviewed with E. K. Marshall at The Johns Hopkins, then the panjandrum of sulfa drugs. The discourse had hardly begun when Marshall stopped me, saying, "Welch, you are a damned fool! Don't you know that sulfamethylthiazole causes peripheral neuropathy and that sulfamethylpyrimidine will do the same? It also causes renal damage; look at the holes in this kidney section!" I asked him why a methyl group should be toxic when substituted on a pyrimidine ring compared with a thiazole ring; it seemed to me a non sequitur. He inquired whether I had heard of CH_3OH! No chemist, Marshall apparently really believed that the methyl group per se is potentially toxic; he suggested that we start over with a sulfaethylpyrimidine! The holes in the kidneys reflected hydronephrosis, of course; they resulted from crystal deposition due to overdosage. I stated that no renal differences would be found with equal blood levels of the two drugs. Marshall remained unconvinced and Feirer was nonplussed, to say the least. To make a very long story short, chicks were used to show that the peripheral neuropathy, readily caused in that species by sulfamethylthiazole, was of minor degree and equal with sulfadiazine and sulfamerazine. Extended studies of many phenomena made clear that the earlier contentions had been correct. With a massive paper ready for publication, we went again to Baltimore. Marshall, really a great man, at last was completely convinced and congratulated us. A very long paper was published in 1943 in the *Journal of Pharmacology and Experimental Therapeutics* without any changes; I suspect that one referee of that manuscript can be identified! Why then did the no-more-costly sulfamerazine not completely displace sulfadiazine, with half the dose given half as often? The reasons were entirely economic. S & D, then a relatively small company, could not afford to out-advertise the developers of sulfadiazine, which by then was so well established that few physicians were interested in altering their memory patterns. Science versus the marketplace!

My career appeared to benefit, at least temporarily, from promotion to assistant director of research (but now with seven departments to supervise), while shortly thereafter Feirer became vice president and I became director of research at age 34. I tried to spend half-time in pharmacology but failed. The then assistant director of the department, Karl Beyer, was given full responsibility for research and went on to a brilliant career. Only my studies that led to folic acid (see below) were continued, then with Lem Wright. At the same time several academic posts became available and in 1944 I decided to move to Western Reserve University, where Torald Sollmann was retiring. Solly had been dean at Western Reserve for fifteen years; the Department of Pharmacology was spatially large but almost without equipment, and with the departure of the last assistant professor, the staff was zero, while my new salary, $7500 per year, now seems inconceivably small.

In addition to my lasting friendships with Bill and Jeanne Feirer, I left S & D with great respect for my many scientific colleagues and for the ethics of the company, then led by John Zinsser. [Incidentally, I began my first major review at S & D; it was the first on the design and use of antimetabolites (4).]

WESTERN RESERVE (WRU) YEARS (1944–1953)

I moved to Cleveland in 1944 during the war. A medical officer in the Army Reserve Corps, I had been rejected for active duty: cardiac hypertrophy, diagnosed erroneously. Two of the men who first moved to the department at Western Reserve were Lawrence (Lawrie) Peters, PhD (now deceased), who had worked with me at S & D for two years (I helped him earn his MD), and Ernest Bueding, MD, who had come from New York University. With army support, we promptly undertook chemotherapeutic studies of filariasis, which the military expected to be a major problem in the South Pacific (it proved not to be). Peters and I were soon chasing vicious wild cotton rats naturally infested with the only practicable source of a filariasis resembling that of man. We had to learn that *Litomosoides carinii* in the pleural cavity of these animals responds differently to drugs than *Wuchereria bancrofti* in the lymphatic system of man. We studied new classes of compounds and found activity among a group of cyanine dyes with resonating systems of bonding. We selected a compound with acceptable toxicity that could kill all adult filarial worms in the cotton rats; however, the microfilaria in the blood-stream (infectious for the vector, a mite) were not directly killed. After extensive studies of toxicity in many animal species, we conducted clinical pharmacological investigations in human volunteers with inoperable neoplastic diseases. We carried out clinical trials in Puerto Rico; these were disappointing. The adult worms in the human lymphatics were not killed, although the *microfilaria* were sensitive; they returned in due course, as might be expected. We developed derivatives, however, for the chemotherapy of other nematodal infestations. In the meantime, the army asked us to study schistosomiasis. Bueding, while studying the mechanism of action of the cyanine dyes, began investigations in mice, using a snail colony to produce the miracidia of *Schistosoma mansoni*. In this and related fields, Bueding is today the world's authority.

Other prominent members of the Department of Pharmacology at Western Reserve included George Bidder, MD, Giulio Cantoni, MD, and Harold Chase, MD, about whom space restrictions preclude discussions.

A major dilemma arose in 1946: I was offered the chairmanship of the Department of Pharmacology at Washington University; Carl Cori had moved to the chair of biological chemistry. Despite my nostalgia for Washington

University, I decided to remain in Cleveland; I wanted to follow up on the two years of hard work I had expended in building something out of almost nothing. In addition, my studies leading to folic acid, begun at S & D, had been reinitiated and were moving forward rapidly.

Lem Wright and I had added poorly absorbed succinylsulfathiazole together with the then-known vitamins to highly purified diets of rats. We hoped to learn whether intestinal microorganisms produce essential nutritional factors that might be disclosed in this way. Elvehjem and his associates had similar ideas using sulfaguanidine and they first identified a factor, not then an entity, termed folic acid. To conserve space, the reader is referred to other articles for the history of this research (5–7).

Much of the work on folic acid, and later on vitamin B_{12}, was done in collaboration with Bob Heinle of the Department of Medicine at Western Reserve. He was a superb colleague who was very even-tempered—always mad. Trained with W. B. (Bill) Castle at the Thorndike in Boston, Heinle was an expert hematologist and internist; we worked effectively together for seven years. After Jack Pritchard, MD, joined us, we fed piglets a purified diet containing succinylsulfathiazole and a crude antagonist of folic acid (supplied by Tom Jukes, by then at Lederle); the piglets became relatively huge swine, so strong that only Jack could successfully wrestle them. Eventually they developed striking bone marrow changes and a macrocytic anemia; their marrow became indistinguishable from that of human pernicious anemia in relapse. This condition responded initially to folic acid, but gradually became insensitive to folate unless we injected purified liver extract, as was used in the treatment of pernicious anemia (later replaced by vitamin B_{12}). Combined system disease did not develop in the deficient animals, but sudden deaths occurred eventually unless liver extract (later vitamin B_{12}) was injected. During subsequent army service, Pritchard became involved in obstetrics and gynecology and has been head of that department at Dallas for many years.

Our studies with swine, coupled with evidence that the purified liver extracts contained no folic acid, led me to suggest that the extrinsic factor, utilized orally by pernicious anemic patients only when administered with Castle's intrinsic factor (i.e. normal human gastric juice), could be identical with the parenterally active antipernicious anemia factor of liver. This was established in 1948 in collaboration with Castle and associates, and was extended to pure vitamin B_{12}, which had just then become available (8). Also in 1948, in collaboration with Stokstad, Jukes, and others (9), we demonstrated the antipernicious anemia efficacy of the microbially produced animal protein factor, given parenterally. This was probably the first reported use of a material derived from a source other than liver for the parenteral treatment of pernicious anemia in relapse.

In 1949, two superb post-docs, C. A. (Chuck) Nichol and W. H. (Bill) Prusoff, joined the group. With the latter, I initiated a program to concentrate the intrinsic factor using desiccated pig stomach as a source, while with Nichol I began studies of the effect of rat liver slices on folic acid. Using *Leuconostoc citrovorum,* which requires for its growth reduced forms of folate, e.g. leucovorin, we soon obtained evidence for a folate reductase. From the standpoint of chemotherapy, it was exciting to find that aminopterin, the forerunner of methotrexate, almost irreversibly inhibits the reductase (10–12), because this was the first clue to the mechanism of action of this invaluable antileukemic agent. Warwick Sakami and I showed the involvement of folate derivatives in the biosynthesis of labile methyl groups (of betaine, methionine, etc) (13).

Some comments concerning the rather ghastly years of anguishing debates about teaching are necessary, because these led to the nearly total (and rather famous) revision of the curriculum of WRU Medical School. Initially, I had inveighed against the examination system that prevailed (frequent regurgitation after memorization), but I knew not whereof I wrought. Major funds were raised by the dean, Joe Wearn (a man with whom I had great personal rapport and who nominated me for membership in the Association of American Physicians); Hale Ham came from Harvard to coordinate the program, and eventually teaching by committees resulted. One participation I will proudly acknowledge: the multidisciplinary student laboratories. Otherwise, I became essentially antipathetic. I believed then, as I do now, that good instruction comes from within; it is a product of knowledgeable individuals who love to stimulate and debate with willing recipients. No committee can do this—or legislate it—only earnest and dedicated individuals. My departure for Yale in 1953 introduced me to a very different teaching system: no examinations except by the National Board. It was a joy to have real rapport with medical students, who studied without built-in fear of their instructors (in most schools then, teachers also were potential executioners). By mid-1952, however, I was able to accept an invitation from Professor J. H. (Josh) Burn to recover at Oxford University.

Other dear old friends at WRU included Normand Hoerr, John Dingle, and Carl Wiggers (deceased) and Harland Wood and Lester Krampitz.

OXFORD DAYS (1952–JANUARY 1953)

Oxford was an unforgettable experience for me; it was a Mecca for pharmacologists, with such stars as Burn, Edith Bülbring, Hugh Blaschko, and many, many others. Initially Burn and I worked together, but discussions with Blaschko soon led us to attempt to determine (again without the possibility of using isotopes) whether dopa and dopamine were converted to noradrenaline and adrenaline by the adrenal medulla. A fresh homogenate was cold-dialyzed against a very small volume of buffered saline suspension of mushroom catechol oxidase to pump out the pressor amines, forming insoluble melanins, by creating a concentration gradient while minimizing the loss of possible cofactors; O_2 was bubbled through the external compartment and N_2 through the homogenate. The level of the pressor amines (as assayed on the blood pressure of the pithed cat) fell rapidly; however, an asymptote was soon reached at 75–80% of the initial concentration in the homogenate. What was causing retention? Could the amines be held within particles? Using Florey's high-speed refrigerated centrifuge, we found the pressor amines in vesicles that sedimented with the mitochondria; from these particles the catecholamines could be readily released. A new field was opened (14) and lasting friendships were made.

Progress toward the end of these experiments was slowed by my hospitalization for a lumbar disc (after a previous laminectomy, I had not anticipated this); during my return to the States from England on the Queen Mary, I was encased in plaster. On an earlier visit to Yale University at the invitation of Joe Fruton I had met the dean-to-be, Vernon Lippard (not yet moved from Charlottesville), and eventually I accepted an offer from Yale. At the same time, 1953, Peters became chairman of pharmacology at Tulane and moved to Kansas two years later, and Cantoni moved to head a lab at the National Institutes of Health. In 1954, Bueding became chairman of pharmacology at Louisiana State University and moved to The Johns Hopkins six years later.

YALE YEARS (1953–1967)

After the death of the previous chairman, Salter, the Department of Pharmacology at Yale had deteriorated somewhat. When I arrived with several colleagues from Western Reserve [e.g. Charles (Nick) Carter, an assistant professor of medicine strongly grounded in biochemistry, Chuck Nichol, Bill Prusoff, Bill Holmes, and Sheldon Greenbaum, as well as several post-docs, including Bernard Langley, and even two graduate students], only two of the former Yale staff members (and too many graduate students) remained. Desmond Bonnycastle, an associate professor, departed when his five-year term-appointment expired. Nicholas (Nick) Giarman, an assistant professor, proved to be an exceptional teacher and a very competent neuropharmacologist; we urged him to remain. Indeed, at the invitation of J. H. Gaddum, Giarman exchanged positions with Henry Adam for a year (to keep it simple, the two men exchanged jobs, salaries, cars, and homes; everything except wives!). Giarman returned as associate professor. In 1963 he succeeded me as American editor of

Biochemical Pharmacology. He died in 1968, a great loss for Yale, science, and his many friends.[6]

In 1953–1954, Blaschko spent six months with us at Yale and work on the adrenal granules resumed, in collaboration with Joe Demis, and later with Paul Hagen. We obtained proof of the precursory role of ^{14}C-dopa in the formation of the pressor amines, and continued studies of the extraordinarily high levels of ATP in the vesicles.

One outstanding recruit of the pharmacology department at Yale was John Vane, D Phil, whom I had known as a graduate student at Oxford. Vane came to Yale as an instructor and was soon promoted. Eventually, however, the tug of his home country became too great and he joined the Department of Pharmacology of the Royal College of Surgeons. Later, he became group research and development director of the Wellcome Laboratories. It is pertinent to mention here, although out of context, that prior to Vane's joining Wellcome he was a very great help to us at Squibb as the senior consultant in pharmacology. For his brilliant work on the prostaglandins and prostacyclin, as well as the mechanism of action of aspirin, Vane shared a Nobel Prize in 1982; he was knighted in 1984 and became a foreign member of the National Academy of Science of the United States. In December 1982 my wife and I were greatly honored by an official invitation, through Vane, of course, to attend the Nobel ceremonies in Stockholm, one of the most memorable experiences of our lives.

The great strengths of the Department of Pharmacology at Yale, which gained worldwide recognition, lay in the many outstanding young scientists who came to work there, either as young faculty members or as post-doctoral fellows. We were able to secure the funds to retain many of these men and women, and gave them encouragement and help in full measure to develop their ideas and intellectual growth. Over the years, many of that group received various honors and special appointments, e.g. Career Development Awards, Scholars in Cancer Research awards, Markle and Burroughs-Wellcome Scholar awards, as well as career professorships. In addition, I shared in memberships and chairmanships of study sections of the NIH and advisory committees of the NSF, the NRC, and the American Cancer Society. The department grew rapidly and in addition to research gained a deserved reputation for good

---

[6]Prior to Giarman's American editorship of *Biochemical Pharmacology,* I (and others) had helped Sir Rudolph Peters in the founding in 1958 of that soon rather prestigious journal. As American editor my initial roles were demanding ones. High standards were set and were maintained by Giarman, while I became a vice chairman of the International Board of Editors. Subsequently, Alan Sartorelli carried the standards of the journal to even greater heights (despite his having much to do with the issue in 1979 that commemorated my seventieth birthday). Subsequent to the death of Sir Rudolph, I became chairman of the editorial board, at the time of a symposium in Oxford (1983) that celebrated the twenty-fifth anniversary of the founding of *Biochemical Pharmacology.*

teaching of medical students (much in small discussion groups), as well as of graduate students, while offering an excellent atmosphere for post-doctoral training. Much of the early financial help came in the form of no-strings grants from either the Squibb Institute for Medical Research or the Upjohn Company, where I was a consultant for about eight years. As research and training grants became more readily available (prior to recent years), funds were relatively easy to obtain. Among the many members of the group were such outstanding men as Bob Handschumacher, a scholar in cancer research and a career professor of the American Cancer Society, who was chairman of the Yale department from 1974 to 1977; Van Canellakis, a career NIH professor; Henry Mautner, chairman of biochemistry and pharmacology at Tufts. Jack Cooper was promoted to professor and remained at Yale, while Julian Jaffe was attracted to the University of Vermont, where he is a professor of pharmacology. Chuck Nichol became head of experimental therapeutics at the Roswell Park Memorial Institute and later director of medicinal biochemistry at the Wellcome Research Laboratories (USA). Another man of distinction who moved to Yale from WRU, Bill Prusoff, became a professor and remained at Yale. Nick Carter returned to WRU as chairman of pharmacology and is now scientific director of NIEHS (NIH). After two years at Cornell, Jack Green became chairman of pharmacology at Mt. Sinai Medical School. Paul Hagen moved to Harvard for three years prior to becoming chairman of biochemistry at Manitoba; he is now dean of graduate studies at the University of Ottawa. Glenn Fischer, after eleven years at Yale, transferred to Brown as a professor of biochemical pharmacology.

Alan C. Sartorelli joined the department as an assistant professor and became a professor in 1967; he was a very distinguished chairman of the department from 1977 to 1984 and is now director of the Yale Comprehensive Cancer Center. Since 1968 the American editor of *Biochemical Pharmacology,* Sartorelli is also the executive editor of *Pharmacology and Therapeutics.* Joe Bertino joined the department (and internal medicine) as assistant professor and later became an American Cancer Society professor. Paul Calabresi left Yale in 1968 for the chairmanship of the Department of Medicine at Brown, but he deserves very special mention because of his various contributions to Yale and to his many co-workers there, including myself; he headed the first section on clinical pharmacology at Yale and was a Burroughs-Wellcome Scholar in that field. Dave Johns, a member of the department for seven years, became chief of two laboratories (medicinal chemistry and biology and chemical pharmacology) at the National Cancer Institute. The two-volume monograph edited by Sartorelli & Johns on antineoplastic and immunosuppressive agents remains a classic in these fields after nearly ten years.

Space does not permit other than brief mention of many other friends and important workers in the department between 1953 and 1967 and subsequently;

these certainly include Pauline Chang, Dave Ludlum, Joe Demis, Bob Levine, Maire Hakala, Zygmunt Zakrzewski, Ming Chu and S.-H. Chu, Arnold Eisenfeld, Richard Schindler, Ron Morris, Norm Gillis, Zoe Canellakis, Bill Creasey, John Perkins, John McCormack, Bill Macmillan, Malcolm Mitchell, Bob Roth, Jack Cramer, Morris Zedeck, Karel Raška, and Ed Coleman, who later joined me at Squibb. A dear friend from Germany, Helmuth Vorherr, with whom I studied the selective embryolethality of 6-azauridine and later, with his wife, Ute, that of N-(phosphonacetyl)-L-aspartate (PALA), is now professor of pharmacology and gynecology at the University of New Mexico. Other dear friends from abroad who worked at Yale included Laszlo Lajtha, until recently director of the MRC unit in the Paterson Labs of the University of Manchester; Ronald Girdwood, professor of therapeutics at the University of Edinburgh; Peter Reichard of the Karolinska Institutet; Tony Mathias; Hamish Keir; Charles Pasternak; Margaret Day; and Margaret and Brian Fox. Warm friends in other departments included Paul Beeson, Joe Fruton and his wife, Sofia Simmonds, Aaron Lerner, Sam Hellman, Dan Freedman, Bob McCollum, Bill Gardner, and Nick Greene. Unintentional omissions of other Yale colleagues I hope will be forgiven.

To discuss the investigations of all these exceptional scientists would require an entire volume. Many of my own studies through early 1966 were summarized in part in my Sollmann oration (15), presented at the time of my Torald Sollmann Award from ASPET; these studies involved many of the fine colleagues referred to above. They and other co-workers enabled me to participate in research and contributed greatly to our efforts to build a strong department that continued to prosper. As I said at the time of the dedication of a newly remodeled wing donated jointly to Yale by the Wellcome Trust and the National Cancer Institute, when I announced my imminent departure for the Squibb Institute for Medical Research, "There is nothing that succeeds like *successors!*" At that time also, my old friend George Hitchings, vice president for research at Burroughs Wellcome, presented me with a most appropriate gift: two large bottles of Empirin Compound, which he correctly predicted I would very soon be needing for my new headaches.

If space permitted, I could present much interesting information concerning the remarkably successful oral therapy of severe psoriasis with azaribine (triacetyl-6-azauridine) initiated by Paul Calabresi, Charlie McDonald, and colleagues. The NDA was approved in 1975 but was withdrawn fifteen months later because of the approximately 4% incidence of thromboses, some intra-arterial. Evidence now suggests that in a few susceptible individuals a deficiency of pyridoxal phosphate may be induced, with resultant homocystinemia (in rabbits, these are prevented by pyridoxine). At present, azaribine is an orphan drug and psoriasis is an orphan disease! The remarkable efficacy of azaribine, not only in psoriasis but also in mycosis fungoides, choriocarcinoma, polycythemia vera, and perhaps as an embryolethal agent, may now be studied in other countries but not in the USA.

After Squibb's initial production of 6-azauridine for us ($\sim$700 g) with the aid of a contract from the National Cancer Institute (NCI), the NCI contracted with Calbiochem to manufacture the substance. Handschumacher and I helped that company to initiate production, using 6-azauracil incubated with *E. coli*, a method devised by our friends in Prague, Jan Škoda et al. Thus, Bob, Jan, and I became close friends of Dr. William (Bill) Drell, then president of Calbiochem. These deep mutual friendships have survived time, distances, and the devastating effect of the loss of azaribine on Calbiochem, now a subsidiary of Hoechst. Handschumacher and I went to Prague to conduct studies with Škoda and Šorm, with each of whom, and with Helena Rašková, warm friendships developed. Toward the end of my second sabbatical, in Frankfurt at the Institut f. Therapeutische Biochemie,[7] where I developed friendships with Helmut Maske, Jürgen Drews, and Bill Pratt, Škoda and I began studies in Prague in March 1965; these were extended in July-August of that year.

This second sabbatical leave (1964–1965) was precipitated by a fall while I was skiing with Tom Jukes in Badger Pass in Yosemite; result: a broken fibula and the man who came to dinner. Later complications of the original break were debilitating, and finally a change in scenery was deemed essential. I must comment that one of the finest personal letters I have ever received had been written by Van Canellakis, who felt I was headed for disaster (presumably attributed to premature aging and overwork [?]); hence, I should slow down and rest on my laurels (i.e. contemplate my navel and admire the wonderful department at Yale that the many great colleagues, he, and I had built). My reactions to these concerns were (*a*) to go to Germany in 1964 to work in the laboratory and write a paper (without coauthors) for the Proceedings of the National Academy of Sciences on the selective inhibition of an enzyme induction; (*b*) to go to Prague in 1965 to work with Škoda; (*c*) to end years of unhappiness through divorce; (*d*) to go to India to study the chemotherapy of smallpox with 5-iododeoxyuridine, (*e*) above all, to be most happily married in Prague in 1966 to Erika (Peter) Martinková; and (*f*) to leave Yale in 1967 to head research and development at Squibb, involving about 1000 scientific

---

[7]While working in Frankfurt, I was invited by my old friends Gustav Born and Sir Alex Haddow to dine with them and Sir Henry Dale, Vane, and several others after a lecture in London. Dale was delighted to learn that I had visited the laboratory of Paul Ehrlich, with whom Dale had worked before I was born. Sir Henry then began to reminisce most fascinatingly about his days with Ehrlich, but in German! Born gently reminded Dale of the German limitations of many of his table companions. Sir Henry commented that if Born, who speaks perfect German, was having difficulty, perhaps he (Dale) should speak English. Within a moment, however, when the old gentleman continued his wonderful anecdotes, he spoke again in German! What I would have given then (as well as on other great occasions) for a tape recorder!

colleagues. Now twenty years later and still working, signs of disintegration have not yet become evident.

5-Iododeoxyuridine (IUdR) was first synthesized by Prusoff and studied by him, others, and me; it was the first specific antiviral drug to be used in man. Its efficacy against corneal keratitis caused by herpes simplex virus had led to studies of other DNA virus–induced diseases. The remarkable efficacy in rabbits of parenteral therapy with IUdR on advanced dermal lesions caused by vaccinia virus led to attempts to treat supposedly terminal human smallpox infections in India. Only three moribund patients became available during an entire year (1965–1966) of observation by David Fedson, then a post-doctoral fellow of Calabresi and mine; by a curious coincidence these patients were admitted during my visit to Madras. Intravenous infusions with IUdR were initiated immediately; result: two of the three patients survived (not reported as a 67% cure rate!). Since the disease probably has now disappeared, it is unlikely that the possible value of IUdR in smallpox therapy will ever be known.

During the last eight of my Yale years, I was a research advisor to Upjohn. There the many good scientists and friends are too numerous to name here, with the exception of Earl Burbidge, one of my closest friends in medical school, Bob Heinle (both died several years ago), and Dave Weisblat, then director of research and development. About Charles G. (Chuck) Smith, Upjohn's then director of biochemical research, much more will be said below.

Only three times prior to 1967 did I even consider offers of positions other than that at Yale: two medical deanships (one also a vice-presidency)[8] and one as vice-president for research and development at a pharmaceutical company other than Squibb. None of these appealed to me, however.

SQUIBB YEARS (1967–1974)

As indicated previously, throughout the years at Yale I had had many contacts with scientists at Squibb, and they had supported Yale's Squibb Fellows for fourteen years.

During the years subsequent to the discovery and development of the fluorocorticoids by Gus Fried and other Squibb scientists, however, Squibb had

---

[8]A memorable incident occurred during an interview for one of these positions: A rather distinguished surgical specialist on the search committee asked, "Dr. Welch, where do you think cardiovascular surgery is going in the next ten years?" My reply, as Paul Calabresi reminded me, was, "That's for you to tell me, and, should I accept this position, for me to help you get there." After a brief pause, I continued, "And if you cannot conceive where it should be, it will soon be time for me to appoint a new Chief of Cardiovascular Surgery." According to Paul, this philosophy, which he had observed during our years at Yale, has become a modus operandi for him and others of my colleagues.

made few contributions to drug discovery. Furthermore, with devastating impact on both morale and productivity, E. R. Squibb & Sons, Inc. had been acquired by the Mathieson Chemical Company, and the latter in turn by the Olin Corporation. In 1967 Squibb research and development was floundering. Then, thanks to the genius of a vice president of Olin then in charge of the E. R. Squibb Division, Richard Furlaud, real vision was introduced to the company. When first approached by Mr. Furlaud, I had no desire to leave Yale; in fact, with an endowed chair (the Eugene Higgins Professorship), it had been agreed at last that after fourteen years I would relinquish the chairmanship and return to my laboratory full-time. Nevertheless, with Mr. Furlaud's assurance that Squibb would shortly be a separate entity again (as indeed it became by a complicated separation from Olin), the challenge to try something very different became irresistible. Accordingly, in 1967 I became vice president for research and development and the director of the Squibb Institute for Medical Research. My first major act was to recruit Chuck Smith from Upjohn, initially as associate director. In 1970 he became a vice president. In 1969, another exceptional man, Dennis Fill, became president of E. R. Squibb & Sons, and Mr. Furlaud took on higher responsibilities. My second major act was to accept the resignation of the then head of pharmacology. John Vane became a senior consultant in pharmacology (three one-week visits annually). In due course, Zola Horovitz was promoted from within to head the department of pharmacology; later he became an associate director and a vice president.

Turning research around was not exactly an easy job for us. Company earnings then did not permit any major new research programs to be launched, except when ongoing programs were terminated. Initially, despite the very complex problems involved in increasing the yield of penicillin, further reducing its cost, and seeking better semi-synthetic derivatives of it, we had few other projects. Great improvements in producing penicillin were accomplished, and a valuable cyclohexadiene derivative of penicillin was developed. With great difficulties we entered the cephalosporin field and developed a new drug, cephradine. Effective new corticosteroids were created to replace those soon to be lost by the expiration of patents. These developments had salutary effects on earnings and therefore on the research and development budget. In addition, we made major efforts in the field of β blockers (β-adrenergic receptor-blocking agents), despite the then antipathy of the Food and Drug Administration toward such valuable drugs. As a result, a major entry into the field was later developed.

At last, however, the long-awaited hot lead appeared and we began research that could genuinely be termed basic. Earlier studies by Professor Rocha e Silva in Brazil had shown that the venom of a poisonous local snake, *Bothrops jararaca,* incubated with plasma led to the formation of a vasodilator polypeptide, bradykinin. Another Brazilian worker, Sergio Ferreira, observed that the venom also contained a factor that potentiated the effects of bradykinin; this was later shown to be the result of inhibition of an enzyme that rapidly inactivates bradykinin. Vane had suspected that this bradykininase might be the same enzyme that activates the polypeptide angiotensin I. (The latter substance, then suspected to be involved in renal hypertension, causes no effect on blood pressure until it is enzymically converted to angiotensin II, the most powerful vasoconstrictor known.) In Vane's lab, Mick Bakhle found that the peptide in the snake venom that inhibited bradykininase was also a powerful inhibitor of the angiotensin-converting enzyme (ACE). ACE catalyzes the removal of two terminal amino acids from both bradykinin and angiotensin I; it was later obtained in a homogeneous state by another good friend, Ervin Erdös, at the University of Texas, Dallas. The inhibitor isolated from the venom by Ferreira and Greene was a pentapeptide, while another potent inhibitory peptide, isolated at Squibb, was a nonapeptide. Management's lack of enthusiasm for research in this area was understandable, when one considers that the peptide inhibitors of course were impracticable as drugs. Indeed, it had not even been firmly established that so-called renal hypertension could be explained entirely by the release of the enzyme renin from hypoxic kidneys, with the final hypertensive state being caused by angiotensin II. To validate this concept required a major gamble. Despite the cost and the difficulties of synthesizing the inhibitory peptide in gram-quantities, I decided to go ahead despite a reluctant management; hence, Dr. Miguel Ondetti, an excellent protein chemist, and Dr. David Cushman, an enzymologist and pharmacologist, continued their now well-known studies. To make a very long story short, their colleagues established that the parenterally administered synthetic nonapeptide could prevent a rise in blood pressure from being caused by the intravenous injection of angiotensin I. Furthermore, studies in patients with malignant hypertension showed that the nonapeptide given intravenously could lead to a normotensive state, without evidence that accumulations of angiotensin I or the plasma precursor or renin in themselves were deleterious. Whereas I had reacted with enthusiasm to the potential for new drug discovery, the then president of the Squibb Corporation (neither Dennis Fill nor Richard Furlaud) could only understand the impracticality of the nonapeptide as a drug. The entire program was regarded as a costly exercise in futility. He ridiculed the idea that the concept of the renin cascade had indeed been validated, and rejected the potential importance, if hypertension was to be attacked rationally, of a key enzyme to inhibit having been identified. Indeed, I was told that the major effort to develop a new and practicable inhibitor of the converting enzyme should be terminated. This, I must state, I refused to do—termination of Welch would have to come first! Fortunately for what was to come, that did not happen. The brilliant work of Ondetti & Cushman continued; they eventually determined the essential inhibitory features and synthesized a modified dipeptide with oral activity! By this time, however, my mandatory retirement at 65 (actually 65.98 years) had occurred. In due course, the then president also left the corporation for reasons other than age and the outstanding Mr. Fill was persuaded by the chairman to become president of the entire Squibb Corporation.

In the meantime, angiotensin II had been shown to be much more than a vasoconstrictor; e.g. it stimulates the secretion of aldosterone and thus affects the retention of both sodium ions and fluid. The ultimate drug, termed captopril and now marketed world-wide, is a modified dipeptide of L-cysteine (free SH) and L-proline. A methyl group adjacent to the imid-linkage renders the compound insusceptible to attack by peptidases; hence, it is orally active. It is used not only in the control of malignant, but also essential, hypertension. In addition, captopril is efficacious (for reasons not yet fully understood) in the therapy of congestive heart failure, while other potential activities (as well as promising new ACE inhibitors), are under investigation, not only by Squibb, but also by other companies.

I like to believe that my approximately 7.5 years as director (or president) of the Squibb Institute for Medical Research did help to turn the company upward. In addition to challenges, headaches, and some successes, Squibb gave me wonderful opportunities for scientific edification as well as for travel. Often my wife was able to accompany me. Frequent trips to the research laboratories of Squibb-Germany (Regensburg) were essential, as were trips to London and Liverpool for pharmaceutical research and to Ireland for production, while for other reasons I traveled to Australia, Austria, Belgium, China, Czechoslovakia, Denmark, Finland, France, Greece, Hawaii, Holland, Hong Kong, Hungary, Italy, Japan, Mexico, Nigeria, Sardinia, Sweden, and Switzerland. These and personal trips to Alaska, the Bahamas, Brazil, East Germany, Egypt, India, Portugal, Puerto Rico, Russia, and Spain bestowed insights that could not have been gained in any other way.

Late in 1974, Chuck Smith, a fine executive and innovative scientist who remains our close friend (as does his wife, Angie), also found the previous president intolerable, and six weeks after Smith's promotion to the presidency of the Squibb Institute for Medical Research, he left the corporation. Chuck is now an executive vice president of Revlon with responsibilities for research and development in such component health-care companies as USV Pharmaceuticals, Armour, and many other subsidiaries. Among my other colleagues at Squibb were also many good friends (some now deceased). I think particularly of Oskar Wintersteiner, Helmut Cords, Naomi Taylor, George Donat, Peter Koerber, Fred Wiselogle, Jack Bernstein, Pat Diassi, Jim Knill, Frank Weisenborn, Bill Brown, Zola Horovitz, Miguel Ondetti, and many others.

Now, ten years later, the Squibb Institute is a very different organization than it was and I know but little about it. A period of my life, which in a great many ways was both exciting and memorable, regretfully came to an end. I am "gone, but not forgotten," or forgotten—I know not which.

ST. JUDE YEARS (1975–1983)

Retirement not being an attractive prospect, I accepted an offer from an outstanding institution, St. Jude Children's Research Hospital in Memphis, on whose board of scientific advisors I had served for three earlier years. My goal was to organize a new Division of Biochemical and Clinical Pharmacology. Many things had changed since my last visit in 1972: a new director, Alvin M. Mauer, MD, had replaced Don Pinkel, of whom I had been fond; a new seven-story building was due to open within three months (the new division was to occupy most of the third floor), while an important change for me was a return to cancer research, none having been possible at Squibb. Indeed, a three-month period in early 1975 offered an excellent opportunity to bore into the two then new superb monographs edited by Alan Sartorelli and David Johns. These massive handbooks, which I had actually commissioned as a senior editor of the handbook series, could not have appeared at a more appropriate time if I had designed it that way. I could afford time for planning as well as for recruiting, particularly in the area of medicinal organic chemistry, which I regarded as a mandatory development for the new division. In this area, I was joined as a full member by an outstanding man, Josef Nemec, whom I lured from the Squibb Institute for Medical Research, where I had known him well. Another chemist joined us, T. L. Chwang, who had worked for several years with Charles Heidelberger, while Bill Beck, who had done his post-doctoral work with Van Canellakis at Yale, came from the University of Southern California. Nahed Ahmed became my research associate; her post-doctoral training with Nicholas Bachur at the Baltimore branch of the NCI had qualified her highly. I began studies of the activity of uridine-cytidine kinase in human colorectal adenocarcinomas. Other studies of this enzyme led to the discovery, with Alan Paterson and colleagues at Alberta, that despite the apparent deletion of this kinase activity from certain 3-deazauridine-resistant mutants of a human B-lymphoblast, their proliferation in culture remained quite sensitive to inhibition by either 6-azauridine or 5-azacytidine (16). We suggested that another nucleoside-phosphorylating enzyme is present in such mutants; my assistants and I have now confirmed and extended this hypothesis (17) using a new method for quantifying acidic nucleosides (18). Judith Belt, a post-doctoral trainee of Efraim Racker, and I found that only the undissociated portion of 6-azauridine (pKa ~6.7), at pH 7.4, is transported by the process of facilitated diffusion (19).

Two post-doctoral fellows from the Chester Beatty, Drs. Janet and Peter Houghton, came to St. Jude after we helped them to immigrate. This was done with almost incredible difficulties, which were finally resolved only with the help of Senator Baker. In addition to those named, four scientists already at St. Jude continued as effective members of the division. These were DeWayne Roberts, a biochemical pharmacologist; Thomas L. Avery, an experienced experimental chemotherapist and colleague with whom I worked very closely and with much friendship; Arnold Fridland, a very competent enzymologist; and Thomas Brent, a specialist in the mechanisms of DNA damage and its enzymic repair.

In 1980, my five-year appointment as member and chairman of the Division of Biochemical and Clinical Pharmacology was extended for a year to enable a search committee and the director to select Raymond L. Blakley to succeed me as chairman. Blakley formerly was professor of biochemistry in the University of Iowa School of Medicine. I became member-emeritus and once again a bench scientist at 72. The subsequent two years were among the happiest of my life, although fifty-hour weeks in the laboratory with two splendid assistants, Jim Panahi, BS, and Glen Germain, MS, gave me little time for my personal life or to write papers.

During my continued studies of resistance to 3-deazauridine in both B- and T-human lymphoblastoid cells, I made the unexpected observation that the cytosolic uridine-cytidine kinase activity is not deleted in CEM(T) cells; indeed, in the parent cells that enzyme has no affinity for the cytotoxic nucleoside. Thus was uncovered a hitherto unrecognized enzyme associated with the nuclei of these (and other) cells that catalyzes the phosphorylation of 3-deazauridine and the activity of which is greatly diminished in the drug-resistant mutants. This enzyme activity can either complement or supplant that of the classical cytosolic enzyme.

At this stage (1983), however, I was approached by three government agencies (the EPA, the FDA, and the NCI), and I decided to accept an offer from the National Cancer Institute. We moved from a lovely home in Memphis to a condominium in Chevy Chase, a suburb of Washington, DC, so that I could start still another career just prior to turning 75.

Before leaving the subject of Memphis and St. Jude, I want to present a few impressions of our eight and a half years there. Memphis provided a rather different atmosphere from those of New Haven and Princeton, particularly for Erika, whose almost unaccented British English, acquired in Prague, had already been transformed to American, although not mid-South American. This new learning period was helped greatly by her linguistic talents (she was formerly a scientific translator). The people of Memphis were warm and friendly, and the city progressed remarkably during our stay there. Today, any individual can and should be able to live happily in Memphis, as we did (with the aid of air-conditioning and a swimming pool!). We have left many dear friends there.

St. Jude Hospital only opened in 1962, and in 1975 it was almost incredible to see what had happened there in only thirteen years. In fact, from our arrival until our departure, the continued growth of the hospital was evident. It is a splendid children's hospital, which provides superb (and completely free) medical care to children with all forms of neoplastic disease. I have only the highest praise for the Board of Governors and Danny Thomas for their dedication and their steadily more efficient fund-raising, especially for the clinical activities at the hospital. St. Jude is now as much the pride of Memphis as is the home of Elvis Presley.

The clinical research accomplishments of St. Jude, e.g. the introduction of cranio-spinal irradiation, which increased the apparent cures in acute lymphoblastic leukemia by tenfold (to now more than 50% of the patients), was a major breakthrough. This occurred during the tenure of Dr. Donald Pinkel, the first medical director, in collaboration with Dr. Joseph Simone. The second director, who departed in 1983, was a dedicated pediatric hematologist and oncologist who made every effort to help St. Jude grow and burnish its image brightly. He had little ability to communicate scientifically, however, or to understand the importance of molecular developments. Thus he could not fully appreciate the reasonable needs for the encouragement and financial support of basic scientists, who are developing many new methods for the treatment of cancer.

St. Jude needs many improvements, and the new director, Joseph Simone, a very experienced oncologist and pediatrician, could institute them with strong advisors in basic areas and with the support of the Board of Governors. The basic science divisions not only need to be more strongly supported financially, they also need to be better oriented toward goals more sensible in terms of modern chemotherapy and immunotherapy (for example, the roles of oncogenes and the great promise of monoclonal antibodies). I am and will continue to be an ardent supporter of the institution, and of the best scientists within it. Finally, I am personally very grateful, despite the very difficult and traumatic struggles we experienced at times, for the many courtesies my colleagues there extended to me. In addition to those in our own division, already mentioned, such splendid colleagues as Charles Pratt, George Cheung, the discoverer of calmodulin, Dave Kingsbury, George Marten, Gaston Rivera, and their respective wives, as well as Dolores Anderson, are among those whom I won't forget as are other wonderful Memphians, especially Dr. Gordon and Nancy Mathes, Dr. Eric and Marie Louise Muirhead, and Dr. Henry and Rosalie Rudner.

One other memorable group in Memphis is the Memphis Medical Seminar, of which I was a member (and once the president). It is largely composed of investigative clinicians, for example, Hall Tacket, our splendid internist; Eric Muirhead, an outstanding investigator and pathologist; and Irv Fleming, a dedicated surgeon. These and all the other members are friends whom I will always remember.

NATIONAL CANCER INSTITUTE (NCI) (1983–   )

In October 1983, I joined the NCI and assumed the rather remarkable title of cancer expert, attached initially to the Office of the Chief of the Drug Evaluation Branch (Dr. John Venditti), Developmental Therapeutics Program, Division of Cancer Treatment. The director of this division, Bruce A. Chabner, MD, is a splendid basic scientist and clinical oncologist as well as a fine administrator. My initial responsibility became the coordination of those National Cooperative Drug Discovery Groups (NCDDG) that were launched in mid-1984. These groups include cooperating academic institutions and in some cases industrial organizations. The admirable and I hope attainable goal of these groups is the discovery and development of essentially new approaches to the treatment of human neoplastic diseases, including new entities and new techniques. For the NCDDG, I function as an intellectual participant and facilitator, not as a director. In the meantime, I have become the acting deputy director of the Division of Cancer Treatment, a relatively huge organization whose total budget, intramural and extramural, is about $318,000,000.

During a long series of careers spanning forty-four years of involvements with the administration of four departments of pharmacology and the research and development activities of two pharmaceutical organizations, inevitably I have gained considerable experience and I hope some wisdom and judgment. If so, my presumably terminal contributions may be of value in the multifaceted areas of research and development of the Division of Cancer Treatment in the fields of biochemical pharmacology, chemotherapy, and drug development, the fields with which I have been deeply concerned for so many years.

Certainly, I am now making many new acquaintances who also will be ne'er forgot as long as the gods see fit to help me, not only to be useful, but also to continue to have a time for remembering.

Literature Cited

1. Davenport, M. 1967. *Too Strong for Fantasy*, p. 6. New York: Scribner
2. Welch, A. D., Bueding, E. 1946. Biochemical aspects of pharmacology. In *Currents in Biochemistry*, ed. D. E. Green, pp. 399–412. New York: Intersciences
3. Welch, A. D., Landau, R. L. 1942. The arsenic analogue of choline as a component of lecithin in rats fed arsenocholine chloride. *J. Biol. Chem.* 144:581–88
4. Welch, A. D. 1945. Interference with biological processes through the use of analogs of essential metabolites. *Phys. Rev.* 25:687–715
5. Welch, A. D. 1983. Folic acid: Discovery and the exciting first decade. *Persp. Biol. Med.* 27:64–75
6. Heinle, R. W., Welch, A. D. 1951. Hematopoietic agents in macrocytic anemias. *Pharmacol. Rev.* 3:345–411
7. Welch, A. D., Nichol, C. A. 1952. Water-soluble vitamins concerned with one- and two-carbon intermediates. *Ann. Rev. Biochem.* 21:633–86
8. Berk, L., Castle, W. B., Welch, A. D., Heinle, R. W., Anker, R., Epstein, M. 1948. Observations on the etiologic relationship of achylia gastrica to pernicious anemia. X. Activity of vitamin B_{12} as food (extrinsic) factor. *N. Engl. J. Med.* 235:911–13
9. Stokstad, E. L. R., Page, A., Franklin, A. L., Jukes, T. H., Heinle, R. W., et al. 1948. Activity of microbial animal protein factor concentrates in pernicious anemia. *J. Lab. Clin. Med.* 33:860–64
10. Nichol, C. A., Welch, A. D. 1950.

Synthesis of citrovorum factor from folic acid by liver slices; augmentation by ascorbic acid. *Proc. Soc. Exp. Biol. Med.* 74:52–55

11. Nichol, C. A., Welch, A. D. 1950. On the mechanism of action of aminopterin. *Proc. Soc. Exp. Biol. Med.* 74:403–11

12. Welch, A. D. 1950. New developments in the study of folic acid. *Trans. Assoc. Am. Physicians.* 63:147–54

13. Sakami, W., Welch, A. D. 1950. Synthesis of labile methyl groups by the rat *in vivo* and *in vitro. J. Biol. Chem.* 187: 379–87

14. Blaschko, H., Welch, A. D. 1953. Localization of adrenaline in cytoplasmic particles of the bovine adrenal medulla. *Arch. Exper. Pathol. Pharmakol.* 219: 17–22

15. Welch, A. D. 1967. The Sollmann oration. *Pharmacologist.* 9:46–52

16. Ahmed, N. K., Germain, G. S., Welch, A. D., Paterson, A. R. P., Paran, J. H., Yang, S. 1980. Phosphorylation of nucleosides catalyzed by a mammalian enzyme other than uridine-cytidine kinase. *Biochem. Biophys. Res. Commun.* 95: 440–45

17. Welch, A. D., Panahi, J., Germain, G. S. 1984. A nucleoside-phosphorylating activity, distinguishable from uridine (Urd)-cytidine (Cyd) kinase, in the nuclei of human lymphoblastoid cells. *Proc. Am. Assoc. Can. Res.* 25:70 (Abstr.)

18. Welch, A. D., Nemec, J., Panahi, J. 1984. Quantitative determination of nucleosides and their phosphate esters. 1. The acidic nucleosides: 3-deazauridine and 6-azauridine. *Intl. J. Biochem.* 16: 587–91

19. Belt, J. A., Welch, A. D. 1983. Transport of uridine and 6-azauridine in human lymphoblastoid cells. Specificity for the uncharged 6-azauridine molecule. *Mol. Pharmacol.* 23:153–58

Ann. Rev. Pharmacol. Toxicol. 1985. 25:27–31

CLINICAL PHARMACOLOGY IN THE UNITED STATES: A PERSONAL REMINISCENCE

Louis Lasagna

Sackler School of Graduate Biomedical Sciences, Tufts University Medical School, Boston, Massachusetts 02111

In 1950, I moved from New York City to Baltimore to start a fellowship in pharmacology and experimental therapeutics at the Johns Hopkins University School of Medicine after completing my residency training in internal medicine. I had opted for Hopkins in part because of the eminence of Dr. E. K. Marshall, Jr., the chairman of the pharmacology department, but also because C. Gordon Zubrod was starting a program in clinical pharmacology with a dual base in the departments of medicine and pharmacology.

When I arrived in Baltimore, I quickly saw that while some excellent trials were being conducted (e.g. studies of antibiotic dosage regimens in the treatment of pneumococcal pneumonia), Zubrod was hampered in developing a full program by the call on his time from a welfare clinic where he functioned as an outpatient physician. (He soon thereafter left for the National Cancer Institute, where for many years he was of crucial importance in the development of that institute's cancer chemotherapy program.)

In 1952, I was assigned to an army project at the Massachusetts General Hospital directed by Henry K. Beecher, Harvard professor and chairman of the hospital's anesthesia department. There I began to learn how to conduct analgesic trials, studied the interaction between psychological variables and the response to placebos and CNS drugs, performed the first modern clinical trial of hypnotics, and became convinced that clinical pharmacology would be a satisfying and exciting career.

27

0362-1642/85/0415-0027$02.00

At the end of that two-year tour of duty, I accepted an offer to return to Johns Hopkins, more or less in the position that Zubrod had filled, except that I had a full-time salary that was not contingent on my duties to a patient clientele. Thus started the first academic division of clinical pharmacology in the world. For the next sixteen years I toiled in the Hopkins vineyard, recruiting our share of superb postdoctoral fellows, many of whom have gone on to distinguished careers in academia, government, or industry, but with relatively modest space and a small core faculty.

In 1970, I moved once more—this time to the University of Rochester, where I assumed the chairmanship of the Department of Pharmacology and Toxicology. Now the home base for clinical pharmacology was a basic science department, although my colleagues and trainees collaborated in research with scientists in clinical departments, and we provided consultation service to all the clinical units at Strong Memorial Hospital. Recently, I have moved to Tufts University in Boston as academic dean of the medical school and dean of the Sackler School of Graduate Biomedical Sciences but with academic titles in psychiatry and pharmacology. Richard Shader and David Greenblatt have developed a division of clinical pharmacology at Tufts in which I hope to play a useful role.

Looking back at the field of clinical pharmacology over the thirty-two years of my own involvement, I see a number of high spots.

In the beginning, funding to encourage training and the creation of new programs came from a variety of sources and played a big role in getting the field off to a good start. Early in the history of our group at Hopkins, E. R. Squibb and Sons and the American Drug Manufacturers Association (later to become the Pharmaceutical Manufacturers Association) contributed fellowship stipends. Over the years, many United States drug companies, as well as the Pharmaceutical Manufacturers Association, have supported academic clinical pharmacology in a variety of ways.

In 1959, a very important support system, clinical pharmacology training grants, was established by the National Heart Institute under the far-sighted leadership of Robert Grant. Over time, a number of the National Institutes of Health have stimulated the discipline in other ways beside training grants. (The era of modern cancer chemotherapy, for example, owes much of its vigor to the cooperative clinical groups whose collaborative research was made possible by National Cancer Institute funds.)

The Burroughs-Wellcome Foundation has also served the field well, giving substantial support to faculty members pursuing careers in clinical pharmacology.

Another program, organized by the Merck Foundation, has stimulated clinical pharmacology both in the United States and abroad by giving two-year fellowships to foreign physicians wishing to study in the United States. The graduates of the program, like those of the Wellcome program, have been of high quality. Many are now pursuing careers of great achievement and promise, either in their homelands or in other countries. While in the United States as trainees, they have often been effective collaborators of United States scientists.

A delightful chapter in the history of United States clinical pharmacology was the establishment of the Non-Society. Several of us were standing on the boardwalk in Atlantic City during the 1962 spring meetings and decided to form a club with no dues, no rules, and no officers whose only purpose was to get together for discussion, drinks, and dinner once a year. The first meeting convened on April 29, 1963. The Non-Society lasted less than a decade, as I recall, but it was fun.

Looking back on these last four decades, I have the strong feeling that the success stories in academic clinical pharmacology have been due to a small number of charismatic, energetic, scientific entrepreneurs who have been able to put together large, successful, well-funded programs. I refer to people like Daniel Azarnoff, Thomas Gaffney, John Oates, and Kenneth Melmon. In Europe the list includes such folks as Colin Dollery, James Crooks, Paul Turner, and Folke Sjöqvist.

The success of these people contrasts with the fate of many other physicians in the field, who toil alone or in a group that lacks both a critical mass and adequate academic support. (The developing countries are in even worse shape.) I believe that this lack of recognition is due to many factors: the heterogeneity of interests of the art's practitioners, the suspicion that academics have of so-called generalists, the failure to take continuing responsibility for a definable body of patients, and the absence of a definite spot in the curricular sun. I find that most deans and clinical chairmen still do not understand either the nature of clinical pharmacology or its potential.

Periodically, some urge that a certifying board be set up, as if somehow board qualifications would convey a respectability now lacking. I doubt this very much. The fact is that a department chairman in medicine who would not dream of doing without a gastrointestinal group or a hematology division feels that he can live comfortably without a clinical pharmacology group.

These problems are not new, nor have they been ignored in the past. In 1965, a first-rate group of clinical pharmacologists met in Basin Harbor, Vermont, to discuss their status and their future. The group bemoaned the lack of stable support of senior faculty and the inadequate space and staffing of most units. The conclusions are as valid today, by and large, as they were then (1).

There is an interesting contrast between the sad state of academic clinical pharmacology in the United States and the burgeoning importance of the discipline in industry and the regulatory agency. The difference is easily explained, in my view: for the Food and Drug Administration and industry, the study of drugs in man is a raison d'etre. One cannot imagine the discipline dying in a given pharmaceutical firm or the FDA because of the loss of a single leader. The same cannot be said of the successful academic units referred to earlier. Indeed, some clinical research wards run by industry are the envy of scientists in academia. So are their budgets.

The failure of academic clinical pharmacology to thrive is a great pity. Such scientists have a great deal to contribute to society: better teaching of undergraduate medical students as well as physicians, improvement in the methodology of clinical trials, expert monitoring of drug usage and of post-registration experience in regard to unsuspected therapeutic benefits and adverse reactions, the providing of appropriate drug information to patients and advice to both regulatory agencies and industry, the facilitation of increased research cooperation between industry and academia, and a source of help to governments as they try to cope with media and other pressures.

What I do not foresee is any fundamental change in the image of clinical pharmacology. Nothing can convert it overnight from a young discipline to an ancient one. It will continue to fuse basic science skills with clinical ones. The field's domain will remain broad, and its practitioners will have great variability in their clinical backgrounds: internal medicine, pediatrics, anesthesiology, psychiatry, oncology, etc. Their research will be—and should be—all over the lot: developing new drugs, investigating mechanisms of action, studying biotransformation, quantifying drug benefits and risks in epidemiologic terms, etc. What must occur, therefore, is a better understanding of all this on the part of university administrators and granting agencies.

Lest this account appear unduly negative, I want to also list some of the positive developments. There are now two United States societies devoted to clinical pharmacology, the American Society for Clinical Pharmacology and Therapeutics and the American College of Clinical Pharmacology, and their membership continues to grow. *Clinical Pharmacology and Therapeutics* is a well-respected and widely read journal. Europe has spawned several other first-class journals. Substantial numbers of competent physicians are engaged in clinical trials. A lot of clinical pharmacology is subsumed under the umbrella of medical specialties: oncology, cardiology, anesthesiology, psychiatry, etc. However, these latter disciplines have constituencies that tend to think of themselves not as clinical pharmacologists but as medical specialists, and they tend to meet separately and to seek to publish for their own colleagues rather than for the clinical pharmacology fraternity.

The achievements of United States clinical pharmacology have been substantial, but they have fallen far short of what could be done. Can we improve the present state of affairs? Will the various segments of society involved recognize the need for outstanding academic programs to train the broadly based clinical pharmacologists of the future? Is it not important for academia to contribute its share of new ideas, new insights, and general intellectual ferment to the field? Will the clinical pharmacologists of today reproduce themselves or will they gradually die out like some sect of scientific Shakers?

Literature Cited

1. Lasagna, L. 1966. Clinical pharmacology: Present status and future development. *Science* 152:388–91

Ann. Rev. Pharmacol. Toxicol. 1985. 25:33–40

PERSPECTIVES IN TOXICOLOGY

Maynard B. Chenoweth

Michigan Molecular Institute, 1910 West St. Andrews Road, Midland, Michigan 48640

Most of the difficulties in the field of toxicology today are not technical but political, psychological, and sociological. Toxicology as a discipline is between a rock and a hard place, to say the least. Very toxic or hazardous materials can be defined promptly, but to prove that a less-obviously toxic material could never do anything, to anybody, any time, is totally impossible. Yet that seems to be what some of the more vociferous public demands, and it is the general public that pays the bills and takes the risks. As a result, far-reaching decisions may be made based on very slender evidence.

Just consider the interaction of diazepam and ethanol. It is generally conceded that the two are positively interactive, but are there any quantitative data? Possibly I have missed them; possibly they lie in Air Force, etc, files. But think about the problem of such research in an open area. First, one must calibrate the subjects against both agents using tests that are agreed upon, and then design a study that combines the two at levels known to be debilitating. What committee would approve such a study? Yet this information is of critical importance in the courts every day!

Today, toxicology is of major social value primarily as a predictive science. We must know, as best we can, what will be: what was is too late. Under these conditions toxicology must do better. The rat is a valuable laboratory reagent but results in this or any other animal species are by no means directly transferable to man, and all kinds of "man" are not necessarily toxicologically equal. The problem of transferring animal data to man in practical terms has been much discussed in the literature and needs no reiteration.

Modern-day measurement on persons during or after mild or moderate industrial environmental exposure has so far produced mostly negative results, a fact that is certainly encouraging. Many studies can be criticized for uncontrolled variables, lack of baseline data, prejudgment and poor design, shifting

33

0362-1642/85/0415-0033$02.00

from one analytical laboratory to another, while the mensuration procedure itself is often insensitive or fatally flawed in principle. The findings often are not usable data, just numbers. The financial cost of doing a human surveillance study as well as is currently possible is extremely high. Furthermore, most of these studies must be made on persons in stable, well-controlled work places where exposures are minimal and documented. Not many managers of this type of organization are willing, let alone anxious, to find that their current operations' practices are harmful, or that such studies often yield more questions than answers.

Government agencies can to some extent overcome this problem by examining many different exposed groups according to an agreed-upon protocol. Determining such a protocol has not been, and will not be, easy. Conditions under which the general public is exposed are so much more complex as to appear to defy analysis, yet many charge in where angels fear to tread.

Epidemiologic studies are important, but only from an historical point of view. Fraught with confounding factors, too small cohorts, biases both known and unknown, etc, they can at best tell us what may have been. Positive findings may be the result of past unknown exposures; negative results are more interpretable and valuable, for they tell us that, no matter what the compound does in the laboratory, recent usage is not hazardous.

Laboratory studies in healthy human volunteers are quite practical and are often used to research the toxicokinetics and metabolic disposition of a test substance. The latest analytic techniques permit biochemical studies that were inconceivable two decades ago. These studies can tell us something about what might be, especially when aided by computer modeling.

But might be is only applicable to the volunteer group: usually male, young, educated, vigorously healthy, and mostly uniracial. All the variables are eliminated as well as possible. A visit to a factory or hospital will reveal only a few of these young men. Studies in other groups are possible, especially with therapeutic materials, but they become somewhat more difficult when non-medicinal chemicals are to be studied, largely for sociological reasons, and have rarely been attempted.

Some of the truly critical studies simply can not be done with human subjects. Yet somehow we must gain a very accurate idea of its effects before a new drug or chemical is offered. How? Detailed studies in a variety of species together with the most sagacious extrapolation of these data seem the only way employed at this time. Such work is very expensive and deters the entrance of many, probably useful, products into agriculture, medicine, and industry. It certainly does not encourage the study of old, generic compounds.

Sagacity is very much improved when toxic mechanisms are well understood. Indeed, in the long run, this may be the least expensive research approach to the problem. For example, the early discovery that man metabolizes a compound differently from most other species could save millions of dollars worth of research, probably still more under application conditions.

Subhuman primate studies are of real value, but unless it is known that they handle a compound as man does they can be more misleading than studies in mice, for there is a natural feeling that primates are sort of a little human. Toxicologically, this is not the case.

Data from accidental poisoning cases are of value, even though they may be described by some as a series of one case. Data from one case are much better than no data at all. Unfortunately, most of these data are difficult to interpret and only rarely reach the scientific literature.

Of late, it seems that we are closing in on the mechanisms of carcinogenesis. The concept that it is often a multi-step process seems promising. The difference between genetic and epigenetic mechanisms is much clearer than it was just a few years ago. The significant difference between excessive experimental doses that overwhelm an animal's metabolic channels and lead to strange metabolities of possibly carcinogenic nature, and more realistic doses that do not, is not yet adequately appreciated by all members of the scientific community. Discoveries progress rapidly, and it may not be many years before toxicology can assert some truly practical rules about chemical carcinogenesis. Much is already known concerning the reactions or forces binding carcinogens to DNA. When all the facts can be put together, toxicologists hope that this most frightening aspect of toxicity will be understood enough to explain or predict adequately for practical purposes.

We should not assume that all the industries promoting materials are beyond reproach. "Playing their cards close to their vest" is the nicest thing that can be said about many. However, confronted by the adversarial attitude underlying US law and the fact that the final presentation to a sensitive agency is often made by persons more attuned to the business world than the scientific, this lack of candor is understandable, though not excusable.

The very largest organizations, with billions of dollars of capital investments, can not pack their bags and run. Their battalions of scientists and regiments of lawyers try to keep them as close to legal perfection as possible, yet things do go wrong in corners of their empires. The smaller organizations are often most blatant in their defiance of laws and regulations, while those intermediate are—intermediate. Frankly criminal operations are not unheard of. Strong federal, state, and local agencies are a necessary element in the control of all.

Perhaps one of the more visible forces to impact toxicology in recent years is the Good Laboratory Practices (GLP) regulation. It has forced sloppy laboratories to improve to a standard or quit. For properly run laboratories it may at times seem to be a nuisance, but it does help assure that they will remain properly running. The financial cost of compliance is considerable, but in the long run it will be well repaid in savings from studies that need not be repeated and from the catastrophe of imaginary or specious data. As most academic laboratories are not interested in research for the record but rather in mechanism and exploratory studies, the GLP regulation should not be a great burden on them. When academic or governmental laboratories do attempt the massive for-the-record studies, it has not been unusual from them to botch them.

Experimental studies in normal humans with industrial chemicals in simulated workplace exposures carried out in non-governmentally supported laboratories seem to fall into a regulatory gap. It seems best that these laboratories follow the Declaration of Helsinki, GLP and *Good Clinical Practices* (GCP), as in the FDA regulations. The protocol should first be reviewed and approved by a stern internal review committee and then sent to an external review committee, such as a cooperating university medical center, for final approval, particularly of the ethical aspects of the proposal. Only upon their approval should volunteers be accepted, informed consent be obtained, and work begin. Physicians other than the investigator should carry out the physical examinations and be on standby with proper equipment during the study. These precautions may seem excessive, but it is better to be safe than sorry.

Does the role of the toxicologist cease once the chemicals are in the total environment? Away with semantics—of course not. Radiation of all kinds, environmental temperature, humidity, heredity, diet, race, age, sex and pregnancy, and, as well, disease, nutritional status, stress, and medication form the background against which all chemicals act and interact. The interaction of chemical with chemical at pharmacological levels in laboratory studies and clinical practice is well recognized. This aspect warrants continued research with non-therapeutic compounds, and this should be done in addition against disease and all the other factors described above. Possible interactions of traces of environmental chemicals are even more difficult to define and study, but it must be attempted.

One aspect of toxicology that probably has always existed is the mass hysteria phenomenon. Only lately has this phenomenon been recognized to be precisely that. This sort of reaction is very apt to confuse the average physician, toxicologist, or industrial hygienist whose groundings are in hard data, but it is nonetheless real and frightening to those caught up in it. Early recognition of its occurrence could save a great many analytical hours and unnecessary ambulance runs, although not much more. It appears to be based on poor working conditions and in general social dissatisfaction. Whether it will increase or decrease in incidence would seem to be quite dependent on such factors. Certain age and sex groupings seem most prone to its occurrence.

An aspect of industrial hygiene that has recently come to the toxicological forefront is the problem of unusual work hours. By no means does everyone work an eight-hour day and a forty-hour week. Yet the threshold limit values

(TLVs) are based on this schedule. We do know that continuous exposure to toxins in the workplace can produce some very nasty results and scraps of experience show that overtime or double shifts can lead to trouble.

The kinetics of excretion and metabolism are useful in developing formulae to calculate the safe odd-hour exposure level, but we know next to nothing about the tissue recovery cycle. A number of compounds spring to mind that still exert a residual effect despite our inability to detect their presence. This is obviously an area crying out for research.

There are some geographic aspects to applications of toxicological information. In one area a low hatch rate of perigrine bird eggs should be regarded seriously. In others, malaria-bearing mosquitoes infect huge numbers of humans. What is appropriate insecticide usage in one area is not appropriate in other areas. In places where it is possible to get reliable analysis in thirty minutes, pesticide levels can be controlled in the environment, food, and feeds. In other areas, insects and rodents uncontrolled can rival the starving human population in consumption of food supplies. Unless they take such local environmental conditions into account, it is impudent for the very advanced countries to make suggestions ridiculous to less-advanced countries with drastic problems.

A considerable amount of money is being spent in an attempt to develop alternatives for whole-animal experiments in the hope that these might be less costly and more humane. To be sure, a 50% solution of NaOH will coagulate egg white as well as corneas. Recently, in preparing the advice to physicians section of an OSHA material safety data sheet for a material of very low systemic toxicity, I found it necessary to write: "ATTENTION. CAUSES *NO* PAIN, CAUSES *SEVERE* CORNEAL BURNS, CAN CAUSE *BLINDNESS*." I cannot conceive how that information could have been obtained from tissue cultures, computers, egg whites or micro-organisms. Furthermore, it could not have been obtained from an anesthetized cornea.

The extreme present pressure to publish or perish together with the shrinkage of the funding base have led scientists into desperate moves. Prepublication publicity, minimum facts, and maximum press confuse the public. The world is not improved by cockamamie scientists who cry wolf at every mouse.

Special interest groups do not trust governmental agencies and exert as much pressure as they can to obtain their way. One such group is often in opposition to another or others. Meanwhile, the general public, which only wants to be protected against unreasonable hazards, does not know where to turn and can panic easily.

Were all the chemical actions and interactions possible to be studied in full detail, toxicology would not become a growth industry, it would be the industry. Everyone wishes to be fully healthy and the medical community has responded with vigor. Already the health industry is under increasing pressure to do more with less, but still it will consume a very large proportion of the GNP. Add to this research on the full toxicological background on all things and 15% of the GNP is not a completely ridiculous estimated expense. Can we keep toxicology from eating itself out of house and home?

The news media in the USA (and probably wherever the news is free) has not been very helpful. In the end, its purpose is to sell itself and its advertising space. This has not escaped the cartoonists (Figure 1). Very recently there have begun to appear editorial self-flagellations and *mea culpas,* as the intoxication with terror becomes a hangover in the light of fact.

People in the USA are not noted for caution. Short tempers, illegal drugs, alcohol and tobacco, tens of millions of guns, automobiles, as well as sports kill or maim more persons in one year than have, in all likelihood, been hurt by identifiable chemicals in all of time. Why then the panicky reaction to a trace of a poisonous material? Perhaps the answer lies in the attitude, "If I kill myself having fun, that's my affair; but why should I be poisoned for someone else's profit?" Add to this the current distrust of government and a kind of paranoia develops. Indeed, there have been enough scandalous occurrences to keep suspicions at a high level. A virtually complete lack of understanding of the usefulness of chemicals in their daily lives, the mystery of maybe regarding possible noxious effects, a total lack of understanding of the dose-response concept, and, finally, their impotence in a sea of incomprehensible chemical names complete the circle. Until the combination of distrust of authority and the tubular vision of litigious and opposed groups can be resolved, toxicologists' work will never end.

What to do? Let us look at some possibilities and their accompanying problems. We cannot ignore toxicology and we can not do every conceivable test. It must be decided what tests are needed and useful. Very reasonable: now who decides? Throwing the question to an electorate is an abdication of duty and may often be tantamount to blackmail. Large units of the bureaucratic

JOHN DARLING   by Armstrong & Batiuk

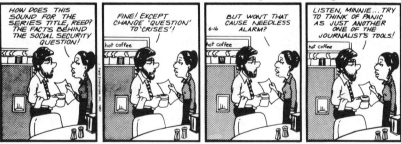

Figure 1 "John Darling," by Tom Armstrong and Tom Batiuk © 1983 Field Enterprises, Inc. Courtesy of Field Newspaper Syndicate.

system are jealous of their power and internally operate on a CYA[1] basis. The record of their cooperation is appalling. It is not difficult to imagine one agency using or approving a material another agency is banning, especially when one considers that a given substance may have toxic and beneficial aspects ranging from human therapeutics and/or toxicity and/or hazard through medicine, agriculture, industrial applications, ecology, environment, and economics.

The excess of lawyers in the USA has helped produce a flood of flimsy law suits, mostly on a contingency basis (i.e. a large percentage of any award goes to the attorney, not the plaintiff). A decision by a judge and jury becomes a precedent and goes to form the corpus of the law. Naturally, most defendants are those with the money and prefer to settle out of court to avoid both establishing a precedent and the high cost of defense, perhaps thus encouraging further suits. While good and wise scientists may differ in their interpretation of the same data, once in court they are forced to express black versus white and not the two shades of gray they really understand. Worst of all, lawyers are now silencing scientists' presentations to scholarly gatherings when sensitive subjects are under discussion.

Judges, no matter how well-chosen, can and do go off half-cocked. Most give decisions based on common sense. Few are technically expert. However, their opinions must be respected or else great wrongs could be done. On this account, we must tolerate the obstructionists who delay necessary or useful actions. Clearly, the courts of law are not the place to formulate an answer to a broad and multifaceted scientific problem.

Possibly an ad hoc blue ribbon panel-like system might work. Twenty-one persons drawn by lot for a specific case from a presidentially approved panel of wise persons, possessing the power to subpoena witnesses from anywhere and the funds to see the matter through to the end, might develop a balanced answer to a specific problem. The public could be assured that the wisest humans available today have done the wisest thing—for the present. We can not know what will be known a century later, for we have to handle today's problems today in order to get to tomorrow.

What does the future hold for a young toxicologist? For full development, a doctorate in an applicable science is almost a prerequisite for a career in research. Some graduates will find a niche deep in the scientific aspects of the discipline, some a place in the combat zone of political toxicology, and some in very ordinary activities. Many will not find employment easily and may be diverted into other areas of bioscience. All scientific fields follow the S-shaped curve of growth, and it is clear that the rapid growth phase is coming to an end

[1]CYA are the initials for a persistent Elizabethan vulgarism elegantly rendered "Protect yourself at all times." Under such conditions, interpretation of all but the most unequivocal data is colored. CYA inevitably means "more work is indicated."

for toxicology, at least with respect to numbers of workers. The opposite is true with regard to the ever-increasing complexity of the subject and the controversies this engenders. As the demand for toxicologists levels off, it seems probable that some of the weaker educational programs will find no students and atrophy—no great loss.

"Of making many books there is no end" (Ecclesiastes XII-12), and much the same could be said of meetings and conferences, most of which also result in a grab-bag volume of proceedings. The proliferation of periodicals bearing "toxicology" in their title also permits the publication of nearly anything, although important negative findings are still largely to be found in letters to the editor or obscure monographs. This liberality of publication is both good and bad. The good is obvious; the bad arises from the fact that many regard the printed word as truth and cannot distinguish between good and bad. The young toxicologist must be highly critical and must take nothing for granted, not even the words of respected names. "Great men are not always wise" (1 Chronicles XXXII-9), and further, "The devil can cite Scripture for his purpose" ("The Merchant of Venice" Act I, Scene 3, line 99).

Now it may seem that I am pressimistic about the future of toxicology—not at all! Toxicology must and will progress, and as time passes and mechanisms are understood, more and better answers will be found. My only complaint is that it will not be I who finds them.

For a century investigators have been working largely with simple materials prepared by the time-honored methods of organic chemistry. While there is yet hope that remarkably non-toxic, biodegradable, specific compounds may be found, the odds are worsening. The movement into fields that use hybridomas of living tissues to prepare super-specific compounds, that use plant products hitherto undetectable, that manufacture more products from biosynthetic sources, and that create complex substances such as unusual polymers, proteins, natural toxins, and who knows what next, is creating new problems that toxicology must address. Cost per gram is meaningless; cost per uninfested crop, cost per day of hospitalization, cost per acre-feet of pure water, are the only valid considerations.

It must not be thought for a moment that this shift will end controversy or placate controversialists. Carbon monoxide and lead are still capable of generating furor as well as illness. Only when avarice and ignorance are eliminated from human kind will toxicology become a dull study. There will be plenty to do!

Ann. Rev. Pharmacol. Toxicol. 1985. 25:41–65
Copyright © 1985 by Annual Reviews Inc. All rights reserved

THE EFFECT OF DRUGS ON RESPIRATION IN MAN

Arthur S. Keats

Division of Cardiovascular Anesthesia, Texas Heart Institute, and Department of Anesthesiology, University of Texas School of Medicine, Houston, Texas 77030

INTRODUCTION

Both previous reviewers (1, 2) of the subject of the effect of drugs on respiration in man noted that respiration may be markedly affected by drugs acting at sites other than the respiratory control center in the brain. Drugs may modify afferent input and transmission to the center or alter the mechanical properties and performance of the effector organ through its airways, circulation, or respiratory muscles. The effects of drugs such as the inhalation anesthetics on respiration are the result of actions on whole body and organ metabolism, on chemoreceptor sensitivity, on mechanical properties of the chest wall and bronchial tree, on volume and distribution of pulmonary blood flow, as well as on the respiratory control center. Of necessity, this review is limited to drugs whose predominant effect is by a mechanism involved in central respiratory control. Its emphasis is on the results of drug administrations rather than on the mechanisms that effect the changes. Because of the ease with which many aspects of respiration are now studied and the abundance of such studies, the data reviewed are limited to those obtained in man except where specifically stated. Further, all data cited were obtained from healthy subjects unless stipulated otherwise. Data reviewed here largely supplement other recent reviews applying to the broad title (3–5).

METHODS OF MEASUREMENT AND THEIR LIMITATIONS

Ideally, the measurement of drug effects on respiration should examine all mechanisms potentially affecting respiration, quantify each, and evolve an

41

0362-1642/85/0415-0041$02.00

integrated picture describing the contribution of each to the net effect observed following a therapeutic dose. The effect of morphine in man, for example, could be described in terms of proportionate changes in CO_2 production, chemoreceptor activity, central chemical sensitivity, altered airway resistance, and pulmonary ventilation/perfusion relationships that follow from a modified pattern of breathing. Such a description has not been attained for any drug. In terms of clinical usefulness and drug safety, the primary questions are: Does the drug act on respiratory control mechanisms leading to hypoventilation (respiratory depression) or hyperventilation (respiratory stimulation)? Is this effect greater or less than some reference drug? Is the effect dose related? To answer these questions, studies have been directed primarily to the measurement of changes in ventilation stimulated by high carbon dioxide or low oxygen in healthy subjects. The stimulus to respiration is expressed in terms of tension, PCO_2 or PO_2. Tensions are usually measured in end tidal gas samples, at times called alveolar gas samples, $P_{ET}CO_2$ or P_ACO_2. Less commonly they are determined from arterial blood ($PaCO_2$). These abbreviations will be used in subsequent descriptions.

The study of drug effects on some aspects of resting ventilation is seriously limited by the relatively small potential range of observed responses. Changes in gas exchange measured as respiratory rate, tidal or minute volume, or their consequence measured as $P_{ET}CO_2$, $PaCO_2$, or PaO_2, are small following doses of drugs that have a profound effect on stimulated respiration. For example, narcotic analgesics or inhalation anesthetics that increase resting $PaCO_2$ only 5 mmHg induce very large changes in the CO_2 response curve. The small range of potential responses decreases sensitivity for quantitative comparisons between drugs and a description of dose-response relationships. By contrast, the range of responses is greatly exaggerated when respiration is stressed by inspiration of high CO_2 or low O_2 tensions.

Response to Carbon-Dioxide Stimulation (CO_2 Response)

In normal subjects, increasing inspired PCO_2 dramatically increases minute volume of ventilation in an almost linear fashion, achieving expired volumes greater than 30 liters per minute at $P_{ET}CO_2$ less than 50 mmHg. Since hypoxia also increases the CO_2 response, 50% or more oxygen is used as the diluent gas to eliminate the chemoreceptor contribution to stimulation. The response to PCO_2 is exquisitely sensitive to drugs acting directly on the respiratory control center, and they alter this response by displacing the curve to the right and by decreasing its slope. No single expression quantifies these two changes. Potent analgesics in therapeutic doses displace curves to the right with small changes in slope, and the change can be quantified by measuring displacements in mmHg P_ACO_2 assuming parallel slopes. High doses of potent analgesics, especially if associated with marked sedation or sleep, as well as inhalation anesthetics exert their predominant effect by decreasing slope, which is usually quantified as percent change from control. It is not unlikely that drugs that displace without changing slope and others that do the converse act at different sites within the intimate structure of the respiratory center. The practical problem is illustrated in Figure 1, which shows the effect of morphine in low dose to be displacement and in high dose to be a decrease in slope. Assumption of parallel slopes for the high dose curves will only measure displacement of the mean of the calculated curve. On the other hand, using change in slope as the measure, the effect of morphine 20 mg is small. At the moment there is no convention for measuring or reporting these changes, permitting easy comparison of drugs, or the construction of dose-effect curves.

A further difficulty in quantifying drug effects on the CO_2 response is that the method influences the curve obtained, leading to uncertainties in comparing results obtained by the two methods. In the rebreathing technique, during which the subject rebreathes from a bag containing oxygen and 6%–7% CO_2, the progressive increase in inspired CO_2 derives from endogenous CO_2 production and excretion into the bag. In this instance, the CO_2 gradient is from the tissues to the lung, and the PCO_2 stimulus in the respiratory center is higher than that measured as $P_{ET}CO_2$. Slopes of curves obtained in this way tend to be greater and displacement less than with curves obtained by breathing discrete CO_2 mixtures to steady-state ventilation without rebreathing. In the latter technique, the CO_2 gradient is from the lungs to the brain. A lower volume ventilation is then measured at a higher $P_{ET}CO_2$, with a decrease in slope of the CO_2 response curve. These differences were well illustrated in a detailed comparison of the two techniques in dogs (6). Problems in quantification of these curves and discussion of techniques and errors have been treated in detail by others (7–12).

CO₂ Stimulation at Constant PCO₂

A sensitive but seldom used method of quantifying drug effects on the CO_2 response is the continuous measurement of minute ventilation at a constant elevated end-tidal PCO_2. The method was first used by Lambertsen (13) to describe the time course of respiratory depression by intramuscular meperidine. He employed a continuous but varied inflow of CO_2 into the inspiratory limb of a non-rebreathing circuit to maintain constant end tidal PCO_2. The method measures continuously one point on the CO_2 response curve and ignores change in slope. It is ideally suited for determining the onset, peak, and duration of drug effect, particularly with drugs whose profile includes rapid onset and peak or short duration. Even the rebreathing method requires so much time that true onset and peak may be missed. A modification of this technique incorporates periodic determinations of the entire CO_2 response curve at intervals during continuous elevated PCO_2 breathing (14). A further modifica-

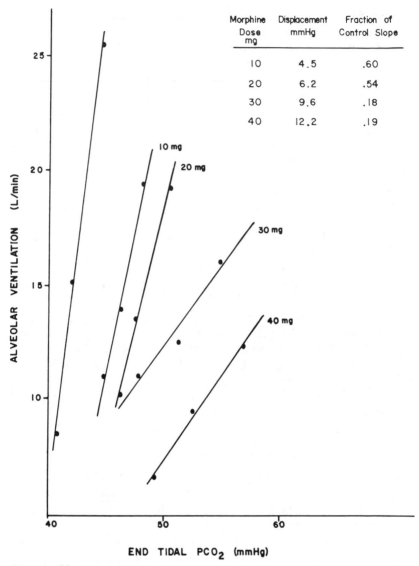

Morphine Dose mg	Displacement mmHg	Fraction of Control Slope
10	4.5	.60
20	6.2	.54
30	9.6	.18
40	12.2	.19

Figure 1 CO$_2$ response curves by the steady-state method from one subject who received four doses of morphine 10 mg intravenously at forty-minute intervals. Displacements were calculated assuming parallel slopes. Low doses primarily displaced the curves, whereas larger doses decreased slope as well.

tion is designed to provide a continuous measure of drugs whose effect is primarily a decrease in slope of the CO$_2$ response curve, for example, the effect of thiopental. Gross, Smith & Smith (15) devised a two-point isohypercapnic technique in which subjects were studied on two separate occasions under identical circumstances during which $P_{ET}CO_2$ was held constant at 46 mmHg on one occasion and at 58 mmHg on the other. Superimposing the data from these studies provides a continuous two-point curve from which slope can be calculated. The disadvantage of these techniques is their prolonged CO_2 inhalation, which may introduce errors by subject discomfort, apprehension, fatigue, and possibly alteration in CO_2 response by altered buffering capacity.

Response to Hypoxic Stimulation (Hypoxic Response)

Healthy subjects breathe progressively lower oxygen tensions until respiratory stimulation occurs through the carotid body chemoreceptors. The hypoxic stimulus is usually limited to 40 mmHg. To test drug effects on chemoreceptor sensitivity isocapnia must be maintained, because PCO_2 itself alters chemoreceptor sensitivity. CO_2 is therefore added to the inspired gas as ventilation increases, and $P_{ET}CO_2$, $P_{ET}O_2$, and minute volume are measured simultaneously. Steady-state techniques are also used and more rapid rebreathing techniques have been proposed to minimize subject exposure to hypoxia. The curve derived from the plot of $P_{ET}O_2$ and minute ventilation has been described as a hyperbola, although when altered by drugs the curve may be exponential or even flat (Figure 2). Drugs alter the hypoxic response by decreasing the $P_{ET}O_2$ at which respiratory stimulation begins and by decreasing the magnitude of ventilation at all levels of $P_{ET}O_2$. As with CO_2 responses, no single expression incorporates both these changes. Even though gross dose-response relationships have been demonstrated for some anesthetics (Figure 2), the lack of easy quantification inhibits comparisons between drugs and the delineation of dose-response relationships. Further, the position and shape of the curve describing the hypoxic response varies with the level of isocapnia selected, and hypercapnia may increase apparent drug-induced depression of the hypoxic response (16). At the moment, there is no uniformity in methods of measurement of the hypoxic response. Techniques and quantification of these curves as applied to the study of drugs have been treated in greater detail elsewhere (11, 12).

A further confounding aspect of stimulated ventilation curves obtained from drugged subjects is that when sufficiently severe both these stimuli, high PCO_2 and low PO_2, depress the respiratory response through their own actions. In healthy subjects, respiratory depression rather than stimulation probably occurs when PaO_2 is less than 35 mmHg and $PaCO_2$ is greater than 100 mmHg. In drugged subjects, these thresholds may not apply. The slope of the CO_2 response of one subject studied by Johnstone et al (18) was negative when $P_{ET}CO_2$ increased from 70 to 110 mmHg after a large dose of morphine. Kroneberg et al (19) observed hypoxic depression of ventilation at PaO_2 40 mmHg in two healthy subjects who received no drugs.

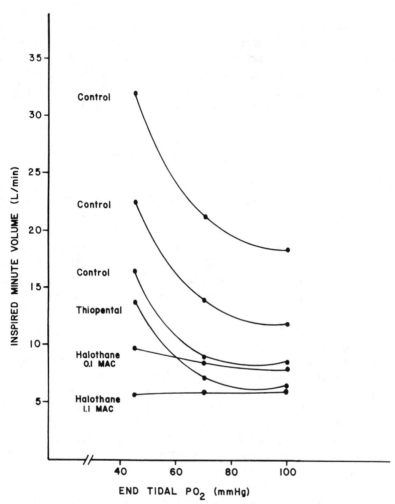

Figure 2   The variety of ventilatory responses to isocapnic hypoxia before and after anesthetics replotted from data of Knill and colleagues (16, 17). The position of control curves is in part related to the level of isocapnia. The topmost curve was the control for the study of thiopental.

SPECIFIC DRUG GROUPS

General Anesthetics

A systematic study of the respiratory and circulatory effects of commonly used inhalation anesthetics was carried out by E. I. Eger II and his colleagues over a period of a decade.

CO_2 RESPONSE   Eger and colleagues employed healthy subjects on whom no operation was performed and obtained quantitative comparisons between drugs

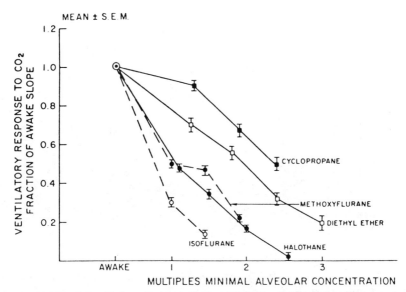

Figure 3 The relationship between doses of various inhaled anesthetic agents and the percent of depression of the slope of the CO_2 response (20, 21). Dose is expressed in multiples of MAC (see text). [Reproduced from (5) with permission.]

and dose-response relationships for each drug. Most of their data were summarized in one publication (20), and subsequently data on isoflurane were added (21). These are summarized in Figures 3 and 4. Dose was expressed as multiples of MAC, the minimal alveolar (end-tidal) concentration of inhaled anesthetic at steady state that prevented movement in response to a surgical skin incision in 50% of patients. The MAC value for each anesthetic had been determined previously in patients undergoing operations. The dose scale is presented linearly and represents multiples of the MAC dose. In equipotent anesthetic doses, isoflurane is the most potent respiratory depressant. Except for diethylether, the increase in $PaCO_2$ during anesthesia with spontaneous ventilation correlated well with depression of the slope of the CO_2 response. The ability of subjects to maintain normocapnia while spontaneously breathing diethylether up to 3 MAC suggests that stimulation of peripheral chemoreceptors or mechanical receptors in the lung or airway, or of those responsive to the irritant properties of diethylether, increases respiratory center input while sensitivity of the center progressively decreases.

HYPOXIC RESPONSE   Recently, the remarkable sensitivity of the chemoreceptor mechanism to depression by inhalation anesthetics was demonstrated by Knill and his colleagues. Their results, together with those of Yacoub et al (22), are summarized in Table 1. Depression of chemoreceptor sensitivity

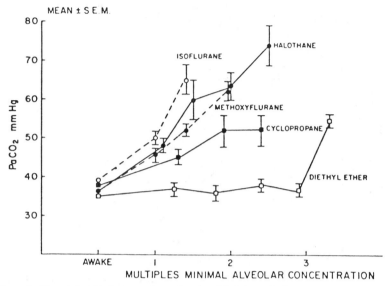

Figure 4   The relationship between doses of various inhaled anesthetic agents and PaCO₂ during spontaneous respiration (20, 21). Note the lack of dose-effect relationship for diethylether. [Reproduced from (5) with permission.]

was almost identical for the three fluorinated hydrocarbons. The site of depression was confirmed by measuring the marked reduction by these anesthetics in the ventilatory response to a small intravenous dose of doxapram, known to stimulate the chemoreceptor mechanism primarily (16, 24). During these studies, responsiveness to the CO_2 stimulus in terms of depression of slope of the CO_2 response was also measured. CO_2 response did not decrease at doses that depressed the hypoxic response (0.1 MAC) and was still present, although decreased, at doses that abolished the hypoxic response (1.1 MAC). An overview of the effect of fluorinated hydrocarbons on respiration is summarized in Figure 5.

INTRAVENOUS ANESTHETICS   Measurement of respiratory effects of intravenous anesthetics has been difficult because of the absence of a steady state owing to rapid drug redistribution. Knill et al (17) studied thiopental given by infusion at rates that maintained either clinical sedation (drowsy, conscious) or anesthesia (loss of eyelid reflex). Sedative doses of thiopental did not alter the CO_2 response or the hypoxic response. However, anesthetic doses depressed both responses, as well as the response to doxapram, to approximately the same degree. The nonspecific depression of responses by thiopental contrasts with the selective chemoreceptor depression by inhaled anesthetics, indicating quantitatively different actions on the components of ventilatory control.

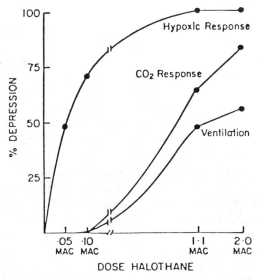

DOSE HALOTHANE

Figure 5   Dose-related effects of halothane on the hypoxic response, the CO_2 response, and on spontaneous ventilation. The lower doses (0.05–0.1 MAC) do not produce unconsciousness, whereas the two higher doses produce general anesthesia. The extreme sensitivity of the hypoxic response to halothane is demonstrated. [Reproduced from (23) with permission.]

Attempts to find alternatives to thiopental as an intravenous induction agent for general anesthesia led to a trial of diazepam and more recently to a trial of a water-soluble benzodiazepine, midazolam, for this purpose. Early studies of changes in resting ventilation or arterial blood gases by diazepam given by mouth or intramuscularly were equivocal on respiratory depressant activity.

Table 1   Effect of anesthetics on ventilatory response to hypoxia

Drug	Dose	Response	Reference
Nitrous oxide	30–50%	Depressed	22
Halothane	0.05 MAC[a]	Depressed	23
	0.1 MAC	Depressed	16, 23
	1.1 MAC	Abolished	16
	2.0 MAC	Abolished	16
Enflurane	0.1 MAC	Depressed	24
	1.1 MAC	Abolished	24
Isoflurane	0.1 MAC	Depressed	25
	1.1 MAC	Abolished	25
Thiopental	Sedation	None	17
	Anesthesia	Depressed	17

[a] Minimal alveolar concentration (see text for definition).

When given intravenously, however, in doses of 0.1–0.4 mg/kg, diazepam showed a consistent decrease of about 50% in the slope of the CO_2 response, with peak effect approximately 30 minutes after administration (15, 26, 27). Forster et al (27) compared diazepam 0.3 mg/kg with midazolam 0.15 mg/kg, both given intravenously, and found that they depressed the CO_2 response equally. Gross et al (28), using the dual isohypercapnic technique, compared midazolam 0.2 mg/kg with thiopental 3.5 mg/kg given intravenously to healthy subjects and to patients with chronic obstructive pulmonary disease. Both drugs significantly depressed the slope of the CO_2 response. Depression was greater after midazolam than after thiopental, and both drugs produced greater depression in patients with obstructive pulmonary disease. Curiously, Power et al (29) were unable to find any significant alteration in the CO_2 response after administering midazolam 0.075 mg/kg or diazepam 0.15 mg/kg intravenously.

Jordan et al (26) claim to have shortened the respiratory depression of diazepam 0.2 mg/kg by giving naloxone 15 mg 60 minutes and again 95 minutes after diazepam compared to similarly administered placebo. Forster et al (30) observed no antagonism when naloxone 1 mg was given five minutes after midazolam in doses up to 0.2 mg/kg intravenously. Clearly, diazepam receptors are different from naloxone receptors.

Narcotic Analgesics

Borison (4) in his review tabulated the available references to drug effects on respiration in man by specific drug, identifying those that studied the CO_2 response and those that studied components of resting ventilation. His table provides a convenient reference source for narcotic analgesics as well as for antagonists. Tilidine can now be added to that list (31).

CO_2 RESPONSE   Most investigations on CO_2 response have been generated by a search for potent analgesics with a lesser side action liability than morphine. The pattern was an initial determination of analgesic potency, usually in postoperative pain, followed by measurement of the respiratory depressant capacity of equianalgesic doses in terms of displacement of the CO_2 response. In contrast to the primary effects of anesthetics and drugs producing sleep on the slope of the CO_2 response, narcotic analgesics primarily displaced response to the right, with statistically insignificant changes in slope. With almost boring consistency, drugs of this type produce equivalent respiratory depression when given in equianalgesic doses (Table 2). Drugs of this type have been identified as μ agonists in opiate receptor terminology.

HYPOXIC RESPONSE   Surprisingly, of the narcotic analgesic compounds only morphine and meperidine have been studied for their effect on the hypoxic response. Weil et al (32) described depression of this response one hour after

Table 2 Doses of clinically used potent analgesics that produce equal analgesia and respiratory depression in man by the intramuscular route

Analgesic	Dosage
Morphine	10 mg
Meperidine	75 mg
Methadone	10 mg
Anileridine	30 mg
Oxymorphone	1 mg
Levorphanol	2.5 mg
Alphaprodine	30 mg
Hydromorphone	1.2 mg
Oxycodone	14 mg
Dihydrocodeine	60 mg
Heroin	5 mg
Fentanyl	0.15 mg
Codeine	~ 120 mg

administering morphine 7.5 mg subcutaneously. The degree of depression was similar to that shown for thiopental in Figure 2. Kryger et al (33) demonstrated a depressed hypoxic response two hours after meperidine 1.2 mg/kg was given by mouth. Like thiopental and unlike the inhalation anesthetics, the magnitude of depression of the hypoxic response and the CO_2 response was approximately equal.

ORAL ADMINISTRATION   The paucity of studies of the respiratory effects of analgesics given by mouth is surprising in view of the abundant studies of analgesic potency by this route. Only Bellville and his associates have pursued this question with any consistency. In a nicely designed study, they determined that the respiratory effect of codeine 100 mg was equal to that of morphine 10 mg when both were given intramuscularly (34). They then determined that oral codeine was 0.72 as potent as intramuscular codeine in terms of respiratory depression. By extrapolation, they estimated codeine 140 mg orally to be the respiratory depressant equivalent of morphine 10 mg intramuscularly. From their companion study on the respiratory effects of oral dextropropoxyphene and codeine, they estimated by extrapolation that 420 mg of dextropropoxyphene would be required by mouth to depress respiration as much as morphine 10 mg intramuscularly (35). Meperidine 1.2 mg/kg by mouth depressed the CO_2 response as well as the hypoxic response (33).

AS AN ANESTHETIC SUPPLEMENT   During the past fifteen years, narcotic analgesics have been increasingly used as supplements during general anesthesia, usually with nitrous oxide. For forty years, meperidine was the traditional drug for this purpose, usually given in 100 to 200 mg doses. Recently, morphine in doses up to 2 mg/kg and fentanyl up to 100 μg/kg have been used to supplement general anesthesia. At times even higher doses, with oxygen alone and with a neuromuscular blocking drug, have been administered as general anesthesia for cardiac operations. The attraction of these techniques, which incorporate very large narcotic doses, is their relative freedom from hemodynamic effects compared to halogenated hydrocarbons. Their drawback is their failure to block the hemodynamic responses to surgical stimulation and, when adequate hypnotic drugs have not been added, the potential of an aware but immobilized patient during operations. Current preference is for fentanyl because of its high milligram potency, rapid onset of action, and short duration. When given as small single doses intravenously to healthy subjects, fentanyl (1.4 μg/kg given over 2.5 minutes) depressed the CO_2 response for a shorter period than alphaprodine or meperidine (14). Time to peak effect, however, was the same for all three drugs, about eight minutes. With a much larger dose of fentanyl (6.4 μg/kg given over 90 seconds) peak respiratory depression in terms of $P_{ET}CO_2$ during spontaneous respiration developed in less than five minutes and returned to control over the next four hours (36). The rate of decrease in $P_{ET}CO_2$ correlated well with the rapid rate of decline in plasma fentanyl levels. Within sixty minutes 98.6% of the fentanyl dose was eliminated from the plasma and terminal half-life was 3.6 hours (37). Recovery from fentanyl-induced respiratory depression occurs primarily by redistribution rather than by drug elimination. As expected with these pharmacokinetic characteristics, the larger the initial dose the more rapid the onset of respiratory depression and the greater its persistence.

Stoeckel et al (38) administered 0.5 mg (approximately 8 ug/kg) to seven healthy subjects, three of whom became apneic for 2–7 minutes. Their CO_2 response did not return to control within the six hours of study. While noting that respiratory depression correlated with plasma fentanyl levels, they found secondary increases in plasma fentanyl 45–90 minutes after intravenous injection. In two subjects, the increase was sufficient to induce a recurrence of severe respiratory depression. This suggested an entero-systemic recirculation of fentanyl as a possible mechanism, since the researchers observed gastric secretion of fentanyl for thirty minutes after the initial dose (39). Adams & Pybus (40) observed severe postoperative respiratory depression in three of their patients after apparent recovery from a general anesthetic that included modest doses of fentanyl. The time course of depression in their patients does not fit the entero-systemic recirculation mechanism described for healthy subjects. The more likely cause of recurrent respiratory depression was the same as that described by Becker et al (41) and inappropriately labeled biphasic respiratory depression. Becker et al (41) noted that patients who received

Table 1 Clinical states often treated with multiple concurrent drugs

Clinical state	Clinical state
infections	rheumatological disorders (e.g., rheumatoid arthritis, gout, degenerative joint disease)
neoplastic diseases	
organ transplantation	allergic disorders (e.g. allergic rhinitis, asthma)
cardiovascular disorders	
hypertension	immunologic disorders (e.g. systemic lupus erythematosus, Wegener's granulomatosis)
congestive heart failure	
angina pectoris	
acute myocardial infarction	
arrhythmias	neurological disorders
hypotension/shock	tension headache
respiratory disorders	migraine headache
bronchospasm (e.g., asthma, chronic bronchitis)	seizure disorders
	Parkinson's disease
cough	psychiatric problems
gastrointestinal diseases	ophthalmologic disease (e.g. glaucoma)
reflux esophagitis	contraception (birth control pills)
peptic ulcer disease	analgesia
inflammatory bowel disease (e.g., regional enteritis, ulcerative colitis)	antipyresis (e.g. sequential alternating of aspirin and acetaminophen to maintain continuous antipyresis and avoid excess use of either drug)
chronic active hepatitis	
constipation	
diarrhea (e.g., Lomotil)	
renal disorders	
nephrotic syndrome	
chronic renal insufficiency	
diuresis	

and combined drug effects on pain is often elusive. Additionally, individual drugs with beneficial actions may be combined but the effectiveness of the combination may never be fully tested (e.g. mixtures used as cold remedies, cough mixtures, and laxatives).

It is not possible to examine all desirable drug interactions in this review. For example, drug combinations used to treat malignancies encompass a vast field in their own right. We have selected examples of beneficial drug-drug combinations that illustrate the mechanisms of desirable interactions and that affect a broad range of clinical problems. These include antimicrobial drug interactions in treating infections, combined drug use in parkinsonism, combined use of diuretics, and antacid mixtures. The mechanism of the interaction will be examined together with its clinical significance. Any drug use, in combination or not, can have adverse effects, but these will only be emphasized as they relate to circumstances under discussion.

ANTIMICROBIAL AGENTS

Since their introduction, antimicrobial drug combinations have been used in an effort to produce enhanced clinical benefits. The rationale for their concurrent use can be divided into four general categories (3): (*a*) to broaden the spectrum of antimicrobial coverage, (*b*) to decrease toxicity by use of lower drug concentrations, (*c*) to prevent emergence of resistant organisms, and (*d*) to produce antimicrobial synergism.

Employing multiple antibiotics to insure broad spectrum coverage is appropriate when there is high suspicion of a serious or grave infection not immediately attributable to a particular microorganism, and when delay in beginning treatment might have an adverse outcome (3). The clinical suspicion of gram-negative bacteremia meets these criteria. Over the years various antibiotic combinations have been recommended for suspected gram-negative bacteremia that depend on the most likely putative organism under given clinical circumstances. This approach is successful if the agents chosen are not antagonistic and are active against the infecting organism. The disadvantages of multiple drug therapy are increased cost, increased risk of adverse drug reactions, and heightened chances of superinfection (4).

The use of multiple antimicrobial agents as a means of reducing the dosage of each to prevent toxicity has little current application, although this was commonplace when sulfonamides were first introduced (3). The limited solubility of early sulfonamides caused renal damage from their crystallization in urine. The solubility of one sulfonamide in solution is essentially independent of the concentration of others. The aggregate therapeutic effect of the mixture is about equal to the sum of individual effects. Because of this, sulfonamide combinations were employed as a way of retaining clinical efficacy while reducing the risk of nephrotoxicity. The most popular sulfonamide combination was the so-called triple sulfa, sulfathiazole, sulfacetamide, and sulfabenzamide. The newer, more soluble sulfonamides have made these mixtures obsolete.

Another erstwhile combination was that of streptomycin and dihydrostreptomycin, each at half strength. Streptomycin causes vestibular damage and dihydrostreptomycin produces cochlea damage. The goal was to reduce toxicity, but the mixture was abandoned when it was found to produce severe hearing loss.

More recently, both beneficial and detrimental effects have been observed from the joint use of amphotericin B and flucytosine in the treatment of patients with cryptococcal meningitis (5). The combination is synergistic and allows for smaller doses of amphotericin B to be used. Although the nephrotoxicity of amphotericin B is reduced, bone marrow toxicity induced by flucytosine has increased. It has been postulated that renal function is impaired even with the use of smaller than usual doses of amphotericin B, which leads to elevated flucytosine blood levels and increased bone marrow toxicity. Amphotericin B combined with flucytosine is recommended as the regimen of choice in the treatment of cryptococcal meningitis (5), but there must be careful monitoring for the adverse effects to both agents.

The use of multiple drugs to prevent the emergence of resistent strains of microorganisms is important in the treatment of tuberculosis and in the clinical use of rifampin (3, 4). There is a theoretical basis for considering that antimicrobial combinations retard or prevent the appearance of resistant organisms. Even when a microorganism develops resistance to one drug in a multiple drug regimen, it should be killed by one of the other drugs. This principle is the basis for using antimicrobial drug combinations to treat mycobacterial infections, since emergence of resistance to streptomycin, isoniazid, or rifampin is rapid when these drugs are used alone. Combination therapy appreciably prevents the emergence of resistant strains.

The use of rifampin is often accompanied by the rapid development of microbial resistance to this drug. In treating methicillin-resistant staphylococcal infections with rifampin, concomitant use of gentamicin or vancomycin averts the appearance of rifampin-resistant organisms. In gram-negative bacterial infections, rifampin has been combined with nalidixic acid and trimethoprim.

Clinically, antibacterial synergism has been the most successful form of combined antimicrobial drug therapy (3, 4). The three major examples of synergism are (a) agents that act on sequential steps in bacterial synthetic pathways, (b) joint use of a drug that impedes bacterial cell-wall synthesis with an aminoglycoside, and (c) a β-lactamase inhibitor combined with a β-lactam antibiotic. The first two types of synergism are exemplified respectively by the combination of trimethoprim and sulfamethoxazole, which blocks two separate sites in the folic acid metabolic pathway of many bacteria, and by the combination of penicillin and streptomycin to treat enterococcal infections. These combinations will be discussed more fully in following sections.

The third type of synergistic interaction, the combination of a β-lactamase inhibitor and a β-lactam antibiotic for treatment of infections due to β-lactamase producing bacteria, may prove to have appreciable clinical significance. This synergism is based on the probability that the administration of a β-lactamase inhibitor will block the action of bacterial β-lactamase, thus enhancing the antibacterial activity of a β-lactam antibiotic. The synergistic effect of these two agents has been shown in vitro against gram-negative bacilli (6). Dicloxacillin was found to inhibit the β-lactamase activity of a strain of *Citrobacter freundii* producing this enzyme. Ampicillin, a β-lactam antibiotic, was then able to exert its antibacterial effect on the cytoplasmic membrane (7). An oxacillin-ampicillin combination was effective in vitro against β–lactamase producing *Escherichia coli* strains with low-level β-lactam resistance but not against strains with high-level resistance (8). Clavulanic acid is a β-lactamase inhibitor, and in vitro and in vivo synergy has been demonstrated when it is combined with a β-lactam antibiotic (9, 10). In combination with amoxicillin, clavulanic acid proved safe and 70% effective in the treatment of urinary-tract infections caused by β-lactamase producing amoxicillin-resistant bacteria (10).

Combinations of agents inducing bacteria to produce β-lactamase and β-lactam antibiotics have been noted to be antagonistic. Cefoxitin can antagonize β-lactam antibiotics in vitro by inducing β-lactamase, which inactivates the β-lactam or serves as a barrier to access to target proteins (11). In experimental infections in mice, cefoxitin has been found to reversibly induce β-lactamases that antagonize carbenicillin and a cefamandole-carbenicillin combination (12). Clinically, the resistance of *Enterobacter* to cefamandole was associated with inducible β-lactamase, which produced cross-resistance to other β-lactam antibiotics given concurrently (13). In vitro and in vivo antagonism also has been demonstrated between cefoxitin and carbenicillin (11).

In vitro data on synergism or antagonism between antibiotics are not always applicable to conditions in vivo, and it is difficult to design studies that will clearly establish the clinical efficacy of some antimicrobial combinations. A group of highly useful antimicrobial combinations will be reviewed (trimethoprim-sulfamethoxazole, penicillin-aminoglycoside for enterococcal infection, penicillin-probenecid for gonorrhea, antibiotic-urease inhibitor for *Proteus* urinary tract infection). Additionally, antibiotic combinations used to treat *Pseudomonas* bacteremia, *Staphylococcus aureus* endocarditis, and *Klebsiella* infections will be examined.

Trimethoprim-Sulfamethoxazole

The development of trimethoprim and sulfamethoxazole in combination was based on the recognized differences between man and bacteria in the metabolism of folic acid (14, 15). The concept of using two drugs, each to inhibit separate steps in an essential bacterial biosynthetic pathway, was first proposed by Hitchings (16). Theoretically, this sequential blockade would produce a synergistic effect.

The concurrent use of a sulfonamide and trimethoprim produces a two-pronged block in the bacterial pathway that leads to the synthesis of tetrahydrofolic acid from its precursors. Sulfonamides are structural analogs of para-aminobenzoic acid (PABA), which is essential for tetrahydrofolate synthesis. Sulfonamides competitively inhibit bacterial utilization of PABA to form dihydropteroic acid, the immediate precursor of pteroylglutamic acid (PGA). Because bacteria are unable to utilize preformed folates, this inhibition results in bacteriostasis (17). Bacteria that are not dependent on folic acid or use preformed folates are not sulfonamide sensitive. Mammals require preformed PGA, and therefore are not adversely affected by sulfonamides.

Trimethoprim is a diaminopyrimidine that strongly inhibits the bacterial enzyme dihydrofolate reductase, which reduces dihydrofolate to tetrahydrofolate (18). Tetrahydrofolate is essential for one-carbon fragment transfer reactions needed for the synthesis of purines, pyrimidines, and some amino acids.

The therapeutic application of trimethoprim was recognized when the inhibition of dihydrofolate reductase by trimethoprim was noted to vary widely according to the species from which the enzyme was derived (19). Trimethoprim has a particularly high affinity for bacterial dihydrofolate reductase, but binds much less tightly to the same enzyme from mammals. There is a high degree of heterogeneity in dihydrofolate reductase from various species. This selective action of trimethoprim on dihydrofolate reductase is based on structural differences in the enzyme isolated from different species and probably is caused by changes in certain amino acids of the enzyme (20).

The use of trimethoprim with sulfamethoxazole produces a much greater antibacterial effect in vitro than the use of either drug alone (17, 21). The folate pathway is probably cyclic rather than linear (22). In microorganisms, tetrahydrofolate is synthesized from PABA. Tetrahydrofolate is reoxidized to dihydrofolate in the synthesis of thymidylate. Dihydrofolate reductase is essential to the maintenance of the tetrahydrofolate pool. Trimethoprim selectively inhibits dihydrofolate reductase, and its effectiveness is markedly enhanced when the synthesis of dihydrofolate is simultaneously blocked by sulfamethoxazole (15). Maximal synergy occurs when bacteria are sensitive to both trimethoprim and sulfamethoxazole, but a synergistic effect still can occur in bacteria resistant to sulfamethoxazole only or resistant to sulfamethoxazole and only moderately sensitive to trimethoprim (17).

Trimethoprim-sulfamethoxazole in vitro has antibacterial activity against numerous gram-positive and gram-negative bacteria (Table 2) (14). Some strains of *Campylobacter fetus* and *Chlamydia* are sensitive but the two drugs together are not synergistic. Although some *Pseudomonas* species are sensitive to trimethoprim-sulfamethoxazole, *Pseudomonas aeruginosa* is not. The drug is also effective in *Pneumocystis carinii* pneumonia. However, trimethoprim-sulfamethoxazole is inactive against *Mycoplasma, Mycobacterium tuberculosis,* and *Treponema pallidum.*

The ratio of trimethoprim to sulfamethoxazole in pharmaceutical preparations is 1:5. This produces a plasma concentration between 1:15 and 1:22, the range in which antibacterial activity is potentiated (14, 23).

Trimethoprim-sulfamethoxazole (co-trimoxazole, Bactrim®, Septra®, and others) is available as tablets formulated with 80 mg trimethoprim and 400 mg sulfamethoxazole or 160 mg and 800 mg of each drug respectively. Suspen-

Table 2 Bacteria sensitive to trimethoprim-sulfamethoxazole

Gram-positive	Gram-negative
Streptococcus pyogenes	*Escherichia coli*
Streptococcus viridans	*Klebsiella-Enterobacter*
Streptococcus pneumoniae	*Proteus* species
Staphylococcus aureus	*Salmonella* species
	Shigella species
	Haemophilus influenzae
	Bordatella pertussis
	Neisseria gonorrhoeae
	Neisseria meningitidis
	Vibrio cholera
	Pseudomonas (but not *P. aeruginosa*)
	Serratia species
	Yersinia species
	Nocardia species

sions, intramuscular, and intravenous preparations also are available. Trimethoprim alone is marketed as Proloprim®, and sulfamethoxazole has been sold as Gantanol®.

Penicillins and Aminoglycosides for Enterococcal Infections

Enterococcal *(Streptococcus faecalis)* endocarditis is best treated with a combination of penicillin and an aminoglycoside, which produces both facilitative and synergistic actions against this microorganism. Although occasional patients with enterococcal endocarditis could be cured with large doses of penicillin alone (24), the cure rate was never greater than 10–20% (4). In vitro and in vivo synergy between penicillin and streptomycin against the enterococcus was noted soon after the introduction of streptomycin.

Early in vitro experiments showed that penicillin alone was bacteriostatic against enterococci and streptomycin alone occasionally delayed growth, but a combination of penicillin and streptomycin was synergistic (i.e. less penicillin was needed) and was bactericidal (25, 26). Similar results have been found in experimental enterococcal endocarditis in the dog (27). Penicillin alone depressed the level of bacteremia, but streptomycin alone had no effect on the level of bacteremia. When penicillin and streptomycin were combined, a more rapid and more sustained decrease in bacteremia occurred.

The intact cell wall of enterococci is relatively impermiable to streptomycin and other aminoglycosides. Penicillins and other inhibitors of cell-wall synthesis enhance the uptake of aminoglycosides by inhibiting cell-wall synthesis and reducing the permeability barrier (28). A similar mechanism accounts for penicillin-streptomycin synergy against *E. coli* (3). Cephalothin alone or in combination with an aminoglycoside, however, is not effective therapy for experimental enterococcal endocarditis (29).

A lack of penicillin-streptomycin synergy occurs in up to 30% of enterococcal strains. Nearly all such strains, however, show in vitro synergy to a penicillin-gentamicin combination. Enterococcal strains not inhibited by the penicillin-streptomycin combination and resistant to streptomycin concentrations of 50,000–150,000 μg/ml were sensitive to a combination of penicillin-gentamicin (30, 31). It has been recommended that penicillin-gentamicin replace penicillin-streptomycin in the treatment of enterococcal infections. In experimental enterococcal endocarditis in rabbits, little difference was found when enterococci sensitive to streptomycin were treated with penicillin and streptomycin and penicillin and gentamicin (32). Clinical cures of enterococcal endocarditis and meningitis have been produced with penicillin and gentamicin, corroborating its in vitro and experimental effectiveness (33). A penicillin-gentamicin combination now often is used routinely to treat enterococcal infections. Ampicillin is more active than penicillin against enterococci in vitro. However, there is no strong evidence that it is any more useful clinically than penicillin. The successful therapy of enterococcal endocarditis requires prolonged administration of synergistic antibiotic combinations (31, 35, 36). Patients with symptoms for more than three months or with mitral valve endocarditis should receive six weeks of therapy to avoid a high recurrence rate (34). Those with a shorter duration of symptoms and aortic valve disease can be treated for four weeks. In patients allergic to penicillin, vancomycin can be substituted. Vancomycin is synergistic with streptomycin and gentamicin (37). These combinations are potentially ototoxic and patients must be carefully observed for hearing loss.

In summary, no single antibiotic combination is completely effective therapy for enterococcal infections (33). A combination of penicillin and an aminoglycoside has proved effective in vitro, in experimental animals, and in clinical studies (35). In most cases of enterococcal endocarditis, combined therapy with penicillin and streptomycin remains effective (35). If the minimal inhibitory concentration of streptomycin for the enterococcus is 2000 μg/ml or greater, gentamicin can be substituted for streptomycin. Determining in vitro bactericidal titers and monitoring serum drug levels are important in guiding therapy. For penicillin-allergic patients, vancomycin is substituted.

Other Antimicrobial Combinations

As corollaries of the synergy between drugs inhibiting cell-wall synthesis and aminoglycosides in the treatment of enterococcal infections, there are three other infections in which this combination may prove useful: *Staphylococcus aureua* endocarditis, *Klebsiella pneumoniae* infections, and *Pseudomonas aeruginosa* bacteremia.

The in vitro combination of a semisynthetic penicillinase-resistant penicillin such as oxacillin or nafcillin with gentamicin is synergistic against most strains of *Staphylococcus aureus*. In patients with penicillin-sensitive *S. aureus* endocarditis, however, those treated with penicillin and gentamicin had the same survival as those treated with penicillin alone (38). When nafcillin alone was compared with nafcillin and gentamicin in treating *S. aureus* endocarditis, the combination produced a more rapid clinical response manifested by defervescence and normalization of the leukocyte count and a reduced duration of bacteremia, but morbidity and mortality were the same in both treatment groups (39). Further studies are needed to accurately assess the efficacy of a penicillin-aminoglycoside combination in treating staphylococcal endocarditis.

The combination of an active antibiotic inhibiting cell-wall synthesis and an aminoglycoside has also been used to treat *Klebsiella pneumoniae* infections. A synergistic effect has been demonstrated in urinary tract infections (40). Similarly, the response to *Klebsiella* causing bacteremia was 92% effective if synergistic antibiotic combinations were used, compared to 61% when non-synergistic combinations were employed. These results did not reach statistical significance (41), however. *Klebsiella* infections also respond to a combination of cefazolin and amikacin (42). In neutropenic rats septicemia due to amikacin-sensitive *K. pneumoniae* responded better to a combination of cefazolin and amikacin than to either antibiotic alone (43).

A combination of cephalothin and gentamicin was found to act synergistically in vitro against more than 80% of *Klebsiella* isolates. Induced intraperitoneal *Klebsiella* infections in rats, however, were not affected differently when treated with gentamicin alone, cephalothin and gentamicin, and gentamicin and chloramphenicol (44).

The in vitro synergy of carbenicillin and an aminoglycoside against most strains of *Pseudomonas aeruginosa* is well documented (45, 46). In addition, the value of carbenicillin-gentamicin against *Pseudomonas* infection has been shown in animal models (47). The combination is most useful in patients with impaired defense mechanisms against infection (42). Whether the combination has value in the uncompromised host is not clear. Cancer patients being treated with antineoplastic drugs often become neutropenic and febrile and may develop *Pseudomonas* bacteremia. The outcome in these patients is better when they are treated with carbenicillin-gentamicin (six of seven patients improved) then with cephalothin-gentamicin (none of five improved) (48). A cephalothin-gentamicin combination is of minimal value against *P. aeruginosa* and in addition is nephrotoxic, especially in the elderly (49).

Current recommendations are that in patients with neutropenia who are suspected of having bacteremia antimicrobial therapy for possible *Pseudomo-*

nas aeruginosa infection should be started promptly. Best results are obtained when at least one antibacterial agent is bactericidal in vitro (49). Presently, a combination of either carbenicillin or ticaricillin with either gentamicin or tobramycin is recommended (48, 49).

Ampicillin/Amoxicillin/Penicillin and Probenecid

Gonococci have become increasingly resistant to penicillin, and larger doses of the antibiotic are now recommended for treatment of gonococcal infections. Even though resistant strains of penicillinase-producing gonococci occur, penicillin therapy remains the intial treatment of choice. The combined use of probenecid plus ampicillin, amoxicillin, or procaine penicillin G on one occasion has made it possible to treat infected patients by using the augmentative effect of probenecid on blood levels of penicillins (50).

Probenecid reduces the rapid renal loss of penicillin and was especially valuable when penicillin was scarce during the 1940s. Probenecid influences proximal renal tubular transport mechanisms for organic molecules and thus affects the excretion and resorption of many compounds. Although mainly used clinically for its uricosuric effect, probenecid also inhibits secretion of penicillins in the proximal tubule and reduces their excretion. Thus, the combined use of probenecid and a penicillin leads to a twofold or higher and more prolonged blood penicillin concentration (51). This allows prophylaxis and treatment of uncomplicated gonorrhea in one session (52, 53). Oral penicillin and intramuscular benzathine penicillin G are not adequate therapy since they do not produce therapeutic blood concentrations. Concurrent administration of probenecid also leads to higher and more prolonged blood levels of ampicillin and amoxicillin. The only difference between ampicillin and amoxicillin is that the latter is more rapidly and more completely absorbed after oral administration, producing higher mean peak serum concentration and a greater area under the curve (54, 55). Tetracycline is used in penicillin-allergic persons, but a week of therapy is required. There is no single-dose tetracycline regimen.

These drug regimens are ineffective against anorectal and pharyngeal gonorrhea and against chlamydial infections, and other treatment regimens are recommended for disseminated and penicillin-resistant gonococcal infections (50).

Chlamydia coexist with gonococci in 27–63% of women with endocervical gonorrhea and 4–32% of men with urethral gonorrhea (56). The best treatment for coexistant gonococcal and chlamydial infection is not clear (50). One of the single-dose amoxicillin or ampicillin regimens, plus probenecid coupled with tetracycline or doxycycline treatment for a week, may be appropriate for combined infection. However, no data on the efficacy of such a regimen is presently available. This type of mixed venereal infection may require the use of additional antibiotic combinations for treatment.

Acetohydroxamic Acid and an Antibiotic

Urinary tract infections due to urea-splitting bacteria can produce struvite and carbonate apatite stones, usually staghorn renal calculi or bladder stones. Nearly all species of *Proteus* and some strains of *Pseudomonas, E. coli,* and *Staphylococcus* produce urease (57). Bacterial urease hydrolyzes urea to ammonia and carbon dioxide, the latter forming carbonate and bicarbonate ions. Increased urinary concentrations of carbonate and bicarbonate and the alkalinity produced by ammonia lead to a urine supersaturated with magnesium ammonium phosphate and calcium phosphate. As a result, there is crystallization of struvite ($MgNH_4PO_4.6H_2O$) and carbonate apatite ($Ca_{10}[PO_4]_6CO_3$) (58).

Acetohydroxamic acid is structurally similar to urea, inhibits urease action, and is relatively nontoxic (59). It inhibits alkalinization of urine, reducing supersaturation and subsequent crystallization of struvite and calcium apatite (60). After oral administration, acetohydroxamic acid is rapidly absorbed and is excreted in the urine (58). With single doses of 1.0 g per day, a reduction of urinary ammonia and pH is regularly achieved (58). Reduction in the size of stones or their dissolution may follow the use of acetohydroxamic acid.

The effectiveness of antimicrobial drugs in treating urinary tract infection in patients forming stones has been increased when acetohydroxamic acid is added to the therapeutic regimen (58). After surgical removal of stones, antibiotics plus urease inhibitors (hydroxyurea or acetohydroxamic acid) eliminates urinary infection more frequently than antibiotics alone (61).

The *Proteus* causing urinary tract infections are active producers of urease (62, 63). In the mouse, however, a urease-negative mutant of *Proteus mirabilis* is just as infectious but produces less renal damage (63). Urease is nephrotoxic and may contribute to the pathogenesis of pyelonephritis. It damages tubular epithelial cells and allows intracellular infection (62). The invasive properties of *Proteus* in the urinary tract appear largely dependent on alkalinization of urine by urease, which results in damage to the renal epithelium (64). In experimental animals, pyelonephritic changes from *Proteus* infection can be prevented by administering a urease inhibitor (57, 64, 65). In vitro, acetohydroxamic acid potentiates the effect of certain antimicrobial agents against several bacterial species (66–68). Although the cause of this synergy is unknown, diverse mechanisms have been suggested. In vitro studies with urease-producing organisms have shown that kanamycin increases cell permeability, allowing urease inhibitors to enter the cell and interact with pyridoxal phosphate, ultimately leading to cell damage (66). Synergy occurred in 17% of instances when twelve antimicrobial agents and acetohydroxamic acid were tested against gram-negative bacteria *(Proteus, Pseudomonas, E. coli, Klebsillas, Enterobacter,* and *Providencia)* (68). In 5%, however, antagonism was noted. Synergy has been observed between methenamine and acetohydroxamic acid against strains of *Proteus*. Reducing alkalinization of the urine may allow formaldehyde to be produced from methenamine, the former being the effective antibacterial substance (67).

Acetohydroxamic acid has only recently been available for clinical use. It may prove a useful adjunct to the treatment of urinary tract infections with urea-splitting organisms. There is evidence that inactivation of urease can make the organism both less virulent and more susceptible to concurrent antimicrobial therapy.

PARKINSONISM

The biochemical basis of parkinsonism is complex and not completely understood, but the primary defect is a decrease in dopaminergic neurons in the basal ganglia. Although viral encephalitis, carbon monoxide exposure, atherosclerosis, and drugs that impede dopamine action in the basal ganglia (phenothiazines, butyrophenones, thioxanthines, metoclopramide, and reserpine) can cause parkinsonism syndromes, the etiology of the neuronal degeneration in idiopathic Parkinson's disease is unknown. The absolute deficit in excitatory dopaminergic neurons is further opposed by the inhibitory activity of cholinergic neurons, leading to a relative cholinergic excess with a resultant imbalance of these neurotransmitter systems. A balance between dopaminergic and cholinergic activity appears necessary for smooth, integrated voluntary movements. This neurochemical disbalance accounts for the cardinal symptoms of parkinsonism: resting tremor, rigidity, bradykinesia, stooped posture, poor balance, and gait disturbances. Symptomatic improvement can be produced pharmacologically either by enhancing dopaminergic activity or by dampening cholinergic activity. Both approaches are clinically useful (69).

Levodopa and Carbidopa

Since parkinsonism is due to central dopamine deficiency, administering exogenous dopamine would be expected to ameliorate symptoms. However, dopamine does not cross the blood-brain barrier and is therefore therapeutically ineffective. Dopamine's immediate precursor, levodopa, does cross the blood-brain barrier, enters the basal ganglia of the brain, and is converted to dopamine by the enzyme dopa decarboxylase located in the remaining dopaminergic nerve terminals. Even though dopaminergic terminals, and hence dopa decarboxylase activity, are diminished in parkinsonism, enough enzyme remains to convert levodopa to adequate amounts of dopamine to produce a therapeutic effect. This has led to the notable success of levodopa in the treatment of parkinsonism. About three-quarters of patients show improvement when treated with levodopa.

Levodopa is well absorbed after oral administration, but about 95% of the drug is rapidly decarboxylated to dopamine, mainly in the liver, by peripheral dopa decarboxylase (70). Probably less than 1% of an administered dose of levodopa enters the brain. In order to insure that an adequate amount of levodopa will reach and cross the blood-brain barrier, large doses must be administered. Many of levodopa's adverse effects, notably anorexia, nausea, vomiting, and hypotension, are due to the large amount of dopamine produced by peripheral decarboxylation. Adverse effects are particularly common in the elderly and in sufferers of postencephalitic parkinsonism (70). Undesirable side effects can be avoided by starting with a small dose of levodopa and gradually increasing it over weeks until the greatest clinical response has been achieved or until unacceptable side effects appear (71).

Dopa decarboxylase is a pyridoxine-dependent enzyme. Small doses of pyridoxine (Vitamin B_6), such as those found in many multivitamin preparations (5 mg or more), enhance dopa decarboxylase activity and the conversion of levodopa to dopamine (72). Consequently, concomitant use of levodopa and pyridoxine can negate the therapeutic effect of levodopa or, conversely, rapidly diminish toxic effects. There is not enough pyridoxine in the average diet to interfere with the action of levodopa. Furthermore, the use of levodopa does not produce pyridoxine deficiency.

The combination of carbidopa, a peripheral dopa decarboxylase inhibitor that does not enter the central nervous system, with levodopa has greatly improved the clinical management of parkinsonism. When these two drugs are given concurrently, decarboxylation of levodopa to dopamine in peripheral tissues is appreciably diminished. This produces higher levodopa plasma concentrations and a prolonged half-life, which allows more drug to cross the blood-brain barrier and reach the nigrostriatal structures for conversion to dopamine (73). Carbidopa also counteracts the antagonistic effect of pyridoxine on levodopa metabolism (74). As a result of dopa decarboxylase blockade, more levodopa is present to enter the brain, and the optimally effective dose can be reduced by about three-quarters. This combination of levodopa and carbidopa is the most effective method available for treating parkinsonism (74). Consequently, adverse effects such as hypotension and vomiting from dopamine stimulation of the emetic center in the medulla, which is not protected by the blood-brain barrier, are largely eliminated or markedly diminished (70, 74). A maximally effective dose can be reached more quickly, since there is less need to develop tolerance to the peripheral effects of levodopa, which are due to peripherally produced dopamine. Apparently large fluctuations in the concentration of dopamine in the brain are dampened and smoother control of symptoms ensues. In addition, the number of patients who improve is somewhat greater than with levodopa alone. About 90% of patients respond to either levodopa or the carbidopa-levodopa combination (75).

Prolonged treatment with levodopa or carbidopa-levodopa has its limitations. After five years of treatment, deterioration occurs in over half of patients (76). The most common difficulties are loss of drug efficacy, abnormal involuntary movements (dyskinesias), the on-off phenomenon, the wearing-off or end-of-dose reaction, and confusion.

Loss of efficacy cannot always be managed by increasing the dose of levodopa. The addition of other drugs, anticholinergics and amantadine and especially bromocriptine, may be helpful.

Dyskinesias may consist of facial grimacing, rhythmic and jerking movements of the hands, head bobbing, chewing and smacking movements of the mouth and lips, and jerking movements extending to the trunk (70). They are decreased by diminishing the dose of levodopa and worsened by increasing levodopa dosage and by anticholinergics.

The on-off phenomenon may occur in up to half the patients. It is characterized by on periods of mobility and off periods of severe akinesia. The on-off phenomenon may occur up to several times in an hour. It generally does not respond to changes in the dose or time of administration of levodopa. The on-off phenomenon may be due to variable plasma levels of levodopa but also to faulty uptake and subsequent synthesis and release of dopamine from this precursor in the basal ganglia.

The wearing-off reaction is a rapid deterioration of symptoms occurring before the next scheduled dose of levodopa. Akinesia becomes more prominent. It results from a short half-life of levodopa and may respond to smaller, more frequent doses.

Confusion, coupled with agitation and impaired recent memory, may progress to delusions and hallucinations. This state has been ascribed to increased central dopaminergic activity resulting from levodopa. The elderly are more susceptible to nocturnal confusion and hallucinations (70).

Carbidopa is combined with levodopa and marketed as Sinemet®. Sinemet 10/100 contains 10 mg of carbidopa and 100 mg of levodopa, while Sinemet 25/250 has 25 mg and 250 mg of these compounds respectively. Sinemet 25/100 provides more carbidopa to block dopa decarboxylase activity and is useful in patients most sensitive to the peripheral toxic effects of dopamine, such as nausea and vomiting (77). This increased ratio of carbidopa to levodopa also produces more rapid symptomatic response than the 1:10 combinations (78).

Treatment with levodopa does not affect the progressive loss of dopaminergic neurons in the basal ganglia. As the process continues, levodopa becomes therapeutically less effective. Other drugs may be helpful at this point, early in the disease, or to ameliorate adverse effects.

Other Drugs

Additional drugs are available to assist in the treatment of parkinsonism (Table 3). They can be used in concert with levodopa to improve the clinical symptoms

Table 3   Drugs used to treat Parkinson's disease

Dopaminergic	Anticholinergics	Antihistamines
levodopa (Larodopa® and others)	benztropine myselate (Cogentin®)	chlorphenoxamine hydrochloride (Phenoxene®)
carbidopa-levodopa (Sinemet®)	biperiden hydrochloride (Akeniton®)	diphenhydramine hydrochloride (Benadryl®)
amantadine hydrochloride (Symmetrel®)	cycrimine hydrochloride (Pagitane®)	orphenadrine hydrochloride (Disipal®)
bromocriptine mesylate (Parlodel®)	ethopropazine hydrochloride (Parsidol®)	
	procyclidine hydrochloride (Kemadrin®)	
	trihexyphenidyl hydrochloride (Artane®)	

of parkinsonism. They fall into three categories: centrally acting dopaminergic drugs, centrally acting anticholinergics, and monoamine oxidase inhibitors.

DOPAMINERGIC DRUGS   Amantadine, originally introduced as a prophylactic drug against influenza A, was found by chance to have antiparkinsonism activity. It is believed to act by causing indirect dopamine release, with some additional direct stimulation of dopamine receptors (79). Amantadine can enhance and smooth out the effects of levodopa. The drugs have an additive effect. However, patients receiving essentially maximal benefit from levodopa receive little additional improvement from amantadine.

The antiparkinsonism effect of amantadine is less than that of levodopa but somewhat more than that of anticholinergics (80). When used together, amantadine and anticholinergic drugs are additive in producing control of parkinsonian symptoms, but confusion is a frequent adverse effect.

Efficacy varies widely from patient to patient. Amantadine exerts its maximal pharmacologic effect after a few days of use, but it is not sustained. Its efficacy diminishes after six to eight weeks of continuous treatment (80, 81). Either increasing the dose or temporarily discontinuing the drug for a few weeks can result in a return of efficacy.

Bromocriptine, an ergot derivative originally used as a prolactin secretion inhibitor, was found to be a striatal dopaminergic agonist as well (82). Bromocriptine and levodopa have an additive effect. Bromocriptine is most useful when given concurrently with levodopa. Treatment with levodopa that is less than optimal may be improved with the addition of small doses of bromocriptine (83). Patients who experience excessive on-off phenomena or wearing-off reactions may be helped by taking bromocriptine. Optimal clinical results may be achieved by levodopa and supplemental doses of bromocriptine, but if bromocriptine is added the use of levodopa should be reduced to prevent more adverse effects. Using bromocriptine results in a reduced dose of levodopa, improved responsiveness, and a decrease in side effects (69, 82–84). Bromocriptine's main disadvantage is the high incidence of untoward mental symptoms, particularly nightmares, hallucinations, and paranoid delusions (85).

Bromocriptine has been used in previously untreated patients with Parkinson's disease in the hope of extending the duration of a favorable therapeutic response in the disease (86). The response rate was less to bromocriptine (56%) than to levodopa (74%), and the pattern of deterioration or diminished responsiveness to bromocriptine was similar to previous experiences with levodopa therapy. Thus, giving bromocriptine before levodopa does not extend the duration of effective drug therapy.

ANTICHOLINERGIC DRUGS   The reduction of dopamine in the basal ganglia in parkinsonism makes the excitatory effects of acetylcholine more prominent. In fact, centrally acting cholinesterase inhibitors such as physostigmine intensify parkinsonism tremor, while centrally acting anticholinergics decrease tremor (87). Anticholinergics were the first drugs used to treat parkinsonism. Centrally acting anticholinergic drugs work well in early or mild parkinsonism and as adjuncts to dopaminergic therapy. In the opinion of some clinicians, they are the preferred drugs for initial treatment. Anticholinergic drugs may be used alone, or when added to levodopa they can further improve symptoms in parkinsonism, especially tremor and rigidity, in about half of patients. Antihistamines have mild anticholinergic effects and are often better tolerated by the elderly.

Large doses of anticholinergic drugs, however, can delay gastric emptying sufficiently to retard small bowel absorption of levodopa. This effect can appreciably diminish the therapeutic effect of levodopa (88). The adverse effects of anticholinergics, particularly confusion and urinary retention, limit their usefulness in the elderly. They may also precipitate or worsen glaucoma, cause dry mouth, constipation, memory defects, and hallucinations. In addition, tricyclic antidepressants are used to treat depression, a frequently encountered problem in patients with parkinsonism. These drugs have notable anticholinergic effects that may at times benefit symptoms of parkinsonism, but they also can produce undesirable anticholinergic side effects as well as sedation and postural hypotension.

MONOAMINE OXIDASE INHIBITORS   Attempts to use monoamine oxidase (MAO) inhibitors with levodopa as a means of enhancing the anti-akinetic properties of levodopa were unsuccessful because hypertensive crises were produced. Later, two types of MAO were discovered: MAO-type A occurs peripherally and MAO-type B occurs predominately in the brain (89). Tyramine and dopamine are substrates for both MAO-type A and MAO-type B, but in the human brain dopamine is metabolized preferentially by MAO-type B. Most MAO inhibitors inhibit both types of MAO indiscriminately, but deprenyl (an experimental drug) preferentially inhibits MAO-type B (90). This has led to clinical trials using deprenyl in patients with Parkinson's disease. By inhibiting the breakdown of dopamine in the brain, deprenyl prolongs and enhances the duration of action of levodopa. Deprenyl's lack of effect on peripheral MAO-type A reduces the chance of producing adverse effects with centrally active amines and with tyramine-containing foods that cause hypertensive crises. Clinical studies have shown favorable results (91). Deprenyl not only increases the duration of levodopa's action but also improves mobility in wearing-off reactions (92). It appears to be a good adjuvant when used with levodopa. At this writing, deprenyl is not available for clinical use.

In summary, in parkinsonism drugs and drug combinations appreciably improve symptoms but do not retard the progress of the underlying disease. The most effective drug is a combination of carbidopa and levodopa, which greatly improves mobility. Other drugs are adjunctive. Drug reactions are not insignificant and occur more frequently in the elderly.

DIURETICS

Diuretic combinations can produce two beneficial effects: prevention of diuretic-induced hypokalemia and enhanced diuresis. The use of a potassium-wasting and a potassium-sparing diuretic combination to prevent hypokalemia is additive and reparative. Enhanced diuresis is synergistic.

Prevention of Hypokalemia

Thiazide diuretics and the structurally different but functionally equivalent chlorthalidone, quinethazone, and metolazone increase urinary excretion of sodium, chloride, and water by inhibiting sodium reabsorption in the early distal tubule. This is accompanied by an appreciable augmentation of potassium excretion, which can lead to hypokalemia. Serum potassium concentrations frequently decrease during long-term diuretic treatment and may be associated with a mild degree of hypochloremic alkalosis. Patients receiving digitalis and those with cirrhosis may be at greater risk from hypokalemia, which can induce digitalis intoxication and hepatic encephalopathy respectively.

Loop diuretics (furosemide, ethacrynic acid, and bumetanide) act on the ascending limb of the loop of Henle. They are potent diuretics with a rapid onset and a short duration of action. Their diuretic effect is much greater than that of the thiazides. An equivalent diuretic effect is produced by 40 mg of furosemide, 50 mg of ethacrynic acid, and 1 mg of bumetanide. Potassium excretion in the distal segment, as with thiazide diuretics, is related to the increased flow rate through this segment of the tubule.

Three potassium-sparing diuretics are available: spironolactone, triamterene, and amiloride. Although mechanisms of action differ, they produce the same final effect, potassium conservation.

Spironolactone is a competitive inhibitor of aldosterone. Aldosterone increases the distal resorption of sodium and chloride while increasing the excretion of potassium. Spironolactone blocks this effect and enhances diuresis while conserving potassium. When spironolactone is used alone, it has a weak diuretic effect.

Triamterene acts directly on the distal segment of the tubule independent of the effect of aldosterone. The rate of potassium secretion is reduced as the result of a primary reduction in sodium resorption. When used alone, triamterene produces only a paltry diuresis.

Amiloride, too, is not an aldosterone antagonist. Amiloride produces natriuresis with either only a slight increase or sometimes an absolute decrease in potassium excretion. This effect is enhanced when a thiazide diuretic is given concurrently. The combination is additive with respect to sodium and chloride excretion but antagnostic with respect to potassium loss.

Kaliuresis is most marked with brisk diuresis and may be negligible during chronic diuretic administration with little diuresis. Potassium deficiency is particularly likely to occur when there is secondary hyperaldosteronism, as in cirrhosis and accelerated hypertension, but also occurs with less marked elevations of aldosterone (congestive heart failure, nephrosis). Diuresis in the face of mineralocorticoid excess can produce marked hypokalemia. Potassium depletion can lead to alkalosis, reduced carbohydrate tolerance (and worsening of diabetes), impaired neuromuscular function (from weakness to paralysis and ileus), abnormal myocardial function, and a renal concentrating deficit with polyuria.

Diuretic-induced potassium deficiency can be prevented or treated with supplemental potassium administration. Oral preparations have drawbacks, however. Liquids taste bad and can cause gastric upset. Tablets can cause ulceration, bleeding, and resultant stricture in the gut. The combination of a thiazide or loop diuretic and a potassium-sparing diuretic obviates the use of oral potassium supplements. In fact, oral potassium supplements can cause severe or fatal hyperkalemia, especially in the elderly, when given in addition to a potassium-sparing diuretic in combination with other diuretics (93). Thiazides are prescribed in combination with potassium-sparing diuretics as a means of obtaining an additive diuretic effect and conserving potassium. This enhanced diuretic effect and the amelioration of potassium loss are both marked in hyperaldosterone states.

Table 4 Fixed-dose thiazide and potassium-sparing diuretic combinations

Name	Ingredients	Dosage
Aldactazide®	spironolactone	25 mg/50 mg
	hydrochlorothiazide	25 mg/50 mg
Dyazide®	triamterene	50 mg
	hydrochlorothiazide	25 mg
Moduretic®	amiloride	5 mg
	hydrochlorothiazide	50 mg

Varying combinations and doses of thiazide and loop diuretics can be used with the potassium-sparing diuretics to achieve maximal clinical benefit in both diuresis and maintenance of potassium balance (94). Fixed-dose combinations of thiazide and potassium-sparing diuretics are available and can be employed to advantage once the ratio of diuretics has been established (Table 4).

These combinations are popular for treating hypertension because they (a) effectively lower blood pressure, (b) avoid the use of potassium supplements, which often are not taken because of their unpleasant taste and their propensity to induce nausea, and (c) can be administered as a single tablet once or twice a day. Regardless of theoretical objections to fixed-dose drug combinations, these preparations have probably done much to enhance compliance to anti-hypertensive regimens and produce the desired effect of lowering blood pressure. In addition, although excess sodium intake has long been regarded as playing an etiologic role in the pathogenesis of hypertension (95), evidence is mounting that increasing body potassium may have a beneficial effect in reducing the level of elevated blood pressure (96). These drug combinations may thus provide triple benefit: loss of sodium, retention of potassium, and lowering of blood pressure.

There is evidence that combinations of potassium-sparing and potassium-losing diuretics provide a useful interaction leading to improved potassium balance. Long-term treatment with triamterene alone, chlorothiazide alone, and both drugs together showed that the drug combination produced the highest incidence of normal plasma potassium values (97). In a study of 1,156 elderly subjects using thiazide diuretics or chlorthalidone, serum potassium concentrations were 3.74 and 3.47 meq per liter respectively. Conversely, in those using a combination of hydrochlorothiazide-triamterene or hydrochlorothiazide-spironolactone, serum potassium concentrations were 3.99 and 4.04 meq per liter respectively (98). An extensive literature review of diuretic-induced hypo-kalemia showed the use of potassium-sparing diuretics to be more effective than potassium supplements (94). A study of elderly veterans using digoxin and various diuretics and diuretic combinations concluded that a potassium-sparing diuretic may be used safely to reduce potassium excretion and the risk of digitalis intoxication and arrhythmias (99). Thus, combining potassium-losing and potassium-sparing diuretics is a practical and effective way of reducing diuretic-induced hypokalemia.

Enhanced Diuresis

No convincing data exist to indicate that combining two thiazide or thiazide-like diuretics will produce any greater diuretic effect than that induced by using maximal dosages of any single agent. However, the efficacy of thiazide and related diuretics can be increased by concomitant use of a potassium-sparing agent or loop diuretic. The beneficial effects of these regimens appear to result from combined actions at different sites in the nephron and differing mechanisms of action.

Thiazide diuretics produce their effects by inhibiting sodium and chloride reabsorption in the cortical diluting segments of the ascending limb of the loop of Henle and distal convoluted tubule, whereas loop diuretics (furosemide, ethacrynic acid, and bumetanide) act on the medullary portion of the ascending limb of the loop of Henle.

Unresponsiveness to the action of loop diuretics can occur from a marked reduction in glomerular filtration rate or the use of sodium-retaining drugs. The combination of a thiazide-type diuretic and a loop diuretic has been found useful in the management of refractory edema (100). Although the addition of a relatively small dose of a thiazide diuretic to a large dose of a loop diuretic in the face of refractory edema would not be expected to produce a vigorous diuresis, it may in fact do so (101). This synergistic effect has been successfully used to treat severe sodium retention in congestive heart failure, renal failure, the nephrotic syndrome, hypertension, and cirrhosis. Effective diuretic combinations have included thiazides, quinethazone, and metolazone used with furosemide, ethacrynic acid, bumetanide, and piretanide (101). It is postulated that the thiazide-type diuretic impedes the increased distal tubular sodium resorption that limits the effect of the loop diuretic (102).

Massive diuresis may produce marked fluid and electrolyte losses (particularly potassium), worsening azotemia, and circulatory collapse and death (101). A potassium-sparing diuretic or supplemental potassium should be used because of large potassium losses (102). Although a high incidence of adverse effects has been noted with this diuretic combination, employing two diuretics can be clinically very useful. It is recommended that the dose of a loop diuretic be reduced and that small amounts of thiazide-type diuretics be used initially to avert excessive fluid and electrolyte losses.

ANTACIDS

Antacids hasten the healing of peptic ulcers, are beneficial for reflux esophagitis, and are used for a number of unrelated gastrointestinal symptoms by both physicians and the public. Large doses of antacids produce healing of duodenal ulcers at a rate superior to that of a placebo (103). Antacids and cimetidine produce similar rates of symptom relief and healing of duodenal ulcers (104). Healed ulcers tend to recur promptly when treatment with antacids or cimetidine is discontinued, with half of patients having a recurrence in six months (105). Cimetidine and ranitidine are comparable in their ability to heal duodenal ulcers (106).

Antacids vary in their ingredients, their acid-neutralizing ability, and probably their clinical effects (107). Antacids generally contain aluminum hydroxide, magnesium hydroxide, calcium carbonate, sodium bicarbonate, or some combination of these ingredients (108). Each ingredient has advantages and disadvantages. Sodium bicarbonate and calcium carbonate are excellent antacids but both are absorbable and can cause systemic alkalosis. Sodium bicarbonate can cause sodium overload and alkalinization of the urine, which can lead to nephrolithiasis. Calcium carbonate can produce hypercalcemia.

Aluminum hydroxide ($Al[OH]_3$) and magnesium hydroxide ($Mg[OH]_2$) are regarded as nonabsorable or nonsystemic antacids; this is because they do not produce systemic alkalosis since the cation forms insoluble basic compounds in the intestine that are nonabsorbable (109). Aluminum hydroxide is constipating and magnesium hydroxide is laxating. They are often combined in the hope that one will cancel out the undesirable effect of the other. In addition, total buffering time is increased by combining fast-acting magnesium hydroxide with slow-acting aluminum hydroxide (109). Although remarkable success is often achieved, great clinical variability occurs from patient to patient, so that a mixture that has no effect on bowel action in one person may lead to constipation in another and more frequent stools in still another. Nonetheless, the combination of aluminum hydroxide and magnesium hydroxide remains a common, useful, and beneficial reparative drug interaction.

The mechanism by which aluminum compounds cause constipation is unknown. Their astringent properties, which are related to reactions with proteins, have been suggested as a mechanism, but the low concentration of the aluminum ion in the intestine makes this an unlikely explanation (109).

Magnesium hydroxide, although a very effective antacid, is better known in its other guise as the cathartic milk of magnesia. Its laxating action is due to the retention of water in the bowel.

Although considered nonabsorbable antacids, small amounts of the metal ions are indeed absorbed. In the presence of renal insufficiency, aluminum can cause encephalopathy. Aluminum antacids bind phosphate in the gut and help ameliorate the hyperphosphatemia of renal failure. This effect can ultimately lead to osteomalacia, however. Greater amounts of magnesium are absorbed than aluminum, and with renal failure hypermagnesemia can occur and, rarely, alkalosis.

An antacid's ability to reduce gastric acidity in vivo is related to its in vitro acid-neutralizing ability (110). Commercially available liquid antacids vary up to seventeenfold in their neutralizing ability per milliliter, but these differences are usually not reflected in the manufacturer's dosage recommendations. Dosage should be determined on milliequivalents of neutralizing capacity rather than by an arbitrary volume or number of tablets.

The composition, neutralizing capacity, and sodium content of commonly used liquid antacids are shown in Table 5 (107, 108, 111). Wide variations exist in the antacid content in 5 ml of liquid antacids. As a result, the acid-neutralizing capacity varies from a low of 1.4 meq/ml for Amphojel® to a high of 4.2 meq/ml for Maalox TC® and Titralac®. These values correlate inversely with the dose in milliliters containing 80 meq of neutralizing capacity. Thus, 61.5 ml of Amphogel but only 15.7 ml of Maalox TC or 20.0 ml of Titralac is needed to neutralize 80 meq of acid.

Even liquid antacids that contain only aluminum hydroxide and magnesium hydroxide show wide variations in amounts and ratios of these ingredients in 5 ml of antacid (Table 5). Simethicone, an antifoaming agent, is present in many antacid mixtures but has no effect on buffering capacity. All currently available antacids are relatively low in sodium content except those that contain sodium bicarbonate (e.g. Bisodol®).

In selecting an antacid, one should aim for the most acid-neutralizing effect with the least degree of gastrointestinal undesirable effects. Individuals may need to test multiple antacids with varying ratios of aluminum hydroxide and magnesium hydroxide to find the one that produces little or no change in intestinal function while requiring a relatively small volume to be effective.

SUMMARY

Controversy has surrounded the use of combinations of different drugs. Most often, this controversy has been about the desirability or appropriateness of combining two or more drugs in the same dosage form, tablet or solution. The administration to a patient of several different drugs at the same time has been common practice, however. Simultaneous administration of different drugs has been used to achieve different therapeutic effects or to achieve beneficial effects from two or more drugs used for the same therapeutic purpose. Some have contended that when two or more drugs are given to enhance a particular therapeutic effect, these drugs should not be combined in the same dosage form but should be given separately. We have not become engaged in this controversy in preparing this paper. We have emphasized, however, that the concurrent administration of two or more drugs in special circumstances can produce beneficial results, and in some instances appears to be quite appropriate.

Table 5 Liquid antacids

Name	Ingredients (5 ml)	Acid-neutralizing capacity (meq/ml)	Dose (ml) containing 80 meq neutralizing capacity	Sodium (mg/5ml)
Aludrox®	aluminum hydroxide, 307 mg magnesium hydroxide, 103 mg	—	29.6	1
Delcid®	aluminum hydroxide, 600 mg magnesium hydroxide, 665	4.1	9.2	1.5
Di-Gel®	aluminum hydroxide, 282 mg magnesium hydroxide, 87 mg simethicone, 20 mg[a]	—	38.1	9
Gelusil®	aluminum hydroxide, 200 mg magnesium hydroxide, 200 mg simethicone, 25 mg[a]	2.2	38.1	0.7
Gelusil-II®	aluminum hydroxide, 400 mg magnesium hydroxide, 400 mg simethicone, 30 mg[a]	3.0	16.7	0.7
Kolantyl®	aluminum hydroxide, 150 mg magnesium hydroxide, 150 mg	—	38.1	< 5
Maalox®	aluminum hydroxide, 225 mg magnesium hydroxide, 200 mg	—	30.8	1
Maalox Plus®	aluminum hydroxide, 225 mg magnesium hydroxide, 200 mg simethicone, 25 mg[a]	2.3		2.5
Maalox T.C.®	aluminum hydroxide, 600 mg magnesium hydroxide, 300 mg	4.2	15.7	< 1–1.2
Mylanta®	aluminum hydroxide, 200 mg magnesium hydroxide, 200 mg simethicone, 20 mg[a]	—	32.0	< 1
Mylanta II®	aluminum hydroxide, 400 mg magnesium hydroxide, 400 mg simethicone, 30 mg[a]	3.6	16.3	1.1
Simeco®	aluminum hydroxide, 365 mg magnesium hydroxide, 300 mg simethicone, 30 mg[a]	—	—	7–14
Bisodol®	sodium bicarbonate, 644 mg magnesium carbonate, 475 mg	—	—	196
Camalox®	aluminum hydroxide, 225 mg magnesium hydroxide, 200 mg calcium carbonate, 250 mg	3.2	23.5	2.5–3
Riopan®	magaldrate, 480 mg	—	36.4	< 1
Titralac®	calcium carbonate, 1000 mg	4.2	20.0	11
AlternaGEL®	aluminum hydroxide, 600 mg	3.4	23.5	2
Amphojel®	aluminum hydroxide, 320 mg	1.4	61.5	7
Basaljel®	aluminum hydroxide, 400 mg	—	—	2
Basaljel Extra Strength®	aluminum hydroxide, 1000 mg	2.0	18.6	23

[a] Not an antacid but an antifoaming agent

Evaluation of the clinical effectiveness of drug combinations for a particular therapeutic effect cannot be determined entirely from in vitro observation. On the other hand, several drug combinations have been developed specifically from an understanding of the pathogenesis of diseases and the application of pharmacologic principles in the design of effective drugs. This has represented one of the most powerful examples of rational drug development.

As we learn more about complex and increasingly common chronic and degenerative diseases, it is likely that single drugs will prove to be less effective than two or more drugs with complementary effects, resulting in beneficial drug interactions. As more and more drugs are administered to a single patient, however, it is important to recognize that this also increases the risk of untoward or adverse drug effects.

ACKNOWLEDGEMENT

This work was supported in part by Public Health Service grants 5 D28 PE14233 and 5 KO7 AG00172.

Literature Cited

1. Prescott, L. F. 1980. Clinically important drug interactions. In *Drug Treatment: Principles and Practice of Clinical Pharmacology and Therapeutics*, ed. G. S. Avery, pp. 236–62. Sydney/New York: ADIS. 1382 pp. 2nd ed.
2. Hansten, P. D. 1979. *Drug Interactions*. Philadelphia: Lea & Febiger. 552 pp. 4th ed.
3. Moellering, R. C. 1983. Rationale for use of antimicrobial combinations. *Am. J. Med.* 75(2A):4–8
4. Eliopoulos, G. M., Moellering, R. C. 1982. Antibiotic synergism and antimicrobial combinations in clinical infections. *Rev. Infect. Dis.* 4:282–93
5. Bennett, J. E., Dismukes, W. E., Duma, R. J., Medoff, G., Sande, M. A., et al. 1979. A comparison of amphoterian B alone and combined with flucytosine in the treatment of cryptococcal meningitis. *N. Engl. J. Med.* 301:126–31
6. Farrar, W. E., Newsome, J. K. 1973. Mechanism of synergistic effects of beta-lactam antibiotic combinations on gram-negative bacilli. *Antimicrob. Agents Chemother.* 4:109–14
7. Mizoguchi, J., Suginaka, H., Kotani, S. 1979. Mechanism of synergistic action of a combination of ampicillin and dicloxacillin against a beta-lactamase-producing strain of *Citrobacter freundii*. *Antimicrob. Agents Chemother.* 16:439–43
8. Neu, H. C. 1969. Effect of beta-lactamase location in *Escherichia coli* on penicillin synergy. *Appl. Microbiol.* 17:783–86
9. Neu, H. C. 1982. Synergistic activity of mecillinam in combination with beta-lactamase inhibitors clavulanic acid and sulbactam. *Antimicrob. Agents Chemother.* 22:518–19
10. Ball, A. P., Geddes, A. M., Davey, P. G., Farrell, I. D., Brooks, G. R. 1980. Clavulanic acid and amoxycillin: A clinical, bacteriological, and pharmacological study. *Lancet* 1:620–23
11. Sanders, C. C., Sanders, W. E., Goering, R. B. 1982. In vitro antagonism of beta-lactam antibiotics by cefoxitin. *Antimicrob. Agents Chemother.* 21:968–75
12. Goering, R. B., Sanders, C. C., Sanders, W. E. 1982. Antagonism of carbenicillin and cefamandole by cefoxitin in treatment of experimental infections in mice. *Antimicrob. Agents Chemother.* 21:963–67
13. Sanders, C. C., Moellering, R. C., Martin, R. R., Perkins, R. L., Strike, D. C., et al. 1982. Resistance to cefamandole: A collaborative study of emerging clinical problems. *J. Infect. Dis.* 145:118–25
14. Salter, A. J. 1982. Trimethoprim-sulfamethoxazole: An assessment of more than 12 years of use. *Rev. Infect. Dis.* 4:196–236
15. Hitchings, G. H. 1973. Mechanism of action of trimethoprim-sulfameth-

oxazole-I. *J. Infect. Dis.* 128:S433–36 (Suppl.)

16. Hitchings, G. H., Burchall, J. J. 1965. Inhibition of folate biosynthesis and function as a basis for chemotherapy. *Adv. Enzymol.* 27:417–68

17. Bushby, S. R. M. 1973. Trimethoprim-sulfamethoxazole: In vitro microbiological aspects. *J. Infect. Dis.* 128:S442–62 (Suppl.)

18. Hitchings, G. H., Falco, E. A., Vanderwerff, H., Russell, P. B., Elion, G. B. 1952. Antagonists of nucleic acid derivatives. VII. 2,4-diaminopyrimidines. *J. Biol. Chem.* 199:43–56

19. Burchall, J. J., Hitchings, G. H. 1965. Inhibitor binding analysis of dihydrofolate reductase from various species. *Mol. Pharmacol.* 1:126–36

20. Burchall, J. J. 1973. Mechanism of action of trimethoprim-sulfamethoxazole-II. *J. Infect. Dis.* 128:S437–41 (Suppl.)

21. Bushby, S. R. M., Hitchings, G. H. 1968. Trimethoprim, a sulfonamide potentiator. *Br. J. Pharmacol. Chemother.* 33:72–90

22. Burchall, J. J. 1979. The development of the diaminopyrimidines. *J. Antimicrob. Chemother.* 5 (Suppl. B):3–14

23. Kremers, P., Duvivier, J., Heusghem, C. 1974. Pharmacokinetic studies of cotrimorxazole in man after single and repeat doses. *J. Clin. Pharmacol.* 14:112–17

24. Hein, G. E., Berg, B. K. 1949. Recovery from subacute bacterial endocarditis *(Streptococcus faecalis)*. *Am. Heart J.* 38:433–37

25. Gunnison, J. B., Jawetz, M. A., Coleman, V. R. 1950. The effect of combinations of antibiotics on enterococci in vitro. *J. Lab. Clin. Med.* 36:900–11

26. Jawetz, M. A., Gunnison, G. B., Coleman, V. R. 1950. The combined action of penicillin with streptomycin or chloromycetin on enterococci in vitro. *Science* 111:254–56

27. Sapico, F. L., Keys, T. F., Hewitt, W. L. 1972. Experimental enterococcal endocarditis. II. Study of in vivo synergism of penicillin and streptomycin. *Am. J. Med. Sci.* 263:128–35

28. Moellering, R. C., Wennersten, C., Weinberg, A. N. 1971. Studies on antibiotic synergism against enterococci. I. Bacteriologic studies. *J. Lab. Clin. Med.* 77:821–28

29. Abrutyn, E., Lincoln, L., Gallagher, M., Weinstein, A. J. 1978. Cephalothin-gentamicin synergism in experimental enterococcal endocarditis. *J. Antimicrob. Chemother.* 4:153–58

30. Watanakunakorn, C. 1971. Penicillin combined with gentamicin or streptomycin: Synergism against enterococci. *J. Infect. Dis.* 124:581–86

31. Hook, E. W., Roberts, R. B., Sande, M. A. 1975. Antimicrobial therapy of experimental enterococcal endocarditis. *Antimicrob. Agents Chemother.* 8:564–70

32. Carrizosa, J., Kaye, D. 1976. Antibiotic synergism in enterococcal endocarditis. *J. Lab. Clin. Med.* 88:132–41

33. Weinstein, A. J., Moellering, R. C. 1973. Penicillin and gentamicin therapy for enterococcal infections. *J. Am. Med. Assoc.* 223:1030–32

34. Wilson, W. R., Wilkowske, C. J., Wright, A. J., Sande, M. A., Ceraci, J. E. 1984. Treatment of streptomycin-susceptible and streptomycin-resistant enterococcal endocarditis. *Ann. Intern. Med.* 100:816–23

35. Sande, M. A., Scheld, W. M. 1980. Combination antibiotic therapy of bacterial endocarditis. *Ann. Intern. Med.* 92:390–95

36. Tompsett, R., Berman, W. 1977. Enterococcal endocarditis: Duration and mode of treatment. *Trans. Am. Clin. Climatol. Assoc.* 89:49–57

37. Watanakunakorn, C., Bakie, C. 1973. Synergism of vancomycin-gentamicin and vancomycin-streptomycin against enterococci. *Antimicrob. Agents Chemother.* 4:120–24

38. Watanakunakorn, C., Baird, I. M. 1977. Prognostic factors in *Staphylococcus aureus* endocarditis and results of therapy with penicillin and gentamicin. *Am. J. Med. Sci.* 273:133–39

39. Korzeniowski, O., Sande, M. A., National Collaborative Endo-Carditis Study Group. 1982. Combination antimicrobial therapy for *Staphylococcus aureus* endocarditis in patients addicted to parenteral drugs and in nonaddicts. *Ann. Intern. Med.* 97:496–503

40. McCabe, W. R., Jackson, G. G. 1975. Treatment of pyelonephritis. *N. Engl. J. Med.* 272:1037–44

41. Anderson, E. T., Young, L. S., Hewitt, W. L. 1978. Antimicrobial synergism in the therapy of gram-negative rod bacteremia. *Chemotherapy* 24:45–54

42. Klastersky, J., Zinner, S. H. 1982. Synergistic combinations of antibiotics in gram-negative bacillary infections. *Rev. Infect. Dis.* 4:294–301

43. Winston, D. J., Sidell, J., Hairston, J., Young, L. S. 1979. Antimicrobial therapy of septicemia due to *Klebsiella*

pneumoniae in neutropenic rats. *J. Infect. Dis.* 139:377–88

44. McNeely, D. J., D'Alessandri, R. M., Kluge, R. M. 1976. In vitro antimicrobial synergy and antagonism against *Klebsiella* species—What does it mean? *Clin. Res.* 24:636A (Abstr.)

45. Kluge, R. M., Standiford, H. C., Tatem, B., Young, V. M., Schimpff, S. C., et al. 1974. The carbenicillin-gentamicin combination against *Pseudomonas aeruginosa*: Correlation of effect with gentamicin sensitivity. *Ann. Intern. Med.* 81:584–87

46. Marks, M. I., Hammerberg, S., Greenstone, G., Silver, B. 1976. Activity of newer aminoglycosides and carbenicillin, alone and in combination, against gentamicin-resistant *Pseudomonas aeruginosa*. *Antimocrob. Agents. Chemother.* 10:399–401

47. Andriole, V. T. 1971. Synergy of carbenicillin and gentamicin in experimental infection with *Pseudomonas*. *J. Infect. Dis.* 124:S46–S55 (Suppl.)

48. EORTC International Antimicrobial Therapy Project Group. 1978. Three antibiotic regimens in the treatment of infections in febrile granulocytopenic patients with cancer. *J. Infect. Dis.* 137:14–29

49. Schimpff, S. C. 1977. Therapy of infections in patients with granulocytopenia. *Med. Clin. N. Am.* 61:1101–18

50. Center for Disease Control. 1982. Sexually transmitted diseases: Treatment guidelines. *Rev. Infect. Dis.* 4:S729–48 (Suppl.)

51. Mudge, G. H.. 1980. Inhibitions of tubular transport of organic compounds. In *Goodman and Gilman's The Pharmacological Basis of Therapeutics*, ed. A. G. Gilman, L. S. Goodman, A. Gilman, pp. 929–34. New York: Macmillan. 1843 pp. 6th ed.

52. Johnson, D. W., Kvale, P. A., Afable, V. L., Stewart, S. D., Halverson, C. W., et al. 1970. Single-dose antibiotic treatment of asymptomatic gonorrhea in hospitalized women. *N. Engl. J. Med.* 283:1–4

53. Kaufman, R. E., Johnson, R. E., Jaffee, H. W., Thornsberry, C., Reynolds, G. H., et al. 1976. National gonorrhea therapy monitoring study: Treatment results. *N. Engl. J. Med.* 294:1–4

54. Gordon, R. C., Regamey, C., Kirby, W. M. M. 1972. Comparative clinical pharmacology of amoxicillin and ampicillin administered orally. *Antimicrob. Agents Chemother.* 1:504–7

55. Robinson, G. N. 1973. Laboratory evaluation of amoxycillin. *Chemotherapy* 18:1–10 (Suppl.)

56. Judson, F. N. 1979. The importance of coexisting syphilitic, chamydial, mycoplasmal, and trichomonal infections in the treatment of gonorrhea. *Sex. Transm. Dis.* 6:112–19 (Suppl.)

57. Griffith, D. P., Musher, D. M. 1973. Prevention of infected urinary stones by urease inhibition. *Invest. Urol.* 11:228–33

58. Griffith, D. P., Gibson, J. R., Clinton, C. W., Musher, D. M. 1978. Acetohydroxamic acid: Clinical studies of urease inhibitor in patients with staghorn renal calculi. *J. Urol.* 119:9–15

59. Kobashi, K., Hase, J., Uehara, K. 1962. Specific inhibition of urease by hydroxamic acids. *Biochem. Biophys. Acta* 65:380–83

60. Griffith, D. P., Musher, D. M., Itin, C. 1976. Urease. The primary cause of infection-induced urinary stones. *Invest. Urol.* 13:346–50

61. Martelli, A., Buli, P., Cortecchia, V. 1981. Urease inhibitor therapy in infected renal stones. *Eur. Urol.* 7:291–93

62. Brande, A. I., Siemienski, J. 1960. Role of bacterial urease in experimental pyelonephritis. *J. Bacteriol.* 80:171–79

63. MacLaren, D. M. 1968. The significance of urease in *Proteus* pyelonephritis: A bacteriological study. *J. Path. Bacteriol.* 96:45–56

64. Musher, D. M., Griffith, D. P., Yawn, D., Rossen, R. D. 1975. Role of urease in pyelonephritis resulting from urinary tract infection with *Proteus*. *J. Infect. Dis.* 131:177–81

65. MacLaren, D. M. 1974. The influence of acetohydroxamic acid on experimental *Proteus* pyelonephritis. *Invest. Urol.* 12:146–49

66. Gale, G. R. 1966. Urease activity and antibiotic sensitivity of bacteria. *J. Bacteriol.* 91:499–506

67. Musher, D. M., Griffith, D. P., Tyler, M., Woelfel, A. 1974. Potentiation of the antibacterial effect of methenamine by acetohydroxamic acid. *Antimicrob. Agents Chemother.* 5:101–5

68. Musher, D. M., Saenz, C., Griffith, D. P. 1974. Interaction between acetohydroxamic acid and 12 antibiotics against 14 gram-negative pathogenic bacteria. *Antimicrob. Agents Chemother.* 5:106–10

69. Calne, D. B. 1977. Development in the pharmacology and therapeutics of parkinsonism. *Ann. Neurol.* 1:111–19

70. Weiner, M. 1982. Update on antiparkinsonian agents. *Geriatrics* 37(9):81–91

71. Cotzias, G. C., Van Woert, M. H.,

Schiffer, L. M. 1967. Aromatic amino acids and modification of parkinsonism. *N. Engl. J. Med.* 276:374–79

72. Duvoisin, R. C., Yahr, M. D., Cote, L. D. 1969. Pyridoxine reversal of l-dopa effects in parkinsonism. *Trans. Am. Neurol. Assoc.* 94:81–84

73. Bianchine, J. R., Shaw, G. M. 1976. Clinical pharmacokinetics of levodopa in Parkinson's disease. *Clin. Pharmacokinet.* 1:313–38

74. Boshes, B. 1981. Sinemet and the treatment of parkinsonism. *Ann. Intern. Med.* 94:364–70

75. Langrall, H. M., Joseph, C. 1972. Evaluation of safety and efficacy of levodopa in Parkinson's disease and syndrome. *Neurology* 22:3–16 (Suppl.)

76. Marsden, C. D., Parkes, J. D. 1976. "On-off" effect in patients with Parkinson's disease on chronic levodopa therapy. *Lancet* 1:292–96

77. Markham, C. H., Diamond, S. G., Treciokas, L. J. 1974. Carbidopa in Parkinson disease and in nausea and vomiting of levodopa. *Arch. Neurol.* 31:128–33

78. Tourtellotte, W. W., Syndulko, K., Potvin, A. R., Hirsch, S. B., Potvin, J. H. 1980. Increased ratio of carbidopa to levodopa in treatment of Parkinson's disease. *Arch. Neurol.* 37:723–26

79. Bailey, E. V., Stone, J. W. 1975. The mechanism of action of amantadine in parkinsonism: A review. *Arch. Int. Pharmacodyn. Ther.* 216:246–62

80. Mawdsley, C., Williams, I. R., Pullar, I. A., Davidson, D. L., Kinlock, N. E. 1972. Treatment of parkinsonism by amantadine and levodopa. *Clin. Pharmacol. Ther.* 13:575–83

81. Timberlake, W. H., Vance, M. A. 1978. Four-year treatment of patients with parkinsonism using amantadine alone or with levodopa. *Ann. Neurol.* 3:119–28

82. Lieberman, A. N., Kupersmith, M., Gopinathan, G., Estey, E., Goodgold, A., et al. 1979. Bromocriptine in Parkinson's disease: Further studies. *Neurology* 29:363–69

83. Lieberman, A., Kupersmith, M., Neophytides, A., Casson, I., Durso, R., et al. 1980. Long-term efficacy of bromocriptine in Parkinson's disease. *Neurology* 30:518–23

84. Goodwin-Austin, R. B., Smith, N. J. 1977. Comparison of the effects of bromocriptine and levodopa in Parkinson's disease. *J. Neurol. Neurosurg. Psychiatr.* 40:479–82

85. Hoehn, M. M. 1981. Bromocriptine and its use in parkinsonism. *J. Am. Geriatr. Soc.* 29:251–58

86. Stern, G. M., Lees, A. J. 1983. Sustained bromocriptine therapy in 50 previously untreated patients with Parkinson's disease. *Adv. Neurol.* 37:17–21

87. Duvoisin, R. C. 1967. Cholinergic-anticholinergic antagonism in parkinsonism. *Arch. Neurol.* 17:124–36

88. Bianchine, J. R., Sunyapridakul, L. 1973. Interactions between levodopa and other drugs: Significance in treatment of Parkinson's disease. *Drugs* 6:364–88

89. Johnston, J. P. 1968. Some observations upon a new inhibitor of monoamine oxidase in brain tissue. *Biochem. Pharmacol.* 17:1285–97

90. Yahr, M. D. 1978. Overview of present day treatment of parkinson's disease. *J. Neurol. Transm.* 43:227–238

91. Birkmayer, W., Riederer, P., Ambrozi, L., Youdim, M. B. H. 1977. Implications of combined treatment with "Madopar" and L-deprenil in Parkinson's disease. *Lancet* 1:439–43

92. Schachter, M., Marsden, C. D., Parkes, J. D., Jenner, P., Testa, B. 1980. Deprenyl in the management of response fluctuations in patients with Parkinson's disease on levodopa. *J. Neurol. Neurosurg. Psychiatry* 43:1016–21

93. Jaffey, L., Martin, A. 1981. Malignant hyperkalaemia after amiloride/hydrochlorothiazide treatment. *Lancet* 1:1272

94. Morgan, D. B., Davidson, C. 1980. Hypokalemia and diuretics: An analysis of publications. *Br. Med. J.* 280:905–8

95. Hunt, J. C. 1983. Sodium intake and hypertension: A cause for concern. *Ann. Intern. Med.* 98(Pt. 2):724–28

96. Tannen, R. L. 1983. Effects of potassium on blood pressure control. *Ann. Intern. Med.* 98(Pt. 2):773–80

97. Hansen, K. B., Bender, A. D. 1967. Changes in serum potassium levels occurring in patients treated with triamterene and triamterene-hydrochlorothiazide combination. *Clin. Pharmacol. Ther.* 8:392–99

98. Stewart, R. B., Hale, W. E., Marks, R. G. 1983. Diuretic use in an ambulatory elderly population. *Am. J. Hosp. Pharm.* 40:409–13

99. Finnegan, T. P., Spence, J. D., Cape, R. D. 1984. Potassium sparing diuretics: Interaction with digoxin in elderly men. *J. Am. Geriatr. Soc.* 32:129–31

100. Wollam, G. L., Tarazi, P. C., Bravo, E. K., Dustan, H. P. 1982. Diuretic potency of combined hydrochlorothiazide and furosemide therapy in patients with azotemia. *Am. J. Med.* 72:929–38

101. Oster, J. R., Epstein, M., Smoller, S. 1983. Combined therapy with thiazide-

type and loop diuretic agents for resistant sodium retention. *Ann. Intern. Med.* 99:405–6

102. Sigurd, B., Olesen, K. H., Wennevold, A. 1975. The supra-additive natriuretic effect addition of bendroflumethiazide and bumetanide in congestive heart failure. *Am. Heart J.* 89:163–70

103. Peterson, W. L., Sturdevant, R. A. L., Frankl, H. D., Richardson, C. T., Isenberg, J. I., et al. 1977. Healing of duodenal ulcer with an antacid regimen. *N. Engl. J. Med.* 297:341–45

104. Ippoliti, A. F., Sturdevant, R. A. L., Isenberg, J. I., Binder, M., Camacho, R., et al. 1978. Cimetidine versus intensive antacid therapy for duodenal ulcer: A multicenter trial. *Gastroenterology* 74: 393–95

105. Ippoliti, A., Elashoff, J., Valenzuela, J., Cano, R., Frankl, H., et al. 1983. Recurrent ulcer after successful treatment with cimetidine or antacid. *Gastroenterology* 85:875–80

106. Brogden, R. N., Carmine, A. A., Heel, R. C., Speight, T. M., Avery, G. S. 1982. Ranitidine: A review of its pharmacology and therapeutic use in peptic ulcer disease and other allied diseases. *Drugs* 24:267–303

107. Drake, D., Hollander, D. 1981. Neutralizing capacity and cost effectiveness of antacids. *Ann. Intern. Med.* 94:215–17

108. Antacids. 1982. *Med. Lett. Drugs Ther.* 24:61–62

109. Harvey, S. C. 1980. Gastric antacids and digestants. See Ref. 51, pp. 988–1001

110. Fordtran, J. S., Marowski, S. G., Richardson, C. T. 1973. In vivo and in vitro evaluation of liquid antacids. *N. Engl. J. Med.* 288:923–28

111. Sherrill, M. C., Rudd, G. D. 1982. In vitro evaluation of liquid antacid products. *Am. J. Hosp. Pharm.* 39:300–2

Ann. Rev. Pharmacol. Toxicol. 1985. 25:97–125

THE PULMONARY UPTAKE, ACCUMULATION, AND METABOLISM OF XENOBIOTICS[1]

John R. Bend, Cosette J. Serabjit-Singh, and Richard M. Philpot

Laboratory of Pharmacology, National Institute of Environmental Health Sciences, National Institutes of Health, Research Triangle Park, North Carolina 27709

INTRODUCTION

Researchers now recognize that the lungs are a site for the uptake, accumulation, and/or metabolism of numerous endogenous and exogenous, or xenobiotic, chemicals and various aspects of these pulmonary processes have recently been reviewed (1–8). Much of the impetus for studying the uptake and metabolism of xenobiotics by lungs is due to their intimate contact with both blood and the external environment and their sensitivity to many chemicals that selectively cause pulmonary damage (9). The lungs have two important characteristics that facilitate the absorption of airborne or blood-borne chemicals. First, the venous drainage from virtually the entire body perfuses through the alveolar-capillary unit, which has an extensive capillary endothelium. Second, the alveolar epithelial and endothelial layers are very thin to facilitate gas exchange. Such an architectural arrangement, which places the epithelial layers in close contact with the blood, allows rapid absorption of unionized lipophilic xenobiotics and metabolism and/or transfer to the circulation.

One important function of lung is to regulate the systemic concentration of biologically active endogenous compounds by selective removal or metabolism. Certain polypeptides (6), prostaglandins (7), and vasoactive amines (8) in venous blood are handled in this manner. Pulmonary endothelial cells are important in the regulation of circulating hormones (10), and consequently it is not surprising that certain xenobiotics, which have physicochemical properties

---

similar to those of the endogenous substrates, also serve as substrates or ligands for the specialized enzymes, receptors, binding sites, and transport mechanisms localized on or in endothelial cells. Similar considerations are relevant for the uptake of chemicals into or transport through the epithelial cells lining the airways of lungs; certain xenobiotics are able to enter these cells by carrier-mediated mechanisms, others enter by nonionic diffusion.

In this review, we describe the classes of xenobiotics known to be taken up by lung and delineate the relative roles, if known, of the endothelium and epithelium. We also discuss the importance of chemical-metabolizing enzymes and their cellular localization in relationship to the clearance of chemicals by the lung and target-cell toxicity. We have taken this particular approach for several reasons. First, we feel it complements several excellent existing reviews in this research area. Second, it emphasizes the structural, functional, and cellular heterogeneity of lungs and the differential contribution of various cell types to the pulmonary uptake, accumulation, and metabolism of chemicals. Finally, it provides a convenient framework for the critical evaluation of recent research in this field, while allowing identification of subject areas that merit additional attention.

HISTORICAL AND GENERAL CONSIDERATIONS

Certain biogenic amines, including 5-hydroxytryptamine (5-HT, serotonin), l-norepinephrine (NE), and β-phenylethylamine (PEA), are removed from pulmonary circulation whereas others, such as histamine, dopamine, and epinephrine, generally are not (11). In perfused lungs, the removal of 5-HT and NE occurs via carrier-mediated transport processes that are saturable and sodium-, energy-, and temperature-dependent. Rapid intracellular metabolism of 5-HT and NE by monoamine oxidases and/or catechol-0-methyltransferases follow, and the metabolites are released into the circulation (12–14). Histochemical localization studies have shown that both 5-HT and NE are transported into pulmonary endothelial cells (15). 5-HT and NE are also known to be removed by saturable processes in vivo, and the endothelial sites for removal of these two amines are distinct (16). On the other hand, PEA enters the lung by passive diffusion and is inactivated by monoamine oxidase activity in lung (17, 18). Although the uptake and metabolism of endogenous compounds by lung remains an active research area, similar studies have been initiated with xenobiotics because many chemicals are concentrated preferentially in lung (19) or cause selective toxicity to the lung (4, 9) after in vivo administration.

Types of Xenobiotics Cleared by the Lungs

BASIC AMINES   Extensive reviews of the types of drugs concentrated in lung are available (3, 19). Although many pharmacological classes are represented (e.g. antihistamines, antimalarials, morphine-like analgesics, anorectics, tricyclic antidepressants, anesthetics), many of the compounds concentrated in the lung are basic amines. Detailed studies of the mechanisms of accumulation of several xenobiotic amines by perfused lungs performed by Eling, Anderson, and collaborators at NIEHS (10–23) have been previously reviewed (3, 24). Similar experiments were also performed by others (e.g. 25). Briefly, the conclusions drawn from these investigations are:

1. To be efficiently removed from the circulation, amines must have a pKa greater than eight and substantial lipophilic character. (Many of the amines removed are amphiphilic in nature, containing both a large hydrophobic region and a charged group, normally cationic, at physiological pH. Examples of such amines include chlorcyclizine (CHLORCY), chlorphentermine (CHLORPH), chlorpromazine (CHLORPR), cyclizine, desipramine, diphenhydramine, fluphenazine, imipramine (IMP), iprindole, methadone (METH), promazine, propranolol, and tripelennamine.

2. The mechanism for the steady-state uptake of basic amines into lung consists of two components, one saturable and one non-saturable. For most basic amines the saturable component is attributed to intracellular binding by facilitated diffusion and not to carrier-mediated transport or metabolism. However, amphetamine appears to be removed by a carrier-mediated transport process (24), and it is conceivable, because of structural similarities, that this compound is a substrate for the NE transport system of pulmonary endothelium. The magnitude of the non-saturable component of uptake is too large to be a reflection of diffusion into the extracellular space.

3. Results of efflux studies of IMP or METH from perfused lungs into drug-free perfusion medium are consistent with at least three different pools of accumulated amine (22, 23). The linear component of lung uptake corresponds to the two components of efflux that have the shortest half-lives, whereas the saturable component of uptake corresponds to the efflux component of longest half-life (18 seconds, 58 seconds, and approximately 8 minutes for IMP efflux respectively). The linear component of uptake is believed to represent the partitioning of amine into membranes in contact with perfusion medium; the saturable component is attributed to intracellular binding to at least two distinct sites, although the cell type or types where this occurs is not precisely known. There is also one pool of IMP or METH that does not efflux during the normal perfusion period (60 minutes). This latter pool, which accounts for approximately 30% of the IMP taken up by lung, is termed the slowly effluxing pool (SEP), and this pool appears to account for the persistence of amphiphilic amines in lung.

A more recent study with IMP in vivo demonstrated that the half-life for the disappearance of the SEP is approximately four hours (26). Subsequent autoradiographic evidence of Wilson et al (27) suggests that intracellular (non-covalent) binding in the alveolar macrophage is the major component of the SEP. This observation has led to the assumption that macrophage removal via the mucociliary clearance mechanism accounts for drug removal from the SEP.

The persistence of certain amines in lung appears important in drug-induced pulmonary phospholipidosis. This condition, characterized by an increased presence of phospholipids in bronchiolar epithelium, type I and type II alveolar epithelial cells, alveolar macrophages, vascular endothelial cells, and pulmonary smooth muscle cells, results after chronic treatment with one of more than twenty drugs, although not all animal species are susceptible (28). It is probable that amphiphilic cationic compounds interact physicochemically with phospholipid (29), leading to decreased catabolism of phospholipid and its accumulation in lung cells (30). Wilson et al (26) have demonstrated that compounds known to induce pulmonary phospholipidosis, such as IMP and CHLORPH, form much larger SEP in vivo than basic amines such as amphetamine, phentermine, and 5-HT, which do not cause this condition.

It follows that drug-endogenous substrate and drug-drug interactions of clinical importance are possible in lung, and this area of research has attracted considerable attention. Most of this work has been performed with perfused lung preparations (3, 24, 31, 32), but recently Gillis and his colleagues (33, 34) adapted the single injection, double or triple indicator-dilution technique (35) for in vivo studies and determined the pulmonary clearance of 5-HT in man (33). They also investigated the effects of IMP or cocaine treatment on the pulmonary clearance of 5-HT and NE in the rabbit (34). With cardiogreen as the reference compound, extraction of 5-HT is decreased significantly when measured 15 minutes, 45 minutes, 75 minutes, and 165 minutes after the administration of IMP (0.5 mg/kg, iv) relative to the 0-hour control value; NE extraction is also decreased by this dose of IMP between 15 minutes (the first time sampled) and 135 minutes after treatment. However, treatment with cocaine (0.5 mg/kg) did not affect NE clearance in vivo, although earlier studies showed that cocaine inhibits the clearance of both 5-HT and NE in perfused rabbit lungs (36, 37). Collectively, these data emphasize that extrapolation of in vitro data to the in vivo situation, particularly where complex interactions are involved, requires caution. For this reason it is encouraging that other authors are now using in vivo approaches (38–40) for investigating drug-endogenous substrate interactions in lung.

Another drug-drug interaction studied recently is the effect of CHLORPH-induced pulmonary phospholipidosis on the clearance of biogenic and non-biogenic amines by perfused rat lungs. Mehendale and his colleagues have shown that, although phospholipidosis decreases the uptake and metabolism of 5-HT (42), it enhances the uptake and accumulation of CHLORPR, IMP, and CHLORPH itself (43, 44). Interactions of these drugs with pulmonary phospholipid, which is increased 60% by CHLORPH, may limit their access to the metabolic sites and thus retard both metabolism (via N-oxidation) and efflux while concomitantly increasing accumulation of amphiphilic amines in perfused lungs. The facts that drug-induced phospholipidosis in rats is accompanied by marked changes in mitochondrial structure and cellular bioenergetics (45) and that the pulmonary clearance mediated by alveolar macrophages is almost totally suppressed in vivo (46) suggest that similar interaction studies should also be conducted in intact animals.

XENOBIOTICS METABOLIZED BY LUNGS   Although lipophilic basic amines are removed from pulmonary circulation, this frequently occurs in the absence of metabolism. There are also many chemicals that are cleared from the circulation by lungs due to metabolism mediated by enzymes present in this tissue. The lung contains, although generally at lower concentrations, virtually all of the hepatic pathways required for the biotransformation of exogenous chemicals. Not all hepatic isozymes are present in lung, however (47). Xenobiotic metabolism by lungs is the subject of several extensive recent reviews (4, 5, 24, 47, 48) and only a few relevant points are repeated here. First, the cytochrome P-450-dependent monooxygenase system is distributed heterogeneously among various pulmonary cell types. Immunochemical localization studies (49), enzymatic studies with freshly isolated lung cells (50, 51), and autoradiographic studies of 4-ipomeanol-derived radioactivity (52) have shown that the nonciliated bronchiolar epithelial (Clara) cell is a major site of cytochrome P-450-dependent activity. However, the alveolar type II cell also contains considerable amounts of monooxygenase activity (50, 51), whereas the alveolar macrophage, at least in the rabbit, is virtually devoid of such activity (53). Recent immunochemical studies in our laboratory have also shown that rabbit aorta and/or its underlying smooth muscle layer contain small amounts of cytochrome P-450 isozymes and their associated enzymatic activity (54). Obviously, these data represent information on only a few of the more than forty cell types found in lung, but they are at least a start in correlating xenobiotic metabolizing activity with pulmonary cell type, a difficult task with such a complex organ.

It must be emphasized that the degree of cellular integrity of the experimental system used for testing can qualitatively and quantitatively affect the results obtained. For example, studies in our laboratory showed (55) that CHLORCY and IMP are not degraded over 60 minutes in a recirculating rabbit lung preparation, whereas these drugs are readily metabolized by rabbit lung homogenate or microsomes. Similarly, Minchin et al (56) found that the kinetically estimated binding capacity for CHLORPH is 0.109 μg/g in perfused rat lungs but 8.3 μg/g in rat lung homogenate (57). It is likely that these experimental differences between the perfused organ and whole homogenate are due to limited substrate access to the sites of metabolism and binding in intact tissue. In any case, we have found that an integrated experimental approach, which incorporates both broken *and* intact cellular preparations, is best suited for the study of xenobiotic metabolism by lung (5). It should be remembered in this context that all chemicals metabolized by lung in vitro have the potential to be cleared from the circulation by this tissue in vivo.

Relationships between xenobiotic metabolism and target cell toxicity in lung, and the use of kinetic parameters of drug-metabolizing enzymes determined in vitro to predict pulmonary clearance of chemicals will be discussed in subsequent sections of this review.

PARAQUAT   Paraquat (PQ) is a widely used quaternary ammonium bipyridyl herbicide (1,1'-dimethyl-4,4-bipyridylium dichloride). The most characteristic feature of PQ toxicity is its pulmonary involvement, and lung damage is observed in rats following systemic (58) or intrabronchial (59) doses. The iv administration of PQ to rats results in the accumulation of unchanged compound in the lung (60), and a recent autoradiographic study showed that PQ is concentrated in discrete areas of mouse lung, presumably in alveolar type II cells, at 3, 9, or 24 hours after iv injection (61). This is interesting because the first phase of PQ-mediated toxicity in the lung is extensive damage to alveolar epithelial cells (62). Other studies showed that PQ is taken up by lung slices by an energy-dependent mechanism (63, 64), and it is now generally accepted that the selective toxicity of this herbicide to lungs is related to the compound accumulated. The characteristics of this transport process, which is believed to be localized in alveolar type I and type II cells (65), is discussed later.

PULMONARY VASCULATURE: ROLE IN XENOBIOTIC UPTAKE, METABOLISM, AND TOXICITY

General Characteristics of the Pulmonary Vasculature

In considering the contribution of this tissue to xenobiotic metabolism and toxicity, one must appreciate the heterogeneity of the vasculature of various organs of an individual as well as differences among species, because relevant data are often derived from tissue homogenates or slices, homogeneous cultures, or isolated perfused organs. Structurally, blood vessels differ in the configuration and proportion of endothelium and smooth muscle between veins and arteries as well as among species (66). Biochemically, differences between veins and arteries and among capillary beds of various organs have been shown: the hexose monophosphate pathway functions in arteries but not in veins (67); receptor and carrier-mediated transport mechanisms of endothelium for endogenous substrates (sugars, amino acids, lipids) are organ specific (68). Given this diversity, the potential for overinterpreting simple qualitative parameters exists. Thus, we shall discuss the uses of various parameters, the suggested mechanisms of toxicity or detoxication, and the limitations of certain approaches in studies of the pulmonary vasculature. In addition, our recent biochemical and immunochemical analyses of rabbit aorta (54) are included because of their potential relevance to the clearance of xenobiotics by the pulmonary vasculature. There are several informative reviews on studies of the uptake and metabolism of biogenic amines, the production of vasoactive peptides, prostaglandins, and hyperoxic or hypoxic response relevant to this tissue (8, 11, 69–73).

Briefly, some previously reviewed characteristics of the pulmonary vasculature are:

1. The lung regulates the concentration of circulating vasoactive peptides. The caveolae of the plasma membrane of endothelial cells (EC's) contain a carboxypeptidase, angiotensin-converting enzyme (ACE) that converts the decapeptide angiotensin I to the potent vasopressor angiotensin II. Although ACE is widely distributed, other tissues significantly degrade angiotensin II, whereas the undamaged lung does not. Bradykinin, a vasoactive peptide, is rapidly degraded during passage through the lungs due to the carboxypeptidase activity (ACE or other peptidases) of the vasculature.

2. The control of vasoactive amines is also a major pulmonary function. The uptake of amines such as 5-HT by the endothelium is a rapid and energy-dependent process, especially in the small vessels, and monoamine oxidases or catechol-0-methyltransferases mediate the deactivation. Thus, monoamine oxidase inhibitors such as tricyclic antidepressants diminish the pulmonary clearance of these vasoactive amines with effects on the cardiovasculature; poor clearance of 5-HT has been associated with carcinoid heart disease, and cardiovascular complications arise from overdoses of antidepressants. The clearance of 5-HT by the lung relative to other tissues may be a reflection of the relative endothelial surface areas rather than a tissue-selective uptake mechanism (74). The uptake sites for all vasoactive amines are not identical, as indicated by the lack of competition between 5-HT and NE and by the differential effects of inhibitors. The specificity of the 5-HT uptake mechanism is further indicated by the lack of competition with polyamines (e.g. spermidine, spermine), which are competitors of the pulmonary uptake of PQ (65).

3. Another aspect of the regulation of vasoactive substances by the lung is the endothelial production of prostacyclin or PGI_2, a potent inhibitor of platelet aggregation and a vasodilator. Although the lung effectively degrades other prostaglandins that stimulate vasoconstriction or platelet aggregation, the role of the vasculature in this process is not clearly established. Prostaglandin synthesis has been indirectly localized in situ to the perivascular cells,

and autoradiographic studies with cultured EC's indicate compartmentalization of prostaglandin synthetase on endoplasmic reticulum. Formation of atherosclerotic plaques is associated with diminished production of PGI_2 (75). The capacity of vascular smooth muscle to produce PGI_2 may correspond to a lower susceptibility to atherosclerosis; thus, the resistance of the rat and the susceptibility of the pig to atherosclerosis. Diminished production of PGI_2 may also facilitate metastasis of tumors that form platelet emboli. Another factor that contributes to the unhindered passage of blood through the lungs appears to be the lack of receptors that lead to immune complex deposition, i.e. bovine EC's in culture lack receptors for the fragment crystallizable (Fc) region of immunoglobulin G and for the 3b component of complement (76, 77). However, injury unmasks these receptors and may lead to deposition of immune complexes, as in the case of certain pulmonary inflammatory diseases.

4. Exposure to inhaled oxidants, oxygen more than ozone or nitrogen dioxide, damages the endothelium with subsequent edema and possibly death. The active species is presumed to be the superoxide anion, and the induction of superoxide dismutase (SOD) by exposure to sublethal doses is associated with the development of tolerance to acute exposures. Production of superoxide radicals and induction of SOD are also associated with exposure to PQ, which during the initial stages of toxicity selectively damages the epithelium. Synergistic acute toxicity of hyperoxia and PQ has been reported (78).

Effects of Xenobiotics on the Pulmonary Vasculature

The biochemical response of the pulmonary vasculature to environmental or therapeutic exposure has been an area of limited study, in spite of the obvious importance of the special functions and size of this vascular bed. Current methods of study include the culturing of EC's from lung or other tissues (79), isolated perfused lungs (31), morphological and immunohistochemical techniques (10), as well as in vivo determinations (74, 80–82). The consequence of exposure to pulmonary toxicants or drugs such as bleomycin, monocrotaline, PQ, oxygen, ozone, IMP, and diesel emissions (9, 24, 80a, 83–90) (Table 1) on the vasculature has been investigated.

Clearly, many physiologically significant functions beside oxygen/carbon dioxide exchange depend on the integrity of the vasculature. Thus, an index of early endothelial damage or disruption may be useful for monitoring the effects of drug therapy or exposure to pollutants. The uptake of 5-HT and NE or ACE activity measured in vivo for this purpose has been proposed (80–82). A radioassay of ACE activity for the diagnosis of sarcoidosis and monitoring the subsequent corticosteroid therapy is a suggested application (82); however, the range of activity in 62 normal subjects varied fourfold, and many clinically

Table 1 Pulmonary vascular toxins

Compound	Source or use	Risk to humans	Mechanism of toxicity	Some parameters of injury				References
				5-HT[a]	NE[a]	ACE[a]	morphology[b]	
Monocrotaline	Plant (*Crotalaria spectabilis*); honey and milk	+	Formation of pyrrole (in liver)	↓	↑→		+	89–92
3-Methylindole	Ruminal fermentation of tryptophan	−	Microsomal mono-pyrrolooxygenase	→			+	93, 94
α-Naphthylthiourea (other aryl-thioureas)	Rat poison	+	Microsomal flavin monooxygenase; cytochrome P-450	→			+	95–97
Bleomycin	Anti-neoplastic drug	+	Free radical formation/ lipid peroxidation	↓	↑→	↑→	+	80a, 98, 99
Oxygen (hyperoxia)	Therapy for respiratory deficiency	+	Free radical formation/ lipid peroxidation	↓←	↓→	↑→	+	85, 100–102
Hypoxia	High altitude	+	Vascular hyperplasia	→			+	103, 104
Ozone[c]	Air pollutant	+	Free radical formation/ lipid peroxidation	→			+	85
Nitrogen dioxide[c]	Air pollutant	+	Free radical formation/ lipid peroxidation	→			+	85
Paraquat[c]	Herbicide	+	Free radical formation/ lipid peroxidation	→			+	84

[a] 5-Hydroxytryptamine, 1-norepinephrine, uptake or accumulation, and angiotensin-converting enzyme activity: (→) no change, (↑) increase, (↓) decrease

[b] + denotes vascular damage/edema

[c] Effect on endothelium secondary to damage of epithelium

diagnosed patients had ACE activities within that range. Thus, a low-serum ACE does not preclude the presence of the disease.

Many types of chemical insult to the endothelium are reflected in diminished uptake of 5-HT, NE, or decreased ACE activity (Table 1) and occur prior to any apparent morphological damage. An example of this is bleomycin, an antineoplastic agent that causes pulmonary fibrosis. A subacute dose in rabbits (i.e. with no morphological evidence or elevated hydroxyproline content indicative of fibrosis) resulted in a sustained decrease in 5-HT uptake and serum ACE activity (80a, 83). The consequence of subnormal enzymatic activity or the critical threshold values of these parameters is not known.

In addition to bleomycin, monocrotaline (a pyrrolizidine alkaloid) and hypoxia induce pulmonary hypertension and have been used for investigating the vascular changes associated with the clinically significant condition (89, 103, 104). Thickening of smooth muscle and EC's concomitant with increased vascular resistance was observed. Further, this research may be directly relevant because of the opportunity for human exposure to pyrrolizidine alkaloids (herbal teas, honey, or milk from bees or cattle that consume the plants that produce these compounds) or hypoxia (high altitude).

Oxidant-Induced Alterations of the Pulmonary Vasculature

The potential for human exposure to oxygen, ozone, or nitrogen dioxide is also recognized, and the resulting endothelial damage and induction of detoxication pathways undoubtedly alter the pulmonary disposition of xenobiotics. Subacute exposure to oxygen, for instance, potentiates the effects of PQ yet provides protection against previously lethal concentrations of oxygen. Increased levels of SOD, glucose-6-phosphate dehydrogenase, glutathione peroxidase, glutathione reductase, or non-protein sulfhydryl groups are associated with exposure to these gases (31, 105). However, the mechanism for development of tolerance and/or toxicity is not yet clear. The lack of complete cross-tolerance, as well as the poor correlation between the time courses of elevated enzyme concentrations and maintenance of tolerance, indicate that the increase in overall levels of deactivating components is not the explanation for tolerance. At least in the case of oxygen toxicity, tolerance does not appear to involve an enhanced rate of induction of these components during exposure (105). Tolerance to acute levels of oxygen appears to provide more protection against acute levels of nitrogen dioxide (106, 107) and other oxidants than vice versa (108). Perhaps the adaptive responses to oxygen occur in more cell types than in the case of ozone or nitrogen dioxide. As changes in content of enzymes or antioxidants have generally been monitored in whole tissue and not in the revelant cell types, the biochemical mechanisms of toxicity and tolerance are not discernable.

The effect of exposure to various levels of oxygen on cultured EC's has been determined, but not with regard to understanding tolerance or mechanisms for xenobiotic uptake and metabolism. Under hypoxic conditions, glycolysis may be favored over oxidative phosphorylation and vice versa under normoxia; the effects of in vitro exposure appear to mimic differences observed in EC's freshly isolated from regions exposed in vivo to different oxygen tensions (109). However, many cautions against artifactual changes have been published. The conditions of isolation (explants or enzymatic digests) and culture (culture medium and cell density) of EC's or smooth muscle cells greatly affect prostaglandin synthesis (110). Although it is tempting to extrapolate from cellular adaptations in vitro to responsiveness to in vivo physiological or pathological changes, restraint is advisable. The dynamic nature of the vasculature presents challenges and obstacles to research; even the method of killing can influence the uptake of 5-HT (111), and the uptake efficiency of the isolated perfused lung is dependent on perfusion flow rates that unfortunately have often been less than the physiological flow rate (112). Correlation of endothelial damage with decreased uptake of 5-HT in the isolated perfused lung (101) excludes the role of platelets in vivo. Platelets contain most of the circulating 5-HT that may be released from platelet thrombi formed in microvascular injury and so increase the pulmonary 5-HT content; thus, the murine pulmonary 5-HT content increases with increasing time of exposure to 100% oxygen (100). It has been suggested that increased 5-HT content may potentiate vascular injury by enhancing interactions between the endothelium and polymorphonuclear leukocytes, which can release harmful oxidants. And, of course, the differences among species are also an important consideration, e.g. the difference between the dog and rabbit lung in their hemodynamic response to acute hypoxia (113). However, species difference in susceptibility to atherosclerosis may be useful for identifying relevant factors in the development of plaques. As previously mentioned, the susceptibility of the pig versus the rat may perhaps be explained by the relative low capacity of porcine vascular smooth muscle cells in culture to produce PGI_2, which in vivo serves to inhibit platelet aggregation at sites of endothelial damage (101).

Vasculature-Associated Xenobiotic Metabolism

The monoclonal proliferation of smooth muscle in the development of atherosclerosis is proposed to be the result of a mutational event. While the ability of vascular tissue to activate potential mutagens/carcinogens has not been studied with pulmonary tissue, the information derived from the aorta is likely relevant. The mitochondrial supernatant fraction of aortal tissue can metabolize benzo(a)pyrene (BP) or 7,12-dimethylbenz(a)anthracene to give a positive reaction in the Ames test or to form metabolite-DNA adducts (114). The increase in these activities following exposure to hydrocarbons such as 3-methylcholanthrene (3-MC) further indicates that a cytochrome P-450 monooxygenase system mediates these reactions. Cytohistochemical studies of pulmonary vasculature suggest that the endothelium may be the cellular site for this enzyme system (115). However, it is possible to recover the majority of the cytochrome P-450, NADPH cytochrome P-450 reductase, and enzymatic activity in microsomes from rabbit aorta after the removal of the endothelium (C. J. Serabjit-Singh, J. R. Bend, R. M. Philpot, unpublished observations). Therefore, whether or not the endothelium contains components of the monooxygenase system, vascular smooth muscle has the necessary enzymes for activation of promutagens that may enhance the development of atherosclerosis. The isozymes of cytochrome P-450 forms 2-, 5-, 6-, and P-450 reductase were detected immunochemically (Western blotting) and enzymatically (activity toward 7-ethoxyresorufin, BP, or cytochrome c) in the microsomal fractions of both intact rabbit aorta (54) and aorta after removing the endothelium (C. J. Serabjit-Singh, J. R. Bend, R. M. Philpot, unpublished observations). The sensitivity of the immunochemical techniques now available provides the means for examining the role of detoxifying or activating enzyme systems in the development of toxicity or disease in the vasculature of various organs. Thus, the contribution of the pulmonary vasculature to the intrinsic metabolic clearance of drugs and pollutants by lung may soon be delineated.

Lymphatic Vasculature

The lymphatic system of the lung plays a major role in alveolar clearance of fluid and particulate matter that may accumulate in the lung (116). Very little data pertaining to mechanisms of cellular damage or biochemical profile of the lymphatic vasculature are available. In α-naphthylthiourea-induced edema, pulmonary lymph flow was shown to increase with increases in extravascular water (117). However, it is difficult to correlate chemically induced edema with lymphatic dysfunction, which is perhaps an indirect effect the study of which would provide little insight into toxic mechanisms.

PULMONARY EPITHELIUM: ROLE IN XENOBIOTIC UPTAKE, METABOLISM, AND TOXICITY

The epithelial lining of the airways and its protective layer of mucus or pulmonary surfactant is in intimate contact with the environment and represents a tremendous surface area for xenobiotic absorption. The organization of the airways is complex, consisting of the trachea, bronchi, and bronchioles, the so-called conducting airways, in addition to the alveolar-capillary unit, the major area for gas exchange. In mammals, the surface area of the alveoli is approximately tenfold greater than that of the conducting airways. There is a heterogeneous distribution of cell types in the pulmonary epithelium (118,

119). For example, the tracheobronchial lining consists of up to eleven epithelial and two mesenchymal cell types, depending upon species; these include the ciliated cell, the goblet cell, the epithelial serous cell, the brush cell, the intermediate cell, the oncocyte, the Kultschitzky-like or K cell, and the nonciliated bronchiolar epithelial (Clara) cell. The epithelial lining layer of the alveoli consists mostly of squamous epithelial, or type I cells, and granular cuboidal cells, called type II cells. There are also a very few brush cells, termed type III cells, present and free alveolar macrophages occur in the alveolar spaces. Because lungs function as organs of gas exchange, their epithelial cells are generally in intimate contact with the vasculature. This is especially true in the alveolar-capillary area. Consequently, it is not surprising that xenobiotics transit the respiratory epithelium, whether exposure is via the air-space or the vasculature. Absorption of drugs such as sulfanilic acid and p-aminohippuric acid through the pulmonary epithelium of the rat is much faster (at least eight to forty-two times faster) than from the rat small intestine (120). Absorption is also more rapid from the alveolar than from the tracheobronchial area (121). Since alveolar type II cells, and especially Clara cells, contain endoplasmic reticulum and its associated xenobiotic-metabolizing enzymes (50), transport through these cell types is likely to be accompanied by partial biotransformation. Volatile xenobiotics and/or their metabolites are also exhaled from the lung across the epithelial lining layer. As a result of recent experiments, quite a bit is known about the transport mechanisms for xenobiotic chemicals in respiratory epithelium.

Diffusion of Xenobiotics Across the Pulmonary Epithelium

Much of the quantitative information concerning xenobiotic absorption from pulmonary airways has come from Schanker's laboratory (122). Due to the complex structure of the lung, it is difficult to evaluate directly the individual permeability of the alveolar and tracheobronchial epithelia in vivo. Routinely, a test compound is added to the airspace in solution or via an aerosol, and passage of the material into blood, lymph, or vascular perfusion fluid follows. Alternatively, unabsorbed chemical remaining in the lungs is assayed, an approach used by Schanker and his colleagues (120). In this case, absorption is equated with passage of the compound across both the epithelial lining layer of the airways and the pulmonary endothelium to enter the circulation. Small volumes (100 μl) of xenobiotic in solution are injected 1 or 2 mm above the bifurcation of the trachea of rats or guinea pigs. A tight-fitting tracheal cannula is employed to prevent clearance of the compound via the mucociliary mechanism. The major advantages of this procedure are that known amounts of chemical are introduced directly into lungs and that there is no interruption of the bronchial circulation or lymph flow, such as occurs in perfused lung preparations. Major disadvantages include the nonuniform distribution of solute throughout the lungs, the fact that the site of solute transport (tracheobronchial versus alveolar epithelium) is unknown, and the inability to detect metabolites formed during passage of a compound through the air-blood barrier.

In spite of these limitations, this methodology has provided valuable information about the permeability of the pulmonary epithelium to xenobiotics (Table 2). For the non-lipid soluble compounds listed, the rate of absorption varies in inverse order with the size of the molecule, and uptake occurs by a non-saturable diffusion process (120, 122). These hydrophilic chemicals pass through paracellular aqueous paths, or pores, in the airway epithelium, and Schanker has suggested that there are at least three populations of different-sized pores in rat lung. It is generally accepted that pores of the alveolar epithelium have a radius of 0.5 to 1.5 nm (127, 128). However, recent studies with canine trachea and bronchi (128, 129) indicate the presence of larger pores (>4 nm) in epithelium of the conducting airways. Thus, there may be a differential distribution of the various-sized pores attributed to rat pulmonary epithelium. In any event, many hydrophilic chemicals are able to enter the circulation from the airways. Of some interest is the observation that pulmonary epithelium of the guinea pig is more permeable to non-lipid soluble compounds than that of the rat. When hydrophilic or lipophilic compounds are administered as a liquid aerosol, absorption is approximately twice as rapid. This phenomenon is presumably due to the delivery of more of the chemical to the alveolar spaces subsequent to administration by aerosol. In rats less than twelve days of age, certain lipid-insoluble xenobiotics are absorbed about twice as fast as in older rats (eighteen days of age to adult). Compounds with a molecular weight of 60 or less, and those of molecular weight 5,250–20,000, are absorbed at similar rates in neonatal and adult animals, but compounds of molecular weight 122–1,355 are absorbed more rapidly in neonatal rats (126). The administration of cortisone (130) or thyroxine (131) accelerates the development of the pulmonary epithelial permeability properties characteristic of adult rats.

However, because many airborne pollutants, toxicants, and drugs that might be administered via the airways are lipophilic in nature, the study of their absorption is more relevant. These lipid-soluble chemicals cross the pulmonary epithelium more rapidly in rats and guinea pigs than hydrophilic compounds of the same molecular weight. Absorption is generally by a non-saturable, passive diffusion process. The higher the lipid/water partition coefficient, the more rapid is the disappearance of compound from the lung. These data are consistent with those illustrating passage through lipid portions of epithelial (and endothelial) cell membranes. As shown in Table 2, there is no significant difference in the rate of absorption of lipid soluble compounds from the airways of neonatal and of adult rat lungs.

An experimental approach that could be used to delineate the alveolar

Table 2 Absorption of several xenobiotics from the airways of lungs of guinea pigs and neonatal and adult rats after drug administration by intratracheal injection or liquid aerosol exposure

Compound	Guinea pig[a]	Neonatal rat[a] (6 days of age)	Adult rat[a]	Adult rat[b]
		Rate of absorption (half-time, minutes)		
Lipid-soluble				
Salicyclic acid	—[c]	—	1.0 (120)[d]	0.67 (121)
Barbital	—	—	1.4 (123)	0.93 (121)
Sulfisoxazole	2.9 (124)	3.2 (125)	3.4 (125)	—
Procainamide	4.5 (124)	5.1 (125)	5.7 (125)	2.3 (121)
Non-Lipid Soluble				
Urea	—	4.1 (126)	4.7 (126)	1.4 (121)
Guanidine	—	5.1 (126)	6.3 (126)	3.1 (121)
p-Aminohippuric acid	22.2 (124)	22 (125)	41 (125)	21.7 (121)
Mannitol	25.8 (124)	32 (125)	60 (125)	26.5 (121)
Tetraethylammonium	22.5 (124)	28 (125)	63 (125)	—
Inulin	—	211 (126)	220 (126)	—
Dextran	—	635 (126)	688 (126)	—

[a] Administered intratracheally (120)
[b] Administered by liquid aerosol (121)
[c] Data not reported
[d] Reference in parentheses

contribution to epithelial transport and to determine the amount of metabolism that occurs during transit through the air-blood barrier is non-recirculating perfused lungs in which known amounts of chemical are administered to the air spaces. In the perfused organ, the bronchial circulation is not functional, so only absorption/metabolism occurring within the alveolar-capillary unit is measured. Such experiments would best be done at short times after the introduction of chemicals into the lung, and this is possible with lipophilic compounds because of their rapid rate of absorption.

There is one metabolically controlled mechanism for the accumulation of xenobiotic metabolites in pulmonary epithelium. Several chemicals are converted to electrophilic products that react covalently with cellular macromolecules, including protein and DNA. The parent chemical reaches the epithelium by diffusion from the vasculature. Metabolic activation is generally catalyzed by the cytochrome P-450-dependent monooxygenase system, known to be concentrated in Clara cells but also present in other epithelial cells (50). For compounds converted to unstable products which then alkylate macromolecules in the cells where they are formed, selective or specific Clara cell toxicity is anticipated. This is observed experimentally with several chemicals, including 4-ipomeanol (132), 3-methylfuran (132), napthalene (133), 2-

methylnapthalene (134), carbon tetrachloride (135), and 1,1-dichloroethylene (136). Other compounds, such as butylated hydroxytoluene (137) and $O,S,S,$-trimethylphosphorothioate (138), also require cytochrome P-450-dependent metabolism, but they cause selective toxicity in the alveolar type I cell. Probable explanations for the latter observation are that the reactive metabolites formed are stable enough to migrate from the site of formation to the site of alkylation, and/or the type I cell is deficient in detoxication enzymes so that only a small amount of intracellular metabolism is required to initiate the deleterious response. It is important to remember that enzyme systems other than the P-450-associated monooxygenases are present in lung and are capable of metabolically activating certain substrates. Moreover, these systems can be distributed unevenly among pulmonary epithelial cells. A recent study from Eling's group (139), for example, demonstrated that freshly isolated rat alveolar type II cells are more efficient than Clara cells at converting, BP 7,8-dihydrodiol to 7β,8α-dihydroxy-9α,10α-epoxy-7,8,9,10-tetra-hydro-benzo(a)pyrene (BPDEI) by the prostaglandin H synthase pathway.

Pulmonary epithelium is an important target for chemical carcinogenesis by some polycyclic aromatic hydrocarbons (PAH), and DNA alkylation by specific PAH metabolites is a required step for the initiation of tumorigenesis. Consequently, relationships between the cellular localization of metabolic activation systems and cell-specific DNA alkylation in tissues, like lung, that are susceptible or resistant to PAH-mediated neoplasia are of interest. A recent study from Anderson's laboratory at NIEHS (140) demonstrated that similar amounts of (+)−BPDEI-DNA adducts are present in tissues of widely divergent monooxygenase activity twenty-four hours after the iv administration of BP (1 mg/kg) to rabbits in vivo. The lung contained the greatest amount (0.06 ± 0.01 pmol/mg DNA, mean ± S.D., N = 5) of (+)−BPDEI-deoxyguanosine, the major DNA adduct formed in each tissue, but tissues deficient in monooxygenase activity such as the muscle (0.03 ± 0.02) and blood (0.03 ± 0.01) had as much of this adduct as liver (0.02 ± 0.002). Subsequently, we conducted a collaborative in vivo-in vitro study to determine the degree of specific DNA alkylation in individual populations of lung and liver cells (141). Treatment conditions identical to those described above (140) were used, except that various cells were isolated from lung and liver twenty-four hours after treatment with BP. BP metabolite-DNA adducts were assayed by HPLC and the values obtained were: alveolar type II cells 0.026 pmol (+)−BPDEI-deoxyguanosine/mg DNA, Clara cells <0.02, alveolar macrophages 0.044, hepatocytes 0.024, and liver non-parenchymal cells 0.030. Collectively, these data demonstrate that there is no obvious correlation between cytochrome P-450-dependent monooxygenase activity and the amount of specific DNA alkylation observed in the various cell types, and this raises the possibility that transport of ultimate carcinogenic metabolites of PAH from one tissue or cell type to another occurs in vivo. Caution must also be exercised with this interpretation, however. Muscle does contain cytochrome P-450, but at a very low concentration (C. J. Serabjit-Singh, J. R. Bend, R. M. Philpot, unpublished observations). Yet low levels of a P-450 isozyme efficient at forming BPDEI could account for the DNA binding observed in muscle. Thus, it is possible that there is a correlation between the relevant parameters, and sensitive immunochemical quantitation techniques are now available to establish this. These recent experiments illustrate how existing technology can be used to study relationships between xenobiotic metabolism and alkylation in lung at the cellular level, but only in a limited number of cell types.

Energy-Dependent Epithelial Transport Systems

PARAQUAT   An interesting recent development is the demonstration by Smith and his colleagues (65, 142, 143) of a high affinity, energy-dependent, sodium-independent, saturable transport system for endogenous diamines and polyamines in rat lung slices. Due to its structural similarity with these diamines, PQ is also transported by this pathway (65, 144), accounting for its accumulation in lung. The diamines putrescine and cadaverine and the polyamines spermine and spermidine are substrates for this transport system, and the apparent K_m values of this first-order process for these compounds are 13.1, 19.0, 14.8, and 10.9 μM respectively (143); the comparable K_m for PQ is 70 μM (63). This transport system is also present in human peripheral lung, where K_m values for putrescine accumulation in four individuals varied from 2–11 μM (145).

The site for PQ uptake has been attributed, at least in part, to the pulmonary epithelium by both autoradiographic (61) and indirect methods. Smith noted that putrescine and PQ accumulation are markedly decreased in lung slices from rats that displayed selective alveolar type I and type II cell damage subsequent to treatment with PQ. In this experiment, 5-HT uptake was the same in lung slices from paraquat-treated and control animals, suggesting that endothelial function is not compromised (62, 142). Further, the administration of PQ to a perfused rat lung preparation via the vasculature did not cause long-term storage, whereas introduction into the airways did (146); the slow component of PQ efflux was about six hours. Some recent experiments with rat alveolar type II cells (granular pneumocytes) cultured for twenty-four hours and alveolar macrophages demonstrated that the type II cells accumulated PQ by an energy-dependent process, presumably carrier-mediated and by diffusion, but the macrophages took up PQ only by diffusion (147). Some experiments performed in our laboratory with Clara cells, alveolar type II cells, and macrophages isolated from rabbit lungs gave complementary information (R.

Brigelius, J. K. Horton, R. P. Mason, J. R. Bend, unpublished observations). Intact Clara cells and type II cells incubated with PQ (1 mM) in an anaerobic ESR sample tube formed PQ radical signal at the earliest times we could scan (4–5 minutes), whereas alveolar macrophages did not produce a detectable ESR signal for this radical even after sixty minutes of repetitive scanning. More ESR signal was generated per Clara cell than per type II cell, consistent with the greater amount of cytochrome P-450 reductase activity present. Subsequent to the lysis of cells by sonication and the addition of NADPH, intense ESR signals of the PQ radical were produced by all three cell types. Collectively, these data are consistent with the facile uptake of PQ by Clara and type II cells but not by alveolar macrophages.

Other biogenic and nonbiogenic amines, including 5-HT (64) and IMP (148), interfere with PQ uptake by lung slices, although they are not substrates for the polyamine transport system. This strongly suggests that the binding sites for various mono-, di-, and polyamines on the plasma membranes of different types of lung cells must have several features in common, even though the processes for substrate transport into the cell or the intracellular binding sites can be quite specific, even demonstrating stereoselectivity (149). Consequently, it seems advisable to conduct interaction studies between PQ and amines, both bio- and nonbiogenic, in highly enriched populations of freshly isolated or cultured lung cells. The use of both broken and intact cells should allow mechanistic studies of extracellular and intracellular transport, binding, and metabolism phenomena.

OTHER XENOBIOTICS   The presence of other energy-dependent transport processes in pulmonary epithelium has also been described. Schanker and his colleagues (150, 151) have shown that phenol red and disodium chromoglycate, organic anions, are transported by a carrier-mediated transport pathway that is saturable and selectively inhibited by low-temperature, anaerobic conditions and metabolic inhibitors (152). Similarly, the nonmetabolized amino acid 1-aminocyclopentanecarboxylic acid is transported across the pulmonary epithelium of the rat by a combination of at least two processes, one a saturable, energy-dependent carrier-type system and the other nonsaturable diffusion (153). Lung epithelia of the mouse, hamster, and guinea pig also transport this amino acid by an active process (154). However, lung epithelium does not actively take up quaternary ammonium compounds, apparently lacking a carrier-mediated system for the absorption of organic cations (155); these compounds are absorbed by diffusion through aqueous membrane channels in the epithelial membranes of lung. We hope these studies will be extended to elucidate the anatomical and cellular localization of the carrier-mediated processes identified and to determine the luminal versus basolateral distribution of these transport systems.

PREDICTION OF CLEARANCE OF XENOBIOTICS BY LUNG

The contribution of the lung to the metabolic clearance of chemicals from the blood has only recently been investigated in detail. Practical and theoretical considerations by Collins & Dedrick (156) and Gillette (157) suggest that in some cases the relative participation of the lung in clearance may be substantially greater than predicted solely on the basis of whole-organ metabolic potentials. In fact, with some chemicals pulmonary clearance may equal or exceed hepatic clearance, even though the metabolic capacity of the liver may be much greater than that of the lung. Two factors make important contributions to this possibility: first, the location of the lung between the arterial and venous branches of the circulatory system, where it is perfused by the entire blood supply; second, limitation of hepatic clearance due to the flow rate of the blood, not metabolic capacity. Attempts to elucidate the precise role of the lung in clearance are being made through the application of predictive mathematical models that can be rationalized by readily obtainable experimental values, by direct measurements of clearance in isolated organs, and by indirect determinations made with intact animals.

In 1973, Rowland et al (158) concluded that clearance (CL) of chemicals from the blood could be described in terms of blood flow (Q), intrinsic clearance (CL_1), and the fraction of the chemical free in the blood (f_b) by the relationship: $CL = Qf_bCL_i/Q + f_bCL_i$. For chemicals whose clearance is a function of metabolism, the results of Rane et al (159) indicate that CL_i can be calculated from the kinetic constants (V_{max} and K_m) of the enzyme(s) involved: $CL_i = V_{max}/K_m$. Limitations on the applicability of the clearance equation include: (a) uptake of the chemical from the blood must be passive (it is assumed that the concentrations of unbound chemical in the blood and tissue are equal); (b) the effective substrate concentration must be low enough to insure that metabolism is a first-order process.

The isolated, perfused lung has been used for the assessment of pulmonary clearance predicted for a number of chemicals. Early studies with this preparation were compromised by flow rates that were much less than physiological. The importance of flow rate, as well as the mode of uptake, is shown by the results of Wiersma & Roth (160), who studied the uptake of 5-HT by isolated rat liver and lung. The predicted clearances at normal blood flows indicated that the efficiency of the liver should exceed that of the lung by about fivefold (7.6 versus 1.34 ml per minute). The predicted relationship between clearance and flow rate was observed with the isolated liver system; at normal flow (11 ml per minute) observed clearance was 6.6 ml per minute. In contrast, predicted pulmonary clearance was substantially less than that observed. At normal flow (44.8 ml per minute) the observed clearance was 19.1 ml per minute. This discrepancy likely reflects a much greater involvement of specific uptake processes in the clearance of 5-HT by lung as compared to liver. The possibility of complete removal by the lung had been suggested by several investigators (161–163) who had examined 5-HT uptake by isolated lungs perfused at low flow rates. Wiersma & Roth (160) did in fact observe nearly complete pulmonary clearance of 5-HT at a flow rate of 10 ml per minute. The effect of flow rate on the pulmonary uptake of 5-HT confirmed earlier findings of Pickett et al (13), who investigated the roles of active transport, flow rate, and concentration on the uptake of 5-HT in the isolated rabbit lung. It should be noted that the effect of flow rate on the clearance of passively transported chemicals ranges from negligible (when CL_i is low with respect to Q) to absolute (when CL_i is much greater than Q, so that the clearance is essentially equal to the flow rate).

In contrast to results with 5-HT, the predicted and observed pulmonary clearances of BP are in agreement (164). For lungs from rats treated with 3-MC, which induces the synthesis of a cytochrome P-450 isozyme that efficiently metabolizes BP, the predicted CL was 7.0 ml per minute and the observed CL was 8.9 ml per minute. The corresponding values for lungs from untreated rats were 0.97 and 0.99 ml per minute. In both cases the major factor in the predicted clearance was CL_i. In contrast, the predominant factor in the prediction of hepatic clearance was flow rate. With livers from treated rats, the predicted clearance was actually equal to the flow rate; however, the observed clearance was significantly less (6.7 versus 10.0 ml per minute). These findings suggest two things: first, the pulmonary clearance of BP in rats treated with 3-MC may be nearly equal to the hepatic clearance; second, values predicted for the hepatic clearance are not realized with the isolated liver. A number of factors associated with binding, distribution, and metabolism could contribute to the discrepancy between the predicted and observed hepatic clearances. In any case, it is not clear that Wiersma & Roth (164) are correct in their conclusion that the differences between the hepatic values are minor. The CL_i calculated from the V_{max} and K_m for the hepatic (3-MC) metabolism of BP was reported to be 28,257 ml per minute; CL_i calculated from the observed clearance is about 15 ml per minute. Therefore, if the inaccuracy of the prediction is a function of an incorrect value for CL_i, the error exceeds a factor of 10^3, an error not likely due to shortcomings in the determinations of the kinetic constants. Unlike the results obtained with livers from treated rats, the observed clearance with liver from untreated rats was reported to be greater than the predicted clearance (5.9 versus 4.6 ml per minute). In this case, however, a value of 0.14 was used for f_b compared to the values of 1.4 used for liver (3-MC), 1.0 for lung (3-MC), and 1.1 for lung (untreated). These values were determined in vitro from the ratios of the rates of microsomal metabolism obtained with 32 or 1 mg BSA/ml in the incubations (the binding of BP could not be measured directly). The relationship between these determinations and the binding of BP to plasma components seems obscure, and the use of different values of f_b for liver and lung is difficult to justify. The predicted clearance by liver, using a value of 1.0 for f_b, is 8.8 ml per minute, which is greater than the observed clearance. In spite of the possible shortcomings in the application of the clearance model to hepatic systems, several important conclusions reached by Wiersma & Roth are strongly supported by their findings. First, the clearance of BP by the isolated, perfused lung can be predicted with a high degree of accuracy. Second, increases in CL_i may have a major effect on pulmonary, but not hepatic, clearance. Third, pulmonary clearance of BP may be equal to or greater than hepatic clearance in rats treated with 3-MC. The results of in vivo experiments appear to confirm the last conclusion, although the observed pulmonary and hepatic clearances appear to be less than those obtained with the isolated organs (165).

Prediction of clearance when metabolism is catalyzed by more than one enzyme requires calculations for each pathway, may be compromised by undetermined competitive effects, and is inherently more prone to error than predictions based on a single enzyme. However, Smith & Bend (166) have examined the pulmonary clearance of BP 4,5-oxide with reasonable success. This arene oxide is metabolized by epoxide hydrolase, a microsomal enzyme, and the glutathione S-transferases, a group of cytosolic enzymes. The predicted extraction ratios ($E = CL/Q$) were 0.25 and 0.74 for the hydrolase and transferase pathways respectively. Therefore, it was predicted that the clearance (20 ml/minute/g) of the oxide would be essentially 100%. A total extraction ratio of 0.64 was calculated from the observed clearance. The difference between the predicted and observed values are accounted for almost entirely by the transferase pathway (observed $E = 0.44$); observed E for the hydrolase pathway (0.20) was in close agreement with the predicted value. The possibility that the transferase activity was limited by the concentration of glutathione in the isolated lung (saturating levels were used for the determination of the kinetic constants) has been suggested. It should be noted that an increase in the flow rate that was used in this study (20 ml/minute/g) to the estimated normal rate (35 ml/minute/g) would be expected to increase the clearance and decrease the extraction efficiency. The predicted values with $Q = 35$ ml/minute/g are 28 and 0.80 ml/minute/g for CL and E respectively.

Because the clearance model appears to estimate pulmonary clearance with reasonable accuracy, it may be of use in predicting the pulmonary toxicity of some chemicals. Therefore, we have analyzed data from a number of studies on the pulmonary toxin, 4-ipomeanol, to determine if predicted clearances are consistent with the observation that covalent binding of metabolites of 4-ipomeanol is about five times greater (per mg tissue protein) in lung than in liver of rats and rabbits (167). The available data include K_m and V_{max} constants for the metabolism of 4-ipomeanol in microsomal preparations from liver and lung of both species (168, 169). The total organ V_{max} and K_m for rat liver are both higher than for lung (twenty and fifteen times respectively). Therefore, the predicted intrinsic clearances for the two tissues are similar, 0.29 ml per minute for liver and 0.20 for lung. These low values relative to Q result in predicted clearances (0.28 and 0.20 ml per minute) that are essentially the same as the intrinsic clearances. Based on these rates, total covalent binding is predicted to be greater in the liver, and binding per mg tissue protein is predicted to be six to eight times greater in the lung.

The difference between the K_m values for the metabolism of 4-ipomeanol in rat liver and lung partially explains why the CL_i values for the two tissues are fairly similar. This difference also suggests that the relevant enzyme(s) in rat liver and lung is dissimilar, which is not the case for the rabbit. The results of antibody inhibition and kinetic studies indicate that the same isozymes of cytochrome P-450 metabolize 4-ipomeanol in rabbit liver and lung (169, 170). However, the concentrations of these enzymes are higher in lung than in liver, and the V_{max} (nmol product/minute/mg microsomal protein) for the lung is about three times that of the liver. The predicted clearances, 7.2 ml per minute for liver and 2.1 ml per minute for lung, are, as with the rat, essentially the same as those predicted for CL_i. These values suggest that binding in the lung (per mg tissue protein) should be three to five times that of the liver. Therefore, we conclude that reasonable estimates of the relative covalent binding of 4-ipomeanol in liver and lung of rats and rabbits can be obtained from predicted clearances.

CONCLUSION

The lung is anatomically complex and contains more than forty different cell types. The macromolecules that are responsible for xenobiotic uptake, accumulation, and/or biotransformation include enzymes for oxidative, reductive, hydrolytic, and biosynthetic metabolism, carriers for energy-dependent transport systems, extracellular and intracellular binding sites of low to high specificity, and receptors. Each of these processes also functions with endogenous chemicals. One of the major problems in pulmonary research is assigning biological activity to a specific anatomical region (tracheobronchiolar, bronchiolar, or alveolar) and/or cell type(s). The integrated experimental approach that is being used by us and others includes immunochemical, biochemical, and metabolic studies in vivo, with perfused lung preparations, whole lung homogenate and its subcellular fractions, homogeneous enzymes purified from lung, and freshly prepared and cultured cells isolated from lungs following mild proteolytic digestion. Each of these procedures used alone has its limitations (5); however, in concert they allow the elucidation of chemical and biochemical mechanisms involved in the uptake and metabolism of chemicals by lungs.

Over the last few years our knowledge of the lungs' contribution to the clearance of xenobiotics from the circulation and their metabolism has increased dramatically, primarily as a result of advances in in vivo and in vitro techniques. Further progress in understanding the contribution of individual pulmonary cell types to these processes is anticipated, especially as methodology for the isolation and culture of lung cells becomes more standardized and widely used, and as highly enriched populations of additional tracheobronchial, bronchiolar, and alveolar cells become available.

ACKNOWLEDGMENT

We are very grateful to those colleagues who participated in studies performed in our laboratory that are discussed in this manuscript. We also acknowledge the excellent assistance of Ms. Debbie Garner, who helped in the preparation of this article.

Literature Cited

1. Bakhle, Y. S., Vane, J. R., eds. 1977. *Metabolic Functions of the Lung*, Vol. 4. New York: Dekker. 353 pp.
2. Witschi, H., Nettesheim, P., eds. 1982. *Mechanisms in Respiratory Toxicology*, Vols. 1, 2. Boca Raton: CRC. 286 pp., 230 pp.
3. Wilson, A. G. E. 1982. Toxicokinetics of uptake, accumulation and metabolism of chemicals by the lung. See Ref. 2, 1:161–85
4. Minchin, R. F., Boyd, M. R. 1983. Localization of metabolic activation and deactivation systems in the lung: Significance to the pulmonary toxicity of xenobiotics. *Ann. Rev. Pharmacol. Toxicol.* 23:217–38
5. Bend, J. R., Serabjit-Singh, C. J. 1984. Xenobiotic metabolism by extrahepatic tissues: Relationship to target organ and cell toxicity. In *Drug Metabolism and Drug Toxicity*, ed. J. R. Mitchell, M. G. Horning, pp. 99–136. New York: Raven. 436 pp.
6. Ryan, J. W. 1982. Processing of endogenous polypeptides by the lungs. *Ann. Rev. Physiol.* 44:241–55
7. Said, S. I. 1982. Pulmonary metabolism of prostaglandins and vasoactive peptides. *Ann. Rev. Physiol.* 44:257–68
8. Gillis, C. N., Pitt, B. R. 1982. The fate of circulating amines within the pulmonary circulation. *Ann. Rev. Physiol.* 44:269–81
9. Witschi, H., Côté, M. G. 1977. Primary pulmonary responses to toxic agents. *CRC Crit. Rev. Toxicol.* 5:23–66
10. Ryan, U. S. 1982. Structural bases for metabolic activity. *Ann. Rev. Physiol.* 44:223–39
11. Gillis, C. N., Greene, N. M. 1977. Possible implications of metabolism of bloodborne substrates by the human lung. See Ref. 1, pp. 173–93
12. Hughes, J., Gillis, C. N., Bloom, F. E. 1969. The uptake and disposition of DL-noradrenaline in perfused rat lung. *J. Pharmacol. Exp. Ther.* 169: 237–48
13. Pickett, R. D., Anderson, M. W., Orton, T. C., Eling, T. E. 1975. The pharmacodynamics of 5-hydroxytryptamine uptake and metabolism by the isolated perfused rabbit lung. *J. Pharmacol. Exp. Ther.* 194:545–53
14. Alabaster, V. A. 1977. Inactivation of endogenous amines in the lungs. See Ref. 1, pp. 3–31
15. Iwasawa, Y., Gillis, C. N., Aghajanian, G. 1973. Hypothermic inhibition of 5-hydroxytryptamine and nonepinephrine uptake by lung: Cellular location of amines after uptake. *J. Pharmacol. Exp. Ther.* 186:498–507
16. Catravas, J. D., Gillis, C. N. 1983. Single pass removal of [14C]-5-hydroxytryptamine and [3H]-norepinephrine by rabbit lung, in vivo: Kinetics and

sites of removal. *J. Pharmacol. Exp. Ther.* 224:28–33

17. Bakhle, Y. S., Youdim, M. B. H. 1976. Metabolism of phenylethylamine in rat isolated perfused lung: Evidence for monoamine oxidase "type B" in lung. *Br. J. Pharmacol.* 56:125–27

18. Bakhle, Y. S., Youdim, M. B. H. 1979. The metabolism of 5-hydroxytryptamine and β-phenylethylamine in perfused rat lung and in vitro. *Br. J. Pharmacol.* 65:147–54

19. Brown, E. A. B. 1974. The localization, metabolism and effects of drugs and toxicants in lung. *Drug Metab. Rev.* 3:33–87

20. Orton, T. C., Anderson, M. W., Pickett, R. D., Eling, T. E., Fouts, J. R. 1973. Xenobiotic accumulation and metabolism by isolated perfused rabbit lungs. *J. Pharmacol. Exp. Ther.* 186:482–97

21. Anderson, M. W., Orton, T. C., Pickett, R. D., Eling, T. E. 1974. Accumulation of amines in the isolated perfused rabbit lung. *J. Pharmacol. Exp. Ther.* 189:456–66

22. Eling, T. E., Pickett, R. D., Orton, T. C. Anderson, M. W. 1975. A study of the dynamics of imipramine accumulation in the isolated perfused rabbit lung. *Drug Metab. Disp.* 3:389–400

23. Wilson, A. G. E., Law, F. C. P., Eling, T. E., Anderson, M. W. 1976. Uptake, metabolism, and efflux of methadone in "single pass" isolated perfused rabbit lungs. *J. Pharmacol. Exp. Ther.* 199:360–67

24. Philpot, R. M., Anderson, M. W., Eling, T. E. 1977. Uptake, accumulation and metabolism of chemicals by the lung. See Ref. 1, pp. 123–71

25. Junod, A. F. 1972. Accumulation of ^{14}C-imipramine in isolated perfused rat lungs. *J. Pharmacol. Exp. Ther.* 183:182–87

26. Wilson, A. G. E., Pickett, R. D., Eling, T. E., Anderson, M. W. 1979. Studies on the persistence of basic amines in the rabbit lung. *Drug Metab. Disp.* 7:420–24

27. Wilson, A. G. E., Sar, M., Stumpf, W. E. 1982. Autoradiographic study of imipramine localization in the isolated perfused rabbit lung. *Drug Metab. Disp.* 10:281–83

28. Lüllmann, H., Lüllmann-Rauch, R., Wassermann, O. 1975. Drug-induced phospholipidoses. *CRC Crit. Rev. Toxicol.* 4:185–218

29. Seydel, J. K., Wassermann, O. 1973. NMR studies on the molecular basis of drug-induced phospholipidosis. *Naunyn-Schmiedeberg's Arch. Pharmacol.* 297:207–10

30. Mitchell, R. H., Allan, D., Bowler, M.,

Brindley, D. N., 1976. A possible metabolic explanation for drug-induced phospholipidosis. *J. Pharm. Pharmacol.* 28:331–32

31. Mehendale, H. M., Angevine, L. S., Ohmiya, Y. 1981. The isolated perfused lung—A critical evaluation. *Toxicology* 21:1–36

32. Bakhle, Y. S., Vane, J. R. 1974. Pharmacokinetic function of the pulmonary circulation. *Physiol. Rev.* 54:1007–45

33. Gillis, C. N., Cronau, L. H., Mandel, S., Hammond, G. L. 1979. Indicator dilution measurement of 5-hydroxytryptamine clearance by human lung. *J. Appl. Physiol.* 46:1178–83

34. Catravas, J. D., Gillis, C. N. 1980. Pulmonary clearance of [^{14}C]-5-hydroxytryptamine and [^{3}H]norepinephrine in vivo: Effects of pretreatment with imipramine or cocaine. *J. Pharmacol. Exp. Ther.* 213:120–27

35. Crone, C. 1963. The permeability of capillaries in various organs as determined by the use of the indicator diffusion method. *Acta Physiol. Scand.* 58:292–305

36. Gillis, C. N., Iwasawa, Y. 1972. Technique for measurement of noradrenaline and 5-hydroxytryptamine uptake by rabbit lung. *J. Appl. Physiol.* 33:404–8

37. Iwasawa, Y., Gillis, C. N. 1974. Pharmacological analysis of norepinephrine and 5-hydroxytryptamine removal from the pulmonary circulation: Differentiation of uptake sites for each amine. *J. Pharmacol. Exp. Ther.* 188:386–93

38. Minchin, R. F., Barber, H. E., Ilett, K. F. 1982. Effect of prolonged desmethylimipramine administration on the pulmonary clearance of 5-hydroxytryptamine and β-phenylethylamine in rats. *Drug Metab. Disp.* 10:356–60

39. Mehendale, H. M., Morita, T., Angevine, L. S. 1983. Effect of chlorphentermine on the pulmonary clearance of 5-hydroxytryptamine in rabbits in vivo. *Pharmacology* 26:274–83

40. Morita, T., Mehendale, H. M. 1983. Effects of chlorphentermine and phentermine on the pulmonary disposition of 5-hydroxytryptamine in the rat *in vivo. Am. Rev. Respir. Dis.* 127:747–50

41. Deleted in proof

42. Angevine, L. S., Mehendale, H. M. 1982. Effect of chlorphentermine pretreatment on 5-hydroxytryptamine disposition in the isolated perfused rat lung. *Fund. Appl. Toxicol.* 2:306–12

43. Ohyima, Y., Angevine, L. S., Mehendale, H. M. 1983. Effect of drug-induced

phospholipidosis on pulmonary disposition of pneumophilic drugs. *Drug Metab. Disp.* 11:25–30

44. Angevine, L. S., Lockhard, V. G., Mehendale, H. M. 1984. Effect of chlorphentermine pretreatment on the distribution of chlorphentermine in isolated perfused rabbit lungs. *Fund. Appl. Toxicol.* 4:202–9

45. Zychlinski, L., Montgomery, M. R., Shamblin, P. B., Reasor, M. J. 1983. Impairment in pulmonary bioenergetics following chlorphentermine administration to rats. *Fund. Appl. Toxicol.* 3:192–98

46. Ferin, J. 1982. Alveolar macrophage mediated pulmonary clearance suppressed by drug-induced phospholipidosis. *Exp. Lung Res.* 4:1–10

47. Philpot, R. M., Wolf, C. R. 1981. The properties and distribution of the enzymes of pulmonary cytochrome P-450-dependent monooxygenase systems. *Rev. Biochem. Toxicol.* 3:51–76

48. Smith, B. R., Bend, J. R. 1981. Metabolic interactions of hydrocarbons with mammalian lung. *Rev. Biochem. Toxicol.* 3:77–122

49. Serabjit-Singh, C. J., Wolf, C. R., Philpot, R. M., Plopper, C. G. 1980. Cytochrome P-450: Localization in rabbit lung. *Science* 207:1469–70

50. Devereux, T. R., Fouts, J. R. 1981. Isolation of pulmonary cells and use in studies of xenobiotic metabolism. *Methods Enzymol.* 77:147–54

51. Jones, K. G., Holland, J. F., Foureman, G. L., Bend, J. R., Fouts, J. R. 1983. Induction of xenobiotic metabolism in Clara cells and alveolar type II cells isolated from rat lungs. *J. Pharmacol. Exp. Ther.* 225:316–19

52. Boyd, M. R. 1977. Evidence for the Clara cell as a site of cytochrome P-450-dependent mixed-function oxidase activity in lung. *Nature* 269:713–14

53. Hook, G. E. R., Bend, J. R., Fouts, J. R. 1972. Mixed-function oxidases and the alveolar macrophage. *Biochem. Pharmacol.* 21:3267–77

54. Serabjit-Singh, C. J., Domin, B. A., Bend, J. R., Philpot, R. M. 1983. Immunochemical and biochemical evidence for the presence of cytochrome P-450 monooxygenase components in rabbit heart and aorta. In *Extraheptic Drug Metabolism and Chemical Carcinogenesis*, ed. J. Rydström, J. Montelius, M. Bengtsson, pp. 253–55. Amsterdam: Elsevier. 630 pp.

55. Law, F. C. P., Eling, T. E., Bend, J. R., Fouts, J. R. 1974. Metabolism of xenobiotics by the isolated perfused lung: Comparison with in vitro incubations. *Drug Metab. Disp.* 2:433–43

56. Minchin, R. F., Ilett, K. F., Madsen, B. W. 1981. A compartmental model for the uptake of chlorphentermine in isolated rat lung. *Eur. J. Drug Metab. Pharmacokin.* 6:127–33

57. Minchin, R. F., Ilett, K. F., Madsen, B. W. 1979. Chlorphentermine binding in rat lung subcellular fractions and its displacement by desmethylimipramine. *Biochem. Pharmacol.* 28:2273–78

58. Murray, R. E., Gibson, J. E. 1972. A comparative study of paraquat intoxication in rats, guinea-pigs and monkeys. *Exp. Mol. Pathol.* 17:317–25

59. Wyatt, I., Doss, A. W., Zavala, D. C., Smith, L. L. 1981. Intrabronchial instillation of parquat in rats: Lung morphology and retention study. *Br. J. Ind. Med.* 38:42–48

60. Sharp, C. W., Ottolenghi, A., Posner, H. S. 1972. Correlation of paraquat toxicity with tissue concentrations and weight loss of the rat. *Toxicol. Appl. Pharmacol.* 22:241–51

61. Waddell, W. J., Marlowe, C. 1980. Tissue and cellular distribution of paraquat in mice. *Toxicol. Appl. Pharmacol.* 56:127–40

62. Sykes, B. I., Purchase, I. F. H., Smith, L. L. 1977. Pulmonary ultrastructure after oral and intravenous dosage of paraquat to rats. *J. Pathol.* 121:233–41

63. Rose, M. S., Smith, L. L., Wyatt, I. 1974. Evidence for the energy dependent accumulation of paraquat into rat lung. *Nature* 252:314–15

64. Lock, E. A., Smith, L. L., Rose, M. S. 1976. Inhibition of paraquat accumulation in rat lung slices by a component of rat plasma and a variety of drugs and endogenous amines. *Biochem. Pharmacol.* 25:1769–72

65. Smith, L. L. 1982. The identification of an accumulation system for diamines and polyamines into the lung and its relevance for paraquat toxicity. *Arch. Toxicol.* 5:1–14 (Suppl.)

66. Tucker, A., McMurtry, I. F., Reeves, J. T., Alexander, A. F., Will, D. H., et al. 1975. Lung vascular smooth muscle as a determinant of pulmonary hypertension at high altitude. *Am. J. Physiol.* 228:762–67

67. Beaconsfield, P. 1962. Metabolism of the normal cardiovascular wall: 2. The pentose phosphate pathway. *Experentia* 18:276–77

68. Syrota, A., Girault, M., Pocidalo, J.-J., Yudilevich, D. L. 1982. Endothelial up-

take of amino acids, sugars, lipids, and prostaglandins in rat lung. *Am. J. Physiol.* 243:C20–26

69. Longnecker, G. L., Huggins, C. G. 1977. Biochemistry of the pulmonary angiotensin-converting enzyme. See Ref. 1, pp. 55–83

70. Gillis, C. N., Catravas, J. D. 1982. Altered removal of vasoactive substances in the injured lung: Detection of lung microvascular injury. *Ann. NY Acad. Sci.* 384:458–74

71. Flower, R. J. 1977. Prostaglandin metabolism in the lung. See Ref. 1, pp. 85–122

72. Weksler, B. B. 1982. Prostacyclin. In *Progress in Hemostasis and Thrombosis,* ed. T. H. Spaet, 6:113–38. New York: Grune & Stratten. 368 pp.

73. Eling, T. E., Alley, A. I. 1984. Pulmonary biosynthesis and metabolism of prostaglandins and related substances. *Environ. Health Perspect.* 55:159–68

74. Pitt, B. R., Hammond, G. L., Gillis, C. N. 1982. Comparison of pulmonary and extrapulmonary extraction of biogenic amines. *J. Appl. Physiol.* 52:545–51

75. Neichi, T., Chang, W.-C., Mitsui, Y., Murota, S. 1982. Comparison of prostaglandin biosynthetic activity between porcine aortic endothelial and smooth muscle cells in culture. *Artery* 11:47–63

76. Ryan, U. S., Schultz, D. R., Del Vecchio, P., Ryan, J. W. 1980. Endothelial cells of bovine pulmonary artery lack receptors for C3b and for the Fc portion of IgG. *Science* 208:748–49

77. Ryan, U. S., Schultz, D. R., Ryan, J. W. 1981. Fc and C3b receptors on pulmonary endothelial cells: Induction by injury. *Science* 214:557–58

78. Wyatt, I. S., Keeling, P. L., Smith, L. L. 1980. The effect of high concentrations of oxygen on paraquat and diquat toxicity in rats. *Arch. Toxicol.* 4:415–18 (Suppl.)

79. Thilo-Körner, D. G. S., Freshney, R. I., eds. 1984. *The Endothelial Cell—A Pluripotent Control Cell of the Vessel Wall.* Basel: Karger. 206 pp.

80. Ryan, J. W. 1983. Assay of peptidase and protease enzymes in vivo. *Biochem. Pharmacol.* 32:2127–37

80a. Catravas, J. D., Lazo, J. S., Dobuler, K. J., Mills, L. R., Gillis, C. N. 1983. Pulmonary endothelial dysfunction in the presence or absence of interstitial injury induced by intratracheally injected bleomycin in rabbits. *Am. Rev. Respir. Dis.* 128:740–46

81. Friedland, J., Silverstein, E. 1976. A sensitive fluorimetric assay for serum angiotensin-converting enzyme. *Am. J. Clin. Pathol.* 66:416–27

82. Rohatgi, F. K., Ryan, J. W. 1980. Simple radioassay for measuring serum activity of angiotensin-converting enzyme in sarcoidosis. *Chest* 78:69–76

83. Lazo, J. S., Catravas, J. D., Dobuler, K. J., Gillis, C. N. 1983. Prolonged reduction in serum angiotensin converting enzyme activity after treatment of rabbits with bleomycin. *Toxicol. Appl. Pharmacol.* 69:276–82

84. Roth, R. A., Wallace, K. B., Alper, R. H., Bailie, M. D. 1979. Effect of paraquat treatment of rats on disposition of 5-hydroxytryptamine and angiotensin I by pefused lung. *Biochem. Pharmacol.* 28:2349–55

85. Mustafa, M. G., Tierney, D. F. 1978. Biochemical and metabolic changes in the lung with oxygen, ozone, and nitrogen dioxide toxicity. *Am. Rev. Resp. Dis.* 118:1061–90

86. McCord, J. M. 1979. Superoxide, superoxide dismutase and oxygen toxicity. *Rev. Biochem. Toxicol.* 1:109–24

87. Stokinger, H. E. 1965. Ozone toxicology. *Arch. Environ. Health* 10:719–31

88. Vostal, J. J., Chan, T. L., Garg, B. D., Lee, P. S., Strom, K. A. 1981. Lymphatic transport in lungs of rats and guinea pigs exposed to diesel exhaust. *Environ. Int.* 5:339–48

89. Huxtable, R. J. 1979. New aspects of the toxicology and pharmacology of pyrrolizidine alkaloids. *Gen. Pharmacol.* 10:159–67

90. Hilliker, K. S., Bell, T. G., Roth, R. A. 1982. Pneumotoxicity and thrombocytopenia after single injection of monocrotaline. *Am. J. Physiol.* 242:H573–79

91. Gillis, C. N., Huxtable, R. J., Roth, R. A. 1978. Effects of monocrotaline pretreatment of rats on removal of 5-hydroxytryptamine and noradrenaline by perfused lung. *Br. J. Pharmacol.* 63:435–43

92. Huxtable, R., Ciaramitaro, D., Eisenstein, D. 1978. The effect of a pyrrolizidine alkaloid, monocrotaline, and a pyrrole, dehydroretronecine, on the biochemical functions of the pulmonary endothelium. *Mol. Pharmacol.* 14:1189–203

93. Atwal, O. S., Persofsky, M. S. 1984. Ultrastructural changes in intraacinar pulmonary veins. Relationship to 3-methylindole-induced acute pulmonary edema and pulmonary arterial changes in cattle. *Am. J. Pathol.* 114:472–86

94. Hammond, A. C., Carlson, J. R., Willett, J. D. 1979. The metabolism and

disposition of 3-methylindole in goats. *Life Sci.* 25:1301–6

95. Block, E. R., Schoen, F. J. 1981. Effect of alpha napthylthiourea on uptake of 5-hydroxytryptamine from the pulmonary circulation. *Am. Rev. Respir. Dis.* 123:69–73

96. Cashman, J. R., Traiger, G. J., Hanzlik, R. P. 1982. Pneumotoxic effects of thiobenzamide derivatives. *Toxicology* 23:85–93

97. Boyd, M. R., Neal, R. A. 1976. Studies on the mechanism of toxicity and of development of tolerance to the pulmonary toxin α-napthylthiourea (ANTU). *Drug Metab. Disp.* 4:314–22

98. Tom, W.-M., Montgomery, M. R. 1980. Bleomycin toxicity: Alteration in oxidative metabolism in lung and liver microsomal fractions. *Biochem. Pharmacol.* 29:3239–44

99. Sugiura, U., Kikuchi, T. 1978. Formation of superoxide and hydroxy radicals in iron (II)-bleomycin-oxygen system: Electron spin resonance detection by spin trapping. *J. Antibiot.* 31:1310–12

100. Mais, D. E., Lahr, P. D., Bosin, T. R. 1982. Oxygen-induced lung toxicity: Effect on serotonin disposition and metabolism. *Toxicol. Appl. Pharmacol.* 64:221–29

101. Block, E. R., Fisher, A. B. 1977. Depression of serotonin clearance by rat lungs during oxygen exposure. *J. Appl. Physiol.* 42:33–38

102. Block, E. R., Cannon, J. K. 1978. Effect of oxygen exposure on lung clearance of amines. *Lung* 155:287–95

103. Meyrick, B., Reid, L. 1978. The effect of continued hypoxia on rat pulmonary arterial circulation: An ultrastructural study. *Lab Invest.* 38:188–200

104. Meyrick, B., Reid, L. 1979. Hypoxia and incorporation of ^{3}H-thymidine by cells of rat pulmonary arteries and alveolar wall. *Am. J. Pathol.* 96:51–70

105. Ospital, J. J., Kasuyama, R. S., Tierney, D. F. 1983. Poor correlation between oxygen toxicity and activity of glutathione peroxidase. *Exp. Lung Res.* 5:193–99

106. Crapo, J. D., Sjostrom, K., Drew, R. T. 1978. Tolerance and cross-tolerance using NO_2 and O_2. I. Toxicology and biochemistry. *J. Appl. Physiol.* 44:364–69

107. Crapo, J. D., Marsh-Salin, J., Ingram, P., Pratt, P. C. 1978. Tolerance and cross-tolerance using NO_2 and O_2. II. Pulmonary morphology and morphometry. *J. Appl. Physiol.* 44:370–79

108. Douglas, J. S., Curry, G., Geffkin, S. A. 1977. Superoxide dismutase and pulmonary ozone toxicity. *Life Sci.* 20:1187–92

109. Cummiskey, J. M., Simon, L. M., Theodore, J., Ryan, U. S., Robin, E. D. 1981. Bioenergetic alterations in cultivated pulmonary artery and aortic endothelial cells exposed to normoxia and hypoxia. *Exp. Lung Res.* 2:155–63

110. Ager, A., Gordon, J. L., Moncada, S., Pearson, J. D., Salmon, J. A., et al. 1982. Effects of isolation and culture on prostaglandin synthesis by porcine aortic endothelial and smooth muscle cells. *J. Cell. Physiol.* 110:9–16

111. Bosin, T. R., Lahr. P. D. 1981. Mechanisms influencing the disposition of serotonin in mouse lung. *Biochem. Pharmacol.* 30:3187–93

112. Roth, R. A. 1982. Flow dependence of norepinephrine extraction by isolated perfused rat lungs. *Am. J. Physiol.* 242:H844–48

113. Catravas, J. D., Gillis, C. N. 1981. Metabolism of [^{3}H]benzoylphenylalanyl-alanyl-proline by pulmonary angiotensin converting enzyme *in vivo*: Effects of bradykinin, SQ 14225 or acute hypoxia. *J. Pharmacol. Exp. Ther.* 217:263–70

114. Bond, J. A., Yang, H.-Y. L., Majesky, M. W., Benditt, E. P., Juchau, M. R. 1980. Metabolism of benzo[a]pyrene and 7,12-dimethylbenz[a]anthracene in chicken aortas: Monooxygenation, bioactivation to mutagens, and covalent binding to DNA in vitro. *Toxicol. Appl. Pharmacol.* 52:323–35

115. Dees, J. A., Masters, B. S. S., Muller-Eberhard, U., Johnson, E. F. 1982. Effect of 2,3,7,8,-tetrachlorodibenzo-*p*-dioxin and phenobarbital on the occurrence and distribution of four cytochrome P-450 isozymes in rabbit kidney, lung, and liver. *Cancer Res.* 42:1423–32

116. Lauweryns, J. M., Baert, J. H. 1977. Alveolar clearance and the role of the pulmonary lymphatics. *Am. Rev. Resp. Dis.* 115:625–83

117. Pine, M. B., Beach, P. M., Cottrell, T. S., Scola, M., Turino, G. M. 1976. The relationship between right duct lymph flow and extravascular lung water in dogs given α-napthylthiourea. *J. Clin. Invest.* 58:482–92

118. Gil, J. 1982. Comparative morphology and ultrastructure of the airways. See Ref. 2, 1: pp. 3-25

119. Breezer, R., Turk, M. 1984. Cellular structure, function and organization in the lower respiratory tract. *Environ. Health Perspect.* 55:3–24

120. Enna, S. J., Schanker, L. S. 1972.

Absorption of drugs from the rat lung. *Am. J. Physiol.* 223:1227–31

121. Brown, R. A., Schanker, L. S. 1983. Absorption of aerosolized drugs from the rat lung. *Drug Metab. Disp.* 11:355–60

122. Schanker, L. S. 1978. Drug absorption from the lung. *Biochem. Pharmacol.* 27:381–85

123. Brown, R. A. Jr., Schanker, L. S. 1983. Sex comparison of pulmonary absorption of drugs in the rat. *Drug Metab. Disp.* 11:392–93

124. Hemberger, J. A., Schanker, L. S. 1983. Pulmonary absorption of drugs in the neonatal and adult guinea pig. *Drug Metab. Disp.* 11:615–16

125. Hemberger, J. A., Schanker, L. S. 1978. Pulmonary absorption of drugs in the neonatal rat. *Am. J. Physiol.* 234:C191–97

126. Hemberger, J. A., Schanker, L. S. 1983. Relation between molecular weight and pulmonary absorption rate of lipid insoluble compounds in neonatal and adult rats. *Biochem. Pharmacol.* 32:2599–601

127. Wangensteen, D., Yankovich, R. 1979. Alveolar epithelium transport of albumin and sucrose: Concentration difference effect. *J. Appl. Physiol.* 47:846–50

128. Gatzy, J. T. 1982. Paths of hydrophilic solute flow across excised bullfrog lung. *Exp. Lung Res.* 3:147–61

129. Boucher, R. C., Stutts, M. J., Gatzy, J. T. 1981. Regional differences in canine airway epithelial ion transport. *J. Appl. Physiol.* 51:706–14

130. Hemberger, J. A., Schanker, L. S. 1981. Effect of cortisone on permeability of the neonatal rat lung to drugs. *Biol. Neon.* 40:99–104

131. Hemberger, J. A., Schanker, L. S. 1978. Effect of thyroxine on permeability of the neonatal rat lung to drugs. *Biol. Neon.* 34:299–303

132. Boyd, M. R. 1980. Biochemical mechanisms in pulmonary toxicity of furan derivatives. *Rev. Biochem. Toxicol.* 2:71–102

133. Warren, D. L., Brown, D. L., Buckpitt, A. R. 1982. Evidence for cytochrome P-450 mediated metabolism in the bronchiolar damage by naphthalene. *Chem.-Biol. Interact.* 40:287–303

134. Griffin, K. A., Johnson, C. B., Breger, R. K., Franklin, R. B. 1981. Pulmonary toxicity, hepatic and extrahepatic metabolism of 2-methylnaphthalene in mice. *Toxicol. Appl. Pharmacol.* 61:185–96

135. Boyd, M. R., Statham, C. N., Longo, N. S. 1980. The pulmonary Clara cell as a target for toxic chemicals requiring metabolic activation; studies with carbon tetrachloride. *J. Pharmacol. Exp. Ther.* 212:109–14

136. Forkert, P.-G., Reynolds, E. S. 1982. 1,1-Dichlorethylene-induced pulmonary toxicity. *Exp. Lung Res.* 3:57–68

137. Adamson, I. Y. R., Bowden, D. H., Côté, M. G., Witschi, H. 1977. Lung injury induced by butylated hydroxytoluene. Cytodynamic and biochemical studies in mice. *Lab Invest.* 36:26–32

138. Aldridge, W. N., Nemery, B. 1984. Toxicology of trialkylphosphorothioates with particular reference to lung toxicity. *Fund. Appl. Toxicol.* 4:S215–23

139. Sivarajah, K., Jones, K. G., Fouts, J. R., Devereux, T., Shirley, J. E., et al. 1983. Prostaglandin synthetase and cytochrome P-450-dependent metabolism of $(\pm)$benzo(α)pyrene 7,8-dihydrodiol by enriched populations of rat Clara cells and alveolar type II cells. *Cancer Res.* 43:2632–36

140. Stowers, S. J., Anderson, M. W. 1984. Ubiquitous binding of benzo(a)pyrene metabolites to DNA and protein in tissues of the mouse and rabbit. *Chem.-Biol. Interact.* 51:151–66

141. Horton, J. K., Rosenoir, J., White, C., Brier, D., Bend, J. R. et al. 1984. Quantitation of metabolite-DNA adducts in selected pulmonary and hepatic cell types isolated from rabbits treated with benzo(a)pyrene. *Pharmacologist* 26:204 (Abstr.)

142. Smith, L. L., Wyatt, I. 1981. The accumulation of putrescine into slices of rat lung and brain and its relationship to the accumulation of paraquat. *Biochem. Pharmacol.* 30:1053–58

143. Smith, L. L., Wyatt, I., Cohen, G. M. 1982. The accumulation of diamines and polyamines into rat lung slices. *Biochem. Pharmacol.* 31:3029–33

144. Ross, J. H., Krieger, R. I. 1981. Structure-activity correlations of amines inhibiting active uptake of paraquat (methyl viologen) into rat lung slices. *Toxicol. Appl. Pharmacol.* 59:238–49

145. Brooke-Taylor, S., Smith, L. L., Cohen, G. M. 1983. The accumulation of polyamines and paraquat by human peripheral lung. *Biochem. Pharmacol.* 32:717–20

146. Charles, J. M., Abou-Donia, M. B., Menzel, D. B. 1978. Absorption of paraquat and diquat from the airways of the perfused rat lung. *Toxicol.* 9:59–67

147. Forman, H. J., Aldrich, T. K., Posner, M. A., Fisher, A. B. 1982. Differential paraquat uptake and redox kinetics of rat granular pneumocytes and alveolar mac-

rophages. *J. Pharmacol. Exp. Ther.* 221:428–33
148. Drew, R., Siddik, Z., Gram, T. E. 1979. The uptake and efflux of ^{14}C-paraquat by rat lung slices: The effect of imipramine and other drugs. *Toxicol. Appl. Pharmacol.* 49:473–78
149. Chi, C. H., Dixit, B. N. 1977. Characterization of (±)-methadone uptake by rat lung. *Br. J. Pharmacol.* 59:539–49
150. Enna, S. J., Schanker, L. S. 1973. Phenol red absorption from the rat lung: Evidence of carrier transport. *Life Sci.* 12:231–39
151. Gardiner, T. H., Schanker, L. S. 1974. Absorption of disodium cromoglycate from the rat lung: Evidence of carrier transport. *Xenobiotica* 4:725–31
152. Gardiner, T. H., Schanker, L. S. 1976. Active transport of phenol red by rat lung slices. *J. Pharmacol. Exp. Ther.* 196:455–62
153. Lin, Y.-J., Schanker, L. S. 1981. Pulmonary absorption of amino acids in the rat: Evidence of carrier transport. *Am. J. Physiol.* 240:C215–21
154. Lin, Y.-J., Schanker, L. S. 1983. Pulmonary absorption and lung slice uptake of a foreign amino acid—species comparison. *Drug Metab. Disp.* 11:75–76
155. Hemberger, J. A., Schanker, L. S. 1983. Mechanism of pulmonary absorption of quaternary ammonium compounds in the rat. *Drug Metab. Disp.* 11:73–74
156. Collins, J. N., Dedrick, R. L. 1982. Contribution of lungs to total body clearance: Linear and nonlinear effects. *J. Pharm Sci.* 71:66–70
157. Gillette, J. R. 1982. Sequential organ first-pass effects: Simple methods for constructing compartmental pharmacokinetic models from physiological models of drug disposition by several organs. *J. Pharm. Sci.* 71:673–77
158. Rowland, M., Benet, L. Z., Graham, G. G. 1973. Clearance concepts in pharmacokinetics. *J. Pharmacokinet. Biopharm.* 1:123–36
159. Rane, A., Wilkinson, G. R., Shand, D. G. 1977. Prediction of hepatic extraction ratio from in vitro measurement of intrinsic clearance. *J. Pharmacol. Exp. Ther.* 200:420–24
160. Wiersma, D. A., Roth, R. A. 1980. Clearance of 5-hydroxytryptamine by rat lung and liver: The importance of relative perfusion and intrinsic clearance. *J. Pharmacol. Exp. Ther.* 212:97–102
161. Iwasawa, Y., Gillis, C. N. 1974. Pharmacological analysis of norepinephrine and 5-hydroxytryptamine removal from the pulmonary circulation: Differentiation of uptake sites for each amine. *J. Pharmacol. Exp. Ther.* 188:386–93
162. Junod, A. F. 1975. Metabolism, production and release of hormones and mediators in the lung. *Am. Rev. Respir. Dis.* 112:93–108
163. Alabaster, V. A., Bakhle, Y. S. 1970. Removal of 5-hydroxytryptamine in the pulmonary circulation of rat isolated lungs. *Br. J. Pharmacol.* 40:468–82
164. Wiersma, D. A., Roth, R. A. 1983. The prediction of benzo[α]pyrene clearance by rat liver and lung from enzyme kinetic data. *Mol. Pharmacol.* 24:300–8
165. Wiersma, D. A., Roth, R. A. 1983. Total body clearance of circulating benzo-(α)pyrene in conscious rats: Effect of pretreatment with 3-methylcholanthrene and the role of liver and lung. *J. Pharmacol. Exp. Ther.* 226:661–67
166. Smith, B. R., Bend, J. R. 1980. Prediction of pulmonary benzo(α)pyrene 4,5-oxide clearance: A pharmacokinetic analysis of epoxide-metabolizing enzymes in rabbit lung. *J. Pharmacol. Exp. Ther.* 214:478–82
167. Dutcher, J. S., Boyd, M. R. 1979. Species and strain differences in target organ alkylation and toxicity by 4-ipomeanol: Predictive value of covalent binding in studies of target organ toxicities by reactive metabolites. *Biochem. Pharmacol.* 28:3367–72
168. Boyd, M. R. 1980. Biochemical mechanisms in pulmonary toxicity of furan derivatives. In *Reviews in Biochemical Toxicology,* ed. E. Hodgson, J. Bend, R. Philpot, pp. 71–102. New York: Elsevier/North Holland. 300 pp.
169. Wolf, C. R., Statham, C. N., McMenamin, M. K., Bend, J. R., Boyd, M. R., Philpot, R. M. 1982. The relationship between the catalytic activities of rabbit pulmonary cytochrome P-450 isozymes and the lung-specific toxicity of the furan derivative, 4-ipomeanol. *Mol. Pharmacol.* 22:738–44
170. Slaughter, S. R., Statham, C. N., Philpot, R. M., Boyd, M. R. 1983. Covalent binding of metabolites of 4-ipomeanol to rabbit pulmonary and hepatic microsomal monooxygenase system. *J. Pharmacol. Exp. Ther.* 224:252–57

Ann. Rev. Pharmacol. Toxicol. 1985. 25:127–46

THE PHARMACOLOGY OF EATING BEHAVIOR[1]

John E. Morley and Allen S. Levine

Neuroendocrine Research Laboratory, Veterans Administration Medical Center, Minneapolis, Minnesota 55417

Fatophobia is rampant throughout America and the Western world. The economic impact of this ubiquitous desire for a lean body image is reflected in the rapid and continued success of diet books. Despite various claims, however, few efficacious pharmacological agents cure obesity. In 1972, the FDA assessed the results of the effects of eleven anorexic agents in over 10,000 patients and found that drugs produced an advantage over placebo of 0.56 pounds of weight loss per week (1). Although such an advantage maintained over months or years would clearly represent a major effect, it has in general failed to satisfy the appetites of those hungry for miracle cures. As a result, over the last decade the pharmaceutical industry has expended a tremendous effort to find the Holy Grail of Satiety.

We will review here much of the recent research on the pharmacology of eating behavior and develop the thesis that the complexities of the regulation of appetite are so great that it is highly unlikely that any single pharmacological agent will produce and maintain the degree of weight loss demanded by worshipers of the body skinny. The closely interwoven nature of the regulatory systems of feeding and other life preserving systems, e.g. temperature and glucoregulation, further suggests that any agent that could truly produce the dramatic alterations in eating behavior demanded of an ideal satiety agent would result in far too many serious side effects to allow it to be marketed.

As already stated, the regulation of food intake is an extremely complex process. It involves the hedonic qualities of food conveyed by olfactory, visual, and gustatory signals, neural and hormonal signals from the gastrointestinal tract, and the physicochemical qualities of the ingested food. In addition, a number of signals relay the overall state of nutrient homeostasis of the organ-

---

[1]The US Government has the right to retain a nonexclusive royalty-free license in and to any copyright covering this paper.

ism, including messages about the status of energy stores and essential nutrients (specific hungers). Superimposed on these biological substrates are psychological factors, such as learned aversions to substances that induce illness and a variety of ecological and sociological factors responsible for determining the availability of food and what is fit (or appropriate) to eat. These multiple inputs eventually must be integrated to determine the timing and quantity of food to be eaten. Much of this integration takes place in the central nervous system, making the brain the most important regulator of digestive processes in the body.

This review focuses mainly on the advances made in our understanding of the pharmacologic control of feeding in the eight years since the publication of Hoebel's article in this series (2). This means a concentration predominantly on the findings concerning the effects of peptides on feeding at the expense of the better established knowledge on the role of monoamines. Those wishing more detail on the monoaminergic regulation of feeding are referred to Hoebel's article (2) or the more recent review by Leibowitz (3).

In view of the complexities of the regulatory systems involved in feeding, it has become convenient to divide the control of feeding into a peripheral satiety system and a central feeding system. The peripheral satiety system appears to send its signals to the brain through both neuronal and hormonal messenger systems. In addition, the processing of foods gives rise to a number of simple nutrients that in turn can themselves act as neuromodulators, the so-called appetostats. The central feeding system(s) responsible for integrating these inputs involves a variety of neurotransmitters. We have suggested that within the central nervous system these interacting neurotransmitters are arranged in a cascade system similar to the classical cascade system regulating clotting and complement fixation (4). Figure 1 illustrates this appetite cascade system. Although the model is grossly oversimplified, it represents a useful malleable matchstick model to aid in understanding the complexities of the system. It also has helped in the design of pharmacological experiments on the nature of appetite control.

Before describing the pharmacological regulation of the peripheral and central feeding systems, we want to briefly discuss an apparent paradox. It is clear that, whereas many agents appear to inhibit feeding in animals, few have proved to be successful longterm modulators of human feeding. There are two major reasons for this discrepancy: first, most of the experiments in animals are carried out over a single meal whereas most human studies are carried out over weeks. In most cases, animals subjected to chronic administration of even the most potent inhibitors of feeding rapidly develop some degree of tolerance. Second, when calculated on a per-kilogram basis, the doses administered to animals are usually much higher and more toxic than those administered to humans. Based on these observations, it appears that the most successful

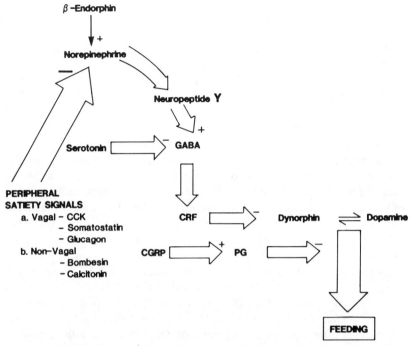

Figure 1 Simplified version of the satiety cascade in the rat. This represents the putative interconnections of the opioid feeding system. Other feeding systems clearly also exist. CCK = cholecystokinin; GABA = gamma amino butyric acid; CRF = corticotropin-releasing factor; CGRP = calcitonin gene-related peptide; PG = prostaglandin.

pharmacological approach for the treatment of obesity may be a sequentially administered, multi-drug approach.

THE PERIPHERAL SATIETY SYSTEM

The Pharmacological Modulation of Taste

Palatability has been suggested to play a role in the pathogenesis of obesity (5). Not surprisingly, all studies have shown that, when the foods are highly palatable, more calories are consumed. In addition, overweight subjects ingest more in response to highly palatable stimuli than do normal-weight people. Cabanac & Duclaux (6) found that in normal-weight people, the ingestion of glucose transforms the normally pleasant sensation of sucrose to an unpleasant sensation, whereas obese subjects continue to perceive the sucrose as pleasant. Occurrence of this alliesthesia has been shown to occur outside the laboratory in Jerba, North Africa, where the premarriage custom of overfeeding young females decreases the rate of pleasantness of sucrose solutions (and presumably increases the appetite for other pleasures!) (7).

Recently a number of studies have explored the possibility of developing pharmacological agents that either substitute for preferred tastes without containing as many calories or that alter the perception of the taste, thus leading to an altered intake.

Studies with the dipeptide aspartame (NutraSweet®; L-aspartyl-L-phenylalanyl-methyl-ester) have suggested that it can satisfactorily mimic sucrose. Brala & Hager (8) found that there was no significant difference in calories ingested after a preload of aspartame compared to sucrose, despite the tremendous difference in the caloric content of the two treatments. In a chronic study, Porikos (9) found that surreptitiously substituting aspartame for sucrose resulted in a decreased caloric intake during the aspartame period compared to when the subjects were ingesting sucrose.

Recently a number of neuropeptides have been demonstrated to modulate taste. The antidipsogenic effect of the opioid antagonist naloxone is enhanced by sweet and salty flavors (10, 11), and naltrexone, a long-acting opioid antagonist, more efficiently reduces the intake of a palatable diet compared to the intake of normal chow (12). In contrast, morphine increases the intake of a relatively preferred saccharin solution (10%) while not affecting lower concentrations (13), and repeated pairings of morphine injections with sucrose or quinine solutions increase both the sucrose preference and the quinine aversion (14). These results suggest that the endogenous opioids may play a role in mediating or producing changes in the incentive values of certain tastes.

Substance P is an undecapeptide present in fibers innervating the circumvallate and fungiform papillae of the rat tongue (15) as well as in the nucleus of the solitary tract (16). Substance P has been shown to have a selective antidipsogenic effect. This effect is markedly attenuated when sucrose or saccharin is added to the drinking water (17). Thus, as is the case for endogenous opioids, flavor can modulate the antidipsogenic effect of substance P.

An established role for substance P in taste is as a mediator of the burning taste of chili pepper. Chili contains capsaicin, a chemical that blocks the re-uptake and promotes the release of substance P at nerve terminals. This produces increased concentrations of substance P in the tongue, leading to the burning sensation associated with chili. Why some acquire a liking for the oral pain sensations produced by chili pepper, why some like it hot, is unclear (18). One psychological theory suggests that the initially negative effect gives rise to an internally generated compensatory positive effect (19). Given our knowledge that the release of substance P results in a compensatory increase in endogenous opioids (20), it may not be unreasonable to speculate that the neurochemical substrate of a liking for chili may be secondary to the reward produced by an increased release of endogenous opioids in the brain.

Cholecystokinin (CCK) is another peptide that has been shown to produce effects on taste perception in addition to its better documented effects on satiety (vide infra). CCK reduces the short-term (three-minute) intake of sucrose solutions (21, 22) and inhibits sham feeding (23), suggesting a pregastric component to its satiety effect. Compatible with this concept, CCK has been shown to inhibit the activity of neurons in the nucleus of the solitary tract (24), and intravenous infusion of CCK-8 increases integrated responses to sucrose from the uncut chorda tympani of the rat (25). Thus, the orosensory qualities of the food appear to play a role in producing the full CCK effect on ingestive behavior.

Gut Hormones as Modulators of Satiety

Studies by Davis et al (26) using cross-perfused rats showed that an unfed rat ate considerably less after being cross-perfused with the blood of a fed rat. This suggests that circulating hormonal factors released during a meal played a role in the satiety syndrome. Cross-perfusion studies with the obese (ob/ob) mouse and with destructive lesions of the ventromedial hypothalamus (VMH) provided further evidence for a circulating satiety factor. When the ob/ob mouse is parabiosed to its lean littermate, it decreases the amount it eats, suggesting that ob/ob mice become obese because of failure to produce a circulating satiety factor (27). On the other hand, when normal rats are parabiosed to rats with VMH lesions, the normal rats decrease their food intake, suggesting overproduction of circulating satiety factors in the rats with VMH lesions (28). These parabiosis experiments have led to an intensive search for these circulating satiety factors. At present the best studied candidate for a circulating satiety factor is cholecystokinin.

Cholecystokinin

Cholecystokinin (CCK) is a polypeptide hormone that was first isolated as a 33-amino acid hormone from the porcine gastrointestinal tract. Subsequently, it has been shown that the active portion of the molecule consists of the eight carboxy terminal amino acids (CCK-8). CCK has subsequently been demonstrated to have a variety of actions both on the gastrointestinal tract and on the central nervous system (29).

In 1973, Gibbs et al (30) proposed that CCK may be a peripheral satiety signal when they found that both a partially purified preparation of CCK and synthetic CCK-8 suppressed solid and liquid food intake in rats. Subsequently, Smith & Gibbs (31) found that L-phenylalanine, a potent releaser of CCK, suppressed food intake in monkeys, whereas its inactive isomer did not. Studies by McLaughlin et al (32) found that the administration of the trypsin inhibitor trasylol decreases food intake in lean and obese rats. Since trypsin inhibitors increase CCK by inhibiting the negative feedback signal for its release, this provides further evidence for a physiological role for CCK in appetite regulation.

Much controversy exists over whether the CCK effect on decreasing food intake represents a true satiety effect or whether its effects are secondary to toxicity or aversion. Studies using classical tests for conditioned taste aversion have given both positive and negative results (33). Recently, we developed the paradigm of different degrees of starvation to measure the satiating effect of peptides (34). Reasoning that a satiety factor should inhibit food intake to a lesser degree as the period of food deprivation is increased, whereas an aversive agent should uniformly inhibit food intake independent of length of deprivation, we studied the effects of CCK at two different degrees of starvation. In this study, CCK reduced intake in the manner we predicted a satiety factor would, whereas lithium chloride effects were those predicted for an aversive agent. Thus, based on the available evidence, it seems that CCK may be a true satiety factor.

Besides decreasing feeding in rats, CCK has been shown to decrease food intake in a variety of species, including humans. Kissileff et al (35) and Pi-Sunyer et al (36) have shown that CCK-8 infusions decreased food intake in lean and obese humans, although previous studies had produced conflicting results (37, 38). Stacher et al (39) confirmed these findings, showing that CCK-8 decreased feeding in humans by about 17%. Our studies in humans have also found that CCK-8 decreases food intake; the data suggest that this effect on food intake may be linked to the ability of CCK to decrease gastric emptying (unpublished observations).

The mechanism by which CCK signals its satiety effect is uncertain and appears to differ in different species. Studies in the rat have shown that peripherally administered CCK-8 acts in the abdomen through vagal fibers and not directly in the brain to produce satiety (40, 41). Both total abdominal vagotomy and selective gastric (but not celiac or hepatic) vagotomy reduce the satiety effect of CCK. Further, Smith et al (40) found no effect of atropine on CCK-induced satiety, suggesting that the effect is mediated by afferent rather than efferent vagal fibers. However, in the dog, vagotomy produces minimal attenuation of the satiety effect of CCK (42).

Although in the rat the major effect of CCK on satiety appears to be through activation of peripheral satiety signals, in the sheep the effect of CCK on feeding seems to involve central mechanisms. Continuous injections of pico-mole quantities of CCK-8 into the cerebral ventricles of sheep decreases feeding (43), and antibody to cholecystokinin injected into the cerebral ventricles stimulates feeding in sheep but not in rats (44). Recently, studies by Denbow & Myers (45) have suggested that in the chicken, like the sheep, the major site of action of CCK in suppressing feeding is within the central nervous system.

Other Gut Hormones That Modulate Feeding

Bombesin is a tetradecapeptide originally isolated from the skin of the frog *Bombina bombina* and subsequently shown to be widely distributed in mammalian systems. In 1979, Gibbs et al (46) reported that peripheral injections of bombesin suppresses food intake in rats. Bombesin was five times less potent at suppressing feeding than cholecystokinin-octapeptide on a molar basis. Bombesin had no effect on water intake and no major effects on locomotor activity, which suggests a fairly specific effect on feeding behavior when administered peripherally. Unlike CCK, peripherally administered bombesin still decreases feeding in the rat following vagotomy (41). Also, bombesin potently decreases feeding after central administration in the rat, suggesting that at least some of its effects may be mediated within the central nervous system (47, 48). Recently, bombesin when infused intravenously has been shown to decrease food intake in humans at doses below those that produce nausea (49). Gastrin-releasing peptide is a 27–amino acid peptide that shares marked structural similarity with bombesin. It too has been shown to decrease feeding in the rat (50, 51).

Somatostatin is another gut hormone that has been shown to decrease feeding after peripheral administration in the rat and the baboon (52, 53). Like CCK, somatostatin appears to produce its effect through a vagal mechanism (53).

Two pancreatic hormones, glucagon and pancreatic peptide, have been suggested to play a role in satiety, at least in some species. In 1957, Schulman et al (54) reported that glucagon decreased caloric intake in humans. It was felt that glucagon's effect was secondary to its effects on glycogenolysis with mobilization of glucose stores from the liver. Subsequently, glucagon was shown to decrease feeding in rats and rabbits; this effect was dependent on an intact vagus (55, 56). Geary & Smith (57) have shown that the glucagon effect on satiety can be blocked by a selective hepatic vagotomy. The most convincing evidence in support of glucagon as a satiety agent is the finding by Langhans et al (58) that intraperitoneal injections of glucagon antibodies increase food intake by increasing both the duration and the length of the meal while at the same time reducing the increases in hepatic portal glucose concentrations normally associated with a meal.

Pancreatic polypeptide is a 36–amino acid peptide secreted predominately from the cephalic part of the pancreas. As its circulating levels rise following a meal, its effects on food intake were tested. Malaisse-Lagae et al (59) reported that peripherally administered pancreatic polypeptide decreases food intake and body weight in the genetically obese (ob/ob) mouse. However, pancreatic polypeptide could not be shown to decrease feeding in the rat (34).

The role of the various peripheral satiety agents is summarized in Figure 2.

Appetostats

The concept that nutrients themselves are directly responsible for producing satiety represents one of the earliest hypotheses concerning weight regulation.

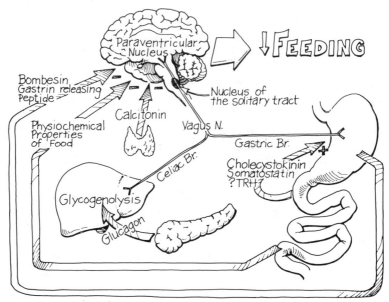

Figure 2   The peripheral satiety system. TRH = thyrotropin-releasing hormone.

As early as 1916, Carlson (60) suggested that falls in circulating glucose levels served as the hunger signal and that eating ceased when glucose levels returned to normal. In 1952, Jean Mayer (61) modified this theory in an attempt to explain why the hyperglycemia of diabetes mellitus was associated with hyperphagia. He suggested that the rate of glucose utilization rather than the absolute glucose concentration was the crucial regulatory mechanism. Further support for glucose as a modulator of neuronal hunger comes from the studies of Oomura (62) showing that iontophoretic application of glucose increases firing of neurons in the medial hypothalamus and lowers the frequency of discharge in the lateral hypothalamus.

There is an inverse relationship between plasma levels of amino acids and food intake. This led Mellinkoff (63) to propose the amino-static hypothesis of feeding. He suggested that excesses and deficiencies of amino acids play a role in the initiation and inhibition of food intake. In view of the fact that certain amino acids, e.g. γ-amino butyric acid (GABA), both act as neurotransmitters and inhibit food intake, this represents an attractive scientific theory of appetite regulation. Wurtman (64) has attempted to link the glucostatic and aminostatic hypotheses by showing that glucose faciliates the transport of tryptophan, the serotonin precursor, across the blood-brain barrier.

Others have suggested that free fatty acids released during lipolysis may signal feeding behavior (65), or that glycerol, which is released into the circulation proportionally to the rate of triglyceride hydrolysis, acts as a signal of the status of body fat stores (66). In 1958, Brobeck (67) proposed that the heat generated by metabolic fuels, i.e. the specific dynamic action of food, was responsible for the regulation of feeding. This concept was supported by studies in goats showing that local cooling or warming of the anterior hypothalamus induced and decreased feeding respectively (68). Recent studies have shown a role for multiple peptides and neurotransmitters in thermoregulation, suggesting that some of the effects of peptides on food intake may be secondary to their effects on central thermoregulatory mechanisms (69).

Both peripheral and central administration of purines decreases feeding (70–72). As there is extensive evidence for a purinergic nervous system, we proposed, somewhat tongue-in-cheek, a purinostatic model of feeding (73). Some of our studies have supported the concept that purinergic modulation of feeding may involve an interaction with the diazepam receptor, and recently we have reported evidence of a close interrelationship between the purinergic feeding system and the opioid feeding system (74). Finally, levels of xanthine in the cerebrospinal fluid are associated with poor appetite in depressed patients, suggesting a possible role for purines in the appetite regulation of humans (75).

Another nutrient-linked theory of longterm appetite regulation suggests that insulin plays a key role as a body-adiposity signal. This hypothesis is based on the impressive correlation between the degree of adiposity and plasma insulin levels (76), and the finding that plasma insulin levels increase proportionately when insulin is infused intravenously (77). Woods et al (77–79) have reported that, in contrast to the effects of peripherally administered insulin, when insulin is administered centrally it markedly decreases feeding in baboons and in lean but not obese (fa/fa) Zucker rats. Instillation of insulin antibodies into the ventromedial hypothalamus of rats results in an increased food intake (80). Tannenbaum et al (81) have found that central administration of a partially purified insulin growth factor is an extremely potent inhibitor of feeding in rats.

The proliferating theories of nutrient control of food intake suggest that the brain possesses multiple mechanisms for modulating the levels of essential nutrients. Such mechanisms are in keeping with the known ability of animals to select a proper balance of macronutrients and micronutrients when feeding freely. Modern knowledge suggests that there are numerous windows on the brain that act as monitors of the milieu interieur. Information from these sensors is then processed within the central nervous system through a cascade system involving multiple neurotransmitters.

THE NEUROPHARMACOLOGY OF THE CENTRAL REGULATION OF APPETITE

A variety of substances have been demonstrated to increase or decrease feeding after central administration (Table 1).

Table 1   Centrally acting neuropharmacological modulators of feeding behavior

	Feeding enhancers	Feeding inhibitors
Monoamines	Norepinephrine (α-agonist)	Epinephrine
		β-agonists
	Dopamine	Dopamine
		Serotonin
		Phenylethylamine
Peptides	Opioid peptides—dynorphin	Corticotropin-releasing factor
	α-neo-endorphin	Thyrotropin-releasing hormone
	β-endorphin	Cyclo-histidyl proline diketopiperazine
	D-Ala^5-d-leu-enkephalin	Neurotensin
	Neuropeptide Y	Bombesin
		Calcitonin
		Calitonin gene-related peptide
		Cholecystokinin (species variability)
		Insulin
		Insulin growth factor
Amino acids	GABA (muscimol)	GABA
		Adenosine
Miscellaneous	Acetylcholine	Acetylcholine
	Benzodiazepines	Adenosine
	Calcium	Prostaglandins

Opioid Feeding Systems

Since the pioneering study by Holtzman (82) demonstrating that the opioid antagonist naloxone decreases feeding in rats, many studies have suggested a role for endogenous opioid peptides in feeding modulation (83). Naloxone decreases feeding in rats under a variety of conditions, including spontaneous (84), starvation-induced (85), norepinephrine-induced (86), muscimol-induced (87), 2-deoxyglucose-induced (88), and stress-induced (88, 89) feeding. However, naloxone poorly antagonizes feeding induced by chronic starvation for three weeks (90), schedule feeding (91) and insulin hypoglycemia (88) suggesting that the opioid feeding system is not the only feeding system. In fact, it has been suggested that the opioid system may play a more important role in macronutrient selection than in the feeding drive per se (92). Also, chronic administration of naloxone, or of the long-acting opioid antagonist naltrexone, produces only small decreases in food intake and body weight in non-obese rats and mice (93, 94). Further, it is clear that the effect of opioid antagonism on feeding is modulated by a variety of hormones (Table 2).

Besides its effects in rodents, naloxone decreases feeding in a variety of other species ranging from wolves (99) to humans (100). Although naloxone clearly decreases feeding over a single meal in humans, chronic naltrexone

Table 2   Effect of hormonal manipulations on opioid antagonism of feeding

Increase effect of naloxone on feeding	Decrease effect of naloxone on feeding	References
Hyperglycemia	Hypoglycemia	88, 95, 96
Ovariectomy	Estradiol	97
Progesterone antagonizes estradiol effect	Adrenalectomy	97, 98

administration to humans has so far yielded equivocal results, with only mild decreases in weight gain in obese females being demonstrated (101). Further, in some species opioid antagonism fails to alter feeding. These species include the golden hamster (102), the Chinese hamster (103), and the racoon (104).

Just as opioid antagonism decreases feeding in rats, a variety of opiate agonists have been shown to increase feeding. The mixed kappa opiate agonists/antagonists, such as ketocyclazocine (105) and butorphanol tartrate (106), appear to be more potent than mu agonists at stimulating feeding. This has led to the suggestion that the kappa opioid receptor plays an integral role in the initiation of feeding. Support for this comes from the finding that the kappa opioid peptide dynorphin is a potent enhancer of feeding after central administration (107). Recent evidence has suggested that the effect of this peptide on feeding involves both the opioid and the non-opioid portion of the molecule (108) (Figure 3). This concept of a double-lock receptor suggests that the non-opioid portion of the dynorphin molecule (5–13) targets the molecule to the receptor and unlocks access to the opioid portion of the receptor. In vitro studies by Chavkin & Goldstein (109) have resulted in a similar concept for the mode of action for dynorphin. Further evidence for a role for dynorphin in feeding comes from studies showing that its levels alter in the central nervous system under conditions that modulate the feeding drive (110, 111).

Although much evidence has accumulated on a primary role for dynorphin and the kappa opioid receptor as the major mediators of the opioid feeding drive, we must point out that other opioid peptides, such as β-endorphin (112) and the delta receptor analog D-ala^{2}D-leu^5-enkephalin (113), also stimulate feeding after central administration. Recently, we obtained preliminary evidence suggesting that more than one opioid receptor and more than one brain site may be involved in the opioid modulation of feeding.

To conclude this section on opioid modulation of feeding, we want to speculate that, from a teleological point of view, the original function of opioids was to stimulate the feeding drive. This forced the animal to go out and forage for food, at times inflicting pain on the animal species; thus, survival would be enhanced by a gene mutation that resulted in a similar peptide subserving the function of analgesia. The fact that opioids also decrease sexual activity (114) makes further teleological sense, as starving animals (increased

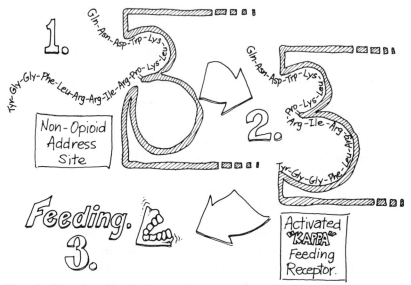

Figure 3   Illustration of the dual nature of the dynorphin-kappa opioid feeding receptor.

opioid activity) are at a disadvantage for procreation and it would be better to procreate at a time when food was readily available.

Monoamines as Feeding Modulators

In 1962, Sebastian Grossman showed that intrahypothalamic injection of norepinephrine induces vigorous feeding and that acetylcholine inhibits feeding (115). Subsequently, Sarah Leibowitz has established that α-adrenergic stimulation in the area of the paraventricular nucleus stimulates feeding and β-adrenergic stimulation in the lateral hypothalamus is inhibitory to feeding (116). The norepinephrine increases in feeding are due to an increase in meal size rather than meal frequency and create a preference for carbohydrate-rich foodstuffs (3). The facilitatory effects of centrally administered norepinephrine on feeding requires an intact vagus (117) and adrenalectomy abolishes the effect, which can be restored by administration of corticosterone (118). As lesions of the paraventricular nucleus result in hyperphagia rather than in decreased eating, while attenuating norepinephrine induces eating (119), it appears that norepinephrine-induced feeding is secondary to inhibition of the release of a satiety factor in this nucleus.

A variety of studies have suggested, but not proven, that serotonin functions as a satiety agent (120). Serotonin agonists and drugs that potentiate serotonin actions, e.g. fenfluramine, decrease feeding, whereas serotonergic antagonists and the serotonergic neurotoxins 5,6- and 5,7-dihydroxytryptamine enhance feeding. Serotonergic stimulants decrease meal size without affecting the initiation of feeding or meal frequency (3). In addition, serotonin results in a decrease in carbohydrate intake while preserving or even potentiating protein intake (3). Serotonin exerts its major site of action in either the paraventricular or ventromedial hypothalamus and inhibits norepinephrine-induced eating (3). Recently, it has been suggested that some of the effects of serotonin stimulators may be mediated through peripheral effects, resulting in a slowing of gastric emptying (121).

Destruction of dopaminergic and other catecholaminergic fibers with the neurotoxin 6-hydroxydopamine can lead to hypophagia and weight loss (122). Dopamine infusion into the hypothalamus can increase or decrease feeding (3). The dopamine agonist bromergocryptine stimulates feeding at low doses after central administration and inhibits it at higher doses, a result associated with stereotypic behaviors (123).

The structures of many of the more widely used anorectic drugs in humans are closely related to the β-phenylethylamine nucleus, e.g. amphetamines, diethylpropion. Multiple studies have demonstrated that amphetamine inhibits eating while leading to hyperactivity and stereotypy (124). The amphetamines' anorectic effect appears to be mediated predominantly in the area of the lateral hypothalamus (116). At present the general consensus is that amphetamine produces its effect by release of catecholamines in the perifornical area, resulting in stimulation of the β-adrenergic satiety system (2).

Peripheral administration of high doses of phenylethylamine inhibits feeding, although the specificity of this effect is unclear (125). Interest in the possibility of a phenylethylamine satiety system was recently stimulated by the study of Paul et al (126), who found highly specific amphetamine receptors in the central nervous system. Phenylethylamine appears to be the endogenous ligand for the amphetamine receptor. In their studies, they found that the anorectic potency of a variety of phenylethylamine derivatives was related to their ability to bind the phenylethylamine receptor.

Neuropeptide Y: A Potent Stimulator of Feeding

Neuropeptide Y is a 36–amino acid peptide isolated by Tatemoto (127) from the porcine hypothalamus. It belongs to the pancreatic polypeptide family and has been shown to co-exist in norepinephrine-containing neurons (128). Neuropeptide Y is the most potent known stimulator of feeding (129; J. Morley, A. Levine, unpublished observations) (Figure 4). Neuropeptide Y also increases water intake. The effect of neuropeptide Y on feeding is not blocked by the α-antagonist phentolamine, but is decreased by naloxone and the dopamine antagonist haloperidol. The discovery of the potent stimulatory effect of neuropeptide Y on feeding may represent one of the more exciting discoveries of the last decade in the study of appetite regulation. Development

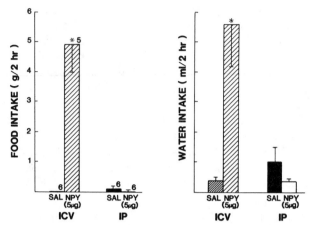

Figure 4 Effect of neuropeptide Y (NPY) on feeding and water intake after central (ICV) administration. Note the lack of effect after the same dose of NPY given peripherally (IP). *p < 0.01 by two-tailed student t-test.

of specific antagonists to neuropeptide Y may represent a potential treatment for the regulation of feeding in obese patients.

Neuropeptides as Satiety Agents

In contrast to neuropeptide Y and the opioid peptides, most other neuropeptides appear to inhibit rather than stimulate feeding. Whether or not this ability of neuropeptides to suppress feeding after central administration represents a true satiety effect or a non-specific disruption of behavior is a subject of intensive debate at the present time.

Calcitonin is a potent inhibitor of feeding after central administration (130). It appears to produce its satiating effects by inhibiting calcium uptake at the hypothalamic level (131). Recently, Rosenfeld et al (132) showed that the calcitonin gene is processed differently in the central nervous system, giving rise to calcitonin gene–related peptide (CGRP). CGRP is distributed in the brain into many anatomical areas connected with the regulation of taste. CGRP suppresses feeding after central administration in rats (133). This effect is less potent than calcitonin on a molar basis. Although CGRP shows some degree of behavioral specificity, it has also been shown to produce a conditioned taste aversion.

Bombesin, a tetradecapeptide originally isolated from the skin of frogs, besides inhibiting feeding after peripheral administration, also decreases feeding when centrally administered (134, 135). It also slows gastric emptying (136) and decreases gastric acid secretion (137). The site of action of bombesin on feeding appears to be in the lateral hypothalamus (138).

Corticotropin-releasing factor (CRF) is a 41–amino acid peptide that releases

ACTH and β-endorphin from the anterior pituitary (139). CRF is a potent inhibitor of feeding after central administration in the rat (140, 141). Animals administered CRF display a marked increase in grooming (140). The effects of CRF on food intake are partially dependent on the presence of an intact adrenal gland (141). We have previously suggested that CRF may play a role in the pathogenesis of anorexia nervosa (142).

Neurotensin is an undecapeptide that has been shown to decrease feeding under a variety of circumstances (143–145). It appears to exert its major action in the region of the paraventricular nucleus (143). Thyrotropin-releasing hormone and its metabolite, cyclohistidyl proline diketopiperazine, have also been demonstrated to decrease feeding under certain circumstances (146–148).

CONCLUSION

The last decade has led to the discovery that a variety of chemical messengers can modulate feeding. Although the physiological significance of these substances remains uncertain, it is clear that the development of pharmacological agonists and antagonists of these substances offers the hope of powerful tools to help modulate appetite control. In view of the multiplicity of factors involved in appetite regulation, it seems clear that no single factor is likely to emerge as the one single regulator of satiety. The etiology of appetite disorders is likely to prove to be multifactorial, with a resulting need to tailor the pharmacotherapy to the individual.

Literature Cited

1. Scoville, B. 1975. Review of amphetamine-like drugs by the Food and Drug Administration. In *Obesity in Perspective, Part 2*, ed. G. A. Bray, pp. 220–25. Washington, DC: GPO
2. Hoebel, B. G. 1977. Pharmacologic control of feeding. *Ann. Rev. Pharmacol. Toxicol.* 17:605–21
3. Leibowitz, S. F. 1980. Neurochemical systems of the hypothalamus in control of feeding and drinking behavior and water and electrolyte excretion. In *Handbook of the Hypothalamus*, ed. P. Morgane, J. Panksepp, 3:299–437. New York: Decker
4. Morley, J. E. 1980. The neuroendocrine control of appetite: The role of the endogenous opiates, cholecystokinin, TRH, gamma-amino butyric acid and the diazepam receptor. *Life Sci.* 27:355–68
5. Spitzer, L., Roden, J. 1981. Human eating behavior: A critical review of studies in normal weight and overweight individuals. *Appetite* 2:293–329

6. Cabanac, M., Duclaux, R. 1970. Obesity: Absence of satiety aversion to sucrose. *Science* 168:496–97
7. Fantino, M., Baigts, F., Cabanac, M., Apfelbaum, M. 1983. Effects of an overfeeding regimen on the affective component of the sweet sensation. *Appetite* 4:155–64
8. Brala, P. M., Hager, R. L. 1983. Effects of sweetness perception and caloric value of a preload on short term satiety. *Physiol. Behav.* 30:1–9
9. Porikos, K. P. 1981. Control of food intake in man: Response to covert caloric dilution of a conventional and palatable diet. In *The Body Weight Regulatory System: Normal and Disturbed Mechanisms*, ed. L. X. Cioffi, W. P. T. James, T. B. Van Itallie, pp. 83–87. New York: Raven
10. LeMagnen, J., Marfaing-Jallut, P., Miceli, D., Devos, M. 1980. Pain modulating and reward systems: A single brain mechanism? *Pharmacol. Biochem. Behav.* 12:729–33

11. Levine, A. S., Murray, S. S., Kneip, J., Grace, M., Morley, J. E. 1982. Flavor enhances the antidipsogenic effect of naloxone. *Physiol. Behav.* 28:23–25
12. Apfelbaum, M., Mandenoff, A. 1981. Naltrexone suppresses hyperphagia induced in the rat by a highly palatable diet. *Pharmacol. Biochem. Behav.* 15:89–91
13. Lynch, W. C., Libby, L. 1983. Naloxone suppresses intake of highly preferred saccharin solutions in food deprived and sated rats. *Life Sci.* 33:1909–14
14. Leshem, M. 1983. Morphine enhances taste preference and aversion: Evidence for opiate mediation in reinforcement or memory. *IRCS Med. Sci.* 11:700
15. Nishimoto, T., Akai, M., Inagaki, S., Shiosaka, S., Shimizu, Y., et al. 1982. On the distribution and origins of substance P in the papillae of the rat tongue: An experimental and immuno-histo-chemical study. *J. Comp. Neurol.* 207:85–92
16. Helke, C. J., Jacobowitz, D. M., Thoa, N. B. 1981. Capsaicin and potassium evoked substance P release from the nucleus tractus solitarius and spinal trigeminal nucleus *in vitro. Life Sci.* 29:1779–85
17. Morley, J. E., Levine, A. S., Murray, S. S. 1981. Flavor enhances the antidipsogenic effect of substance P. *Brain Res.* 226:334–38
18. Rozin, P., Ebert, L., Schull, L. 1982. Some like it hot: A temporal analysis of hedonic responses to chili peppers. *Appetite* 3:13–22
19. Solomon, R. L. 1977. An opponent process theory of motivation. V. Affective dynamics of eating. In *Learning Mechanisms in Food Selection,* ed. L. Barker, M. R. Best, M. Domjon, pp. 255–69. Waco, TX: Baylor Univ. Press
20. Del Rio, J., Naranjo, J. R., Yang, H.-Y. T., Costa, E. 1983. Substance P induced release of met-5-enkephalin from striatal and periaqueductal gray slices. *Brain Res.* 279:121–26
21. Gosnell, B. A., Hsiao, S. 1981. Cholecystokinin satiety and orosensory feedback. *Physiol. Behav.* 27:153–56
22. Waldbillig, R. J., Bartness, T. J. 1982. The suppression of sucrose intake by cholecystokinin is scaled according to the magnitude of the orosensory control over feeding. *Physiol. Behav.* 28:591–95
23. Antin, J., Gibbs, J., Smith, G. P. 1978. Cholecystokinin interacts with pregastric food stimulation to elicit satiety in the rat. *Physiol. Behav.* 20:67–70
24. Morin, M. P., DeMarchi, P., Champagnat, J., Vanderhaeghen, J. J., Rossier, J., Denavit-Saubie, M. 1983. Inhibitory

effect of cholecystokinin octapeptide on neurons in the nucleus of tractus solitarius. *Brain Res.* 265:333–38
25. Gosnell, B. A., Hsaio, S. 1984. The effects of cholecystokinin on taste preference and sensitivity in rats. *Behav. Neurosci.* 98:452–60
26. Davis, W. J., Mpitsos, G. J., Pinneo, J. M. 1974. The behavioral hierarchy of the mollusk, Pleurobranchea. II. Hormonal suppression of feeding associated with egg laying. *J. Comp. Physiol.* 95:225–43
27. Coleman, D. L. 1973. Effects of parabiosis of obese with diabetes and normal mice. *Diabetologia* 9:294–98
28. Hervey, G. R. 1959. The effects of lesions in the hypothalamus in parabiotic rats. *J. Physiol.* 145:336–52
29. Morley, J. E. 1982. The ascent of cholecystokinin (CCK): From gut to brain. *Life Sci.* 30:479–93
30. Gibbs, J., Young, R. C., Smith, G. P. 1973. Cholecystokinin decreases food intake in rats. *J. Comp. Physiol. Psychol.* 84:488–91
31. Smith, G. P., Gibbs, J. 1977. Cholecystokinin and satiety in rats and rhesus monkeys. *Am. J. Clin. Nutr.* 30:758–61
32. McLaughlin, C. L., Peikin, S. R., Baile, C. A. 1983. Trypsin inhibitor effects on food intake and weight gain in Zucker rats. *Physiol. Behav.* 31:487–91
33. Deutsch, J. A. 1982. Controversies in food intake regulation. In *The Neural Basis of Feeding and Reward,* ed. B. G. Hoebel, D. Novin. Brunswick, ME: Haer Inst.
34. Billington, C. J., Levine, A. S., Morley, J. E. 1983. Are peptides truly satiety agents? A method of testing for neurohumoral satiety effects. *Am. J. Physiol.* 245:R920–26
35. Kissileff, H. R., Pi-Sunyer, F. X., Thornton, J., Smith, G. P. 1981. C-terminal octapeptide of cholecystokinin decreases food intake in man. *Am. J. Clin. Nutr.* 34:154–60
36. Pi-Sunyer, F. X., Kissileff, H. R., Thornton, J., Smith, G. P. 1982. C-terminal octapeptide of cholecystokinin decreases food intake in obese men. *Physiol. Behav.* 29:627–30
37. Greenway, F. L., Bray, G. A. 1977. Cholecystokinin and satiety. *Life Sci.* 21:769–71
38. Sturdevant, R., Goetz, H. 1976. Cholecystokinin both stimulates and inhibits human food intake. *Nature* 261:713–15
39. Stacher, G., Steinringer, H., Schnierer, G., Schneider, C., Winklehner, S. 1982. Cholecystokinin octapeptide decreases

intake of solid food in man. *Peptides* 3:133–36

40. Smith, G. P., Jerome, C., Cushin, B. J., Eterno, R., Simansky, K. J. 1981. Abdominal vagotomy blocks the satiety effect of cholecystokinin: A progress report. *Peptides* 2:57–59

41. Morley, J. E., Levine, A. S., Kneip, J., Grace, M. 1982. The effect of vagotomy on the satiety effects of neuropeptides and naloxone. *Life Sci.* 30:1943–47

42. Levine, A. S., Sievert, C. E., Morley, J. E., Gosnell, B. A., Silvis, S. E. 1984. Peptidergic regulation of feeding in the dog *(Canis familiaris)*. *Peptides.* 5:675–78

43. Della-Fera, M. A., Baile, C. A. 1979. Cholecystokinin octapeptide: Continuous picomole injections into the cerebral ventricles suppress feeding. *Science* 206:471–73

44. Della-Fera, M. A., Baile, C. A., Schneider, B. S., Grinker, J. A. 1981. Cholecystokinin-antibody injected in cerebral ventricles stimulates feeding in sheep. *Science* 212:687–89

45. Denbow, D. M., Myers, R. D. 1982. Eating, drinking and temperature responses to intracerebroventricular cholecystokinin in the chick. *Peptides* 3:739–43

46. Gibbs, J., Fauser, D. J., Rowe, E. A., Rolls, B. J., Rolls, E. T., Maddison, S. P. 1979. Bombesin suppresses feeding in rats. *Nature* 282:208–10

47. Morley, J. E., Levine, A. S. 1981. Bombesin inhibits stress-induced eating. *Pharmacol. Biochem. Behav.* 14:149–51

48. Stuckey, J. A., Gibbs, J. 1982. Lateral hypothalamic injection of bombesin decreases food intake in rats. *Brain Res. Bull.* 8:617–21

49. Muurahainen, N. E., Kissileff, H. R., Thornton, J., Pi-Sunyer, F. X. 1983. Bombesin: Another peptide that inhibits feeding in man. *Soc. Neurosci. Abstr.* 9:183

50. Stein, L. J., Woods, S. C. 1982. Gastrin releasing peptide reduces meal size in rats. *Peptides* 3:833–35

51. Morley, J. E., Levine, A. S., Kneip, J., Grace, M., Billington, C. J. 1983. The effect of peripherally administered satiety substances on feeding induced by butorphanol tartrate. *Pharmacol. Biochem. Behav.* 19:577–82

52. Lotter, E. C., Krinsky, R., McKay, J. M., Treneer, C. M., Porte, D., Woods, S. C. 1981. Somatostatin decreases food intake in rats and baboons. *J. Comp. Physiol. Psychol.* 95:278–87

53. Levine, A. S., Morley, J. E. 1982.

Peripherally administered somatostatin reduces feeding by a vagal mediated mechanism. *Pharmacol. Biochem. Behav.* 16:897–902

54. Schulman, J. C., Carleton, J. L., Whitney, G., Whitehorn, J. C. 1957. Effect of glucagon on food intake and body weight in man. *J. Appl. Physiol.* 11:419–21

55. Martin, T. R., Novin, D., Van der Weele, D. A. 1978. Loss of glucagon suppression of feeding following vagotomy in rats. *Am. J. Physiol.* 3:E314–18

56. Van der Weele, D. A., Haraczkiewicz, E., Di Conti, M. 1980. Pancreatic glucagon administration, feeding, glycemia and liver glycogen in rats. *Brain Res. Bull.* 4:17–21

57. Geary, N., Smith, G. P. 1983. Selective hepatic vagotomy blocks pancreatic glucagon's satiety effect. *Physiol. Behav.* 31:391–94

58. Langhans, W., Zieger, U., Scharrer, E., Geary, N. 1982. Stimulation of feeding in rats by intraperitoneal injection of antibodies to glucagon. *Science* 218:894–95

59. Malaisse-Lagae, F., Carpenter, J. L., Patel, Y. C., Malaisse, W. J., Orci, L. 1977. Pancreatic polypeptide: A possible role in the regulation of food intake in the mouse. *Hypoth. Exp.* 33:915–17

60. Carlson, A. J. 1916. *The Control of Hunger in Health and Disease.* Chicago: Univ. Chicago Press

61. Mayer, J. 1952. The glucostatic theory of regulation of food intake. *Bull. New York Med. Ctr.* 14:43–49

62. Oomura, Y. 1976. Significance of glucose, insulin and free fatty acid on the hypothalamic feeding and satiety neurons. In *Hunger: Basic Mechanisms and Clinical Applications,* ed. D. Novin, W. Wyrwicka, G. A. Bray, pp. 145–51. New York: Raven

63. Mellinkoff, S. M., Frankland, M., Boyle, D., Greipel, M. 1956. Relationship between serum amino acid concentrations and fluctuations in appetite. *J. Appl. Physiol.* 8:535–38

64. Wurtman, R. J. 1983. Behavioral effects of nutrients. *Lancet* 1:1145–47

65. Kennedy, G. C. 1972. The regulation of food intake. *Adv. Psychosom. Med.* 7:91–99

66. Glick, Z. 1980. Food intake of rats administered with glycerol. *Physiol. Behav.* 25:621–26

67. Brobeck, J. R. 1958. Food intake as a mechanism of temperature regulation. *Yale J. Biol. Med.* 20:545–52

68. Andersson, B., Larsson, B. 1961. Influence of local temperature changes in the preoptic area and the rostral hypothala-

mus on the regulation of food and water intake. *Acta Physiol. Scand.* 52:75–89

69. Morley, J. E., Levine, A. S., Oken, M. M., Grace, M., Kneip, J. 1982. Neuropeptides and thermoregulation: The interactions of bombesin, neurotensin, TRH, somatostatin, naloxone and prostaglandins. *Peptides* 3:1–6

70. Capogrossi, M. C., Francendese, A., DiGirolama, M. 1979. Suppression of food intake by adenosine and inosine. *Am. J. Clin. Nutr.* 32:1762–68

71. Levine, A. S., Morley, J. E. 1982. Purinergic regulation of food intake. *Science* 217:77–79

72. Levine, A. S., Morley, J. E. 1983. Effect of intraventricular adenosine on food intake in rats. *Pharmacol. Biochem. Behav.* 19:23–26

73. Levine, A. S., Srdar, S., Morley, J. E. 1983. Purines and the regulation of food intake. *Integr. Psych.* 1:4–14

74. Wager-Srdar, S. A., Levine, A. S., Morley, J. E. 1984. Food intake: Opioid/purine interactions. *Pharmacol. Biochem. Behav.* 21:33–38

75. Agren, H., Nikalsson, F., Hallgren, R. 1983. Brain purinergic activity linked with depressive symptomatology: Hypoxanthine and xanthine in CSF of patients with major depressive disorders. *Psychiat. Res.* 9:179–89

76. Woods, S. C., Decek, E., Vasselli, J. R. 1974. Metabolic hormones and regulation of body weight. *Psychol. Res.* 81:26–35

77. Woods, S. C., Porte, D. Jr. 1977. Relationship between plasma and cerebrospinal fluid insulin levels of the dog. *Am. J. Physiol.* 233:E331–36

78. Woods, S. C., Lotter, E. C., McKay, L., Porte, D. Jr. 1979. Chronic intracerebroventricular intake and body weight of baboons. *Nature* 282:503–5

79. Stein, L. J., Dorsa, D. M., Baskin, D. G., Figliwicz, D. P., Ikeda, H., et al. 1983. Immunoreactive insulin levels are elevated in the cerebrospinal fluid of genetically obese Zucker rats. *Endocrinology* 113:2299–301

80. Strubbe, J. H., Mein, C. G. 1977. Increased feeding in response to bilateral injection of insulin antibodies in the VMH. *Physiol. Behav.* 17:309–14

81. Tannenbaum, G. S., Guyda, H. J., Posner, B. I. 1983. Insulin-like growth factors: A role in growth hormone negative feedback and body weight regulation. *Science* 220:777–79

82. Holtzman, S. G. 1974. Behavioral effects of separate and combined administration of naloxone and d-amphetamine. *J. Pharmacol. Exp. Ther.* 189:51–60

83. Morley, J. E., Levine, A. S., Yim, G. K. W., Lowy, M. T. 1983. Opioid modulation of appetite. *Neurosci. Biobehav. Rev.* 7:281–305

84. Jaloweic, J. E., Panksepp, J., Zolovick, A. J., Najam, N., Herman, B. 1981. Opioid modulation of ingestive behavior. *Pharmacol. Biochem. Behav.* 15:477–84

85. Brands, B., Thornhill, J. A., Hirst, M., Gowdey, C. W. 1979. Suppression of food intake and body weight gain by naloxone in rats. *Life Sci.* 24:1773–78

86. Morley, J. E., Levine, A. S., Murray, S. S., Kneip, J. 1982. Peptidergic regulation of norepinephrine induced feeding. *Pharmacol. Biochem. Behav.* 16:225–28

87. Morley, J. E., Levine, A. S., Kneip, J. 1981. Muscimol induced feeding: A model to study the hypothalamic regulation of appetite. *Life Sci.* 29:1213–18

88. Lowy, M. T., Maickel, R. P., Yim, G. K. W. 1980. Naloxone reduction of stress-related feeding. *Life Sci.* 26:2113–18

89. Morley, J. E., Levine, A. S. 1980. Stress induced eating is mediated through endogenous opiates. *Science* 209:1259–61

90. Morley, J. E., Levine, A. S., Gosnell, B. A., Billington, C. J. 1984. Which opioid receptor mechanism modulates feeding? *Appetite.* 5:61–68

91. Sanger, D. J., McCarthy, P. S. 1981. The anorectic effect of naloxone is attenuated by adaptation to a food-deprivation schedule. *Psychopharmacology* 74:217–20

92. Marks-Kaufman, R., Kanarek, R. B. 1980. Morphine selectively influences macronutrient intake in the rat. *Pharmacol. Biochem. Behav.* 12:427–30

93. Mandenoff, A., Fumeson, F., Appelbaum, M., Margules, D. L. 1982. Endogenous opiates and energy balance. *Science* 215:1536–38

94. Shimonura, Y., Oku, J., Glick, Z., Bray, G. A. 1982. Opiate receptors, food intake and obesity. *Physiol. Behav.* 28:441–43

95. Levine, A. S., Morley, J. E. 1981. Peptidergic control of insulin-induced feeding. *Peptides* 2:261–64

96. Levine, A. S., Morley, J. E., Brown, D. M., Handwerger, B. S. 1982. Extreme sensitivity of diabetic mice to naloxone-induced suppression of food intake. *Physiol. Behav.* 28:987–89

97. Morley, J. E., Levine, A. S., Grace, M., Kneip, J., Gosnell, B. A. 1984. The effect of ovariectomy, estradiol and pro-

gesterone on opioid modulation of feeding. *Physiol. Behav.* 33:237–41

98. Levine, A. S., Morley, J. E. 1983. Adrenal modulation of opiate induced feeding. *Pharmacol. Biochem. Behav.* 19:403–6

99. Morley, J. E., Levine, A. S., Plotka, E. D., Seal, U. S. 1983. The effect of naloxone on feeding and spontaneous locomotion in the wolf. *Physiol. Behav.* 30:331–34

100. Atkinson, R. L. 1982. Naloxone decreases food intake in obese humans. *J. Clin. Endocrinol. Metab.* 55:196–98

101. Atkinson, R. L. 1983. Naltrexone for weight loss in obesity. *Abstr. 4th Intl. Congr. Obesity* 30A:81

102. Lowy, M. T., Yim, G. K. W. 1982. Drinking, but not feeding is opiate sensitive in hamsters. *Life Sci.* 30:1639–44

103. Billington, C. J., Morley, J. E., Levine, A. S., Gerritsen, G. C. 1984. Feeding systems in Chinese hamsters. *Am. J. Physiol.* 247:R408–11

104. Nizielski, S. E., Levine, A. S., Morley, J. E., Plotka, E. D., Seal, U. S. 1982. Lack of feeding suppression with naloxone in torpid hibernating animals. *Fed. Proc.* 42:5259

105. Sanger, D. J., McCarthy, P. S. 1981. Increased food and water intake produced in rats by opiate receptor agonists. *Psychopharmacology* 74:217–20

106. Levine, A. S., Morley, J. E. 1983. Butorphanol tartrate induces feeding in rats. *Life Sci.* 32:781–85

107. Morley, J. E., Levine, A. S. 1981. Dynorphin-(1–13) induces spontaneous feeding in rats. *Life Sci.* 29:1901–3

108. Morley, J. E., Levine, A. S. 1983. Involvement of dynorphin and the kappa opioid receptor in feeding. *Peptides* 4:797–800

109. Chavkin, C., Goldstein, A. 1981. Specific receptor for the opioid peptide dynorphin: Structure-activity relationships. *Proc. Natl. Acad. Sci. USA* 78:6543–47

110. Morley, J. E., Elson, M. K., Levine, A. S., Shafer, R. B. 1982. The effects of stress on central nervous system concentrations of the opioid peptide, dynorphin. *Peptides* 3:901–6

111. Reid, L. D., Konecka, A. M., Prezewlocki, R., Millan, M. H., Millan, M. J., Herz, A. 1982. Endogenous opioids, circadian rhythms, nutrient deprivation, eating and drinking. *Life Sci.* 31:1829–32

112. Leibowitz, S. F., Hor, L. 1982. Endorphinergic and α-noradrenergic systems in the paraventricular nucleus: Effects on eating behavior. *Peptides* 3:421–28

113. Tepperman, F. S., Hirst, M. 1983.

Effects of intrahypothalamic injection of D-ala^2, D-Leu^5-enkephalin on feeding and temperature in the rat. *Eur. J. Pharmacol.* 96:243–49

114. Morley, J. E. 1983. Neuroendocrine effects of endogenous opioid peptides in human subjects: A review. *Psychoneuroendocrinology* 8:361–79

115. Grossman, S. P. 1962. Direct adrenergic and cholinergic stimulation of hypothalamic mechanisms. *Am. J. Physiol.* 303:872–82

116. Leibowitz, S. F. 1975. Amphetamine: Possible site and mode of action for producing anorexia in the rat. *Brain Res.* 84:160–65

117. Sawchenko, P. E., Gold, R. M., Leibowitz, S. F. 1981. Evidence for vagal involvement in the eating elicited by adrenergic stimulation of the paraventricular nucleus. *Brain Res.* 225:249–69

118. Leibowitz, S. F., Roland, C. R., Hor, L., Squillari, V. 1984. Noradrenergic feeding elicited via the paraventricular nucleus is dependent upon circulating corticosterone. *Physiol. Behav.* 32:857–64

119. Leibowitz, S. F., Hammer, N. J., Chang, K. 1983. Feeding behavior induced by central norepinephrine injection is attenuated by discrete lesions in the hypothalamic paraventricular nucleus. *Pharmacol. Biochem. Behav.* 19:945–50

120. Blundell, J. E. 1979. Serotonin and feeding. In *Serotonin in Health and Disease,* ed. W. B. Esmon, 5:403–50. New York: Spectrum

121. Davies, R. F., Rossi, J. III, Panksepp, J., Bean, N. J., Zolovik, A. J. 1983. Fenfluramine anorexia: A peripheral locus of action. *Physiol. Behav.* 30:723–30

122. Ungerstedt, U. 1971. Stereotaxic mapping of the monoamine pathways in the rat brain. *Acta Physiol. Scand. Suppl.* 367:1–48

123. Morley, J. E., Levine, A. S., Grace, M., Kneip, J. 1982. Dynorphin-(1–13), dopamine and feeding in rats. *Pharmacol. Biochem. Behav.* 16:701–5

124. Blundell, J. E., Burridge, S. L. 1980. Control of feeding and the psychopharmacology of anorexic drugs. In *Obesity and Its Treatment,* ed. J. Munro, pp. 53–81. Lancaster, PA: MTP

125. Dourish, C. T. 1982. Phenylethylamine-induced anorexia in the albino rat. See Ref. 33, pp. 543–49

126. Paul, S. M., Hulihan-Giblin, B., Skolnick, P. 1982. (+)-Amphetamine binding to rat hypothalamus: Relation to anorexic potency of phenylethylamines. *Science* 218:487–90

127. Tatemoto, K. 1982. Neuropeptide Y:

Complete amino acid sequence of the brain peptide. *Proc. Natl. Acad. Sci. USA* 79:5485–89

128. Emson, P. C., Dequidt, M. E. 1984. NPY—A new member of the pancreatic polypeptide family. *Trends Neurosci.* 7:31–35

129. Clark, J. J., Kalra, P. S., Crowley, W. R., Kalra, S. P. 1984. Neuropeptide Y and human pancreatic polypeptide stimulate feeding behavior in rats. *Endocrinology.* 115:427–29

130. Freed, W. J., Perlow, M. J., Wyatt, R. D. 1979. Calcitonin: Inhibitory effect on eating in rats. *Science* 206:850–52

131. Levine, A. S., Morley, J. E. 1981. Reduction of feeding in rats by calcitonin. *Brain Res.* 222:187–91

132. Rosenfeld, M., Mermod, J.-J., Amara, S. G., Swanson, L. W., Sawchenko, P. E., Rivier, J., Vale, W. W., Evans, R. M. 1983. Production of a novel neuropeptide encoded by the calcitonin gene via tissue specific RNA processing. *Nature* 304:129–35

133. Krahn, D. D., Gosnell, B. A., Levine, A. S., Morley, J. E. 1984. Effect of calcitonin gene-related peptide on feeding. *Peptides* 5:861–64

134. Morley, J. E., Levine, A. S. 1981. Bombesin inhibits stress-induced eating. *Pharmacol. Biochem. Behav.* 14:149–51

135. Gibbs, J., Kulkosky, P. J., Smith, G. P. 1981. Effects of peripheral and central bombesin on feeding behavior of rats. *Peptides* 2:179–83

136. Porreca, F., Burks, T. F. 1983. Centrally administered bombesin effects gastric emptying and small and large bowel transit in the rat. *Gastroenterology* 85:313–17

137. Tache, Y., Vale, W., Rivier, J., Brown, M. 1980. Brain regulation of gastric secretion: Influence of neuropeptides. *Proc. Natl. Acad. Sci. USA* 77:5515–19

138. Stuckey, J. A., Gibbs, J. 1982. Lateral hypothalamic injection of bombesin de-

creases food intake in rats. *Brain Res. Bull.* 8:617–21

139. Vale, W., Spiess, J., Rivier, C., Rivier, J. 1981. Characterization of a 41-residue ovine hypothalamic peptide that stimulates secretion of corticotropin and β-endorphin. *Science* 213:1394–97

140. Morley, J. E., Levine, A. S. 1982. Corticotropin releasing factor, grooming and ingestive behavior. *Life Sci.* 31:1459–64

141. Gosnell, B. A., Morley, J. E., Levine, A. S. 1983. Adrenal modulation of the inhibitory effect of corticotropin releasing factor on feeding. *Peptides* 4:807–12

142. Morley, J. E., Levine, A. S., Gosnell, B. A., Billington, C. J., Krahn, D. D. 1984. Control of food intake. In *Neuroendocrine Perspectives,* ed. R. M. McLeod, E. Muller. Amsterdam: Elsevier Biomed. In press

143. Stanley, B. G., Hoebel, B. G., Leibowitz, S. F. 1983. Neurotensin: Effects of hypothalamic and intravenous injections on eating and drinking in rats. *Peptides* 4:493–500

144. Luttinger, D., King, R. A., Shippard, D., Strup, J., Nemeroff, C. B., Prange, A. J. Jr. 1981. The effect of neurotensin on food consumption in the rat. *Eur. J. Pharmacol.* 81:699–703

145. Levine, A. S., Kneip, J., Grace, M., Morley, J. E. 1983. Effect of centrally administered neurotensin on multiple feeding paradigms. *Pharmacol. Biochem. Behav.* 18:19–23

146. Vijayan, E., McCann, S. M. 1977. Suppression of feeding and drinking activity in rats following intraventricular injection of thyrotropin releasing hormone (TRH). *Endocrinology* 100:1727–30

147. Morley, J. E., Levine, A. S. 1980. Thyrotropin releasing hormone (TRH) suppresses stress induced eating. *Life Sci.* 27:269–74

148. Morley, J. E., Levine, A. S., Prasad, C. 1981. Histidyl-proline diketopiperazine decreases food intake in rats. *Brain Res.* 210:475–78

Ann. Rev. Pharmacol. Toxicol. 1985. 25:147–70

PHOSPHATIDYLINOSITOL TURNOVER IN RECEPTOR MECHANISM AND SIGNAL TRANSDUCTION

Keisuke Hirasawa

Department of Cell Biology, National Institute for Basic Biology, Okazaki 444, Japan

Yasutomi Nishizuka

Department of Biochemistry, Kobe University School of Medicine, Kobe 650, Japan, and Department of Cell Biology, National Institute for Basic Biology, Okazaki 444, Japan

INTRODUCTION

The activation of cellular functions and proliferation are frequently initiated by the interaction of external stimuli with their specific cell-surface receptors. Early events of the intracellular response include a metabolic cascade of membrane phospholipids. Investigations of the target site of biochemical changes in cell membranes have focused particularly on the immediate breakdown of inositol phospholipids and the accumulation of phosphatidic acid.

As early as 1953, Hokin & Hokin (1) observed that one effect of acetylcholine on pancreas slices was the rapid enhancement of phospholipid metabolism, specifically, the incorporation of $^{32}P_i$ into phosphatidylinositol (PtdIns) and phosphatidic acid. Later, the physiological significance of this original observation was found in the cholinergic release of amylase from pancreatic acinar cells (2). A specific increase in the turnover of PtdIns has since been documented repeatedly in a number of tissues in response to stimulation by a wide variety of neurotransmitters, hormones, and many other biologically active substances [for reviews, see (3–6)]. The activation of the receptors involved, for example, muscarinic rather than nicotinic and α- rather than

147

β-adrenergic, which constitute a class distinct from those acting through cyclic AMP, results in the increased availability of other second messengers such as Ca^{2+} (7). In no system does cyclic AMP or its derivatives elicit such phospholipid metabolic effects. The precise consequences and physiological significance of these effects are not yet fully understood. However, many functions for the stimulated PtdIns turnover thus far have been proposed: e.g. membrane fusion (8,9), early events in cell proliferation (10, 11), elevation of intracellular Ca^{2+} concentration, arachidonic acid release (12–14), increases in cyclic GMP levels (15–17), and visual signal transduction (18, 19).

In recent years, polyphosphoinositides, particularly phosphatidylinositol 4,5-bisphosphate (PtdIns4,5P$_2$), which represent less than a few percent of the total inositol phospholipids (20) and are relatively enriched in the nervous system (21), have been studied with renewed interest. Rapid disappearance of the phospholipid has been observed in stimulated cells, and more recently the water soluble product, inositol 1,4,5-trisphosphate, has been proposed by Berridge and his colleagues (22,23) to be an intracellular mediator for the release of Ca^{2+} from internal stores. On the other hand, Nishizuka and colleagues (24,25) have demonstrated that a small amount of another product, diacylglycerol, acts as a novel intracellular mediator and stimulates a unique Ca^{2+}-activated, phospholipid-dependent protein kinase (protein kinase C). Thus, the receptor-mediated turnover of inositol phospholipid appears to represent a multifunctional second messenger–transducing mechanism (Figure 1).

THE ASSOCIATION OF CYTOSOLIC Ca^{2+} ELEVATION

The stimulation of the receptors relating to inositol phospholipid breakdown is usually accompanied by an elevation of intracellular Ca^{2+}. The second-messenger function for Ca^{2+} has been proposed in many stimulated tissues (26–28). The intracellular Ca^{2+} can be raised both by external influx and by release from its internal stores. When blowfly salivary gland is stimulated with 5-hydroxytryptamine in Ca^{2+}-free media, the decline in secretion is not immediate, but there is a short initial period during which a normal secretory response may be observed. Prince & Berridge (29) have suggested that this temporary independence of external Ca^{2+} is probably maintained by the internal mobilization of this divalent cation. In addition, in the liver, the glycogenolytic action of α_1-adrenergic agonists and vasoactive peptide hormones is mediated by an initial increase in the cytosolic Ca^{2+} concentration that is probably released from intracellular compartments (30, 31). Farese et al (2) have reported that in rat pancreatic slices the removal of Ca^{2+} from the media abolishes both the cholinergic release of amylase and the chemically measurable loss of PtdIns. Thus, in some tissues at least, external Ca^{2+} influx appears to have a role in the long-term potential of physiological cell responses.

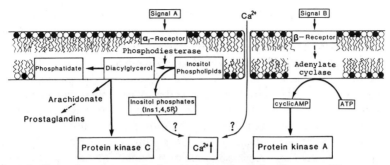

Figure 1   Two major receptor mechanisms in transmembrane signaling. α_1- and β-receptors are used as representatives. Ins1,4,5P$_3$: inositol 1,4,5-trisphosphate; protein kinase A: cyclic AMP-dependent protein kinase.

In 1975, Michell (4) proposed that breakdown of inositol phospholipids is responsible for opening the Ca^{2+} gate. Some of the implications of this proposal have been reviewed by Cockcroft (32) and Hawthorne (33). Many studies have been made as to whether Ca^{2+}-ionophores provoke the degradation of inositol phospholipids. Creba et al (34) have reported that disappearance of ^{32}P-labeled phosphatidylinositol 4-phosphate (PtdIns4P) and PtdIns4,5P$_2$ is not observed when cells are incubated with the Ca^{2+} ionophore A23187. In Ca^{2+}-depleted cells, hormone-stimulated polyphosphoinositide disappearance is reduced but not abolished.

However, to date there has been no conclusive agreement among previous reports, probably because the phosphodiesterase must be activated not only by Ca^{2+} but also by unknown mechanisms such as proteolytic activation (35). Unless the phosphodiesterase is activated, the inositol phospholipids will not be hydrolyzed, even if the intracellular Ca^{2+} is increased by the addition of a Ca^{2+} ionophore. The question of what is responsible for opening channels for external Ca^{2+} still remains to be resolved. Recently, Cachelin et al (36) have proposed that in some tissues cyclic AMP–dependent phosphorylation of Ca^{2+} channels primarily promotes the forward rate constants that lead to the open state of Ca^{2+} channels during depolarization.

INOSITOL PHOSPHOLIPID TURNOVER AND POLYPHOSPHOINOSITIDES

In pancreas, an enhanced turnover of PtdIns in response to acetylcholine is accompanied by the formation of phosphatidic acid, which can be approximately equal to the decrease in the level of PtdIns (37). In stimulated tissues the lipid-soluble products of inositol phospholipid breakdown appear as phosphatidic acid, CDP-diacylglycerol, or diacylglycerol (38). The overall pathway of PtdIns turnover is known as the PtdIns-resynthesis cycle. The first step of this cycle is initiated by a Ca^{2+}-dependent phospholipase C-type phosphodiesterase(s) that hydrolyzes inositol phospholipids to produce diacylglycerol and inositol phosphates (39–42). The diacylglycerol is then immediately phosphorylated to phosphatidic acid with ATP by the reaction of diacylglycerol kinase (43). The measurement of enhanced $^{32}P_i$ incorporation into PtdIns and phosphatidic acid is therefore a secondary effect of external stimuli on inositol phospholipids breakdown. Results obtained using this method have lead to considerable confusion over the stimulated PtdIns turnover, for example, over the important question of which inositol phospholipids are really hydrolyzed by the phosphodiesterase in response to external stimuli. Earlier reports do not appear to support a primary role for polyphosphoinositides in stimulated phosphatidic acid and PtdIns labeling (44–46), possibly because the changes seen are relatively small and rapid. However, two polyphosphoinositides, PtdIns4P and PtdIns4,5P$_2$, are potentially more interesting as membrane constituents because of their unique physicochemical properties. Particularly PtdIns4,5P$_2$ is a multiply-charged anion that has a very high affinity for Ca^{2+} (greater than that of EDTA) and exhibits a rapid turnover in vivo. Its hydrophilic/hydrophobic solubility partition coefficient is markedly altered when Ca^{2+} replaces monovalent phosphate counterions (47–49).

The phosphorylated PtdIns-derivatives PtdIns4P and PtdIns4,5P$_2$ are synthesized by the stepwise phosphorylation of PtdIns by the enzyme PtdIns kinase and PtdIns4P kinase. PtdIns kinase has been described in a variety of tissues, erythrocytes (50), brain (51–54), liver (55, 56), and kidney (57), where subcellular fractionation studies have suggested that it is localized in the plasma membrane. One area of recent interest has been the relationship between the transforming genes and phosphorylation of PtdIns and diacylglycerol (58, 59). Phosphomonoesterases that degrade PtdIns4,5P$_2$ to PtdIns4P and thence to PtdIns are also present (Figure 2).

THE DISAPPEARANCE OF INOSITOL PHOSPHOLIPIDS

PtdIns4P and PtdIns4,5P$_2$, very minor phospholipids in the inner leaflet of cell membranes, have been considered alternative candidates to PtdIns in the early breakdown of inositol phospholipids by receptor-mediated hydrolysis (60). Like PtdIns, these phospholipids may be degraded by phosphodiesterase action to inositol phosphates and diacylglycerol (41, 61).

It has recently been suggested that the breakdown of PtdIns4P and PtdIns4,5P$_2$ may precede the previously known PtdIns response. Rapid signal-induced breakdown of PtdIns4P and PtdIns4,5P$_2$ has been reported in a variety of tissues [for a review, see (62)]. For example, results from iris smooth muscle have shown that the activation of muscarinic cholinergic and α_1-adrenergic receptors results in the immediate breakdown of PtdIns4,5P$_2$ but not of PtdIns

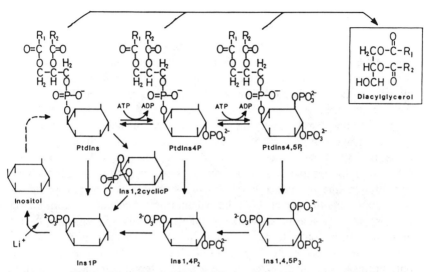

Figure 2   Production of diacylglycerol and inositol phosphates in inositol phospholipid metabolism. PtdIns: phosphatidylinositol; PtdIns4P: phosphatidylinositol 4-phosphate; PtdIns4,5P$_2$: phosphatidylinositol 4,5-bisphosphate; Ins1P: inositol 1-phosphate; Ins1,2 cyclic P: inositol 1,2-cyclic phosphate; Ins1,4P$_2$: inositol 1,4-bisphosphate; Ins1,4,5P$_3$: inositol 1,4,5-trisphosphate.

or PtdIns4P (63–65). Michell and his colleagues have also observed that Ca^{2+}-mobilizing hormones such as vasopressin, angiotensin II, and epinephrine active at the α_1-receptor provoke rapid degradation of ^{32}P-labeled PtdIns4P and PtdIns4,5P$_2$ in hepatocytes (34, 66). The maximum disappearance of PtdIns4,5P$_2$ is detected one minute after the addition of vasopressin. Similar results have been obtained in the early actions of thyrotropin-releasing hormone on hormone-responsive clonal GH$_3$ pituitary cells (67), carbachol and pancreozymin on pancreatic acinar cells (68), and thrombin on platelets (69). Addition of these stimulators results in the rapid disappearance of labeled polyphosphoinositide(s), whereas levels of PtdIns and other phospholipids remain unchanged. Litosch et al (70) have observed the breakdown of both PtdIns and PtdIns4,5P$_2$ in response to vasopressin in hepatocytes within 30 seconds. More recently, Orchard et al (71) have described the stimulation by carbachol or pancreozymin of ^{32}P-labeled rat pancreas acinar cells, which causes a decrease of PtdIns4,5P$_2$ by 30–50% within 10–15 seconds; this decrease is followed by the sequential increase in ^{32}P$_i$ incorporation into phosphatidic acid and PtdIns. This signal-induced disappearance of PtdIns4,5P$_2$ is not dependent on external Ca^{2+}. These authors of this study have suggested that the disappearance may initiate the Ca^{2+}-independent labeling of phosphatidic acid and PtdIns. Ca^{2+} mobilization may follow these responses and subsequently cause Ca^{2+}-dependent hydrolysis of PtdIns and exocytosis.

These observations raise the possibility that the initial action of various extracellular messengers involves the hydrolysis of polyphosphoinositides. At present, it is still not absolutely clear which inositol phospholipid is specifically cleaved by the phosphodiesterase. Michell (72) has speculated that PtdIns is never hydrolyzed by phospholipase C-type enzyme but disappears due to sequential phosphorylation by the specific kinases. If this is correct, a continuous increase of PtdIns4,5P$_2$ may be expected during stimulation. The kinase probably has to be activated in order to replenish the polyphosphoinositides, since disappearance of PtdIns continues over rather a long period. Using carbamyl-choline injection as the cholinergic stimulation of polyphosphoinositide metabolism, Soukup et al (73) have demonstrated enhanced incorporation of phosphate as well as inositol into polyphosphoinositides in regions of the rat brain in vivo. In contrast, the stimulation of hepatocytes by vasopressin does not result in an increase of PtdIns4,5P$_2$ (34). It seems still early to conclude that only PtdIns4,5P$_2$ is hydrolyzed in response to external stimuli. It is possible that the three inositol phospholipids are hydrolyzed by the phosphodiesterase(s) at different times in different rates, or, as Hokin-Neaverson & Sadeghian (74) have speculated, that polyphosphoinositide and PtdIns responses occur at different sites within the cell.

THE PHOSPHOLIPASE C-TYPE CLEAVAGE

Since the discovery of specific phosphodiesterase in pancreas (39) and liver (75), it has been proposed that the phospholipase C-type cleavage of inositol phospholipids is responsible for the receptor-mediated PtdIns turnover. Until recently this hypothesis has not been fully substantiated, but researchers now agree that the putative initial step of increased PtdIns turnover following receptor stimulation is due to the hydrolysis of inositol phospholipids by specific phosphodiesterase(s). This is supported by recent studies that used direct chemical measurement of the water soluble products, inositol 1-phosphate and inositol cyclic 1,2-phosphate from PtdIns, or inositol 1,4-bisphosphate and inositol 1,4,5-trisphosphate from PtdIns4P and PtdIns4,5P$_2$, respectively. Durell et al (76) have observed that the primary effect of acetylcholine is to stimulate the hydrolysis of the inositol phospholipids. This reaction has been best observed over a short period; a trace of inositol 1,4,5-trisphosphate and the accumulation of inositol 1,4-bisphosphate and inositol 1-phosphate are measured. The enhanced incorporation of $^{32}P_i$ into the phospholipids subsequently observed is thus a secondary synthetic reaction that occurs due to the increased concentration of diacylglycerol bound to active membranes. In addition, when platelets are stimulated to aggregate by thrombin (13), diacylglycerol is observed as an early product of inositol phospholipid catabolism. In their serial experiments with insect salivary gland stimulated by 5-hydroxytryptamine, a very short time after stimulation Berridge and his colleagues (77, 78) saw a large and rapid increase in the levels of inositol 1,4,5-trisphosphate and inositol 1,4-bisphosphate but no change in the amount of inositol 1-phosphate or inositol present. Similar results have been reported in rat parotid gland after muscarinic stimulation (79) and in GH_3 pituitary cell following stimulation by thyrotropin-releasing hormone (67).

It is known that the inhibitory effect of lithium ion on *myo*-inositol 1-phosphate phosphatase, which is different from $PtdIns4,5P_2$ phosphomonoesterase, causes an increase in the level of *myo*-inositol 1-phosphate both in vivo (80) and in vitro (81, 82). This may be related to the control of manic-depressive illness. A recent study by Hokin-Neaverson & Sadeghian (74) has shown lithium-induced accumulation of inositol 1-phosphate during cholecystokinin octapeptide and acetylcholine stimulation of mouse pancreas acinar cells. These authors have noted that inositol 1,4,5-trisphosphate and inositol 1,4-bisphosphate can not be detected for 15 minutes following stimulation.

These reports support the disappearance of inositol phospholipids by the phospholipase C-type cleavage as a very early event in the receptor-mediated cell responses. However, results to date do not allow us to conclude that only $PtdIns4,5P_2$ is hydrolyzed, with PtdIns and PtdIns4P in turn disappearing by the sequential action of PtdIns kinase and PtdIns4P kinase to $PtdIns4,5P_2$. Lithium ion appears to be a specific inhibitor of inositol 1-phosphate phosphatase, but not of inositol 1,4,5-trisphosphate or inositol 1,4-bisphosphate phosphatases. However, lack of inhibition of the latter phosphatases by lithium ion needs to be more clearly demonstrated. To test the hypothesis that $PtdIns4,5P_2$ but not PtdIns is hydrolyzed by the phosphodiesterase, a specific inhibitor for inositol 1,4,5-trisphosphate phosphatase must be developed. If, as a result, inositol 1,4,5-trisphosphate accumulation occurs in stimulated cells, and if it is correct that PtdIns disappears by the sequential action of kinases to $PtdIns4,5P_2$, then a continuous elevation of intracellular Ca^{2+} should be seen, as discussed below.

On the other hand, PtdIns is decreased over rather a long time, and it may be required for the long-term potentiation of the physiological cell responses. Hokin-Neaverson & Sadeghian (74) have speculated that stimulated $PtdIns4,5P_2$ breakdown and stimulated PtdIns breakdown may be separate processes. In mouse pancreas these authors have observed that the breakdown of PtdIns in response to 10 μM acetylcholine continues in a linear fashion for much longer than it does in response to lower concentrations of acetylcholine. This may suggest an alternative hypothesis: that enhanced breakdown of $PtdIns4,5P_2$ and PtdIns are two separate processes that may serve different, as yet unknown, functions. The enhanced breakdown of $PtdIns4,5P_2$ seems to be an event that is initiated and terminated rapidly, whereas the enhanced break-down of PtdIns appears to persist for a much longer period of time. When three inositol phospholipids are attacked by the phosphodiesterase in stimulated cells, obviously the ratio of the products, diacylglycerol/inositol 1,4,5-trisphosphate, is largely increased. Because the content of $PtdIns4,5P_2$ in plasma membrane is so small compared to the other inositol phospholipids, this different amount of production of the second messengers may contribute to the uneven activation of protein kinase C and Ca^{2+} release from an internal store (see below). It would be interesting to know how the cells rearrange such uneven activations into the appropriate intracellular responses.

Ca^{2+}-DEPENDENT INOSITOL PHOSPHOLIPID PHOSPHODIESTERASES

It has now been clearly demonstrated that a Ca^{2+}-dependent phosphodiesterase that hydrolyzes inositol phospholipids plays a central role in receptor-mediated PtdIns turnover.

This phosphodiesterase was first found in sheep pancreas (39) and has since been demonstrated in various tissues, such as rat liver (75), guinea-pig intestinal mucosa (83), rat brain (84), pig lymphocytes (85, 86), and blowfly salivary gland (87, 88). Dawson and colleagues (42, 89) have identified the cleavage products of PtdIns phosphodiesterase as diacylglycerol, D-inositol 1-phosphate, and D-inositol 1,2-cyclic phosphate. The latter can be further hydrolyzed to D-inositol 1-phosphate by a specific phosphatase. As yet no specific physiological function for these water-soluble products has been demonstrated. $PtdIns4,5P_2$ phosphodiesterase could be involved in the breakdown of $PtdIns4,5P_2$, since it has been shown to be activated by Ca^{2+} and Mg^{2+} in brain tissue (40, 41) and human erythrocytes (90, 91). However, it has not been clearly resolved whether PtdIns phosphodiesterase and PtdIns4P and $PtdIns4,5P_2$ phosphodiesterases exist as different enzymes. To date, in vitro studies indicate that the phosphodiesterase(s) seems to attack all three inositol phospholipids; there is not one specific substrate. Rittenhouse (92) has reported that partially purified phospholipase C from human platelets is maximally active in the presence of 0.1 mM Ca^{2+} and displays substrate affinities in the order PtdIns > PtdIns4P > $PtdIns4,5P_2$ and maximum rates in the order PtdIns4P > $PtdIns4,5P_2$ > PtdIns. Irvine et al (93) have reported that an enzymological study of the phosphodiesterase using $PtdIns4,5P_2$ as a substrate has shown very similar profiles of PtdIns phosphodiesterase activity in terms of the Ca^{2+} requirement and the pH response curve. At present, it is not known how the phosphodiesterase is controlled so that a specific substrate, for instance only $PtdIns4,5P_2$ among all the inositol phospholipids, is hydrolyzed when the cells are stimulated.

Normally the enzyme extracted from various tissues is virtually inactive under physiological Ca^{2+} concentrations (10^{-7}–10^{-6} M) and at neutral pH. When the cytosolic supernatant is assayed at a concentration of 1 μM free Ca^{2+}, a low level of activity with an optimum of pH 6.0 is detected; complete activation is achieved by increasing Ca^{2+} concentration to 1 mM (94, 95). Furthermore, if choline-containing phospholipids are present in a lipid bilayer (96, 97) or monolayer (94), the PtdIns phosphodiesterase cannot attack its substrate even at high Ca^{2+} concentrations (10^{-3} M). These observations seem to suggest that the enzymatic hydrolysis of inositol phospholipids requires activation factors that remove or overcome the various inhibitory effects on enzyme activity and alter its requirement for Ca^{2+} concentrations. Researchers have made one suggestion based on the observation that PtdIns breakdown under physiological Ca^{2+} concentrations (10^{-7}–10^{-6} M at pH 7.25) is stimulated by trypsin (98). Hirasawa (35) has proposed that the modification of the enzyme molecule, for example, limited proteolysis, may be essential for the long-term cell responses. A similar characteristic of Ca^{2+} and phospholipid-dependent protein kinase (protein kinase C) is shown after cleavage of the molecule by the proteases. The kinase becomes fully active without Ca^{2+}, phospholipids, and diacylglycerol. A recent report from Tapley & Murray (99) has shown that incubation of intact human platelets with exogenous phospholipase C from *Clostridium perfringens* induces such a proteolytic cleavage of protein kinase C. Interestingly, the possible involvement of proteolytic enzymes in the receptor-mediated triggering mechanism has often been proposed, since protease inhibitors frequently block receptor-linked physiological cell responses such as IgE-mediated histamine release from rat mast cells (100), acetylcholine-stimulated catecholamine release from bovine adrenal medullary cells (101), and antibody secretion from B lymphocytes (102). At present, however, the protease involvement has not been unequivocally clarified in terms of the receptor mechanisms.

On the other hand, Irvine et al (93) have proposed that the initial activation of the phosphodiesterase that acts against PtdIns4,5P_2 can be achieved by a change of the substrate microenvironment, such as the presence of phosphatidylethanolamine near the inositol phospholipid.

HETEROGENEITY AND THE Ca^{2+}-SENSITIVITY OF PHOSPHODIESTERASE

Although some inconsistencies appear in the enzymological characterization of the phosphodiesterase(s), at least two distinct pH optima have been obtained for PtdIns phosphodiesterase from lymphocytes (86) and rat brain (95, 103) if the enzyme is assayed at 0.4 mM and 1 mM Ca^{2+} respectively. However, only one peak is observed when the Ca^{2+} concentration is buffered to 1 μM. These observations can be resolved on the basis of the enzyme molecules' Ca^{2+} sensitivity at different pH. Kemp et al (75) have also reported some evidence for two pH optima in the enzyme from liver, a major one at 5.7 and a minor one at 6.9. Dawson et al (104) have recently extended these observations to a sheep pancreas supernatant fraction, where strong PtdIns phosphodiesterase activity is seen up to pH 8.5. Similar results have been obtained in rat liver and kidney (105). The activity at an alkaline pH is relatively unstable if the enzyme is submitted to ammonium sulphate fractionation and dialysis, as has been the case in the enzyme preparations of rat brain (84), guinea-pig intestinal mucosa (83), ox brain (61), rabbit smooth muscle (106), and rat liver (107). However, the activity can be maintained by the addition of an SH-residue protector such as dithiothreitol into the enzyme preparation.

In addition, the apparent heterogeneity of the phosphodiesterase has been examined by a standard isoelectrofocusing technique and by a new chromatofocusing technique, both of which have been proven to be valuable aids in probing the heterogeneity of the enzyme. Highly reproducible patterns of enzyme elution have been obtained from the brain (108), liver, and kidney (105). Hirasawa et al (108) have suggested that the brain cytosolic supernatant has at least four different forms of the phosphodiesterase according to their isoelectric points. Takenawa & Nagai (107) presumably have isolated one of these fractions, which is activated under 2 mM Ca^{2+} at neutral pH, from rat liver supernatant. Similarly, two distinct PtdIns phosphodiesterases have been purified from sheep seminal vesicular glands by Hofmann & Majerus (109). Nevertheless, the exact nature of this heterogeneity is not yet unequivocally understood.

It has been reported that the Ca^{2+}-dependent soluble PtdIns phosphodiesterase obtained from pig lymphocytes is fully active in the presence of 1 μM Ca^{2+} at pH 7.0, and such a characteristic is similar to those of certain peaks obtained by chromatofocusing of the trypsinized or the long-term preincubated cytosolic supernatant from rat brain (98). The enzyme forms in lymphocytes, separated by using the chromatofocusing technique, are two different Ca^{2+}-sensitive forms that appear at isoelectric points almost identical to those of the Ca^{2+}-sensitive forms produced in trypsin-treated and preincubated brain supernatants (K. Hirasawa, unpublished data). It is possible that there are active and inactive forms of the phosphodiesterases in physiological Ca^{2+} concentrations and that these can be obtained without artificial treatments such as trypsinization. These observations suggest that one early step in the signal-induced hydrolysis of inositol phospholipids may be an activation of the phosphodiesterase(s). The possibility that there are receptor-sensitive enzymes responsible for activating the phosphodiesterase needs serious consideration in the light of these results.

It is also worth noting that the receptor-mediated breakdown of inositol phospholipids appears to be a complicated process, since recent evidence suggests that GTP-binding protein(s) may be involved in this stimulus-response coupling (110, 111).

INOSITOL 1,4,5-TRISPHOSPHATE AND Ca^{2+} MOBILIZATION

The stimulation of the α_1-adrenergic receptor increases the intracellular concentration of Ca^{2+} to between 10^{-7} and 10^{-6} M. This increase can be the result of both external Ca^{2+} influx and release from internal stores. The release of Ca^{2+} from internal stores appears to be important for very early cell responses in the liver (27), pancreas (112), cockroach salivary gland (113), and blowfly salivary gland (114). On the other hand, the external Ca^{2+} influx appears to be responsible for long-term cell responses. The most recent suggestion, based on results with permeabilized leaky pancreatic acinar cells (22) and saponin-treated hepatocytes (23, 115, 116), is that the addition of inositol 1,4,5-trisphosphate into media similar to cytosol induces the release of Ca^{2+}, which is previously taken up by nonmitochondrial stores in an ATP-dependent manner. Streb et al (22) have suggested that this Ca^{2+}, released from an internal store by inositol 1,4,5-trisphosphate, is the same as the Ca^{2+} released by acetylcholine. This finding has given biochemical significance to $PtdIns4,5P_2$ hydrolysis by the phosphodiesterase.

Berridge (117) has proposed that the role of very rapid signal-dependent $PtdIns4,5P_2$ hydrolysis by the phosphodiesterase may be in the release of intracellular Ca^{2+}, which acts as a mediator for subsequent cellular responses. This reaction would not be limited by the intracellular level of ATP, whereas enhanced PtdIns turnover has an energy-requiring step that can be identified as the sequential phosphorylation of PtdIns into $PtdIns4,5P_2$. Thus, the synthesis of $PtdIns4,5P_2$ must be inhibited by depression of the internal ATP level. Presumably, the release of Ca^{2+} from the internal store is a part of the initial trigger system. Although the depletion of Ca^{2+} from the bathing media causes the termination of long-term cell responses, the initial trigger response or short-time cell responses could be completed.

The other water-soluble products from the hydrolysis of inositol phospholipids, inositol 1-phosphate, inositol 1,2-cyclic phosphate, and inositol 1,4-bisphosphate, do not appear to show any effect on the elevation of Ca^{2+} release (22). $PtdIns4,5P_2$, however, is able to chelate Ca^{2+} even more strongly than EDTA. The phospholipid can hold more than one Ca^{2+} in the hydrophilic head group of the inositol ring, the 1,4, and 5 positions of which are occupied by phosphates. It seems likely that the $PtdIns\,4,5P_2$ molecule could exist in vivo as a $Ptd4,5P_2$-Ca^{2+} complex. ^{31}P NMR studies have shown that Ca^{2+} interacts simultaneously with the 4 and 5 positions of phosphate in the $Ptd4,5P_2$ molecule (118). If both $PtdIns4,5P_2$-Ca^{2+} and $PtdIns4,5P_2$ molecules are hydrolyzed by a specific phosphodiesterase, the negative charge of the inositol 1,4,5-trisphosphate would be increased to some degree, since the 1 position of the inositol ring would become free. It is possible that inositol 1,4,5-trisphosphate can attract Ca^{2+} from the internal Ca^{2+} store. The less Ca^{2+} bound to the inositol 1,4,5-trisphosphate molecule, the stronger the attraction of Ca^{2+}. The preparation of the inositol 1,4,5-trisphosphate employed for the experiments is therefore very important in identifying which form of inositol 1,4,5-trisphosphate, Ca^{2+}-bound or free form, actually works on the release of Ca^{2+}.

The role of the inositol 1,4,5-trisphosphate in this effect has been discussed as that of an internal stimulus acting on the intracellular organelle. Prentki et al (119) have reported that this highly negatively charged compound causes a rapid release of Ca^{2+} from isolated microsomal fractions of rat insulinoma. At present, it is not clear whether the effect is a direct stimulation of the organelle surface or whether there are several steps involved in the release of Ca^{2+} from its internal store.

DIACYLGLYCEROL AND THE ACTIVATION OF PROTEIN KINASE C

The rapid appearance of diacylglycerol-containing arachidonic acid has been observed in plasma membranes as a result of the concomitant phospholipase C–type cleavage of inositol phospholipids in response to external signals (13, 120–23). It is important to note that normally diacylglycerol is almost absent from membranes; it only appears transiently due both to its rapid phosphorylation to phosphatidic acid by diacylglycerol kinase and/or to its further degradation to monoacylglycerol and arachidonic acid by diacylglycerol lipase for the synthesis of prostaglandin and thromboxane. The diacylglycerol produced in this way initiates the activation of a unique protein kinase C, so that the information from extracellular signals can be directly translated across the membrane to protein phosphorylation (124). This finding has given new biochemical significance to the enhanced turnover of inositol phospholipids.

In the case of human platelets, the two endogenous proteins with approximate molecular weights of 40,000 daltons (40K) and 20,000 daltons (20K) are rapidly and heavily phosphorylated by natural stimuli such as thrombin (121, 123, 125), collagen (123), or platelet-activating factor (122). Protein kinase C is responsible for phosphorylation of the 40K protein (123). Recently, Imaoka et al (126) have confirmed this reaction using a highly purified 40K protein, which they found to have a 47K component with some microheterogeneity shown with isoelectrofocusing. The function of the 40K protein remains unknown. On the other hand, the 20K protein, a myosin light chain, is phosphorylated by a calmodulin-dependent protein kinase, which has an absolute requirement for Ca^{2+} mobilization.

The ability of various synthetic diacylglycerols to be intercalated into the membrane and to directly activate protein kinase C without inositol phospholipid breakdown has been tested in intact cell systems. 1-Oleoyl-2-acetylglycerol is most effective in activating the enzyme in platelets (15, 127, 128). In intact platelets, the enzyme activity may be monitored by measuring the phosphorylation of the 40K protein. The synthetic diacylglycerol is then rapidly converted in situ to 1-oleoyl-2-acetyl-3-phosphorylglycerol by the action of diacylglycerol kinase.

Enzymological studies have shown that the activity of protein kinase C is induced by the addition of membrane fractions containing phospholipids, especially phosphatidylserine, and Ca^{2+}. A small amount of diacylglycerol dramatically increases the apparent affinity of protein kinase C for Ca^{2+} (129). Apparently, one of the fatty acid chains of the diacylglycerol must be unsaturated for activation of the enzyme both in vivo and in vitro (130, 131). In mammalian tissues, inositol phospholipids are usually a rich source of arachidonic acid at the 2 position (132, 133). Ohki et al (134) have suggested that the effect of diacylglycerol on protein kinase activation may be the enhancement of Ca^{2+}-induced phase separation in the phosphatidylserine-containing membranes. Acidic phospholipids are indispensable for full protein kinase C activity, with phosphatidylserine the most effective. This phospholipid possesses a strong affinity for Ca^{2+}. Unimolecular films of the lipid are able to complex with Ca^{2+} through coordination-chelation binding (135). It is well known that the stimulatory and inhibitory effects of solvents and surface active lipids on many lipolytic enzymes may often be dependent on the physicochemical status of the lipid substrate (136). A common feature of phospholipases is that their activities are markedly affected by the ζ potential, which is influenced by the electrostatic charge of membrane components or by the binding of metal ions to the membrane substrate.

Protein kinase C and Ca^{2+}-dependent inositol phospholipid phosphodiesterase have very similar characteristics in terms of the sensitivity of their activities to other phospholipids (96, 137); choline-containing phospholipids are inhibitory and acidic phospholipids are stimulatory. It is probable that the Ca^{2+} dependency of both enzymes is associated with these effects. Therefore, it is attractive to suggest that these two receptor-mediated enzymes are both partly controlled by modification of the microenvironment of the inner leaflet of cell membranes. Several other aspects of protein kinase C system have been reviewed elsewhere (25, 138).

PROTEIN KINASE C AS A MOBILE RECEPTOR FOR A TUMOR PROMOTER

Recent studies from this laboratory have provided evidence about the transmembrane signaling of phorbol esters. Protein kinase C is a prime target for the action of phorbol esters such as 12-O-tetradecanoylphorbol-13-acetate (TPA), which is known as a potent tumor promoter (139). TPA, which possesses a diacylglycerol-like structure in its molecule, is able to substitute for diacyl-glycerol at extremely low concentrations and directly activates the enzyme both in vivo and in vitro (139, 140). As observed in the diacylglycerol requirement for protein kinase C activation, TPA also dramatically increases the affinity of this enzyme for Ca^{2+} to the 10^{-7} M range (140), resulting in its full activation without detectable cellular mobilization of Ca^{2+} (140, 141).

Kinetic analysis (142) indicates that the binding of ^{3}H-labeled phorbol-12, 13-dibutyrate to purified protein kinase C also has an absolute requirement for Ca^{2+} and phospholipid. The phorbol ester does not appear to bind directly to the enzyme; all four components combine together to form a strong quaternary complex, contributing to the activation of the protein kinase. This idea has been supported by recent reports that Ca^{2+} and phospholipids are needed for the binding of the tumor promoter to a specific direct binding site of the membrane. Delclos et al (143) have reported that the phorbol ester interacts primarily with phospholipid but not with protein in membranes. The tumor promoter presum-ably activates the enzyme by modifying its phospholipid microenvironment.

It is possible that, in intact cells where phospholipid and Ca^{2+} are sufficient-ly available, each molecule of the tumor-promoting phorbol ester intercalated into the plasma membrane phospholipid bilayer intracts with one molecule of protein kinase C. The movement of the enzyme toward the complex of Ca^{2+}, phospholipid, and tumor promoter in the plasma membrane is just like a mobile receptor (144). The protein kinase is usually recovered in the cytosolic soluble fraction before the tumor promoters are added, but after its addition protein kinase C is tightly associated with the membrane fraction. Supporting evidence for this hypothesis comes from Niedel et al (145) and Leach et al (146), who have partially co-purified a TPA binding protein with protein kinase C from brain tissues.

In physiological processes, it is possible that one molecule of diacylglycerol produced from inositol phospholipid hydrolysis in the stimulated plasma mem-brane can activate one molecule of protein kinase C. If so, it may be that, even though PtdIns4,5P$_2$ is a very minor membrane component, its breakdown provides sufficient diacylglycerol to activate all the protein kinase C within the cell.

SYNERGISM OF Ca^{2+} AND DIACYLGLYCEROL

Stimulation of the receptors relating to the turnover of inositol phospholipids often causes an increase of Ca^{2+} mobilization as well as a transient accumula-tion of diacylglycerol. The activation of protein kinase C by diacylglycerol appears to be a prerequisite but not a sufficient requirement for physiological responses of target cells, because the cellular responses to synthetic diacylglycerol or to tumor promoter per se are always incomplete. Under appropriate conditions it is possible to demonstrate that in an intact cell system the independent induction of both protein kinase C activation and Ca^{2+} mobilization can be obtained by the exogenous addition of synthetic diacylglycerol or TPA and a Ca^{2+} ionophore respectively (15, 127, 128, 140). Attempts have thus been made to obtain full physiological cellular responses by replacing the natural stimuli with synthetic diacylglycerols or TPA and Ca^{2+} ionophores. When the platelets are incubated with thrombin, collagen, and platelet-activating factor, especially two endogenous proteins with approximate molecular weights of 40K and 20K are rapidly and heavily phosphorylated concomitantly, in association with the release of various constituents of platelet granules such as serotonin (121–123). If only the synthetic diacylglycerol, 1-oleoyl-2-acetylglycerol, is added to the media, the 40K protein is phosphory-lated, indicating activation of protein kinase C. On the other hand, if a Ca^{2+} ionophore is added separately the 20K protein (myosin light chain) is phos-phorylated, indicating that calmodulin-dependent phosphorylation of this pro-tein absolutely requires the mobilization of Ca^{2+}. In neither case does serotonin secretion from the platelets occur (127, 128, 140). However, when these cells are incubated with diacylglycerol or TPA in the presence of a low concentration of A23187, the release reactions are dramatically enhanced. The Ca^{2+} ionophore alone at the same concentration has little effect. Again, it is plausible that protein phosphorylation by protein kinase C and mobilization of Ca^{2+}, both of which are evoked by a single extracellular messenger, are equally indispensable and synergistically effective for causing full physiological re-sponses (Figure 3). Tumor-promoting phorbol esters at low concentration, by inducing the activation of protein kinase C alone, may leave the cell ready to function once Ca^{2+} becomes available.

The involvement of the two synergistic pathways for release reactions may explain, at least in part, the signal-selectivity that is often observed during release reactions. For instance, in platelets, serotonin and adenine nucleotides are released from dense bodies in response to a variety of signals such as thrombin, collagen, ADP, epinephrine, and platelet-activating factor (PAF), while the release of lysosomal enzymes are observed only at higher concentra-tions of thrombin and collagen. By using permeabilized platelets, Knight et al (147) have elegantly shown that such signal selectivity of secretion is not related to Ca^{2+} concentrations because there is no difference in their sensitivity to Ca^{2+}. It is possible that the two signal pathways may exert differential control over release reactions from different granules within a single activated platelet.

This synergism of protein kinase C activation and Ca^{2+} mobilization has been recently extended to many other systems, such as the release of lysosomal enzymes from neutrophils (148), catecholamine release from bovine adrenal

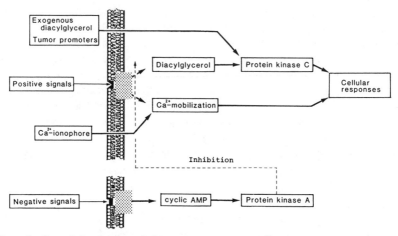

Figure 3 Synergistic role of protein kinase C activation and Ca^{2+}-mobilization for eliciting full cellular responses. Protein kinase A: cyclic AMP-dependent protein kinase.

medullary cells (149), aldosterone secretion from porcine adrenal glomerulosa cells (150), amylase secretion from pancreatic acinar cells (151), acetylcholine release from ileal nerve endings (152), histamine release from mast cells (153), insulin secretion from rat pancreatic islets (154), glycogenolysis in rat hepatocytes (155, 156), and concanavalin A–induced activation of bovine lymphocytes (157, 158). However, for the proliferation of macrophage-depleted peripheral lymphocytes, a very low concentration of phytohaemagglutinin is required in addition to both internal Ca^{2+} elevation and protein kinase C activation (158). This suggests that an additional receptor may also be involved in producing the cell-proliferation responses. These observations have confirmed that protein kinase C and Ca^{2+} mobilization act synergistically to elicit the physiological responses.

CONCLUSION

Enhanced PtdIns turnover is an early event in the cell receptor mechanism and is initiated by the hydrolysis of inositol phospholipids by the phospholipase C-type phosphodiesterase. This has been demonstrated by the large accumulation of a water-soluble product, inositol 1-phosphate, when lithium ion is used as an inhibitor of inositol 1-phosphate phosphatase. Recently, it has been suggested that two phosphorylated derivatives of PtdIns, PtdIns4P and PtdIns4,5P$_2$, rather than PtdIns are responsible for the receptor-mediated inositol phospholipid breakdown; PtdIns may disappear due to sequential phosphorylation by PtdIns kinase. However, this hypothesis has not yet been fully supported by the experimental evidence. The development of an inhibitor of inositol 1,4,5-trisphosphate phosphatase is urgently required to substantiate it.

Since an elevation of internal Ca^{2+} is observed together with enhanced PtdIns turnover, interest in Ca^{2+}-mobilization has recently focused on the role of inositol 1,4,5-trisphosphate as an internal second messenger for the release of Ca^{2+} from nonmitochondrial internal stores, such as the endoplasmic reticulum. If this hypothesis is correct, then one cycle of inositol phospholipid turnover may generate two intracellular mediators, diacylglycerol and inositol 1,4,5-trisphosphate, for subsequent signal transduction at the expense of four molecules of ATP. The evidence presented thus far appears to be plausible, but this attractive hypothesis is yet to be substantiated. On the other hand, the control of external Ca^{2+} influx essential for the long-term potentiation of physiological responses is still not understood.

The role of diacylglycerol in the receptor mechanism has been well established as that of a second messenger for the activation of novel protein kinase C, which can also act as the mobile receptor for tumor-promoting phorbol esters. Moreover, a synergism of Ca^{2+} and diacylglycerol has been demonstrated in various tissues as causing full physiological responses such as secretion, exocytosis, and glycogenolysis, as well as cell proliferation. At present, it is not known how the Ca^{2+}-dependent inositol phospholipid phosphodiesterase is activated once the receptor is stimulated. The mechanism may involve modification of the enzyme molecule itself or it may involve a change in the membrane physicochemical properties surrounding the substrate. In addition, some still-unknown event involving a GTP-requiring process probably occurs before inositol phospholipid hydrolysis.

ACKNOWLEDGEMENTS

The authors thank Dr. P. J. Lumsden for reading the manuscript and Miss T. Kamiya for skillful secretarial assistance. This work has been supported in part by research grants from the Research Fund of the Ministry of Education, Science, and Culture, the Intractable Diseases Division, Public Health Bureau, and the Ministry of Health and Welfare; by a grant-in-aid from the New Drug Development division of the Ministry of Health and Welfare; and by the Special Coordination Funds of the Science and Technology Agency, Japan.

Literature Cited

1. Hokin, M. R., Hokin, L. E. 1953. Enzyme secretion and the incorporation of ^{32}P into phospholipids of pancreas slices. *J. Biol. Chem.* 203:967–77

2. Farese, R. V., Larson, R. E., Sabir, M. A. 1980. Effects of Ca^{2+} ionophore A23187, Ca^{2+} deficiency on pancreatic phospholipids and amylase release in vitro. *Biochim. Biophys. Acta* 633:479–84

3. Hokin, M. R., Hokin, L. E. 1964. Interconversions of phosphatidylinositol and phosphatidic acid involved in the response to acetylcholine in the salt gland. In *The Metabolism and Physiological Significance of Lipids,* ed. R. M. C. Dawson, D. N. Rhodes, pp. 423–34. London/New York/Sydney: Wiley

4. Michell, R. H. 1975. Inositol phospho-

lipids and cell surface receptor function. *Biochim. Biophys. Acta* 415:81–147
5. Hawthorne, J. N., Pickard, M. R. 1979. Phospholipids in synaptic function. *J. Neurochem.* 32:5–14
6. Irvine, R. F., Dawson, R. M. C., Freinkel, N. 1982. Stimulated phosphatidylinositol turnover: A brief appraisal. In *Contemporary Metabolism,* ed. N. Freinkel, 2:301–42. New York: Plenum
7. Berridge, M. J. 1981. Phosphatidylinositol hydrolysis: A multifunctional transducing mechanism. *Mol. Cell Endocr.* 24:115–40
8. Hokin, L. E. 1968. Dynamic aspects of phospholipids during protein secretion. *Intl. Rev. Cytol.* 23:187–208
9. Pickard, M. R., Hawthorne, J. N. 1978. The labelling of nerve ending phospholipids in guinea-pig brain *in vivo* and the effect of electrical stimulation on phosphatidylinositol metabolism in prelabelled synaptosomes. *J. Neurochem.* 30:145–55
10. Fisher, D. B., Mueller, G. C. 1971. Studies on the mechanism by which phytohemagglutinin rapidly stimulates phospholipid metabolism of human lymphocytes. *Biochim. Biophys. Acta* 248:434–48
11. Masuzawa, Y., Osawa, T., Inoue, K., Nojima, S. 1973. Effects of various mitogens on the phospholipid metabolism of human peripheral lymphocytes. *Biochim. Biophys. Acta* 326:339–44
12. Dawson, R. M. C., Irvine, R. F. 1978. Possible role of lysosomal phospholipases in inducing tissue prostaglandin synthesis. *Adv. Prostagl. Thromb. Res.* 3:47–54
13. Rittenhouse-Simmons, S. 1979. Production of diglyceride from phosphatidylinositol in activated human platelets. *J. Clin. Invest.* 63:580–87
14. Bell, R. L., Kennerly, D. A., Stanford, N., Majerus, P. W. 1979. Diglyceride lipase, a pathway for arachidonate release from human platelets. *Proc. Natl. Acad. Sci. USA* 76:3238–41
15. Nishizuka, Y. 1983. Calcium, phospholipid turnover and transmembrane signalling. *Phil. Trans. R. Soc. London Ser. B* 302:101–12
16. Takai, Y., Kaibuchi, K., Matsubara, T., Nishizuka, Y. 1981. Inhibitory action of guanosine 3',5'-monophosphate on thrombin-induced phosphatidylinositol turnover and protein phosphorylation in human platelets. *Biochem. Biophys. Res. Commun.* 101:61–67
17. Knight, D. E., Scrutton, M. C. 1984. Cyclic nucleotides control a system

which regulates Ca^{2+} sensitivity of platelet secretion. *Nature* 309:66–68
18. Anderson, R., Hollyfield, J. G. 1981. Light stimulates the incorporation of inositol into phosphatidylinositol in the retina. *Biochim. Biophys. Acta* 665:619–22
19. Schmidt, S. Y. 1983. Light enhances the turnover of phosphatidylinositol in rat retinas. *J. Neurochem.* 40:1630–38
20. Michell, R. H., Kirk, C. J., Jones, L. M., Downes, C. P., Creba, J. A. 1981. The stimulation of inositol lipid metabolism that accompanies calcium mobilization in stimulated cells: Defined characteristics and unanswered questions. *Phil. Trans. R. Soc. London Ser. B* 296:123–37
21. Dawson, R. M. C., Eichberg, J. 1965. Diphosphoinositide and triphosphoinositide in animal tissues. *Biochem. J.* 96:634–43
22. Streb, I., Irvine, R. F., Berridge, M. J., Schulz, I. 1983. Release of Ca^{2+} from a nonmitochondrial intracellular store in pancreatic acinar cells by inositol-1,4,5-trisphosphate. *Nature* 306:67–69
23. Burgess, G. M., Godfrey, P. P., McKinney, J. S., Berridge, M. J., Irvine, R. F., Putney, J. W. Jr. 1984. The second messenger linking receptor activation to internal Ca release in liver. *Nature* 309:63–66
24. Takai, Y., Kishimoto, A., Inoue, M., Nishizuka, Y. 1977. Studies on a cyclic nucleotide-independent protein kinase and its proenzyme in mammalian tissues. *J. Biol. Chem.* 252:7603–9
25. Nishizuka, Y. 1984. The role of protein kinase C in cell surface signal transduction and tumour promotion. *Nature* 308:693–98
26. Rasmussen, H. 1970. Cell communication, calcium ion and cyclic adenosine monophosphate. *Science* 170:404–12
27. Exton, J. H. 1981. Molecular mechanisms involved in α-adrenergic responses. *Mol. Cell. Endocr.* 23:233–64
28. Williamson, J. R., Cooper, R. H., Hoek, J. B. 1981. Role of calcium in the hormonal regulation of liver metabolism. *Biochim. Biophys. Acta* 639:243–95
29. Prince, W. T., Berridge, M. J. 1973. The role of calcium in the action of 5-hydroxytryptamine and cyclic AMP on salivary glands. *J. Exp. Biol.* 58:367–84
30. Blackmore, P. F., Hughes, B. P., Shuman, E. A., Exton, J. H. 1982. α-Adrenergic activation of phosphorylase in liver cells involves mobilization of intracellular calcium without influx of extracellular calcium. *J. Biol. Chem.* 257:190–97

31. Joseph, S. K., Williamson, J. R. 1983. The origin, quantitation, and kinetics of intracellular calcium mobilization by vasopressin and phenylephrine in hepatocytes. *J. Biol. Chem.* 258:10425–32

32. Cockcroft, S. 1981. Does phosphatidylinositol breakdown control the Ca^{2+}-gating mechanism? *Trends Pharmacol. Sci.* 2:340–42

33. Hawthorne, J. N. 1982. Is phosphatidylinositol now out of the calcium gate? *Nature* 195:281–82

34. Creba, J. A., Downes, C. P., Hawkins, P. T., Brewster, G., Michell, R. H., Kirk, C. J. 1983. Rapid breakdown of phosphatidylinositol 4-phosphate and phosphatidylinositol 4,5-bisphosphate in rat hepatocytes stimulated by vasopressin and other Ca^{2+}-mobilizing hormones. *Biochem. J.* 212:733–47

35. Hirasawa, K. 1984. Possible involvement of proteases in phosphatidylinositol turnover. *Proc. 7th Intl. Taniguchi Symp., Transmembrane Signaling and Sensation, OHTSU, 1984.* Tokyo: Jpn. Sci. Soc. In press

36. Cachelin, A. B., de Peyer, J. E., Kokubun, S., Reuter, H. 1983. Ca^{2+} channel modulation by 8-bromocyclic AMP in cultured heart cells. *Nature* 304:462–64

37. Hokin-Neaverson, M. 1974. Acetylcholine causes a net decrease in phosphatidylinositol and a net increase in phosphatidic acid in mouse pancreas. *Biochem. Biophys. Res. Commun.* 58:763–68

38. Hokin-Neaverson, M., Sadeghian, K., Harris, D. W., Merrin, J. S. 1977. Synthesis of CDP-diglyceride from phosphatidylinositol and CMP. *Biochem. Biophys. Res. Commun.* 78:364–71

39. Dawson, R. M. C. 1959. Studies on the enzymic hydrolysis of monophosphoinositide by phospholipase preparations from *P. notatum* and ox pancreas. *Biochim. Biophys. Acta* 33:68–77

40. Thompson, W., Dawson, R. M. C. 1964. The hydrolysis of triphosphoinositide by extracts of ox brain. *Biochem. J.* 91:233–36

41. Thompson, W., Dawson, R. M. C. 1964. The triphosphoinositide phosphodiesterase of brain tissue. *Biochem. J.* 91:237–43

42. Dawson, R. M. C., Freinkel, N., Jungalwala, F. B., Clarke, N. 1971. The enzymic formation of *myo*inositol 1:2-cyclic phosphate from phosphatidylinositol. *Biochem. J.* 122:605–7

43. Hokin, L. E., Hokin, M. R. 1959. The mechanism of phosphate exchange in phosphatidic acid in response to acetylcholine. *J. Biol. Chem.* 243:1387–90

44. Hokin-Neaverson, M., Sadeghian, K., Majumder, A. L., Eisenberg, F. 1975. Inositol is the water-soluble product of acetylcholine-stimulated breakdown of phosphatidylinositol in mouse pancreas. *Biochem. Biophys. Res. Commun.* 67:1537–44

45. Yagihara, Y., Hawthorne, J. N. 1972. Effects of acetylcholine on the incorporation of $[^{32}P]$orthophosphate *in vitro* into the phospholipids of nerve-ending particles from guinea pig brain. *J. Neurochem.* 19:355–67

46. Schacht, J., Agranoff, B. W. 1972. Effects of acetylcholine on labeling of phosphatidate and phosphoinositides by $[^{32}P]$orthophosphate in nerve ending fractions of guinea pig cortex. *J. Biol. Chem.* 247:771–77

47. Dawson, R. M. C. 1954. The measurement of ^{32}P labelling of individual kephalins and lecithin in a small piece of tissue. *Biochim. Biophys. Acta* 14:374–79

48. Brockerhoff, H., Ballou, C. E. 1961. The structure of the phosphoinositide complex of beef brain. *J. Biol. Chem.* 236:1907–11

49. Dawson, R. M. C. 1965. "Phosphatidopeptide"-like complexes formed by the interaction of calcium triphosphoinositide with protein. *Biochem. J.* 97:134–8

50. Downes, C. P., Hawkins, P. T., Michell, R. H. 1982. Measurement of the metabolic turnover of the 4-and 5-phosphates of phosphatidylinositol 4,5-bisphosphate in erythrocytes. *Biochem. Soc. Trans.* 10:250–51

51. Kai, M., Salway, J. G., Michell, R. H., Hawthorne, J. N. 1966. The biosynthesis of triphosphoinositide by rat brain *in vitro*. *Biochem. Biophys. Res. Commun.* 22:370–75

52. Kai, M., Salway, J. G., Hawthorne, J. N. 1968. The diphosphoinositide kinase of rat brain. *Biochem. J.* 106:791–801

53. Harwood, J. L., Hawthorne, J. N. 1969. Metabolism of the phosphoinositides in guinea-pig brain synaptosomes. *J. Neurochem.* 16:1377–87

54. Colodzin, M., Kennedy, E. P. 1965. Biosynthesis of diphosphoinositide in brain. *J. Biol. Chem.* 240:3771–80

55. Michell, R. H., Hawthorne, J. N. 1965. The site of diphosphoinositide synthesis in rat liver. *Biochem. Biophys. Res. Commun.* 21:333–38

56. Michell, R. H., Harwood, J. L., Coleman, R., Hawthorne, J. N. 1967. Characteristics of rat liver phosphatidylinositol kinase and its presence in the plasma membrane. *Biochim. Biophys. Acta* 144:649–58

57. Tou, J. S., Hurst, M. W., Huggins, C. C., Foor, W. E. 1979. Biosynthesis of triphosphoinositide in rat kidney cortex. *Arch. Biochem. Biophys.* 140:492–502

58. Sugimoto, Y., Whitman, M., Cantley, L. C., Erikson, R. L. 1984. Evidence that the Rous sarcoma virus transforming gene product phosphorylates phosphatidylinsitol and diacylglycerol. *Proc. Natl. Acad. Sci. USA* 81:2117–21

59. Macara, I. G., Marinetti, G. V., Balduzzi, P. C. 1984. Transforming protein of avian sarcoma virus UR2 is associated with phosphatidylinositol kinase activity: Possible role in tumorigenesis. *Proc. Natl. Acad. Sci. USA* 81:2728–32

60. Michell, R. H. 1982. Stimulated inositol lipid metabolism: An introduction. *Cell Calc.* 3:285–94

61. Keough, K. M. W., Thompson, W. 1972. Soluble and particulate forms of phosphoinositide phosphodiesterase in ox brain. *Biochim. Biophys. Acta* 270:324–36

62. Fisher, S. K., Van Rooijen, L. A. A., Agranoff, B. W. 1984. Renewed interest in the polyphosphoinositides. *Trends Biochem. Sci.* 9:53–56

63. Abdel-Latif, A. A., Akhtar, R. A., Hawthorne, J. N. 1977. Acetylcholine increases the breakdown of triphosphoinositide of rabbit iris muscle prelabelled with [^{32}P]phosphate. *Biochem. J.* 162:61–73

64. Akhtar, R. A., Abdel-Latif, A. A. 1978. Calcium ion requirement for acetylcholine-stimulated breakdown of triphosphoinositide in rabbit iris smooth muscle. *J. Pharmacol. Exp. Ther.* 204:655–68

65. Akhtar, R. A., Abdel-Latif, A. A. 1980. Requirement for calcium ions in acetylcholine-stimulated phosphodiesteratic cleavage of phosphatidyl-*myo*-inositol 4,5-bisphosphate in rabbit iris smooth muscle. *Biochem. J.* 192:783–91

66. Kirk, C. J., Michell, R. H., Hems, D. A. 1981. Phosphatidylinositol metabolism in rat hepatocytes stimulated by vasopressin. *Biochem. J.* 194:155–65

67. Martin, T. F. J. 1983. Thyrotropin-releasing hormone rapidly activates the phosphodiester hydrolysis of polyphosphoinositides in GH$_3$ pituitary cells. *J. Biol. Chem.* 258:14816–22

68. Weiss, S. J., McKinney, J. S., Putney, J. W. Jr. 1982. Receptor-mediated net breakdown of phosphatidylinositol 4,5-bisphosphate in parotid acinar cells. *Biochem. J.* 206:555–60

69. Billah, M. M., Lapetina, E. G. 1982. Rapid decrease of phosphatidylinositol

70. Litosch, I., Lin, S.-H., Fain, J. N. 1983. Rapid changes in hepatocyte phosphoinositides induced by vasopressin. *J. Biol. Chem.* 258:13727–32

71. Orchard, J. L., Davis, J. S., Larson, R. E., Farese, R. V. 1984. Effects of carbachol and pancreozymin (cholecystokinin-octapeptide) on polyphosphoinositide metabolism in the rat pancreas *in vitro*. *Biochem. J.* 217:281–87

72. Michell, R. H. 1982. Is phosphatidylinositol really out of calcium gate? *Nature* 296:492–93

73. Soukup, J. F., Friedel, R. O., Schanberg, S. M. 1978. Cholinergic stimulation of polyphosphoinositide metabolism in brain *in vivo*. *Biochem. Pharmacol.* 27:1239–43

74. Hokin-Neaverson, M., Sadeghian, K. 1984. Lithium-induced accumulation of inositol 1-phosphate during cholecystokinin octapeptide- and acetylcholine-stimulated phosphatidylinositol breakdown in dispersed mouse pancreas acinar cells. *J. Biol. Chem.* 259:4346–52

75. Kemp, P., Hübscher, G., Hawthorne, J. N. 1961. Phosphoinositides. 3: Enzymic hydrolysis of inositol-containing phospholipids. *Biochem. J.* 79:193–200

76. Durell, J., Sodd, M. A., Friedel, R. O. 1968. Acetylcholine stimulation of the phosphodiesteratic cleavage of guinea pig brain phosphoinositides. *Life Sci.* 7:363–68

77. Berridge, M. J., Dawson, R. M. C., Downes, C. P., Heslop, J. P., Irvine, R. F. 1983. Changes in the levels of inositol phosphates after agonist-dependent hydrolysis of membrane phosphoinositides. *Biochem. J.* 212:473–82

78. Berridge, M. J. 1983. Rapid accumulation of inositol trisphosphate reveals that agonists hydrolyse polyphosphoinositides instead of phosphatidylinositol. *Biochem. J.* 212:849–58

79. Downes, C. P., Wusteman, M. M. 1983. Breakdown of polyphosphoinositides and not phosphatidylinositol accounts for muscarinic agonist-stimulated inositol phospholipid metabolism in rat parotid glands. *Biochem. J.* 216:633–40

80. Allison, J. H., Boshans, R. L., Hallcher, L. M., Packman, P. M., Sherman, W. R. 1980. The effects of lithium on *myo*-inositol levels in layers of frontal cerebral cortex, in cerebellum, and in corpus callosum of the rat. *J. Neurochem.* 34:456–58

81. Hallcher, L. M., Sherman, W. R. 1980. The effects of lithium ion and other

agents on the activity of *myo*-inositol-1-phosphatase from bovine brain. *J. Biol. Chem.* 255:10896–901

82. Berridge, M. J., Downes, C. P., Hanley, M. R. 1982. Lithium amplifies agonist-dependent phosphatidylinositol responses in brain and salivary glands. *Biochem. J.* 206:587–95

83. Atherton, R. S., Hawthorne, J. N. 1968. The phosphoinositide inositolphosphohydrolase of guinea-pig intestinal mucosa. *Eur. J. Biochem.* 4:68–75

84. Thompson, W. 1967. The hydrolysis of monophosphoinositide by extracts of brain. *Can. J. Biochem.* 45:853–61

85. Allan, D., Michell, R. H. 1974. Phosphatidylinositol cleavage catalysed by the soluble fraction from lymphocytes. *Biochem. J.* 142:591–97

86. Allan, D., Michell, R. H. 1974. Phosphatidylinositol cleavage in lymphocytes, requirement for calcium ions at a low concentration and effects of other cations. *Biochem. J.* 142:599–604

87. Fain, J. N., Berridge, M. J. 1979. Relationship between hormonal activation of phosphatidylinositol hydrolysis, fluid secretion and calcium flux in the blowfly salivary gland. *Biochem. J.* 178:45–58

88. Irvine, R. F., Berridge, M. J., Letcher, A. J., Dawson, R. M. C. 1982. Phosphatidylinositol-hydrolysing enzymes in blowfly salivary glands. *Biochem. J.* 204:361–64

89. Dawson, R. M. C., Clarke, N. 1972. D-*myo*Inositol 1:2-cyclic phosphate 2-phosphohydrolase. *Biochem. J.* 127:113–18

90. Downes, C. P., Michell, R. H. 1981. The polyphosphoinositide phosphodiesterase of erythrocyte membranes. *Biochem. J.* 198:133–40

91. Downes, C. P., Michell, R. H. 1982. The control by Ca^{2+} of the polyphosphoinositide phosphodiesterase and the Ca^{2+}-pump ATPase in human erythrocytes. *Biochem. J.* 202:53–58

92. Rittenhouse, S. E. 1983. Human platelets contain phospholipase C that hydrolyzes polyphosphoinositides. *Proc. Natl. Acad. Sci. USA* 80:5417–20

93. Irvine, R. F., Letcher, A. J., Dawson, R. M. C. 1984. Phosphatidylinositol-4,5-bisphosphate phosphodiesterase and phosphomonoesterase activities of rat brain. *Biochem. J.* 218:177–85

94. Hirasawa, K., Irvine, R. F., Dawson, R. M. C. 1981. The hydrolysis of phosphatidylinositol monolayers at an air/water interface by the calcium ion–dependent phosphatidylinositol phosphodiesterase of pig brain. *Biochem. J.* 193:607–14

95. Hirasawa, K., Irvine, R. F., Dawson, R. M. C. 1981. The catabolism of phosphatidylinositol by an EDTA-insensitive phospholipase A_1 and calcium-dependent phosphatidylinositol phosphodiesterase in rat brain. *Eur. J. Biochem.* 120:53–58

96. Irvine, R. F., Hemington, N., Dawson, R. M. C. 1979. The calcium-dependent phosphatidylinositol-phosphodiesterase of rat brain. *Eur. J. Biochem.* 99:525–30

97. Dawson, R. M. C., Hemington, N., Irvine, R. F. 1980. The inhibition and activation of Ca^{2+}-dependent phosphatidylinositol phosphodiesterase by phospholipids and blood plasma. *Eur. J. Biochem.* 112:33–38

98. Hirasawa, K., Irvine, R. F., Dawson, R. M. C. 1982. Proteolytic activation can produce a phosphatidylinositol phosphodiesterase highly sensitive to Ca^{2+}. *Biochem. J.* 206:675–78

99. Tapley, P. M., Murray, A. W. 1984. Platelet Ca^{2+}-activated, phospholipid-dependent protein kinase: Evidence for proteolytic activation of the enzyme in cells treated with phospholipase C. *Biochem. Biophys. Res. Commun.* 118:835–41

100. Ishizaka, T., Ishizaka, K. 1983. Activation of mast cells for mediator release through IgE receptors. *Prog. Allergy* 34:188–235

101. Nishibe, S., Ogawa, M., Murata, A., Nakamura, K., Hatanaka, T., Kambayashi, J., Kosaki, G. 1983. Inhibition of catecholamine release from isolated bovine adrenal medulla cells by various inhibitors: Possible involvement of protease, calmodulin and arachidonic acid. *Life Sci.* 32:1613–20

102. Kishimoto, T., Kikutani, H., Nishizawa, Y., Sakaguchi, N., Yamamura, Y. 1979. Involvement of anti-Ig-activated serine protease in the generation of cytoplasmic factor(s) that are responsible for the transmission of Ig-receptor-mediated signals. *J. Immunol.* 123:1504–10

103. Dawson, R. M. C., Irvine, R. F., Hirasawa, K. 1982. The hydrolysis of phosphatidylinositol in nervous tissue. *Phospho. Nerv. Syst.* 1:241–49

104. Dawson, R. M. C., Irvine, R. F., Hirasawa, K., Hemington, N. L. 1982. Hydrolysis of phosphatidylinositol by pancreas and pancreatic secretion. *Biochim. Biophys. Acta* 710:212–20

105. Hirasawa, K., Irvine, R. F., Dawson, R. M. C. 1982. Heterogeneity of the calcium-dependent phosphatidylinositol-phosphodiesterase of rat liver and kidney, as revealed by column chromatofo-

cusing. *Biochem. Biophys. Res. Commun.* 107:533–37

106. Abdel-Latif, A. A., Luke, B., Smith, J. P. 1980. Studies on the properties of a soluble phosphatidylinositol-phosphodiesterase of rabbit iris smooth muscle. *Biochim. Biophys. Acta* 614:425–34

107. Takenawa, T., Nagai, Y. 1981. Purification of phosphatidylinositol-specific phospholipase C from rat liver. *J. Biol. Chem.* 256:6769–75

108. Hirasawa, K., Irvine, R. F., Dawson, R. M. C. 1982. Heterogeneity of the calcium-dependent phosphatidylinositol phosphodiesterase in rat brain. *Biochem. J.* 205:437–42

109. Hofmann, S. L., Majerus, P. W. 1982. Identification and properties of two distinct phosphatidylinositol-specific phospholipase C enzymes from sheep seminal vesicular glands. *J. Biol. Chem.* 257: 6461–69

110. Gomperts, B. D. 1983. Involvement of guanine nucleotide-binding protein in the gating of Ca^{2+} by receptors. *Nature* 306:64–66

111. Haslam, R. J., Davidson, M. L. 1984. Guanine nucleotides decrease the free $[Ca^{2+}]$ required for secretion of serotonin from permeabilized blood platelets. *FEBS Lett.* 174:90–95

112. Renckens, B. A. M., Schrijen, J. J., Swarts, H. G. P., de Pont, J. J. H. H. M., Bonting, S. L. 1978. Role of calcium in exocrine pancreatic secretion. IV: Calcium movements in isolated acinar cells of rabbit pancreas. *Biochim. Biophys. Acta* 544:338–50

113. House, C. R., Ginsborg, B. L. 1982. Properties of dopamine receptors at a neuroglandular synapse. *Ciba Found. Symp.: Neuropharmacol. Insects* 88:32–47

114. Berridge, M. J. 1982. 5-Hydroxytryptamine stimulation of phosphatidylinositol hydrolysis and calcium signalling in blowfly salivary gland. *Cell Calc.* 3:385–97

115. Joseph, S. K., Thomas, A. P., Williams, R. J., Irvine, R. F., Williamson, J. R. 1984. *myo*-Inositol 1,4,5-trisphosphate. *J. Biol. Chem.* 259:3077–81

116. Thomas, A. P., Alexander, J., Williamson, J. R. 1984. Relationship between inositol polyphosphate production and the increase of cytosolic free Ca^{2+} induced by vasopressin in isolated hepatocytes. *J. Biol. Chem.* 259:5574–84

117. Berridge, M. J. 1984. Inositol triphosphate and diacylglycerol as second messengers. *Biochem. J.* 220:345–60

118. Hayashi, F., Inoue, H., Amakawa, T., Yoshioka, T. 1980. ^{31}P NMR study of neomycin toxicity. *Proc. Jpn. Acad.* 56: 597–602

119. Prentki, M., Biden, T. J., Janjic, D., Irvine, R. F., Berridge, M. J., Wollheim, C. B. 1984. Rapid mobilization of Ca^{2+} from rat insulinoma microsomes by inositol-1,4,5-trisphosphate. *Nature* 309:562–64

120. Bell, R. L., Majerus, P. W. 1980. Thrombin-induced hydrolysis of phosphatidylinositol in human platelets. *J. Biol. Chem.* 255:1790–92

121. Kawahara, Y., Takai, Y., Minakuchi, R., Sano, K., Nishizuka, Y. 1980. Phospholipid turnover as a possible transmembrane signal for protein phosphorylation during human platelet activation by thrombin. *Biochem. Biophys. Res. Commun.* 97:309–17

122. Ieyasu, H., Takai, Y., Kaibuchi, K., Sawamura, M., Nishizuka, Y. 1982. A role of calcium-activated, phospholipid-dependent protein kinase in platelet-activating factor-induced serotonin release from rabbit platelets. *Biochem. Biophys. Res. Commun.* 29:1701–8

123. Sano, K., Takai, Y., Yamanishi, J., Nishizuka, Y. 1983. A role of calcium-activated phospholipid-dependent protein kinase in human platelet activation. *J. Biol. Chem.* 258:2010–13

124. Nishizuka, Y. 1983. Phospholipid degradation and signal translation for protein phosphorylation. *Trends Biochem. Sci.* 8:13–16

125. Haslam, R. J., Salama, S. E., Fox, J. E. B., Lynham, J. A., Daridson, M. M. L. 1980. Roles of cyclic nucleotides and of protein phosphorylation in regulation of platelet function. In *Platelets: Cellular Response Mechanisms and their Biological Significance*, ed. A. Rotman, F. A. Meyer, C. Gitler, A. Silderberg, pp. 213–31. New York: Wiley

126. Imaoka, T., Lynham, J. A., Haslam, R. J. 1983. Purification and characterization of the 47,000-dalton protein phosphorylated during degranulation of human platelets. *J. Biol. Chem.* 258:11404–14

127. Kaibuchi, K., Sano, K., Hoshijima, M., Takai, Y., Nishizuka, Y. 1982. Phosphatidylinositol turnover in platelet activation; calcium mobilization and protein phosphorylation. *Cell. Calc.* 3:323–35

128. Kaibuchi, K., Takai, Y., Sawamura, M., Hoshijima, M., Fujikura, T., Nishizuka, Y. 1983. Synergistic functions of protein phosphorylation and calcium mobilization in platelet activation. *J. Biol. Chem.* 258:6701–4

129. Takai, Y., Kishimoto, A., Iwasa, Y., Kawahara, Y., Mori, T., Nishizuka, Y. 1979. Calcium-dependent activation of a multifunctional protein kinase by membrane phospholipids. *J. Biol. Chem.* 254:3692–95

130. Takai, Y., Kishimoto, A., Kikkawa, U., Mori, T., Nishizuka, Y. 1979. Unsaturated diacylglycerol as a possible messenger for the activation of calcium-activated, phospholipid-dependent protein kinase system. *Biochem. Biophys. Res. Commun.* 91:1218–24

131. Kishimoto, A., Takai, Y., Mori, T., Kikkawa, U., Nishizuka, Y. 1980. Activation of calcium and phospholipid-dependent protein kinase by diacylglycerol, its possible relation to phosphatidylinositol turnover. *J. Biol. Chem.* 255:2273–76

132. Baker, R. R., Thompson, W. 1972. Positional distribution and turnover of fatty acid in phosphatidic acid, phosphoinositides, phosphatidylcholine and phosphatidylethanolamine in rat brain *in vivo. Biochim. Biophys. Acta* 270:489–503

133. Marcus, A. J. 1978. The role of lipids in platelet function: With particular reference to the arachidonic acid pathway. *J. Lipid Res.* 19:794–826

134. Ohki, K., Yamauchi, T., Banno, Y., Nozawa, Y. 1981. A possible role of stimulus-enhanced phosphatidylinositol turnover: Calcium-sparing effect of diacylglycerol in inducing phase separation of phosphatidylcholine/phosphatidylserine mixtures. *Biochem. Biophys. Res. Commun.* 100:321–27

135. Bangham, A. D., Papahadjopoulos, D. 1966. Biophysical properties of phospholipids. I: Interaction of phosphatidylserine monolayer with metal ions. *Biochim. Biophys. Acta* 126:181–84

136. Dawson, R. M. C., Hemington, N. L., Miller, N. G. A., Bangham, A. D. 1976. On the question of an electrokinetic requirement for phospholipase C action. *J. Membr. Biol.* 29:179–84

137. Kaibuchi, K., Takai, Y., Nishizuka, Y. 1981. Cooperative roles of various membrane phospholipids in the activation of calcium-activated, phospholipid-dependent protein kinase. *J. Biol. Chem.* 256:7146–49

138. Nishizuka, Y. 1984. Turnover of inositol phospholipids and signal transduction. *Science.* 225:1365–70

139. Castagna, M., Takai, Y., Kaibuchi, K., Sano, K., Kikkawa, U., Nishizuka, Y. 1982. Direct activation of calcium-activated, phospholipid-dependent pro-

tein kinase by tumor-promoting phorbol esters. *J. Biol. Chem.* 257:7847–51

140. Yamanishi, J., Takai, Y., Kaibuchi, K., Sano, K., Castagna, M., Nishizuka, Y. 1983. Synergistic functions of phorbol ester and calcium in serotonin release from human platelets. *Biochem. Biophys. Res. Commun.* 112:778–86

141. Rink, T. J., Sanchez, A., Hallam, T. J. 1983. Diacylglycerol and phorbol ester stimulate secretion without raising cytoplasmic free calcium in human platelets. *Nature* 305:317–19

142. Kikkawa, U., Takai, Y., Tanaka, Y., Miyake, R., Nishizuka, Y. 1983. Protein kinase C as a possible receptor protein of tumor-promoting phorbol esters. *J. Biol. Chem.* 258:11442–45

143. Delclos, K. B., Yeh, E., Blumberg, P. M. 1983. Specific labeling of mouse brain membrane phospholipids with [20-^{3}H]phorbol 12-*p*-azidobenzoate 13-benzoate, a photolabile phorbol ester. *Proc. Natl. Acad. Sci. USA* 80:3054–58

144. Nishizuka, Y. 1984. Protein kinases in signal transduction. *Trends Biochem. Sci.* 9:163–66

145. Niedel, J. E., Kuhn, L. J., Vandenbark, G. R. 1983. Phorbol diester receptor copurifies with protein kinase C. *Proc. Natl. Acad. Sci. USA* 80:36–40

146. Leach, K. L., James, M. L., Blumberg, P. M. 1983. Characterization of a specific phorbol ester aporeceptor in mouse brain cytosol. *Proc. Natl. Acad. Sci. USA* 80:4208–12

147. Knight, D. E., Hallam, T. J., Scrutton, M. C. 1982. Agonist selectivity and second messenger concentration in Ca^{2+}-mediated secretion. *Nature* 296:256–57

148. Kajikawa, N., Kaibuchi, K., Matsubara, T., Kikkawa, U., Takai, Y., Nishizuka, Y. 1983. A possible role of protein kinase C in signal-induced lysosomal enzyme release. *Biochem. Biophys. Res. Commun.* 116:743–50

149. Knight, D. E., Baker, P. F. 1983. The phorbol ester TPA increases the affinity of exocytosis for calcium in "leaky" adrenal medullary cells. *FEBS Lett.* 160:98–100

150. Kojima, I., Lippes, H., Kojima, K., Rasmussen, H. 1983. Aldosterone secretion: Effect of phorbol ester and A23187. *Biochem. Biophys. Res. Commun.* 116:555–62

151. de Pont, J. J. H. H. M., Fleuren-Jakobs, A. M. M. 1984. Synergistic effect of A23187 and a phorbol ester on amylase secretion from rabbit pancreatic acini. *FEBS Lett.* 170:64–68

152. Tanaka, C., Taniyama, M., Kusunoki,

M. 1984. A phorbol ester and A-23187 act synergistically to release acetylcholine from the guinea pig ileum. *FEBS Lett.* 175:165–69

153. Katakami, Y., Kaibuchi, K., Sawamura, M., Takai, Y., Nishizuka, Y. 1984. Synergistic action of protein kinase C and calcium for histamine release from rat peritoneal mast cells. *Biochem. Biophys. Res. Commun.* 121:573–78

154. Zawalich, W., Brown, C., Rasmussen, H. 1983. Insulin secretion: Combined effects of phorbol ester and A23187. *Biochem. Biophys. Res. Commun.* 117: 448–55

155. Fain, J. N., Li, S.-Y., Litosch, I., Wallace, M. 1984. Synergistic activation of rat hepatocyte glycogen phosphorylase by A23187 and phorbol ester. *Biochem. Biophys. Res. Commun.* 119:88–94

156. Garrison, J. C., Johnsen, D. E., Campanile, C. P. 1984. Evidence for the role of phosphorylase kinase, protein kinase C, and other Ca^{2+}-sensitive protein kinases in the response of hepatocytes to angiotensin II and vasopressin. *J. Biol. Chem.* 259:3283–92

157. Mastro, A. M., Smith, M. C. 1983. Calcium-dependent activation of lymphocytes by ionophore, A23187, and a phorbol ester tumor promoter. *J. Cell. Physiol.* 116:51–56

158. Kaibuchi, K., Sawamura, M., Kikkawa, U., Takai, Y., Nishizuka, Y. 1984. Calcium and inositol phospholipid degradation in signal transduction. In *Inositol and Phosphoinositides*, ed. J. E. Bleasdale, J. Eichberg, J. Hauser, Dallas: Humana. In press

Ann. Rev. Pharmacol. Toxicol. 1985. 25:171–91

THE PHARMACOLOGICAL AND PHYSIOLOGICAL ROLE OF CYCLIC GMP IN VASCULAR SMOOTH MUSCLE RELAXATION

Louis J. Ignarro and Philip J. Kadowitz

Department of Pharmacology, Tulane University School of Medicine, New Orleans, Louisiana 70112

INTRODUCTION

The biological role of cyclic GMP in vascular smooth muscle regulation is a relatively new concept that had its debut at a time when the biological significance of alterations in cellular levels of cyclic GMP was itself a controversial issue. Indeed, even today the physiological importance of this cyclic nucleotide remains unclear, although recent studies may be on the verge of providing important new insights. Information on the regulatory role of cyclic AMP, on the other hand, is far more prevalent, probably because such studies commenced about fifteen years prior to those on cyclic GMP, and many more investigators are presently studying cyclic AMP than are studying cyclic GMP.

Progress in cyclic GMP research seems to have been thwarted somewhat because certain concepts developed in the mid-1970s no longer appear to be tenable. Due in part to the paucity of basic information on cyclic GMP at the time, incompletely tested hypotheses were forwarded that suggested that cyclic GMP might be involved in the contraction of smooth muscle, including vascular smooth muscle. This was an attractive hypothesis because other studies had suggested that cyclic AMP was involved in smooth muscle relaxation, thereby providing the intriguing concept that by their opposing actions cyclic nucleotides could regulate smooth muscle function. However, surprising reports appeared illustrating that some clinically employed vasodilator drugs

171

0362-1642/85/415-0171$02.00

caused a marked accumulation of cyclic GMP, but not cyclic AMP, in vascular tissue. The initial message from these studies was that cyclic GMP might not be involved in the expression of smooth muscle contraction. Then a new insight into the significance of these early observations emerged, along with the question: could cyclic GMP possibly be involved in smooth muscle relaxation?

The objective of this review is to focus attention on the possibility that cyclic GMP is involved in vascular smooth muscle relaxation brought about not only pharmacologically but also by physiological means.

EARLY STUDIES ON CYCLIC GMP

The first reports on the role of cyclic GMP in smooth muscle function leaned toward the possibility that tissue cyclic GMP accumulation and contraction were closely related events. Several autacoids, muscarinic receptor agonists, and related calcium-dependent agents that caused smooth muscle contraction also caused cyclic GMP accumulation in these tissues (1–5). Both cellular responses were dependent on calcium, but contraction usually preceded any significant increase in tissue levels of cyclic GMP. Later, the subsequent accumulation of cyclic GMP was suggested to be the result of indirect actions of intracellular calcium on intracellular guanylate cyclase (6). In any event, this temporal relationship between contraction and cyclic GMP accumulation suggested that the latter event was a consequence rather than a cause of the former. Such a view was no longer consistent with the earlier concept that cyclic GMP was involved in smooth muscle contraction.

A further clue that cyclic GMP was not likely to be involved in contraction developed in 1975 when nitroglycerin, a potent vasodilator, was reported to elevate cyclic GMP levels in arterial and other tissues (7, 8). At about the same time, other reports appeared showing that sodium azide, hydroxylamine, and sodium nitrite activated soluble guanylate cylcase and stimulated tissue cyclic GMP accumulation (9–11). These chemical agents were well known to cause smooth muscle relaxation. Subsequently, sodium nitroprusside, nitroglycerin, and related smooth muscle relaxants were reported to increase muscle levels of cyclic GMP (12–14). The above studies were suggestive of the possibility that cyclic GMP might be involved in smooth muscle relaxation. However, other studies (15, 16) revealed that if this hypothesis were correct, it might not generally be applied to all smooth muscles. Thus, the interpretation of these data was unclear.

The first experiments in our laboratory on this subject were designed to test a relatively straightforward concept. Chemical agents known to activate soluble guanylate cyclase should cause vascular smooth muscle relaxation if cyclic GMP is involved in the relaxation process. In addition, since sodium nitroprusside is unstable in aqueous solution and releases nitric oxide and because nitric oxide is a potent activator of guanylate cyclase, then nitric oxide itself should be a vasodilator. Moreover, unstable organic nitroso compounds, which release nitric oxide, should also cause relaxation. In our first series of experiments, nitric oxide gas and nitrosoguanidine compounds were demonstrated to cause potent and marked relaxation of precontracted helical strips of bovine coronary artery (17, 18). This was a novel observation that was extended to include other chemical agents related to nitric oxide (19–22). The concomitant observations that nitric oxide, nitroso compounds, and compounds capable of forming or releasing nitric oxide all activated soluble guanylate cyclase from vascular smooth muscle and elevated arterial levels of cyclic GMP but not cyclic AMP led us to believe that cyclic GMP is somehow involved in vascular smooth muscle relaxation elicited by pharmacological intervention (20, 21, 23, 24). Reports from other laboratories on the close relationship between arterial relaxation and cyclic GMP accumulation in the presence of standard vasodilators such as sodium nitroprusside and nitroglycerin soon followed (25–30). These observations indicated that vascular and nonvascular smooth muscle may differ in regard to the role of cyclic GMP. Tracheal smooth muscle, however, appears to respond similarly to vascular smooth muscle with respect to the effects of nitroso compounds that elevate tissue levels of cyclic GMP (13).

NITRIC OXIDE AS A VASCULAR SMOOTH MUSCLE RELAXANT

Keeping in mind the earlier observations inconsistent with a role for cyclic GMP in smooth muscle relaxation, several groups nevertheless made the decision to continue studies designed to test the hypothesis that cyclic GMP is involved in the relaxation of smooth muscle. In view of the clear indication that the most consistent data were obtained with known vasodilator drugs, we elected to restrict our studies to vascular smooth muscle. At this point, what was needed was a better understanding of the relationship between nitric oxide and certain vasodilators and a selective antagonist of this class of vascular smooth muscle relaxant.

An earlier suggestion that nitric oxide probably was the common factor involved in the activation of soluble guanylate cyclase by sodium nitroprusside, nitrites, organic nitrates, and nitroso compounds (9–11, 31–33) seemed very plausible. Moreover, the fact that nitric oxide is very lipophilic and unstable was consistent with the well-known transient hypotensive actions of the latter vasodilators. Thus, the attractive hypothesis that nitric oxide is responsible for the vascular effects of this class of vasodilator drug was set forth (17, 18, 20). Additional studies were consistent with this view. The direct release or formation of nitric oxide from sodium nitroprusside, sodium nitrite, amyl nitrite, nitroglycerin, nitrosoguanidines, and related agents was demonstrated (34–39). The transient relaxant effects of nitric oxide in both arteries and veins were associated with equally transient increases in vascular cyclic GMP levels, whereas nitroglycerin elicited longer-lasting effects on both cellular events (20, 24). Nitroglycerin produces a much longer-lasting response, probably because once this highly lipophilic ester permeates the cell continual formation of nitric oxide occurs within the cell (21). The same appears true for sodium nitroprusside, nitroso compounds, other organic nitrate esters, and organic nitrite esters (21).

Several years ago, we suggested the use of the term *nitrogen oxide–containing vasodilators* for those hypotensive agents that possess, generate, or release nitric oxide (21). These drugs include inorganic and organic nitroso compounds and organic nitrite and nitrate esters. This terminology, or a related one, should be used instead of the older *direct-acting vasodilators* or *direct-acting spasmolytics* because much more information is now available on how these drugs work. It appears no longer necessary to employ the older and more ambiguous terminology.

METHYLENE BLUE AS A SELECTIVE ANTAGONIST

In an attempt to find antagonists of the relaxant effects of nitric oxide, the authors took advantage of previous reports that hemoglobin and methylene blue were inhibitors of guanylate cyclase activation by nitric oxide (40). Hemoglobin, myoglobin, related hemoproteins, and methylene blue were found to inhibit coronary arterial relaxation elicited by nitric oxide but not catecholamines (17–22). Hemoproteins, however, failed to inhibit the relaxant effects of sodium nitroprusside, organic nitrates, and nitrosoguanidines, whereas methylene blue was still an effective antagonist. At first, these observations were puzzling, but further experimentation cleared up the apparent enigma. High molecular–weight hemoproteins have a high affinity for nitric oxide and react with the latter to form relatively stable nitrosylhemoprotein complexes that cannot penetrate cells. Organic nitrates and nitrites and nitroso compounds are lipophilic substances and release or form nitric oxide within cells. Methylene blue is a vital biological stain that by definition permeates cell membranes. Therefore, hemoproteins cannot antagonize the effects of nitric oxide liberated intracellularly, whereas methylene blue can (17–22). Similarly, the highly charged inorganic species ferricyanide, which is an oxidant and inhibits guanylate cyclase activation by nitric oxide, as does methylene blue (40), cannot inhibit the relaxant effect of nitric oxide because the ferricyanide cannot enter the cell to interact with soluble guanylate cyclase (17). Since methylene blue inhibits vascular smooth muscle relaxation elicited by all of the nitric oxide–forming or nitric oxide–releasing vasodilator drugs without influencing relaxation elicited by other drugs such as isoproterenol, certain prostaglandins, and calcium antagonists (17, 19; L. J. Ignarro, P. J. Kadowitz, unpublished information), methylene blue is a very useful selective antagonist of the former class of vascular smooth muscle relaxant (19, 41). Chemically related vital biological stains (brilliant cresyl blue) are similarly effective.

Methylene blue inhibits not only the relaxant effect of the nitrogen oxide–containing vasodilators but also their stimulatory effects on vascular cyclic GMP accumulation (20, 21, 24). These observations are important for several reasons. First, these actions of methylene blue greatly strengthened our initial belief that cyclic GMP is involved in vascular smooth muscle relaxation. Second, these data illustrate the potential utility of methylene blue and related agents as pharmacological probes to discern other biological roles of cyclic GMP in cellular function. Third, the studies suggest strongly that the nitrogen oxide–containing vasodilators interact with intracellular receptors, the most apparent candidate being guanylate cyclase, to stimulate the formation of cyclic GMP and thereby generate the intracellular signal for initiating the relaxation process. More recent studies from this laboratory, based on the original observations by Craven & DeRubertis (33, 42), suggest that the intracellular receptor for nitric oxide is soluble guanylate cyclase-bound heme (43–45).

Methylene blue has also been employed to demonstrate unequivocally that cyclic GMP is not responsible for causing or promoting vascular smooth muscle contraction elicited by certain hormonal-like agents. Employing methylene blue as a pharmacological probe, Kukovetz and co-workers (46) showed that vascular smooth muscle contraction caused by acetylcholine is markedly enhanced by methylene blue and that this is associated with decreased tissue levels of cyclic GMP. Contrariwise, the cyclic GMP phosphodiesterase inhibitor M&B-22,948 elevates cyclic GMP levels and inhibits contractions caused by acetylcholine. By lowering resting tissue levels of cyclic GMP, methylene blue raises vascular smooth muscle tone (20, 21; L. J. Ignarro, P. J. Kadowitz, unpublished information). The cyclic GMP phosphodiesterase inhibitor, on the other hand, potentiates relaxation and cyclic GMP accumulation elicited by relaxants (28). These findings indicate clearly that cyclic GMP accumulation and vascular smooth muscle contraction can be completely dissociated. Moreover, the data further support the view that cyclic GMP accumulation and vascular smooth muscle relaxation are closely associated biological processes.

S-NITROSOTHIOLS AS ACTIVE INTERMEDIATES

Discussions of the original observations on S-nitrosothiols as active intermediates and the rationale behind their design were reported previously (41). Briefly, thiols have been consistently found to enhance or unmask the activation of vascular soluble guanylate cyclase (21). Additional studies revealed that the nitrogen oxide–containing vasodilators react with thiols to generate chemically unstable S-nitrosothiols (21, 23, 38, 39). Organic nitrates reacted only with cysteine and formed S-nitrosocysteine, which is consistent with the observations that only cysteine enabled three different organic nitrates to activate purified soluble guanylate cyclase (21). A series of S-nitrosothiols were tested and found to elicit potent and marked relaxation of coronary artery, intrapulmonary artery and vein, and mesenteric artery (21, 22, 24). These observations, together with those that thiols react with nitrogen oxide–containing vasodilators to rapidly generate the corresponding S-nitrosothiols, suggested that S-nitrosothiols could serve as intracellular active intermediates of the parent drugs in the expression of vascular smooth muscle relaxation.

Subsequent experiments revealed that S-nitrosothiols caused a rapid accumulation of arterial and venous levels of cyclic GMP, which clearly preceded the onset of relaxation (21, 24). Moreover, both cellular responses were inhibited by methylene blue but not by propranolol, indomethacin, atropine, or antihistamines. The results of these in vitro experiments were confirmed in several in vivo studies. Intravenous injections of S-nitrosothiols in the anesthetized cat caused transient but marked decreases in systemic arterial pressure without appreciably altering cardiac output (21). Thus, a marked decrease in systemic vascular resistance had occurred. We have also shown that sodium nitroprusside, nitroglycerin, and S-nitrosothiols decrease pulmonary vascular resistance by dilating intrapulmonary veins and upstream segments when pulmonary vascular resistance is increased by an active process (47; H. L. Lippton, L. J. Ignarro, A. L. Hyman, P. J. Kadowitz, unpublished information). The latter observations are strikingly consistent with the clinical impressions and experimental findings (24) that veins are generally more sensitive than arteries to the relaxant and cyclic GMP accumulating effects of S-nitrosothiols, organic nitrates, and sodium nitroprusside. Thus, studies in the intact animal correlate closely with results obtained in isolated vessel segments, suggesting that isolated vessels provide a good model system with which to study relationships between vasodilatation and cyclic GMP accumulation. The hypotensive actions of these agents are unaltered by propranolol, atropine, or indomethacin. Additional in vivo studies showed that S-nitroso-N-acetyl-penicillamine, nitroglycerin, and sodium nitroprusside produce almost identical qualitative hypotensive response in the feline mesenteric and intrapulmonary arterial vascular beds (H. L. Lippton, P. J. Kadowitz, L. J. Ignarro, unpublished information).

In all the in vivo experiments in which agents were injected systemically (iv), it was clear that the hemodynamic properties of the S-nitrosothiols are remarkably similar, if not identical, to those of sodium nitroprusside and nitroglycerin. All vasodilators displayed similar onset times of several seconds, similar durations of action of 45–90 seconds, and little or no effect on cardiac output. That the half-lives of the S-nitrosothiols in oxygenated aqueous media are very short (21) is consistent with the transient effects not only of S-nitrosothiols but also of sodium nitroprusside and nitroglycerin on systemic arterial pressure.

On the basis of all of these observations, we offered the view that nitrogen oxide–containing vasodilators caused vascular smooth muscle relaxation by permeating smooth muscle cells and generating intracellular S-nitrosothiols, which rapidly decompose to liberate nitric oxide, resulting in the stimulation of cyclic GMP formation and consequent vascular smooth muscle relaxation (21). This hypothesis encompasses all of the observations that we and others have made during the past six years and is illustrated schematically in Figure 1.

THE MECHANISM OF TOLERANCE

Tolerance to the hypotensive action of organic nitrates in man is well known but little understood. Needleman and colleagues (48, 49) suggested earlier that vascular smooth muscle relaxation caused by organic nitrates may be dependent on free −SH groups in the tissue. Depletion of −SH groups by chemical agents, including nitroglycerin, caused a marked decrease in relaxation responses to organic nitrates but not to other vasodilators. Responsiveness was restored by treatment of vessels with sulfhydryl reducing agents. This earlier conclusion is consistent with more recent observations that organic nitrates may elicit vascular smooth muscle relaxation by first reacting with tissue −SH groups to generate highly active S-nitrosothiol intermediates that are responsible for the effects of the organic nitrates (21). Moreover, recent studies indicate clearly that arterial strips rendered tolerant to nitroglycerin also display equal tolerance to the arterial cyclic GMP accumulating effects of organic nitrates but not to these effects of sodium nitroprusside or cyclic GMP itself (29, 50, 51). Preliminary studies indicate that arterial and venous segments made tolerant to nitroglycerin are still fully responsive to S-nitrosothiols.

These observations suggest three things. First, the persistent close association between cyclic GMP accumulation and relaxation further supports the view that cyclic GMP is involved in vascular smooth muscle relaxation elicited through pharmacological intervention by nitrogen oxide–containing vasodilators. Second, organic nitrates are likely metabolized within vascular smooth muscle cells to S-nitrosothiols, which, because of their instability, liberate nitric oxide and stimulate cyclic GMP formation. Third, vascular tolerance to organic nitrates may be attributed to the loss of formation of S-nitrosothiols, thereby resulting in less cyclic GMP accumulation and decreased vascular smooth muscle relaxation.

A recent clinical study supports the above interpretations (52). Patients who

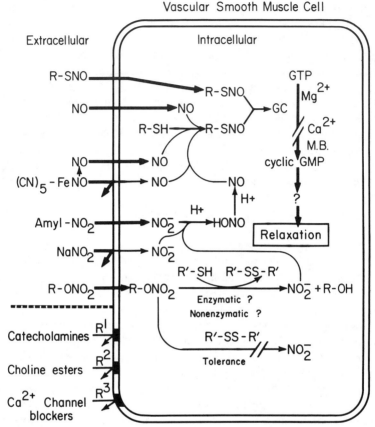

Figure 1 Schematic illustration of proposed mechanism of vascular smooth muscle relaxation produced by nitrogen oxide–containing vasodilators. Lipophilic substances permeate cells and form or release NO, either directly or through NO_2^-, which then reacts with thiol(s) to generate R-SNO. R-SNO, or NO released from R-SNO, activates GC to generate cyclic GMP. $NaNO_2$ is hydrophilic and is a very weak vasodilator. Nitroprusside (nitrosoferricyanide) is somewhat lipophilic, but is unstable in solution and liberates NO. Abbreviations: R-SNO, S-nitrosothiol; NO, nitric oxide; HONO, nitrous acid; $(CN)_5$-FeNO, nitroprusside; $R-ONO_2$, organic nitrate; R-OH, denitrated organic nitrate; R-SH low/high molecular weight thiol; R'-SH, thiol distinct from R-SH; GC, guanylate cyclase; M.B., methylene blue; R^1, R^2, R^3, extracellular receptors. [Reproduced with permission from (21).]

experienced varying degrees of tolerance to the hypotensive effects of nitroglycerin were given intravenous injections of N-acetylcysteine. The latter drug is a sulfhydryl reducing agent that can be administered systemically in relatively large doses without causing overt effects. Patients receiving N-acetylcysteine showed marked potentiation of the hypotensive effects of acutely administered nitroglycerin. These important clinical observations support the views that tolerance to organic nitrates is due to tissue −SH depletion and that S-nitrosothiols are the active intracellular intermediates of organic nitrates.

THE MECHANISM OF VASODILATATION BY ACETYLCHOLINE

Until the recent discovery by Furchgott and co-workers (53) that arterial smooth muscle relaxation by acetylcholine is dependent on a functioning endothelial cell layer, acetylcholine was known to contract isolated vessels, although vasodilatation was the principal effect in vivo. Prior to this important advance, acetylcholine-elicited contractions were reported to be associated with a concomitant accumulation of tissue cyclic GMP (discussed above). These early observations prompted the premature conclusion that cyclic GMP was involved in the contractile process. Upon learning that acetylcholine can in fact relax vascular smooth muscle in vitro provided the endothelium remains intact, several groups of investigators began to elucidate the relationship between cyclic GMP and relaxation in response to acetylcholine and related vasodilators.

The first reports illustrated the close relationship between vascular smooth muscle relaxation and cyclic GMP accumulation elicited by acetylcholine on arterial segments possessing a functioning endothelium (54–57). Acetylcholine elicits concentration- and time-dependent increases in arterial cyclic GMP levels that correlate well with relaxation (54–57). A comprehensive time-course analysis revealed that cyclic GMP accumulation clearly precedes the onset of relaxation (57). Atropine, a muscarinic receptor antagonist, and methylene blue, a guanylate cyclase inhibitor, each abolished both cellular responses to acetylcholine (54, 57). Cyclic AMP levels were not altered by acetylcholine. Cyclic GMP phosphodiesterase inhibitors enhanced responses to acetylcholine (54).

The inhibition of acetylcholine-elicited cyclic GMP accumulation by atropine and methylene blue provides evidence that a link exists between muscarinic receptors and guanylate cyclase (57). As acetylcholine is well known not to directly activate guanylate cyclase, the stimulation of cyclic GMP formation inside vascular smooth muscle cells must be an indirect consequence of muscarinic receptor stimulation. The finding that endothelium-damaged arteries and endothelium-intact veins both contract and show small but significantly elevated cyclic GMP levels in response to acetylcholine indicates that vascular endothelium is not obligatory for stimulated cyclic GMP formation by acetylcholine (57). In bovine intrapulmonary arteries, the endothelium greatly enhances the capacity of acetylcholine to stimulate cyclic GMP formation, and this is accompanied by marked relaxation (57). Thus, arterial endothelial cells may generate one or more factors that either directly or indirectly activate guanylate cyclase. This endothelium-derived factor(s) may be the same as or similar to that suggested for endothelium-dependent, acetylcholine-elicited, arterial smooth muscle relaxation (53, 58). The possible mechanisms by which acetylcholine elicits vascular smooth muscle relaxation are illustrated in Figure 2.

It may be of importance that endothelium-intact arteries relax to acetylcholine but endothelium-intact veins rarely undergo relaxation (57, 58). The reasons for this are unknown and may reflect the inability of venous endothelium to respond to acetylcholine with the generation of factors capable of causing relaxation. Alternatively, such factors may be generated but are less active in relaxing venous smooth muscle. The use of intrapulmonary arteries and the closely associated veins to compare the effects of acetylcholine and related agents shows promise in better understanding the differences in responsiveness of arteries and veins to endothelium-dependent vasoactive substances. The use of this technique in evaluating the effects of arachidonic acid and prostaglandins is described in the next section.

ARACHIDONIC ACID AND PROSTAGLANDINS

We have examined the effects of arachidonic acid and prostaglandins on intrapulmonary arteries and veins (59). The objective of these studies was to compare and contrast responses to acetylcholine and arachidonic acid because of suggestions that acetylcholine elicits relaxation by generating an endothelium-derived, lipoxygenase metabolite of arachidonic acid (53, 60, 61). Arachidonic acid causes relaxation of precontracted rings of endothelium-intact intrapulmonary artery by two distinct mechanisms (59). Extensive unpublished observations from this laboratory indicate that arachidonic acid stimulates the formation of both cyclic AMP and cyclic GMP. One component of relaxation and cyclic AMP production is inhibited by indomethacin, and methylene blue inhibits the second component of relaxation and cyclic GMP production. Endothelium-damaged arterial rings only contract in response to arachidonic acid or acetylcholine and show no changes in cyclic AMP levels. The contraction by arachidonic acid, but not by acetylcholine, is abolished by indomethacin. These data indicate that intrapulmonary arterial endothelium can generate at least two substances that elevate cyclic AMP and cyclic GMP levels. The endothelium-derived substance that causes cyclic AMP formation and relaxation in response to arachidonic acid appears to be prostacyclin, because PGE_2 elicits negligible effects and $PGF_{2\alpha}$ contracts, whereas prostacyclin markedly relaxes and elevates cyclic AMP levels in intrapulmonary artery. Veins with intact endothelium contract to both PGE_2 and $PGF_{2\alpha}$ and show little or no response to prostacyclin. The findings that arachidonic acid–elicited contractions of veins are abolished by indomethacin indicate that cyclooxy-

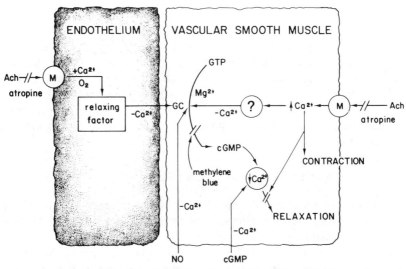

Figure 2   Schematic illustration of possible mechanism of vascular (arterial) smooth muscle relaxation produced by acetylcholine. Ach interacts with endothelial muscarinic receptors to generate a relaxing factor(s) in a Ca^{2+}- and O_2-dependent manner, which then permeates the smooth muscle cell to activate GC. The resulting elevated levels of cGMP promote intracellular Ca^{2+} sequestration, leading to muscle relaxation. Ach can also interact with smooth muscle muscarinic receptors to raise intracellular Ca^{2+} concentrations and cause contraction along with a small rise in cGMP levels. Abbreviations: Ach, acetylcholine; M, muscarinic receptor; NO, nitric oxide or nitrogen oxide–containing vasodilators; GC, guanylate cyclase; cGMP, cyclic GMP; $+Ca^{2+}$, calcium-dependent mechanism; $-Ca^{2+}$, calcium-independent mechanism; ?, unknown intermediate or mechanism. [Reproduced with permission from (57).]

genase products such as PGE_2 or $PGF_{2\alpha}$ may be responsible for this venous contraction. This view is supported by recent studies that microsomes isolated from intrapulmonary vein can synthesize significant quantities of PGE_2 (62). Moreover, both human (62) and bovine (D. B. McNamara, P. J. Kadowitz, unpublished information) intrapulmonary venous microsomes can generate significant amounts of PGI_2.

Since bovine intrapulmonary veins do not respond to prostacyclin in vitro, although they are clearly capable of forming it, it appears that arachidonic acid does not relax veins because these vessels are insensitive to prostacyclin. On the other hand, arteries markedly relax to both prostacyclin and its precursor arachidonic acid, and this is consistent with the observations that microsomes prepared from intrapulmonary artery can generate prostacyclin (62).

In view of the observations that acetylcholine relaxes endothelium-intact arterial rings in a cyclic AMP-independent manner, it appears inconceivable that acetylcholine elicits its marked relaxant response merely by releasing free arachidonic acid within endothelial cells. At concentrations that do not non-selectively depress smooth muscle function, quinacrine does not inhibit cyclic GMP accumulation elicited by acetylcholine (57). Moreover, whereas arterial contractions by arachidonic acid are abolished by indomethacin, contractions to acetylcholine are not at all affected (53, 58). Endothelium-dependent arterial relaxation by acetylcholine may occur through activation of the lipoxygenase pathway or by mechanisms unrelated to arachidonic acid metabolism. The isolation and unequivocal identification of the proposed acetylocholine-stimulated, endothelium-derived relaxing factor(s) is essential prior to drawing any further conclusions.

PROBLEMS WITH NONSELECTIVE ANTAGONISTS

In general, experimentation on vascular smooth muscle employing relatively selective antagonists such as atropine, certain β-receptor blockers, methylene blue, and even indomethacin has yielded data that can be intrepreted unambiguously and with confidence. Other types of antagonists have been employed, however, and these data must be interpreted with caution. For example, quinacrine (also known as mepacrine) is an inhibitor of phospholipase A_2 activity and thereby reduces the liberation of arachidonic acid from phospholipid stores. Unfortunately, quinacrine possesses many other actions as well, including inhibition of certain effects of cyclic GMP (63) and nonselective depression of smooth muscle contractions through its local anesthetic action (41). In a recent study, the use of quinacrine to elucidate the mechanism of endothelium-dependent, acetylcholine-elicited, arterial relaxation proved fruitless (57). The same frustrations were experienced with several lipoxygenase and epoxygenase inhibitors (59). For example, in bovine intrapulmonary artery, nordihydroguiaretic acid elicits indomethacin-like effects on responses to arachidonic acid. The cytochrome P-450 inhibitor SKF 525-A also behaves like indomethacin, whereas another cytochrome P-450 inhibitor, metyrapone, is without effect.

A detailed and careful analysis of the effects of such enzyme inhibitors on vascular smooth muscle functions is mandatory before these chemicals can be used to assess the mechanisms of action of relaxing agents. Premature and incorrect conclusions will almost certainly result if such precautions are not followed. Nonselective inhibitors may not prove useful in assessing the nature of endothelium-derived relaxing substances.

THE PHYSIOLOGICAL IMPORTANCE OF CYCLIC GMP

Some of the most difficult questions to answer in the biological sciences pertain to the physiological relevance of proposed second messengers. Only after many years of research have the biological roles of cyclic AMP and calcium, for example, become clearer. The possible physiological role of cyclic GMP constitutes a very recent development from only a limited number of laboratories. Recent evidence suggests that cyclic GMP is involved in the regulation of platelet aggregation (64, 65) and vascular smooth muscle relaxation (17–30, 41, 50, 51, 54–59). This chapter addresses the latter supposition.

Until recently, almost all the published work related to a possible second messenger role of cyclic GMP in expressing vascular smooth muscle relaxation elicited by exogenous chemicals, the nitrogen oxide–containing vasodilators. More recent work, however, hints that vasodilatation by endogenous neurotransmitters and autacoids may also be mediated by cyclic GMP. If this is true, then at least one physiological role for cyclic GMP becomes clear. Although endothelium-dependent relaxation by acetylcholine appears to involve cyclic GMP, several problems with the significance of these observations still exist. First, what is the source of acetylcholine in contact with endothelium in arteries that are at best only poorly innervated with cholinergic fibers, usually at the adventiomedial junction, a considerable distance from the endothelial cells? Second, what metabolic events occur in endothelial cells to render cyclic GMP accumulation in and relaxation of smooth muscle cells? Third, what is the mechanism by which intracellular cyclic GMP elicits vascular smooth muscle relaxation?

The importance of endothelial cells in arterial vasodilatation after parasympathetic nerve stimulation is unknown. Indeed, the contribution of neuronally released acetylcholine to vasodilatation has been debated in the past. Although responses to cholinergic stimulation appear to be modest in systemic vascular beds such as skeletal muscle (66), responses in the pulmonary vascular bed can be substantial under certain circumstances (67). Moreover, when pulmonary vascular tone is actively increased and the influence of adrenergic nerves in the vagosympathetic trunk are blocked, efferent vagal stimulation elicits marked frequency-dependent vasodilation (67), which is blocked by atropine but not by 5,8,11,14-eicosatetraynoic acid (67). Therefore, the physiological relevance of the in vitro observations that acetylcholine-elicited relaxation is endothelium-dependent is still uncertain. The only published study that comes close to addressing this problem is the recent observation that electrical field stimulation of norepinephrine-precontracted segments of intrapulmonary artery results in an endothelium-dependent relaxation (68). However, this relaxation was not affected by atropine, quinacrine, indomethacin, 5,8,11,14-eicosatetraynoic acid, tetrodotoxin, or procaine. Moreover, not only arteries but also veins relaxed in response to stimulation. Thus, a diffusible endothelium-derived relaxing factor is released by mechanisms unrelated to classical neurotransmitter release or arachidonic acid metabolism. Since acetylcholine is not involved here, the original question of the physiological importance of acetylcholine-elicited vasodilatation is even more important.

The nature of the endothelium-derived relaxing factor(s) generated by acetylcholine, electrical field stimulation, arachidonic acid, and various autocoids is unknown. Where studied, however, it is clear that cyclic GMP is involved in the relaxation process. It would be of great interest to know whether or not electrical field stimulation–elicited vascular smooth muscle relaxation is associated with concomitant increases in tissue cyclic GMP accumulation. In addition, it is clearly essential that the endothelium-derived factor(s) be isolated, purified, and characterized with respect to their capacity to stimulate cyclic GMP formation and relax vascular smooth muscle.

The mechanism by which cyclic GMP relaxes vascular smooth muscle needs to be understood prior to attempting to link cyclic GMP and relaxation in a cause-and-effect manner. At least one laboratory is currently attacking this problem by studying the properties of cyclic GMP–dependent protein kinase (69). Cyclic GMP itself relaxes vascular smooth muscle (70, 71), and sodium nitroprusside, a guanylate cyclase activator, leads to activation of cyclic GMP–dependent protein kinase in these tissues (72, 73). Cyclic GMP appears to antagonize the accumulation of free cytosolic calcium by intracellular mechanisms rather than by blocking extracellular influx of calcium (73). The first suggestion that cyclic GMP may regulate cellular calcium concentrations came as early as 1973 (2). One plausible theory is that cyclic GMP decreases intracellular free calcium concentrations in order to preserve normal cellular function (69). Other hypotheses are not ruled out. The mechanism by which cyclic GMP may elicit these effects could involve cyclic GMP–dependent protein kinase because large amounts of the kinase, as well as substrates for the kinase, exist in particulate material from vascular smooth muscle (74).

Certain autacoids and related substances now shown to require a functional endothelium in order to relax vascular smooth muscle have also been shown to stimulate the formation of cyclic GMP in these vessels. In addition to acetylcholine, researchers found that histamine and the calcium ionophore A23187 elevated cyclic GMP levels in rat thoracic aorta and that this was closely associated with relaxation (55). In other preliminary studies, A23187 and ultraviolet (UV) light were shown to elevate rabbit aortic levels of cyclic GMP and to elicit relaxation, both of which were dependent on endothelial cells (75, 76). It will be important to learn whether other autacoids that elicit endothelium-dependent relaxation also stimulate cyclic GMP formation in a temporally related manner.

Excellent correlations between vascular smooth muscle relaxation and cyclic GMP accumulation have been reported by several laboratories studying both nitrogen oxide–containing vasodilators and acetylcholine (see above). A recent report, however, suggested a poor correlation between relaxation and cyclic GMP accumulation when responses to nitroglycerin and acetylcholine were compared (56). That is, nitroglycerin caused more relaxation for a given increment in cyclic GMP levels than did acetylcholine. Based on these and other observations, the authors of the report concluded that nitroglycerin may relax rabbit aorta by more than one mechanism. Perhaps a better and more obvious explanation for these apparently discrepant findings is simply that the concentration of intracellular calcium is a critical determinant of the degree of relaxation but not of cyclic GMP accumulation. It is fairly widely appreciated that nitroglycerin elicits relaxation and cyclic GMP accumulation in a calcium-independent manner, whereas acetylcholine has an absolute requirement for calcium. Acetylcholine raises intracellular calcium concentrations whereas nitroglycerin does not, and elevated calcium ion may tend to attenuate the relaxations to acetylcholine or any other relaxant. It is important to appreciate that acetylcholine still partially elevates cyclic GMP levels while contracting endothelium-damaged arteries (57). Thus, nitroglycerin and related agents would be expected to elicit greater relaxation at a given degree of cyclic GMP accumulation than would acetylcholine. This interpretation is supported by observations that lowering calcium concentrations in vascular smooth muscle results in the enhancement of relaxation by sodium nitroprusside and 8-bromo-cyclic GMP (73).

Over the years, good experimental evidence has accumulated to suggest that cyclic AMP is a second messenger in expressing the relxant effects of agents that activate hormone-sensitive adenylate cyclase. These agents include epinephrine, isoproterenol, other catecholamines, prostacyclin, other prosta-glandins, and related neurohormonal substances and autacoids (27, 28). One unresolved question is why do both cyclic AMP and cyclic GMP seem to be involved in mediating or modulating vascular smooth muscle relaxation? Figure 3 attempts to illustrate schematically the possible complementary phys-iological roles of both cyclic nucleotides in vasodilatation.

CONCLUSIONS, HYPOTHESIS, AND EVIDENCE

Based on the available experimental evidence, discussed above, we offer the working hypothesis that cyclic GMP plays an essential physiological role in modulating vascular smooth muscle tone. The evidence that cyclic GMP is intimately involved in vascular smooth muscle relaxation elicited by a variety of vasodilators can be summarized as follows.

1. Nitrogen oxide–containing vasodilators, as well as acetycholine and certain related agents, produce concentration- and time-dependent increases in vascular cyclic GMP levels that are associated temporally with relaxation;
2. Activators of soluble guanylate cyclase cause both cyclic GMP accumula-tion in and relaxation of arteries and veins;
3. Inhibitors of guanylate cyclase (which permeate cells, i.e. methylene blue)

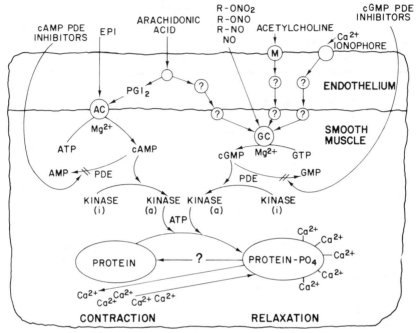

Figure 3 Schematic illustration of the possible physiological role of cyclic AMP and cyclic GMP in vascular smooth muscle relaxation. cAMP levels are increased by activation of AC in smooth muscle or by inhibition of PDE. Similarly, cGMP levels are increased by activation of GC (by endothelium-dependent or independent mechanisms) or by inhibition of PDE. Arachidonic acid can stimulate formation of both cAMP and cGMP by endothelium-dependent mechanisms. cAMP and cGMP activate their own specific, cyclic nucleotide–dependent protein kinases, resulting in the phosphorylation of one or more similar proteins. The phosphorylated form of the protein(s) rapidly binds intracellular Ca^{2+}, thereby leading to smooth muscle relaxation. Dephosphorylation of protein-PO$_4$ may release bound Ca^{2+} and enhance tone (or attenuate relaxation). Abbreviations: EPI, epinephrine; R-ONO$_2$, organic nitrates; R-ONO, organic nitrites; R-NO, organic nitroso compounds; NO, nitric oxide, cAMP, cyclic AMP; cGMP, cyclic GMP; AC, hormone-sensitive adenylate cyclase; GC, soluble guanylate cyclase; ?, unknown intermediate or mechanism.

cause marked inhibition or abolition of both cyclic GMP accumulation and relaxation elicited by nitrogen oxides or acetycholine;

4. Cyclic GMP phosphodiesterase inhibitors potentiate both cyclic GMP accumulation and relaxation in response to the above vasodilators;

5. Cyclic GMP itself or more lipophilic analogs directly relax vascular smooth muscle.

Additional evidence is amassing that cyclic GMP may be important for regulating vascular smooth muscle tone. This is summarized as follows.

1. The guanylate cyclase inhibitor methylene blue (also brilliant cresyl blue), when used in concentrations exceeding 0.1 mM, lowers resting levels of

cyclic GMP and causes vascular smooth muscle contraction, both of which are readily reversed by inhibitors of cyclic GMP phosphodiesterase;

2. Guanylate cyclase inhibitors markedly enhance contractions in response to α-receptor agonists, KCl and acetylcholine in veins or in endothelium-damaged arteries, whereas cyclic GMP phosphodiesterase inhibitors attenuate such contractions;

3. Guanylate cyclase activators stimulate cyclic GMP–dependent protein kinase in smooth muscle, and these tissues contain substrates for the kinase;

4. Relaxants that elevate cyclic GMP levels also stimulate phosphorylation of endogenous proteins;

5. Lowering calcium concentrations in vascular smooth muscle enhances relaxation responses to added cyclic GMP or guanlyate cyclase activators.

The successful design and execution of the following experiments could add considerable support to the hypothesis that cyclic GMP modulates, and may be obligatory for, vasodilatation by nitrogen oxide–containing drugs, acetylcholine, and closely related vasodilators.

1. The isolation, identification, and characterization of endothelium-derived relaxing factors, which may be different for different hormone-like, calcium-dependent vasodilators;

2. The isolation and characterization of calcium-binding proteins from vascular smooth muscle, which may be the principal substrates for cyclic GMP–dependent protein kinase in these tissues;

3. The development of specific antibodies to soluble guanylate cyclase and/or cyclic GMP-dependent protein kinase in order to ascertain the absolute involvement of these metabolic pathways in vasodilatation under a variety of test conditions.

ACKNOWLEDGMENTS

We are indebted to Jan Ignarro for her expert assistance in editing and typing this review. This work was supported in part by US Public Health Service grants HL27713, AM17692, HL15580, and HL18070.

Literature Cited

1. Lee, T. P., Kuo, J. F., Greengard, P. 1972. Role of muscarinic cholinergic receptors in regulation of guanosine 3',5'-cyclic monophosphate content in mammalian brain, heart muscle, and intestinal smooth muscle. *Proc. Natl. Acad. Sci. USA* 69:3287–91

2. Schultz, G., Hardman, J. G., Sutherland, E. W. 1973. Cyclic nucleotides and smooth muscle function. In *Asthma, Physiology, Immunopharmacology, and Treatment*, ed. K. F. Austen, L. M. Lich-tenstein, pp. 123–38. New York: Academic

3. Dunham, E. W., Haddox, J. K., Goldberg, N. D. 1974. Alteration of vein cyclic 3',5'-nucleotide concentrations during changes in contractility. *Proc. Natl. Acad. Sci. USA* 71:815–19

4. Andersson, R., Nilsson, K., Wikberg, J., Johansson, S., Mohme-Lundholm, E., Lundholm, L. 1975. Cyclic nucleotides and the contraction of smooth muscle. *Adv. Cyclic Nucl. Res.* 5:491–518

5. Clyman, R. I., Sandler, J. A., Manganiello, V. C., Vaughan, M. 1975. Guanosine 3',5'-monophosphate and adenosine 3',5'-monophosphate content of human umbilical artery. *J. Clin. Invest.* 55:1020–25

6. Spies, C., Schultz, K. D., Schultz, G. 1980. Inhibitory effects of mepacrine and eicosatetraynoic acid on cyclic GMP elevations caused by calcium and hormonal factors in rat ductus deferens. *Naunyn-Schmiedeberg's Arch. Pharmacol.* 311:71–77

7. Diamond, J., Holmes, T. G. 1975. Effects of potassium chloride and smooth muscle relaxants on tension and cyclic nucleotide levels in rat myometrium. *Can. J. Physiol. Pharmacol.* 53:1099–107

8. Diamond, J., Blisard, K. S. 1976. Effects of stimulant and relaxant drugs on tension and cyclic nucleotide levels in canine femoral artery. *Mol. Pharmacol.* 12:688–92

9. Kimura, H., Mittal, C. K., Murad, F. 1975. Increases in cyclic GMP levels in brain and liver with sodium azide an activator of guanylate cyclase. *Nature* 257:700–2

10. Kimura, H., Mittal, C. K., Murad, F. 1975. Activation of guanylate cyclase from rat liver and other tissues by sodium azide. *J. Biol. Chem.* 250:8016–22

11. Katsuki, S., Arnold, W., Mittal, C., Murad, F. 1977. Stimulation of guanylate cyclase by sodium nitroprusside, nitroglycerin and nitric oxide in various tissue preparations and comparison to the effects of sodium azide and hydroxylamine. *J. Cyclic Nucl. Res.* 3:23–35

12. Schultz, K. D., Schultz, K., Schultz, G. 1977. Sodium nitroprusside and other smooth muscle relaxants increase cyclic GMP levels in rat ductus deferens. *Nature* 265:750–51

13. Katsuki, S., Murad, F. 1977. Regulation of adenosine cyclic 3',5'-monophosphate and guanosine cyclic 3'5'-monophosphate levels and contractility in bovine tracheal smooth muscle. *Mol. Pharmacol.* 13:330–41

14. Bohme, E., Graf, H., Schultz, G. 1978. Effects of sodium nitroprusside and other smooth muscle relaxants on cyclic GMP formation in smooth muscle and platelets. *Adv. Cyclic Nucl. Res.* 9:131–43

15. Diamond, J. 1978. Role of cyclic nucleotides in control of smooth muscle contraction. *Adv. Cyclic Nucl. Res.* 9:327–40

16. Diamond, J. 1983. Lack of correlation between cyclic GMP elevation and relaxation of nonvascular smooth muscle by nitroglycerin, nitroprusside, hydroxylamine and sodium azide. *J. Pharmacol. Exp. Ther.* 225:422–26

17. Gruetter, C. A., Barry, B. K., McNamara, D. B., Gruetter, D. Y., Kadowitz, P. J., Ignarro, L. J. 1979. Relaxation of bovine coronary artery and activation of coronary arterial guanylate cyclase by nitric oxide, nitroprusside and a carcinogenic nitrosoamine. *J. Cyclic Nucl. Res.* 5:211–24

18. Gruetter, C. A., Barry, B. K., McNamara, D. B., Kadowitz, P. J., Ignarro, L. J. 1980. Coronary arterial relaxation and guanylate cyclase activation by cigarette smoke, N'-nitrosonornicotine and nitric oxide. *J. Pharmacol. Exp. Ther.* 214:9–15

19. Gruetter, C. A., Kadowitz, P. J., Ignarro, L. J. 1981. Methylene blue inhibits coronary arterial relaxation and guanylate cyclase activation by nitroglycerin, sodium nitrite and amyl nitrite. *Can. J. Physiol. Pharmacol.* 59:150–56

20. Gruetter, C. A., Gruetter, D. Y., Lyon, J. E., Kadowitz, P. J., Ignarro, L. J. 1981. Relationship between cyclic GMP formation and relaxation of coronary arterial smooth muscle by glyceryl trinitrate, nitroprusside, nitrite and nitric oxide: Effects of methylene blue and methemoglobin. *J. Pharmacol. Exp. Ther.* 219:181–86

21. Ignarro, L. J., Lippton, H. L., Edwards, J. C., Baricos, W. H., Hyman, A. L., et al. 1981. Mechanism of vascular smooth muscle relaxation by organic nitrates, nitrites, nitroprusside and nitric oxide: Evidence for the involvement of S-nitrosothiols as active intermediates. *J. Pharmacol. Exp. Ther.* 218:739–49

22. Lippton, H. L., Gruetter, C. A., Ignarro, L. J., Meyer, R. L., Kadowitz, P. J. 1982. Vasodilator actions of several N-nitroso compounds. *Can. J. Physiol. Pharmacol.* 60:68–75

23. Ignarro, L. J., Gruetter, C. A. 1980. Requirement of thiols for activation of coronary arterial guanylate cyclase by glyceryl trinitrate and sodium nitrite: Possible involvement of S-nitrosothiols. *Biochim. Biophys. Acta* 631:221–31

24. Edwards, J. C., Ignarro, L. J., Hyman, A. L., Kadowitz, P. J. 1984. Relaxation of intrapulmonary artery and vein by nitrogen oxide–containing vasodilators and cyclic GMP. *J. Pharmacol. Exp. Ther.* 228:33–42

25. Axelsson, K. L., Wikberg, J. E. S., Andersson, R. G. G. 1979. Relationship

between nitroglycerin, cyclic GMP and relaxation of vascular smooth muscle. *Life Sci.* 24:1779–86

26. Kukovetz, W. R., Holzmann, S., Wurm, A., Poch, G. 1979. Evidence for cyclic GMP-mediated relaxant effects of nitro-compounds in coronary smooth muscle. *Naunyn-Schmiedeberg's Arch. Pharmacol.* 310:129–38

27. Kukovetz, W. R., Poch, G., Holzman, S., Wurm, A., Rinner, I. 1979. Cyclic nucleotides and coronary flow. In *Cyclic Nucleotides and Therapeutic Perspectives,* ed. G. Cehovic, G. A. Robison, pp. 109–25. Oxford: Pergamon

28. Kukovetz, W. R., Poch, G., Holzmann, S. 1981. Cyclic nucleotides and relaxation of vascular smooth muscle. In *Vasodilatation,* ed. P. M. Vanhoutte, I. Leusen, pp. 339–53. New York: Raven

29. Keith, R. A., Burkman, A. M., Sokoloski, T. D., Fertel, R. H. 1982. Vascular tolerance to nitroglycerin and cyclic GMP generation in rat aortic smooth muscle. *J. Pharmacol. Exp. Ther.* 221:525–31

30. Galvas, P. E., DiSalvo, J. 1983. Concentration and time-dependent relationships between isosorbide dinitrate-induced relaxation and formation of cyclic GMP in coronary arterial smooth muscle. *J. Pharmacol. Exp. Ther.* 224:373–78

31. Arnold, W. P., Mittal, C. K., Katsuki, S., Murad, F. 1977. Nitric oxide activates guanylate cyclase and increases guanosine $3',5'$-cyclic monophosphate levels in various tissue preparations. *Proc. Natl. Acad. Sci. USA* 74:3203–7

32. DeRubertis, F. R., Craven, P. A. 1976. Calcium-independent modulation of cyclic GMP and activation of guanylate cyclase by nitrosoamines. *Science* 193:897–99

33. Craven, P. A., DeRubertis, F. R. 1978. Restoration of the responsiveness of purified guanylate cyclase to nitrosoguanidine, nitric oxide, and related activators by heme and heme proteins: Evidence for the involvement of the paramagnetic nitrosyl-heme complex in enzyme activation. *J. Biol. Chem.* 253:8433–43

34. Schoental, R., Rive, D. J. 1965. Interaction of N-alkyl-N-nitrosourethanes with thiols. *Biochem. J.* 97:466–74

35. McCalla, D. R., Reuvers, A., Kitai, R. 1968. Inactivation of biologically active N-methyl-N-nitroso compounds in aqueous solution: Effect of various conditions of pH and illumination. *Can. J. Biochem.* 46:807–11

36. Schulz, U., McCalla, D. R. 1969. Reactions of cysteine with N-methyl-N-nitroso-p-toluenesulfonamide and N-methyl-N'-nitro-N-nitrosoguanidine. *Can. J. Chem.* 47:2021–27

37. Lawley, P. D., Thatcher, C. J. 1970. Methylation of deoxyribonucleic acid in cultured mammalian cells by N-methyl-N'-nitro-N-nitrosoguanidine. *Biochem. J.* 116:693–707

38. Ignarro, L. J., Edwards, J. C., Gruetter, D. Y., Barry, B. K., Gruetter, C. A. 1980. Possible involvement of S-nitrosothiols in the activation of guanylate cyclase by nitroso compounds. *FEBS Letts.* 110:275–78

39. Ignarro, L. J., Barry, B. K., Gruetter, D. Y., Edwards, J. C., Ohlstein, E. H., et al. 1980. Guanylate cyclase activation by nitroprusside and nitrosoguanidine is related to formation of S-nitrosothiol intermediates. *Biochem. Biophys. Res. Commun.* 94:93–100

40. Murad, F., Mittal, C. K., Arnold, W. P., Katsuki, S., Kimura, H. 1978. Guanylate cyclase activation by azide, nitro compounds, nitric oxide, and hydroxyl radical and inhibition by hemoglobin and myoglobin. *Adv. Cyclic Nucl. Res.* 9:145–58

41. Ignarro, L. J., Gruetter, C. A., Hyman, A. L., Kadowitz, P. J. 1983. Molecular mechanisms of vasodilatation. In *Dopamine Receptor Agonists,* ed. G. Poste, S. T. Crooke, pp. 259–88. New York: Plenum

42. Craven, P. A., DeRubertis, F. R., Pratt, D. W. 1979. Electron spin resonance study of the role of NO-catalase in the activation of guanylate cyclase by NaN_3 and NH_2OH: Modulation of enzyme responses by heme protein and their nitrosyl derivatives. *J. Biol. Chem.* 254:8213–22

43. Ignarro, L. J., Degnan, J. N., Baricos, W. H., Kadowitz, P. J., Wolin, M. S. 1982. Activation of purified guanylate cyclase by nitric oxide requires heme: Comparison of heme-deficient, heme-reconstituted and heme-containing forms of soluble enzyme from bovine lung. *Biochim. Biophys. Acta* 718:45–59

44. Wolin, M. S., Wood, K. S., Ignarro, L. J. 1982. Guanylate cyclase from bovine lung: A kinetic analysis of the regulation of the purified soluble enzyme by protoporphyrin IX, heme and nitrosyl-heme. *J. Biol. Chem.* 257:13312–20

45. Ignarro, L. J., Wood, K. S., Wolin, M. S. 1984. Regulation of purified soluble guanylate cyclase by porphyrins and metalloporphyrins: A unifying concept. *Adv. Cyclic Nucl. Res.* 17:267–74

46. Kukovetz, W. R., Holzmann, S., Poch,

G. 1982. Function of cyclic GMP in acetylcholine-induced contraction of coronary smooth muscle. *Naunyn-Schmiedeberg's Arch. Pharmacol.* 319: 29–33

47. Kadowitz, P. J., Nandiwada, P., Gruetter, C. A., Ignarro, L. J., Hyman, A. L. 1981. Pulmonary vasodilator responses to nitroprusside and nitroglycerin in the dog. *J. Clin. Invest.* 67:893–902

48. Needleman, P., Johnson, E. M. 1973. Mechanism of tolerance development to organic nitrates. *J. Pharmacol. Exp. Ther.* 184:709–15

49. Needleman, P., Jakschik, B., Johnson, E. M. 1973. Sulfhydryl requirement for relaxation of vascular smooth muscle. *J. Pharmacol. Exp. Ther.* 187:324–31

50. Axelsson, K. L., Andersson, R. G. G., Wikberg, J. E. S. 1982. Vascular smooth muscle relaxation by nitro compounds: Reduced relaxation and cyclic GMP elevation in tolerant vessels and reversal of tolerance by dithiothreitol. *Acta Pharmacol. Toxicol.* 50:350–57

51. Axelsson, K. L., Andersson, R. G. G. 1983. Tolerance towards nitrogylcerin, induced in vivo, is correlated to a reduced cGMP response and an alteration in cGMP turnover. *Eur. J. Pharmacol.* 88:71–79

52. Horowitz, J. D., Antman, E. M., Lorell, B. H., Barry, W. H., Smith, T. W. 1982. Potentiation of cardiovascular effects of nitroglycerin by N-acetylcysteine. *Circulation* 66(2):II-264

53. Furchgott, R. F., Zawadzki, J. V. 1980. The obligatory role of endothelial cells in the relaxation of arterial smooth muscle by acetylcholine. *Nature* 288:373–76

54. Holzmann, S. 1982. Endothelium-induced relaxation by acetylcholine associated with larger rises in cyclic GMP in coronary arterial strips. *J. Cyclic Nucl. Res.* 8:409–19

55. Rapoport, R. M., Murad, F. 1983. Agonist-induced endothelium-dependent relaxation in rat thoracic aorta may be mediated through cGMP. *Circ. Res.* 52:352–57

56. Diamond, J., Chu, E. B. 1983. Possible role for cyclic GMP in endothelium-dependent relaxation of rabbit aorta by acetylcholine. Comparison with nitroglycerin. *Res. Commun. Chem. Pathol. Pharmacol.* 41(3):369–81

57. Ignarro, L. J., Burke, T. M., Wood, K. S., Wolin, M. S., Kadowitz, P. J. 1984. Association between cyclic GMP accumulation and acetylcholine-elicited relaxation of bovine intrapulmonary artery. *J. Pharmacol. Exp. Ther.* 228:682–90

58. Furchgott, R. F. 1984. The role of endothelium in the responses of vascular smooth muscle to drugs. *Ann. Rev. Pharmacol. Toxicol.* 24:175–97

59. Ignarro, L. J., Harbison, R., Burke, T., Wolin, M., Kadowitz, P. J. 1984. Endothelium-dependent relaxation of bovine intrapulmonary artery by arachidonic acid. Involvement of two distinct mechanisms. *Fed. Proc.* 43:737

60. Furchgott, R. F., Zawadzki, J. V., Cherry, P. D. 1981. Role of endothelium in the vasodilator response to acetylcholine. See Ref. 28, pp. 49–66

61. Furchgott, R. F. 1983. Role of endothelium in responses of vascular smooth muscle. *Circ. Res.* 53:557–73

62. McMullen-Laird, M., McNamara, D. B., Kerstein, M. D., Hyman, A. L., Kadowitz, P. J. 1982. Human lung metabolism of prostaglandin endoperoxide. *Circulation* 66(2):II-166

63. Greenberg, R. N., Guerrant, R. L., Chang, B., Robertson, D. C., Murad, F. 1982. Inhibition of *Escherichia coli* heat-stable enterotoxin effects on intestinal guanylate cyclase and fluid secretion by quinacrine. *Biochem. Pharmacol.* 31: 2005–9

64. Mellion, B. T., Ignarro, L. J., Ohlstein, E. H., Pontecorvo, E. G., Hyman, A. L., Kadowitz, P. J. 1981. Evidence for the inhibitory role of cylic GMP in ADP-induced human platelet aggregation in the presence of nitric oxide and related vasodilators. *Blood* 57:946–55

65. Mellion, B. T., Ignarro, L. J., Meyers, C. B., Ohlstein, E. H., Ballot, B. A., et al. 1983. Inhibition of human platelet aggregation by S-nitrosothiols: Heme-dependent activation by soluble guanylate cyclase and stimulation of cyclic GMP accumulation. *Mol. Pharmacol.* 23:653–64

66. Brody, M. J., Shaffer, R. A. 1970. Distribution of vasodilator nerves in the canine hindlimb. *Am. J. Physiol.* 218: 470–74

67. Nandiwada. P. A., Hyman, A. L., Kadowitz, P. J. 1983. Pulmonary vasodilator responses to vagal stimulation and acetylcholine in the cat. *Circ. Res.* 53:86–95

68. Frank, G. W., Bevan, J. A. 1983. Electrical stimulation causes endothelium-dependent relaxation in lung vessels. *Am. J. Physiol.* 244:H793–98

69. Lincoln, T. M., Corbin, J. D. 1983. Characterization and biological role of the cGMP-dependent protein kinase. *Adv. Cyclic Nucl. Res.* 15:139–92

70. Schultz, K. D., Bohme, E., Kreye, V. A.

W., Schultz, G. 1979. Relaxation of hormonally stimulated smooth muscular tissues by the 8-bromo derivative of cyclic GMP. *Naunyn-Schmiedeberg's Arch. Pharmacol.* 306:1–9

71. Napoli, S. A., Gruetter, C. A., Ignarro, L. J., Kadowitz, P. J. 1980. Relaxation of bovine coronary arterial smooth muscle by cyclic GMP, cyclic AMP and analogs. *J. Pharmacol. Exp. Ther.* 212:469–73

72. Rapoport, R. M., Draznin, M. B., Murad, F. 1982. Sodium nitroprusside-induced protein phosphorylation in intact rat aorta is mimicked by 8-bromo cyclic GMP. *Proc. Natl. Acad. Sci. USA* 79:6470–74

73. Lincoln. T. M. 1983. Effects of nitro-

prusside and 8-bromo-cyclic GMP on the contractile activity of the rat aorta. *J. Pharmacol. Exp. Ther.* 224:100–7

74. Casnellie, J. E., Schlichter, D. J., Walter, U., Greengard, P. 1978. Photoaffinity labeling of a guanosine 3':5'-monophosphate-dependent protein kinase from vascular smooth muscle. *J. Biol. Chem.* 253:4771–76

75. Martin, W., Villani, G. M., Furchgott, R. F. 1984. Hemoglobin and methylene blue selectively inhibit relaxation of rabbit aorta by agents which increase cyclic GMP levels. *Fed. Proc.* 43:737

76. Furchgott, R. F., Jothianandan, D. 1984. Relaxation of rabbit aorta by light is associated with an increase in cyclic GMP. *Fed. Proc.* 43:737

Ann. Rev. Pharmacol. Toxicol. 1985. 25:193–223

AFFINITY LABELS FOR OPIOID RECEPTORS

A. E. Takemori

Department of Pharmacology, University of Minnesota Medical School, Minneapolis, Minnesota 55455

P. S. Portoghese

Department of Medicinal Chemistry, University of Minnesota College of Pharmacy, Minneapolis, Minnesota 55455

INTRODUCTION

The concept of multiple opioid receptors and multiple modes of interaction with a single receptor emanated from two convergent lines of research. This proposal was based originally on a detailed analysis of a wide spectrum of structure-activity relationships among analgesic ligands (1, 2). Very soon, pharmacological studies complemented and provided a more detailed framework for this concept (3–5). More recently, the multiple receptor concept has been advanced through a number of in vitro and in vivo biological assays and the opioid receptor binding assay. Data from such studies have been summarized in a number of reviews (6–13).

Based on a wide range of pharmacological tests in the chronic spinal dog, Martin and coworkers (14, 15) suggested the designation μ, κ, or σ for those receptors at which morphine, ketazocine, and SKF 10,047 (N-allyl-normetazocine) respectively are postulated to interact. The notion of different receptors for morphine-like and ketazocine- or nalorphine-like compounds has been strengthened by the use of the pA_2 concept (16) both in vitro (17–19) and in vivo (5) and by various other testing methods in vivo (20–22). The δ and ϵ receptor through which the enkephalins and β-endorphin respectively are thought to mediate their effects have been identified in vitro (19, 23, 24). The δ receptor in vivo has been implicated in a number of physiological functions

193

0362-1642/85/415-0193$02.00

(25–27). In addition, recent evidence suggests that there may be subtypes of certain of these types of opioid receptors (28–30).

While opioid antagonists such as naloxone and naltrexone have been used extensively as pharmacologic tools (31, 32), these agents are not highly selective for the types of opioid receptors they block. Despite their vast utility in opioid-receptor research, a great deal more useful information might be obtained if more highly selective ligands were available. In some instances ligands of the nonequilibrium type would be preferable for use as pharmacologic tools in vitro and in vivo. For example, the use of a compound that bonds covalently and specifically with opioid receptors would be far more advantageous than a reversible ligand for receptor-isolation studies. The advantage would be increased further if the ligand were specific for a particular type of opioid receptor. Such specific, nonequilibrium ligands could be used in sorting out the various opioid receptor types. The interaction of a ligand with a specific type of receptor would avoid cross-reactivity with other types of receptors, as is the case with the presently available reversible antagonists. Precise information can be obtained by the use of specific ligands in receptor binding experiments as well as in mapping the location and distribution of type-specific sites. Specific agonists and antagonists could also be used to determine the relative involvement of a certain receptor type in a particular opiate-induced pharmacologic effect. Finally, nonequilibrium ligands are inherently long-acting and as such may find clinical utility, e.g. an ultralong-lasting narcotic antagonist.

It is the purpose of this article to review the availability of affinity labels for opioid receptors, discuss their selectivity for the various types of opioid receptors, and point out their utility as pharmacologic tools in opioid-receptor research.

Nomenclature

It is important at the outset to define the manner in which certain nomenclature is used in this review. Affinity labels refer to ligands that have very high affinity for receptors such that the interaction is essentially nonequilibrium. The ligands may or may not be covalently bonded to receptors.

As suggested by Avram Goldstein and Hans Kosterlitz (personal communication), opioid receptors such as μ, κ, and δ are designated as receptor types. Subclassifications of these types of receptors are called subtypes. It should be borne in mind, however, that the designation of different receptors as subtypes of a population rather than of types can be quite arbitrary in the absence of definitive criteria for classification. Ultimately, whether different opioid receptors (e.g. μ_1 and μ_2) are more correctly designated as types or subtypes awaits their chemical and biochemical characterization. Presently, it appears that the chemical reaction of μ-type receptors with the μ-specific affinity label, β-funaltrexamine (β-FNA) (33), is diagnostic for this opioid-receptor system.

A distinction between selectivity and specificity deserves comment. A selective ligand possesses a preferential affinity for a certain type or subtype of receptor, but will have affinity for one or more other types or subtypes. The selectivity of these agents may be relatively high or low at the various receptor types or subtypes. On the other hand, a specific ligand has exclusive affinity for one particular type or subtype of receptor. An agent may possess such high selectivity for a certain type of receptor that interactions at other types are undetectable, in which case the agent could be considered specific.

FACTORS CONTRIBUTING TO SELECTIVITY

By definition, affinity labels take part in a recognition process that leads to a selectively or specificially bound recognition site (34). Their usefulness as pharmacologic and biochemical tools resides with their extremely low degree of dissociation from the site. For these reasons, many affinity labels for opioid receptors possess chemical groups that are sufficiently reactive to form covalent linkages. These groups may be intrinsically reactive and are usually electrophilic in nature, or they may require an activation step that leads to a reactive chemical species. The most common example of the latter involves the photoconversion of the reversibly bound photoaffinity label to a highly reactive intermediate, most often a nitrene or carbene, that covalently binds the opioid receptor.

A ligand with exceptionally high affinity, but without covalent binding capacity, may also meet the criteria for an affinity label if it is sufficiently selective. In this regard, a K_d of not greater than 1×10^{-12}M might be required (assuming an association rate of 10^6M^{-1} sec^{-1}) for such a ligand to remain firmly attached to the receptor for a useful duration (35).

With affinity labels that contain an electrophilic moiety, high selectivity for opioid receptors is dependent on four parameters. These are: (*a*) the affinity of the receptor for the ligand, (*b*) the receptor selectivity of the ligand, (*c*) location of the electrophilic center in the ligand, and (*d*) the reactivity and chemical selectivity of the electrophile. If any one of these parameters is unfavorable, it may have a profound effect on the usefulness of the affinity label as a probe. The studies of Baker (36) on the design of active site–directed irreversible inhibitors of enzymes have considered the importance of some of these parameters.

In considering each of these parameters, it is evident that electrophilic affinity labels are involved in two consecutive recognition processes that lead to the covalent binding of its receptor (33). The first recognition step is reflected by receptor affinity, and the second recognition step involves the proper alignment of the electrophilic center (attached to the reversibly bound ligand) with a compatible, proximal, receptor-based nucleophile. Because two recognition steps rather than one lead to the covalent binding of the affinity label, enhanced receptor selectivity (recognition amplification) is attainable. This recognition amplification may be particularly evident with chemically selective electrophiles.

When the affinity label contains a highly reactive electrophilic group, such recognition amplification is either minimal or absent. The promiscuous nature of such an electrophile (e.g. aziridinium ion derived from a nitrogen mustard group) enables it to alkylate almost any nucleophile within covalent bonding distance on the opioid receptor. In such cases, the covalent binding selectivity is determined primarily by its affinity for the receptor (first recognition step).

This is particularly the case for photoaffinity labels where there is essentially one recognition step due to the high reactivity of the photolyzed intermediate. Such intermediates are so reactive that they can bind covalently to any amino acid sidechain. Consequently, the ability of a photoaffinity label to covalently bind to a particular opioid receptor type is conferred by its selectivity as a reversible ligand. Because the high reactivity of the intermediate ensures covalent binding to a variety of groups on the receptor, the location of the activated center in the photoaffinity label is not critical. It therefore follows that the covalent selectivity of a photoaffinity label is no better than its reversible binding selectivity. This is not the case for affinity labels that contain a chemically selective electrophile.

In view of the very high selectivity, and perhaps specificity, that can be conferred by the intervention of a second recognition step leading to covalent bonding, an electrophilic affinity label is more capable of sorting out a single opioid receptor type among multiple types than are other classes of affinity labels. Thus, if each opioid receptor type contains an unique array of nucleophiles that differ with respect to reactivity and accessibility, then specific covalent binding will depend upon the nature and orientation of the electrophilic center in the reversibly bound affinity label (33). This is illustrated schematically in Figure 1, where three types of receptors (**A, B, C**) with similar topographic features all are capable of associating reversibly with the affinity label. The electrophilic group **X** is sufficiently chemically selective to permit a reaction with the receptor nucleophile G^1 only when it is within covalent bonding distance. This occurs with type **A** receptors, but not with types **B** and **C**. This is because the nucleophiles in the latter are either within covalent bonding distance but insufficiently reactive (type **B**), or beyond the distance required for an efficient reaction (type **C**). As can be noted, an electrophilic affinity label need not form a highly selective, reversible receptor complex to ensure specific covalent binding. Receptor type **A** is specifically covalently

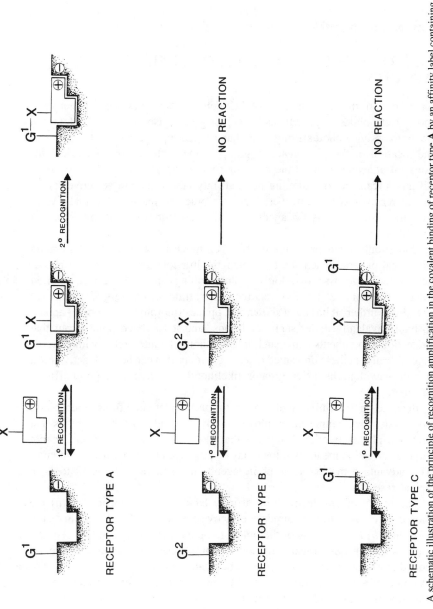

Figure 1 A schematic illustration of the principle of recognition amplification in the covalent binding of receptor type **A** by an affinity label containing a group-selective electrophile **X**. Note that receptor types **A–C** have similar topographic features that lead to reversible binding (1° recognition). However, the receptor types differ with respect to the reactivity (**G**¹ versus **G**² in **A** and **B**) and location (**G**¹ in **A** and **C**) of nucleophiles. Only in **A** is the nucleophile **G**¹ reactive with respect to **X** and within covalent binding distance (2° recognition).

bound, despite recognition of the ligand by types **B** and **C**. Of course, the efficiency with which covalent binding takes place at receptor **A** also is dependent on the residence time (affinity) of the ligand at that site.

PHOTOAFFINITY VERSUS ELECTROPHILIC AFFINITY LABELS

On account of the high reactivity of the photoactivated intermediate relative to most electrophiles (e.g., Michael acceptor groups, isothiocyanate, etc), it is easier to design a photoaffinity label than an electrophilic affinity label. Thus, the location of the photoreactive group in the molecule is not critical for covalent attachment, as is the case for an electrophilic group. This offers a distinct advantage to designing photoaffinity labels that are selective for an opioid receptor type. However, there are practical reasons that make electrophilic affinity labels the agents of choice as probes to investigate opioid receptors.

One should be aware of the effect of modest fluxes of irradiation on biological material when short-wavelength ultraviolet light is used for photoactivation. Large losses of opioid receptor–binding capacity have been reported after irradiation at 254 nm for relatively short time periods (e.g. 7.5 minutes) (37, 38). Further, it has been shown that opiates (morphine, etorphine) appear to bind covalently under such conditions, and it has been pointed out that protection experiments using such ligands should be interpreted with extreme care. Because of these unwanted reactions, groups that can be photoactivated at longer wavelengths offer greater likelihood of success in photoaffinity labeling.

Because photoaffinity labels are useful only under conditions amenable to photolysis, they cannot be employed in vivo or under other conditions that preclude photoactivation. The fact that electrophilic affinity labels do not require activation means that they may be employed both in vitro and in vivo. This advantage makes electrophilic agents much more versatile as tools in opioid research.

The utility of an electrophilic affinity label in vivo depends on (*a*) the biophase concentration required for effective covalent binding to opioid receptors, and (*b*) ready access of the ligand to opioid receptors. The first requirement is met if a significant fraction of opioid receptors become covalently bound at a concentration of affinity label that is not toxic to the animals. For example, if a concentration in the μM range is required for covalent binding within a time-frame of one half hour in vitro, it seems unlikely that this can occur in vivo without toxic effects. With regard to the second requirement, the distribution of the affinity label should be sufficiently favorable to penetrate the opioid receptor compartment.

PHOTOAFFINITY LABELS

The earliest attempt at making a photoaffinity label for opioid receptors was that of Winter & Goldstein (39), who synthesized a [^{3}H]norlevorphanol derivative (APL) (Figure 2). APL acted as a typical reversible agonist in mice and in the guinea pig ileum longitudinal muscle preparation (GPI) before photoactivation. When APL was photolyzed in the presence of either mouse brain particulate fraction or the GPI, irreversible binding occurred, but levorphanol failed to effectively block the binding. As the authors suggest, extensive nonspecific binding probably occurred with this agent. Indeed, even bovine serum albumin was readily bound by APL. The N-methyl quaternary derivative of APL, MAPL, was subsequently synthesized and tested on the GPI (40). Upon photoactivation, MAPL displayed irreversible activity in decreasing acetylcholine output from the preparation. Although the selectivity of this agent was not examined, this agonist effect did show that the rate of ligand-receptor dissociation (41) was not important for agonist activity in the GPI.

A number of fentanyl derivatives (Figure 3) have been synthesized (42). These compounds were generally unsuccessful as affinity labels, although the diazoketone **3** and the arylazide **5** appeared upon photolysis to produce a moderate irreversible inhibition of [^{3}H]naloxone binding to opioid receptors. Related ligands with electrophilic R^1 substituents similarly were unsuccessful as affinity labels.

In another attempt at obtaining useful photoaffinity probes, the synthesis and properties of a nitro-azido derivative of 14β-aminonormorphinone (NAM)

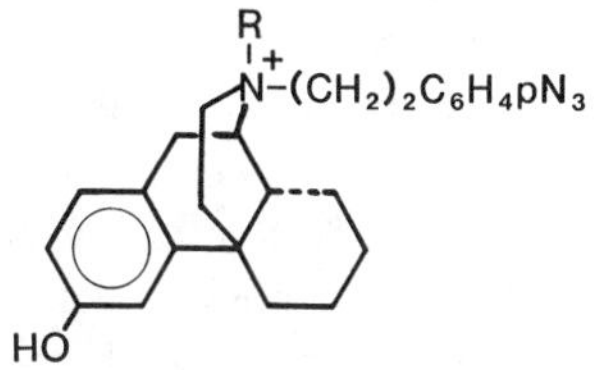

	R
APL	H
MAPL	CH$_3$

Figure 2

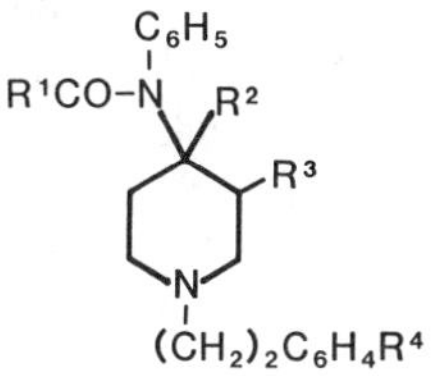

	R^1	R^2	R^3	R^4
1	CHN$_2$	H	H	H
2	CHN$_2$	CO$_2$Me	H	H
3	CHN$_2$	H	CH$_3$	H
4	CH$_2$N$_3$	H	H	H
5	Et	CH$_2$OMe	H	p–N$_3$

Figure 3

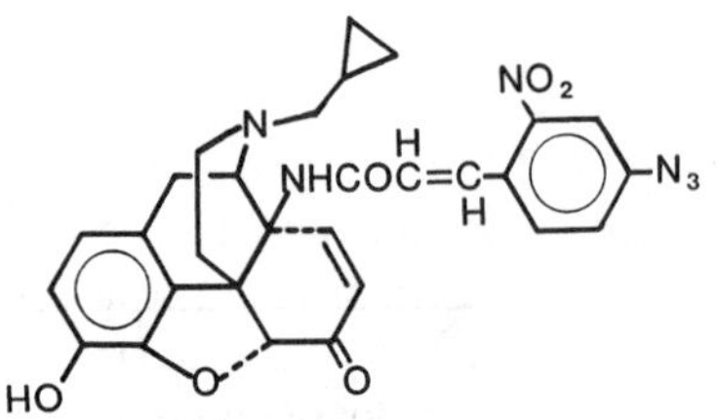

Figure 4

(Figure 4) has been reported (43). NAM was a pure antagonist in both the GPI and the mouse vas deferens preparation (MVD) with a slow association and dissociation rate from opioid receptors. In binding studies, photoactivation of NAM in the presence of rat brain membranes inhibited irreversibly the binding of [^{3}H][D-Ala^2,MePhe^{4}Gly-ol^5]enkephalin (DAGO). Although NAM appeared to bind selectively to μ opioid receptors, it has been deemed unsuitable for labeling opioid receptors due to its slow receptor kinetics. An important observation from this study was that ultraviolet irradiation of rat brain membranes alone decreased their binding activity, as reported earlier by others (37).

Attempts to photoaffinity label opioid receptors also have been carried out with enkephalin analogues (Table 1). Photolysis of analogue 1 (44) inhibited irreversibly the binding of [^{3}H][D-Ala^2,Met^5]enkephalinamide (DAME) to membrane fractions of neuroblastoma × glioma hybrid cells (NG 108–15), which are known to contain only δ opioid receptors (45). Although δ receptors are implicated in this interaction, no further experiments on the selectivity of this ligand have been performed. Analogue 2 (46) inhibited [^{125}I][D-Ala^2,D-Leu^5]enkephalin (DADLE) binding to brain membranes, and upon photoactivation it appeared to bind covalently. The selectivity of the covalent association has not been examined. In a related series of azide enkephalin analogs (3–5) (38), the results of the receptor binding assay showed that opioid receptors in bovine caudate nucleus were inactivated. Since [^{3}H]etorphine was used in the opiate binding assay and etorphine is known to possess equal affinity at most types of opioid receptors (47), the selectivity of these photo-affinity labels has not been established. These peptides possessed agonist activity in the GPI, but photoactivation was not possible because ultraviolet irradiation alone eliminated completely and irreversibly the electrically stimulated contractions of the GPI. Recently, two other photoaffinity labels (6, 7) that contain a 2-nitro-4-azidophenyl group linked to [D-Ala^2,Leu^5]enkephalin by ethylenediamine or ethylenediamine-β-alanine spacers have been described (48, 49). Both compounds had high affinity in displacing [^{3}H]DAME from rat brain membranes, in inhibiting contractions of the MVD, and in inhibiting opiate-sensitive adenylate cyclase of NG 108-15 hybrid cell membranes. The latter two effects were reversed by naloxone. When photoactivated in the presence of brain membranes, both compounds bound irreversibly to about

Table 1 Photoaffinity enkephalin analogues

Compound number	Analogue
1	Tyr·D-Ala·Gly·Phe·Met·Tyr-NH$(CH_2)_2$NH-C_6H_4(2-NO$_2$,4-N$_3$)
2	Tyr·D-Ala·Gly·Phe·Leu-NHCH(CO$_2$H)$(CH_2)_4$NH-C_6H_4(2-NO$_2$,4-N$_3$)
3	Tyr·D-Ala·Gly-NH$(CH_2)_3C_6H_4$$p$-N$_3$
4	Tyr·D-Ala·Gly·Phe-NH$(CH_2)_3C_6H_4$$p$-N$_3$
5	Tyr·D-Ala·Gly·DL-(m-N$_3$)Phe·Leu-NH$_2$
6	Tyr·D-Ala·Gly·Phe·Leu-NH$(CH_2)_2$NH-C_6H_4(2-NO$_2$,4-N$_3$)
7	Tyr·D-Ala·Gly·Phe·Leu-NH$(CH_2)_2$NH·CO$(CH_2)_2$NH-C_6H_4(2-NO$_2$,4-N$_3$)
8	Tyr·D-Thr·Gly·(p-N$_3$)Phe·Leu·Thr
9	Tyr·D-Ala·Gly·Me-(p-N$_3$)Phe·Gly-ol

50% of the binding sites. However, when membranes of NG 108-15 cells were used, up to 80% of the receptors were inactivated. Since DAME binds equally well to μ and δ receptors present in brain membranes, and NG 108-15 cells are known to contain only δ receptors, the investigators concluded that these ligands were relatively selective for δ receptors. They also found with [^{3}H]7 that much of the label bound selectively to opioid receptors, although this labeling of brain membranes was not specific. An important departure in the photoactivation procedure in this study was the use of purely visible light for photolysis rather than the usual ultraviolet irradiation. Thus, these investigators avoided the destruction of opioid receptors associated with short-wavelength ultraviolet irradiation (37). More recently, the azido derivatives of two selective peptides have been synthesized (50). They are derivatives of DAGO (a μ-selective ligand) and Tyr·D-Thr-Gly·Phe·Leu·Thr (DTLET) (a δ-selective ligand). Upon photoirradiation of brain membranes in the presence of azido-DTLET (**8**), binding of [^{3}H]DTLET was inhibited without any effect on the binding of [^{3}H]DAGO. Excess DTLET was capable of completely protecting δ binding sites from alkylation by azido-DTLET. At high concentrations of azido-DTLET, photoinactivation of some μ sites also occurred. The authors did not rule out the possibility of inactivating κ sites with azido-DTLET. Analogous photoactivation experiments with azido-DAGO (**9**) have not been described. If azido-DTLET proves to have high selectivity in receptor binding as well as in biological systems, it may find utility in characterizing δ receptors in the future.

ELECTROPHILIC AFFINITY LABELS

Agonists

May et al (51) have described the first attempt to design electrophilic ligands for opioid receptors. These compounds, which are two N-2-bromoalkyl substituted benzomorphans (**1–3**) (Figure 5), produced prolonged central depression together with a low degree of analgesic activity in mice. However, the opioid nature and the irreversibility of the pharmacologic effects have not been demonstrated. Thus, it is uncertain whether these derivatives interacted with opioid receptors in a nonequilibrium manner. Very recently, another potential benzomorphan affinity label (**4**) (52) has been reported to inhibit irreversibly the binding of [^{3}H]DAME to opioid receptors on NG 108-15 hybrid cells. Although δ receptors are implicated here, the extent of its selectivity has not been explored.

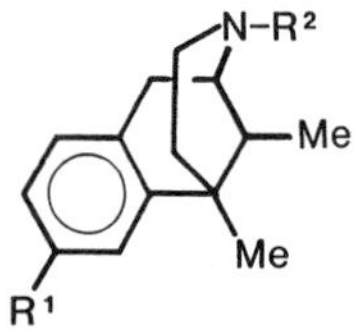

	R^1	R^2	
1	H	CH_2CH_2Br	
2	H	$CH_2CHBrCH_3$	
3	H	$CH_2CHBrC_6H_5$	
4	OH	$(CH_2)_2C_6H_4pNHCOCH_2Br$	*Figure 5*

An early effort to design affinity labels with the anileridine pharmacophore afforded equivocal results (53). Derivatives containing electrophilic moieties attached to the anilino nitrogen (Figure 6) all possessed analgesic activity in mice, but only the fumaramido ethyl ester (**2**) appeared to cause fairly long-lasting (> 6 hours) blockade of morphine analgesia. Pretreatment of mice with naloxone prevented the analgesic activity of **2** and protected opioid receptors from long-lasting blockade. It was suggested that the initial interaction of **2** with opioid receptors gave rise to a reversible complex that resulted in analgesia, while the subsequent interaction arose from the alkylation and inactivation of opioid receptors. Further studies on the GPI indicated that compounds in this series interacted with μ opioid receptors (54). Unexpectedly, however, **2** did not display any antagonist activity in this preparation. This observation suggests that central opioid receptors may differ from those in the ileum.

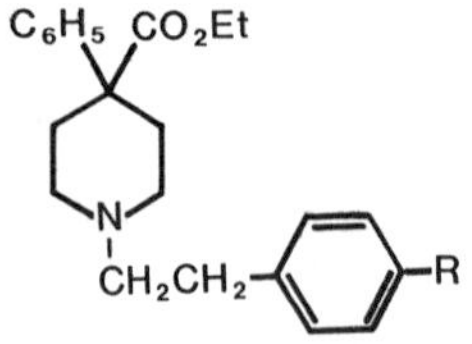

	R
1	$NHCOCH_2X$, X = Br or I
2	NHCOC=CCOOEt (H; H)
3	NHCOC=CCOOEt (H H; H H)
4	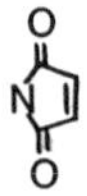

Figure 6

A similar rationale has been employed in the utilization of 3-hydroxy-morphinan as a pharmacophore (Figure 7) (55). Many of these derivatives exhibited analgesic activity in mice and some have been found to be modest inhibitors of morphine-induced analgesia. The most potent antagonist among these compounds was the maleimide derivative (4). Studies with naloxone revealed that it blocked the analgesic action of 4 and protected the receptors from interaction with this ligand. Although this compound contained an electrophilic moiety, additional pharmacologic data suggested that the blockage of opioid receptors in vivo may not involve covalent association.

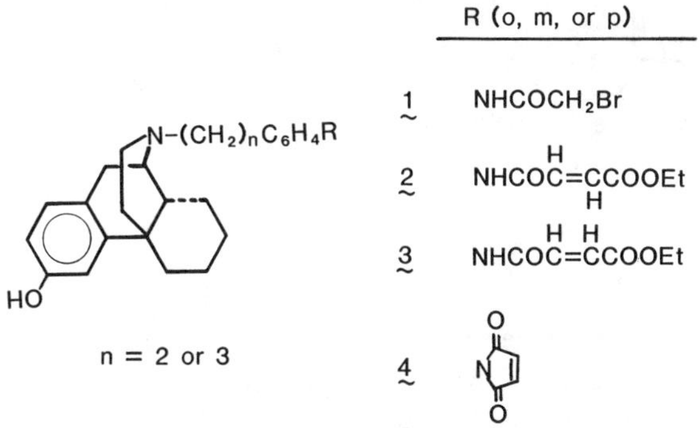

Figure 7

In another effort to obtain selective affinity labels, the isothiocyanate derivatives of fentanyl (FIT) and etonitazene (BIT) and the fumaramido derivative of endoethenotetrahydrooripavine (FAO) have been synthesized (Figure 8) (56). In the opioid receptor binding assay using both rat brain membranes and NG 108-15 hybrid cells, FIT and FAO appeared to be highly selective alkylators of δ receptors and BIT appeared to alkylate μ receptors selectively. These labels have been reported to possess no cross-reactivity between these two types of receptors. The possible interaction of these ligands with κ receptors and their activities in biological systems in vitro or in vivo have not been investigated. Employing NG 108-15 hybrid cells, [^{3}H]FIT has been used to identify a Mr 58,000 subunit of opioid receptors (57). The binding of [^{3}H]FIT to this subunit withstood extensive washing, and levorphanol, but not dextrorphan, prevented this binding. From its adsorption on and specific elution from wheat germ agglutinin, the subunit has been thought to be a glycoprotein. [^{3}H]FIT also labels a number of proteins and phospholipids nonspecifically.

Morphinone (1) (Figure 9) has been reported to irreversibly inhibit [^{3}H]naloxone binding to opioid receptors in brain membranes (58). Since dihydromorphinone did not inhibit binding, it is possible that the α,β-unsaturated ketone system in morphinone may not react with a receptor nucleophile. The authors of this report have also demonstrated that the parenteral

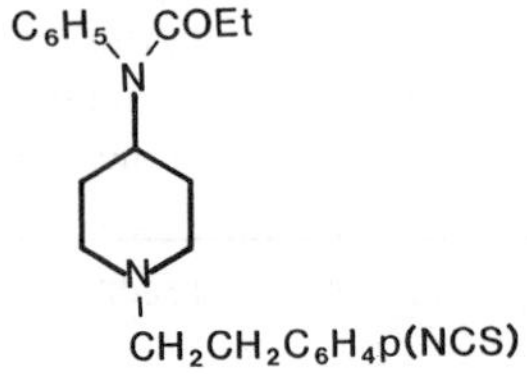

C$_6$H$_5$ COEt
N

CH$_2$CH$_2$C$_6$H$_4$p(NCS)

FIT

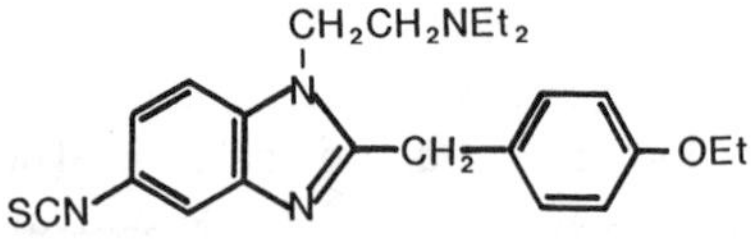

CH$_2$CH$_2$NEt$_2$
N

SCN— —CH$_2$— —OEt
N

BIT

N—Me

'''NHCO-$\overset{H}{\underset{H}{C=C}}$-CO$_2$Me

HO   OMe

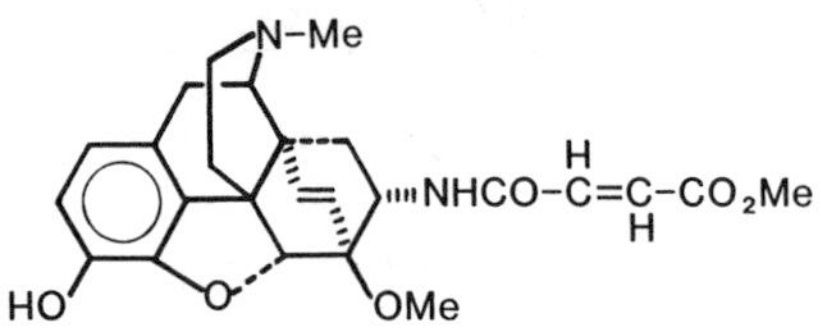

FAO   *Figure 8*

administration of morphinone to mice for 1–3 days inhibited markedly the analgesic effect of morphine. Recently, cyclopropylmethylnormorphinone (**2**) as well as morphinone have been prepared and tested on the GPI, MVD, and in mice (59). Morphinone behaved as a reversible agonist and cyclopropylmethyl-normorphinone as a reversible antagonist in the in vitro and in vivo assays. No evidence for sustained agonism or antagonism has been observed with either compound. Since in the earlier report, morphinone was administered parenter-ally and the latter study employed the intracerebroventricular (icv) route, a direct comparison of the two studies is difficult with regard to antagonism of morphine analgesia. However, if morphinone were capable of antagonizing morphine analgesia, it would have been more easily detected by the icv route. Another morphinone derivative **3** and its morphine derivative have been de-scribed (60). Both compounds had modest irreversible inhibitory activity against [^{3}H]naloxone binding to opioid receptors in brain membranes. A rigorous test for selectivity or experiments in biological systems have not been performed.

The nitrogen mustard derivative of oxymorphone, β-chloroxymorphamine

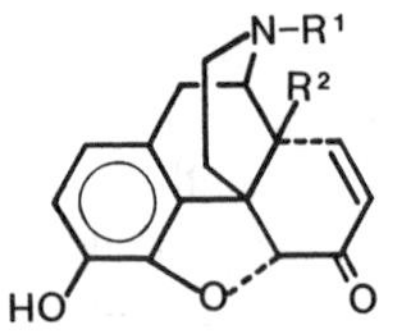

N—R^1
R^2

HO   O   O

	R^1	R^2
1	Me	H
2	CH$_2$—◁	H
3	Me	NHCOCH$_2$Br

Figure 9

(β-COA) (Figure 10) has been shown to be an irreversible agonist in the GPI (61, 62). This observation suggests that receptor occupation rather than rate of ligand-receptor dissociation (41) is important for agonist activity in the GPI (40). β-COA also appeared to bind irreversibly opioid receptor sites in brain membranes, as indicated by the fact that exhaustive washing and eight hours of dialysis of β–COA treated membranes did not eliminate the inhibition of [³H]naltrexone binding. In mice, β-COA produced analgesia with a duration four times that of its reversible analogue, oxymorphone. This β–COA induced analgesia was inhibited by pretreatment of mice with naloxone. In addition, β-COA given icv had long-lasting antagonist effect (~ 6 days) against morphine-induced analgesia. The antagonism of morphine-induced analgesia at spinal sites was even more pronounced when β-COA was given intrathecally (it), as the antagonism in this case lasted more than 21 days (63). The inhibition of [³H]naltrexone binding to brain membranes of β–COA treated animals also persisted for about six days. These results indicated that β-COA was covalently bound to opioid receptors in vivo.

| Oxymorphone | β-COA | Figure 10 |

With the success of obtaining the irreversible agonist β-COA, which has the nitrogen mustard group at the 6β position of the opiate, placement of the electrophilic group at other positions in the opiate molecule, such as at the C-8 position, has been investigated in order to explore the accessibility of other nucleophiles on opioid receptors to alkylation (64). An opiate with the nitrogen mustard group in the C-8 position (Figure 11) has been found to be a weak, reversible, partial agonist in both the GPI and MVD without any significant irreversible agonist or antagonist activity. It also has been found that a small moiety, such as an azide substitution at C-8, did not seriously impair reversible agonist activity, but a larger moiety, such as the precursor diol of the nitrogen mustard derivative, was devoid of any reversible agonist or antagonist activity. These observations led the authors to conclude that this nitrogen mustard derivative has low affinity for opioid receptors and that the C-8 position cannot accommodate large electrophilic groups without compromising the primary recognition step for ligand-receptor interaction.

The first reported peptide electrophilic affinity label was the chloromethyl ketone derivative of [D-Ala²Leu⁵]enkephalin (DALECK) (Figure 12), which

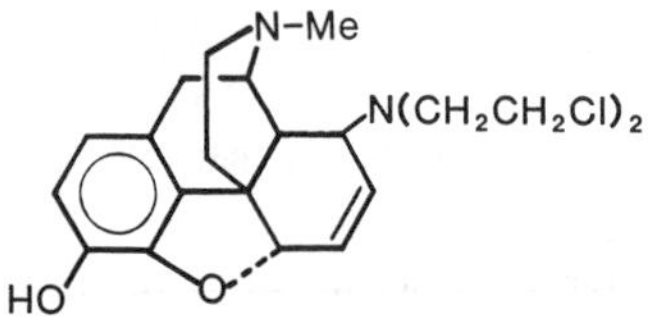

Figure 11

was initially synthesized by Pelton et al (65) and subsequently by two other groups (66, 67). The binding of this agent to opioid receptors in the receptor binding assay using [³H]DADLE, [³H]etorphine, or [³H]naloxone appeared to be irreversible. However, the agonist effects of DALECK in the GPI, MVD, and analgesic assays were all fully reversible by naloxone. Thus, it is uncertain whether DALECK possesses selectivity or if covalent association of opioid receptors is possible with this agent in biological systems. In another approach to obtain a potential peptide label, [D-Ala²,Leu⁵]enkephalin (DALA) was extended with the methyl ester of the nitrogen mustard drug melphalan (Mel) at the C-terminus (68). This compound, DALA-Mel-OMe, displayed high affinity in displacing [³H]DALA and [³H]naloxone from brain membranes. Although DALA-Mel-OMe appeared to block irreversibly the binding of [³H]naloxone, the fact that naloxone and DALA afforded only partial protection suggests that nonspecific labeling also occurred.

Tyr·D-Ala·Gly·Phe·Leu-R

	R
DALA	OH
DALECK	CH_2Cl
DALA-Mel-OMe	$NHCH(COOH)CH_2C_6H_5pN(CH_2CH_2Cl)_2$

Figure 12

Antagonists

It is obvious from the preceding discussion that agonist electrophilic affinity labels in general have not yielded compounds with wide utility. In investigations of pharmacologic effects and characterizations of opioid receptor types, antagonists, especially those without agonist activity, have been extremely useful, as exemplified by the contribution that naloxone and naltrexone have made in this field as pharmacologic tools. However, the reversible nature of such antagonists and their cross-reactivity with the various opioid receptor types are inherent limitations to their use as receptor probes. Thus, there have been a number of efforts to develop highly selective antagonists of the non-equilibrium type.

The first successful antagonist affinity label synthesized was a nitrogen mustard derivative of naltrexone, β-chlornaltrexamine (β-CNA) (Figure 13) (69, 70). β-CNA proved to be a potent affinity label highly selective for opioid receptors both in vitro and in vivo. β-CNA inhibited irreversibly the binding of either [^{3}H]naloxone or [^{3}H]naltrexone to brain membranes. Support for opioid receptor alkylation by β-CNA has been indicated by the fact that neither exhaustive washing nor eight hours of dialysis dissociated β-CNA from opioid receptors, while the reversible ligands, naltrexone and oxymorphone, were completely removed by these procedures. Nonopioid nitrogen mustards, chlorambucil and phenoxybenzamine, had no affinity for specific opioid sites in this regard (62). In both the GPI and the MVD preparations, β-CNA produced irreversible antagonism that could be prevented but not reversed by naloxone (61, 71). β-CNA displayed classical nonequilibrium antagonism in that the agonist concentration-response curve was shifted to the right with a decrease in the maximum effect. Although β-CNA blocked all opioid receptor types, i.e. antagonism of the effects of morphine (μ) and ethylketazocine (κ) in the GPI and additionally DADLE (δ) in the MVD, it did not antagonize the effects of norepinephrine in the GPI. The observation that β-CNA failed to block cholinergic, prostaglandin, or benzodiazepine binding sites (72) provided further evidence for the selectivity of β-CNA for opioid receptors. The nonopioid nitrogen mustards, chlorambucil and phenoxybenzamine, possessed no antagonist activity against morphine in the GPI. The facility with which β-CNA irreversibly blocked different receptor types was μ > κ > δ, which parallels its affinity for these sites in the reversible association phase preceding covalent binding. This is in accordance with the idea that little or no secondary recognition is operative in affinity labels that contain highly reactive and indiscriminate electrophiles (73).

In mice, β-CNA produced ultralong antagonism (> 3 days) of morphine-induced analgesia after a single icv injection. By comparison, antagonism by naltrexone icv lasted less than two hours (62). β-CNA displayed very weak analgesia that dissipated within 30 minutes. In line with the long duration of action, a single icv administration of β-CNA to mice inhibited the development of physical dependence on morphine during the 72-hour observation period. When given it, β-CNA produced even longer antagonism against it morphine analgesia (> 13 days) (63). The antagonism by β-CNA could be prevented by prior administration of naloxone, indicating that opioid receptors were involved. Significantly, the specific [^{3}H]naltrexone binding capacity of brain membranes of animals treated with β-CNA was significantly decreased for the same length of time as β-CNA antagonism, which suggests that covalent bonding had occurred in vivo as well.

[^{3}H]β-CNA has been used to isolate opioid receptor components from brain membranes (74). Covalently bound [^{3}H]β-CNA complex has been solubilized,

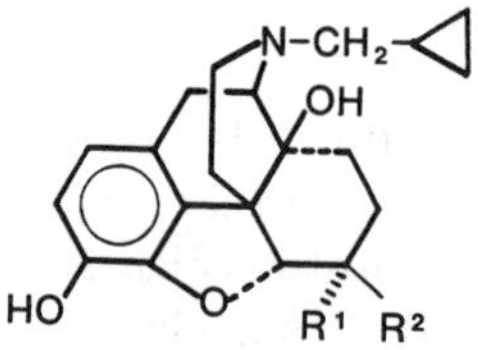

		R¹	R²
1	β–CNA	H	$N(CH_2CH_2Cl)_2$
	α–CNA	$N(CH_2CH_2Cl)_2$	H
2	β–FNA	H	NHCOC=CCOOMe (with H, H on double bond)
	α–FNA	NHCOC=CCOOMe (with H, H on double bond)	H
3		H	NCS
		NCS	H
4		H	NHCOC=CCOOMe (with H, H)
5		H	$NHCOCH=CH_2$
6		H	$NHCOC=CH_2$ (with Cl)
7		H	NHCOC=CCOMe (with H, H)
8		H	NHCOC≡CH
9		H	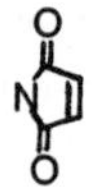 (maleimide N-linked)
10		H	$NHCOCH_2$–(maleimide) 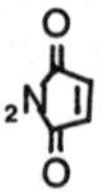
11		H	$NHCOCH_2$–S–S–$C_6H_5O(NO_2)$
12		H	$NHCOCH_2HgCl$
13		H	$NHCOCH_2I$
14		H	$NH–COCO–C_6H_5$

Figure 13

dialyzed, and chromatographed. The elution profile suggests four selective [^{3}H]β-CNA complexes. At least two of these complexes migrated in a single large peak, which has been calibrated to be 590,000 daltons. One of the complexes eluted at the elution volume and was dialyzable, while putative aggregates of these complexes eluted at the void volume. Because of the high reactivity of β-CNA, these complexes may represent multiple forms of opioid receptors.

Since β-CNA is highly selective for opioid receptors, it has been used for typical protection studies. For example, in the MVD, β-CNA has been used with Tyr·D-Ser·Gly·Phe·Leu·Thr (DSLET), a highly selective δ agonist, as the protector to irreversibly block μ and κ receptors. Such preparations contain a near-homogeneous population of δ receptors and have been used in assessing the δ activity of agonists (75). In the GPI, β-CNA has been used with DADLE, which interacts with μ receptors in this preparation, and dynorphin$_{(1-13)}$ as protectors to selectively alkylate κ and μ receptors respectively (76, 77). Further studies using ethylketazocine and normorphine as additional protectors suggested that the relative potencies of dynorphin$_{(1-13)}$ in these blocked preparations are very similar to those of ethylketazocine. This observation, together with the fact that naloxone had similar K_e values in antagonizing dynorphin$_{(1-13)}$ and ethylketazocine, has led investigators to conclude that dynorphin is a specific endogenous κ agonist. Further work in the GPI has revealed that low concentrations of β-CNA selectively alkylated μ and κ receptors without inactivating δ receptors (78). In addition, increasing concentrations of β-CNA have been employed to progressively block dynorphin receptors in the GPI and MVD (79). A concentration of β-CNA that lowered substantially the maximum effect of dynorphin in the MVD caused a parallel shift of the concentration-response curve in the GPI. It has been concluded that the difference in potency of dynorphin in the two preparations is due to the presence of more spare receptors in the GPI than in the MVD. The dissociation constant of the normorphine-receptor complex in the GPI has been estimated by using β-CNA to partially block a fraction of the receptor population (80). The estimate of the dissociation constant has been accomplished by the principle laid down by Furchgott & Bursztyn (81). Since the dissociation constants of normorphine in naive and morphine-tolerant ilea were not significantly different, the authors concluded that changes in affinity at opioid receptors do not occur with the development of tolerance and that tolerance may be related to events after the receptor interaction. However, in relating this to the whole animal, it has already been demonstrated that in chronic studies opioid receptors in the GPI may not be an appropriate model for those in the central nervous system (82).

Using the protection procedure, β-CNA has been used to enrich specific binding sites in brain membranes (83). Sufentanil, DADLE, and dynorphin A have been used as protectors for μ, δ, and κ sites respectively. However, as in all protection studies, the protection of selected receptor sites is only as good as the selectivity of the protector. Thus, except for the dynorphin-protected sites, the enriched preparations were still not completely homogeneous. Nevertheless, β-CNA pretreatment procedure affords better estimates of binding selectivity than the conventional method. Highly selective agonists for the various opioid receptor types have been identified: DAGO, sufentanil, and morphiceptin for μ sites; [D-Pen^2,D-Pen^5]enkephalin and [D-Pen^2,L-Pen^5]enkephalin for δ sites; and tifluadom and Trans-($\pm$)-3,4-dichloro-N-methyl-N-[2-(1-pyrrolidinyl) cyclohexyl]benzeneacetamide (U50,488) for κ sites.

β-CNA also has been used in vivo as a pharmacologic tool in a variety of studies. In an early study, β-CNA was used to study the opiate nature of the effects of Δ^9-tetrahydrocannabinol (THC) in rats (84). After a single icv injection of β-CNA, the analgesia, hypothermia, hypothermic tolerance, and physical dependence produced by THC were all inhibited. The results suggested that there are some common features between THC and opiates and that some actions of THC may be mediated by an opioid-related mechanism. β-CNA has been employed in several behavioral studies. The long-lasting opioid antagonism of β-CNA has been confirmed in studies involving climbing behavior in mice (85), suppression of autoshaped behavior in rats (86), and separation-induced distress vocalization in chicks (87). Opioid selectivity of β-CNA also has been demonstrated by the ability of β-CNA to antagonize morphine, but not amphetamine, in suppressing autoshaped behavior (86). In an effort to study the role of the spinal cord in the development of tolerance and physical dependence, β-CNA has been used to block spinal opioid receptors (88). β-CNA treatment it antagonized the analgesic action of morphine, blocked the development of tolerance, and attenuated several characteristic signs of precipitated withdrawal. The authors concluded that opioid receptors in the spinal cord play a significant role in the development of tolerance and physical dependence induced by systemically administered opiates.

Although β-CNA has proved to be selective for opioid receptors, it was not able to distinguish readily between various receptor types. The very high reactivity of the aziridinium ion generated from β-CNA facilitates the alkylation of opioid receptors but has made this step less selective because this electrophile can react with a variety of nucleophiles. As discussed earlier, the selectivity of the probe for a given opioid receptor type may depend on the reactivity of the attached electrophile and the proximity of the correct nucleophile within that opioid receptor type. In an effort to obtain affinity labels that have more selectivity, electrophilic groups that are less reactive and more selective than the nitrogen mustard group have been attached to the C-6 position of naltrexone (73, 89). One of the most selective ligands in this series was the fumaramate methyl ester derivative β-funaltrexamine (β-FNA) (Figure

14) (90). The analogous derivative of oxymorphone, β-fuoxymorphamine (β-FOA), also has been synthesized in order to compare the interaction of an antagonist with a closely related agonist affinity label. In the GPI, both β-FNA and β-FOA were reversible agonists (90, 91). Using naloxone as the antagonist, pA$_2$ analyses revealed that β-FOA interacted with μ receptors, whereas β-FNA interacted with κ receptors to manifest agonism. Remarkably, in the case of β-FNA but not β-FOA, a concurrent irreversible blockage of μ sites occurred. Thus, after the agonism of β-FNA was terminated by thorough washing of the GPI, a persistent antagonism of the effect of morphine was observed. The degree of irreversible antagonism was concentration- and time-dependent. That this antagonism was selective for μ sites was revealed by the lack of inhibition of κ agonists such as nalorphine and ethylketazocine. In addition, β-FNA antagonized the agonist effect of β-FOA (μ sites) but not its own agonist effect (κ sites). In contrast to β-CNA, which displayed a typical irreversible antagonism, the inhibition of morphine by β-FNA was manifested as a parallel shift of the concentration-response curve. No diminution of the maximum response has been observed because morphine also is a full agonist at κ receptors (75). In the MVD, β-FNA also displayed a reversible agonist action that upon pA$_2$ analysis with naloxone appeared to be mediated through κ receptor interaction (71). β-FNA displayed all the irreversible antagonist features that it exhibited in the GPI. In addition to having little or no effect on the activity of the κ-agonists, nalorphine and ethylketazocine, β-FNA did not inhibit the effects of the δ-agonists, met-enkephalin, leu-enkephalin, and DADLE. Moreover, IC$_{50}$ of μ-agonists, morphine and methadone, were increased substantially, and the IC$_{50}$ of δ-agonists, leu- and met-enkephalin, were unchanged in vas deferentia taken from mice treated with β-FNA forty-eight hours prior to testing. These observations showed the specificity of β-FNA for μ receptors in this preparation. However, as with any affinity label, at very high concentrations, β-FNA may interact with receptors other than the μ type.

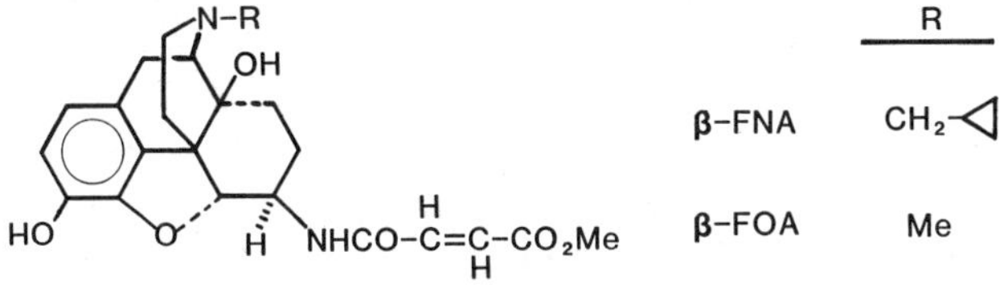

	R
β-FNA	CH$_2$-◁
β-FOA	Me

Figure 14

In the opioid receptor binding assay, β-FNA bound to mouse brain membranes in both a reversible and irreversible manner (92). When membranes were treated with β-FNA followed by thorough washing, the binding capacity for [^{3}H]morphine and [^{3}H]naltrexone was reduced markedly, whereas binding of [^{3}H]met-enkephalin, [^{3}H]DADLE, and [^{3}H]ethylketazocine was decreased to a lesser extent. In brain membranes from mice treated with β-FNA forty-eight hours prior to sacrifice, the binding sites for [^{3}H]morphine were reduced by about 50%, whereas those for [^{3}H]met-enkephalin were unaffected. The receptors in the NG 108-15 hybrid cells were also unaffected by treatment with β-FNA (K.-J. Chang, personal communication). The ability of various un-labeled ligands to inhibit the reversible binding of [^{3}H]β-FNA resembled the relative ability of the same ligands to inhibit the binding of [^{3}H]ethylketazocine (92). The binding characteristics of β-FNA appeared to be consistent with its profile in isolated tissues in that the irreversible portion of β-FNA binding demonstrated selectivity for μ over δ binding sites, while the reversible portion of β-FNA binding exhibited a selectivity for κ over μ or δ binding sites.

In vivo, β-FNA demonstrated analgesic activity in mice of short duration (93). This analgesic effect was antagonized by naloxone and upon pA$_2$ analysis appeared to be mediated by κ opioid receptors. In contrast, the antagonist action of β-FNA was of remarkably long duration and selective toward μ agonists. For example, antagonism of morphine-induced analgesia by β-FNA subcutaneously (sc) lasted over four days. The locus of action of β-FNA has been thought to be central because sc administration of β-FNA antagonized the action of morphine given icv and vice versa. The selectivity of the antagonism of β-FNA was exemplified by its lack of antagonism of analgesia elicited by either nalorphine or β-FNA when mice were tested forty-eight hours after β-FNA treatment. This activity profile is consistent with that in vitro.

One of the initial uses of β-FNA has been to deplete the GPI of functional μ receptors (75). Under appropriate conditions, all the μ receptors can be irre-versibly blocked by β-FNA, thereby affording a near homogeneous population of κ receptors. This preparation is useful in assessing the κ activity of agonists. It has been shown in this blocked preparation that morphine was a full agonist at κ receptors, i.e. the pA$_2$ value of morphine-naloxone changed to that resem-bling ethylketazocine-naloxone. A whole range of so-called μ agonists have been tested in this β-FNA-treated GPI and they all exhibited κ activity at high concentrations (A.E. Takemori, P. S. Portoghese, unpublished data). The use of a specific irreversible antagonist such as β-FNA obviates the necessity for protection experiments involving μ receptors. This is particularly advan-tageous in view of the cross-reactivity to κ receptors by μ agonists at the high concentrations used for protection. In this connection, the β–FNA treated GPI has been used to characterize dynorphin as a κ agonist (94). β-FNA also has been used in the tolerant GPI to demonstrate that selective opiate tolerance is not associated with selective dependence, i.e. induction of a selective tolerance at μ receptors produces cross-dependence at κ receptors and vice versa (95). Although μ agonists (normorphine and morphine) and δ agonists such as the enkephalins and their derivatives are presumed to interact at μ receptors in the

GPI (pA_2 values with naloxone are similar), recently it has been reported that in the β–FNA treated GPI the pA_2 values of the μ agonists decreased to values resembling κ agonists, whereas the pA_2 values of the peptides remained unaltered (96, 97). One group has suggested that the peptides were interacting with δ sites uncovered by β-FNA, while another investigator has proposed that the peptides interacted with a μ receptor subtype. Very recently, in a protection experiment involving the same conditions under which the MVD was converted into a relatively pure δ preparation (DSLET + β-CNA) (75), DSLET failed to protect against alkylation by β-CNA in the GPI (A. E. Takemori, P. S. Portoghese, unpublished data). Thus, whatever these β-FNA insensitive sites are called, they do not appear to be of the δ type found in the MVD.

Since β-FNA interacts reversibly at κ receptors and irreversibly at μ receptors, and β-FOA interacts reversibly only at μ receptors, the GPI has been used to study the possibility that μ agonists and antagonists may interact at different sites (98). A series of opioid agonists and antagonists have been evaluated for their ability to protect against the irreversible antagonism of the action of morphine by β-FNA. Antagonists afforded excellent protection against irreversible blockage by β-FNA, whereas most of the agonists were relatively poor protectors. Moreover, the ability of the compounds to protect against β-FNA antagonism appeared to correlate with their antagonist potencies (K_e) but not with their agonist activities (IC_{50}). These results suggest that agonists and antagonists may interact at separate sites on the μ receptor system. Additionally, the fact that both β-FNA and β-FOA contain an identical electrophilic moiety at the C-6 position, with only β-FNA alkylating opioid receptors, suggests that β-FOA and β-FNA may interact at different sites as an agonist and antagonist respectively. This is supported by the fact that β-FOA was unable to protect against β–FNA induced irreversible antagonism. A model consistent with the above findings has been proposed that consists of a μ subunit with which agonists have high affinity and a regulatory ρ subunit with which antagonists have high affinity (98). Occupation of the ρ site has been proposed to produce an unidirectional coupling (allosteric coupling) to the μ site such that a decrease in affinity of agonist interaction at the μ site occurs. The ρ site may be occupied by agonists but only after the μ site is occupied, whereas antagonists interact selectively at the ρ site. The ρ sites are envisaged as regulatory sites for some endogenous μ agonist ligand. A similar dual site opioid receptor model has been proposed by others (99).

A number of studies in vivo have made use of β-FNA to study the relative involvement of μ receptors in various opiate actions. The μ receptor involvement in opiate-induced respiratory depression (100), decrease in gastrointestinal transit (101), cardiovascular effects (102, 103), prolactin secretion (104; L. Krulich, personal communication), spinal analgesia (105, 106), and antidiuresis (107) has been investigated. β-FNA also has been used to demonstrate the noninvolvement of μ receptors in certain opioid actions such as endotoxic shock (108) and post-ictal analgesia (109), which are thought to be mediated by δ receptors, and diuresis (107), which is thought to involve κ receptors. The μ receptor involvement in analgesia produced by κ and δ agonists has also been investigated using β-FNA (110–114).

An important use of β-FNA has been to determine if the phenomena of tolerance and physical dependence are associated with μ opioid receptors. In rats, the physical dependence produced by a continuous intraperontoneal (ip) infusion of morphine was completely blocked by β-FNA (115). When β-FNA was given it, the tolerance and dependence produced by sc morphine pellets was markedly inhibited (116). These results suggest that μ receptors in the central nervous system, including the spinal cord, play a prominent role in the development of tolerance and physical dependence in rodents. β-FNA sc promptly precipitated withdrawal signs in morphine-dependent monkeys that were still evident thirty hours later in spite of the fact that morphine was being administered every six hours (115). In contrast, naloxone-precipitated withdrawal lasted ninety minutes. In another study, β-FNA sc precipitated withdrawal in morphine-dependent monkeys that lasted seventy-two hours (117). When β-FNA was administered icv it was much more potent in precipitating withdrawal, and the syndrome was more severe and longer-lasting than that produced upon abrupt withdrawal of morphine. It is evident that these findings strongly implicate μ opioid receptors in the development of physical dependence in primates. It is also important to note that β-FNA was about 20,000 times more effective when administered icv than sc, indicating that β-FNA may have encountered some difficulty distributing to the brain (117). These investigators also have studied the surmountability by morphine of the antagonist-induced withdrawal in morphine-dependent monkeys. Naltrexone-precipitated withdrawal and abrupt withdrawal were completely suppressed by a relatively moderate dose of morphine sc. However, extremely high doses of morphine did not completely alleviate the monkeys from β-FNA precipitated withdrawal, which strongly suggests the covalent nature of the binding of β-FNA to opioid μ receptors.

In order to determine whether the orientation of the electrophile is important for covalent bonding to opioid receptors, a series of epimeric pairs of naltrexone derivatives (1–3) that contain an electrophilic group at the 6α- or 6β-position have been investigated (73) (Figure 13). All compounds were active as reversible agonists in the GPI, but only the 6β-isomers of the fumaramate ester (β-FNA) and isothiocyanate (3) displayed selective irreversible antagonism of the μ agonist, morphine, without affecting κ agonist activity. The 6α-isomer (α-FNA) acted reversibly and was able to protect the receptors against irreversible blockage by β-FNA, indicating that the two epimers bind to the same μ site. These results suggest that proper orientation of the electrophilic substituent with a proximal nucleophile in μ receptors is necessary for covalent bonding to occur. Moreover, the lack of covalent bonding to κ receptors by ligands in this series indicated that sufficiently reactive nucleophiles were not within covalent bonding distance at the κ site. In the MVD, β-FNA, but not α-FNA, irreversibly antagonized morphine, whereas neither isomer antagonized the δ agonist, DADLE. In contrast, both isothiocyanate epimers (3) irreversibly blocked μ and δ receptors. Because a more reactive electrophile is less efficient in its ability to distinguish between different types of nucleophiles, the isothiocyanate epimers, which are presumably more reactive and less selective than the fumaramates, displayed less of a difference in their capacity to covalently bind receptors. With an extremely reactive electrophile such as the nitrogen mustard group in α- and β-CNA, the difference between the receptor covalent-binding capacity of the two epimers was even less pronounced. Thus, in cases of highly reactive electrophiles, the chirality at C-6 becomes less important in the secondary recognition process.

In addition to the importance of the 6β stereochemistry in ligands that contain moderately reactive and relatively selective electrophiles, it appears that trans geometry of the double bond in the Michael acceptor group is required for irreversible blockage of μ receptors. Thus, it has been found that ligands that contain cis double bonds (4 and 9) (Figure 13) do not irreversibly block the effects of morphine, while β-FNA and 7 are effective in this regard (73). It is conceivable that the role of geometry is one of orienting the electrophilic center within covalent bonding distance of a compatible (e.g. sulfhydryl group) receptor-bound nucleophile. In this connection, the lack of correlation between irreversible μ antagonism and the chemical reactivity of the Michael acceptor ligands supports this notion. Several of these compounds (6, 7) (Figure 13) acted like β-FNA in the GPI and MVD, i.e. reversible agonism at κ receptors and irreversible antagonism at μ, but not κ or δ receptors. Some derivatives (8, 14) were considerably more potent as κ agonists than was β-FNA. These compounds, as well as the maleimidoacetamide (10) and chloromercuriacetamide (12) derivatives, exhibited irreversible agonism. It is noteworthy that 10 and the iodoacetamide (13) were very different from β-FNA in that the irreversible μ antagonism that they displayed was substantially greater in the MVD than in the GPI. α-CNA, in addition to covalently binding μ, κ, and δ receptors, also displayed concurrent irreversible agonist activity in the GPI but not in the MVD (118). These observations suggest that the two preparations contain different proportions of opioid μ receptor subtypes.

MISCELLANEOUS AFFINITY LABELS

It sometimes may be difficult to distinguish between tight noncovalent association and covalent binding of a ligand with its receptor. In the case of ligands that do not contain intrinsically reactive groups, apparent nonequilibrium binding is most likely a consequence of very high affinity, but other mechanisms also are possible. For example, entrapment of a ligand in a tissue compartment or membrane domain that interfaces with opioid receptors might lead to apparent irreversible binding or sustained activity if washing does not readily remove the ligand (89). This mechanism implies that the ligand-receptor interaction is comprised of two consecutive steps: i.e. the partitioning of ligand into a tissue compartment followed by association with the receptor (119). In this case, a locally high concentration may result in an apparent high affinity. Sustained activity can arise from inefficient removal of ligand from the compartment rather than from high receptor affinity. A combination of entrapment and high affinity also will afford sustained activity. It is conceivable that the slow offset of action of the μ partial agonist, buprenorphine (120), in the GPI and its slow dissociation from rat brain receptors arise from such factors.

Nonequilibrium binding and ultralong actions have been reported for hydrazone derivatives of naloxone, naltrexone, and oxymorphone (Figure 15) (121, 122). However, subsequent studies (123) have suggested that the nonequilibrium actions of these hydrazones are due wholly or in part to the corresponding azines as the result of a disproportionation reaction of the hydrazone in solution. Presently, the mechanism of the persistent effect of the azines at opioid receptors is not known. These azines blocked opiate binding in vitro 20–40 times more potently than did their corresponding hydrazones. It is therefore possible that the irreversible action of the hydrazones might be due to conversion of a small fraction of the hydrazone to azine. These azines appear to block a high affinity morphine binding site, designated as μ_1, in brain membranes. A low affinity site, named μ_2 by the researchers, was not permanently blocked. Since it was found that the effects of the azines were reversible in both binding and pharmacologic assays on the GPI, it has been suggested that morphine mediates its effects through a different μ receptor subtype (μ_2) in this preparation (124). More recently, the fact that naloxonazine inhibited the high affinity binding sites for [^{3}H]dihydromorphine and [^{3}H]DADLE far more potently than for the lower affinity sites prompted the proposal for a common high affinity binding site for opiates and opioid peptides (125). Naloxazone and naloxonazine have been employed as biochemical and pharmacological tools in a variety of studies to sort out different opioid receptor types and subtypes (126).

Still another mechanism that may lead to nonequilibrium binding of an unreactive ligand is enzymatic bioactivation. Because of the noncatalytic nature of the opioid receptor, such bioactivation would occur in the biophase. The reactive ligand then would covalently bind after recognition by the receptor. Rice et al have attempted the design of such a compound (127) in the synthesis of N(2,4,5-trihydroxyphenethyl)normetazocine (Figure 16). Their rationale was based on 6-hydroxydopamine, which is known to undergo facile

hydrazones   azines

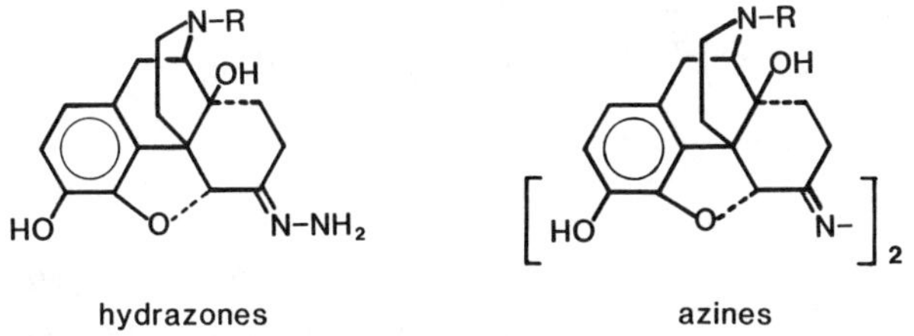

R
CH$_2$CH=CH$_2$
CH$_2$-◁
CH$_3$

Figure 15

oxidation to an electrophilic intermediate that reacts covalently with catechol-amine receptors. However, the normetazocine analogue was not active, possibly because of its low affinity for opioid receptors.

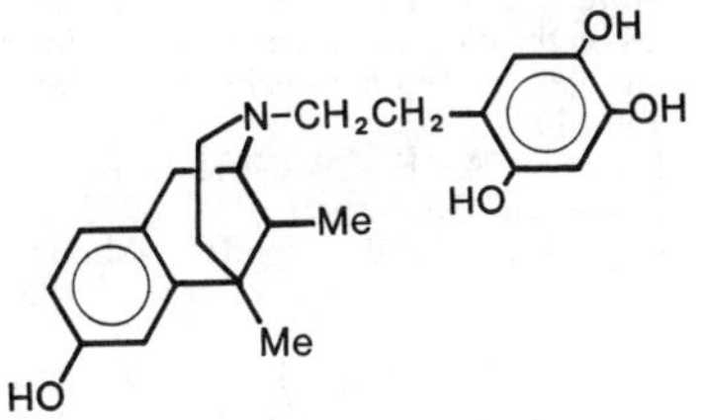

Figure 16

SUMMARY AND CONCLUSIONS

A variety of affinity labels have been synthesized as pharmacologic and biochemical probes for opioid receptors. Their usefulness as affinity labels is related to their receptor selectivity and pharmacologic characteristics. High selectivity or, better still, specificity for a single receptor type or subtype is an important feature. The potential for obtaining specific electrophilic affinity labels is greater than for other classes of affinity labels because two consecutive recognition steps lead to the amplification of selectivity (Figure 1). Indeed, of the presently available affinity labels, the electrophilic antagonist affinity labels have proved to be the most useful opioid receptor probes for pharmacologic studies. The fact that electrophilic affinity labels can be employed in studies both in vitro and in vivo represents a distinct advantage over photoaffinity labels, which can be activated only in vitro.

ACKNOWLEDGEMENTS

The research in the authors' laboratories was supported by US Public Health Service Grants DA-01533 and DA-00289 from the National Institute on Drug Abuse.

Literature Cited

1. Portoghese, P. S. 1965. A new concept on the mode of interaction of narcotic analgesics with receptors. *J. Med. Chem.* 8:609–16
2. Portoghese, P. S. 1966. Stereochemical factors and receptor interactions associated with narcotic analgesics. *J. Pharm. Sci.* 55:865–87
3. Martin, W. R. 1967. Opioid antagonists. *Pharmacol. Rev.* 19:463–521
4. Takemori, A. E., Kupferberg, H. J., Miller, J. W. 1969. Quantitative studies of the antagonism of morphine by nalorphine and naloxone. *J. Pharmacol. Exp. Ther.* 169:39–45
5. Smits, S. E., Takemori, A. E. 1970. Quantitative studies on the antagonism by naloxone of some narcotic and narcotic-antagonist analgesics. *Br. J. Pharmacol.* 39:627–38
6. Snyder, S. H., Goodman, R. R. 1980. Multiple neurotransmitter receptors. *J. Neurochem.* 35:5–15
7. Kosterlitz, H. W. 1980. Enkephalins, endorphins and their receptors. In *Neuropeptides and Neural Transmission,* ed. C. A. Marsan, W. Z. Traczyk, pp. 191–97. New York: Raven. 391 pp.
8. Smith, A. P., Loh, H. H. 1980. Heterogeneity of opiate-receptor interaction. *Pharmacology* 20:57–63
9. Simon, E. J. 1981. Opiate receptors and endorphins: Possible relevance to narcotic addiction. *Adv. Alcohol Subst. Abuse* 1:13–31
10. Zukin, R. S., Zukin, S. R. 1981. Multiple opiate receptors: Emerging concepts. *Life Sci.* 29:2681–90
11. Wüster, M., Schulz, R., Herz, A. 1981. Multiple opiate receptors in peripheral tissue preparations. *Biochem. Pharmacol.* 30:1883–87
12. Iwamoto, E. T., Martin, W. R. 1981. Multiple opioid receptors. *Med. Res. Rev.* 1:411–40
13. Martin, W. R. 1983. Pharmacology of opioids. *Pharmacol. Rev.* 35:283–323
14. Martin, W. R., Eades, C. G., Thompson, J. A., Huppler, R. E., Gilbert, P. E. 1976. The effects of morphine- and nalorphine-like drugs in the nondependent and morphine-dependent chronic

spinal dog. *J. Pharmacol. Exp. Ther.* 197:517–33
15. Gilbert, P. E., Martin, W. R. 1976. The effects of morphine- and nalorphine-like drugs in the nondependent, morphine-dependent and cyclazocine-dependent chronic spinal dog. *J. Pharmacol. Exp. Ther.* 198:66–82
16. Schild, H. O. 1957. Drug antagonism and pAx. *Pharmacol. Rev.* 9:242–46
17. Hutchinson, M., Kosterlitz, H. W., Leslie, F. M., Waterfield, A. A., Terenius, L. 1975. Assessment of the guinea pig ileum and mouse vas deferens of benzomorphans which have strong antinociceptive activity but do not substitute for morphine in the dependent monkey. *Br. J. Pharmacol.* 55: 541–46
18. Ward, A., Takemori, A. E. 1976. Studies on the narcotic receptor in the guinea pig ileum. *J. Pharmacol. Exp. Ther.* 199:117–23
19. Lord, J. A. H., Waterfield, A. A., Hughes, J., Kosterlitz, H. W. 1977. Endogenous opioid peptides: Multiple agonists and receptors. *Nature* 267:495–99
20. Herling, S., Woods, J. H. 1981. Discriminative stimulus effects of narcotics: Evidence for multiple receptor-mediated actions. *Life Sci.* 28:1571–84
21. Adler, M. W. 1981. The *in vivo* differentiation of opiate receptors: Introduction. *Life Sci.* 28:1543–45
22. Cowan, A. 1981. Simple *in vivo* tests that differentiate prototype agonists at opiate receptors. *Life Sci.* 28:1559–70
23. Lemaire, S., Magnan, J., Regoli, D. 1978. Rat vas deferens: A specific bioassay for endogenous opioid peptides. *Br. J. Pharmacol.* 64:327–29
24. Schulz, R., Faase, E., Wüster, M., Herz, A. 1979. Selective receptors for β-endorphin on the rat vas deferens. *Life Sci.* 24:843–50
25. Way, E. L., Glasgow, C. 1978. The endorphins: Possible physiological roles and therapeutic application. *Clin. Ther.* 1:371–86
26. Olson, G. A., Olson, R. D., Kastin, A. J., Coy, D. H. 1979. Endogenous opi-

ates: Through 1978. *Neurosci. Biobehav. Rev.* 3:285–99

27. Jacob, J. 1979. Physiological and pathophysiological relevance of endogenous ligands of the opiate receptors. In *Advances in Pharmacology and Therapeutics* ed. J. Jacob, 1:57–69. Oxford: Pergamon. 294 pp.

28. Sayre, L. M., Portoghese, P. S., Takemori, A. E. 1983. Difference between μ-receptors in the guinea pig ileum and the mouse vas deferens. *Eur. J. Pharmacol.* 90:159–60

29. Pasternak, G. W., Gintzler, A. R., Houghten, R. A., Ling, G. S. F., Goodman, R. R., et al. 1983. Biochemical and pharmacological evidence for opioid receptor multiplicity in the central nervous system. *Life Sci.* 33 (Suppl. 1):167–73

30. Pilapil, C., Wood, P. L. 1983. [³H]-SKF10047 binding to rat brain membranes: Evidence for kappa isoreceptors. *Life Sci.* 33(Suppl. 1):263–65

31. Sawyonk, J., Pinsky, C., LaBella, F. S. 1979. On the specificity of naloxone as an opiate antagonist. *Life Sci.* 25:1621–32

32. Gold, M. S., Dackis, C. A., Pottash, A. L. C., Sternbach, H. H., Annitto, W. J. 1982. Naltrexone, opiate addiction and endorphins. *Med. Res. Rev.* 2(3):211–46

33. Portoghese, P. S., Takemori, A. E. 1982. Highly selective affinity labels for investigation of opioid receptor subtypes. In *The Chemical Regulation of Biological Mechanisms*, ed. A. M. Creighton, S. Turner, pp. 180–99. London: Burlington House. 319 pp.

34. Jacoby, W. B., Wilchek, M., eds. 1977. *Affinity Labelling, Methods in Enzymology*, Vol. 46. New York: Academic. 774 pp.

35. Bennett, J. P. Jr. 1978. Methods in binding studies. In *Neurotransmitter Receptor Binding*, ed. H. I. Yamamura, S. J. Enna, M. J. Kuhar, p. 65. New York: Raven. 195 pp.

36. Baker, B. R. 1967. *Design of Active-Site-Directed Irreversible Enzyme Inhibitors.* New York: Wiley. 325 pp.

37. Glasel, J. A., Venn, R. F. 1981. The sensitivity of opiate receptors and ligands to short wavelength ultraviolet light. *Life Sci.* 29:221–28

38. Smolarsky, M., Koshland, D. E. Jr. 1980. Inactivation of the opiate receptor in bovine caudate nucleus by azide enkephalin analogs. *J. Biol. Chem.* 255:7244–49

39. Winter, B. A., Goldstein, A., 1972. A photochemical affinity-labelling reagent

for the opiate receptor(s). *Mol. Pharmacol.* 8:601–11

40. Schulz, R., Golstein, A. 1975. Irreversible alteration of opiate receptor function by a photoaffinity labelling reagent. *Life Sci.* 16:1843–48

41. Paton, W. D. M. 1961. A theory of drug action based on the rate of drug-receptor combination. *Proc. R. Soc. London Ser. B* 154:21–69

42. Maryanoff, B. E., Simon, E. J., Gioannini, T., Gorissen, H. 1982. Potential affinity labels for the opiate receptor based on fentanyl and related compounds. *J. Med. Chem.* 25:913–19

43. Peers, E. M., Rance, M. J., Barnard, E. A., Haynes, A. S., Smith, C. F. 1983. Photoaffinity probes for opiate receptors: Synthesis and properties of a nitro-azido-derivative of 14-β-aminomorphinone. *Life Sci.* 33(Suppl. 1):439–42

44. Lee, T. T., Williams, R. E., Fox, C. F. 1979. Photoaffinity inactivation of the enkephalin receptor. *J. Biol. Chem.* 254:11787–90

45. Chang, K.-J., Cuatrecasas, P. 1979. Multiple opiate receptors. *J. Biol. Chem.* 254:2610–18

46. Hazum, E., Chang, K.-J., Shecter, Y., Wilkinson, S., Cuatrecasas, P. 1979. Fluorescent and photo-affinity enkephalin derivatives: Preparation and interaction with opiate receptors. *Biochem. Biophys. Res. Commun.* 88:841–46

47. Gillian, M. G. C., Kosterlitz, H. W., Paterson, S. J. 1980. Comparison of the binding characteristics of tritiated opiates and opioid peptides. *Br. J. Pharmacol.* 70:481–90

48. Zioudrou, C., Varoucha, D., Loukas, S., Streaty, R. A., Klee, W. A. 1982. Photolabile ligands for opiate receptors. *Life Sci.* 31:1671–74

49. Zioudrou, C., Varoucha, D., Loukas, S., Nicolaou, N., Streaty, R. A., Klee, W. A. 1983. Photolabile opioid derivatives of D-Ala²-Leu⁵-enkephalin and their interactions with the opiate receptor. *J. Biol. Chem.* 258:10934–37

50. Garbay-Jaureguiberry, C., Robichon, A., Roques, B. P. 1983. Selective photoinactivation of δ-opiate binding sites by azido DTLET: Tyr-D-Thr-Gly-pN₃Phe-Leu-Thr. *Life Sci.* 33(Suppl. 1):247–50

51. May, M., Czoncha, L., Garrison, D. R., Triggle, D. J. 1968. The analgesic, hypothermic and depressant activities of some N-substituted α-5,9-dimethyl-6,7-benzomorphans. *J. Pharm. Sci.* 57:884–87

52. Hallermayer, K., Harmening, C., Merz, H., Hamprecht, B. 1983. Irreversible

activation of the opiate receptor of neuroblastoma × glioma hybrid cells by an alkylating benzomorphan derivative. *J. Neurochem.* 41:1761–65

53. Portoghese, P. S., Telang, V. G., Takemori, A. E., Hayashi, G. 1971. Potential nonequilibrium analgetic receptor inactivators. Synthesis and biological activities of N-acylanileridines. *J. Med. Chem.* 14:144–48

54. Takemori, A. E., Ward, A., Portoghese, P. S., Telang, V. G. 1974. Potential nonequilibrium analgetic receptor inactivators. Further pharmacologic studies of N-acylanileridines. *J. Med. Chem.* 17: 1051–54

55. Portoghese, P. S., Hanson, R. N., Telang, V. G., Winger, J. L., Takemori, A. E. 1977. 3-Hydroxy-17-aralkylmorphinans as potential opiate receptor-site-directed alkylating agents. *J. Med. Chem.* 20:1020–24

56. Rice, K. C., Jacobson, A. E., Burke, T. R. Jr., Bajwa, B. S., Streaty, R. A., Klee, W. A. 1983. Irreversible ligands with high selectivity toward δ or μ opiate receptors. *Science* 220:314–16

57. Klee, W. A., Simonds, W. F., Sweat, F. W., Burke, T. R. Jr., Jacobson, A. E., Rice, K. C. 1982. Identification of a Mr 58000 glycoprotein subunit of the opiate receptor. *FEBS Lett.* 150:125–28

58. Nagamatsu, K., Kido, Y., Terao, T., Ishida, T., Toki, S. 1982. Effect of morphinone on opiate receptor binding and morphine-elicited analgesia. *Life Sci.* 31:1451–57

59. Fang, S., Takemori, A. E., Portoghese, P. S. 1984. Activities of morphinone and N-cyclopropylmethylnormorphinone at opioid receptors. *J. Med. Chem.* 27:1361–63

60. Archer, S., Seyed-Mozaffari, A., Osei-Gyimah, P., Bidlack, J. M., Abood, L. G. 1983. 14β-(2-bromoacetamido)morphine and 14β-(2-bromoacetamido)morphinone. *J. Med. Chem.* 26:1775–77

61. Caruso, T. P., Takemori, A. E., Larson, D. L., Portoghese, P. S. 1979. Chloroxymorphamine, an opioid receptor site-directed alkylating agent having narcotic agonist activity. *Science* 204:316–18

62. Caruso, T. P., Larson, D. L., Portoghese, P. S., Takemori, A. E. 1980. Pharmacological studies with an alkylating narcotic agonist chloroxymorphamine and antagonist, chlornaltrexamine. *J. Pharmacol. Exp. Ther.* 213:539–44

63. Larson, A. A., Armstrong, M. J. 1980. Morphine analgesia after intrathecal administration of a narcotic agonist, chloroxymorphamine and antagonist, chlornaltrexamine. *Eur. J. Pharmacol.* 68:25–31

64. Fang, S., Bell, K. H., Portoghese, P. S. 1984. Synthesis and pharmacological evaluation of an 8β-bis(2-chloroethyl) amino opiate as a nonequilibrium opioid receptor probe. *J. Med. Chem.* 27:1090–92

65. Pelton, J. T., Johnson, R. B., Balk, J. L., Schmidt, C. J., Roche, E. B. 1980. Synthesis and biological activity of chloromethyl ketones of leucine enkephalin. *Biochem. Biophys. Res. Commun.* 97: 1391–98

66. Venn, R. F., Barnard, E. A. 1981. A potent peptide affinity reagent for the opiate receptor. *J. Biol. Chem.* 256:1529–32

67. Szücs, M., Benyhe, S., Borsodi, A., Wollemann, M., Jancsó, G., et al. 1983. Binding characteristics and analgesic activity of D-Ala^2-Leu^5-enkephalin chloromethyl ketone. *Life Sci.* 32:2777–84

68. Szücs, M., DiGleria, K., Medzihradszky, K. 1983. A new potential affinity label for the opiate receptor. *Life Sci.* 33 (Suppl. 1):435–38

69. Portoghese, P. S., Larson, D. L., Jiang, J. B., Takemori, A. E., Caruso, T. P. 1978. 6β - [N,N - Bis(2 - chloroethyl) amino] - 17 - (cyclopropylmethyl) - 4,5α-epoxy-3,14 dihydroxymorphinan (Chlornaltrexamine), a potent opioid receptor alkylating agent with ultralong narcotic antagonist activity. *J. Med. Chem.* 21: 598–99

70. Portoghese, P. S., Larson, D. L., Jiang, J. B., Caruso, T. P., Takemori, A. E. 1979. Synthesis and pharmacologic characterization of an alkylating analogue (chlornaltrexamine) of naltrexone with ultralong-lasting narcotic antagonist properties. *J. Med. Chem.* 22:168–73

71. Ward, S. J., Portoghese, P. S., Takemori, A. E. 1982. Pharmacological profiles of β-funaltrexamine (β-FNA) and β-chlornaltrexamine (β-CNA) on the mouse vas deferens preparation. *Eur. J. Pharmacol.* 80:377–84

72. Fantozzi, R., Mullikin-Kilpatrick, D., Blume, A. J. 1981. Irreversible inactivation of the opiate receptors in the neuroblastoma × glioma hybrid NG108-15 by chlornaltrexamine. *Mol. Pharmacol.* 20: 8–15

73. Sayre, L. M., Larson, D. L., Fries, D. S., Takemori, A. E., Portoghese, P. S. 1983. Importance of C-6 chirality in conferring irreversible opioid antagonism to naltrexone-derived affinity labels. *J. Med. Chem.* 26:1229–35

74. Caruso, T. P., Larson, D. L., Portoghese, P. S., Takemori, A. E. 1980. Isolation of selective ^{3}H-chlornaltrexamine-bound complexes, possible opioid receptor components in brains of mice. *Life Sci.* 27:2063–69

75. Ward, S. J., Portoghese, P. S., Takemori, A. E. 1982. Improved assays for the assessment of κ- and δ-properties of opioid ligands. *Eur. J. Pharmacol.* 85: 163–70

76. Chavkin, C., James, I. F., Goldstein, A. 1982. Dynorphin is a specific endogenous ligand of the κ opioid receptor. *Science* 215:413–15

77. Chavkin, C., Goldstein, A. 1981. Demonstration of a specific dynorphin receptor in guinea pig ileum myenteric plexus. *Nature* 291:591–93

78. Goldstein, A., James, I. F. 1984. Site-directed alkylation of multiple opioid receptors: II. Pharmacological selectivity. *Mol. Pharmacol.* 25:343–48

79. Cox, B. M., Chavkin, C., 1983. Comparison of dynorphin-selective *kappa* receptors in mouse vas deferens and guinea pig ileum. *Mol. Pharmacol.* 23:36–43

80. Porreca, F., Burks, T. F. 1983. Affinity of normorphine for its pharmacologic receptor in the naive and morphine-tolerant guinea pig isolated ileum. *J. Pharmacol. Exp. Ther.* 225:688–93

81. Furchgott, R. F., Bursztyn, P. 1967. Comparison of dissociation constants and of relative efficacies of selected agonists acting on parasympathetic receptors. *Ann. NY Acad. Sci.* 144:882–99

82. Ward, A., Takemori, A. E. 1976. Studies on the narcotic receptor in the guinea pig ileum. *J. Pharmacol. Exp. Ther.* 199:117–23

83. James, I. F., Goldstein, A., 1984. Site-directed alkylation of multiple opioid receptors. I. Binding selectivity. *Mol. Pharmacol.* 25:337–42

84. Tulunay, F. C., Ayhan, I. H., Portoghese, P. S., Takemori, A. E. 1981. Antagonism by chlornaltrexamine of some effects of Δ^9-tetrahydrocannabinol. *Eur. J. Pharmacol.* 70:219–24

85. Quock, R. M., Lucas, T. S. 1981. Enhancement of apomorphine-induced climbing in mice by reversible and irreversible narcotic antagonist drugs. *Life Sci.* 28:1421–24

86. Messing, R. B., Portoghese, P. S., Takemori, A. E., Sparber, S. B., 1982. Antagonism of morphine-induced behavioral suppression by opiate receptor alkylators. *Pharmacol. Biochem. Behav.* 16:621–26

87. Panksepp, J., Siviy, S., Normansell, L.,

White, K., Bishop, P. 1982. Effects of β-chlornaltrexamine on separation distress in chicks. *Life Sci.* 31:2387–90

88. DeLander, G. E., Takemori, A. E. 1983. Spinal antagonism of tolerance and dependence induced by systemically administered morphine. *Eur. J. Pharmacol.* 94:35–42

89. Sayre, L. M., Larson, D. L., Takemori, A. E., Portoghese, P. S. 1984. Design and synthesis of naltrexone-derived affinity labels with nonequilibrium opioid agonist and antagonist activities. Evidence for the existence of different *mu* receptor subtypes in different tissues. *J. Med. Chem.* 27:1325–35

90. Portoghese, P. S., Larson, D. L., Sayre, L. M., Fries, D. S., Takemori, A. E. 1980. A novel opioid receptor site directed alkylating agent with irreversible narcotic antagonistic and reversible agonistic activities. *J. Med. Chem.* 23:233–34

91. Takemori, A. E., Larson, D. L., Portoghese, P. S. 1981. The irreversible narcotic antagonistic and reversible agonistic properties of the fumaramate methyl ester derivative of naltrexone. *Eur. J. Pharmacol.* 70:445–51

92. Ward, S. J., Fries, D. S., Larson, D. L. Portoghese, P. S., Takemori, A. E. 1984. Opioid receptor binding characteristics of the nonequilibrium μ antagonist, β-funaltrexamine (β-FNA). *Eur. J. Pharmacol.* In press

93. Ward, S. J., Portoghese, P. S., Takemori, A. E. 1982. Pharmacological characterization *in vivo* of the novel opiate, β-funaltrexamine. *J. Pharmacol. Exp. Ther.* 220:494–98

94. Huidobro-Toro, J. P., Yoshimura, K., Way, E. L. 1982. Application of an irreversible opiate antagonist (β-FNA, β-funaltrexamine) to demonstrate dynorphin selectivity for κ-opioid sites. *Life Sci.* 31:2409–16

95. Seidl, E., Schulz, R., 1983. Selective opiate tolerance in the guinea pig ileum is not associated with selective dependence. *Life Sci.* 33 (Suppl. 1):357–60

96. Gintzler, A. R., Hyde, D. 1983. Unmasking myenteric delta receptors. *Life Sci.* 33(Suppl. 1):323–25

97. Ward, S. J. 1983. Differential properties of *mu* receptors in the guinea pig ileum (GPI) and mouse vas deferens (MVD) preparations. *Abstr. Soc. Neurosci.* 9: 327

98. Portoghese, P. S., Takemori, A. E. 1983. Different receptor sites mediate opioid agonism and antagonism. *J. Med. Chem.* 26:1341–43

99. Sarne, Y., Itzhak, Y., Keren, O. 1982.

Differential effect of humoral endorphin on the binding of opiate agonists and antagonists. *Eur. J. Pharmacol.* 81:227–35

100. Ward, S. J., Takemori, A. E. 1983. Determination of the relative involvement of μ-opioid receptors in opioid-induced depression of respiratory rate by use of β-funaltrexamine. *Eur. J. Pharmacol.* 87: 1–6

101. Ward, S. J., Takemori, A. E. 1983. Relative involvement of receptor subtypes in opioid-induced inhibition of gastrointestinal transit in mice. *J. Pharmacol. Exp. Ther.* 224:359–63

102. Holaday, J. W., Ward, S. J. 1982. Morphine-induced bradycardia is predominantly mediated at *mu* sites, whereas morphine-induced hypotension may involve both *mu* and *delta* opioid receptors. *Abstr. Soc. Neurosci.* 8:389

103. Pfeiffer, A., Kopin, I. J., Shimohigashi, Y., Faden, A. I., Feuerstein, G. 1984. On the involvement of opiate receptor subtypes in cardiovascular actions of opiate agonists. *Peptides* In press

104. Holaday, J. W., Pennington, L., Ward, S. J. 1983. Selective μ and δ receptor antagonists and neuroendocrine response to morphine: Evidence for μ receptors in prolactin release. *Abstr. Soc. Neurosci.* 9:744

105. Hylden, J. K., Wilcox, G. L. 1983. Intrathecal opioids block a spinal action of substance P in mice: Functional importance of both μ- and δ-receptors. *Eur. J. Pharmacol.* 86:95–98

106. Hylden, J. K., Wilcox, G. L. 1983. Pharmacological characterization of substance P-induced nociception in mice: Modulation by opioid and noradrenergic agonists at the spinal level. *J. Pharmacol. Exp. Ther.* 226:398–404

107. Zimmerman, D. M., Hart, J. C., Reel, J. K., Leander, J. D. 1984. Effects of β-funaltrexamine (β-FNA) on the diuretic actions of *kappa* agonists and the antidiuretic actions of *mu* agonists. *Fed. Proc.* 43:966

108. Holaday, J. H., D'Amato, R. J. 1983. Multiple opioid receptors: Evidence for μ-δ binding site interactions in endotoxic shock. *Life Sci.* 33 (Suppl. 1):703–6

109. Belenky, G. L., Gelinas-Sorell, D., Kenner, J. R., Holaday, J. W. 1983. Evidence for δ-receptor involvement in the post-ictal antinociceptive responses to electroconvulsive shock in rats. *Life Sci.* 33 (Suppl. 1):583–85

110. Hynes, M. D., Henderson, J. K., Zimmerman, D. M. 1984. Pretreatment with the opioid receptor antagonist β-

funaltrexamine (β-FNA) markedly alters the analgesic activity of opioid mixed agonist-antagonist analgesics. *Fed. Proc.* 43:965

111. Dykstra, L. 1984. Effects of buprenorphine and morphine alone and in combination with naloxone, diprenorphine or β-funaltrexamine (β-FNA) in squirrel monkeys. *Fed. Proc.* 43:965

112. Frederickson, R. C. A., Zimmerman, D. M., Hynes, M. D. 1984. Comparative effects of the opioid antagonist β-funaltrexamine (β-FNA) on analgesia produced by morphine and metkephamid. *Fed. Proc.* 43:965

113. Leander, J. D., Hart, J. C., Zimmerman, D. M. 1984. β-Funaltrexamine (β-FNA) blocks mu-opioid agonists on shock-titration in the squirrel monkey. *Fed. Proc.* 43:965

114. Schafer, J. T., France, C. P., Wood, J. H. 1984. Comparison of the antimorphine actions of narcotic antagonists in the pigeon. *Fed. Proc.* 43:967

115. Aceto, M. D., Dewey, W. L., Portoghese, P. S., Takemori, A. E. 1984. β-funaltrexamine (β-FNA) and morphine dependence. *Fed. Proc.* 43:741

116. DeLander, G. E., Portoghese, P. S., Takemori, A. E. 1984. The role of spinal *mu* opioid receptors in the development of morphine tolerance and dependence. *J. Pharmacol. Exp. Ther.* 231:91–96

117. Gmerek, D. E., Woods, J. H. 1984. Effects of β-FNA in drug naive and morphine dependent rhesus monkeys. *Proc. Prob. Drug Dep.* In press

118. Sayre, L. M., Takemori, A. E., Portoghese, P. S. 1983. Alkylation of opioid receptor subtypes by α-chlornaltrexamine produces concurrent irreversible agonistic and irreversible antagonistic activities. *J. Med. Chem.* 26:503–6

119. Perry, D. C., Mullis, K. B., Oie, S., Sadee, W. 1980. Opiate antagonist receptor binding *in vivo*: Evidence for a new receptor binding model. *Brain Res.* 199:49–61

120. Rance, M. J. 1979. Animal and molecular pharmacology of mixed agonist-antagonist analgesic drugs. *Br. J. Clin. Pharmacol.* 7:281S–86S

121. Pasternak, G. W., Hahn, E. F. 1980. Long acting opiate agonists and antagonists: 14-hydroxydihydromorphinones. *J. Med. Chem.* 23:674–77

122. Pasternak, G. W., Childers, S. R., Snyder, S. H. 1980. Naloxazone, a long-acting opiate antagonist: Effects on analgesia in intact animals and in opiate receptor binding in vitro. *J. Pharmacol. Exp. Ther.* 214:455–62

123. Hahn, E. F., Carroll-Buatti, M., Pasternak, G. W. 1982. Irreversible opiate agonists and antagonists: The 14-hydroxydihydromorphinone azines. *J. Neurosci.* 2:572–76

124. Gintzler, A. R., Pasternak, G. W. 1983. Multiple mu receptors: Evidence for mu_2 sites in the guinea pig ileum. *Neurosci. Lett.* 39:51–56

125. Nishimura, S. L., Recht, L. D., Pasternak, G. W. 1984. Biochemical characterization of high affinity ^{3}H-opioid binding: Further evidence for mu_1 sites. *Mol.*

Pharmacol. 25:20–37

126. Pasternak, G. W., Gintzler, A. R., Houghten, R. A., Ling, G. S. F., Goodman, R. R., et al. 1983. Biochemical and pharmacological evidence for opioid receptor multiplicity in the central nervous system. *Life Sci.* 33:167–73

127. Rice, K. C., Shiotani, S., Creveling, C. R., Jacobson, A. E., Kee, W. A. 1977. N - (2,4,5 - trihydroxyphenethyl)normetazocine, a potential irreversible inhibitor of the narcotic receptor. *J. Med. Chem.* 20:673–75

Ann. Rev. Pharmacol. Toxicol. 1985. 25:225–47

PERSPECTIVES ON ALTERNATIVES TO CURRENT ANIMAL TESTING TECHNIQUES IN PRECLINICAL TOXICOLOGY

Andrew N. Rowan

Tufts University School of Veterinary Medicine, 203 Harrison Avenue, Boston, Massachusetts 02111

Alan M. Goldberg

Division of Environmental Health Sciences, Johns Hopkins University School of Hygiene and Public Health, Baltimore, Maryland 21205

INTRODUCTION

In ancient times, knowledge of the biological properties of natural substances, both medicinal and lethal, was a vital source of power for witch doctors and magician priests. Today, given the steady increase in public concern about the possible deleterious effects of chemicals in our environment, the information the toxicologist possesses is once again an important influence in society. Toxicologists are being asked to provide answers to ever more complex questions. Unfortunately, the knowledge base and the techniques currently being used to acquire that knowledge are often unequal to the task.

In the early 1960s, both the thalidomide disaster (1) and the publication of *Silent Spring* by Rachel Carson (2) dramatized the possible negative impact of potent new pharmaceuticals and pesticides. As a result, government authorities throughout Europe, North America, and Japan responded to public concern by demanding a dramatic increase in the requirements for premarket testing of new products. Existing animal tests were refined and more animal tests were developed in an attempt to evaluate the safety of drugs, food additives,

225

0362-1642/85/0415-0225$02.00

pesticides, and other chemicals. Between 1965 and 1979, one company reported that the costs of toxicology testing increased by a factor of 3.2, even after correcting for the effects of inflation (3). One factor contributing to these costs is the enormous numbers of animals now consumed in routine toxicology testing, accounting for an estimated 20% of the 50–70 million laboratory animals used every year in the United States (4).

Public authorities undoubtedly bear a responsibility to attempt to ensure that individuals in society are protected from harm. Given the current state of our knowledge, this necessitates some testing in animals and extrapolating the results, no matter how difficult, to predict likely human responses. We are still far too ignorant to know the toxic effects of a compound from first principles (via theoretical toxicology?). Therefore, we must fall back on appropriate models of the human system to identify possible hazards. By necessity, this leads to the use of mammals or other species that respond in a manner sufficiently similar to humans to provide an index of the potential hazard. Nevertheless, the problems of extrapolation and evaluation are formidable. Thousands of new chemicals must be investigated every year, while only a fraction of the estimated 65,000 chemicals (5) in common use have been subject to testing according to available public information (6). In addition, the present animal testing technologies are generally crude, cumbersome, and costly, and there is growing public criticism of animal use.

Among toxicologists, there are some who see animal testing as an unsatisfactory answer to toxicology's problems. In 1971, Rofe (7), in an excellent but little-cited review on the use of tissue culture in toxicology, stated: "In seeking to bridge the gap between the effects of foreign substances on animals and their effects on man, it seems unlikely that a substantial contribution to the problem can be made by prolonging the conventional toxicological procedures or including additional organ function tests."

Others, scientific and non-scientific, have also criticized animal testing (7–13), commenting variously that in the last decade toxicology has sometimes created more problems than it has solved, that toxicology is a science without scientific underpinning, and that toxicologists should move toward the development of an appropriate battery of short-term tests, using both in vitro and in vivo approaches, to assess product safety.

Since 1975, criticism of animal testing from another source, the animal welfare movement, has grown considerably. For the most part, the bulk of this criticism has been targeted against the Draize eye irritancy (14) and the LD50 tests (15). The animal welfare campaigns have been effective. Campaigns have not only brought about a reevaluation of the rationale for Draize eye irritancy and LD50 testing, they have also spurred a reassessment of the entire animal-testing approach. In general, the animal activists advocate the elimination of the use of animals in toxicity testing and the establishment of non-animal alternatives, in particular tissue culture and computer modeling. The most effective campaigners recognize that these are long-term goals and in the short term seek to reduce animal use as much as is feasible by eliminating unnecessary animal tests or developing, validating, and using potential alternatives as fast as possible.

The combination of these two forces, internal toxicological self-criticism and external animal welfare pressure, has begun to have an impact. Numerous workshops, plenary sessions, and full-scale symposia have been organized in the last three to four years to discuss testing on animals and the development of alternatives (cf. 16–20). Over four million dollars from private sources has been allocated to support research on potential new approaches, and government authorities also are beginning to recognize the appropriateness and necessity for in vitro methods of toxicological evaluation (21).

Given these changes, it is important that the concept of alternatives be clearly explained and that the potential for developing and using appropriate alternatives be carefully considered. This review attempts to introduce the reader to the concept of alternatives and its implications in toxicology testing. Recent relevant research advances will also be briefly discussed. The authors have catalogued alternative approaches to the subject rather than attempting a thorough critical evaluation. The use of animals and alternatives in mutagenicity and carcinogenicity testing will not be covered in any detail. There is already an extensive literature on in vitro tests for carcinogenicity and mutagenicity, and the reader is referred to several recent reviews (22–25) for discussion of these topics.

WHAT ARE ALTERNATIVES?

The term *alternatives* is a relatively recent addition to the campaign literature of the animal-protection movement, and there is still widespread disagreement over its precise definition. Some organizations use the term to refer only to techniques that replace completely the use of animals in a particular area, for example, a computer model to predict LD50 values. However, others follow the definition developed by Russell & Burch in 1959 (26); they defined an alternative as any technique that replaces the use of animals, that reduces the need for animals in a particular test, or that refines a technique in order to reduce the amount of suffering endured by the animal. Thus, use of the up-down method to determine an acute toxicity value (27) is an alternative to the classical LD50 test because fewer animals are required. These three R's represent the common definition of alternatives; we define the term this way in this article.

One of the key features of the concept of alternatives is that it refers to techniques used in biomedical research. Thus, a discussion of alternatives in toxicology testing is really only a review of the merits of different methodological approaches with a particular focus on ways to reduce animal use and suffering. The alternatives most commonly considered are cell and organ culture, computer modeling, and the use of minimally invasive procedures and endpoints that produce little stress or suffering. A number of reviews of the use of cell and organ culture in toxicology investigations have already been published, beginning with a seminal paper by Pomerat & Leake in 1954 (28), followed by a number of reviews after 1970 (7, 29–38). However, judging from the number of citations to these papers, none has had impact. According to the records of the *Science Citation Index,* Rofe's 1971 review has been cited less than twenty times in the following twelve years, with a high of three citations each in 1976 and 1980. Although more and more toxicological research is being conducted in vitro, the potential of cell culture in toxicological evaluation and hazard assessment is only now beginning to be tested and evaluated. This is the result of public pressure, the availability of funds for such studies, and increased concern among scientists.

However, the use of cell cultures must be developed and implemented cautiously in toxicology testing and hazard assessment. Obviously, a single cell culture cannot mimic the complex interactions of all cell types in the body, no matter how exquisite the experimental design. In vivo metabolism may be simulated to some extent but not completely (39), and integrating functions such as hormones, immune reactions, and phagocytosis cannot be duplicated. In addition, a cell culture is a relatively static system in which the dose of the test chemical reaching the target system and the duration of contact may not be the same as those that occur in the in vivo test. Cell cultures also present physical problems regarding the solubility, stability, and biophysical effects of the test compound.

On the other hand, cell culture technique has great potential once investigators have acquired the background knowledge to ask highly focused and specific questions. The static nature of cell culture is also an advantage in that the dose and duration of contact of a test chemical can be precisely determined. Far less of the test chemical is required for cell culture investigations than in in vivo tests. Therefore, one can easily set up replicate cultures and generate more data in a short time.

One of the most exciting aspects of cell culture studies in toxicology is that one can use human tissue. Such studies have been limited in the past because of the difficulty of growing and maintaining differentiated human cell types in culture. But technical problems are being steadily overcome. Important developments in the last years include improvements in the quality control of media and the plasticware provided by manufacturers, improved quality control in the laboratory, better media formulations (40) for the growth of normal cells as well as for cells exhibiting specialized functions (e.g. heart cell contractility and melanin production by melanocytes), and improvements in cell separation and cloning techniques (cf. 41).

Nardone & Bradlaw (41) describe four interfaces between in vitro methodology and animal toxicology: screening tests, mechanistic studies, personnel monitoring, and considerations for risk assessment. Screening tests are the most developed and are likely to remain the major focus of in vitro toxicology. However, mechanistic studies probably will become increasingly more important, both in toxicological evaluations and for risk assessment. One could also classify in vitro methodology according to whether the approach is empirical, model development, or mechanistic (42).

The empirical approach to the development of methodology is problematic. The questions asked are generally not focused and correlations develop prior to fundamental understandings. Additionally, the results tend to be somewhat unpredictable. Should this be the case in the development of in vitro toxicological methods, we will unfortunately have provided supplementary testing strategies but not replacement testing strategies. This will leave us with the dilemma of attempting to use the in vitro methodologies without being able to rely on them.

Model development utilizes systems that try to mimic in vivo systems. Generally, the model system is neither complete nor faithful in all aspects of the system being modeled, but it tends to provide useful information if the data are not overinterpreted. In those model systems where a single aspect of an integrated response is examined and the data are interpreted in that single system, this technique can provide meaningful inferences for the evaluation of chemical effects.

The mechanistic approach to the development of in vitro methodologies should be based on a thorough knowledge of the metabolism, kinetics, and biology of the system or species to be examined. If the metabolic pathways are understood, or if it is known that the parent compound produces the toxicological insult, then one can develop a system to examine the mechanisms by which the chemical(s) works. That is, one can examine the adverse chemical or physical effects that lead to a significant functional loss in the tissue or system. This approach allows the in vitro system to be derived from the species under study. It also provides a better understanding of chemical-biological interaction and the consequences of that interaction. Once a mechanism has been identified, it may then be possible to develop appropriate, interpretable, simple, and reliable in vitro methodologies.

From a scientific viewpoint, the mechanistic approach is not only preferable but necessary. In vitro methods will be more acceptable and will develop rapidly when the knowledge base has advanced far enough to permit a focus on mechanisms.

ALTERNATIVES IN TOXICOLOGY

Toxicity testing on animals may be divided into acute, subacute, and chronic tests. Acute tests are those in which the animals are dosed with one or a few doses of the test compound and kept for at most a few weeks. Such tests include protocols for determining various LD50's as well as eye and skin irritancy tests. Up to 50% of all animals used in toxicology testing are killed in acute tests (4). Subchronic tests last from a few weeks to several months. Chronic tests last for more than three months and include tests for reproductive and carcinogenic effects, among others. The search for alternatives in all these areas will continue to evolve. However, at the present time our lack of knowledge about the mechanisms of possible toxic insults is such that some animal testing is going to be required.

Acute Toxicity Testing

In acute tests, the investigator observes an immediate response in which the organism's defense mechanisms are rapidly overwhelmed. Where specific endpoints are being determined (e.g. eye irritancy), it may be possible to develop an adequate in vitro alternative based on one or more screening systems. However, one of the functions of acute testing is the identification of unexpected toxic effects. The empiricism of this approach requires that a relatively good model for the whole human being be used. This generally means using a whole mammal, because the metabolism and response of other mammals is at least sufficiently similar to human responses to provide an index of hazard. However, there are acute tests for which the prospect of either reducing the number of animals used or for developing an adequate in vitro test is relatively good. These are discussed below.

LD50 TESTING   The calculation of median lethal dose (LD50) for the measurement of toxicity was introduced in 1927 (43). At that time, determination of the LD50 was used to standardize such potent biologicals as digitalis, insulin, and diphtheria toxin. With time, however, the LD50 came to be used as a standard measure by which the toxicity of all chemicals was assessed. In 1968, Morrison, Quinton, and Reinert questioned this use of the LD50 (44), arguing that the classical test used too many animals and that the statistical figure resulting was meaningless. They contended that a figure generated from the use of six to ten animals was the best that could be achieved given the inadequacies of the test system (45). More recently, several others have also criticized the LD50 approach (46–48). As a result of scientific criticism coupled with political pressure from the animal welfare movement, the classical LD50 test (with a few specific exceptions) appears to be on its way out as a regulatory requirement. For example, the German authorities have said that they will accept acute toxicity test data using small numbers of animals (49, 50), and the Food and Drug Administration has explicitly stated that it no longer requires LD50 tests and that acute toxicity data from alternative tests may be acceptable (51).

Alternative tests for acute toxicity all require far fewer animals than the traditional methods. Bruce (27) has proposed the use of six to ten animals in the up-down method (52), although this technique cannot be recommended for testing materials where delayed deaths (more than a few days) are the rule. Several simplifications of the standard method, all of which require fewer animals, have been proposed (53–56), and the most recent (56), which recommends the use of only thirteen animals, is claimed to be suitable for industrial use where a variety of chemicals of widely differing toxicities must be assessed. Where only an estimate is required, the method proposed by Deichmann & LeBlanc offers yet another choice (57).

Another suggested approach is the use of a structure-activity computer model to estimate LD50's (58, 59). This approach has been criticized because the chemicals used to design the models were not congeneric and because the biological endpoint (death) used is not the function of a single active site in a well-defined system (60). The developers of the model argue that there is no question that the use of a congeneric set of chemicals would produce tighter estimates but that this is insufficient reason not to explore a model based on heterogenous collections of chemicals. As this field of quantitative structure-toxicity relationships (QSTR) develops, one can anticipate major strides in the use of these systems as predicters of toxicity (61).

Several papers have correlated the results of cytotoxicity assays with animal LD50's (62–66), but the development of an adequate cell culture alternative is very unlikely. There are many different toxic effects, and a crude cytotoxicity assay is unlikely to be successful as a general screen for acute toxicity. In addition, these nonmechanistic tests may result in the identification of an excessive number of false-positives and false-negatives, and efforts to correlate cytotoxicity data with questionable LD50 figures are unlikely to yield significant toxicological insights. Nevertheless, good cytotoxicity data and the development of reliable measures of cytotoxicity (cf. 63, 66) are clearly needed.

The present state of alternatives development for the classical LD50 test is focused on the use of fewer animals (up to a 90% reduction), with more attention being paid to morbidity and symptoms than to a statistical estimate of the median lethal dose. For most purposes, the use of small numbers of animals to estimate the median lethal dose appears to be a satisfactory alternative. Cell culture systems have been investigated, but they cannot provide the breadth of coverage of possible toxic insults of a simple in vivo mammalian organism. A computer model for estimating LD50's has been developed (58). While it allows one to estimate the toxicity of a new substance quickly, it suffers limitations as a possible replacement for animal tests.

OPHTHALMIC IRRITANCY TESTING   The classic method for assessing the potential for the ophthalmic irritancy of chemicals is the Draize eye irritancy test (67, 68). In recent years, this test has been criticized by both scientists (69, 70) and by animal welfare groups (71). In fact, in 1978, Smyth commented that the Draize eye irritancy test is one area where a search for a non-animal alternative has a real chance of success (72). A recent review of eye irritation testing outlines some of the difficulties in identifying eye irritants, as well as the specific historical background of and problems with the Draize eye irritancy test (73). For example, one of the main difficulties with this test as a regulatory tool is the subjective nature of scoring and evaluating the response.

Pressure from animal welfare campaigns in recent years has led to support for a number of projects seeking an alternative to the Draize eye irritancy test, with promising results. Some attempt to modify the test to reduce animal distress, and others are investigating in vitro and protozoan systems as possible replacements for it (cf. 41).

Refinements to the classical Draize eye irritancy test   Proposed test modifications to the Draize eye irritancy test include the use of smaller volumes (70), which would reduce the severity of the reaction as well as permit the development of dose-response curves; the use of local anesthetics (73); the use of an exfoliative cytology test, which is reportedly more sensitive and more easily quantified than the classic test (74); and the identification of all severe dermal irritants as eye irritants without further testing. Griffith and his colleagues have argued, with some justification, that the use of a single 100 μl aliquot for eye irritation testing is inappropriate. They suggest that a 10 μl aliquot (and higher multiples) is retained in the eye better and that dose-response curves can be developed if necessary (70). In most cases, the use of smaller quantities of material in the eye will result in less irritation and therefore less animal distress.

In recent years, there have been several investigations of the use of local anesthetics in the eye during ophthalmic testing as a means of reducing animal suffering. Ulsamer has reported that butacaine sulfate provides adequate anesthesia without notably affecting the irritancy scores (75). Hoheisel (personal communication) indicates that two doses of tetracaine (separated by ten minutes) are more effective in abolishing pain and interfere less with the irritant response, although Walberg disputes this (74). Johnson reports that amethocaine HCl is also effective. In a trial of thirty-one substances, the anesthetic either had no effect or produced an increase in the irritant response and did not therefore mask irritancy (76).

Walberg has developed a very promising modification to the Draize eye irritancy test that is less stressful to the animal, more sensitive, and more easily quantified than the classic test (74). The eye is exposed to the test substances; then at standard intervals after exposure exfoliated cells are retrieved from the conjunctival sac via a distilled water rinse. The number of cells retrieved is a very sensitive index of irritancy and correlates well with published Draize eye irritancy test scores. The approach needs further validation, but it appears to be a more sensitive and more objective approach to eye irritancy testing. The greater sensitivity of the exfoliative cytology test means that smaller or more dilute doses of irritant substances can be used, thereby causing less trauma and distress.

Some researchers have suggested that a simple and rapid approach to the elimination of most severe eye irritant tests that would also reduce the number of rabbits required is to pretest materials for primary skin irritation or other properties. However, Williams (77) investigated sixty materials for primary eye irritancy that were also severe primary skin irritants or corrosive to the skin. Of these, only thirty-four were severe eye irritants; fifteen of the sixty were only mildly irritating or were not irritating at all. Williams cautions, therefore, that it may be misleading to classify a substance as an eye irritant solely on the basis of dermal irritancy. He suggests that the twenty-four hour occlusion method used in skin testing may well overwhelm physiological defense mechanisms. The lack of correlation between dermal and ophthalmic scores may be due to an overestimation of the dermal response by current test procedures.

Substances with a pH of 12 or more are usually regarded as eye irritants. However, Murphy and colleagues (78) caution that there is no simple rule for predicting irritancy from pH. Acetic acid (5%) with a pH of 2.7 produces substantial corneal opacity, while 0.3% hydrochloric acid (pH 1.3) causes no corneal opacity. At the other end of the scale, 2.5% ammonium hydroxide (pH 11.8) produces corneal opacity, while 0.3% sodium hydroxide (pH 12.8) does not. Nevertheless, Walz (79) reports a clear relation between irritation (edematous reaction after intracutaneous injection) and pH in a mouse skin test of tissue compatible buffers. Buffers with a pH of below 3 and above 11.5 caused irritation. The boundary for the alkalis was very sharp.

Replacement methods for the classical Draize eye irritancy test   A wide range of in vitro and protozoan systems have been proposed as possible alternatives (at least as preliminary screens) for the Draize eye irritancy test. Nardone & Bradlaw (41) have already reviewed many of these systems, including those using enucleated eyes of rabbit, human or rabbit corneal cell cultures, other types of cell culture, and the chorioallantois of chick embryos. Some of the first attempts to devise a specific alternative to the Draize eye irritancy test were undertaken in Britain using mouse (80) or human buccal mucosa cells (81). The authors of both reports indicate that the in vitro approach shows promise but that much more work is needed to develop and validate an adequate test system. While there have been a spate of recent research reports (82–94) from investigators seeking an alternative to the Draize eye irritancy test, there is still no clear indication of which approach or approaches will be the most effective.

Cytotoxicity and cell morphology studies appear to be the favored approach in this regard, but few of them have gone beyond a characterization of the in vitro system. Douglas & Spilman chose to develop a human ocular cell culture as an in vitro assay, since it retains species-specific and organ-specific characteristics (91). They chose corneal tissue since corneal damage is the most heavily weighted in the scores of the Draize eye irritancy test. They further required that the test system be practical for routine use and that the assay be based on cell perturbations relevant to in vivo irritation [e.g. ^{51}Cr release, LDH release, uptake of AIB (a nonmetabolized amino acid), and rhodamine uptake as an index of mitochondrial function]. Although the preliminary results from ^{51}Cr release were promising, the project was unfortunately not completed.

While Douglas and others have favored the idea of using corneal cells to match, as far as is possible, organ-specific characteristics, Borenfreund (87) reports that cells from different organs and species appear to give very similar results, indicating that it may not be that important to match cell culture type with the target organ. The results of Borenfreund's cytotoxicity and morphology assay indicate reasonable correlation with Draize eye irritancy test scores as well as with another possible alternative based on a cellular uridine-transport assay developed in the same laboratory (86).

Another approach has involved the use of whole enucleated rabbit (85) or bovine (93) eyes. Burton et al (85) report that enucleated eyes remain viable for at least four hours and that there is good correlation of the results from this system, using a measurement of corneal swelling, with in vivo eye irritancy. However, although whole eye systems may be useful as predictors of human eye irritation, Douglas argues that they are poorly suited to the screening of a large number of compounds or of many replicate samples (91).

It has been suggested that cell culture systems are not well suited to predicting how fast the eye might recover from the toxic insult. However, Chan (83) is working with a corneal cell culture system that might predict recovery from injury and Jumblatt & Neufeldt (95) have described a cell culture model for wound closure studies.

Two other in vitro models using the chick chorioallantoic membrane (88) and excised guinea pig ileum (89, 90) have also been reported recently. Leighton is developing the chorioallantoic membrane (CAM) from the chick embryo as a nonsentient but intact organ that can be used to evaluate irritation and inflammation (88). The initial reports are based on tests conducted with fairly strong acid and alkali solutions that measure the size of the resultant lesion. This is an endpoint that requires refinement. In addition, background irritation caused by shell fragments falling on the CAM when the aperture is cut has also caused problems. Nevertheless, the CAM system could be a very promising method for modeling inflammatory responses provided a simple but elegant endpoint can be developed.

Many new model systems have been investigated in the past few years and some already show considerable promise as improvements on the Draize eye irritancy test or as the basis for rapid screening systems. However, at the present time, none of the in vitro systems has yet been sufficiently validated or evaluated to be considered as replacements to the classical or modified Draize test.

DERMAL TOXICITY TESTING   As mentioned above, Williams's (77) analysis of the skin and eye irritancy of a range of substances indicates that severe skin irritancy does not reliably predict severe eye irritancy. In discussing this result, he raises the possibility that the twenty-four hour occlusion used in the standard skin test may be too severe. For example, better correlation was found between skin and eye irritation when only a four-hour occlusion period was used in the skin test. The Organization for Economic Cooperation and Development (OECD) guidelines also call for only a four-hour occlusion. This is not the only question that has been raised about skin irritancy tests. Marks (96) notes that there are many differences between the skin of common test animals (rats, guinea pigs, rabbits, and mice) and human skin. Kligman (97) points out that the dose-response relationship for irritants is flat in animal skin and as a result discriminative ability is low. Furthermore, animal testing appears to be of little value for detecting mild human skin irritants. Marks (96) suggests that one way to overcome this difficulty is to test substances of low and moderate toxicity in human volunteers (with suitable safeguards), although he recognizes that such testing may be limited by ethical and regulatory restrictions.

Very little research into possible in vitro systems for identifying skin irritants has so far been undertaken. There have been isolated reports of the use of in vitro skin cultures to study toxic reactions or mechanisms (cf. 98–100), but no concerted program to seek an in vitro screening test for irritancy and cutaneous toxicity has been carried out. Part of the problem is the lack of a reliable supply of human skin samples, and it is probably desirable to use human material rather than animal tissues in these tests. However, adequate supplies of rudimentary human epidermal sheets may become available for toxicity studies as a result of work being done to develop an artificial epidermal substitute for burn victims (101, 102). In addition, some of the irritancy test systems now being developed as alternatives to the Draize test may also be suitable for testing possible skin irritancy. For example, if the problems with the chick chorioallantoic membrane system (88) can be resolved, it could become a useful system for identifying inflammatory responses. Another approach to the assessment of dermal absorption in animals may be the use of a lipid-impregnated filter (103).

Phototoxicity is now routinely evaluated in animals, but the methods are time-consuming, expensive, and not always good predictors of the human response. Several publications evaluate possible in vitro assays for phototoxicity. For example, a number of authors have used yeast growth inhibition (cf. 104, 105) and have reported good correlation between this inhibition and acute, nonphotoallergic phototoxicity. Another recent approach has employed human peripheral blood monocytes, with inhibition of mitogen-stimulated thymidine incorporation as an endpoint (106, 107). Investigators using this approach argue that their test avoids the problem of false-negative results and note that preliminary data from a human lymphoblastoid cell line indicate that these cells perform well in the assay (106). Use of human lymphoblastoid cells would simplify the problem of cell supply and standardization if the test is found to be sufficiently reliable to use as a standard screening system.

The investigation of in vitro tests for dermal toxicity has not progressed as far as that for ophthalmic toxicity tests. Nevertheless, the principles in each case are the same, and we are therefore optimistic about the potential for developing a dermal irritancy alternative.

OTHER ORGANS   One area of acute toxicity where alternative methods may contribute to our understanding of potential chemical insult is the acute reactions of isolated organs or cell cultures to large doses such as might occur during unintentional exposure. The setting of public emergency limits and the development of appropriate therapies for acute poisoning cases could find data from in vitro organotypic systems to be invaluable. Little attention has been paid to this area of acute organ toxicity. Some in vitro work relevant to these issues is discussed in the section on chronic toxicity below.

Chronic Toxicity Testing

In chronic toxicity testing that assesses the likelihood of both targeted (e.g. carcinogenicity) and nontargeted (e.g. disorder in lipid metabolism) effects, we are much more likely to be able to predict human hazards if we understand the mechanism of the toxic insult than if we continue to rely on empirical testing approaches. In the acute toxicity field discussed above, there has been a focused, funded effort to find alternatives that follow both empirical and mechanistic lines. In chronic toxicity testing, a similar effort is underway to develop short-term tests to identify mutagens, carcinogens, and teratogens but not to investigate organ-specific effects. We will discuss some of the issues in developing alternatives in chronic toxicity testing, specifically for hepatotoxicity, neurotoxicity, and teratogenicity. We will not discuss carcinogenicity and mutagenicity.

HEPATOTOXICITY   The liver is particularly vulnerable to injury by ingested chemicals because it receives higher concentrations of chemicals absorbed from the intestine than do other organs and it plays a major role in the biotransformation, concentration, and excretion of xenobiotics or their metabolites. The liver is therefore an important target organ in any evaluation of the toxic potential of a chemical. Liver function is generally assessed by hepatic excretion measurements and chemical and histological analyses (108). The development of a simple in vitro test system to evaluate hepatotoxicity would be very useful.

Several in vitro approaches for the evaluation of hepatotoxicity have already been investigated, including perfused liver (109), liver cell suspensions (110), and various types of liver cell cultures (110–113). However, all these systems have disadvantages that limit their usefulness (112). Perfused liver preparations are viable for only a few hours, are technically complicated, and show limited reproducibility from one laboratory to another. Liver cell lines lose many of the differentiated functions of normal hepatocytes in vitro. Freshly prepared hepatocyte suspensions usually demonstrate cell damage and impaired enzyme functions, while primary hepatocyte cultures usually contain only a fraction of in vivo levels of microsomal drug-metabolizing enzymes such as cytochrome P-450. However, several investigators have recently demonstrated that one can maintain good levels of cytochrome P-450 by manipulating the culture medium (114–116). Omitting cystine (and cysteine) and adding 5-aminolevulinic acid and nicotinamide (or metarypone) to the usual cell culture media maintains cytochrome P-450 at levels close to in vivo ones for up to seven days (112, 115).

Liver cell cultures show considerable promise for the investigation of the mechanism of action of hepatotoxins and, as culture methods are improved and differentiated liver cell functions are maintained longer in vitro (117), the research and testing potential of such systems will expand. Hepatocyte cultures have been used successfully in detailed toxicological studies in relatively few laboratories around the world (cf. 111, 112), and then they have been used to study mechanisms of toxicity. Only limited attention has been given to their potential usefulness in routine screening tests.

NEUROTOXICITY   Although the development of in vitro systems to investigate hepatotoxicity may appear a daunting task, the development of systems for the routine investigation of neurotoxicity in vitro is likely to be even more difficult. The nervous system is extremely complex and it is composed of many different cell types. Many neurotoxins affect only one specific cell type in the nervous system, and the full range of potential neurotoxic effects cannot be evaluated in any single in vitro system. Nevertheless, some in vitro and invertebrate test systems have potential as screens for specific neurotoxins (118, 119).

Damstra & Bondy (120) discuss the usefulness of neurochemical approaches, in vivo and in vitro, in neurotoxicological studies. However, they caution the unwary investigator of the many pitfalls of such tests. For example, changes in body temperature, such as those caused by amphetamine or chlorpromazine, may affect neurochemistry, while food deprivation causes an increased turnover of 5-hydroxytryptamine as a result of increases in free-serum tryptophan. Nevertheless, recent advances in neurochemistry permit analysis of an ever-increasing range of specific processes in nerve cells affected by neurotoxins.

Another approach to the development of rapid and reliable neurotoxicity screens is the use of invertebrates whose relatively simple nervous systems still possess sufficient complexity to be of use. Best (121) argues that fresh-water planaria fit these requirements and that they could prove to be very useful in neurotoxicological studies.

The culture of nervous system tissues of various types has now become commonplace, ranging from organotypic cultures through primary cell cultures to the cultures of the various tumor cell lines such as neuroblastomas, gliomas, and pheochromocytomas. Schrier (122) discusses the advantages and disadvantages of various cell and organ cultures in neurotoxicology studies and emphasizes that the greatest potential for cell culture systems is in investigations of mechanisms. Nevertheless, some believe that cell cultures can be used as general screening systems. For example, Fedalei & Nardone (123) report that they have developed a neuroblastoma (N1E-115) assay for organophosphate toxicity that might be used as an in vitro alternative to the hen brain assay for neurotoxic esterase, the usual test for organophosphate toxicity. Nardone is also investigating the development of a neuroblastoma screening test for acrylamides (124).

Despite these developments, Dewar, in a comprehensive review of neurotoxicity studies (125), emphasizes that in all probability no single technique will ever be able to detect all possible neurotoxic endpoints. Nevertheless, he urges that more effort be put into the development of in vitro biochemical tests for certain well-defined neurotoxic endpoints. He also argues that nervous cell cultures should be further investigated and developed and that efforts to validate lower vertebrate models, such as Xenopus tadpoles, as neurotoxicological screens should be encouraged.

FETOTOXICITY   After the thalidomide disaster, more stringent requirements for animal tests of fetal toxicity were established. However, the routine animal test systems have not proved particularly reliable predictors of hazards to the human fetus. For example, the human fetus is fifty times more sensitive to thalidomide than the rabbit but is totally insensitive to corticosteroid-induced cleft palate, to which rabbits and rodents are very susceptible. The standard animal tests using rodents or rabbits are not only relatively poor predictors of human hazard, they are also expensive and time-consuming. As a result, a number of investigators have attempted to develop an in vitro screening test for teratogenicity.

One of the problems with the search for a satisfactory in vitro screen is that a number of different mechanisms appear to lead to one of a range of different outcomes, all of which result in some feature of fetotoxicity (e.g. living or dead terata, resorption or spontaneous abortion of embryos, functional impairment of offspring, or underweight offspring). Wilson (126) suggests that certain key aspects of reproductive success need to be tested, including mutagenesis, epigenesis, and organogenesis. He also describes the essential criteria for an ideal in vitro teratogenicity screen; it must be a system that uses large numbers of subjects, that is relevant to mechanisms of teratogenesis, that is easy to use, and that yields uniform and repeatable responses. Wilson (126) favors the use of fish embryos, Drosophila larva, sea urchin embryos, or chick embryos, although he cautions that only the chick embryo has been sufficiently investigated to offer promise for early validation as a preliminary screen for teratogenicity.

In the last few years, a number of other systems have been proposed as possible screening tests for teratogenicity. The available in vitro systems may be broadly classified into the following categories.

Mammalian embryo or embryo organ culture   The maintenance and development in culture of whole rodent embryos from day 9.5 to day 12.5 has been described and developed by New (127), who suggests using the system for screening teratogens (128). Several groups have begun to employ the technique for this purpose (129, 130, 132), and one group (131) has cultured the embryos in human serum to identify the possible teratogenicity of drugs being taken by human subjects. This system could be very useful as a screen as it is further refined and developed.

Use of other veterbrate embryos   The most studied of the other vertebrate embryos is the chick embryo, which has been extensively investigated as a possible teratogen screen (cf. 133, 134). However, the chick embryo is very sensitive to a wide range of experimental and chemical treatments, and this reduced discrimination may limit its usefulness for a single-purpose test. On the other hand, recent modifications to the shell-windowing procedure (135) may help reduce the embryo's sensitivity to experimental manipulations and thus render it more useful.

Birge and co-workers (136) have proposed that fish and amphibians in the embryo-larval stages constitute simple and effective models to investigate teratogenesis and to screen for environmental compounds that may be of concern to human health. They report large differences in sensitivity to test chemicals among six different amphibians. For example, bullfrog larva have an LC50 for atrazine of 0.41 mg/l, while larva of the American toad have an LC50 greater than 48 mg/l. Dumont & Schultz (137) also promote an amphibian system using Xenopus for screening environmental mixtures.

Invertebrate systems   Several invertebrate systems have been proposed as suitable for teratogen screening, including Drosophila (138), the cricket *(Acheta domesticus)* (139), and hydra (140). The Drosophila test has been more extensively investigated than the cricket system. In a recent trial using Drosophila (the system detects interference with muscle and/or neuron differentiation in embryo cell cultures), researchers reported that the test correctly identified all but six of the one hundred chemicals investigated (138). The authors also researched strain differences and dose-responses of a few selected chemicals and suggested that the system might be useful in studying teratogenic mechanisms. Johnson & Gabel (140), however, argue that one cannot classify substances as being teratogenic or non-teratogenic, since the terms have little meaning in terms of hazard to the conceptus. It is more important to establish whether there is a large difference between the dose that produces toxicity in the adult (A) and the dose that affects development (D). Where the A/D ratio is close to unity, the test substance has no specific developmental toxicity, but when the ratio is large (for thalidomide the ratio is 60), this indicates substantial risk to the conceptus.

   Johnson & Gabel (140) propose that an artificial embryo system composed of dissociated and pelleted hydra cells be used to study the effects on development and that the adult hydra be used to study general toxicity. They report agreement between the A/D ratios for mammals compared to the ratios for their hydra system.

Cell culture systems   Several investigators have proposed using differentiating cells (141–144, 147) or non-differentiating cells (145, 146) in culture as a teratogen screen. They variously suggest that cell cultures could be useful screening systems because they assess sensitivity to cell-cell interactions (146), cell killing and reduction in cell proliferation (142, 145), and disruption of cellular anabolism involved in morphogenesis and organogenesis (141, 143–144). Some of these systems (142, 146) are currently being validated in a trial sponsored by the National Toxicology Program, while others are still being developed. Nevertheless, some of the published results are encouraging, especially in comparison to the early days of short-term mutagen test development.

Braun and his colleagues (146) have developed an assay that discriminates between teratogens and non-teratogens on the basis of their ability to inhibit attachment of ascites cells to concanavalin A–coated surfaces. This test shows qualitative agreement between animal data and in vitro activity for eighty-one of the 102 (79%) chemicals tested. Mummery and co-workers report that thirty-five of thirty-nine teratogenic and four of eighteen non-teratogenic chemicals interfered with the growth and differentiation of cultured neuroblastoma cells. Eighty-six percent of the chemicals were correctly identified (143).

As is apparent, a number of possible teratogen screening systems can be used for the rapid identification of potential teratogens. At present, no single in vitro system is likely to supersede animal testing, but one can foresee the development of a successful battery of tests for identifying compounds for further in vivo testing. Logistically, it will never be possible to test chemicals in widespread use if we have to rely solely on the mammalian bioassay, which uses small treatment populations and takes six to ten months to complete.

CONCLUSION

It has not been possible in this review to consider thoroughly all possible methods of alternative toxicology testing, but the examination of acute toxicity tests, eye irritancy testing, and fetal toxicity testing should provide a reasonable introduction to the meaning and scope of the concept of alternatives in the field. Greater attention to and support for alternatives to animal testing will not only provide ways to alleviate animal stress and societal pressures, but will in addition bring major benefits to the science of toxicology.

An empirical search for in vitro tests that correlate with various toxic endpoints will not only be insufficient, it will be detrimental. Developing superior methods for safety evaluation will be much more possible if in vitro tests are investigated mechanistically. Cell cultures, both animal and human, will be used to their full potential only when culture techniques are considerably improved. Fully defined growth media that will support the growth of a wide range of defined cells must be developed. It is now possible to maintain and grow many different types of cells that express differentiated function in vitro. For example, changing culture conditions allowed one group of investigators to establish a thyroid cell line that expressed differentiated thyroid cell characteristics even after three years of continuous culture (148). Beating heart cells can be maintained for a week in good condition and have been used to investigate anesthetic (149) and isoproterenol (150) cardiotoxicity.

Computer-assisted structure-activity relationships in toxicology have not yet been developed. As toxicology data bases and our understanding of mechanisms improve, so will the potential applicability of quantitative structure-toxicity relationships (61, 151, 152).

Current techniques are slowly being improved, refined, and applied where appropriate. Yet even as new tests or approaches become available, a lack of general acceptance can retard their use. In toxicology testing, established methods tend to be set in stone. Even where new approaches seem an improvement and have widespread scientific support, explicit or implicit guidelines are slow to change. Replacing the classic LD50 test with an acute test using fewer animals was proposed in 1968 (44) and has been reproposed many times since, for example.

With the exciting advances now taking place in the disciplines that contribute to toxicology (e.g. molecular biology, cell biology), the time is opportune for academic, industrial, and regulatory toxicologists to explore new avenues for safety evaluation. This will mean discarding tests that no longer do what they are meant to and developing new ones that provide better assessments of potential human hazards.

Literature Cited

1. The Insight Team of the Sunday Times of London. 1979. *Suffer the Children: The Story of Thalidomide*. New York: Viking
2. Carson, R. 1962. *Silent Spring*. Boston: Houghton Mifflin
3. Weatherall, M. 1982. An end to the search for new drugs? *Nature* 296:387–90
4. Rowan, A. N. 1984. *Of Mice, Models and Men: a Critical Analysis of Animal Research*. Albany: State Univ. NY Press
5. Maugh, T. M. 1978. Chemicals: How many are there? *Science* 199:162
6. National Research Council. 1984. *Toxicity Testing: Strategies to Determine Needs and Priorities*. Washington, DC: Natl. Acad. Sci.
7. Rofe, P. C. 1971. Tissue culture and toxicology. *Food Cosmet. Toxicol.* 9:683–96
8. Zbinden, G. 1976. A look at the world from inside the toxicologist's cage. *Eur. J. Clin. Pharmacol.* 9:33–38
9. Heywood, R. 1978. Animal studies in drug safety evaluation. *J. R. Soc. Med.* 71:686–89
10. Melmon, K. L. 1976. The clinical pharmacologist and scientifically unsound regulations for drug development. *Clin. Pharmacol. Ther.* 20:125–29
11. Muul, I., Hegyeli, A. F., Dacre, J. C., Woodard, G. 1976. Toxicological testing dilemma. *Science* 193:834
12. Stevenson, D. E. 1979. Current problems in the choice of animals for toxicity testing. *J. Toxicol. Environ. Health* 5:9–15
13. Efron, E. 1984. *The Apocalyptics: Politics, Science and the Big Cancer Lie*. New York: Simon & Schuster
14. See Ref. 4, pp. 222–28
15. Rowan, A. N. 1983. The LD50—The beginning of the end. *Int. J. Study Animal Prob.* 4:4–7
16. Rowan, A. N., Stratmann, C. J., eds. 1980. *The Use of Alternatives in Drug Research*. London: Macmillan
17. Balls, M., Riddell, R. J., Worden, A. N., eds. 1983. *Animals and Alternatives in Toxicity Testing*. London: Academic
18. Goldberg, A. M., ed. 1983. *Product Safety Evaluation. Alternative Methods in Toxicology*, Vol. 1. New York: Liebert
19. Goldberg, A. M., ed. 1984. *Acute Toxicity Testing: Alternative Approaches. Alternative Methods in Toxicology*, Vol. 2. New York: Liebert
20. Lindgren, P., Thelestam, M., Lindquist, N. G., eds. 1983. LD50 and possible alternatives. *Acta Pharmacol. Toxicol.* 52(Suppl. 2):3–293
21. Holden, C. 1982. New focus on replacing animals in the lab. *Science* 215:35–38
22. Hollstein, M., McCann, J., Angelosanto, F. A., Nichols, W. W. 1979. Short-term tests for carcinogens and mutagens. *Mutat. Res.* 65:133–226
23. Weisburger, J. H., Williams, G. M. 1981. Carcinogen testing: Current problems and new approaches. *Science* 214:401–7
24. Heidelberger, C., Freeman, A. E., Pienta, R. J., Sivak, A., Bertram, J. S., et al. 1983. Cell transformation by chemical

agents—A review and analysis of the literature. *Mutat. Res.* 114:283–385

25. Bartsch, H., Malaveille, C., Camus, A. M., Martel-Planche, G., Brun, G., et al. 1980. Validation and comparative studies on 180 chemicals with S. typhimurium strains and V79 Chinese hamster cells in the presence of various metabolizing systems. *Mutat. Res.* 76:1–50

26. Russell, W. M. S., Burch, R. L. 1959. *The Principles of Humane Experimental Technique.* London: Methuen

27. Bruce, R. D. 1984. An up-and-down procedure for acute toxicity testing. *Fund. Appl. Toxicol.* 4:In press

28. Pomerat, C. M., Leake, C. D. 1954. Short-term cultures for drug assays. *Ann. NY Acad. Sci.* 58:1110–28

29. Worden, A. N. 1974. Tissue culture. In *Modern Trends in Toxicology,* ed. E. Boyland, R. Goulding, 2:216–49. London: Butterworth

30. Dawson, M. 1972. *Cellular Pharmacology.* Springfield: Thomas

31. Berky, J., Sherrod, C., eds. 1978. *In Vitro Toxicity Testing 1975–1976.* Philadelphia: Franklin Inst.

32. Deutsch Pharmakologische Gesellschaft, Toxicology Symposium. 1980. Isolated cell systems as a tool in toxicology research. *Arch. Toxicol.* 44:1–210

33. Zucco, F., Hooisma, J., eds. 1982. Proceedings of the second international workshop on the application of tissue culture in toxicology. *Toxicology* 25:1–74

34. Tardiff, R. G. 1978. In vitro methods of toxicity evaluation. *Ann. Rev. Pharmacol. Toxicol.* 18:357–69

35. Nardone, R. M. 1977. Toxicity testing *in vitro.* In *Growth, Nutrition and Metabolism of Cells in Culture,* ed. R. M. Rothblatt, V. J. Cristofala, 3:471–96. New York: Academic

36. Stammatti, A. P., Silano, V., Zucco, F. 1981. Toxicology investigations with cell culture systems. *Toxicology* 20:91–153

37. Ekwall, B. 1983. Screening of toxic compounds in mammalian cell cultures. *Ann. NY Acad. Sci.* 407:64–77

38. Grisham, J. W., Smith, G. J. 1984. Predictive and mechanistic evaluation of toxic responses in mammalian cell culture systems. *Pharmacol. Rev.* 36:151S–71S

39. Fry, J. R., Bridges, J. W. 1977. The metabolism of xenobiotics in cell suspension and cell culture. In *Progress in Drug Metabolism,* ed. J. W. Bridges, L. F. Chasseaud, 2:71–118. London: Wiley

40. Barnes, D., Sato, G. 1980. Serum-free culture: A unifying approach. *Cell* 22: 649–55

41. Nardone, R. M., Bradlaw, J. A. 1983. Toxicity testing with *in vitro* systems: I. Ocular tissue culture. *J. Toxicol. Cut. Ocul. Toxicol.* 2:81–98

42. Goldberg, A. M. 1984. Approaches to the development of in vitro toxicological methods. *Pharmacol. Rev.* 36:173S–75S

43. Trevan, J. W. 1927. The error of determination of toxicity. *Proc. R. Soc. Lond. Ser. B* 101:483–514

44. Morrison, J. K., Quinton, R. M., Reinert, M. 1968. The purpose and value of LD 50 determinations. In *Modern Trends in Toxicology,* ed. E. Boyland, R. Goulding, 1:1–17. Chichester: Wiley

45. Hunter, W. J., Lingk, W., Recht, P. 1978. Intercomparison study on the determination of single administration toxicity in rats. *J. Assoc. Off. Anal. Chem.* 62:864–73

46. Zbinden, G., Flury-Roversi, M. 1981. Significance of the LD50-test for the toxicological evaluation of chemical substances. *Arch. Toxicol.* 47:77–99

47. Rowan, A. N. 1983. Shortcomings of LD-50 values and acute toxicity testing in animals. *Acta Pharmacol. Toxicol.* 52(Suppl. 2):52–64

48. See Ref. 19

49. Bass, R., Gunzel, P., Henschler, D., Konig, J., Lorke, D., et al. 1982. LD50 versus acute toxicity: Critical assessment of the methodology currently in use. *Arch. Toxicol.* 51:183–86

50. Uberla, K., Schnieders, B. 1982. LD50 versus acute toxicity: Clinical assessment of the methodology currently in use. *Arch. Toxicol.* 51:187

51. Food and Drug Administration. 1984. *Final Rep. Acute Studies Workshop, Feb. 23.* Washington, DC: Off. Sci. Coord. US Food Drug Adm.

52. Dixon, W. J., Mood, A. M. 1948. A method of obtaining and analysing sensitivity data. *J. Am. Stat. Assoc.* 43:109–26

53. Tattersall, M. L. 1982. Statistics and the LD50 study. *Arch. Toxicol.* 5:267–70 (Suppl.)

54. Schutz, E., Fuchs, H. 1982. A new approach to minimizing the numbers of animals used in acute toxicity testing and optimizing the information of test results. *Arch. Toxicol.* 51:197–200

55. Muller, H., Kley, H. P. 1982. Retrospective study of the reliability of an "approximate LD50" determined with a small number of animals. *Arch. Toxicol.* 51:189–96

56. Lorke, D. 1983. A new approach to prac-

tical acute toxicity testing. *Arch. Toxicol.* 54:275–87

57. Deichmann, W. B., LeBlanc, T. J. 1943. Determination of the approximate lethal dose with about six animals. *J. Ind. Hyg. Toxicol.* 25:415–17

58. Enslein, K., Lander, T. R., Tomb, M. E., Craig, P. N. 1983. A predictive model for estimating rat oral LD50 values. *Benchmark Papers in Toxicology,* Vol. 1. Princeton: Princeton Sci.

59. Enslein, K., Craig, P. N. 1978. A toxicity prediction system. *J. Environ. Toxicol.* 2:115–21

60. Rekker, R. F. 1980. LD50 values: Are they about to become predictable? *Trends Pharmacol. Sci.* 1:383–84

61. Golberg, L., ed. 1983. *Structure-Activity Correlation as a Predictive Tool in Toxicology: Fundamentals, Methods, and Applications.* Washington, DC: Hemisphere. 330 pp.

62. Barile, M. F., Hardegree, M. 1970. A cell culture assay to evaluate the toxicity of Arlacel. *Proc. Soc. Exp. Biol. Med.* 133:222–28

63. Autian, J., Dillingham, E. O. 1978. Overview of general toxicity testing with emphasis on special tissue culture tests. See Ref. 31, pp. 23–49

64. Sako, F., 1977. Effects of food dyes on *Paramecium caudatum:* toxicity and inhibitory effects on leucine aminopeptidase and acid phosphatase activity. *Toxicol. Appl. Pharmacol.* 39:111–17

65. Ekwall, B. 1980. Screening of toxic compounds in tissue culture. *Toxicology* 17:127–42

66. Balls, M., Bridges, J. W. 1984. The FRAME research program on *in vitro* cytotoxicology. See. Ref. 19, pp. 61–79

67. Draize, J. H., Woodard, G., Clavery, H. O. 1944. Methods for the study of irritation and toxicity of substances applied topically to the skin and mucous membranes. *J. Pharmacol. Exp. Ther.* 82:377–90

68. Friedenwald, J. S., Hughes, W. F., Herrmann, H. 1944. Acid-base tolerance of the cornea. *Arch. Ophthalmol.* 31:279–83

69. Weil, C. S., Scala, R. A. 1971. Study of intra- and inter-laboratory variability in the results of rabbit eye and skin irritation tests. *Toxicol. Appl. Pharmacol.* 19:276–360

70. Griffith, J. F., Nixon, G. A., Bruce, R. D., Reer, P. J., Bannan, E. A. 1980. Dose-response studies with chemical irritants in the albino rabbit eye as a basis for selecting optimum testing conditions for predicting hazard to the human eye. *Toxicol. Appl. Pharmacol.* 55:501–13

71. Rowan, A. N. 1981. The Draize test: political and scientific issues. *Cosmet. Technol.* 3(7):32–37

72. Smyth, D. H. 1978. *Alternatives to Animal Experiments,* p. 68. London: Scolar

73. Falahee, K. J., Rose, C., Olin, S. S., Seifried, H. E. 1981. *Eye Irritation Testing: An Assessment of Methods and Guidelines for Testing Materials for Eye Irritancy.* Washington, DC: Off. Pest. Toxic Subst., US Environ. Protect. Agen. (EPA-560/11-82-001)

74. Walberg, J. 1983. Exfoliative cytology as a refinement of the Draize eye irritancy test. *Toxicol. Lett.* 18:49–55

75. Ulsamer, A. G., Wright, P. L., Osterberg, R. E. 1977. A comparison of the effects of model irritants on anesthetized and nonanesthetized rabbit eyes. 16th Annual Meet. *Soc. Toxicol.* Abstr. 143. Akron, OH: Soc. Toxicol.

76. Johnson, A. W. 1980. Use of small dosage and corneal anaesthetic for eye testing *in vivo.* In *Proc. CTFA Ocular Safety Testing Workshop: In Vivo and In Vitro Approaches, October 6–7.* Washington, DC: Cosmet., Toil. Fragr. Assoc.

77. Williams, S. J. 1984. Prediction of ocular irritancy potential from dermal irritation test results. *Food Chem. Toxicol.* 22:157–61

78. Murphy, J. C., Osterberg, R. E., Seabaugh, V. M., Bierbower, G. W. 1982. Ocular irritancy responses to various pH's of acids and bases with and without irritation. *Toxicology* 23:281–91

79. Walz, D. 1984. Towards an animal-free assessment of topical irritancy. *Trends Pharmacol. Sci.* 5:221–24

80. Simons, P. J. 1980. An alternative to the Draize test. See Ref. 16, pp. 147–51

81. Bell, M., Holmes, P. M., Nisbet, T. M., Uttley, M., Van Abbe, N. J. 1979. Evaluating the potential eye irritancy of shampoos. *Intl. J. Cosmet. Sci.* 1:123–31

82. Scaife, M. C. 1982. An investigation of detergent action on cells *in vitro* and possible correlations with *in vivo* data. *Int. J. Cosmet. Sci.* 4:179–83

83. Chan, K. Y., Haschke, R. H. 1983. Epithelial-stromal interactions: Specific stimulation of corneal epithelial cell growth *in vitro* by a factor (s) from cultured stromal fibroblasts. *Exp. Eye Res.* 36:231–46

84. McCormack, J. 1981. A procedure for the *in vitro* evaluation of the eye irritation potential of surfactants. In *Trends in Bioassay Methodology: In Vivo, In Vitro*

and Mathematical Approaches, pp. 177–86. Washington, DC: NIH Publ. 82-2382

85. Burton, A. B. G., York, M., Lawrence, R. S. 1981. The *in vitro* assessment of severe eye irritants. *Food Cosmet. Toxicol.* 19:471–80

86. Shopsis, C., Sathe, S. 1984. Uridine uptake inhibition as a cytotoxicity test: Correlations with the Draize test. *Toxicology* 29:195–206

87. Borenfreund, E., Borrero, O. 1984. *In vitro* cytotoxicity assays: Potential alternatives to the Draize ocular irritancy test. *Cell Biol. Toxicol.* 1:33–39

88. Leighton, J., Nassauer, J., Tchao, R., Verdone, J.. 1983. Development of a procedure using the chick egg as an alternative to the Draize rabbit test. See Ref. 18, pp. 163–77

89. Muir, C. K., Flower, C., Van Abbe, N. J. 1983. A novel approach to the search for *in vitro* alternatives to *in vivo* eye irritancy testing. *Toxicol. Lett.* 18:1–5

90. Muir, C. K. 1984. Further investigations on the Ileum model as a possible alternative to *in vivo* eye irritancy testing. *Alt. Lab. Animals* 11:129–34

91. Douglas, W. H. J., Spilman, S. D. 1983. *In vitro* ocular irritancy testing. See Ref. 18, pp. 205–30

92. Silverman, J. 1983. Preliminary findings on the use of protozoa (Tetrahymena thermophila) as models for ocular irritation testing in rabbits. *Lab. Animal Sci.* 33:56–59

93. Carter, L. M., Duncan, G., Rennie, G. K. 1973. Effects of detergents on the ionic balance and permeability of isolated bovine cornea. *Exp. Eye Res.* 17:409–16

94. North-Root, H., Yackovitch, F., Demetrulias, J., Gracula, M., Heinze, J. E. 1982. Evaluation of an *in vitro* cell toxicity test using rabbit corneal cells to predict the eye irritation potential of surfactants. *Toxicol. Lett.* 14:207–12

95. Jumblatt, M. M., Neufeldt, A. H. 1983. Corneal epithelial wound closure: A tissue culture model. *Invest. Ophthalmol. Vision Sci.* 24:44(Suppl.)

96. Marks, R. 1983. Testing for cutaneous toxicity. See Ref. 17, pp. 313–27

97. Kligman, A. M. 1982. Assessment of mild irritants. In *Principles of Cosmetics for the Dermatologist,* ed. P. Frost, S. N. Horwitz, pp. 265–73. St. Louis, Mo: Mosby

98. Imokawa, G., Okamoto, K. 1983. The effect of zinc pyrithione on human skin cells *in vitro. J. Soc. Cosmet. Chem.* 34:1–11

99. Kao, J., Hall, J., Holland, J. M. 1983. Quantitation of cutaneous toxicity: An *in vitro* approach using skin organ culture. *Toxicol. Appl. Pharmacol.* 68:206–17

100. Fouts, J. R. 1982. The metabolism of xenobiotics by isolated pulmonary and skin cells. *Trends Pharmacol. Sci.* 3:164–66

101. Hansbrough, J. F., Boyce, S. T. 1984. Current status of artificial skin replacements for burn wounds. *J. Trauma.* In press

102. Ryan, S. R., Norris, D. A., Fritz, K. A., Boyce, S. T., Weston, W. L. 1983. Comparison of mechanisms of epidermal cytotoxicity *in vitro. Clin. Res.* 31:150A

103. Guy, R. H., Fleming, R. 1981. Transport across a phospholipid barrier. *J. Coll. Interf. Sci.* 83:130–37

104. Weinberg, E. H., Springer, S. T. 1981. The evaluation *in vitro* of fragrance materials for phototoxic activity. *J. Soc. Cosmet. Chem.* 32:303–15

105. Tenenbaum, S., Dinardo, J., Morris, W. E., Wolf, B. A., Schnetzinger, R. W. 1984. A quantitative *in vitro* assay for the evaluation of phototoxic potential of topically applied materials. *Cell Biol. Toxicol.* 1:1–6

106. McAuliffe, D. J., Morison, W. L., Parrish, J. A. 1983. An *in vitro* test for predicting the photosensitizing potential of various chemicals. See Ref. 18, pp. 285–307

107. Morison, W. L., McAuliffe, D. J., Parrish, J. A., Bloch, K. J. 1982. *In vitro* assay for phototoxic chemicals. *J. Invest. Dermatol.* 78:460–63

108. Plaa, G. L., Hewitt, W. R. 1984. Detection and evaluation of chemically induced liver injury. In *Principles and Methods of Toxicology,* ed. A. W. Hughes, pp. 407–45. New York: Raven

109. Thurman, R. G., Reinke, L. A. 1979. The isolated perfused liver: A model to define biochemical mechanisms of chemical toxicity. In *Reviews in Biochemical Toxicology,* ed. E. Hodgson, J. R. Bend, R. M. Philpot, 1:249–85. New York: Elsevier

110. Fry, J. R., Bridges, J. W. 1977. The metabolism of xenobiotics in cell suspensions and cell cultures. See Ref. 39, 2:71–118

111. Grisham, J. W. 1979. Use of hepatic cell cultures to detect and evaluate the mechanisms of action of toxic chemicals. *Intl. Rev. Exp. Pathol.* 20:123–210

112. Acosta, D., Sorensen, E. M. B. 1983. Role of calcium in cytotoxic injury of cultured hepatocytes. *Ann. NY Acad. Sci.* 407:78–92

113. Schwarz, L. R., Greim, H. 1981. Isolated hepatocytes: An analytical tool in

hepatotoxicology. In *Frontiers in Liver Disease*, ed. P. D. Berk, T. C. Chalmers, pp. 61–79. New York: Thieme–Stratton

114. Paine, A. J., Williams, L. J., Legg, R. F. 1979. Apparent maintenance of cytochrome P-450 by nicotinamide in primary cultures of rat hepatocytes. *Life Sci.* 24:2185–92

115. Paine, A. J., Hockin, L. J., Allen, C. M. 1982. Long term maintenance and induction of cytochrome P-450 in rat liver cell culture. *Biochem. Pharmacol.* 31:1175–78

116. Nelson, K. F., Acosta, D. 1982. Long-term maintenance and induction of cytochrome P-450 in primary cultures of rat hepatocytes. *Biochem. Pharmacol.* 31:2211–14

117. Fry, J. R. 1983. A review of the value of isolated hepatocyte systems in xenobiotic metabolism and toxicity studies. In *Animals in Scientific Research: An Effective Substitute for Man?* ed. P. Turner, pp. 81–88. London: Macmillan

118. Goldberg, A. M. 1980. Mechanisms of neurotoxicity as studied in tissue culture systems. *Toxicology* 17:201–8

119. Brookes, N., Goldberg, A. M. 1979. Choline acetyltransferase activity of spinal cord cell cultures is increased by diisopropylphosphoro-fluoridate. *Life Sci.* 24:889–94

120. Damstra, T., Bondy, S. C. 1982. Neurochemical approaches to the detection of neurotoxicity. In *Nervous System Toxicology*, ed. C. L. Mitchell, pp. 349–73. New York: Raven

121. Best, J. B., Morita, M., Ragin, J., Best, J. Jr. 1981. Acute toxic responses of the freshwater planarian, *Dugesia dorotocephala*, to methylmercury. *Bull. Environ. Contam. Toxicol.* 27:49–54

122. Schrier, B. K. 1982. Nervous system cultures as toxicologic test systems. See Ref. 120, pp. 337–48

123. Fedalei, A., Nardone, R. M. 1983. An in vitro alternative for testing the effect of organophosphates on neurotoxic esterase activity. See Ref. 18, pp. 251–69

124. Krause, D., Nardone, R. M. 1982. Effect of acrylamide on acetylcholinesterase and neuron specific enolase activity in mouse neuroblastoma cells. *In Vitro* 18:235

125. Dewar, A. J. 1983. Neurotoxicity. See Ref. 17, pp. 229–84

126. Wilson, J. G. 1978. Review of in vitro systems with potential for use in teratogenicity screening. *J. Environ. Pathol. Toxicol.* 2:149–67

127. New, D. A. T. 1978. Whole embryo culture and the study of mammalian embryos during organogenesis. *Biol. Rev.* 53:81–122

128. New, D. A. T. 1976. Techniques for the assessment of teratologic effects: Embryo culture. *Environ. Health Perspect.* 18:105–10

129. Kitchin, K. T., Ebron, M. T. 1984. Further development of rodent whole embryo culture: Solvent toxicity and water insoluble compound delivery system. *Toxicology* 30:45–57

130. Warner, C. W., Sadler, T. W., Shockey, J., Smith, M. K. 1983. A comparison of the *in vivo* and *in vitro* response of mammalian embryos to a teratogenic insult. *Toxicology* 28:271–82

131. Sadler, T. W., Warner, C. W. 1984. Use of whole embryo culture for evaluating toxicity and teratogenicity. *Pharmacol. Rev.* 36:145S–50S

132. Chatot, C. L., Klein, N. W., Piatek, J., Pierro, L. J. 1980. Successful culture of rat embryos on human serum: Use in the detection of teratogens. *Science* 207:1471–73

133. Gebhardt, D. O. E. 1972. The use of the chick embryo in applied teratology. In *Advances in Teratology*, ed. D. H. M. Woollam, 5:97–111. London: Academic

134. Jelinek, R. 1982. Use of chick embryo in screening for embryotoxicity. *Teratogen. Carcinogen. Mutagen.* 2:255–61

135. Fisher, M., Schoenwolf, G. C. 1983. The use of early chick embryos in experimental embryology and teratology: Improvements in standard procedures. *Teratology* 27:65–72

136. Birge, W. J., Black, J. A., Westerman, A. G., Ramey, B. A. 1983. Fish and amphibian embryos—a model system for evaluating teratogenicity. *Fund. Appl. Toxicol.* 3:237–42

137. Dumont, J. N., Schultz, T. W. 1983. Frog embryo teratogenesis assay, Xenopus (FETAX): A short term assay applicable to complex environmental mixtures. *Environ. Sci. Res.* 27:393–405

138. Bournias-Vardiabasis, N., Teplitz, R. L., Chernoff, G. F., Seecof, R. L. 1983. Detection of teratogens in the Drosophila embryonic cell culture test: Assay of 100 chemicals. *Teratology* 28:109–22

139. Walton, B. T. 1983. Use of the cricket embryo (Acheta domesticus) as an invertebrate teratology model. *Fund. Appl. Toxicol.* 3:233–36

140. Johnson, E. M., Gabel, B. E. G. 1983. An artificial embryo for detection of abnormal developmental biology. *Fund. Appl. Toxicol.* 3:243–49

141. Wilk, A. L., Greenberg, J. H., Morigan, E. A., Pratt, R. M., Martin, G. R. 1980.

Detection of teratogenic compounds using differentiating embryonic cells in culture. *In Vitro* 16:269–76

142. Pratt, R. M., Grove, R. I., Willis, W. D. 1982. Prescreening for environmental teratogens using cultured mesenchymal cells from the human embryonic palate. *Teratogen. Carcinogen. Mutagen.* 2: 313–18

143. Mummery, C. L., Van den Brink, C. E., Van der Saag, P. T., De Laat, S. W. 1984. A short-term screening test for teratogens using differentiating neuroblastoma cells *in vitro*. *Teratology* 29:271–79

144. Guntakatta, M., Matthews, E. J., Rundell, J. O. 1984. Development of a mouse embryo limb bud cell culture system for screening for teratogenic potential. *Teratogen. Carcinogen. Mutagen.* 5:(In press)

145. Francis, B. M., Metcalf, R. L. 1982. Percutaneous teratogenicity of nitrofen. *Teratology* 25:41A

146. Braun, A. G., Buckner, C. A., Emerson, D. J., Nichinson, B. B. 1983. Quantitative correspondence between the *in vivo* and *in vitro* activity of teratogenic agents. *Proc. Natl. Acad. Sci. USA* 79:2056–60

147. Clayton, R. M. 1980. An *in vitro* system for teratogenicity testing. See Ref. 16, pp. 153–73

148. Ambesi-Impiombato, F. S., Parks, L. A. M., Coon, H. G. 1980. Culture of hormone-dependent functional epithelial cells from rat thyroids. *Proc. Natl. Acad. Sci. USA* 77:3455–59

149. Miletich, D. J., Khan, A., Albrecht, R. F., Jozefiak, A. 1983. Use of heart cell cultures as a tool for the evaluation of halothane arrhythmia. *Toxicol. Appl. Pharmacol.* 70:181–87

150. Ramos, K., Combs, A. B., Acosta, D. 1983. Cytotoxicity of isoproterenol to cultured heart cells: Effects of antioxidants on modifying membrane damage. *Toxicol. Appl. Pharmacol.* 70:317–23

151. Wold, S., Hellberg, S., Dunn, W. J. 1983. Computer methods for the assessment of toxicity. *Acta Pharmacol. Toxicol.* 52(Suppl. 2):158–89

152. Craig, P. N. 1983. Mathematical models for toxicity evaluation. *Ann. Rep. Med. Chem.* 18:303–6

Ann. Rev. Pharmacol. Toxicol. 1985. 25:249–73

THE CENTRAL AND PERIPHERAL INFLUENCES OF OPIOIDS ON GASTROINTESTINAL PROPULSION

Luciano Manara and Alberto Bianchetti

Groupe SANOFI, Research Center MIDY S.p.A., Via Piranesi 38, 20137 Milan, Italy

INTRODUCTION

The constipating effects of extracts of the poppy plant *Papaver somniferum* are among the oldest known pharmacological actions, and their application as antidiarrheal remedies preceded the use of opium preparations for analgesia. However, we are still far from a thorough understanding of how opioids[1] influence the gut in spite of considerable recent advances, including the discovery of specific binding sites and their endogenous ligands (65). While the mechanism of pain relief by morphine-like natural alkaloids and related synthetic narcotic analgesics is currently assumed to involve exclusively the central nervous system (CNS), both their direct effects on the bowel and their centrally elicited actions are believed to account for constipation (66). Opioid receptors and endorphins are widely distributed in the CNS and throughout the gastrointestinal (GI) tract, implying possible participation of the endogenous opiate system at either level in the regulation of gut functions, including motility.

This article represents an effort to lay out a framework against which to assess the relative roles of central and peripheral opioid–specific mechanisms affecting gastrointestinal propulsion. Our sights have been kept on subjects of

---

[1]Throughout this paper, the word *opioid,* according to its currently prevailing use, is used interchangeably with morphine-like plant alkaloids, their synthetic analogues and animal peptides mimicking their effects.

249

0362-1642/85/415-0249$02.00

clinical significance, like the well-recognized selectivity of newer synthetic antidiarrheal agents for the gut (3) and the unwanted intestinal spasm and constipation that are virtually inevitable complications associated with pain relief by narcotic analgesics (85).

Space limitations do not permit exhaustive coverage of the available literature, so we concentrated on summarizing, correlating, and interpreting mostly recent and some older experimental studies selected primarily in terms of the above aim. Our reference to reviews, without necessarily endorsing the opinions expressed therein, is intended as a useful complement to the present compact overview.

EXPERIMENTAL CONDITIONS

Anyone wishing to provide a coherent picture of the imposing amount of data on gastrointestinal motility as affected by opioids is faced with the initial obstacle of variation in results depending on experimental conditions. These include animal species, techniques, and drugs.

Considerable species differences have long been known in the effects of morphine and similar drugs, excitation versus sedation, for example, and myosis versus mydriasis (66). To some extent this also applies to the gastrointestinal tract. The mode of opioid action on the motility of all intestinal portions of different animals and the related neurochemical factors have been reviewed elsewhere (21, 35, 36, 166). The variety of mechanisms, which range from inhibition of tone and acetylcholine release in the guinea pig ileum to spasmogenic action and increased release of serotonin and/or acetylcholine in most other species, all produce constipation in the mammalian gut. This is the key aspect in the present context, where slowing of the propulsion of intestinal contents is dealt with as the main functional consequence of altered gut movement by opioids.

The propulsive performance of the intestine in vivo is usually assessed by measuring the transit of nonabsorbable markers along the alimentary canal of animals (100) and man (16). Clearly, these relatively coarse techniques preclude any detailed analysis of opioid influences on distinct but integrated events underlying gastrointestinal motor function at different levels. Thus, myogenic and neural events are studied through mechanical or electrical recordings from isolated preparations either in situ or in vitro (36, 39). These kinds of studies have often been considered merely model systems to clarify typical problems of CNS opioid pharmacology like tolerance and dependence, but of course they also provide extensive evidence that specific responses to opioids can be elicited locally throughout the gut. However, several questions persist regarding the relevance of the responses observed in isolated gut preparations to the possible local functional role of endogenous opioids in animals under physiological conditions or to the direct intestinal origin of the constipating action of morphine-like drugs, as seen in therapeutics. How does local application of substances compare to their reaching the gut through the bloodstream upon systemic administration or to neuronal release at discrete sites? Does removal of other controlling mechanisms as a consequence of isolation of preparations show up responses to opioids otherwise absent and/or of little or no significance in the interplay of the many factors concurring in gastrointestinal propulsion in the intact organism? Are anesthesia or other medications a source of artifacts?

These outstanding questions apart, this review considers mostly in vivo studies measuring transit along the intestine of intact animals, because it is essentially under such conditions that the balance between central and peripheral opioid specific mechanisms of constipation can best be assessed. Most available data have been produced by different laboratories using rats and mice and the long-established charcoal meal test (58) or related methods[2]; for review see (100). Some meaningful extrapolations to man should be possible judging from the results obtained with these animal models, which have been instrumental in the development of the newer, gut-selective, clinically effective antidiarrheal opioids (3). While these animal models essentially reflect the propulsive performance of the small intestine, in humans only about a quarter of the constipating action of morphine is believed to take place there, half being attributed to delayed gastric emptying and the remaining quarter to large intestine and anal sphincter spasms plus inattention to sensory stimuli for the defecation reflex (66).

Differences in constipating action among morphine-like drugs have been generally regarded as quantitative rather than qualitative (66). Narcotic analgesics reportedly less constipating than morphine include mixed agonists like pentazocine (17), nalbuphine (80), butorphanol (59) and buprenorphine (60). Mixed agonists are also relatively free from respiratory depression, a side effect of exclusively central origin. This suggests that a common factor possibly inherent in receptor mechanisms might account for the lower frequency of either undesirable action. Pethidine is also indicated from therapeutic experi-

---

[2]In these methods, transit along the small intestine of a nonabsorbable marker fed by stomach tube is generally measured from the percentage of the total length reached by the marker in a given time. The marker may be introduced through a duodenal cannula in chronically implanted animals (48, 145); the presence or absence of the marker in the cecum can be taken as an all-or-none response (101); the slope produced by linear regression analysis of the cumulative percentage of radioactive marker passing through each of several intestinal segments or the geometric center of the distribution of radioactivity throughout the intestine are the scored endpoints (96); cathartic-primed rather than normal animals may be used (145). Additional factors influencing the results are: observation times in relation to drug treatment and to marker progression kinetics (151); fasted versus freely feeding animals (58); drug administration routes and techniques, particularly intraperitoneal injection, which, at least in rats, might be regarded as local intestinal application (151).

ence as less constipating than morphine (97), this being consistent with precise animal findings that pethidine doses producing analgesia are lower than those required for inhibition of intestinal transit (58).

Whether differences exist between narcotic analgesics other than morphine in the extent to which central or local intestinal mechanisms underlie their constipating action does not seem to have been investigated; for a beginning see (110).

RECEPTOR ASPECTS OF THE INTESTINAL MOTOR EFFECTS OF OPIOIDS

Throughout the modern era of research on opioids, considerable efforts have been made to explain their action in terms of receptor pharmacology. The existence of specific opioid receptors was postulated in the mid-50s by Beckett & Casy, who formulated theoretical opiate receptor models based on stereochemical considerations for synthetic narcotic analgesics (5). The characterization of such receptors has since proceeded mainly by pharmacological and biochemical approaches in vitro in isolated tissue preparations and tissue homogenates.

In the gut, opioid receptors were first identified by classical pharmacological methods. After the pioneering work of Paton on the action of morphine on the electrically stimulated contraction of guinea pig ileum and associated acetylcholine-release inhibition (108), this in vitro preparation was extensively studied by Kosterlitz and his group (70). They found that the concentration-response relation of morphine and other narcotic agonists in the presence and absence of specific antagonists conformed to the law of mass action and calculated kinetic parameters for agonists and antagonists.

Biochemical evidence for opioid receptors was later provided by several investigators, who identified specific, stereoselective binding sites in isolated tissues by in vitro techniques using radiolabelled opioid agonists and antagonists as ligands (56, 111, 141, 156). With these techniques, the presence of opioid binding sites could be confirmed, not only in brain but also in intestinal tissues such as the myenteric plexus of the guinea pig (155) and, more recently, of the rat (98). The most convincing evidence that the guinea pig ileum binding sites represent pharmacological receptors comes from the close correlation between binding affinities and potencies in influencing electrically induced contraction for a variety of opioid drugs (33); it was also suggested that these receptors are similar to those located centrally, after comparison of the rank order of potencies of agonists and antagonists in this preparation and in the CNS (33).

Attempts to identify and characterize opioid receptors on the basis of pharmacological responses in vivo have also been described (90, 148, 149). Despite the apparent difficulties of establishing precise, reliable receptor-kinetic constants (119, 150), the in vivo approach has the considerable advantage of correlating the pharmacological effects to receptor occupancy in an integrated system—the whole animal. As to the specific receptors involved in opioid constipation, several investigators have measured either dissociation constants for narcotic agonists or pA_2 values for antagonists in rodents treated by different administration routes. In mice injected subcutaneously, Takemori et al (148) found that the pA_2 value of naloxone for antagonism of morphine constipation (6.6) was lower than for antagonism of morphine analgesia (7.0) and even lower than that reported in the isolated guinea pig ileum (8.7) by Kosterlitz & Watt (70). These findings suggest that the receptors for analgesia and inhibition of intestinal motility may not be the same and that different mechanisms of inhibition of intestinal motility by morphine may apply in vitro and in vivo.

Opposite conclusions may be drawn from the results of Raffa et al, who measured the receptor dissociation constant (K_a) of morphine for inhibition of gastrointestinal transit in subcutaneously treated rats and found it similar to that for antinociception (124). However, from theoretical considerations, the authors excluded the applicability of the classical drug-receptor theory to their system. To obtain reliable pA_2 values from in vivo experiments, it has been recommended that antagonist concentrations at the sites of action should be determined; alternatively, the antagonist should be given by a route ensuring drug delivery in the proximity of the presumed loci of action (119). Accordingly, a pA_2 value of 8.8 was obtained for naloxone against morphine constipation in intraperitoneally treated rats (90), this being remarkably close to that (8.7) obtained in vitro on the guinea pig ileum (70). In contrast to a previous study in subcutaneously treated mice (148), this supports the notion of functional similarity of intestinal opioid receptors in vivo and in vitro. Since direct intracranial administration of morphine is known to induce constipation in rodents (see below), the estimated pA_2 for morphine-naloxone, both administered intracerebroventricularly to rats, yielded a value of 7.1, which agrees substantially with pA_2 values in various analgesia tests, but in systemically treated animals (107). Nonetheless, these results have led their authors to advocate the primary importance of centrally located receptors, similar to those inducing antinociception, for mediation of the effects of systemic morphine on the gut (107).

A recent different in vivo approach in localizing and characterizing opioid receptors involved in the constipating action of morphine consisted of monitoring the drug's intestinal effects and its tissue levels in the same rats; morphine levels in small intestine longitudinal muscle, but not in plasma or brain, presented a striking correlation with gastrointestinal transit inhibition scores as predicted by a currently accepted equation describing drug-receptor kinetics

(10). Consistently, narcotic antagonists antagonized morphine's antipropulsive action and under the same experimental conditions prevented in vivo labelling of binding sites in the gut with the radiolabelled opioid buprenorphine, further supporting the presence and relevance to motor function of specific receptor mechanisms in the rat intestine (11).

Opioid receptors are currently classified as several subtypes [for review, see (93, 140)] whose relative importance in influencing gastrointestinal function is still uncertain. Most work on this subject has been carried out in vitro on isolated intestinal segments, where the presence of a given receptor subtype may be inferred from the different sensitivity of the preparation to various agonists and antagonists presumably selective with regard to postulated multiple opioid receptors. Thus, the GI tract was shown to contain the putative receptor subtypes μ, κ, and δ, but their distribution along the gut presented broad variability depending on the species and intestinal segment considered (105). Only a few in vivo studies have so far attempted to ascribe opioid effects on intestinal propulsion and/or mechanical activity to activation of a particular receptor subtype. Based on the effects of several opioid-agonists injected in the esophageal branch of the left gastric artery in anesthetized opossums, it was concluded that the lower esophageal sphincter (LES) contains μ, κ, σ, and δ opioid receptors (126). In order to identify and localize the receptor subtypes involved in inhibition of intestinal transit in mice, Ward & Takemori (162) utilized β-funaltrexamine (β-FNA) as a specific, irreversible μ antagonist, and morphine, D-Ala^2 D-Leu^5 enkephalin (DADL) and nalorphine as selective agonists for μ, δ, and κ sites respectively. A full dose-response curve was obtained with morphine given either intracerebroventricularly or subcutaneously, while DADL and nalorphine only partially inhibited transit. Since β-FNA antagonizes morphine and DADL but not nalorphine, the authors supported the existence of central and peripheral μ-mediated components and of a peripheral κ component accounting for limited inhibition of GI transit; furthermore, from the outcome of the combined administration of agonists and antagonists by the intracerebroventricular and/or subcutaneous routes, they concluded that the effects of subcutaneous morphine are mediated predominantly at peripheral sites. Whether there are any κ receptors instrumental in the slowing of GI transit by opioids in rodents is doubtful in view of the inconsistent results in intact rats (54, 153) with benzomorphans or other compounds proposed as acting on κ sites in vitro. Porreca et al (118) found that ketazocines, considered κ agonists, slow intestinal transit in both mice and rats when administered subcutaneously, but, unlike morphine, not when injected intracerebroventricularly; they suggested an anatomically distinct distribution of μ and κ sites mediating intestinal function. However, the intestinal activity of ketazocines in rodents is likely to consist of poor discrimination between μ and κ receptors, since cross tolerance between ethylketocyclazocine and morphine on the intestine has been reported (117). In the anesthetized dog, the contractions of duodenum circular muscle are increased by normorphine and Met-enkephalin but not by the putative κ agonists dynorphin 1-13, bremazocine, and U-50,488H, which shows that in these conditions, too, no κ component of intestinal action can be detected (158). Data supporting the involvement of enkephalin (δ) receptors in the constipating action of opioids have been presented by Cowan & Gmerek, who showed intestinal transit inhibition in mice by the opioid peptide metkephamid and its prevention by the reportedly selective antagonist ICI 154,129 (32). Likewise, in anesthetized cats, Met-enkephalin was a hundred times more potent than morphine in inducing phasic ileal contractions associated with ileocecal sphincter closure (106). In addition, based on in vitro findings, it has been suggested that a δ opioid receptor might mediate permeability changes across the guinea pig ileal mucosa and thereby account for antidiarrheal action consisting of an antisecretory effect more than actual inhibition of propulsive activity (67).

CNS-ELICITED OPIOID INFLUENCES ON GUT MOTILITY

Evidence for central opioid-sensitive sites of inhibition of gastrointestinal transit comes primarily from animal studies consisting of administering morphine-like drugs or endogenous peptides directly into the CNS. This approach can be traced back to the work of Margolin (91), who reported delay in the transit of a charcoal suspension through the small intestine of unanesthetized mice given intracranial (subdural) morphine at doses considerably lower than the intravenous ones required to produce comparable constipation; this author reported similar findings in rats and guinea pigs. Subsequent observations by different laboratories in mice (8, 137, 162), rats (51, 53, 58, 89, 107, 137, 143, 145), guinea pigs (137), ewes (19), and cats (144) have provided more adequate evidence that morphine applied intracranially with several techniques produces centrally initiated intestinal motor responses.

Very little is known of the precise cerebral sites involved in these intestinal responses. Conceivably, morphine could more easily, via the circulating cerebrospinal fluid, reach the periventricular regions currently indicated as the loci of CNS-mediated analgesia (66). The periaqueductal gray matter has been consistently associated with inhibition of gastrointestinal propulsion in rats (133). A nervous (vagal) pathway seems to link central opioid–specific mechanisms to the gut (44, 145). The original suggestion by Margolin et al postulating release by morphine from the brain of an unknown humoral agent that inhibits gastrointestinal propulsion through the circulation (92, 113) has been recently reexamined in the light of its possible opioid peptidergic nature, but the results are not compatible with this hypothesis (137).

Narcotic drugs other than morphine may not all share its ability to affect gastrointestinal transit after central administration. Thus, putative κ agonists ketazocines slowed transit of a suitable marker through the small intestine of rodents when administered subcutaneously, but not by the intracerebroventricular route, whereas phenazocine, a benzomorphan supposedly acting at μ receptors, delayed marker transit after intracerebroventricular injection (118) and so did heroin and etorphine (112). Likewise, different results have been obtained by intraventricular injection to rats (castor oil–primed) of opioid peptides: β-endorphin and [D-Ala^2, Met^5] enkephalinamide reduced transit along the small intestine of intraduodenally administered radiochromium, but [D-Ala^2, Leu^5] enkephalinamide and dynorphin 1–13 did not (52). Other opioid peptides with constipating action when injected intracerebroventricularly to mice tested with the charcoal meal procedure are Leu-enkephalin and Met-enkephalin (31) and the enkephalin-like pentapeptide FK 33824 (137).

The results of studies showing effects on enteric functions of opioids directly administered into the CNS are of considerable interest for supporting specific action sites, therein influencing the gut. However, this does not justify assigning a definite role in gastrointestinal physiology to central endogenous opioids. In addition, an essential caveat is that centrally elicited effects on the bowel of narcotic drugs directly injected into the CNS are by no means a precise reflection of their mechanism of intestinal action on systemic administration. On these questionable grounds, in fact, a primarily central component affecting gut peristalsis has been attributed to parenterally administered morphine (107, 137). Yet the following important aspects seriously undermine this conclusion. Because of possible biotransformation and different distribution kinetics, generally great caution is required in extrapolating the responses evoked by local application of drugs to the effects presumably associated with their reaching the same site via the general circulation. With intracranial morphine, the delivered amounts that produce constipation in rats largely exceed the lower than microgram per gram brain concentrations[3] recovered even after a subtoxic intravenous dose (88). Therefore, not surprisingly: (a) in the early report by Green describing rats given morphine intracisternally, the dose-response curves for charcoal meal intestinal transit inhibition and respiratory depression were superposable and stood to the right of that for antinociception (58); (b) later studies clarified that test meal transit inhibition in rats by a standard intracerebroventricular morphine dose was constantly associated with severe catatonia that persisted in naloxone subcutaneously pretreated animals whose transit had fully recovered to control values (89). More importantly, a lower

---

[3]Regional distribution of morphine in the rat brain is reportedly fairly uniform (20, 34), which makes it unlikely that drug concentrations are higher at cerebral sites involved in the constipating action of opioids.

dose of morphine that substantially slowed gastrointestinal transit when injected intraperitoneally failed to do so upon intracerebroventricular administration, although it produced sustained catatonia in all treated rats (151).

Since only small amounts of systemically administered morphine pass the blood brain barrier (66), reasonable doses cannot be expected to have a predominantly central component of intestinal action (see below).

An apparently less questionable approach to ascertaining whether systemically administered opioids have central effects on the gut consists in checking their reversibility in animals given a narcotic antagonist intracerebroventricularly. Naloxone, the best tolerated,[4] is more readily diffusible across the blood brain barrier than is morphine, thus requiring careful titration of the intracerebral dose plus adequate controls of its exclusively local effectiveness. Several narcotic analgesics were compared at subcutaneous doses producing about 50% inhibition of gastrointestinal transit in rats; intracerebroventricular naloxone failed to antagonize morphine but fully antagonized etorphine and pethidine and partly antagonized heroin and methadone (110). These results are reinforced by the outcome of a twin experiment in which intracerebroventricular naloxone was replaced by intraperitoneally administered, peripherally selective quaternary ammonium antagonists (see below) and suggest that, unlike morphine, other narcotics act largely, if not exclusively, in the brain to affect the gut (110).

Recently, the spinal cord, which is currently indicated as an important site for pain relief by narcotic analgesics (78, 170), has been considered a potential locus of opioid action in the production of gastrointestinal motor effects. Morphine and some of a number of narcotic analgesics and opioid peptides directly administered (intrathecally) in the spinal cord of mice effectively inhibit the passage of a radiolabel maker through the gastrointestinal tract (116, 120, 121), but a similar study including rats did not confirm spinally elicited constipating effects in this species (159). In this connection, the rat may be a more predictive model for humans than mice, because constipation does not seem to occur in patients receiving spinal analgesia with morphine (28, 171).

THE LOCAL INTESTINAL MOTOR EFFECTS OF OPIOIDS

The presence throughout the gastrointestinal tract of opioid receptors whereby specific responses can be elicited in a variety of isolated gut preparations strongly suggests that in vivo, too, the intestinal motor effects of systemically

---

[4]Quaternary narcotic antagonists (see below) given intracranially may cause animals to convulse (24, 55).

administered morphine-like drugs may be initiated locally. However, undisputed evidence for CNS-originated inhibition of gut peristalsis following intracranial application of opioids (see above) poses the question of whether and to what extent this central component of intestinal action contributes to the effects produced in intact animals treated by a systemic route. Different approaches can be taken to answer this question.

Since resection of the vagus nerve in rats abolished the antidiarrheal action of intracerebroventricular but not of subcutaneous morphine, the latter action was considered free of any central component (145).

Assuming no major differences, as allowed in the light of current knowledge, between centrally and peripherally located opioid receptors influencing bowel movements, clearly pharmacokinetic factors (i.e. the drug distribution in the CNS and gut after systemic treatment) should account mainly for the central and/or peripheral modes of the constipation action of any given opioid drug (89, 110). This is best demonstrated with agents that are virtually completely excluded from the CNS like the peripherally selective opioids and antagonists (see below), but conceivably morphine-like drugs poorly passing the blood-brain barrier may also act primarily, or perhaps even solely, at local intestinal opioid receptors. Thus, in mice the constipating intravenous dose of the stabilized enkephalin derivative FK 33824 amounts to only 2% of the corresponding analgesic dose, but the drug is equipotent in producing analgesia and constipation when given intracerebroventricularly; on these grounds, it was inferred that the drug has considerable direct action on the intestine (137). In rats pretreated with a dose of naloxone sufficient to completely prevent analgesia by intravenous FK 33824, its inhibition of gastrointestinal transit is consistently only slightly relieved (47).

Only small amounts of morphine pass the blood-brain barrier after systemic administration (10, 66). Moreover, the clinical notion that "it requires considerably less morphine to affect the gut than to produce analgesia" (66) agrees with experimental animal data. As an example, the rat subcutaneous ED_{50} for morphine analgesia (14) is about four times[5] that for reduction of charcoal meal gastrointestinal transit (47, 110) and the difference for the oral route is much larger (89). The latter difference seems particularly to suggest the local intestinal nature of the constipating side effects of oral morphine in pain therapy of terminal patients, a currently recommended measure (2).

---

[5]The ratio between subcutaneous analgesic and constipating doses of morphine found by Green in rats is also very close to four (58). Subcutaneous morphine doses (5–10 mg/kg) considerably larger than those slowing the progression of a charcoal meal in normal rats have been required in the work of Stewart et al to antagonize castor oil diarrhea (145), but clearly this is a less sensitive model for prediction of clinical constipation as a side effect of narcotic analgesia. However, about 20 times less morphine is needed to antagonize castor oil diarrhea than to produce analgesia in orally treated mice (100).

Recently, the intraperitoneal route was reported as by far the most effective for producing morphine inhibition of the progression of a stomach tube fed charcoal meal along the rat small intestine (10, 89, 90, 151). Reasons have been presented (151) for previous failures (107, 137) to show the remarkable potency of the constipating action by intraperitoneal morphine under mostly comparable conditions (7, 151), and it has been clarified that this exclusively local intestinal action (90) consists of inhibition of small bowel propulsion rather than a direct effect on the stomach, delaying gastric emptying (48). More interestingly, comparison of morphine tissue levels and the effects on charcoal meal transit of intraperitoneally and intravenously dosed rats shows that higher intestinal morphine concentrations account for greater potency with the former injection route (10). These concentrations, irrespective of different doses, administration routes, and observation times, largely exceeded those in brain and, contrary to the latter, were closely correlated with the observed constipating effects so as to fit computer-generated curves described by equations complying with the receptor occupation theory of drug response (10). All together, these recent observations in rats, starting from pharmacokinetic considerations, render the animal model consistent with a primary role of a gut-located action site in morphine-induced constipation.

Peripherally Selective Opioids and Antagonists

In principle, opioids unable to pass through the blood-brain barrier offer an ideal means for acting selectively on their specific receptors outside the CNS, thereby revealing in vivo peripherally elicited effects.

QUATERNARY AMMONIUM COMPOUNDS   Foster et al pioneered this approach[6] and showed that morphine and its N-methyl quaternary derivative given at the same intravenous dose to mice had comparable constipating effects scored as frequency of scybala output (49). Limitations of this early study for supporting an exclusively local intestinal action of morphine include the absence of dose-response analysis; the assumption that N-methyl morphine was unable to penetrate the CNS because of its failure to produce antinociception in a different experimental protocol (intraperitoneally dosed rats); the lack of control of the opioid-specific nature of the constipating effect based on reversal by a narcotic antagonist.

More recently, a growing number of studies have focused on quaternary ammonium salts of narcotic antagonists as a tool for differentiation between the central and peripheral components of opioid effects on the gut.

The N-allyl quaternary analog of nalorphine [diallylnormorphine (DANM)],

---

[6]As early as 1933, N. B. Eddy demonstrated the ability of quaternarized morphine and codeine to depress motility of the rabbit intestine in vivo [quoted in (49)].

unlike its parent tertiary amine and consistent with previous in vitro results (69), behaves like a pure narcotic antagonist, since by itself it does not slow gastrointestinal transit of a charcoal test meal fed to rats. Unlike naloxone, DANM does not reduce in vivo binding of buprenorphine in cerebrum, nor does it prevent gastrointestinal transit inhibition by intracerebroventricular morphine. DANM under comparable conditions substantially relieves the constipating action of a supramaximal analgesic dose of intravenous morphine, preserving at least part of its antinociceptive action in the same rats (89, 152). Other investigators have observed partial antagonism of the inhibition of intestinal propulsion of radioactive chromium after subcutaneous morphine in rats given an intracerebroventricular dose of DANM that had no such effect when given intravenously (24). In spite of apparent discrepancies due to different test conditions, these and an additional study with DANM in rats (12) agree in supporting a major, locally elicited component of slowing of intestinal transit by systemic morphine given even at larger than analgesic doses. However, DANM completely prevents the marked inhibition of gastrointestinal transit produced in rats by lower systemic doses of morphine (89).

The quaternary N-methyl analog of naloxone given intraperitoneally to mice at doses presumably lacking CNS action, as indicated by the lack of effect on morphine analgesia, antagonizes the constipating action of the peripherally acting opioid loperamide, but not that of intravenous morphine (137). Doses of N-methyl naloxone higher than those preventing morphine antinociception do antagonize its slowing action on gastrointestinal transit when given systemically to mice (38, 137). Conversely, in rats quaternary naloxone restores gastrointestinal transit, nearly blocked by intravenous morphine, to about 70% of drug-free controls with no detectable impairment of analgesia tested concurrently in the same animals (12, 47). Near-maximal inhibition of gastrointestinal transit after either morphine or the enkephalin-like peptide FK 33824 given intraperitoneally to rats is virtually fully prevented by N-methyl naloxone at doses about one tenth those with no effect on morphine analgesia under comparable conditions (47). In rats given any of several narcotic analgesics subcutaneously at approximately equipotent doses inhibiting gastrointestinal transit by about 50%, intraperitoneal quaternary naloxone fails to antagonize etorphine and pethidine but fully antagonizes morphine and partly antagonizes heroin and methadone (110). Therefore, central and peripheral inhibition of gastrointestinal transit seems to differ depending on the narcotic tested, which may act at one or both levels.

Russel et al (132) showed that the N-methyl quaternary analog of naltrexone, at doses well below those that failed to precipitate behavioral signs (central) in morphine-dependent dogs, attenuates morphine-induced spike potentials recorded from chronically implanted canine duodenum. In the same study (132), intraperitoneal quaternary naltrexone in mice reversed antinociception by morphine but not its attenuation of prostaglandin-diarrhea, while in rats antinociception was not reversed and diarrhea attentuation was only inconsistently prevented. Gmerec et al (55) reported full antagonism of gastrointestinal transit inhibition by subcutaneous morphine in rats given quaternary naltrexone subcutaneously that only slightly attenuated the constipating action of intracerebroventricular morphine.

The N-methyl quaternary analogs of nalorphine, naloxone, and naltrexone, and DANM, all given subcutaneously over a wide dose range, were compared by rating their abilities to prevent antinociception and gastrointestinal transit inhibition in individual rats receiving morphine intravenously. All four quaternary antagonists proved gut-selective when given shortly before morphine and started to antagonize antinociception only at doses up to 60 times those restoring test meal transit to 50% of drug-free controls. However, a time factor proved critical for peripheral selectivity, which was virtually lost within 80 minutes in the case of the most selective compound, quaternary naltrexone (12). Different laboratories have confirmed the short-lived peripheral selectivity of N-methyl naltrexone (18, 125).

These limitations of the available quaternary antagonists have prompted the search for better compounds. The first one tested was N-allyl levallorphan bromide (CM 32191). In mice treated subcutaneously, it did not interfere with morphine analgesia at a dose five times that reducing constipation by 50%, and its peripheral selectivity did not decrease with time; a 1.7 ratio between the anti-analgesic and anticonstipating doses was found for N-methyl naloxone tested in the same way (8). In rats, extensive tests over a range of doses and time intervals have shown that CM 32191 selectively prevented morphine's antipropulsive action and buprenorphine's in vivo binding in the intestine without impairing CNS binding and analgesia (11).

Despite its superiority over similar compounds in terms of peripheral selectivity, CM 32191 still presented the shortcoming of limited potency. Further efforts to clarify the stereochemical requirements at the chiral nitrogen for in vitro and in vivo activity of quaternary narcotic antagonist (9) yielded levallorphan methyl iodide (SR 58002), currently the best available peripheral antagonist (38).

These recent developments are providing more reliable research tools for characterizing opioid effects outside the CNS, including those arising locally in the gut. In addition, newer peripheral antagonists may yet render clinically applicable the dissociation of morphine analgesia from its direct intestinal side effects, as has already been done successfully in animal models (12, 47, 89, 152).

GUT-SELECTIVE ANTIDIARRHEAL OPIOIDS   The potential of gut-located action sites for the production of clinically important opioid constipating effects is best illustrated by the recently developed antidiarrheal agents selective for the intestine. These agents, including diphenoxylate (157), loperamide (101, 102), and SC 27166 (83, 102), reportedly have little or no analgesic or euphoriant action at doses largely exceeding those required for constipation and have been extensively reviewed (3, 36, 157). Here we will only briefly mention just a few aspects of special interest and/or closer relevance to the present context.

The selectivity of newer antidiarrheal opioids for the gut is proposed as a significant advance in therapeutics compared to previously available related agents that might produce central side effects, like analgesia, if not acute poisoning (respiratory depression) or physical dependence on repeated use (3). Gut selectivity apparently does not involve different drug-opioid receptor interactions in the CNS and at local intestinal sites (84), but simply reflects the drug's virtual inability to reach the CNS (61).

Loperamide, the most selective antidiarrheal opioid currently available for clinical use (160), has been shown to have narcotic antagonist reversible constipating action in that it delays the transit of a test meal along the gastrointestinal tract of normal animals (137) and man (4), like the traditional remedy codeine (123). This is the principal aspect for discussion here, because it stands as unequivocal evidence of an important, exclusively local, antipropulsive opioid action. However, interest is growing in alternative interpretations of the mechanism whereby antidiarrheal opioids are therapeutically effective (122, 134).

Abnormalities of intestinal water and electrolyte transport besides motility alterations are recognized factors in the pathophysiology of diarrhea (122, 134). The classic view has been that inhibition of muscle propulsive activity by opioids holds back the intestinal content, allowing more efficient absorption (13). Data supporting direct stimulation of intestinal water and electrolyte absorption by opioids have recently attracted more attention (45, 67, 94, 95, 163). Representative data (67) and concern about smooth muscle paralysis as a potentially dangerous complication when using opioids to treat secretory diarrhea have even led researchers to envisage the development of synthetic opioids specific for epithelial ion transport (27). Yet recent clinical studies with loperamide indicate that it relieves diarrhea by influencing motor function rather than the rate of absorption by intestinal mucosal cells (135). Therefore, at the moment this is only a challenging area for future research that inter alia must be addressed in any case to clarify the relationship between intestinal motility, blood flow, and absorption of luminal content as affected by opioids (6, 29, 41, 79, 86, 109, 161).

ENDOGENOUS OPIOIDS AND GASTROINTESTINAL PROPULSION

Endogenous opioid peptides originally isolated from the CNS (65) are present throughout the gastrointestinal tracts of several animal species and man, as demonstrated by immunocytochemical and radioimmunological methods; for reviews see (104, 115, 129). Met-enkephalin and Leu-enkephalin immunoreactive-like material has been localized mainly in the neurons of the myenteric plexus (1, 114), but it has also been detected in the endocrine cells of the gut (1, 77). More recently, substances immunoreactive to dynorphin antibodies have been found in intestinal tissues (74, 164).

If the gut contains these opioid peptides plus their precursors (87) and putative inactivating enzymes (81), they should play a role in gastrointestinal physiology, inasmuch as specific intestinal receptors have already been identified (see above). Indeed, exogenously administered enkephalins and β-endorphin influence gastrointestinal motility and other gut functions and mimic the action of morphine-like drugs in several in vitro and in vivo conditions, as reviewed (68). These are pharmacological actions of endogenous opioid peptides. In the search for better evidence for their postulated natural function in the bowel: (a) the observed effects of pure opioid antagonists like naloxone may be tentatively attributed to the suppression of a physiological tonic action of endogenous opioid peptides; (b) biochemical events pertaining to endorphins (e.g. release) may be detected and monitored at the same time as functional recordings in order to assess the underlying relationship.

This dual approach has been followed to ascertain whether endogenous opioids are involved in the modulation of peristalsis. In guinea pig isolated ileal segments, Kromer & Pretzlaff (75) found that naloxone significantly increases the frequency of peristaltic waves and concluded that intestinal-borne opioids, whose release from myenteric plexus was reported (138), participate in the control of peristalsis. These authors with the same in vitro technique showed that periodicity rather than efficacy of peristaltic waves (76) may be under the control of an endogenous opioid mechanism located in the intestinal wall. By a different in vivo method, in the anesthetized guinea pig, Clark & Smith (30) demonstrated that blockade of opioid receptors by naloxone facilitates induction of the peristaltic reflex evoked by luminal infusion of saline. However, several investigators have shown that naloxone had no effect on intestinal propulsion when given intravenously (152), subcutaneously (12) or intraperitoneally (107) to conscious rats, intraperitoneally to conscious mice (137), and intravenously to anesthetized dogs (84). Thus, we still do not know whether peristalsis might be inhibited by endogenous opioids under more physiological experimental conditions.

As regards the upper GI tract, various findings suggest either involvement or no participation of endogenous opioids in the regulation of gastric emptying, depending on the species studied and the experimental conditions. Edin et al (42) found that the atropine-resistant contraction of the pyloric sphincter induced by vagal stimulation in the anesthetized cat is blocked by naloxone dose-dependently. Considering that local intra-arterial injection of enkephalins also elicits pyloric contraction and gastric relaxation, the authors proposed the existence of a vagal control of the pylorus and stomach mediated via enkephalinergic neurons in the cat. It has, in fact, been recently reported that in the same species pyloric contraction in response to duodenal acidification involves local neural pathways that may be mediated through an opioid peptide (128). Evidence for endogenous opioid involvement in digestive motility has also been obtained in ruminants. Maas (82) reported that intravenous injection of naltrexone and naloxone to conscious goats significantly increases the frequency of ruminal contractions, possibly by unmasking an inhibitory opioid system controlling forestomach motility. Identification of these mechanisms is important with a view to improving physiological functions or correcting pathological alterations in veterinary pharmacology with opioid antagonists (130, 131).

Other studies did not support a function of endorphins in the upper GI tract. For instance, Shea-Donohue et al (139) found that in conscious primates doses of naloxone sufficient to prevent the effects of exogenously administered opioid peptides on the stomach do not affect gastric emptying; these authors were thus led to assume that endogenous opioids play no major role in this connection. In humans, too, unequivocal evidence that endogenous opioids intervene as physiological mediators of the normal motricity of the GI tract is currently lacking. Feldman et al (46) found that intravenous infusion of naloxone to healthy subjects has no effect on the rate of gastric emptying of a liquid meal, even though gastric emptying is significantly reduced by morphine (46) or exogenously administered opioid peptides (146). Conversely, in recent experiments on healthy volunteers by different research groups, naloxone infusion was found to reduce antroduodenal contractile activity (127) and to inhibit the gastrocolonic response to eating (147).

Since specific receptors are present in the gastrointestinal tract along with their endogenous opioid ligands, their physiological function, whatever it is, should be primarily local. However, because of intestinal motor effects after direct intracranial application of opioid peptides (see above), and considering the good bioavailability of parenteral naloxone to the brain, its aforementioned effects might be interpreted as supporting an unidentified central endogenous opioid mechanism of gastrointestinal regulation. A related aspect is that of presumed peptidergic-mediated neural connections between gut and brain, supported by recent work in rats showing the modulation of central representation of gastric mechanoreceptor activity on application of opioid peptides or naloxone to the dorsal vagal nucleus (44).

If available information is still largely inadequate for assigning endogenous opioid peptides a definite physiological regulatory role in the enteric system, even less can be said of their involvement in gastrointestinal disease. Inhibition of ileal peristalsis in rats after laparotomy and cecum ablation was considered an experimental model representative of paralytic ileus in humans after intestinal surgery (64); naloxone did not reverse peristaltic inhibition, so no support was obtained for increased release of endorphins under surgical stress as a causative factor in decreased intestinal motility. Subcutaneous administration of the enkephalin analog FK 33824 to human volunteers inhibited relaxation of the lower esophageal sphincter (LES), this inhibition being abolished by naloxone, which, given alone, had no influence on normal LES function; it was speculated that nonetheless naloxone might improve acalasia as a possible endogenous opioid–mediated disorder (63). Concurrent elevations in plasma β-endorphin (immunoreactive-material) and norepinephrine in healthy volunteers submitted to cold pain and labyrinthine stimulation suggest that these substances may be involved in stress-induced gastroduodenal motor disturbances (142). On the basis of two case-histories, Kreek and colleagues reported chronic constipation in humans to benefit from naloxone treatment (73), which implies that this condition might be sustained by hyperactivity of the endogenous opiate system; interestingly enough, naloxone relieved constipation even when given orally, its negligible central bioavailability upon oral administration suggesting an exclusively local intestinal mode of action. Improvement in eight aged constipated subjects after four days of treatment with oral naloxone, but not with placebo, on a double-blind, random, crossover protocol, has now been preliminarily reported by the same group (72). In this connection, food-derived opioid-like peptides (exorphins) may be mentioned for their potential effects on bowel movements, as suggested by the finding that hydrolyzed gluten prolongs intestinal transit time in man, this action being antagonized by concomitant oral naloxone (99). Quite recently, low doses of intracerebroventricular naloxone inactive intravenously were seen to prevent the inhibitory effect of *Escherichia coli* endotoxin on forestomach and antro-duodenal motility in ewes, and it was therefore suggested that a central endogenous opioid mechanism might account for the intestinal troubles (40), but whether this merely depends on the reversal of cardiovascular shock by naloxone (62) has not been clarified.

ADDITIONAL ASPECTS AND CONCLUSIONS

The effects of opioids on gut motility are still incompletely understood. While highlighting current developments in this area, we intend as well to call attention to some aspects of the gastrointestinal pharmacology of opioids that seem worthy of further work.

The recent significant advance in therapeutic utility consisting of the availability of gut-selective antidiarrheal agents without undesirable central actions clearly indicates that this kind of work can be highly rewarding, in terms of practical application among other things. These synthetic antidiarrheals unequivocally attest that local intestinal opioid-specific mechanisms are largely sufficient for the production of important drug-induced motor effects in animals and man. The same local mechanisms have been classically advocated as the only ones accounting for morphine's constipating action (57), which, after the updated analysis presented in this review, can still be regarded as primarily if not exclusively peripheral. If the above holds for man, the undesirable constipation complicating morphine pain relief could be prevented by concurrent administration of a peripherally selective opioid antagonist, as already demonstrated in animal models (12, 47, 89, 152). This is reminiscent of the quite successful therapeutic combination of levodopa and a decarboxylase inhibitor unable to enter the CNS for treating Parkinson's disease, with lower incidence of peripheral side effects (25). Constipation as a troublesome complication of methadone maintenance in heroin addicts (37, 71) could possibly be managed by coadministration of suitable peripherally selective opioid antagonists, whose additional clinical potential might include replacement of naloxone for emergency reversal of delay in gastric emptying by narcotic analgesics during the induction of anesthesia (50, 103).

The pharmacological relevance of specific sites in the CNS inhibiting gut peristalsis, as evidenced by direct intracranial application of opioids, needs to be clarified. Narcotic analgesics such as etorphine that, unlike morphine (10), seem to be more readily available to the brain than to the gut (154), might act predominantly if not exclusively in the CNS to produce constipation (110). But information on distribution in intestinal tissues and CNS is scanty for most opioid drugs. Currently we are witnessing a boom in opioid receptor research, mostly in vitro, although the pharmacokinetic aspects of these agents appear to be somewhat neglected. Yet one of the most meaningful recent therapeutic examples of selectivity in opioid action, loperamide, is accounted for only pharmacokinetically, a factor that was fully considered in the sound in vivo pharmacological tests instrumental in developing this drug (157). Whether opioid receptor subtypes subserve any specific function affecting gut motility may well be ascertained in the light of future experiments.

The paucity of reports on in vivo studies on bowel function as affected by repeated administration of opioids [for representative work, see (22, 23, 26, 112, 117, 136, 154, 165, 167–169)] does not enable us to attempt an evaluation of the involvement of central and peripheral mechanisms in the development of intestinal tolerance and dependence.

Most of the arguments in favor of a role for endogenous opioids in gastrointestinal physiology are based on observations following either their administration or their presumed blockade by naloxone, with all the limitations of these approaches in studying gastrointestinal or other body systems (15). Better research tools—and we hope that newer, peripherally selective narcotic antagonists will provide some—are certainly needed for improving our knowledge of endogenous opioid function. However, this, like any other area of research, relies on critical attitudes of investigators as well as more sharply honed tools.

ACKNOWLEDGMENTS

We are grateful to Judy Baggott for style editing and to Monique Bibou for editorial assistance and for typing the manuscript.

Literature Cited

1. Alumets, J., Hakanson, R., Sundler, F., Chang, K. J. 1978. Leuenkephalin-like material in nerves and enterochromaffin cells in the gut. *Histochemistry* 56:187–96

2. American College of Physicians. 1983. Drug therapy for severe, chronic pain in terminal illness. *Ann. Int. Med.* 99:870–73

3. Awouters, F., Niemegeers, C. J. E., Janssen, P. A. J. 1983. Pharmacology of antidiarrheal drugs. *Ann. Rev. Pharmacol. Toxicol.* 23:279–301

4. Basilisco, G., Bozzani, A., Camboni, G., Recchia, M., Quatrini, M., et al. 1985. Effect of loperamide and naloxone on mouth-to-cecum transit time evaluated by lactulose hydrogen breath test. *Gut.* In press

5. Beckett, A. H., Casy, A. F. 1954. Synthetic analgesics: Stereochemical considerations. *J. Pharm. Pharmacol.* 6:986–99

6. Bennett, S., Shepherd, P., Simmonds, W. J. 1962. The effect of alterations in intestinal motility induced by morphine and atropine on fat absorption in the rat. *Austr. J. Exp. Biol.* 40:225–32

7. Bianchetti, A., Giudice, A., Ferrarese, N., Picerno, N., Moulineaux, C., et al. 1981. Selective effects of the opioid antagonist naloxone methylsulfate on the gastrointestinal motility of morphine-treated mice. *J. Pharmacol.* 13:96–97

8. Bianchetti, A., Giudice, A., Picerno, N., Carminati, P. 1982. Pharmacological actions of levallorphan allyl bromide (CM 32191), a new peripheral narcotic antagonist. *Life Sci.* 31:2261–64

9. Bianchetti, A., Nisato, D., Sacilotto, R., Dragonetti, M., Picerno, N., et al. 1983. Quaternary derivatives of narcotic antagonists: Stereochemical requirements at the chiral nitrogen for in vitro and in vivo activity. *Life Sci.* 33(Suppl. 1):415–18

10. Bianchi, G., Ferretti, P., Recchia, M., Rocchetti, M., Tavani, A., Manara, L. 1983. Morphine tissue levels and reduction of gastrointestinal transit in rats: Correlation supports primary action site in the gut. *Gastroenterology* 85:852–58

11. Bianchi, G., Fiocchi, R., Peracchia, F., Petrillo, P., Tavani, A., Manara, L. 1984. The peripheral narcotic antagonist N-allyl levallorphan-bromide (CM 32191) selectively prevents morphine antipropulsive action and buprenorphine in vivo binding in the rat intestine. *J. Pharm. Pharmacol.* 32:326–30

12. Bianchi, G., Fiocchi, R., Tavani, A., Manara, L. 1982. Quaternary narcotic antagonists' relative ability to prevent antinociception and gastrointestinal transit inhibition in morphine-treated rats as an index of peripheral selectivity. *Life Sci.* 30:1875–83

13. Binder, H. J. 1977. Pharmacology of laxatives. *Ann. Rev. Pharmacol. Toxicol.* 17:355–67

14. Blane, G. F., Boura, A. L. A., Fitzgerald, A. E., Lister, R. E. 1967. Actions of etorphine hydrochloride, (M99): A potent morphine-like agent. *Br. J. Pharmacol. Chemother.* 30:11–22

15. Bloom, F. E. 1983. The endorphins: A growing family of pharmacologically pertinent peptides. *Ann. Rev. Pharmacol. Toxicol.* 23:151–70

16. Bond, J. H., Levitt, M. D. 1975. Investigation of small bowel transit time in man utilising pulmonary hydrogen (H_2) measurement. *J. Lab. Clin. Med.* 85:546–55

17. Brogden, R. N., Speight, T. M., Avery, G. S. 1973. Pentazocine: A review of its pharmacological properties, therapeutic efficacy and dependence liability. *Drugs* 5:6–91

18. Brown, D. R., Robertson, M. J., Goldberg, L. I. 1983. Reversal of morphine-induced catalepsy in the rat by narcotic antagonists and their quaternary derivatives. *Neuropharmacology* 22:317–21

19. Bueno, L., Ruckebusch, Y. 1978. Origine centrale de l'action excitomotrice de l'intestin par la morphine. *C. R. Soc. Biol.* 172(5):972–77

20. Bullock, P., Spanner, S., Ansell, B. 1977. Distribution of morphine and morphine metabolites in rat brain. *Biochem. Soc. Trans.* 5:166–68

21. Burks, T. 1976. Gastrointestinal pharmacology. *Ann. Rev. Pharmacol. Toxicol.* 16:15–31

22. Burks, T. F., Castro, G. A., Weisbrodt, N. W. 1976. Tolerance to intestinal stimulatory actions of morphine. In *Opiates and Endogenous Opioid Peptides,* ed. H. W. Kosterlitz, pp. 369–76. Amsterdam: Elsevier. 456 pp.

23. Burks, T. F., Jaquette, D. L., Grubb, M. N. 1974. Development of tolerance to the stimulatory effect of morphine in dog intestine. *Eur. J. Pharmacol.* 25:302–7
24. Burleigh, D. E., Galligan, J. J., Burks, T. F. 1981. Subcutaneous morphine reduces intestinal propulsion in rats partly by a central action. *Eur. J. Pharmacol.* 75:283–87
25. Calne, D. B., Reid, J. L., Vakil, S. D., Rao, S., Petrie, A., et al. 1971. Idiopathic parkinsonism treated with an extracerebral decarboxylase inhibitor in combination with levodopa. *Br. Med. J.* 3:729–32
26. Chang, E. B., Brown, D. R., Field, M., Miller, R. J. 1984. An antiabsorptive basis for precipitated withdrawal diarrhea in morphine-dependent rats. *J. Pharmacol. Exp. Ther.* 228:364–69
27. Chang, E. B., Field, M. 1983. Intestinal electrolyte transport and diarrheal disease. In *The Gastroentorology Annual*, ed. F. Kern Jr., A. L. Blum, pp. 148–80. Amsterdam/New York/Oxford: Elsevier. 481 pp.
28. Chirubasik, J. 1984. Epidural, on-demand, low-dose morphine infusion for postoperative pain. *Lancet* 1:107–8
29. Chou, C. C. 1982. Relationship between intestinal blood flow and motility. *Ann. Rev. Physiol.* 44:29–42
30. Clark, S. J., Smith, T. W. 1981. Modulation of the peristaltic reflex in vivo by endogenous opioids. *Br. J. Pharmacol.* 74:953P–54P
31. Cowan, A., Doxey, J. C., Metcalf, G. 1976. A comparison of pharmacological effects produced by leucine-enkephalin, methionine-enkephalin, morphine and ketocyclazocine. See Ref. 22, pp. 95–102
32. Cowan, A., Gmerek, D. E. 1982. In vivo studies with ICI 154,129, a putative delta receptor antagonist. *Life Sci.* 31:2213–16
33. Creese, I., Snyder, S. H. 1975. Receptor binding and pharmacological activity of opiates in the guinea pig intestine. *J. Pharmacol. Exp. Ther.* 194:205–19
34. Dahlström, B. E., Paalzow, L. K. 1975. Pharmacokinetics of morphine in plasma and discrete areas of the rat brain. *J. Pharmacokinet. Biopharm.* 3:293–302
35. Daniel, E. E. 1968. Pharmacology of the gastrointestinal tract. In *Handbook of Physiology, Alimentary Canal*, Sec. 6, ed. C. F. Code. 4:2267–324. Washington: Am. Physiol. Soc. 758 pp.
36. Daniel, E. E. 1982. Pharmacology of adrenergic, cholinergic, and drugs acting on other receptors in gastrointestinal muscle. In *Handbook of Experimental Pharmacology, Mediators and Drugs in Gastrointestinal Motility II*, ed. G. Bertaccini, 59/II:249–322. Berlin/Heidelberg/New York: Springer-Verlag. 386 pp.
37. Dobbs, W. H. 1971. Methadone treatment of heroin addicts: Early results provide more questions than answers. *J. Am. Med. Assoc.* 218:1536–41
38. Dragonetti, M., Bianchetti, A., Sacilotto, R., Giudice, A., Ferrarese, N., et al. 1983. Levallorphan methyl iodide (SR 58002), a potent narcotic antagonist with peripheral selectivity superior to that of other quaternary compounds. *Life Sci.* 33(Suppl. 1):477–80
39. Duggan, A. W., North, R. A. 1984. Electrophysiology of opioids. *Pharmacol. Rev.* 35:220–81
40. Duranton, A., Buéno, L. 1984. Central opiate mechanism involved in gastrointestinal motor disturbances induced by E. coli endotoxin in sheep. *Life Sci.* 34:1795–99
41. Eckenhoff, J. E., Oech, S. R. 1960. The effects of narcotics and antagonists upon respiration and circulation in man. A review. *Clin. Pharmacol. Ther.* 1:483–524
42. Edin, R., Lundberg, L., Terenius, L., Dahlström, A., Hökfelt, T., Kewenter, J., Ahlman, H. 1980. Evidence for vagal enkephalinergic neural control of the feline pylorus and stomach. *Gastroenterology* 78:492–97
43. Deleted in proof
44. Ewart, W. R., Wingate, D. L. 1983. Central representation and opioid modulation of gastric mechanoreceptor activity in the rat. *Am. J. Physiol.* 244:G27–32
45. Farack, U. M., Loeschke, K. 1984. Inhibition by loperamide of deoxycholic acid induced intestinal secretion. *Naunyn-Schmiedebergs Arch. Pharmakol.* 325:286–89
46. Feldman, M., Walsh, J. H., Taylor, I. L. 1980. Effect of naloxone and morphine on gastric acid secretion and on serum gastrin and pancreatic polypeptide concentrations in humans. *Gastroenterology* 79:294–98
47. Ferretti, P., Bianchi, G., Tavani, A., Manara, L. 1981. Inhibition of gastrointestinal transit and antinociceptive effects of morphine and FK 33-824 in rats are differently prevented by naloxone and by its N-methyl quaternary analog. *Res. Commun. Subst. Abuse* 2:1–11
48. Fiocchi, R., Bianchi, G., Petrillo, P., Tavani, A., Manara, L. 1982. Morphine inhibits gastrointestinal transit in the rat primarily by impairing propulsive activ-

ity of the small intestine. *Life Sci.* 31:2221–23

49. Foster, R. S., Jenden, D. J., Lomax, P. 1967. A comparison of the pharmacologic effects of morphine and N-methyl morphine. *J. Pharmacol. Exp. Ther.* 157:185–95

50. Frame, W. T., Alison, R. H., Moir, D. D., Nimmo, W. S. 1984. Effect of naloxone on gastric emptying during labour. *Br. J. Anaesth.* 56:263–66

51. Galligan, J. J., Burks, T. F. 1982. Inhibition of gastric and intestinal motility by centrally and peripherally administered morphine. *Proc. W. Pharmacol. Soc.* 25:307–11

52. Galligan, J. J., Burks, T. F. 1982. Opioid peptides inhibit intestinal transit in the rat by a central mechanism. *Eur. J. Pharmacol.* 85:61–68

53. Galligan, J. J., Burks, T. F. 1983. Centrally mediated inhibition of small intestinal transit and motility by morphine in the rat. *J. Pharmacol. Exp. Ther.* 226:356–61

54. Gambino, M. C., Petrillo, P., Tavani, A. 1983. Agonist and antagonist properties of some benzomorphans on nociceptive reaction and intestinal transit in rats. *Life Sci.* 33(Suppl. 1):461–64

55. Gmerek, D. E., Cowan, A., Woods, J. H. 1983. Distinct peripheral and central sites for morphine-induced inhibition of gastrointestinal transit in rats. *Pharmacologist* 25:208 (Abstr.)

56. Goldstein, A., Lowney, L. I., Pal, B. K. 1971. Stereospecific and nonspecific interactions of the morphine congener levorphanol in subcellular fractions of mouse brain. *Proc. Natl. Acad. Sci. USA* 68:1742–47

57. Goodman, L. S., Gilman, A. 1955. Natural and synthetic narcotics. In *The Pharmacological Basis of Therapeutics,* ed. A. Goodman, L. Goodman, pp. 216–80. New York: Macmillan. 1831 pp. 2nd ed

58. Green, A. F. 1959. Comparative effects of analgesics on pain threshold, respiratory frequency and gastrointestinal propulsion. *Br. J. Pharmacol.* 14:26–34

59. Heel, R. C., Brogden, R. N., Speight, T. M., Avery, G. S. 1978. Butorphanol: A review of its pharmacological properties and therapeutic efficacy. *Drugs* 16:473–505

60. Heel, R. C., Brogden, R. N., Speight, T. M., Avery, G. S. 1979. Buprenorphine: A review of its pharmacological properties and therapeutic efficacy. *Drugs* 17:81–110

61. Heykants, J., Michiels, M., Knaeps, A.,

Brugmans, J. 1974. Loperamide (R 18 553), a novel type of antidiarrheal agent. Part 5: The pharmacokinetics of loperamide in rats and man. *Arzneim. Forsch.* 24:1649–53

62. Holaday, J. W. 1983. Cardiovascular effects of endogenous opiate systems. *Ann. Rev. Pharmacol. Toxicol.* 23:541–94

63. Howard, J. M., Belsheim, M. R., Sullivan, S. N. 1982. Enkephalin inhibits relaxation of the lower oesophageal sphincter. *Br. Med. J.* 285:1605–6

64. Howd, R. A., Adamovics, A., Palekar, A. 1978. Naloxone and intestinal motility. *Experentia* 34:1310–11

65. Hughes, J., ed. 1983. Opioid peptides. *Br. Med. Bull.,* Vol. 39. New York: Churchill Livingstone. 106 pp.

66. Jaffe, J. H., Martin, W. R. 1980. Opioid analgesics and antagonists. In *The Pharmacological Basis of Therapeutics,* ed. A. Goodman, L. Goodman, A. Gilman, pp. 494–534. New York: Mcmillan. 1843 pp. 6th ed.

67. Kachur, J. F., Miller, R. J., Field, M. 1980. Control of guinea pig intestinal electrolyte secretion by a δ-opiate receptor. *Proc. Natl. Acad. Sci. USA* 77:2753–56

68. Konturek, S. J. 1980. Opiates and the gastrointestinal tract. *Am. J. Gastroenterol.* 74:285–91

69. Kosterlitz, H. W., Leslie, F. M., Waterfield, A. A. 1975. Rates of onset and offset of action of narcotic analgesics in isolated preparations. *Eur. J. Pharmacol.* 32:10–16

70. Kosterlitz, H. W., Watt, A. J. 1968. Kinetic parameters of narcotic agonists and antagonists, with particular reference to N-allylnoroxy-morphone (naloxone). *Br. J. Pharmacol. Chemother.* 33:266–76

71. Kreek, M. J. 1973. Medical safety and side effects of methadone in tolerant individuals. *J. Am. Med. Assoc.* 223:665–68

72. Kreek, M. J., Paris, P., Bartol, M. A., Mueller, D. 1984. Effects of short term oral administration of the specific opioid antagonist naloxone on fecal evacuation in geriatric patients. *Gastroenterology* 86:1144 (Abstr.)

73. Kreek, M. J., Shaefer, R. A., Elliot, F. H., Fishman, J. 1983. Naloxone, a specific opioid antagonist, reverses chronic idiopathic constipation. *Lancet* 1:261–62

74. Kromer, W., Höllt, V., Schmidt, H., Herz, A. 1981. Release of immunoreactive-dynorphin from the isolated guinea pig small intestine is reduced during

peristaltic activity. *Neurosci. Lett.* 25: 53–56

75. Kromer, W., Pretzlaff, W. 1979. In vitro evidence for the participation of intestinal opioids in the control of peristalsis in the guinea pig small intestine. *Naunyn-Schmiedebergs Arch. Pharmakol.* 309: 153–57

76. Kromer, W., Pretzlaff, W., Woinoff, R. 1980. Opioids modulate periodicity rather than efficacy of peristaltic waves in the guinea pig ileum in vitro. *Life Sci.* 26:1857–65

77. Larsson, L. I., Stengaard-Pedersen, K. 1981. Enkephalin endorphin-related peptides in antropyloric gastrin cells. *J. Histochem. Cytochem.* 29:1088–98

78. LeBars, D., Besson, J. M. 1981. The spinal site of action of morphine in pain relief: From basic research to clinical applications. *Trends Pharmacol. Sci.* 2: 323–25

79. Lee, J. 1983. Relationship between intestinal motility, tone, water absorption and lymph flow in the rat. *J. Physiol.* 345:489–99

80. Lewis, J. R. 1980. Evaluation of new analgesics: Butorphanol and nalbuphine. *J. Am. Med. Assoc.* 243:1465–67

81. Llorens, C., Schwartz, J. C. 1981. Enkephalinase activity in rat peripheral organs. *Eur. J. Pharmacol.* 69:113–16

82. Maas, C. L. 1982. Opiate antagonists stimulate ruminal motility of conscious goats. *Eur. J. Pharmacol.* 77:71–74

83. Mackerer, C. R., Brougham, L. R., East, P. F., Bloss, J. L., Dajani, E. Z., Clay, G. A. 1977. Antidiarrheal and central nervous system activities of SC-27166 (2 - [3 - 5 - methyl - 1,3,4 - oxadizol - 2 - yl)-3,3 - diaphenylpropyl] - 2 - azabicyclo-[2.2.2] octane), a new antidiarrheal agent, resulting from binding to opiate receptor sites of brain and myenteric plexus. *J. Pharmacol. Exp. Ther.* 203: 527–38

84. Mackerer, C. R., Clay, G. A., Dajani, E. Z. 1976. Loperamide binding to opiate receptor sites of brain and myenteric plexus. *J. Pharmacol. Exp. Ther.* 199:131–40

85. Maguire, L. C., Yon, J. L., Miller, E. 1981. Prevention of narcotic-induced constipation. *N. Engl. J. Med.* 305:1651

86. Mailman, D. 1980. Effects of morphine on canine intestinal absorption and blood flow. *Br. J. Pharmacol.* 68:617–24

87. Makhlouf, G. M. 1983. Hormones and neuropeptides of the gut. See Ref. 27, pp. 181–97

88. Manara, L., Aldinio, C., Cerletti, C., Coccia, P., Luini, A., Serra, G. 1978. In vivo tissue levels and subcellular distribution of opiates with reference to pharmacological action. In *Factors Affecting the Action of Narcotics*, ed. M. L. Adler, L. Manara, R. Samanin, pp. 271–96. New York: Raven. 744 pp.

89. Manara, L., Bianchi, G., Ferretti, P., Monferini, E., Strada, D., Tavani, A. 1980. Local and CNS-mediated effects of morphine and narcotic antagonists on gastrointestinal propulsion in rats. In *Endogenous and Exogenous Opiate Agonists and Antagonists*, ed. E. L. Way, pp. 143–46. New York: Pergamon. 570 pp.

90. Manara, L., Bianchi, G., Fiocchi, R., Notarnicola, A., Peracchia, F., Tavani, A. 1982. Inhibition of gastrointestinal transit by morphine and FK 33-824 in the rat and comparative narcotic antagonist properties of naloxone and its N-methyl quaternary analog. *Life Sci.* 31:1271–74

91. Margolin, S. 1954. Decreased gastrointestinal propulsive activity after intracranial morphine. *Fed. Proc.* 13:383–84

92. Margolin, S. 1963. Centrally mediated inhibition of gastrointestinal propulsive motility by morphine over a non-neural pathway. *Proc. Soc. Exp. Biol. Med.* 112:311–15

93. Martin, W. R. 1984. Pharmacology of opioids. *Pharmacol. Rev.* 35:283–323

94. McKay, J. S., Linaker, B. D., Higgs, N. B., Turnberg, L. A. 1982. Studies of the antisecretory activity of morphine in rabbit ileum in vitro. *Gastroenterology* 82:243–47

95. McKay, J. S., Linaker, B. D., Turnberg, L. A. 1981. Influence of opiates on ion transport across rabbit ileal mucosa. *Gastroenterology* 80:279–84

96. Miller, M. S., Galligan, J. J., Burks, T. F. 1981. Accurate measurement of intestinal transit in the rat. *J. Pharmacol. Methods* 6:211–17

97. Miller, R. R., Jick, H. 1978. Clinical effects of meperidine in hospitalized medical patients. *J. Clin. Pharmacol.* 18:180–89

98. Monferini, E., Strada, D., Manara, L. 1981. Evidence for opiate receptor binding in rat small intestine. *Life Sci.* 29:595–602

99. Morley, J. E., Levine, A. S., Yamada, T., Gebhard, R. L., Frigge, W. F., et al. 1983. Effect of exorphins on gastrointestinal function, hormonal release and appetite. *Gastroenterology* 84:1517–23

100. Niemegeers, C., Lenaerts, F., Awouters, F. 1976. Preclinical animal studies of modern antidiarrheals: In vivo pharmacology. See Ref. 157, pp. 65–114

101. Niemegeers, C. J. E., Lenaerts, F. M.,

Janssen, P. A. J. 1974. Loperamide (R 18 553) a novel type of antidiarrheal agent. Part 2: In vivo parenteral pharmacology and acute toxicity in mice. Comparison with morphine, codeine and diphenoxylate. *Arzneim. Forsch.* 24: 1636–41

102. Niemegeers, C. J. E., McGuire, J. L., Heykants, J. J. P., Janssen, P. A. J. 1979. Dissociation between opiate-like and antidiarrheal activities of antidiarrheal drugs. *J. Pharmacol. Exp. Ther.* 210:327–33

103. Nimmo, W. S., Heading, R. C., Wilson, J., Prescott, L. F. 1979. Reversal of narcotic-induced delay in gastric emptying and paracetamol absorption by naloxone. *Br. Med. J.* 2:1189

104. North, R. A., Egan, T. M. 1983. Actions and distributions of opioid peptides in peripheral tissues. *Br. Med. Bull.* 39:71–75

105. Oka, T. 1981. Enkephalin (opiate) receptors in the intestine. *Trends Pharmacol. Sci.* 2:328–30

106. Ouyang, A., Clain, C. J., Snape, W. J. Jr., Cohen, S. 1982. Characterization of opiate-mediated responses of the feline ileum and ileocecal sphincter. *J. Clin. Inv.* 69:507–15

107. Parolaro, D., Sala, M., Gori, E. 1977. Effect of intracerebroventricular administration of morphine upon intestinal motility in rat and its antagonism with naloxone. *Eur. J. Pharmacol.* 46:329–38

108. Paton, W. D. M. 1957. The action of morphine and related substances on contraction and on acetylcholine output of coaxially stimulated guinea pig ileum. *Br. J. Pharmacol.* 11:119–27

109. Pawlik W. W., Walus, K. M., Fondacaro, J. D. 1980. Effects of methionine-enkephalin on intestinal circulation and oxygen consumption. *Proc. Soc. Exp. Biol. Med.* 165:26–31

110. Peracchia, F., Bianchi, G., Fiocchi, R., Petrillo, P., Tavani, A., Manara, L. 1984. Central and peripheral inhibition of gastrointestinal transit in rats: Narcotics differ substantially by acting at either or both levels. *J. Pharm. Pharmacol.* 36: 699–701

111. Pert, C. B., Snyder, S. H. 1973. Opiate receptor: Demonstration in nervous tissue. *Science* 179:1011–14

112. Petersen, D. W., Fujimoto, J. M. 1983. Differential tolerance to the intestinal inhibitory effect of opiates in mice. *Eur. J. Pharmacol.* 95:225–30

113. Plekss, O. J., Margolin, S. 1968. Further evidence for an unique neurohumoral agent released from brain by morphine

given intracerebrally. *Proc. Soc. Exp. Biol. Med.* 128:317–21

114. Polak, J. M., Sullivan, S. N., Bloom, S. R., Facer, P., Pearse, A. G. E. 1977. Enkephalin-like immunoreactivity in the human gastrointestinal tract. *Lancet* 1:972–74

115. Polak, J. M., Sullivan, S. N., Buchan, A. M. J., Bloom, S. R., Facer, P., et al. 1978. Endorphins. In *Gut Hormones,* ed. S. R. Bloom, pp. 501–6. Edinburgh: Churchill Livingstone. 650 pp.

116. Porreca, F., Burks, T. F. 1983. The spinal cord as a site of opioids effects on gastrointestinal transit in the mouse. *J. Pharmacol. Exp. Ther.* 227:22–27

117. Porreca, F., Cowan, A., Raffa, R. B., Tallarida, R. J. 1982. On the criteria for classifying opiate agonists in rats. *J. Pharm. Pharmacol.* 34:525–26

118. Porreca, F., Cowan, A., Raffa, R. B., Tallarida, R. J. 1983. Ketazocines and morphine: Effects on gastrointestinal transit after central and peripheral administration. *Life Sci.* 32:1785–90

119. Porreca, F., Cowan, A., Tallarida, R. J. 1981. Time course of antagonism of morphine antinociception intracerebroventricularly administered naloxone in the rat. *Eur. J. Pharmacol.* 76:55–59

120. Porreca, F., Filla, A., Burks, T. F. 1983. Studies in vivo with dynorphin-(1-9): Analgesia but not gastrointestinal effects following intrathecal administration to mice. *Eur. J. Pharmacol.* 91:291–94

121. Porreca, F., Filla, A., Burks, T. F. 1983. Spinal cord-mediated opiate effects on gastrointestinal transit in mice. *Eur. J. Pharmacol.* 86:135–36

122. Powell, W. 1981. Muscle or mucosa: The site of action of antidiarrheal opiates? *Gastroenterology* 80:406–7

123. Pressman, J., Hofmann, A. F., Witztum, K. F., Gertler, S., Steinbach, J. H., Dharmsathaphorn, K. 1984. Use of ^{14}C-lactulose breath test to show that codeine, but not clonidine, slows small intestinal transit in man. *Gastroenterology* 86:1213 (Abstr.)

124. Raffa, R. B., Porreca, F., Cowan, A., Tallarida, R. J. 1982. Morphine-receptor dissociation constant and the stimulus-effect relation for inhibition of gastrointestinal transit in the rat. *Eur. J. Pharmacol.* 79:11–16

125. Ramabadran, K. 1982. Effects of N-methylnaloxone and N-methylnaltrexone on nociception and precipitated abstinence in mice. *Life Sci.* 33:1253–56

126. Rattan, S., Goyal, R. K. 1983. Identification and localization of opioid receptors in the opossum lower esophageal

sphincter. *J. Pharmacol. Exp. Ther.* 224:391–97

127. Rees, W. D. W., Sharpe, G. R., Christofides, N. D., Bloom, S. R., Turnberg, L. A. 1983. The effects of an opiate agonist and antagonist on the human upper gastrointestinal tract. *Eur. J. Clin. Invest.* 13:221–25

128. Reynolds, J. C., Ouyang, A., Cohen, S. 1984. Evidence for an opiate-mediated pyloric sphincter reflex. *Am. J. Physiol.* 246:G130–36

129. Rozé, C., Dubrasquet, M. 1983. Endorphines, enképhalines et tube digestif. *Gastroenterol. Clin. Biol.* 7:177–88

130. Ruckebusch, Y. 1983. Pharmacology of reticulo-ruminal motor function. *J. Vet. Pharmacol. Ther.* 6:245–72

131. Ruckebusch, Y., Bueno, L. 1983. La naloxone: Pharmacologie et intérêt thérapeutique. *Revue Méd. Vét.* 134:77–82

132. Russel, J., Bass, P., Goldberg, L. I., Schuster, C. R., Merz, H. 1982. Antagonism of gut, but not central effects of morphine with quaternary narcotic antagonists. *Eur. J. Pharmacol.* 78:255–61

133. Sala, M., Parolaro, D., Crema, G., Spazzi, L., Giagnoni, G., et al. 1983. Involvement of periaqueductal gray matter in intestinal effect of centrally administered morphine. *Eur. J. Pharmacol.* 91:251–54

134. Schiller, L. R., Davis, G. R., Santa Ana, C. A., Morawski, S. G., Fordtran, J. S. 1982. Studies of the mechanism of the antidiarrheal effect of codeine. *J. Clin. Invest.* 70:999–1008

135. Schiller, L. R., Santa Ana, C. A., Morawski, S. G., Fordtran, J. S. 1984. Mechanism of the antidiarrheal effect of loperamide. *Gastroenterology* 86:1475–80

136. Schrier, W. A., Burks, T. F. 1980. Site of morphine withdrawal diarrhea in the rat. *Fed. Proc.* 39:301 (Abstr.)

137. Schulz, R., Wüster, M., Herz, A. 1979. Centrally and peripherally mediated inhibition of intestinal motility by opioids. *Naunyn-Schmiedebergs Arch. Pharmakol.* 308:255–60

138. Schulz, R., Wüster, M., Simantov, R., Snyder, S., Herz, A. 1977. Electrically stimulated release of opiate-like material from the myenteric plexus of the guinea pig ileum. *Eur. J. Pharmacol.* 41:347–48

139. Shea-Donohue, P. T., Adams, N., Arnold, J., Dubois, A. 1983. Effects of met-enkephalin and naloxone on gastric emptying and secretion in rhesus monkeys. *Am. J. Physiol.* 245:G196-200

140. Simon. E. J., Hiller, J. M. 1984. Multiple opioid receptors. In *Opioid Past, Present and Future*, ed. J. Hughes, H. O. J. Collier, M. J. Rance, M. B. Tyers, pp. 33–52. London: Taylor & Francis. 352 pp.

141. Simon, E. J., Hiller, J. M., Edelman, I. 1973. Stereospecific binding of the potent narcotic analgesic ³H-etorphine to rat brain homogenate. *Proc. Natl. Acad. Sci. USA* 70:1947–49

142. Stanghellini, V., Malagelada, J. R., Zinsmeister, A. R., Go, V. L. W., Kao, P. C. 1983. Stress-induced gastroduodenal motor disturbances in humans: Possible humoral mechanisms. *Gastroenterology* 85:83–91

143. Stewart, J. J. 1982. Neostigmine antagonism of morphine's effects on intestinal transit. *J. Pharm. Pharmacol.* 34:405–7

144. Stewart, J. J., Weisbrodt, N. W., Burks, T. F. 1977. Centrally mediated intestinal stimulation by morphine. *J. Pharmacol. Exp. Ther.* 202:174–81

145. Stewart, J. J., Weisbrodt, N. W., Burks, T. F. 1978. Central and peripheral actions of morphine on intestinal transit. *J. Pharmacol. Exp. Ther.* 205:547–55

146. Sullivan, S. N., Lamki, L., Corcoran, P. 1981. Inhibition of gastric emptying by enkephalin analogue. *Lancet* 2:86–87

147. Sun, E. A., Snape, W. J. Jr., Cohen, S., Renny, A. 1982. The role of opiate receptors and cholinergic neurons in the gastrocolonic response. *Gastroenterology* 82:689–93

148. Takemori, A. E., Kupferberg, H. J., Miller, J. W. 1969. Quantitative studies of the antagonism of morphine by nalorphine and naloxone. *J. Pharmacol. Exp. Ther.* 169:39–45

149. Tallarida, R. J., Cowan, A., Adler, M. W. 1979. pA₂ and receptor differentiation: A statistical analysis of competitive antagonism. *Life Sci.* 25:637–54

150. Tallarida, R., J., Jacob, L. 1979. *The Dose-Response Relation in Pharmacology,* 3:49–84. New York: Springer-Verlag. 207 pp.

151. Tavani, A., Bianchi, G., Ferretti, P., Manara, L. 1980. Morphine is most effective on gastrointestinal propulsion in rats by intraperitoneal route: Evidence for local action. *Life Sci.* 27:2211–17

152. Tavani, A., Bianchi, G., Manara, L. 1979. Morphine no longer blocks gastrointestinal transit but retains antinociceptive action in diallylnormorphine-pretreated rats. *Eur. J. Pharmacol.* 59:151–54

153. Tavani, A., Gambino, M. C., Petrillo, P. 1984. The opioid k-selective compound

U-50,488H does not inhibit intestinal propulsion in rats. *J. Pharm. Pharmacol.* 36:343–44

154. Tavani, A., Luini, A., Manara, L. 1979. Time course of etorphine levels in tissues of opiate tolerant and nontolerant rats. *J. Pharmacol. Exp. Ther.* 211:140–44

155. Terenius, L. 1972. Specific uptake of narcotic analgesics by subcellular fractions of the guinea pig ileum. *Acta Pharmacol. Toxicol.* 31(Suppl. 1):50

156. Terenius, L. 1973. Stereospecific interaction between narcotic analgesics and a synaptic plasma membrane fraction of rat cerebral cortex. *Acta Pharmacol. Toxicol.* 32:317–20

157. Van Bever, W., Lal, H., eds. 1976. *Synthetic Antidiarrheal Drugs: Synthesis-Preclinical and Clinical Pharmacology.* New York/Basel: Dekker. 284 pp.

158. Vaught, J. L., Cowan, A., Jacoby, H. I. 1983. In vivo differentiation between mu, delta and kappa opioid receptors. *Pharmacologist* 25:261 (Abstr.)

159. Vaught, J. L., Cowan, A., Gmerek, D. E. 1983. A species difference in the slowing effect of intrathecal morphine on gastrointestinal transit. *Eur. J. Pharmacol.* 94:181–84

160. Verhaegen, H., De Cree, J., Schuermans, V. 1974. Loperamide (R 18 553), a novel type of antidiarrheal agent. Part 7: Clinical investigation. Efficacy and safety of loperamide in patients with severe chronic diarrhea. *Arzneim. Forsch.* 24:1657–60

161. Walus, K. M., Jacobson, E. D. 1981. Relation between small intestinal motility and circulation. *Am. J. Physiol.* 241:G1–15

162. Ward, S. J., Takemori, A. E. 1983. Relative involvement of receptor subtypes of opioid-induced inhibition of gastroin-

testinal transit in mice. *J. Pharmacol. Exp. Ther.* 224:359–63

163. Warhust, G., Smith, G., Tonge, A., Turnberg, L. 1983. Effects of morphine on net water absorption, mucosal adenylate cyclase activity and PGE$_2$ metabolism in rat intestine. *Eur. J. Pharmacol.* 86:77–82

164. Watson, S. J., Akil, H., Ghazarossian, V. E., Goldstein, A. 1981. Dynorphin immunocytochemical localization in brain and peripheral nervous system: Preliminary studies. *Proc. Natl. Acad. Sci. USA* 78:1260–63

165. Wei, E. T. 1981. Enkephalin analogs and physical dependence. *J. Pharmacol. Exp. Ther.* 216:12–18

166. Weinstock, M. 1971. Sites of action of narcotic analgesic drugs-peripheral tissues. In *Narcotic Drugs: Biochemical Pharamcology,* ed. D. H. Clouet, pp. 394–407. New York: Plenum. 506 pp.

167. Weisbrodt, N. W., Badial-Aceves, F., Dudrick, S. J., Burks, T. F., Castro, G. A. 1977. Tolerance to the effect of morphine on intestinal transit. *Proc. Soc. Exp. Biol. Med.* 154:587–90

168. Weisbrodt, N. W., Thor, P. J., Copeland, E. M., Burks, T. F. 1980. Tolerance to the effects of morphine on intestinal motility of unanesthetized dogs. *J. Pharmacol. Exp. Ther.* 215:515–21

169. Wong, C. L., Roberts, M. B., Wai, M. K. 1980. Effect of morphine and naloxone on intestinal transit in mice. *Eur. J. Pharmacol.* 64:289–95

170. Yaksh, T. L., Rudy, T. A. 1976. Analgesia mediated by a direct spinal action of narcotics. *Science* 192:1357–58

171. Zenz, M., Schappler-Scheele, B., Neuhaus, R., Piepenbrock, S., Hilfrich, J. 1981. Long-term peridural morphine analgesia in cancer pain. *Lancet* 1:91

Ann. Rev. Pharmacol. Toxicol. 1985. 25:275–305

DRUG-EXERCISE INTERACTIONS

David T. Lowenthal

Likoff Cardiovascular Institute, Hahnemann University, Philadelphia, Pennsylvania 19102

Zebulon V. Kendrick

Biokinetics Laboratory, College of Health, Physical Education, Recreation, and Dance, Temple University, Philadelphia, Pennsylvania 19122

INTRODUCTION

The bulk of the studies performed to investigate the effects of drugs on exercise and of exercise on drug biotransformation have dealt with the antihypertensive class of medications. However, complicating the understanding of drug-exercise interactions are the confounding contributions of caffeine, salicylates, anabolic steroids, and alcohol consumed as ergogenic aids in normals and those with cardiovascular diseases. In patients with hypertensive and other forms of cardiovascular disease who exercise or who are undergoing cardiac rehabilitation, it is beneficial to allow activity without the adverse effects of extreme increases in pulse rate, blood pressure, catecholamines, and potassium. As a result, laboratories are seeking drugs that will allow a patient to exercise while keeping this expected rise in exercise parameters modest, protecting an oftentimes compromised and vulnerable myocardium.

In general, all the drugs consumed by patients with cardiovascular disease, with the exception of β–adrenergic blocking agents, permit a normal exercise response. This normal response acutely is an increase in systolic and no change or fall in diastolic blood pressure and an increase in heart rate, stroke index, and cardiac index. Following a conditioning program, the various regulatory responses result in the appropriate increases during physical activity but at a lower level.

The majority of the studies reported have investigated the effects of drugs

275

0362-1642/85/415-0275$02.00

during acute episodes of exercise. The literature contains short-term chronic studies but they are scant in number. Within the context of this paper, we will show some evidence for the long-term effect on patients receiving propranolol and performing dynamic physical activity, citing the training capability even when on a β–adrenergic blocking agent. Thus, when the majority of anti-hypertensives, calcium–channel blocking drugs, digitalis preparations, anti-arrhythmic agents, and nitrates are prescribed, there is no embarrassment to the acute response during stress testing or beyond the initial exercise period, wherein training effects would be blunted.

Review material will be presented that relates the biochemical and physio-logic responses to exercise in people taking ergogenic acids. The paper will also attempt to elucidate the effects of drugs on the hemodynamic and/or biochemical responses during stress testing and where possible refer to the long-term effects of training under the influence of such drugs taken for cardiovascular disease.

DRUGS USED IN CARDIOVASCULAR DISEASES AND THE EFFECT OF EXERCISE

Diuretics

The hemodynamics of diuretic effect have been studied by Lund-Johansen (1), who found that not all diuretics have similar actions during exercise. Thiazides bring about a drop in exercise blood pressure via a decrease in peripheral resistance and plasma volume. Thiazide-like diuretics, specifically chlorthali-done 100 mg daily, were shown to reduce blood pressure during exercise by decreasing cardiac output. However, at dosages of 200 mg per day, there was a paradoxical increase in diastolic blood pressure and heart rate (2), probably a reflection of marked volume contraction. Long-term thiazide dosing does not cause a drop in cardiac output. Although studies involving drug effects on exercise have included patients with heart failure who are taking furosemide, no studies dealing with this drug's direct effects on exercise parameters have been carried out. Additionally, as with any diuretic therapy, hypokalemia can become significant, resulting in moderate ST segment depression, cardiac irritability, and skeletal muscle fatigue.

During vigorous exercise serum potassium increases. The source is skeletal muscle. This can occur in the setting of diuretic-induced hypokalemia, and the response indicates that total body potassium is not depleted (3). However, to insure against potassium loss, patients on diuretics should receive potassium supplements.

Thus, diuretics result in a moderate decrease in the blood pressure response to exercise, and, with adequate potassium supplementation, should not invoke any drug-related risks during physical activity.

Central α Agonists

Many studies dealing with the central α-agonist antihypertensives have been recently performed. Both clonidine and α-methyldopa (methyldopa) decrease central and/or peripheral outflow of catecholamines. This results in reductions of plasma norepinephrine at rest and during exercise (4, 5). Although both of these drugs can blunt the sympathetic response during exercise, they have significantly different hemodynamic effects.

During bicycle ergometry in mild hypertensives, methyldopa may decrease the blood pressure and heart rate response (6). Total peripheral resistance and cardiac output may (7) or may not (8) decrease. On the contrary, work in our laboratory with normals taking methyldopa in multiple doses for one week demonstrated no decrease in heart rate at rest or at peak exercise, yet systolic pressure was reduced at these times after one week of treatment (9). Differences between this and clonidine's response may result from the peripheral effects of the false neurotransmitters of methyldopa.

Clonidine differs from methyldopa in that, in addition to reducing blood pressure and heart rate during exercise, it decreases both resting blood pressure and pulse rate (10, 11). The decrease in heart rate through central vagal stimulation results in a drop in cardiac output (12). This, however, is not considered a negative inotropic property, since after chronic use cardiac output is normalized.

In several studies (5, 9, 11), the exercise-associated changes seen in serum potassium, renin, and aldosterone have been observed in normal volunteers following single and multiple doses of clonidine and methyldopa. Increases in potassium during dynamic exercise in subjects taking clonidine or methyldopa were parallel to the response on placebo. With both α agonists, plasma renin concentration was suppressed at rest and the expected increase was blunted during exercise at maximum dosages. Plasma aldosterone apparently had no significant differences in value with the drugs when compared to placebo, increasing during exercise in all groups. No significant ST-T changes have been shown to occur during exercise using these drugs. The rise in diastolic blood pressure (DBP) induced by isometric activity, i.e. 50% handgrip, may be decreased with methyldopa or clonidine, especially if the resting DBP is reduced. However, the mean change is not different from rest to peak handgrip during placebo and with multiple doses of these drugs (Figures 1, 2; Tables 1, 2).

β Blockers

The hemodynamic changes during exercise have been intensively studied in association with β-blockade. Response mechanisms as they relate to isometric and dynamic activity lead to a reduction in cardiac output without any peripheral vascular effects. A reduction in myocardial contractility and heart rate are the

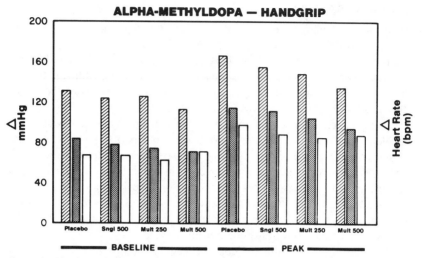

Figure 1 50% handgrip systolic and diastolic blood pressure and heart rate response under the influence of placebo, methyldopa 500 mg, methyldopa 250 mg bid for one week, and 500 mg bid for one week. Patients were studied at rest and at peak levels of activity. The change from baseline to peak is no different from placebo through maxiumum dosage. Resting diastolic pressure is apparent with the chronic dosing regimen and thus peak response is blunted.

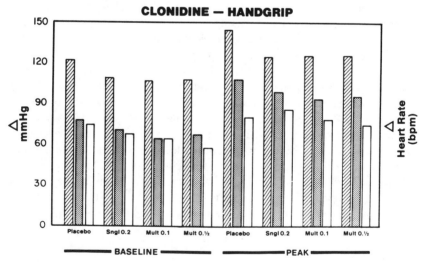

Figure 2 50% handgrip systolic and diastolic blood pressure and heart rate response under the influence of placebo, clonidine 0.2 mg single, 0.1 mg bid, and 0.1 mg AM and 0.2 mg PM each times one week. Patients were studied at rest and at peak levels of activity. The change from baseline to peak is no different from placebo through maximum dosage. Resting diastolic pressure is apparent with the chronic dosing regimen and thus peak response is blunted.

Table 1   Antihypertensives that do not blunt cardiovascular response during dynamic physical activity (bicycle ergometer or treadmill)

Clonidine
Diuretics
Guanabenz
Methyldopa
Nifedipine
Prazosin
Verapamil

Table 2   Antihypertensives that obtund the diastolic pressor response to static exercise (handgrip 50%)

Atenolol
Clonidine
Methyldopa
Prazosin
Propranolol

basis for these alterations. Both bring about a longer diastolic phase that allows for better coronary perfusion. This observation lends itself best to patients with coronary artery disease who undergo cardiac rehabilitation. Many of these subjects have increased dynamic exercise duration, less angina, and fewer incidents of ST depression (13). Indeed, it has been shown that up to a 31% improvement in exercise capacity as a direct result of training can occur in patients with ischemic heart disease on propranolol (14). It has been postulated that since cardiac output is reduced to a greater extent than is blood pressure, peripheral resistance must increase (15, 16). This results from the fact that α receptors are not blocked and can give rise to vasoconstriction with catecholamine release during exercise (15). However, this increased vascular resistance is thought to be obtunded by chronic β-blockade, leading to lower blood pressure (17, 18).

It has been demonstrated that in patients with ischemic heart disease receiving β–adrenergic blocking drugs (BABD), a training effect can be observed even though there is an obtundation of the normal cardiovascular response. This implies an increase in the duration of activity over a period of time as well as an increase in the workload being performed. Studies in our laboratory (19) have confirmed this data and have extended them into a consideration of whether the elderly are capable of achieving a similar training effect on and off the β–adrenergic blocking drugs. The data in Tables 3 and 4 show that

Table 3 Relationship between age and dynamic training[a]

	≤ 54 years		> 54 years	
	Pre-training	Post-training	Pre-training	Post-training
Total exercise duration (min)	11 ± 3	15 ± 4[b]	8 ± 2	13 ± 2[b]
Exercise workload (kpm)	678 ± 295	1163 ± 393[b]	386 ± 222	713 ± 179[b]

[a] Values are mean ± SD
[b] p ≤ .001

Table 4 Relationship between β-adrenergic blocking drugs (BABD) and dynamic training[a]

	On BABD		No BABD	
	Pre-training	Post-training	Pre-training	Post-training
Total exercise duration (min)	9 ± 3	14 ± 4[b]	10 ± 3	14 ± 3[b]
Exercise workload (kpm)	474 ± 279	933 ± 337[b]	592 ± 313	1020 ± 375[b]

[a] Values are mean ± SD
[b] p ≤ .001

regardless of age, i.e. greater or less than age 54, and regardless of β-blocker regimen, patients can have a training response. The factors of age and BABD considered independently demonstrated significant increases in the pre- and post-training values of exercise duration and workload. Training in this particular study totaled eight weeks, three times per week, 45 minutes per session, using treadmill, bicycle ergometer, arm ergometry, rowing machine, steps, wall pulleys, and light weights.

In regard to isometric and isotonic physical activity, propranolol and the cardioselective β-blockers atenolol and metroprolol have been studied in normal volunteers against placebo (5, 9, 20, 21). In a study comparing propranolol, metoprolol, and placebo in a graded treadmill exercise, it was shown that both heart rate and systolic blood pressure are reduced at maximum exercise (20). There were no significant changes in diastolic blood pressure, oxygen consumption, or anaerobic threshold (that point at which oxygen consumption fails to increase in proportion to minute ventilation) (20). According to Sklar et al (20), this indicates blood flow to the active muscles is unaltered.

Pharmacodynamically there may be some small differences between cardioselective and nonselective β–adrenergic blocking drugs (22). Following nine months' administration of chronic atenolol, metoprolol, pindolol, and sustained-release propranolol, researchers found that atenolol and metoprolol reduced exercise-induced increases in systolic blood pressure significantly whereas pindolol and propranolol did not. Cardioselective β blockers therefore appear to be more effective than nonselective agents in blunting the increase in systolic blood pressure with dynamic physical activity. On the other hand, there is marked interindividual variability of β blocking effects on heart rate and blood pressure during exercise (23). Normal volunteers given parenteral metroprolol or placebo in intraindividual cross-over design using bicycle ergometry showed comparable plasma levels of metoprolol after each intravenous dose, but the extended inhibition of exercise-induced tachycardia or increase in systolic blood pressure varied considerably among the subjects (23). There was never any correlation between the extended inhibition of heart rate and systolic blood pressure increase during exercise on β blockade. The extent of a β-blocking effect on these parameters is an individual constant in acute as well as in chronic conditions.

Studies in our laboratory (21) dealing with isometric exercises in which normal volunteers are dosed with atenolol and propranolol indicated that both resting and peak exercise diastolic blood pressures are reduced at maximum dosages when compared to placebo. This is due to a reduction in rest DBP and the ensuing lower pressor response to handgrip. The mean change from rest to peak is no different with placebo or with single or multiple doses of the drugs (Figures 3, 4). Although disputed by investigations indicating the failure of antihypertensives to attenuate blood pressure rises during isometric exercise (7, 10), the data (21) imply that persons with cardiovascular disease receiving antihypertensive therapy may be at decreased risk for pressor response when performing arm labor.

Similar results have been discovered in research with hypertensive patients on β-blocking drugs (4). In these subjects, both metoprolol and propranolol reduced heart rate and systolic blood pressure at rest and at peak exercise over placebo controls. Concurrently, similar decreases in heart rate and diastolic blood pressure at rest and at peak activity were seen when the patients used a 30% hand grip exercise. However, it was shown that in patients with borderline hypertensive heart failure as defined by radiologic criteria, i.e. cardiac enlargement, M-mode echocardiography, and ECG findings, metoprolol, with and without prazosin vasodilatory treatment, does not safely abolish dangerous increases in blood pressure during isometric activity (24–27).

The studies on the metabolic effects of β blockade during exercise have produced a number of provocative results. Propranolol in single and multiple doses has been reported to cause an increase in serum potassium significantly greater than placebo during dynamic exercise. However, it has more recently

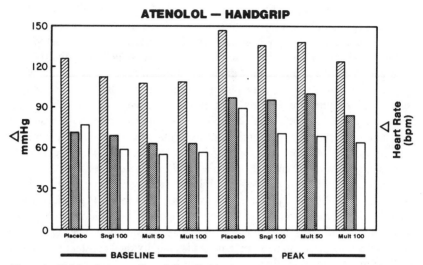

Figure 3   50% handgrip systolic and diastolic blood pressure and heart rate response under the influence of placebo, atenolol 100 mg single, 50 mg bid for one week, and 100 mg bid for one week. Patients were studied at rest and at peak levels of activity. The change from baseline to peak is no different from placebo through maximum dosage. Resting diastolic pressure is apparent with the chronic dosing regimen and thus peak response is blunted.

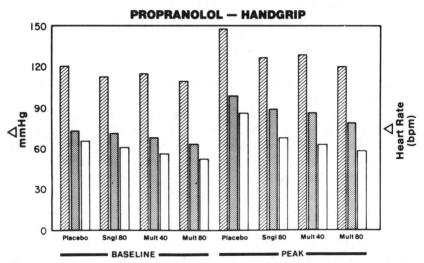

Figure 4   50% handgrip systolic and diastolic blood pressure and heart rate response under the influence of placebo, propranolol 80 mg single, 40 mg bid for one week, and 80 mg bid for one week. Patients were studied at rest and at peak levels of activity. The change from baseline to peak is no different from placebo through maxiumum dosage. Resting diastolic and pressure is apparent with the chronic dosing regimen and thus peak response is blunted.

been shown that this hyperkalemic effect may occur only upon initial treatment with the drug (5). In addition, Lowenthal et al (5) revealed that β blockade results in significantly decreased levels of renin at rest and at peak exercise. Despite this, when compared to placebo, no changes in plasma aldosterone values have been seen, most likely because of a lag time in the suppression of the renin-aldosterone axis or because of too low a dosage of propranolol (40 mg bid for one week). Unlike the central α agonists, propranolol and metoprolol either increase plasma norepinephrine (28) or give rise to expected normal increases in plasma values (5, 29) during physical activity. The latter observation has been attributed to the hypothesis that during light exercise vagal withdrawal occurs yet sympathetic activity does not increase until the heart rate rises beyond 30 beats per minute (30).

In order to determine the origin of β-receptor antagonist-induced exercise fatigue seen in normal, active individuals (in contrast to drug-induced exercise longevity in cardiac patients), Lundborg (29) undertook a study to examine specific metabolic effects of β blockade. After the disruption of neuromuscular transmission and decreased blood flow to working muscles were ruled out as causes of subject fatigue, investigators targeted exercise substrate limitation, i.e. glucose and nonesterified fatty acid availability. In fact, blood glucose, nonesterfied fatty acid, and glycerol levels were found to be significantly reduced during bicycle activity on propranolol and metoprolol. This was followed by more rapid rises in glucagon levels on the drugs and most likely results from decreased muscle glycogenolysis, a β–adrenoreceptor mediated process.

Conflicting metabolic studies involving β blockade during exercise include the finding that neither propranolol nor metoprolol decreases the ventilatory response to CO_2 during physical activity (30). This would be significant for the management of COPD patients, in whom these drugs will not worsen CO_2 retention at rest or during exercise. On the contrary, following 80 mg of propranolol given in single oral dosage to normal volunteers, the response to submaximal and maximal bicycle ergometry revealed a reduction in oxygen consumption at both submaximal and maximal efforts (31). These changes were not related to any difference in muscle fiber type distribution (32–34). It has been suggested that individuals with muscles made up of high proportions of slow twitch fibers and possessing a great capillary supply were most impeded by β-adrenergic blockade.

Similar results have been obtained at submaximal workloads of 50% and 70% wherein ventilation (VE), CO_2 (VCO_2), and O_2 uptake (VO_2) were measured. Propranolol effected an early reduction in all of these parameters at 50% and 70% maximum by five minutes (35). Ventilation was greater at five minutes owing to an increase in venous lactate, and the initial reductions in VO_2 and VCO_2 were related to reduction in cardiac output and muscle perfusion induced by the propranolol. Since anaerobic metabolism is increased early during heavy exercise, the increase in ventilation could be explained on this basis. These results could not necessarily be extrapolated to individuals with impaired cardiac function (35).

Finally, another unrelated investigation pointed out that plasma levels of both propranolol and acebutolol increase significantly during exercise; this occurrence is possibly related to pH changes during physical activity (36) or possibly attributable to the decrease in hepatic blood flow during activity that would affect those drugs with a high hepatic-extraction ratio.

Vasodilators

The vasodilators, used adjunctively with other drugs in the treatment of hypertension, include hydralazine, minoxidil, and prazosin (more of an atypical α antagonist than a direct-acting vasodilator) for which a number of exercise-related investigations have been performed.

In normal volunteers, hydralazine acts to decrease arterial pressure with a resultant reflex tachycardia. This tends to increase cardiac output through an increase in sympathetic drive, which in a compromised heart may lead to myocardial ischemia, e.g. angina and/or infarction, in cardiac patients (37). However, the drug is useful as an afterload reducer in chronic heart failure (38). Prazosin, an atypical α blocker, similarly has been shown to decrease mean arterial blood pressure and total peripheral resistance at rest and at dynamic workloads (39). In contrast to hydralazine, during arm-cycle ergometry using single and multiple prazosin doses, there is no reflex increase in heart rate or pressor response greater than that seen when compared to placebo (40). During isometric activity, hydralazine neither improves skeletal muscle oxygen delivery during exercise in patients with heart failure (41) nor adequately attenuates isometric-induced increases in sympathetic activity (24, 42).

Prazosin therapy results in reduction in both baseline and peak exercise values of diastolic and systolic blood pressure during 50% hand-grip activity at single and multiple doses (42). Since upper-extremity activity confers a greater heart rate-blood pressure product than the type of work seen with lower extremity activity, the blood-pressure response to prazosin during graded arm ergometry exercise reveals that prazosin does significantly lower systolic blood pressure at rest and at peak exercise; however, no change in heart rate has been observed. There is a fall in diastolic blood pressure, as would be anticipated with any form of dynamic physical activity. This data is based on studies in normal volunteers and may not necessarily be extrapolated to draw conclusions of safety in patients with ischemic heart disease and/or heart failure.

As a result of the increasing use of vasodilators in cardiac patient management, a great deal of interest in the effects of these drugs during exercise of heart-failure subjects has arisen. While increasing cardiac output with reduction in afterload, hydralazine reduces both arterial and pulmonary wedge pressure and increases stroke volume at rest and to a lesser degree during bicycle exercise in patients with chronic heart failure (38). The reduced effect during physical activity is thought to reflect initial impaired pump function and may also give rise to the observation of unimproved exercise tolerance despite improved hemodynamic parameters with oral hydralazine. In addition, hydralazine does not increase compromised blood flow to peripheral musculature during hand-grip activity in patients with heart failure, indicating that its vasodilatory effect does not add to that of local metabolic effects (41), the significance of which may also limit improvement in exercise tolerance of these individuals treated with the drug. Prazosin has been tested in patients with borderline hypertensive heart failure (25), giving rise to the observation that the drug similarly improves hemodynamics (cardiac output) and obtunds the increases in diastolic blood pressure associated with isometric activity. Minoxidil, a most potent direct vasodilator, may improve exercise tolerance in patients with chronic heart failure due to its afterload-reducing properties.

Angiotensin–Converting Enzyme Inhibitors

Captopril is an angiotensin–converting enzyme inhibitor. Data on its effects on dynamic exercise vary among investigators. Although Pickering and coworkers (43) found no changes in blood pressure or heart rate during graded treadmill activity, other studies indicate a significant reduction in systolic and diastolic blood pressure during bicycle exercise (44), seen to be even more pronounced during physical activity than at rest (45). Similar decreases in blood pressure with dynamic activity have been seen with saralasin, an angiotensin II partial antagonist (46). The reduction in angiotensin II with captopril and saralasin, coupled with an unaltered blood-pressure response to exercise, indicates that angiotensin II is not a major determinant of blood-pressure regulation during exercise in hypertensive patients.

Manhem and colleagues (44) investigated the metabolic effects of captopril during dynamic exercise, measuring the drug's effect on catecholamines, renin activity, angiotensin II levels, and plasma aldosterone. After 4–5 days of high-dose captopril, both angiotensin II and plasma-aldosterone levels were reduced significantly at rest and during physical activity. Plasma-renin activity underwent increases over placebo at baseline and peak exercise, while concentration of norepinephrine and epinephrine remained unchanged.

Calcium Antagonists

The calcium antagonists verapamil and nifedipine have differing clinical usages, the former as an antiarrhythmic agent particularly in paroxysmal atrial tachycardia, the latter in treatment of angina and in post-MI and CABG management to prevent further ischemia and augment collateral myocardial flow (47). However, both drugs are equally effective as antianginal agents and useful in post-MI and CABG management. The understanding of their effects on physical activity is important in terms of rehabilitating cardiac patients while on these drugs.

In normal, active volunteers, both nifedipine and verapamil have little effect on resting and treadmill or on systolic and diastolic blood pressure, although verapamil appears to have a slight obtunding effect on diastolic blood pressure increases during isometric exercise (48). In patients with chronic angina, however, studies have shown consistent improvement in patients on both verapamil (49) and nifedipine (50). The reductions in exercise-induced angina and ST-depression seen in these patients is thought to be due to a reduction in myocardial oxygen demand, and this is associated with a decrease in afterload with both drugs (50, 51). An enhancement of left ventricular diastolic filling seen with verapamil may also explain some of the beneficial effects with its usage in the angina syndrome. Although serum potassium levels were seen to rise in isometric activity with placebo in a recent study (48), no significant variance from this increase could be seen in either isometric or dynamic activity with these calcium antagonists. Thus, verapamil and nifedipine may be used during training programs with cardiac patients without risk of dangerous increases in blood pressure or serum potassium when compared to placebo.

Nitrates

In normal men, nitrates, represented by nitroglycerine and isosorbide dinitrate, have a number of hemodynamic effects, most attributable to their venodilatory actions. These include reduced mean arterial pressure, decreased cardiac filling and increased heart rate (52). During dynamic activity, these parameters balance out to produce an unchanged cardiac output as determined by exercise radionuclide angiography (53). More important, however, are changes resulting from the drug in patients with coronary artery disease and/or heart failure. It is well known that nitroglycerine is effective in controlling angina pectoris, and it follows that it also increases exercise duration limited by chest pain in most patients. These actions are thought to result from a decrease in preload that gives rise to a reduction in left ventricular end-diastolic pressure (LVEDP) (53). An earlier theory involving the redistribution of blood flow to ischemic myocardium is apparently less valid (54).

The long-acting nitrate isosorbide dinitrate is similar in its effects on exercise. In patients with congestive heart failure these changes are not seen during initial treatment, but improvement in cardiac output, oxygen consumption, and exercise duration occur after three months of treatment when compared to placebo (55). This is thought to be due possibly to a time-related enhancing of peripheral utilization of oxygen by the drug. Isosorbide dinitrate does not improve vasodilation in exercising muscle of patients with congestive heart failure in short-term drug administration (41). With individual dosages of isosorbide dinitrate and compared to placebo, the mean exercise time of patients with angina due to coronary heart disease increases 54% at one hour following drug dosing, 36% at three hours, and 13% at five hours (56).

The acute administration of 20–50 mg of isosorbide dinitrate to 21 patients with the angina syndrome resulted in a significant reduction in resting systolic pressure from a half hour to five hours after drug dosing. It also produced a marked increase in heart rate within the same time frame after drug dosing. These changes were significant when compared to placebo. Other studies have demonstrated an increase in net exercise time of at least 25% at one hour after isosorbide dinitrate dosing, with similar results at three hours and at five hours (57). These results have been reproduced by others wherein an enhanced exercise tolerance has been demonstrated in patients with angina receiving large doses of oral isosorbide dinitrate. In patients undergoing exercise, nitrates will not bring about any worsening in ST-segment changes during physical activity (56). In fact, reduced ECG evidence of myocardial ischemia after exercise has been observed in patients with angina after they have received large doses of isosorbide dinitrate (58).

Digitalis

A great deal of research involving digitalis and exercise has been performed. In normal volunteers, digitalis causes a reduction in heart rate and cardiac output with no change in blood pressure (50). It has also been shown to produce ST-segment depression during exercise in persons with normal coronary vessels (13). In patients with congestive heart failure, digitalization brings about a reduction in ventricle size and oxygen consumption at baseline (60) and decreases left ventricular end diastolic pressure during exercise (61). Unfortunately, however, no changes in exercise tolerance have been noted in these patients (62). Arrhythmias associated with the drug can be provoked by exercise, especially with concurrent diuretic-induced potassium depletion (63). As a result, patients who take digitalis should be monitored carefully in any training program with regard to electrolyte values as well as for ectopy.

Antiarrhythmics

Studies by Gey and co-workers (64, 65) have shown that procainamide and quinidine exhibit no change in heart rate or oxygen uptake during dynamic exercise, yet a slight drop in systolic blood pressure may be observed. Exercise-induced arrhythmias were seen to decrease in number and to be of less severity in most patients in the study. Others have pointed out that both procainamide and quinidine can mask exercise-induced ST-segment depression-producing false negative stress tests (66, 67). Thus, in patients with demonstratable ectopy during physical activity not corrected by overdrive suppression, these drugs may be used effectively to reduce the risk of exercise-induced arrhythmias.

Conclusion

The graded treadmill or cycle ergometry exercise must be interpreted in the context of the drug regimen the patient is following. An appreciation of the hemodynamic and/or biochemical changes induced by drugs is critical for a logical critique of the performance of the patient during exercise and for the projected exercise prescription that the patient is being asked to follow. Drug therapy is clearly not a contraindication to acute or chronic exercise as long as the principles of basic exercise physiology in the unmedicated can be translated and understood in the medicated patient.

ERGOGENIC AIDS TO PERFORMANCE

In spite of physicians' efforts to provide rational and individualized therapy for patients and despite warnings to healthy participants in sports, the consumption of caffeine, salicylates, nonsteroidal antiinflammatory drugs (used to decrease colonic motility in runners), alcohol, anabolic steroids, and amphetamines to improve performance is rampant.

The following will amplify on the salient effects of a number of these drugs and their interaction during exercise.

Caffeine

Caffeine has long been considered an ergogenic aid and/or doping agent (68) that can elicit physiological changes to enhance work or athletic performance (69, 70, 72, 73). However, the ergogenic effects of caffeine and related methylxanthine compounds are often unclear and equivocal. The lack of a well-defined understanding of caffeine's influence on work or athletic performance enhancement may be due to caffeine-induced physiological responses that are influenced by dose (74, 75), differ between habitual and nonhabitual users (75–79), and elicit both direct and indirect effects.

EFFECTS ON THE CENTRAL NERVOUS SYSTEM   Caffeine and related methylxanthines have been documented to exert a stimulating action on the central nervous system (80, 81) because of the ability of these compounds to pass the blood-brain barrier (82). Caffeine increases locomotor activity (81), increases spontaneously firing units in the sensorimotor cortex (80), and may act directly on the medullary vasomotor and vagal centers (83).

Caffeine has been demonstrated to decrease the perception of drowsiness while increasing the perception of alertness (76) and possibly to reduce the perception of fatigue during prolonged work (69, 71, 77). The exact mechanisms responsible for the decreased perception of fatigue during prolonged work after caffeine ingestion are unclear but possibly occur by reducing neuronal thresholds (84), by influencing central catecholamine receptors, and/ or by a direct effect on the adrenal medulla (85).

Caffeine may exert its influence in part as an antagonist to adenosine receptors in the brain (86). Adenosine has depressant, anticonvulsant, and hypnotic properties in the central nervous system. Adenosine antagonism occurs at lower caffeine concentrations than are needed for peripheral actions (87). This observation suggests that caffeine increases arousal and thereby decreases the perception of fatigue by its antagonistic effect on adenosine receptors. Potentiation of adenosine-elicited inhibition in the central nervous system may occur through norepinephrine, which rises with caffeine administration, suggesting that caffeine alters some of the neural actions of this transmitter. Certainly, considerable research remains to elucidate the mechanism(s) of caffeine on the reduced perceptors of fatigue by the central nervous system during prolonged work.

EFFECTS ON SKELETAL MUSCLE   Caffeine and related methylxanthines may potentiate the con'ractile activity of skeletal muscle by the following mechanism(s): (a) facilitation of neurotransmitter release and impulse transmission; (b) potentiation of twitch responses in both rested and fatigued muscle.

Caffeine and related methylxanthines have been reported to have an effect on neuromuscular impulse transmission (88). The enhancement of neuromuscular impulse transmission may be due to a prejunctional action via increased acetylcholine release (89). Expanding the work by Waldeck (84) to the myoneural junction, the possibility exists that caffeine increases neuronal excitability by reducing neuronal threshold.

Caffeine will rapidly distribute to skeletal muscle mass whether administered in vivo (90) or in vitro (91), and the physiological response to caffeine is proportional to its concentration (74). Enhanced in vitro muscle tension production has been observed when caffeine is added to normal Ringer's solution (92). Caffeine has been shown to induce shortening of the muscle resting length (91); the degree of shortening may be due in part to fiber types (91, 93). In these studies, high doses of caffeine result in "contractures" and loss of ability to respond to electrical stimulation with a twitch. Researchers have proposed that changes in muscle length are mediated by calcium release and independent of electrical activity at the sarcolemma (94). The phenomenon known as *escalation* (95) is related to caffeine-induced local release of calcium from the sarcoplasmic reticulum that in turn induces further release along the sarcoplasmic reticulum. However, this calcium release is not enough to induce a full twitch. Caffeine's ability to induce a release of calcium suggests that caffeine may enhance muscle contraction, thereby reducing the state of fatigue in working muscle. Caffeine's enhancement of contractile state during times of muscle fatigue is suggested to be due in part to an increase in calcium permeability of the sarcolemma (96) and/or vesicles (97), a more rapid calcium release (98), and/or a decrease in calcium uptake (99) by the sarcoplasmic reticulum, and in part to an increase in cyclic AMP levels by the inhibition of phosphodiesterase (100) or mediated by all the forecited proposed mechanisms (101). Metabolically, the accumulation of glucose-6-phosphate may enhance contractility (102). The increase of glucose-6-phosphate is due to caffeine's stimulation of glycogenolysis (81, 103).

SUBSTRATE MOBILIZATION AND UTILIZATION   Fuel availability, in particular muscle glycogen, is related to exhaustion during prolonged exercise in which glycogen is significantly degraded (104–106). Caffeine may exert a pronounced influence on substrate mobilization and utilization during prolonged work by stimulating adipocyte lipolysis (69, 77, 107) via the activation of lipase (108); by altering glucose homeostasis, inducing a hyperglycemic action (81); by activation of liver phosphorylase (109); and/or by affecting muscle triglyceride utilization (110–112) and fatty acid availability. Caffeine is proposed to alter these substrates via inhibition of phosphodiesterase, which alters the concentration of cyclic AMP (100) and/or increases plasma catecholamine levels (75, 85, 113).

The stimulation by caffeine of adipocyte lipolysis (via lipase) may be due to either direct inhibition of phosphodiesterase (114, 115), which increases the activity of cyclic AMP, or by an indirect effect of increased catecholamine. Catecholamines may activate adenyl cyclase, thereby increasing cyclic AMP activity (116). The indirect effect of catecholamine stimulation is probably the primary mechanism, since phosphodiesterase inhibition requires caffeine levels several-fold greater than levels required to stimulate catecholamine-induced lipolysis (69, 77, 107, 117). Exercise stress itself increases circulating catecholamines (116), which in the presence of caffeine should markedly stimulate lipolysis (115).

The profile and the time course of plasma free fatty–acid elevation are altered by caffeine dose (71, 75, 77, 118). However, the increased mobilization of adipose free–fatty acids would make more free fatty acids available to working muscle. Free fatty acid uptake by muscle increases with the duration of exercise and free fatty acid oxidation progressively increases with time (119, 120). Increased oxidation of free fatty acids for the same intensity of work would in turn suppress glycogen degradation, thereby "sparing" glycogen (69, 71, 120). The sparing of muscle glycogen would be due in part to the high rates of fatty acid oxidation, which may inhibit the activities of phosphofructokinase and pyruvate dehydrogenase reactions (121–123).

The increased turnover of free fatty acids in man cannot account for all of the fat oxidized during prolonged work (112, 124, 125). Therefore, local triglyceride stores must be oxidized in working muscle (126). Caffeine influences muscle triglyceride utilization (77, 127). In his study, Crass estimated that endogenous triglyceride utilization increased by about 60% during 30 minutes of exercise. Theophylline, a methylxanthine, has also been demonstrated to stimulate endogenous utilization of triglycerides (110).

CAFFEINE AND EXERCISE PERFORMANCE   Caffeine has been demonstrated to significantly improve work production in trained cyclists and cross-country skiers (71, 128). It is interesting to note that in the cycling study (71) perception of the intensity of the activity remained unchanged from the control conditions, even though oxygen consumption increased with the additional work. Another study from the same laboratory demonstrated that caffeine administration prolongs the time to voluntary exhaustion by about 12% when working at 80% of maximum oxygen consumption (69). In this study, the perceived exertion was lower with caffeine administration. These findings are supported by earlier investigations in which caffeine was reported to increase an individual's work output on a bicycle ergometer work time to exhaustion (73, 129). Enhancement of work performance only occurs during prolonged cycling ergometry work and not during short-term work episodes (129) (Table 5).

Caffeine administration has no apparent influence on work performance of short-duration exercise (129). Speed enhancement for a 100-yard swim was found to be unaffected by caffeine administration (130). Likewise, caffeine has been shown to have no effect on short-duration tasks such as work capacity on the Balke walking treadmill test (131), short-term cycling to exhaustion (132), and running to exhaustion on a treadmill (133). In cardiac patients, caffeine administration has resulted in no effect on isometric grip and cardiovascular parameters during a stress test (134).

Salicylates

Salicylates and similar nonnarcotic analgesic and antiinflammatory agents are often used by athletes, athletic trainers and team physicians for a variety of musculoskeletal disorders. The availability and the numerous therapeutic applications of salicylates and other nonnarcotic analgesic compounds make them one of the most commonly used groups of agents worldwide. Aspirin, the best known nonnarcotic analgesic, is commonly used therapeutically by athletes for its potent analgesic and antiinflammatory properties.

Table 5 Selected caffeine and exercise interactions

Amount of caffeine	Time after ingestion	Subjects	Exercise	Results	Reference
250 mg	90 min.	Untrained	100-yd. swim	No time difference	130
200 mg	?	Untrained	Balke test	No difference	131
390 mg	30 min.	Cardiac patients	3 min. isometric grip	No difference in dysrrhythmias	134
			25 min. arm and leg cycling	No difference in heart rate and blood pressure	134
330 mg	60 min.	Trained cyclist	80% VO_2 max. cycling to exhaustion	Increased work time, FFA, 19.5% glycerol, lipid oxidation. Decreased RQ. No difference. VO_2 max., HR, lactate, glucose	69
5 mg/kg	60 min.	Volunteers	70% VO_2 max. cycling	Increased FFA, 18% increase in TG utilization. Decreased glycogen utilization by 42%. No difference in caloric expenditure.	77
4 mg/kg	60 min.	Trained cross-country skiers	7 mile race; 3 mile race	Decreased time of race at high altitude. Decrease time for 7 mile race at low altitude.	128
250 mg twice	60 min.	Trained cyclist	Variable cycling for 2 hours	Increase total work by 7.4%, and VO_2 max. by 7.3%. Increased FFA by 31%. Increased total fat oxidation.	71

Intolerance to aspirin has been well documented. Commonly cited toxic manifestations include angioedema and rhinitis and bronchial asthma and gastrointestinal complications (135, 136). The severity of these disturbances may be age-dependent (137, 138). Disturbances of acid-base balance and respiratory alkalosis resulting from altered respiratory stimulation have been reported (125, 136, 139). Aspirin intoxication may result in a pronounced pyrogenic effect, which may be due to an uncoupling of oxidative phosphorylation, resulting in paradoxical hyperthermia (140–145).

Exercise increases the metabolic rate and thereby heat production. In hot environments, the physiological responses to exercise are dependent on the intensity of the exercise, the ambient temperature, and the humidity (146, 147). Exercise and aspirin (heat producers) and hot environments (diminish passive avenues of heat dissipation) may result in an increased susceptibility to heat injury.

Paradoxical Hyperthermia

Salicylates have been demonstrated to increase total energy and heat production in healthy resting canines (141, 148), rodents (138, 149), and man (140, 145). In the study by Wood & Reichert (148), heat production in canines increased by about 40% following salicylate administration. This increased heat production, coupled with increased oxygen consumption, has been observed by others (141). Locus of the increased energy production has been thought to be of skeletal muscle origin.

Paradoxical hyperthermia is of clinical importance since severe hyperthermia results when the rate of heat production exceeds the capacity of heat-dissipating mechanisms (150). An increase in total heat production is not the sole cause of hyperpyrexia, however. Severe hyperpyrexia cannot develop unless the normal heat-regulating mechanisms are impaired (151, 152). Passive means of heat loss are attenuated when blood is shunted to the skin (153, 154) to equilibrate the heat-production and heat-dissipation mechanisms. If the ambient temperature is greater than skin temperature, heat cannot be lost through convection and radiation, necessitating the activation of the sweating mechanism for evaporative heat loss (155). Salicylate's direct action of inducing sweating at rest may enhance heat loss, thereby maintaining a constant body temperature. However, during long-duration exercise the efficiency of sweating is important in thermoregulation. Inefficient sweating in hot environments may lead to dehydration and electrolyte and acid-base disturbances (156–158). We have demonstrated 62% and 69% increases in salicylate-induced sensitivity to sweating during exercise bouts for two hours at 25° C and 35° C respectively (150). These findings suggest that sweating occurs at lower rectal temperatures. In a case study (160), researchers suggested that therapeutic doses of aspirin may have resulted in severe heat disturbances during a 100-mile race.

Profuse sweating occurred and symptoms of heat illness, such as chills and loss of thirst, were observed.

In exercise studies where salicylates were administered, varying results have been observed (159, 161). In the study by Troup, oxygen consumption was significantly increased after salicylate administration during the neutral ambient environment. The subjects in this study exercised approximately four times longer than in the two aforementioned studies. Although Downey & Darling (162) did not find a difference in exercise oxygen consumption and rectal temperature, they did report an increase in rectal temperatures during recovery after salicylate administration.

Alcohol

Recently there has been a furor over the supposedly salutary effects of beer consumption for electrolyte replacement during long-distance races, especially marathons (42 km). In long-distance races, runners depend on free fatty acids and triglycerides for energy utilization during the exercise (see caffeine section above) (163–166). Alcohol will raise the levels of circulating fatty acids but will also inhibit the oxidation of this substrate (167, 168). Metabolizing the ethanol-oxidation system accounts for 20%–30% of alcohol metabolism without generating any energy source (167). Alcohol plus an accumulation of reduced NADH may prevent gluconeogenesis, thereby resulting in hypoglycemia (167). Work performed in our laboratory demonstrated a marked decrease in blood glucose after the consumption of 25 ml of ethanol (169). The ethanol was administered in grapefruit juice in two equal volumes of 12.5 ml at 10 minutes prior to and at 30 minutes of a one-hour treadmill run. Blood glucose decreased by 11% between 30 minutes and the termination of exercise, while blood glucose remained constant for the placebo treatment.

Assuming the steady consumption of an alcohol beverage prior to and during a race, the metabolic consequences of alcohol ingestion are impaired gluconeogenesis, hyperuricemia, an increase in free fatty acids, an increase in ketones, and an increase in lactate (167). The rate of liver and muscle glycogen degradation is of paramount importance during a marathon or long-duration race, since glycogen depletion is related to metabolic exhaustion (163–166). Endurance-trained athletes utilize lipids to a greater extent than carbohydrates for energy sources, and untrained athletes depend more on carbohydrate, in particular muscle glycogen, for substrate (163). The low free fatty acid utilization in untrained individuals is associated with high serum lactate concentrations. The fact that ethanol impairs liver gluconeogenesis and fatty acid oxidation should qualify this drug for exclusion during athletic performance.

As a result of training, the skeletal muscle of endurance-trained athletes responds to increased plasma concentrations of free fatty acids by increasing the activity of cytochrome c and the rate of lipid oxidation (170). The consumption of alcohol is related to an increase in lactate, a depression of free fatty acid oxidation, and consequently hypertriglyceridemia (168, 169). Coincidentally, carbohydrate loading stimulates insulin release. Insulin inhibits lipolysis (163). Thus, the fashionable practice of carbohydrate loading coupled with alcohol consumption may result in poor lipid utilization even in the trained athlete.

Lactate accumulation secondary to alcohol will block uric acid secretion. In the state of volume contraction and renal hypoperfusion experienced by distance runners, uric acid retention with or without alcohol may be a consequence of muscle catabolism and may play a pathogenic role in rhabdomyolysis (171).

Exercise in hot, humid environments has been reported to be a significant cause of rhabdomyolysis and acute renal failure (171, 172). Exercise-induced rhabdomyolysis occurs in part as a result of potassium deficiency (173). Potassium deficiency diminishes potassium release and blunts the normal exercise-induced increase in skeletal muscle blood flow and produces necrosis of muscle cells. The necrosis may lead to increased hematin, a product toxic to renal tubular cells (174) and uric acid via released muscle purines (175). Uric acid competes with lactic acid for excretion. Blood lactate increases with the increasing intensity of exercise, which may be potentiated after alcohol consumption. This could in turn lead to dangerously high levels of uric acid in renal interstitial fluid, favoring uric acid precipitation and acute renal failure. Since beer consumption while racing is proposed to replenish electrolytes, one would expect higher levels of alcohol consumption in hot environments. The greater levels of alcohol consumption in hot environments may precipitate severe renal problems.

Alcohol is also a myocardial depressant. Impaired myocardial performance parameters, such as a decrease in stroke work with concomitant increase in LVEDP and in the left ventricular work and tension time index, have been reported after alcohol ingestion (176–178). Alcohol consumption has been demonstrated to increase skin blood flow and sweating (179, 180). Heart rate and cardiac output at rest and during submaximal exercise are reported to be higher after ingestion of alcohol, whereas the total arteriovenous oxygen difference and total peripheral resistance decrease. During maximal work, pulmonary ventilation is reduced but circulatory responses are not affected (181, 182).

Thus, alcohol does not have a salubrious and/or ergogenic effect beneficial during exercise.

Anabolic Steroids

The Press sisters from the Soviet Union were the first athletes in Olympic competition, at Melbourne in 1956, alleged to have been primed with androgenic agents. Twenty years later, in Montreal in 1976, the International Olympic Committee (IOC) inaugurated tests for anabolic steroids using urine specimens submitted for specific radioimmunoassay (183, 184). The IOC began testing for doping drugs at the winter and summer Olympic games of 1968.

Androgens have been given to victims of starvation and to debilitated patients with chronic disease to help induce a state of positive nitrogen balance. The anabolic steroids are less virilizing drugs than pure testosterone and are used today by weight lifters, shot putters, discus throwers, wrestlers, and football players. The rationale for their use is that they enhance performance by increasing muscle mass, strength, and body weight, especially if consumed with a diet high in protein (185–188). Since many of the studies reaching this conclusion were poorly controlled, there is ample evidence that negates these contentions (189, 190). It has been demonstrated that no change occurs in body weight or strength with dianabol whether or not it is accompanied by high dietary protein (191). Casner (192) demonstrated that the increase in weight is due primarily to water retention (188). Carefully controlled studies in male albino rats (193) found no change in body weight or performance, but did find an increase in SGOT with high doses of nandrolone deconate.

Several factors may account for the conflicting data. Testosterone is the only androgen capable of enhancing muscle mass, strength, and body weight. The type and degree of response to synthetic anabolic steroids depend largely on the age of the subject. Increased muscle strength occurs to a greater extent when the drugs are administered before puberty or after the age of 50, as a result of decreased testosterone production in both instances. The dosage of the drug and the regularity with which it is administered also influence the results. The usual recommended dosage of methandrostenolone (methandienone, Dianabol®) is 10 mg per day for 6–12 weeks. Ill-advised athletes may enormously exceed this dosage by two or three times (194, 195). Is it any wonder that there is a conflict between subjective impressions of an increase in strength and the lack of confirmation by scientific evidence?

Body weight, total body potassium and nitrogen, muscle size, leg performance, and strength increased significantly in men taking methandinone but not during placebo (196). The increase in total body nitrogen implies that the weight gain is not only intracellular fluid. The increases in body potassium and nitrogen are too great in proportion to weight gain for this to be attributed to gain of normal muscle or other lean tissue. Thus, the appearance may be anabolic but the weight gain produced is not normal muscle.

The adverse effects of anabolic steroids should suffice to keep athletes from using them. Most notable among these adverse effects are the following: hepatic dysfunction, including cirrhosis of the liver and hepato-cellular carcinoma (seen in aplastic anemia); decreased libido, testicular atrophy; gynecomastia; salt and water retention; and hypertension. Anabolic steroids may also cause premature closure of the epiphyses (189, 197).

In women, anabolic agents may produce such signs of virilization as beard, increased body hair, male escutcheon, increased musculature, and receding hair line. Amenorrhea and sterility have also been noted. Therefore, anabolic steroids play no role in maintaining the health of the athlete and are of questionable benefit as aids to enhanced performance (195).

Amphetamines and Related Stimulants

It is well known that athletes consume amphetamines and related stimulants in large dosages, but their effects are controversial and dangerous (198, 199). Their original medical indication was for weight control, but they are no longer recommended for this purpose. They have been found more useful in the treatment of narcolepsy and hyperactivity in children. The customary dosage of benzadrine or dexadrine is 15 mg, but professional football players allegedly consume 150 mg of amphetamines per game (200). The short-term effects of the average dose (15 mg) include a decrease in appetite, a dramatic increase in alertness and confidence, an elevation in mood, an improvement in physical performance and concentration, and a decrease in the sense of fatigue; yet associated with these is a feeling of anxiousness or of generally being on a high.

On the other hand, the short-term effects of large amounts (150 mg) of amphetamines are profound overstimulation, acute paranoia, agitation, insomnia, fear, irritability, a sharp rise in blood pressure, fever, chest pain, headaches, chills, stomach distress, rhabdomyolysis due to a direct toxic effect of the amphetamine on the skeletal muscle, and, rarely, death. For those who depend on the long-term effects of chronic abuse, tolerance develops rapidly. Psychological dependence on and preoccupation with these drugs is customary. The user may suffer from paranoia, auditory and visual hallucinations, and formication. Withdrawal syndrome is very well appreciated. It would be senseless to belabor the issue that amphetamines are in fact deleterious to the athlete as well as to the nonathlete when improperly consumed.

Cocaine has an effect similar to amphetamines, but the subjective symptoms of the drug are more intensely felt. This may be due to the fact that the way in which cocaine is taken results in a more rapid onset of action and a shorter duration of effect for the average dosage. Short-term effects of large amounts of cocaine are similar to amphetamines; however, an initial tachycardia may become slow and weak and the tachypnea may become shallow and slow.

Conclusion

An example of the principles of clinical exercise physiology and pharmacology is demonstrated clinically wherein the relationships between diuretic-induced hypokalemia, water loss from diuretics and lack of heat acclimatization, alcohol, amphetamines, and salicylates can have adverse effects on skeletal muscle, resulting in rhabdomyolysis and renal failure.

We have attempted to review significant developments in the burgeoning area of exercise pharmacology. The incorporation of the precepts of clinical pharmacology and of exercise physiology are herein woven into a scenario of cardiovascular pharmacology and ergogenic aids to performance.

Literature Cited

1. Lund-Johansen, P. 1970. Hemodynamic changes in long-term diuretic therapy of essential hypertension. A comparative study of chlorthalidone, polythiazide and hydrochlorothiazide. Acta Med. Scand. 187:509–18
2. Ogilvie, R. I. 1976. Cardiovascular response to exercise under increasing doses of chlorthalidone. Eur. J. Clin. Pharmacol. 9:339–44
3. Falkner, B., Onesti, G., Lowenthal, D. T., Affrime, M. B. 1982. Effectiveness of centrally acting drugs and diuretics in adolescent hypertension. Clin. Pharm. Ther. 32:577–83
4. Virtanen, K., Janne, J., Frick, M. H. 1982. Response of blood pressure and plasma norepinephrine to propranolol, metoprolol and clonidine during isometric and dynamic exercise. Eur. J. Clin. Pharmacol. 21:275–79
5. Lowenthal, D. T., Affrime, M. B., Falkner, B., Saris, S., Hakki, H., et al. 1982. Potassium disposition and neuroendocrine effects of propranolol, methyldopa and clonidine during dynamic exercise. Clin. Exp. Hypertens.-Theory Pract. A4(9–10):1895–911
6. Sannerstedt, R., Varnanskes, E., Werko, L. 1962. Hemodynamic effects of methyldopa (Aldomet) at rest and during exercise in patients with arterial hypertension. Acta Med. Scand. 171:75–82
7. Lund-Johansen, P. 1972. Hemodynamic changes in long-term alpha methyldopa therapy of essential hypertension. Acta Med. Scand. 192:221–26
8. Chamberlain, D. A., Howard, J. 1964. Guanethidine and methyldopa: A haemodynamic study. Br. Heart J. 26:528–36
9. Rosenthal, L., Affrime, M. B., Lowenthal, D. T., Falkner, B., Saris, S., et al. 1982. Biochemical and dynamic responses to single and repeated doses of methyldopa and propranolol during dynamic physical activity. Clin. Pharm. Ther. 32:701–10
10. Lund-Johansen, P. 1974. Hemodynamic changes at rest and during exercise in long-term clonidine therapy of essential hypertension. Acta Med. Scand. 195:111–17
11. Lowenthal, D. T., Affrime, M. B., Rosenthal, L., Gould, A. B., Borruso, J., et al. 1982. Dynamic and biochemical responses to single and repeated doses of coinidine during dynamic physical activity. Clin. Pharm. Ther. 32:18–24
12. Onesti, G., Schwartz, A. B., Kim, K. E., Paz-Martinez, V., Swartz, C. 1971. Antihypertensive effect of clonidine. Circ. Res. 28(Suppl. 2):53–69
13. Ellestad, M. H. 1980. Ischemic S-T segment depression: Hemodynamic, electrophysiologic, and metabolic factors in its genesis. Stress Testing. Principles and Practice, ed. M. H. Ellestad, pp. 77–96. Philadelphia: Davis. 2nd ed.
14. Pratt, C. M., Welton, D. E., Squires, W. G. Jr., Kirby, T. E., Hartung, G. H., et al. 1981. Demonstration of training effect during chronic beta-adrenergic blockade in patients with coronary artery disease. Circulation 64:1125–129
15. Epstein, S. E., Robinson, B. F., Kahler, R. L., Braunwald, E. 1965. Effects of beta-adrenergic blockade on the cardiac response to maximal and submaximal exercise in man. J. Clin. Invest. 44:1745–53
16. Hamer, J., Sowton, E. 1965. Cardiac output after beta-adrenergic blockade in ischaemic heart disease. Br. Heart J. 27:892–95
17. Hannson, L. 1975. Hemodynamic effects of acute and prolonged beta-adrenergic blockade in essential hypertension. Scand. J. Clin. Lab. Invest. 35(Suppl. 143):59 (Abstr.)
18. Tarazi, R. D., Dustan, H. P. 1972. Beta-adrenergic blockade in hypertension. Practical and theoretical implications of long-term hemodynamic variations. Am. J. Cardiol. 29:633–40
19. Hare, T. W., Lowenthal, D. T., Hakki, H. H., Goodwin, M. 1984. The effect of exercise training in older patients on beta adrenergic blocking drugs. Ann. Sports Med. In press
20. Sklar, J., Johnston, D. G., Overlie, P., Gerber, J. G., Brammell, H. L., et al. 1982. The effects of a cardioselective (metoprolol) and a nonselective (propranolol) beta-adrenergic blocker on the

response to dynamic exercise in normal men. *Circulation* 65:894–99

21. Lowenthal, D. T., Saris, S. D., Packer, J., Haratz, A., Conry, K. 1984. The mechanisms of action and the clinical pharmacology of beta adrenergic blocking drugs. *Am. J. Med.* 77(4A):119–27

22. Floras, J., Hassan, M. O., Jones, J. V., Sleight, P. 1983. Contrasting effects of cardioselective and non-selective beta blockers on changes in blood pressure during bicycle exercise in subjects with essential hypertension. *J. Am. Coll. Cardiol.* 1:611 (Abstr.)

23. Kramer, B., Kramer, G., Walz, G., Stankov, G., Welsch, M., et al. 1983. Analysis of inter-individual variability of beta blocking effects on heart rate and blood pressure during exercise. *J. Am. Coll. Cardiol.* 1:625 (Abstr.)

24. O'Hare, J. A., Murnaghan, D. J. 1981. Failure of antihypertensive drugs to control blood pressure rise with isometric exercise in hypertension. *Post-Grad. Med. J.* 57:552–55

25. Nelson, G. I. C., Donnelly, G. L., Hunyor, S. N. 1982. Haemodynamic effects of sustained treatment with prazosin and metoprolol, alone and in combination, in borderline hypertensive heart failure. *J. Cardiovasc. Pharm.* 4:240–45

26. Hansson, B. G., Dymling, J. F., Manhem, P., Hokfelt, B. 1977. Long-term treatment of moderate hypertension with the beta$_1$-receptor blocking agent metoprolol. II. Effect of submaximal work and insulin-induced hypoglycaemia on plasma catecholamines and renin activity, blood pressure and pulse rate. *Eur. J. Clin. Pharmacol.* 11:247–54

27. Lijnen, P. G., Amery, A. K., Fagard, R. H., Reybrouck, T. M., Moerman, E. F., et al. 1979. The effect of beta-adrenoceptor blockade on renin, angiotensin, aldosterone and catecholamines at rest and during exercise. *Br. J. Clin. Pharmacol.* 7:175–81

28. Christensen, N. J., Brandsborg, O. 1973. The relationship between plasma catecholamine concentration and pulse rate during exercise and standing. *Eur. J. Clin. Invest.* 3:299–306

29. Lundborg, P., Astrom, H., Bengtsson, C., Fellenius, E., Von Schenck, H., et al. 1981. Effect of beta-adrenoceptor blockade on exercise performance and metabolism. *Clin. Sci.* 61:299–305

30. Leitch, A. G., Hopkin, J. M., Ellis, D. A., Clarkson, D. M., Merchant, S., et al. 1980. Failure of propranolol and metoprolol to alter ventilatory responses to car-

bon dioxide and exercise. *Br. J. Clin. Pharmacol.* 9:493–98

31. Twentyman, O. P., Disley, A., Gribbin, H. R., Alberti, K. M. G. G. 1981. Effect of beta adrenergic blockade on respiratory and metabolic responses to exercise. *J. Appl. Physiol.* 51:788–93

32. Kaiser, P., Rossner, S., Karlsson, J. 1981. Effects of beta adrenergic blockade on endurance and short time performance in respect to individual muscle fiber composition. *Intl. J. Sport Med.* 2:37–42

33. Holmberg, E., Waldeck, B. 1980. The effect of insulin on skeletal muscle contraction and its relation to the effect produced by beta adrenoceptor stimulation. *Acta Physiol. Scand.* 109:225–29

34. Petrofsky, J. S., Phillips, C. A., Lind, A. R. 1981. The influence of fiber composition, recruitment order and muscle temperature on the pressor response to isometric contractions and skeletal muscle of the cat. *Circ. Res.* 48(Suppl. 1):138–48

35. Tesch, P. A., Kaiser, P. 1983. Effects of beta adrenergic blockade on O_2 uptake during submaximal and maximal exercise. *J. Appl. Physiol.* 54:901–5

36. Henry, J. A., Iliopoulou, A., Kaye, C. M., Sankey, M. G., Turner, P. 1981. Changes in plasma concentrations of acebutolol, propranolol and indomethacin during physical exercise. *Life Sci.* 28:1925–29

37. Moyer, J. H. 1953. Hydralazine (apresoline) hydrochloride. Pharmacological observations and clinical results in the therapy of hypertension. *Arch. Int. Med.* 91:419–39

38. Ginks, W. R., Redwood, D. R. 1980. Haemodynamic effects of hydralazine at rest and during exercise in patients with chronic heart failure. *Br. Heart J.* 44:259–64

39. Lund-Johansen, P. 1975. Hemodynamic changes at rest and during exercise in long-term prazosin therapy for essential hypertension. In *Postgrad. Med. Symp. Prazosin.* New York: McGraw-Hill. 45 pp.

40. Lowenthal, D. T., Broderman, S. 1984. Hypertension and exercise. In *Exercise Medicine: Physiologic Principles and Clinical Applications*, ed. A. A. Bove, D. T. Lowenthal, pp. 291–303. New York: Academic

41. Wilson, J. R., Untereker, W., Hirshfeld, J. 1981. Effects of isosorbide dinitrate and hydralazine on regional metabolic responses to arm exercise in patients with heart failure. *Am. J. Cardio.* 48:934–38

42. Lowenthal, D. T., Dickerman, D., Saris,

S. D., Falkner, B., Hare, T. W. 1984. The effect of pharmacological interaction on central and peripheral alpha-receptors and pressor response to static exercise. *Ann. Sports Med.* 1(3):100–4

43. Pickering, T. G., Base, D. B., Sullivan, P. A., Laragh, J. H. 1982. Comparison of anti-hypertensive and hormonal effects of captopril and propranolol at rest and during exercise. *Am. J. Cardiol.* 49:1566–68

44. Manhem, P., Bramnert, M., Hulthen, U. L., Hokfelt, B. 1981. The effect of captopril on catecholamines, renin activity, angiotensin II and aldosterone in plasma during physical exercise in hypertensive patients. *Eur. J. Clin. Invest.* 11:389–95

45. Fagard, R., Lijnen, P., Amery, A. 1982. Hemodynamic response to captopril at rest and during exercise in hypertensive patients. *Am. J. Cardiol.* 49:1569–71

46. Fagard, R., Amery, A., Reybrouck, T., Lijnen, P., Moerman, E., et al. 1977. Effects of angiotensin antagonism on hemodynamics, renin and catecholamines during exercise. *J. Appl. Physiol.* 43:440–44

47. Stone, P. H., Antman, E. M., Muller, J. E., Braunwald, E. 1980. Calcium channel blocking agents in the treatment of cardiovascular disorders. Part II: Hemodynamic effects of clinical applications. *Ann. Int. Med.* 93:886–904

48. Stein, D. T., Lowenthal, D. T., Porter, R. S., Falkner, B., Bravo, E. L., Hare, T. W. 1984. Effects of nifedipine and verapamil on isometric and dynamic exercise in normal subjects. *Am. J. Cardiol.* 54:386–89

49. Subramanian, B., Bowles, M. H., Davies, A. B., Raftery, E. B. 1982. Combined therapy with verapamil and propranolol in chronic stable angina. *Am. J. Cardiol.* 49:125–32

50. Moskowitz, R. M., Piccini, P. A., Nacarelli, G. V., Zelis, R. 1979. Nifedipine therapy for stable angina pectoris: Preliminary results of effects on angina frequency and treadmill exercise response. *Am. J. Cardiol.* 44:811–16

51. Bonow, R. O., Leon, M. B., Rosing, D. R., Kent, K. M., Lipson, L. C., et al. 1982. Effects of verapamil and propranolol on left ventricular function and diastolic filling in patients with coronary artery disease: Radionuclide angiographic studies at rest and during exercise. *Circulation* 65:1337–50

52. Goldstein, R. E., Rosing, D. R., Redwood, D. R., Beiser, G. D., Epstein, S. E. 1971. Clinical and circulatory effects of isosorbide dinitrate: Comparison with nitroglycerine. *Circulation* 43:629–40

53. Sorensen, S. G., Ritchie, J. L., Caldwell, J. H., Hamilton, G. W., Kennedy, J. W. 1980. Serial exercise radionuclide angiography. Validation of count-derived changes in cardiac output and quantitation of maximal exercise ventricular volume change after nitroglycerine and propranolol in normal men. *Circulation* 61(3):600–9

54. Fam, W. M., McGregor, M. 1964. The effect of coronary vasodilator drugs on retrograde flow in areas of chronic myocardial ischemia. *Circ. Res.* 15:355–65

55. Franciosa, J. A., Goldsmith, S. R., Cohn, J. N. 1980. Contrasting immediate and long-term effects of isosorbide dinitrate on exercise capacity in congestive heart failure. *Am. J. Med.* 69:559–66

56. Danahy, D. T., Burwell, D. T., Aronow, W. S., Prakash, R. 1977. Sustained hemodynamic and anti-anginal effect of high dose oral isosorbide dinitrate. *Circulation* 55:381–87

57. Glancy, D. L., Richter, M. A., Ellis, E. V., Johnson, W. 1977. Effect of swallowed isosorbide dinitrate on blood pressure, heart rate and exercise capacity in patients with coronary artery disease. *Am. J. Med.* 62:39–46

58. Lee, G., Mason, D. T., Amsterdam, E., DeMaria, A., Davis, V. C. 1976. Improved exercise tolerance for six hours following isosorbide dinitrate capsules in patients with ischemic heart disease. *Am. J. Cardiol.* 37:150 (Abstr.)

59. Williams, M. H. Jr., Zohman, L. R., Ratner, A. C. 1958. Hemodynamic effects of cardiac glycosides on normal human subjects during rest and exercise. *J. Appl. Physiol.* 13:417–21

60. Gross, G. J., Warltier, D. C., Hardman, H. F., Somani, P. 1977. The effect of ouabain on nutritional circulation and regional myocardial blood flow. *Am. Heart J.* 93:487–95

61. Parker, J. O., West, R. O. Jr., Ledwich, J. R., DiGiorgi, S. 1969. The effect of acute digitalization on the hemodynamic response to exercise in coronary artery disease. *Circulation* 40:453–62

62. Glancy, D. L., Higgs, L. M., O'Brien, K. P., Epstein, S. E. 1971. Effects of ouabain on the left ventricular response to exercise in patients with angina pectoris. *Circulation* 43:45–57

63. Gooch, A. S., Natarajan, G., Goldberg, H. 1974. Influence of exercise on arrhythmias induced by digitalis-diuretic

therapy in patients with atrial fibrillation. *Am. J. Cardiol.* 33:230–37

64. Gey, G. P., Levy, R. H., Fisher, L., Pettet, G., Bruce, R. A. 1974. Plasma concentration of procainamide and prevalence of exertional arrhythmias. *Ann. Int. Med.* 80:718–22

65. Gey, G. P., Levy, R. H., Pettet, G., Fisher, L. 1975. Quinidine plasma concentration and exertional arrhythmia. *Am. Heart J.* 90:19–24

66. Surawicz, B., Lasseter, K. C. 1970. Effects of drugs on the electrocardiogram. *Prog. Cardiovasc. Dis.* 13:26–55

67. Freedberg, A. S., Riseman, J. E. F., Speigel, E. D. 1941. Objective evidence of the efficiency of medical therapy in angina pectoris. *Am. Heart J.* 22:494–518

68. Venerando, A. 1963. Doping: Pathology and ways to control it. *Med. Sport* 3:972–93

69. Costill, D. L., Dalsky, G., Fink, W. 1978. Effects of caffeine ingestion on metabolism and exercise performance. *Med. Sci. Sports* 10:155–58

70. Grollman, A. 1930. The action of alcohol, caffeine and tobacco on the cardiac output (and its related functions) of normal man. *J. Pharmacol. Exp. Ther.* 39:313–27

71. Ivy, J. L., Costill, D. L., Fink, W. J., Lower, R. W. 1979. Influence of caffeine and carbohydrate feedings on endurance performance. *Med. Sci. Sports Exer.* 11:6–11

72. Rivers, W., Webber, H. 1907. The action of caffeine on the capacity for muscular work. *J. Physiol.* 36:33–47

73. Schirlitz, K. 1930. Uber caffein bei ermiidender mUskelarbeit. *Int. Z. Angew. Physiol. Einschl. Arbeitsphysiol.* 2:273–77

74. Axelrod, J., Reichenthal, J. 1953. The fate of caffeine in man and a method for its estimation in biological material. *J. Pharmacol. Exp. Ther.* 107:519–23

75. Van Handel, P. J., Burke, E., Costill, D. L., Cote, R. 1977. Physiological responses to cola ingestion. *Res. Q.* 48:436–44

76. Goldstein, A., Warren, R., Kaizer, S. 1965. Psychotropic effects of caffeine in man. I. Interindividual differences in sensitivity to caffeine-induced wakefulness. *J. Pharmacol. Exp. Ther.* 149:156–59

77. Essig, D., Costill, D. L., Van Handel, P. J. 1980. Effects of caffeine injestion on utilization of muscle glycogen and lipid during leg ergometer cycling. *Intl. J. Sports Med.* 1:86–90

78. Robertson, D., Johnson, G. A., Robertson, R. M., Nies, A. S., Shand, D. G., Oates, J. A. 1979. Comparative assessment of stimuli that release neuronal and adrenomedullary catecholamines in man. *Circulation* 59:637–43

79. Victor, B. S., Lubetsky, M., Greden, J. F. 1981. Somatic manifestations of caffeinism. *J. Clin. Psych.* 42:185–88

80. Arushanyan, E. B., Belozertsev, Y. A., Arvazov, K. G. 1974. Comparative effect of amphetamine and caffeine on spontaneous activity of sensomotor cortical units and their responses to stimulation of the caudate nucleus. *Bull. Exp. Biol. Med.* 78:776–79

81. Thithapandha, A., Maling, H. M., Gillette, J. R. 1972. Effects of caffeine and theophylline on activity of rats in relation to brain xanthine concentrations. *Proc. Exp. Biol. Med.* 139:582–86

82. Oldendorg, W. H. 1971. Brain uptake of metabolites and drugs following carotid arterial injections. *Trans. Am. Neural. Assoc.* 96:46–50

83. Syed, I. B. 1976. The effects of caffeine. *J. Am. Pharm. Assoc.* 16:568–72

84. Waldeck, B. 1973. Sensitization by caffeine of central catecholamine receptors. *J. Neural Transm.* 34:61–72

85. Berkowitz, B., Spector, S. 1971. Effect of caffeine and theophylline on peripheral catecholamines. *Eur. J. Pharmacol.* 13:193–96

86. Fredholm, B. B. 1980. Are methylxanthine effects due to antagonism of endogenous adenosine? *Pharmacol. Res.* 1:129–32

87. Second International Caffeine Workshop. 1980. Special report. *Nutr. Rev.* 38:196–200

88. Breckenridge, B. M., Burn, J. H., Matschinsky, F. M. 1967. Theophylline, epinephrine and neostigmine facilitation on neuromuscular transmission. *Proc. Natl. Acad. Sci. USA* 57:1893–97

89. Varagic, V. M., Zugic, M. 1971. Interactions of xanthine derivatives, catecholamines and glucose-6-phosphate on the isolated phrenic nerve diaphragm preparation of the rat. *Pharmacology* 5:275–86

90. Berg, A. W. 1975. Physiological disposition of caffeine. *Metab. Rev.* 4:199–228

91. Bianchi, C. P. 1962. Kinetics of radiocaffeine uptake and release in frog sartorius. *J. Pharmacol.* 138:41–47

92. Hartree, W., Hill, A. V. 1924. The heat production of muscles treated with caffeine or subjected to prolonged discon-

tinuous stimulation. *J. Physiol.* 58:441–54

93. Connett, R. J., Ugol, L. M., Hammack, M. J., Hays, E. T. 1981. Caffeine contractures in rat soleus muscle. *Fed. Proc.* 40:513

94. Issacson, A., Sandow, A. 1967. Quinine and caffeine effects on 45 Ca movements in from sartorius muscle. *J. Phys.* 50:2109–28

95. Coleman, A. W., Coleman, J. R. 1980. Characterization of the methylxanthine-induced propagated wave phenomenon in striated muscle. *J. Exp. Zool.* 212:403–13

96. Kavaler, F., Anderson, T. W., Fisher, V. J. 1978. Sarcolemmal site of caffeine's inotropic action on ventricular muscle of the frog. *Circ. Res.* 42:285–90

97. Blayney, L., Thomas, H., Muir, J., Henderson, A. 1978. Action of caffeine on calcium transport by isolated fractions of myofibrils, mitochondria, and sarcoplasmic reticulum from rabbit heart. *Circ. Res.* 43:520–26

98. Fabiato, A., Fabiato, F. 1975. Dependence of the contractile activation of skinned cardiac cells on the sarcomere length. *Nature* 256:54–56

99. Weber, A., 1968. The mechanism of the action of caffeine on sarcoplasmic reticulum. *J. Gen. Physiol.* 52:760–72

100. Butcher, R. W., Sutherland, E. W. 1962. Adenosine 3',5'-phosphate in biological materials. *J. Biol. Chem.* 237:1244–50

101. Chuck, L. H. S., Parmley, W. W. 1980. Caffeine reversal of length-dependent changes in myocardial contractile state in the cat. *Circ. Res.* 47:592–98

102. Bowman, W. C., Raper, C. 1964. The effects of adrenalin and other drugs affecting carbohydrate metabolism on contractions of the rat diaphragm. *Br. J. Pharmacol.* 23:184–200

103. Strubelt, O. 1969. The influence of reserpine, propranolol and adrenal medullectomy on the hyperglycemic actions of theophylline and caffeine. *Arch. Int. Pharmacodyn. Ther.* 179:215–24

104. Ahlborg, G., Felig, P. 1977. Substrate utilization during prolonged exercise preceded by ingestion of glucose. *Am. J. Physiol.* 233:188–94

105. Costill, D. L., Jansson, E., Gollnick, P. D., Saltin, B. 1974. Glycogen utilization in leg muscles of men during level and uphill running. *Acta Phys. Scand.* 91:475–81

106. Essen, B. 1977. Intramuscular substrate utilization during prolonged exercise. *Ann. NY Acad. Sci.* 301:30–44

107. Bellet, S., Kershbaum, A., Finck, E.

1968. Response of free fatty acids to coffee and caffeine. *Metabolism* 17:702–7

108. Dole, V. P. 1961. Effect of nucleic acid metabolites on lipolysis in adipose tissue. *J. Biol. Chem.*, 236:3125–30

109. Berthet, J., Sutherland, E. W., Rall, T. W. 1957. The assay of glucagon and epinephrine with use of liver homogenates. *J. Biol. Chem.* 229:351–54

110. Crass, M. F. 1972. Exogenous substrate effects of endogenous lipid metabolism in the working rat heart. *Biochem. Biophys. Acta* 280:71–81

111. Froberg, S. O., Rossner, S., Ericsson, M. 1978. Relation between triglycerides in human skeletal muscle and serum and the fractional elimination rate of exogenous plasma triglycerides. *Eur. J. Clin. Invest.* 8:93–97

112. Froberg, S. O., Mosefeldt, F. 1971. Effect of prolonged strenuous exercise on the concentration of triglycerides, phospholipids and glycogen in muscle of man. *Acta Physiol. Scand.* 82:167–71

113. Bellet, S., Roman, L., DeCastro, O., Kim, K. E., Kershbaum, A. 1969. Effect of coffee ingestion on catecholamine release. *Metabolism* 18:288–91

114. Davis, I. 1968. In vitro regulation of the lipolysis of adipose tissue. *Nature* 218:349–52

115. Butcher, R. W., Baird, C. E. 1969. The regulation of cAMP and lipolysis in adipose tissue by hormones and other agents. In *Drugs Affecting Lipid Metabolism*, ed. W. Holmes, L. A. Carlson, R. Paoletti. New York: Plenum

116. Goldfarb, A. H., Kendrick, Z. V., 1981. Effect of an exercise run to exhaustion on cAMP in the rat heart. *J. Appl. Physiol.* 51:1539–42

117. Cheung, W. Y. 1967. Properties of cyclic 3',5' nucleotide phosphodiesterase from rat brain. *Biochemistry* 6:1079–87

118. Patwardhan, R. V., Desmond, P. V., Johnson, R. F., Dunn, G. D., Robertson, D. H., et al. 1980. Effects of caffeine on plasma free fatty acids, urinary catecholamines and drug binding. *Clin. Pharm. Ther.* 28:398–403

119. Carlson, L. A., Liljedahl, S. W., Wirsen, C. 1965. Blood and tissue changes in the dog during and after excessive free fatty acid mobilization: A biochemical and morphological study. *Acta Med. Scand.* 178:81–107

120. Paul, P., Issekutz, B. 1967. Role of extra muscular energy sources in the metabolism of exercising dogs. *J. Appl. Physiol.* 22:615–22

121. Mansour, T. E. 1972. Phosphofructokinase. *Curr. Top. Cell. Reg.* 5:1–46

122. Neely, J. R., Bowman, R. H., Morgan, H. E. 1968. Conservation of glycogen in the perfused rat heart developing intraventricular pressure. In *Control of Glycogen Metabolism*, ed. W. J. Whelan. New York: Academic

123. Randle, P. J. 1963. Endocrine control of metabolism. *Ann. Rev. Physiol.* 25:291–324

124. Fink, W. J., Costill, D. L., Van Handel, P. J. 1975. Leg muscle metabolism during exercise in the heat and cold. *Eur. J. Appl. Physiol.* 34:183–90

125. Reitman, J., Baldwin, K. M., Holloszy, J. O. 1973. Intramuscular triglyceride utilization by red, white and intermediate skeletal muscle and heart during exhausting exercise. *Proc. Soc. Exp. Biol. Med.* 143:628–31

126. Georg, J. C., Vallyathan, N. V. 1964. Effects of exercise on fatty acid levels in the pigeon. *J. Appl. Physiol.* 19:619–22

127. Essig, D. A., White, T. P. 1981. Effects of caffeine on glycogen and triglyceride concentration in the soleus and plantaris muscles of the exercising rat. *Fed. Proc.* 40:513 (Abstr.)

128. Temples, T. E., Haymes, E. M. 1982. The effects of caffeine on substrates in a cold and neutral environment. *Med. Sci. Sports* 14:176 (Abstr.)

129. Asmussen, E., Boje, O. 1948. The effects of alcohol and some drugs on the capacity to work. *Acta Physiol. Scand.* 15:109–18

130. Haldi, J., Wynn, W. 1946. Action of drugs on the efficiency of swimmers. *Res. Q.* 17:96–101

131. Ganslen, R. V., Balke, B., Nagle, F., Phillips, E. 1964. Effects of some tranquilizing analeptic and vasodilating drugs on physical work capacity and orthostatic tolerance. *Aerosp. Med.* 35:630–33

132. Perkins, R., Williams, M. H. 1975. Effect of caffeine upon maximum muscular endurance of females. *Med. Sci. Sports* 7:221–24

133. Margaria, R., Aghemo, P., Rovelli, E. 1964. The effect of some drugs on the maximal capacity of athletic performance in men. *Int. Z. Angew. Physiol. Einschl. Arbeitsphysiol.* 20:281–87

134. Brink, L. S., McKirnan, M. D., O'Connell, R. S., Motto, R. E., Froelicher, V. F. 1980. Caffeine ingestion by cardiac patients prior to ECG monitored exercise training. *Med. Sci. Sports Exer.* 12:117

135. Ali Abrishami, M., Thomas, J. 1977. Aspirin intolerance, a review. *Ann. Allergy* 39:28–37

136. Goodman, A., Gillman, A., Goodman, L., eds. *The Pharmacological Basis of Therapy*, p. 693. New York: Macmillan. 6th ed.

137. Baskin, S. I., Goldfarb, A. H. 1983. Age associated changes of nonnarcotic analgesic. In *The Handbook of Pharmacology of Aging*, ed. J. Roberts. Boca Raton, Fla.: CRC

138. Kendrick, Z. V., Baskin, S. I., Goldfarb, A. H., Lowenthal, D. T. 1984. The influence of age and salicylate on rectal temperature of Fischer 344 rats during hot ambient temperature exposures. *Age* (In press)

139. Samter, M., Beers, R. F. 1968. Intolerance to aspirin, clinical studies and consideration of its pathogenesis, *Ann. Int. Med.* 68:975

140. Barbour, H. G., Devenis, M. M. 1919. Antipyreties. II Acetylsalicylic acid and heat regulations in normal individuals. *Arch. Int. Med.* 24:617–23

141. Levin, S. 1976. Ventilatory stimulation by sodium salicylate: Role of thoracic receptors. *J. Appl. Physiol.* 41:498–503

142. Paulus, H. E., Whitehouse, M. W. 1973. Nonsteroid anti-inflammatory agents. 1973. *Ann. Rev. Pharmacol.* 13:107–25

143. Miller, R. H., Tenney, S. M. 1956. Action of sodium salicylate on tissue gas tensions. *Proc. Soc. Exp. Biol. Med.* 92:791–93

144. Tenney, S. M., Miller, R. M. 1955. Respiratory and circulatory actions of salicylate. *Am. J. Med.* 19:498–508

145. Segar, W. E., Holliday, M. A. 1958. Physiologic abnormalities of salicylate intoxication. *N. Engl. J. Med.* 259:1191–98

146. Consolazio, C. F., Matoush, L. O., Nelson, R. A., Torres, J. B., Issac, G. J. 1963. Environmental temperature and energy expenditures. *J. Appl. Phys.* 18:65–68

147. Wyndham, G. H., Morrison, J. F., Williams, C. G. 1965. Heat reactions of male and female Caucasians. *J. Appl. Phys.* 20:357–64

148. Wood, H. C., Reichert, E. T. 1882. Contribution to our knowledge of action of certain drugs upon bodily temperature. *J. Physiol.* 3:321–26

149. Kendrick, Z. V., Troup, J. T., Rumsey, W. L., Qualey, D., Lowenthal, D. T., Affrime, M. B. 1982. The influence of salicylate on rectal temperature at high ambient temperatures. *Med. Sci. Sports Exer.* 14:126 (Abstr.)

150. Nielson, B. 1968. Thermoregulatory responses to arm work, leg work, and intermittent leg work. *Acta Phys. Scand.* 72:25–32

151. Irion, G., Wailgum, T. D., Stevens, C., Kendrick, Z.V., Paolone, A. M. 1984. The effect of age on the hemodynamic response to thermal stress during exercise. In *Altered Endocrine States During Aging*, ed. J. Roberts, R. Adelman, V. Cristofalo, pp. 187–95. New York: Liss (In press)

152. Wyndham, C. H., Strydom, H. B., Morrison, J. F., DuToit, F. D., Kraan, J. G. 1954. Responses of unacclimatized men under stress of heat and work. *J. Appl. Phys.* 6:681–86

153. Chen, W. Y., Elonzondo, R. S. 1974. Peripheral modification of thermoregulatory function during heat acclimation. *J. Appl. Phys.* 37:367–73

154. Saltin, B. 1964. Circulatory response to submaximal and maximal exercise after thermal dehydration. *J. Appl. Phys.* 19(6):1125–32

155. Folk, G. E. Jr. 1974. *Textbook of Environmental Physiology*. Philadelphia: Lea & Febingar

156. Davison, C. 1971. Salicylate metabolism in man. *Ann. NY Acad. Sci.* 179:249–68

157. Elkington, J. R., Singer, R. B., Barker, E. S., Clark, J. R. 1955. Effects in man of acute experimental respiratory alkalosis and acidosis on ionic transfers in the total body fluids. *J. Clin. Invest.* 34:1671–75

158. Senay, L. C. Jr., Christensen, M. L. 1968. Changes in blood plasma during progressive dehydration. *J. Appl. Phys.* 24(3):302–9

159. Troup, J. T. 1983. *The effect of acetylsalicylic acid administration on metabolic, cardiovascular and thermoregulatory function in young males during acute exercise in hot and neutral environments.* PhD dissertation. Temple Univ., Pa. 134 pp.

160. Fred, H. L. 1980. Reflections on a 100 mile run: Effects of aspirin therapy. *Med. Sci. Sports Exer.* 12(3):212–15

161. Zambraski, E. J., Rofrano, T. A., Ciccone, C. D. 1982. Effects of aspirin treatment on kidney function in exercise man. *Med. Sci. Sports Exer.* 14:419–23

162. Downey, J. A., Darling, R. C. 1962. Effect of salicylates on elevation of body temperatures during exercise. *J. Appl. Phys.* 17:323–25

163. Felig, P., Wahren J. 1978. Fuel homeostasis in exercise. *N. Engl. J. Med.* 293:1078–84

164. Costill, D. L., Dalsky, G. P., Fink, W. J. 1978. Effects of caffeine ingestion on metabolism and exercise performance. *Med. Sci. Sports* 10:155–58

165. Ivy, J. L., Costill, D. L., Fink, W. J., Lower, R. W. 1979. Influence of caffeine and carbohydrate feedings on endurance performance. *Med. Sci. Sports and Exer.* 11:6–11

166. Essig, D., Costill, D. L., Van Handel, P. J. 1980. Effects of caffeine ingestion on utilization of muscle glycogen and lipid during leg ergometer cycling. *Intl. J. Sports Med.* 1:86–90

167. Lieber, C. S., Robinson, S. H., Glickman, R. 1978. Pathogenesis and early diagnosis of alcoholic liver injury. *N. Engl. J. Med.* 298:888–93

168. Fleming, C. R., Higgins, J. A. 1977. Editorial. Alcohol: Nutrient and poison. *Ann. Int. Med.* 87(4):492–93

169. Kendrick, Z. V., Lowenthal, D. T. 1984. The effect of caffeine and alcohol on metabolic and blood parameters during a one hour run in highly trained athletes. *Intl. J. Sports Med.* Submitted

170. Van Handel, P. J., Sandel, W. R., Mole, P. A. 1977. Effects of exogenous cytochrome c on respiratory capacity of heart and skeletal muscle. *Biochem. Biophys. Res. Commun.* 74:1213–19

171. Knochel, J. P. 1976. Renal injury in muscle disease. In *The Kidney in Systemic Disease*, 3:129–40 New York: Wiley.

172. Schrier, R. W., Henderson, H. S., Tisher, C. C., Tannen, R. L. 1967. Nephropathy associated with heat stress and exercise. *Ann. Int. Med.* 67:356–76

173. Knochel, J. P., Schlein, E. M. 1972. On the mechanism of rhabdomyolysis in potassium depletion. *J. Clin. Invest.* 51:1750–58

174. Knochel, J. P., Carter, N. W. 1976. The role of muscle cell injury in the pathogensis of acute renal failure after exercise. *Kidney Int.* 10 (4, Suppl.6):58–64

175. Cathurt, E. P., Kernanny, E. L., Leather, J. B. 1908. On the origin of endogenous uric acid. *Quart. J. Med.* 1:416

176. Regan, T. J., Weisse, A. B., Moschos, C. B., et al. 1965. The myocardial effects of acute and chronic usage of ethanol in man. *Trans. Assoc. Am. Phys.* 78:282–91

177. Blomquist, G., Saltin, B., Mitchell, J. H. 1970. Acute effects ethanol ingestion on the response to submaximal and maximal exercise in man. *Circulation* 42:463–70

178. Conway, N. 1968. Haemodynamic effects of ethyl alcohol in patients with coronary heart disease. *Br. Heart J.* 30:638–44

179. Gillespie, J. A. 1967. Vasodilator properties of alcohol. *Br. Med. J.* 2:274–77

180. Fewings, J. D., Hanna, M. J. D., Walsh,

J. A., et al. 1966. The effects of ethyl alcohol on the blood vessels of the hand and in man. *Br. J. Pharmacol.* 27:93–106

181. Riff, D. P., Jain, A. C., Doyle, J. T. 1969. Acute hemodynamic effects of ethanol on normal human volunteers. *Am. Heart J.* 78:592–97

182. Garlind, T., Goldberg, L., Graf, K., Perman, E., Strandell, T., Stram, G. 1960. Effects of ethanol on circulatory, metabolic, and neurohumoral function during muscular work in man. *Acta Pharmacol. Toxicol.* 17:106–14

183. Percy, E. C. 1977. Athletic aids: Fact or fiction. *Can. Med. Assoc. J.* 117:601–5

184. Dugal, R., Dupuis, C., Bertrand, M. J. 1977. Radioimmunoassay of anabolic steroids: An evaluation of three antisera for the detection of anabolic steroids in biological fluids. *Br. J. Sports Med.* 11:162–69

185. Tahmindjis, A. J. 1976. The use of anabolic steroids by athletes to increase body weight and strength. *Med. J. Austr.* 1:991–93

186. Johnson, L. C., Fisher, G., Silvester, L. J., Hofheins, C. C. 1972. Anabolic steroids: Effect on strength, body weight, oxygen uptake and spermatogenesis upon mature males. *Med. Sci. Sports* 4:43–45

187. Johnson, L. C., O'Shea, J. P. 1969. Anabolic steroids—Effects on strength development. *Science* 164:957–59

188. O'Shea, J. P., Winkler, W. 1970. Biochemical and physical effects of an anabolic steroid in competitive swimmers and weight lifters. *Nutr. Rep. Intl.* 6:351–54

189. Shepard, R. J., Killinger, D., Fried, T. 1977. Responses to sustained use of anabolic steroids. *Br. J. Sports Med.* 11:170

190. Hervey, G. R., Hutchinson, I., Knibbs, A. V. 1976. "Anabolic" effects of methandienone in men undergoing athletic training. *Lancet* 2:699–702

191. American College of Sports Medicine. 1977. Position statement on the use and abuse of anabolic-androgenic steroids in sports. *Med. Sci. Sports* 9:xi-xii

192. Casner, S. W., Early, R. G., Carlson, B. R. 1971. Anabolic steroid effects on body composition in normal young men. *J. Sports Med. Phys. Fit.* 11:98

193. Young, M., Crookshant, H. R., Ponder, L. 1977. Effects of an anabolic steroid on selected parameters in male albino rats. *Res. Quart. Am. Assoc. Health Phys. Educ.* 48:653–56

194. News and comment. 1972. Anabolic steroids: Doctors denounce them but athletes aren't listening. *Science* 176:1399–401

195. Darden, E. 1972. Drugs and athletic performance: Facts and fallacies. *Clin. Med.* 79:25–29

196. Harvey, G. R., Knibbs, A. V., Burkinshaw, L., Morgan, D. B., Jones, P. R., et al. 1981. Effects of methandienone on the performance and body composition of men undergoing athletic training. *Clin. Sci.* 60:457–61

197. Johnson, F. L., Feagler, J. R., Lerner, K. G. 1972. Association of adrenergic anabolic steroid therapy with development of hepatocellular carcinoma. *Lancet* 2:1273–78

198. Smith, G. M., Beecher, H. K. 1959. Amphetamine sulfate and athletic performance. *J. Am. Med. Assoc.* 170:542

199. Karpovich, P. V. 1959. Effect of amphetamine sulfate on athletic performance. *J. Am. Med. Assoc.* 170:558

200. Underwood, J. 1978. Brutality: Part 3. Speed is all the rage. *Sports Illus.* (Aug. 28) 49:30–41

Ann. Rev. Pharmacol. Toxicol. 1985. 25:307–23

SYNTHETIC AND FERMENTATION-DERIVED ANGIOTENSIN-CONVERTING ENZYME INHIBITORS

Marlene L. Cohen

Lilly Research Laboratories, Eli Lilly and Company, Indianapolis, Indiana 46285

INTRODUCTION

Interest in the development of inhibitors of angiotensin-converting enzyme (EC 3.4.15.1) (ACE) has exploded since the announced discovery in 1977 of captopril (1), an orally effective inhibitor of ACE, by Cushman & Ondetti of the Squibb Institute for Medical Research. Following extensive clinical studies, ACE inhibitors have been heralded as a "major therapeutic advance" (2) and a "new approach to the therapy of hypertension" (3). ACE inhibitors have been the subject of numerous review articles (3–9), many symposia (10–12), editorials (13), and texts (14) during the last two years.

Based primarily on clinical studies with captopril, the utility of ACE inhibitors in most forms of hypertension has been established. In addition, the beneficial effect of captopril in congestive heart failure (15–17) has led to its recent approval for this use. Because of the ubiquitousness of ACE and the expanding research to identify those diseases associated with elevations in ACE activity (sarcoidosis, Gaucher's disease, diabetes mellitus, and hyperthyroidism), clinical studies with ACE inhibitors may expand into other pathological states (8, 18, 19). That ACE inhibitors may be useful in limiting experimental infarct size has also been reported (20).

Recently, a focal point in the research on ACE inhibitors has been the mechanism(s) by which ACE inhibitors exert their antihypertensive effects. This topic has been addressed in several excellent recent reviews (7, 9, 21–23) and will only be briefly mentioned here. In this regard, it is generally accepted that the inhibition of plasma angiotensin-converting enzyme, although known

307

0362-1642/85/0415-0307$02.00

to occur with ACE inhibitors, does not sufficiently explain their antihypertensive effects. Because of this, several theories have been advanced to explain the antihypertensive activity of ACE inhibitors. These include (a) inhibition of angiotensin II-induced facilitation of sympathetic neurotransmission in blood vessels, (b) tissue-specific inhibition of ACE, possibly within the central nervous system, kidney, or vasculature, (c) other actions of ACE inhibitors unrelated to the inhibition of the direct effects of angiotensin II. These latter actions include potential postsynaptic α-blocking activities, potential elevations in bradykinin or other peptides (substance P, enkephalins, etc) degraded by ACE, and possible indirect effects of angiotensin II mediated via prostaglandin derivatives. Clarification of this controversy awaits additional comparative data on the actions of multiple ACE inhibitors with regard to each of the mechanisms specified above.

We are currently entering an era that will see a rapidly expanding armamentarium of ACE inhibitors. The race to develop such inhibitors has begun in earnest, and over the next few years we shall no doubt see an emerging literature on subtle differences in the pharmacological activity of the newer ACE inhibitors. Such differences will help to ellucidate the precise mechanism for their antihypertensive activity and may provide a rational basis for specific clinical implications for some of the newer agents.

This review focuses on the development of these newer ACE inhibitors, their structural relationship to captopril, and their current clinical status. Although I have attempted to present all of the ACE inhibitors under development, the rapid and dramatic growth in the plethora of available ACE inhibitors makes this task a formidable one. I have chosen to discuss only compounds on which published data, including recent abstracts, are available, and with only minor exceptions to review data generated within the last two years. No attempt has been made to review the voluminous patent literature.

ACE INHIBITORS FROM NATURAL PRODUCTS

The evolution of synthetic ACE inhibitors (Figure 1) began with the discovery that certain peptides isolated from the venom of the snake *Bothrops jararaca* were inhibitors of ACE (24). Of the several peptides isolated and examined for ACE inhibitory activity, the nonapeptide, later known as teprotide (SQ 20,881), was the most potent inhibitor [for reviews see (25–27)]. Since that discovery in the early 1970s, structure-activity correlations developed with the snake venom peptides have been used to synthesize small molecular-weight compounds with even greater bioavailability and affinity for ACE, and hence greater clinical utility. However, more recently, interest in the possibility of discovering novel structures (unrelated to teprotide or captopril) from natural products has been renewed.

COMPOUND	SOURCE	STRUCTURE	REFERENCE
TEPROTIDE	BOTHROPS JARARACA	NONAPEPTIDE	25
ANCOVENIN	STREPTOMYCES	HEXADECAPEPTIDE	28
ASPERGILLOMARASMINE	ASPERGILLUS COLLETOTRICHUM FUSARIUM PYRENOPHORA	A	29

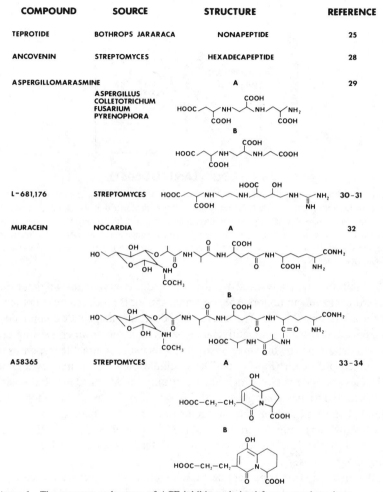

Figure 1   The structure and source of ACE inhibitors derived from natural products.

Ancovenin (28) is a hexadecapeptide isolated from streptomyces. It has been found to be approximately six-fold less potent than captopril as an ACE inhibitor. Other microorganism-derived peptide inhibitors (Figure 1) with even lower ACE inhibitory activity include the aspergillomarasmines (29), L-681,176 (30–31), and muramyl peptides (muraceins) (32). Clearly, the low inhibitory activity and minimal bioavailability of such agents precludes any direct therapeutic or clinical utility for them.

The utility of natural products produced from microorganisms to provide small molecular-weight structural leads for the future development of novel

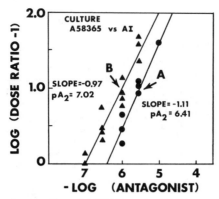

Figure 2 Schild plot for the effect of A58365A and A58365B to antagonize angiotensin I contractile responses in the isolated guinea pig ileum. Plot of the logarithm of dose ratio −1 against the negative logarithm of the molar concentration of antagonists yielded a straight line whose slope approximated one, indicating a competitive interaction of the antagonists with ACE. The intercept along the abcissa is the pA_2 value, which is equal to the negative logarithm of the dissociation constant (*i.e.* −log K_B).

ACE inhibitors was advanced by the recent discovery of the angiotensin-converting enzyme inhibitors A58365A and A58365B produced by streptomyces chromofuscus (33–34). These natural products are nonpeptide compounds. A58365A and B were competitive antagonists of angiotensin-converting enzyme as determined by the antagonism of angiotensin I contractile responses in the guinea pig ileum (Figure 2). These simple bicyclic dicarboxcylic acid molecules showed relatively high in vitro affinity for ACE and may be considered natural product analogues of the newer bicyclic ACE inhibitors (see below). The identification of these agents supports the contention that efforts directed toward isolating microbially derived ACE inhibitors may well provide an avenue for the development of second and third generation ACE inhibitors of novel structures.

Other naturally occurring peptide ACE inhibitors have been identified from mammalian sources. These include a peptide derived from fibrin (35), ACTH-related peptides (36), and metabolites of thyrotropin-releasing hormone (37). The physiological function of such endogenous peptide inhibitors is a subject of current research and remains to be clarified.

SULFUR-CONTAINING ACE INHIBITORS

Based on the ACE inhibitory activity of the nonapeptide, teprotide, and the contention that an orally effective ACE inhibitor would find utility in hypertension, Cushman & Ondetti generated an elegant SAR that led to the discovery of the first potent and orally active ACE inhibitor, captopril (25–27). This discovery was soon followed by the demonstration that captopril was effective in many animal models of hypertension and in almost all clinical forms of hypertension, including essential hypertension associated wth low or normal plasma renin levels.

The fact that the clinical use of captopril exceeded initial expectations spurred interest in the development of other ACE inhibitors. Initially, synthesis was directed toward compounds structurally similar to captopril (Figure 3). These included YS980 (36–39), SA446 (40–44), pivalopril (RHC 3659) (45–47), CL242,817 (48–50), and zofenopril (51), all sulfur-containing structures with an affinity for ACE lower than or similar to that of captopril. YS980 and SA446 are more lipophilic structures than captopril; hence, they may distribute to the central nervous system (CNS) to inhibit brain ACE to a greater extent than captopril. Pivalopril, CL242,817, and zofenopril contain protected sulfhydryl groups and may serve as prodrugs. More recently, chemists from both Ciba-Geigy (52) and Wyeth Laboratories (53, 54) independently reported on the synthesis of the bicyclic molecule WY-44,221, a compound shown to be 10–20 times more potent than captopril. It is interesting to note that such a minor chemical change could result in a marked improvement in ACE inhibition. In general, however, little novel chemistry and only minor pharmacological advantage emerged with these new sulfur-containing compounds.

Using computer graphics to postulate the favored spatial orientation of functional groups for ACE inhibition, Hassall and co-workers (55) designed the bicyclic rigid molecule compound III, which had in vitro activity close to that of captopril. Also using computer modeling to generate energy minimized conformations, Thorsett and colleagues (56) investigated a series of mercaptomethyl lactams similar to those previously reported by Klutchko and colleagues (57) and found that seven or eight membered lactam rings optimized ACE inhibitory activity. The mercapto lactam 5d compared favorably with captopril in terms of ACE inhibition in vitro. Both these latter sulfhydryl-containing compounds served as prototypes for the development of non-sulfhydryl rigid lactam ACE inhibitors (see below).

Of the sulfur-containing ACE inhibitors that followed in the wake of captopril, clinical studies have been reported only for pivalopril (47). These studies suggest that pivalopril has a rapid onset of action with a short duration based on serum ACE inhibition. No clinical data are reported on pivalopril in hypertensive patients or on the other sulfur-containing compounds, although zofenopril has been selected for clinical study (51).

During this flurry of chemical activity, captopril continued to be evaluated clinically. Initial clinical tests used relatively high doses of captopril to insure clinical efficacy. As clinical experience expanded, side effects attributed to captopril emerged (58–60). These included skin rashes and loss of taste, along with proteinurea and alterations in the haematopoietic system. Although the

COMPOUND	STRUCTURE	REFERENCE
CAPTOPRIL	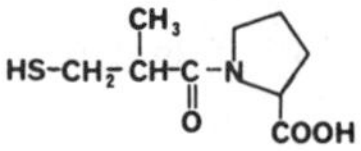	25-27
YS 980		36-39
SA 446	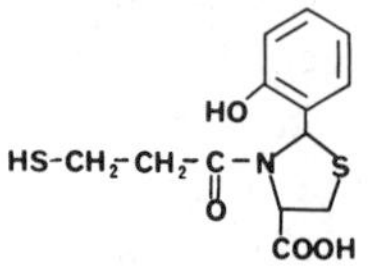	40-42
PIVALOPRIL (RHC 3659)	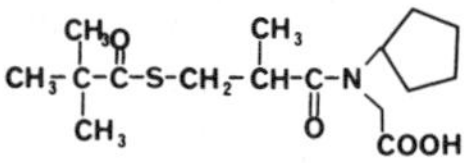	45-47
CL 242,817	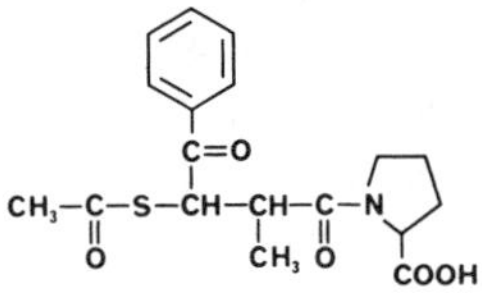	48-50
ZOFENOPRIL (SQ 26,991)	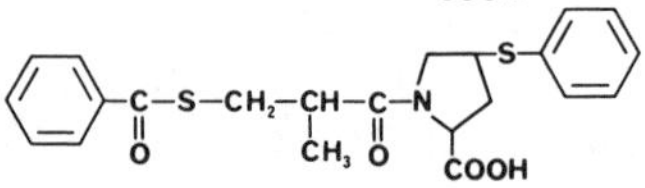	51
WY-44,221	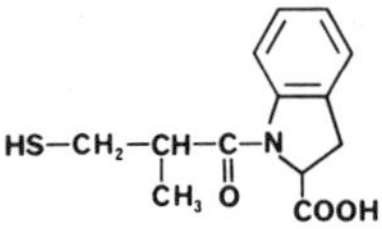	52-54
III	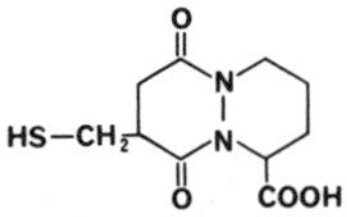	55
MERCAPTOLACTAM (5d)	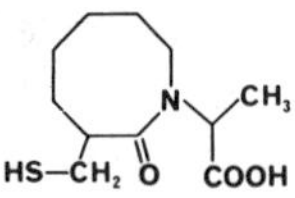	56

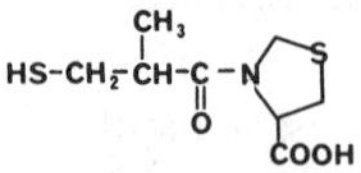

Figure 3   The structures of ACE inhibitors that contain sulfur.

cause of these side effects remains unclear, their resemblance to side effects produced by penicillamine, another sulfhydryl-containing molecule, led some to implicate captopril's sulfhydryl moiety as a causative factor (60). This possibility, coupled with the potential for multiple interactions of sulfur-containing molecules, led to a rapid redirection of synthetic effort in the development of ACE inhibitors, although reduced dosage has minimized the occurrence of side effects in the use of captopril (61, 62).

NON-SULFHYDRYL ACE INHIBITORS

Patchett and co-workers elegantly accomplished the replacement of the sulf-hydryl moiety in captopril by designing a series of substituted N-carboxymethyl-dipeptides (63) (Figure 4). The dicarboxylic acid compound, enalaprilic acid (MC422), was a potent inhibitor of ACE with approximately ten times greater affinity for ACE than captopril (64, 65). Although enalaprilic acid showed high affinity for ACE, oral bioavailability was poor in both animals (65) and man (66). This problem was partially overcome by the development of the ethyl ester, enalapril (MK421). Enalapril has become a prototype for a generation of ACE inhibitors that are prodrugs that must be hydrolyzed for ACE inhibition. Relative to captopril, enalapril has a slower onset of action (65, 67), which may be related both to the need for hydrolysis to the active moiety and to poor oral absorption (although oral absorption is improved compared to enalaprilic acid) (68). The major clinical advantage of enalapril resides in its relatively long duration of action (69, 70), which should permit once or at most twice daily dosing for maintenance of blood pressure reduction. In addition, unlike captopril, plasma ACE inhibition can be used as a rough index of plasma levels of enalapril, since enalapril-induced ACE inhibition was stable on storage whereas captopril-induced ACE inhibition was not (23). Although developed to minimize captopril-like side effects, mucocutaneous reactions (71, 72) and reversible leucopenia have been reported with enalapril (73). The occurrence of such side effects will be placed in perspective as the clinical use of enalapril expands pending its approval by the Food and Drug Administration.

During the development of enalapril, the lysine derivative of enalaprilic acid (lisinopril, MK521) was found to be a potent ACE inhibitor with affinity for ACE similar to enalaprilic acid. Lisinopril offered the singular advantage of oral activity similar to enalapril, in spite of the fact that it was a dicarboxylic acid (66, 74, 75). Blood pressure after lisinopril (2.5 and 5 mg) was significantly reduced for more than twenty-four hours in hypertensive patients, indicating that once daily dosing will be likely with this agent (76, 77).

The development of these two novel ACE inhibitors has opened a new era in the synthesis of ACE inhibitors. Shortly after the identification of enalapril and lisinopril, researchers at both Schering Corporation (78, 79) and Warner-Lambert/Parke-Davis Research Laboratories (80–82) independently reported on the synthesis and development of indolapril (SCH31846, CI907), a close analog of enalapril. Like enalapril, indolapril is a prodrug that must be hydrolyzed to the diacid for ACE inhibition. Indolapril's duration of action appears similar to that of enalapril. The ethyl ester, CI-906, is an analog of both enalapril and indolapril (80, 81). However, unlike these other ethyl ester derivatives, CI906 showed relatively high affinity for ACE, an affinity that was

COMPOUND	STRUCTURE	REFERENCE
ENALAPRIL (MK-421)	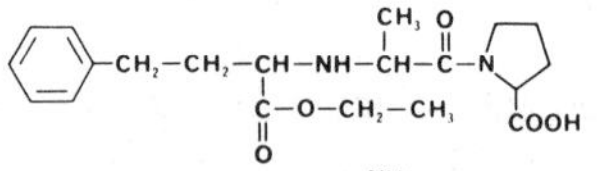	63
LISINOPRIL (MK-521)	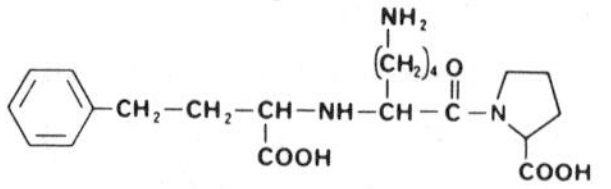	74-77
INDOLAPRIL (CI 907) (SCH 31846)	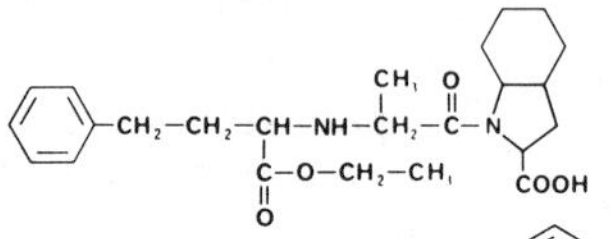	78-82
CI 906	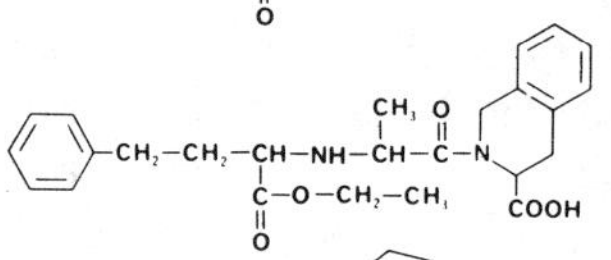	80-81
RO31-2848	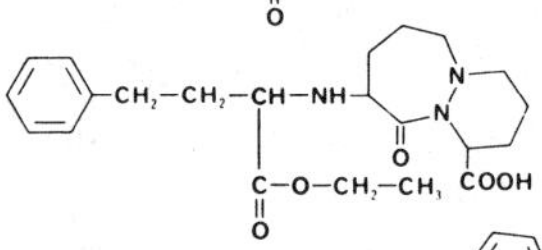	83
CGS 14824A	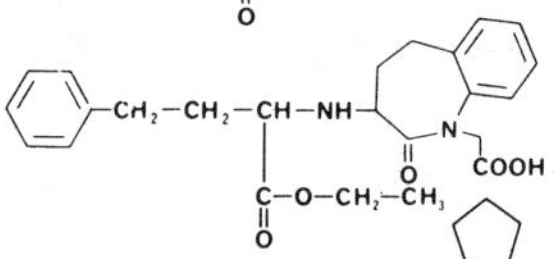	84-85
HOE 498	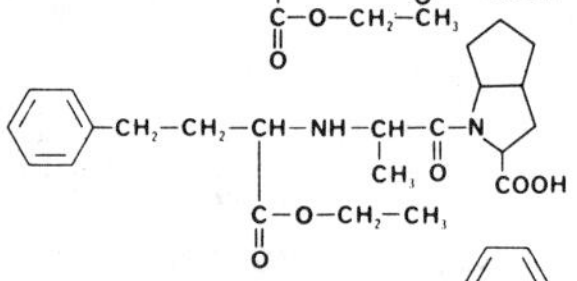	86-88
CGS13945	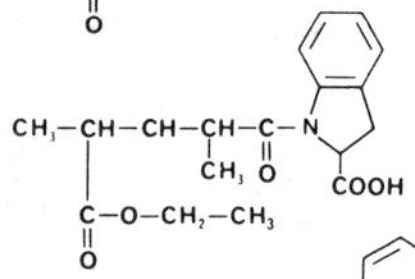	89-93
20	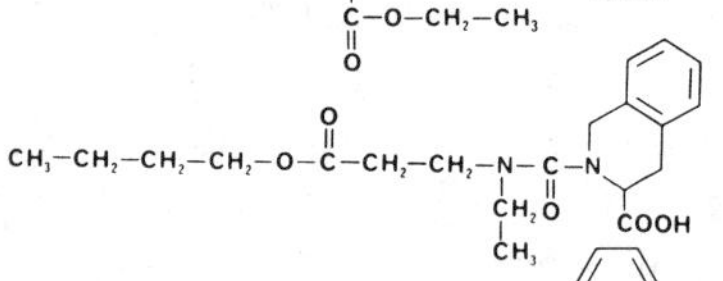	94
REV6000-A	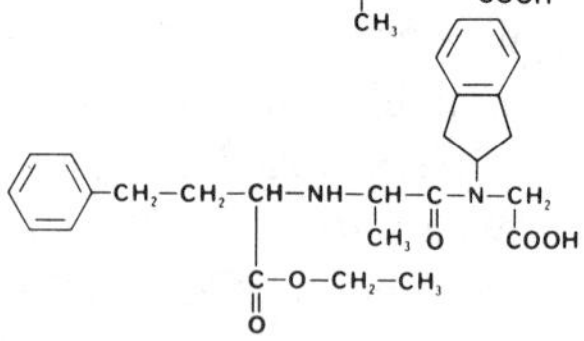	95-96

Figure 4 The structures of ACE inhibitors that do not contain sulfur or sulfhydryl moieties.

only three-fold less than that of its diacid metabolite (81). Why CI-906 showed such high affinity for ACE relative to enalapril and indolapril remains to be determined. Should this in vitro activity be translated to the in vivo situation, CI-906 might have a more rapid onset of action (due to activity of the parent compound) and a longer duration of action (due to activity of the diacid) than enalapril or CI-907. However, initial preclinical data evaluating inhibition of an angiotensin I pressor response in conscious rats and dogs did not reveal any major differences in the time course among these three ACE inhibitors (80). Clinically, CI-906 (5 and 10 mg, p.o.) lowered blood pressure for twelve to twenty-four hours without adverse effects in hypertensive patients (82), effectiveness similar to enalapril and lisinopril. CI-925, the dimethoxy derivative of CI-906, has a rapid onset and long duration of ACE inhibition in preclinical studies and is currently also undergoing clinical evaluation (H. Kaplan, personal communication).

Following the identification of indolapril and CI-906, several additional bicyclic ACE inhibitors have been synthesized. These include bicyclic lactam derivatives that possess a seven-membered lactam ring as in R031-2848 (83) and CGS14824A (84), the active isomer of the seven-membered lactams reported by Parsons et al (85). The increase in lactam ring size from five and six carbons improved affinity for ACE.

The bicyclic ACE inhibitor HOE-498 is a structural variant of enalapril and indolapril. Based on blockade of angiotensin I (AI) pressor response, intravenously administered HOE 498 showed similar potency to enalapril, yet oral or intraduodenal administration of HOE-498 resulted in approximately ten-fold greater potency than enalapril (86). Thus the bioavailability of HOE-498 was greater than that of enalapril, consistent with previous observations suggesting the relatively poor oral bioavailability of enalapril. The greater oral activity of HOE-498 relative to enalapril was also reflected in a better reduction in blood pressure and inhibition of plasma and tissue ACE following oral administration to stroke-prone, spontaneously hypertensive rats (87). Initial reports (87) with HOE-498 also suggest a different distribution of tissue ACE inhibitory effectiveness (heart, adrenal, and brain ACE were markedly inhibited by HOE-498 and not by MK-421 at 10 mg/kg, p.o.). Furthermore, clinical data with HOE-498 confirm the high potency and long duration of activity with regard to plasma ACE inhibition in normal volunteers (88). Should these differences observed with HOE-498 relative to indolapril or enalapril be maintained with further scrutiny, the dramatic effect on pharmacological activity produced by minor structural modification of ACE inhibitors will become obvious.

As a departure from the phenethylamine ester side chain in previously discovered ACE inhibitors, scientists at Ciba-Geigy and Tanabe Seiyaku Company have synthesized bicyclic ACE inhibitors with markedly different side chains (Figure 4). This modification resulted in a disappointing reduction in activity. Both these compounds, CGS 13945 (89–93) and compound 20 (94), are esters that must be hydrolyzed for in vivo ACE inhibitory activity. In vitro affinity for ACE of the diacid forms of these molecules, as well as in vivo activity of the esters, was lower than that reported for compounds with the phenethylamine side chain, such as in enalapril. In fact, CGS 13945, although possessing a long duration of action, was less effective than captopril in inhibiting the AI pressor response in both rats and dogs after intravenous and oral administration (90). Likewise, CGS 13945 was less potent in inhibiting human plasma ACE activity after oral administration than was captopril (92, 93). The effectiveness of CGS 13945 in hypertensive patients has not yet been reported.

Lastly, REV 6000A is a newly revealed ACE inhibitor of a nonrigid bicyclic structure in which the proline nitrogen is not enclosed in a ring structure. Although REV 6000A possesses a long duration of action, it appears to be less potent than enalapril after oral administration to animals (95, 96). Clinical data on this compound are not yet available.

PHOSPHOROUS-CONTAINING ACE INHIBITORS

In a search for ACE inhibitors with novel properties, Holmquist & Vallee (97) and Galardy (98–100) were the first to demonstrate that the carboxyl or mercapto moiety proposed as the ligand for the active site zinc ion on ACE could be replaced by a phosphorous group with the retention of reasonable ACE inhibitory activity (Figure 5). This observation paved the way for Thorsett and colleagues (101) in the Merck Sharp & Dohme Laboratories and Powell and colleagues (102) from the Squibb Institute for Medical Research to design phosphorous-containing molecules as potential candidates for clinical therapy.

As with other described ACE inhibitors, SQ 28,555 is a prodrug with in vitro ACE inhibitory activity similar to that of captopril. SQ 28,555 was orally effective in animal studies and had a relatively long duration of action based on reductions in mean arterial pressure following oral administration in animals (102). Although clinical data on phosphorous-containing ACE inhibitors has not yet been reported, this new class of ACE inhibitors, when studied in more detail, may produce a new profile of pharmacological activity.

MISCELLANEOUS INHIBITORS

On route to the discovery of the potent ACE inhibitors previously mentioned, several other compounds have been reported (Figure 6). Reports of di-peptide and tri-peptides as weak inhibitors of angiotensin-converting enzyme have prompted Almquist and colleagues (103–106) to direct a synthetic effort toward the development of potent and orally effective tri-peptide analogs as inhibitors of ACE. In general, this effort has not met with great success. However, the most recent preclinical demonstration of antihypertensive activity following the oral administration of peptides that inhibit ACE may prompt further synthetic effort in this area (107). The possibility of success here must be

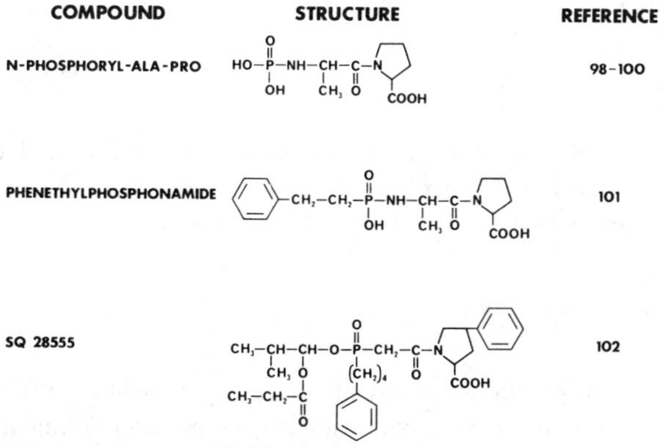

COMPOUND	STRUCTURE	REFERENCE
N-PHOSPHORYL-ALA-PRO		98-100
PHENETHYLPHOSPHONAMIDE		101
SQ 28555		102

Figure 5 The structure of ACE inhibitors that contain phosphorous.

tempered by the suggestion that, although such peptides possess ACE inhibitory activity, the antihypertensive activity may result from other actions of these peptides.

Replacement of the amide moiety in compounds such as captopril with a ketone has resulted in active ACE inhibitors, although activity was somewhat lower than that found for the corresponding amide analogs (108). In vivo and clinical data on such compounds are not available.

Harris and colleagues (109) have demonstrated that hydroxamate derivatives of di-peptides, known to be inhibitors of other zinc-containing enzymes, are

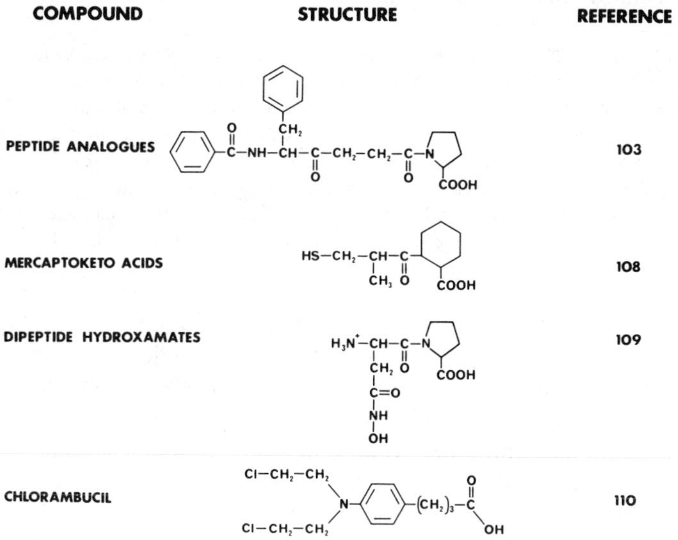

COMPOUND	STRUCTURE	REFERENCE
PEPTIDE ANALOGUES		103
MERCAPTOKETO ACIDS		108
DIPEPTIDE HYDROXAMATES		109
CHLORAMBUCIL		110

Figure 6 The structure of miscellaneous ACE inhibitors.

also relatively weak inhibitors of angiotensin-converting enzyme. Such inhibitors appear less potent than captopril and may lack specificity for angiotensin-converting enzyme. Furthermore, no in vivo data are reported on di-peptide hydroxamates.

Chlorambucil and its proline derivative have been reported to produce irreversible inhibition of ACE (110). Because this anticarcinogenic agent is a nitrogen mustard alkylating agent, specificity of action may be minimal.

SUMMARY AND CONCLUSIONS

The availability of potent and orally effective angiotensin-converting enzyme inhibitors will no doubt have a major impact on the future clinical therapy of hypertension and probably other disease states. It remains the challenge of the pharmacologist to decipher the subtle differences in the pharmacological profile of activity of these various ACE inhibitors and to capitalize on that information in order to determine the precise mechanism or mechanisms responsible for the antihypertensive activity of this class of agents. With the availability of these agents, this will be the challenge of the next few years.

The area of research involving ACE inhibitors, from their synthesis to the unravelling of their pharmacological activities, is a major example of a therapeutic breakthrough and benefit resulting entirely from the dedication and motivation of research accomplished within the pharmaceutical industry. Irvine H. Page has made this point before with reference to the overall development of antihypertensive agents (111). In his words:

> It must be evident that this was an extraordinary period in the history of the treatment of hypertension. Within about fifteen years, a panoply of highly effective drugs had been made available wholly through the skills of chemists in the pharmaceutical industry. These scientists have received little or no recognition by the medical community for this amazing achievement. . . . It is important to realize that drug innovation begins with investigators who work in the chemical laboratories in cooperation with pharmacologists, is followed by studies in patients by clinicians, and results in large-scale government finance and committee-directed studies. Each of these steps has its importance, but to date the first has been generally ignored.

The perceived importance of this group of antihypertensive agents has fostered considerable competition within the pharmaceutical industry. This is perhaps best reflected in the number of patents filed on ACE inhibitors and in the dual development of chemical compounds by different pharmaceutical companies (i.e. indolapril, WY44,221 and CGS14824A). This healthy competition will undoubtedly result in the improved therapy of hypertension, congestive heart failure, and other disease states.

ACKNOWLEDGEMENTS

I am grateful to Dr. Jon Mynderse for his helpful discussion and assistance, to Ms. Kathryn Schenck for preparing the chemical structures, to Ms. Laura Wittenauer for compiling the references, and to Ms. Elaine Gardner for her expert typing of the manuscript.

Literature Cited

1. Ondetti, M. A., Rubin, B., Cushman, D. W. 1977. Design of specific inhibitors of angiotensin-converting enzyme: New class of orally active antihypertensive agents. *Science* 196:441–43
2. Stronger role forecast for ACE inhibitors. 1984. *Practitioner* 228:368–69
3. Johnston, C. I., Arnolda, L., Hiwatari, M. 1984. Angiotensin-converting enzyme inhibitors in the treatment of hypertension. *Drugs* 27:271–77
4. Ondetti, M. A., Cushman, D. W. 1982. Enzymes of the renin-angiotensin system and their inhibitors. *Ann. Rev. Biochem.* 51:283–308
5. Antonaccio, M. J. 1982. Angiotensin-converting enzyme (ACE) inhibitors. *Ann. Rev. Pharmacol. Toxicol.* 22:57–87
6. Petrillo, E. W. Jr., Ondetti, M. A. 1982. Angiotensin-converting enzyme inhibitors: Medicinal chemistry and biological actions. *Med. Res. Rev.* 2(1):1–41
7. Van Zwieten, P.A., DeJonge, A., Timmermans, P. B. 1983. Inhibitors of the angiotensin-I converting enzyme as antihypertensive drugs. *Pharmaceut. Wklbd. Sci. Ed.* 5:197–204
8. Studdy, P. R., Lapworth, R., Bird, R. 1983. Angiotensin-converting enzyme and its clinical significance—A review. *J. Clin. Pathol.* 36:938–47
9. Antonaccio, M. J. 1983. Development and pharmacology of angiotensin converting enzyme inhibitors. *J. Pharmacol.* 14:29–45
10. Doyle, A. E., ed. 1982. Symposium on angiotensin converting enzyme inhibition. *Clin. Exp. Pharmacol. Physiol.* 6(Suppl. 7):1–144
11. Zanchetti, A., Tarazi, R. C., eds. 1982. Symposium on angiotensin converting enzyme inhibition: A developing concept. *Am. J. Cardiol.* 49:1381–580
12. Abrams, W. B. 1984. Research forum: Angiotensin-converting enzyme inhibitors. *Fed. Proc.* 43:1313–50
13. Dargie, H. J., Ball, S. G., Atkinson, A. B., Robertson, J. I. S. 1983. Converting enzyme inhibitors in hypertension and heart failure. *Br. Heart J.* 49:305–8
14. Doyle, A. E., Bearn, A. G., eds. 1984. *Hypertension and the Angiotensin System Therapeutic Approaches.* New York: Raven. 304 pp.
15. Awan, N. A., Massie, B. M. 1982. Therapy of severe chronic congestive heart failure. *Am. Heart J.* 104: 1125–26
16. Sullivan, J. M. 1983. Drug suppression of the angiotensin system in congestive heart failure. *Ann. Rev. Med.* 34:169–77
17. Romankiewicz, J. A., Brogden, R. N., Heel, R. C., Speight, T. M., Avery G. S. 1983. Captopril: An update review of its pharmacological properties and therapeutic efficacy in congestive heart failure. *Drugs* 25:6–40
18. Rohatgi, P. K. 1982. Serum angiotensin converting enzyme in pulmonary disease. *Lung* 160:287–301
19. Smallridge, R. C., Rogers, J., Verma, P. S. 1983. Serum angiotensin-converting enzyme. Alterations in hyperthyroidism, hypothyroidism, and subacute thyroiditis. *J. Am. Med. Assoc.* 250:2489–93
20. Ertl, G., Kloner, R. A., Alexander, R. W., Braunwald, E. 1982. Limitation of experimental infarct size by an angiotensin-converting enzyme inhibitor. *Circulation* 65:40–8
21. Unger, T., Ganten, D., Lang, R. E. 1983. Converting enzyme inhibitors: Antihypertensive drugs with unexpected mechanisms. *Trends Pharmacol. Sci.* 4:514–19
22. Unger, T., Ganten, D., Lang, R. E. 1983. Pharmacology of converting enzyme inhibitors: New aspects. *Clin. Exper. Hyper.* A5:1333–54
23. Cohen, M. L., Kurz, K. 1983. Captopril and MK-421: Stability on storage, distribution to the central nervous system, and onset of activity. *Fed. Proc.* 42:171–75
24. Bakhle, Y. S. 1968. Conversion of angiotensin I to angiotensin II by cell-free extracts of dog lung. *Nature* 220:919–20
25. Cushman, D. W., Ondetti, M. A. 1980. Inhibitors of angiotensin-converting enzyme for treatment of hypertension. *Biochem. Pharmacol.* 29:1871–77

26. Cushman, D. W., Ondetti, M. A. 1982. Inhibitors of angiotensin-converting enzyme. *Chemtech* 12:620–24

27. Cushman, D. W., Cheung, H. S., Sabo, E. F., Ondetti, M. A. 1982. Development and design of specific inhibitors of angiotensin-converting enzyme. *Am. J. Cardiol.* 49:1390–94

28. Kido, Y., Hamakado, T., Yoshida, T., Anno, M., Motoki, Y. 1983. Isolation and characterization of ancovenin, a new inhibitor of angiotensin I converting enzyme, produced by actinomycetes. *J. Antibiot.* 36:1295–99

29. Mikami, Y., Suzuki, T. 1983. Novel microbial inhibitors of angiotensin-converting enzyme, aspergillomarasmines A and B. *Agric. Biol. Chem.* 47:2693–95

30. Huang, L., Rowin, G., Dunn, J., Sykes, R., Dobna, R., et al. 1983. Discovery of an angiotensin converting enzyme inhibitor, L-681,176 in the culture filtrate of *streptomyces sp. 83rd Ann. Meet. Am. Soc. Microbiol. New Orleans, 6–11 March 1983*, p. 244 (Abstr.)

31. Huang, L., Rowin, G., Dunn, J., Sykes, R., Dobna, R., et al. 1984. Discovery, purification and characterization of the angiotensin converting enzyme inhibitor, L-681,176, produced by *streptomyces sp.* MA 5143a. *J. Antibiot.* 37:462–68

32. Singh, P. D., Johnson, J. H. 1984. Muraceins—Muramyl peptides produced by *nocardia orientalis* as angiotensin-converting enzyme inhibitors. *J. Antibiot.* 37:336–43

33. Dubus, R., Fukuda, D., Samlaska, S., Baker, P., Hunt, A. et al. 1984. Isolation of A58365A and A58365B, angiotensin converting enzyme inhibitors produced by streptomyces chromofuscus. *84th Ann. Meet. Am. Soc. Microbiol., St. Louis, 4–9 March 1984*, p. 198 (Abstr.)

34. Hunt, A. H., Mynderse, J. S., Maciak, G. M., Jones, N. D., Samlaska, S., et al. 1984. Structure elucidation of A58365A and A58365B, angiotensin converting enzyme inhibitors produced by streptomyces chromofuscus. *187th Natl. Meet. Am. Chem. Soc., St. Louis, 8–13 April 1984*, p. 145 (Abstr.)

35. Saldeen, T., Ryan, J. W., Berryer, P. 1981. A peptide derived from fibrin-(ogen) inhibits angiotensin converting enzyme and potentiates the effects of bradykinin. *Thrombosis Res.* 23:465–70

36. Verma, P. S., Miller, R. L., Taylor, R. E., O'Donohue, T. L., Adams, R. G. 1982. Inhibition of canine lung angiotensin converting enzyme by ACTH and

structurally related peptides. *Biochem. Biophys. Res. Commun.* 104:1484–88

37. MacGregor, J. S., Resnick, L. M., Laragh, J. H. 1982. Metabolites of thyrotropin releasing hormone inhibit angiotensin converting enzyme *in vitro*. *Biochem. Biophys. Res. Commun.* 109:556–61

38. Unger, T., Rockhold, R. W., Schaz, K., Vescei, P., Bonner, G., et al. 1979. A novel orally active converting-enzyme inhibitor YS 980: Effects on blood pressure in spontaneously hypertensive rats. *Clin. Sci.* 57:157s–60s

39. Funae, Y., Komori, T., Sasaki, D., Yamamoto, K. 1980. Inhibitor of angiotensin I converting enzyme: (4R)-3-[(2S)-3-mercapto-2-methylpropranoyl]-4-thiazolidinecarboxylic acid (YS-980). *Biochem. Pharmacol.* 29:1543–47

40. Abe, Y., Miura, K., Imanishi, M., Yukimura, T., Komori, T., et al. 1980. Effects of an orally active converting enzyme inhibitor (YS-980) on renal function in dogs. *J. Pharmacol. Exp. Ther.* 214:166–70

41. Komori, T., Yamamoto, K. 1981. Effects of YS-980, an orally active converting enzyme inhibitor, on blood pressure in normotensive and hypertensive rats. *Jpn. J. Pharmacol.* 31:401–7

42. Iso, T., Yamauchi, H., Suda, H., Nakata, K., Nishimura, K., et al., 1981. A new potent inhibitor of converting enzyme: (2R,4R)-2-(2-hydroxyphenyl)-3-(3-mercaptopropionyl)-4-thiazolidinecarboxylic acid (SA446). *Jpn. J. Pharmacol.* 31:875–82

43. Unger, T., Yukimura, T., Marin-Grez, M., Lang, R. E., Rascher, W., et al. 1982. SA446, a new orally active converting enzyme inhibitor: Antihypertensive action and comparison with captopril in stroke-prone spontaneously hypertensive rats. *Eur. J. Pharmacol.* 78:411–20

44. Takata, Y., DiNicolantonio, R., Hutchinson, J. S., Mendelsohn, F. A. O., Doyle, A. E. 1982. *In vivo* comparison of three orally active inhibitors of angiotensin-converting enzyme. *Am. J. Cardiol.* 49:1502–4

45. Schwab, A., Weinryb, I., Macerata, R., Rogers, W., Suh, J., et al. 1983. Inhibition of angiotensin-converting enzyme by derivatives of 3-mercapto-2-methylpropanoyl glycine. *Biochem. Pharmacol.* 32:1957–60

46. Wolf, P. S., Mann, W. S., Suh, J. T., Loev, B., Smith, R. D. 1984. Angiotensin-converting enzyme inhibitory and antihypertensive activities of pivalopril [RHC 3659-(S)]. *Fed. Proc.* 43:1322–25

47. Burnier, M., Turini, G. A., Brunner, H. R., Porchet, M., Kruithof, D., Vukovich, R. A., Gavras, H. 1981. RHC 3659: A new orally active angiotensin converting enzyme inhibitor in normal volunteers. *Br. J. Clin. Pharmacol.* 12:893–99

48. Lai, F. M., Chan, P. S., Cervoni, P., Tanikella, T., Shepherd, C., et al. 1982. Antihypertensive activity of [S-(R*,S*)]-1-[3-(acetylthio)-3-benzoyl-2-methylpropionyl] - L - proline (CL 242,817), an inhibitor of angiotensin converting enzyme (ACE). *Fed. Proc.* 41:1647

49. McEvoy, F. J., Lai, F. M., Albright, J. D. 1983. Antihypertensive agents: Angiotensin converting enzyme inhibitors. 1-[3-(acylthio)-3-aroylpropionyl]-L-prolines. *J. Med. Chem.* 26:381–93

50. Lai, F. M., Cervoni, P., Tanikella, T., Shepherd, C., Quirk, G., et al. 1983. Some *in vitro* and *in vivo* studies of a new angiotensin I-converting enzyme inhibitor [[S - (R*,S*)] - 1 - [(3 - Acetylthio) - 3 - benzoyl - 2 - methylpropionyl] - L - proline] (CL 242,817) in comparison with captopril. *Drug Develop. Res.* 3:261–69

51. Dean, A. V., Kripalani, K. J., Migdalof, B. H. 1984. Disposition of SQ 26,991 (zofenopril) and SQ 26,900, new angiotensin converting enzyme (ACE) inhibitors in rats. *Fed. Proc.* 43:349

52. Stanton, J. L., Gruenfeld, N., Babiarz, J. E., Ackerman, M. H., Friedmann, R. C., et al. 1983. Angiotensin converting enzyme inhibitors: N-substituted monocyclic and bicyclic amino acid derivatives. *J. Med. Chem.* 26:1267–76

53. Kim, D. H., Guinosso, C. J., Buzby, G. C. Jr., Herbst, D. R., McCaully, R. J., et al. 1983. (Mercaptopropanoyl)indoline-2-carboxylic acids and related compounds as potent angiotensin converting enzyme inhibitors and antihypertensive agents. *J. Med. Chem.* 26:394–403

54. Lappe, R. W., Kocmund, S., Todt, J. A., Wendt, R. L. 1984. Effects of Wy-44,221, a new angiotensin converting enzyme inhibitor, on regional vascular resistance in the conscious SHR. *Fed. Proc.* 43:554

55. Hassall, C. H., Krohn, A., Moody, C. J., Thomas, W. A. 1982. The design of a new group of angiotensin-converting enzyme inhibitors. *FEBS Letts.* 147:175–79

56. Thorsett, E. D., Harris, E. E., Aster, S., Peterson, E. R., Taub, D., Patchett, A. A. 1983. Dipeptide mimics. Conformationally restricted inhibitors of angiotensin-converting enzyme. *Biochem. Bio-phys. Res. Commun.* 111:166–71

57. Klutchko, S., Hoefle, M. L. 1981. Synthesis and angiotensin-converting enzyme inhibitory activity of 3-(mercaptomethyl)-2-oxo-1-pyrrolidineacetic acids and 3-(mercaptomethyl)-2-oxo-1-piperidineacetic acids. *J. Med. Chem.* 24:104–9

58. Wilkin, J. K., Hammond, J. J., Kirkendall, W. M. 1980. The captopril-induced eruption. A possible mechanism: Cutaneous kinin potentiation. *Arch. Dermatol.* 116:902–5

59. Waeber, B., Gavras, I., Brunner, H. R., Gavras, H. 1981. Safety and efficacy of chronic therapy with captopril in hypertensive patients: An update. *J. Clin. Pharmacol.* 21:508–16

60. Rotmensch, H. H., Vlasses, P. H., Ferguson, R. K. 1982. Inhibition of angiotensin-converting enzyme: Therapeutic implications. *Israel. J. Med. Sci.* 18:981–85

61. Veterans Administration Cooperative Study Group on Antihypertensive Agents. 1982. Captopril: evaluation of low doses, twice-daily doses and the addition of diuretic for the treatment of mild to moderate hypertension. *Clin. Sci.* 63:443s–45s

62. Drayer, J. I. M., Weber, M. A. 1983. Monotherapy of essential hypertension with a converting-enzyme inhibitor. *Hypertension* 5:III–108–13

63. Patchett, A. A., Harris, E., Tristram, E. W., Wyvratt, M. J., Wu, M. T., et al. 1980. A new class of angiotensin-converting enzyme inhibitors. *Nature* 288:280–83

64. Gross, D. M., Sweet, C. S., Ulm, E. H., Backlund, E. P., Morris, A. A. et al. 1981. Effect of N-[(S)-1-carboxy-3-phenylpropyl]-L-Ala-L-Pro and its ethyl ester (MK-421) on angiotensin converting enzyme *in vitro* and angiotensin I pressor responses *in vivo*. *J. Pharmacol. Exp. Ther.* 216:552–57

65. Sweet, C. S. 1983. Pharmacological properties of the converting enzyme inhibitor, enalapril maleate (MK-421). *Fed. Proc.* 42:167–70

66. Biollaz, J., Burnier, M., Turini, G. A., Brunner, D. B., Porchet, M., et al. 1981. Three new long-acting converting-enzyme inhibitors: Relationship between plasma converting-enzyme activity and response to angiotensin I. *Clin. Pharmacol. Ther.* 29:665–70

67. Cohen, M. L., Kurz, K. D. 1982. Angiotensin converting enzyme inhibition in tissues from spontaneously hypertensive rats after treatment with

captopril or MK-421. *J. Pharmacol. Exp. Ther.* 220:63–69

68. Cohen, M. L., Kurz, K. D., Schenck, K. W. 1983. Tissue angiotensin converting enzyme inhibition as an index of the disposition of enalapril (MK-421) and metabolite MK-422. *J. Pharmacol. Exp. Ther.* 226:192–96

69. Abrams, W. B., Davies, R. O., Ferguson, R. K. 1984. Overview: The role of angiotensin-converting enzyme inhibitors in cardiovascular therapy. *Fed. Proc.* 43:1314–21

70. Gavras, H., Waeber, B., Gavras, I., Biollaz, J., Brunner, H. R., Davies, R. O. 1981. Antihypertensive effect of the new oral angiotensin converting enzyme inhibitor "MK-421". *Lancet* 2:543–46

71. Kubo, S. H., Cody, R. J. 1984. Enalapril, a rash, and captopril. *Ann. Int. Med.* 100:616

72. Vlasses, P. H., Rotmensch, H. H., Ferguson, R. K., and Sheaffer, S. L. 1982. "Scalded mouth" caused by angiotensin-converting enzyme inhibitors. *Br. Med. J.* 284:1672–73

73. Studer, A., Vetter, W. 1982. Reversible leucopenia associated with angiotensin-converting-enzyme inhibitor MK-421. *Lancet* 1:458

74. Brunner, D. B., Desponds, G., Biollaz, J., Keller, I., Ferber, F., et al. 1981. Effect of a new angiotensin converting enzyme inhibitor MK 421 and its lysine analogue on the components of the renin system in healthy subjects. *Br. J. Clin. Pharmac.* 11:461–67

75. Ulm, E. H., Hichens, M., Gomez, H. J., Till, A. E., Hand, E., et al. 1982. Enalapril maleate and a lysine analogue (MK-521): Disposition in man. *Br. J. Clin. Pharmac.* 14:357–62

76. Rotmensch, H. H., Vincent, M., Vlasses, P. H., Swanson, B. N., Irvin, J. D., et al. 1984. Initial evaluation of the non-sulfhydryl-containing converting enzyme inhibitor MK-521 in hypertensive humans. *Fed. Proc.* 43:1333–35

77. Rotmensch, H. H., Vlasses, P. H., Swanson, B. N., Irvin, J. D., Harris, K. E., et al. 1984. Antihypertensive efficacy of once daily MK-521, a new nonsulfhydryl angiotensin-converting enzyme inhibitor. *Am. J. Cardiol.* 53:116–19

78. Baum, T., Sybertz, E. J., Watkins, R. W., Ahn, H. S., Nelson, S., et al. 1983. Antihypertensive activity of SCH 31846, a non-sulfhydryl angiotensin-converting enzyme inhibitor. *J. Cardiovasc. Pharmacol.* 5:655–67

79. Sybertz, E. J., Baum, T., Ahn, H. S., Nelson, S., Eynon, E., et al. 1983. Angiotensin-converting enzyme inhibi-

tory activity of SCH 31846, a new non-sulfhyrdryl inhibitor. *J. Cardiovasc. Pharmacol.* 5:643–54

80. Ryan, M. J., Boucher, D. M., Cohen, D. M., Olszewski, B. J., Singer, R. M., et al. 1984. Antihypertensive profile of the angiotensin-converting enzyme inhibitors CI-906 and CI-907. *Fed. Proc.* 43:1330–32

81. Kaplan, H. R., Cohen, D. M., Essenburg, A. D., Major, T. C., Mertz, T. E., et al. 1984. CI-906 and CI-907: New orally active nonsulfhydryl angiotensin-converting enzyme inhibitors. *Fed. Proc.* 43:1326–29

82. Gavras, I., Vlahakos, D., Melby, J. C., Gavras, H. 1984. Effects of the angiotensin converting enzyme inhibitor CI-906 on patients with essential hypertension. *Clin. Res.* 32:480A

83. Attwood, M. R., Francis, R. J., Hassall, C. H., Krohn, A., Lawton, G., et al. 1984. New potent inhibitors of angiotensin converting enzyme. *FEBS Letts.* 165:201–6

84. Miller, D., Hopkins, M. F., Tonnesen, S. T., Watkins, B. E. 1983. Antihypertensive assessment of CGS 14824A, an orally effective angiotensin-converting enzyme (ACE) inhibitor. *Pharmacologist* 25:102

85. Parsons, W. H., Davidson, J. L., Taub, D., Aster, S. D., Thorsett, E. D., Patchett, A. A. 1983. Benzolactams. A new class of converting enzyme inhibitors. *Biochem. Biophys. Res. Commun.* 117:108–13

86. Becker, R. H. A., Scholkens, B. A., Unger, T., Linz, W. 1983. HOE 498: An orally active non-sulfhydryl ACE-inhibitor. *Naunyn-Schmiedeberg's Arch. Pharmacol.* 324:R42

87. Unger, T., Scholkens, B. A., Ganten, D., Lang, R. E. 1983. Chronic administration of the novel converting enzyme inhibitor HOE 498 in spontaneously hypertensive rats (SHRSP): Comparison with MK 421. *Naunyn-Schmiedeberg's Arch. Pharmacol.* 324:R43

88. Witte, P. U., Metzger, H., Irmisch, R. 1983. Pharmacodynamics of a new orally active long acting angiotensin converting enzyme inhibitor (HOE 498) in healthy subjects. *IRCS Med. Sci.* 11:1053

89. Gruenfeld, N., Stanton, J. L., Yuan, A. M., Ebetino, F. H., Browne, L. J., et al. 1983. Angiotensin converting enzyme inhibitors: 1-glutarylindoline-2-carboxylic acid derivatives. *J. Med. Chem.* 26:1277–82

90. Chen, D. S., Watkins, B. E., Ku, E. C., Dotson, R. A., Burrell, R. D. Jr. 1984. Pharmacological profiles of two new

angiotensin-converting enzyme (ACE) inhibitors: CGS 13945 and CGS 13934. *Drug Develop. Res.* 4:167–78

91. Miller, D., Watkins, B. E., Hopkins, M. F., Tonnesen, S. T., Van Orsdell, D. 1984. Antihypertensive assessment of two new angiotensin-converting enzyme (ACE) inhibitors: CGS 13945 and CGS 13934. *Drug Develop. Res.* 4:179–89

92. Chen, D. S., Brunner, H. R., Waeber, B. 1984. *In vitro* response of plasma angiotensin converting enzyme to precursors and active forms of converting enzyme inhibitors. *Curr. Ther. Res.* 35:253–62

93. des Combes, B. J., Turini, G. A., Brunner, H. R., Porchet, M., Chen, D. S., et al. 1983. CGS 13945: A new orally active angiotensin-converting enzyme inhibitor in normal volunteers. *J. Cardiovasc. Pharmacol.* 5:511–16

94. Hayashi, K., Nunami, K. I., Sakai, K., Ozaki, Y., Kato, J., et al. 1983. Studies on angiotensin converting enzyme inhibitors. II. Syntheses and angiotensin converting enzyme inhibitory activities of carboxyethylcarbamoyl-1,2,3,4-tetrahydroisoquinoline-3-carboxylic acid derivatives. *Chem. Pharm. Bull.* 31:3553–61

95. Mann, W. S., Samuels, A. I., Bauer, K., Schwab, A., Wolf, P. S., et al. 1984. Indalapril (I), a new non-sulfur containing ACE inhibitor: Pharmacological characterization in rats and dogs. *Fed. Proc.* 43:733

96. Town, C., Knipe, J. O., Freiler, L., Tantillo, N., Magnien, E., et al. 1984. The disposition of indalapril (REV 6000-A(SS)), an orally active, non-sulfhydryl angiotensin-converting enzyme inhibitor, in animals. *Fed. Proc.* 43:958

97. Holmquist, B., Vallee, B. L. 1979. Metal-coordinating substrate analogs as inhibitors of metalloenzymes. *Proc. Natl. Acad. Sci. USA* 76:6216–20

98. Galardy, R. E. 1980. Inhibition of angiotensin converting enzyme with N^{α}-phosphoryl-L-alanyl-L-proline and N^{α}-phosphoryl-L-valyl-L-tryptophan. *Biochem. Biophys. Res. Commun.* 97:94–99

99. Galardy, R. E. 1982. Inhibition of angiotensin converting enzyme by phosphoramidates and polyphosphates. *Biochemistry* 21:5777–81

100. Galardy, R. E., Kontoyiannidou-Ostrem, V., Kortylewicz, Z. P. 1983. Inhibition of angiotensin converting enzyme by phosphonic amides and phosphonic acids. *Biochemistry* 22:1990–95

101. Thorsett, E. D., Harris, E. E., Peterson, E. R., Greenlee, W. J., Patchett, A. A., et al. 1982. Phosphorous-containing inhibitors of angiotensin-converting enzyme. *Proc. Natl. Acad. Sci. USA* 79:2176–80

102. Powell, J. R., DeForrest, J. M., Cushman, D. W., Rubin, B., Petrillo, E. W. 1984. Antihypertensive effects of a new angiotensin converting enzyme (ACE) inhibitor, SQ 28,555. *Fed. Proc.* 43:733

103. Almquist, R. G., Chao, W. R., Ellis, M. E., Johnson, H. L. 1980. Synthesis and biological activity of a ketomethylene analogue of a tripeptide inhibitor of angiotensin converting enzyme. *J. Med. Chem.* 23:1392–98

104. Almquist, R. G., Crase, J., Jennings-White, C., Meyer, R. F., Hoefle, M. L., et al. 1982. Derivatives of the potent angiotensin converting enzyme inhibitor 5(S)-Benzamido-4-oxo-6-phenylhexanoyl-L-proline: Effect of changes at positions 2 and 5 of the hexanoic acid portion. *J. Med. Chem.* 25:1292–99

105. Meyer, R. F., Essenburg, A. D., Smith, R. D., Kaplan, H. R. 1982. Angiotensin converting enzyme inhibitors: Modifications of a tripeptide analogue. *J. Med. Chem.* 25:996–99

106. Almquist, R. G., Christie, P. H., Chao, W. R., Johnson, H. L. 1983. Synthesis and biological activity of an amino analogue of a tripeptide inhibitor of angiotensin-converting enzyme. *J. Pharm. Sci.* 72:63–67

107. Morikawa, T., Takada, K., Kimura, T., Sakakibara, S., Kurauchi, M., et al. 1984. Novel peptides with orally active and long-lasting antihypertensive activity. *Biochem. Biophys. Res. Commun.* 119:1205–10

108. Condon, M. E., Petrillo, E. W. Jr., Ryono, D. E., Reid, J. A., Neubeck, R., et al. 1982. Angiotensin-converting enzyme inhibitors: Importance of the amide carbonyl of mercaptoacyl amino acids for hydrogen bonding to the enzyme. *J. Med. Chem.* 25:250–58

109. Harris, R. B., Strong, P. D. M., Wilson, I. B. 1983. Dipeptide-hydroxamates are good inhibitors of the angiotensin I-converting enzyme. *Biochem. Biophys. Res. Commun.* 116:394–99

110. Harris, R. B., Wilson, I. B. 1982. Irreversible inhibition of bovine lung angiotensin I-converting enzyme with p-[N,N-Bis(chloroethyl)amino]phenylbutyric acid (chlorambucil) and chlorambucyl L-proline with evidence that an active site carboxyl group is labeled. *J. Biol. Chem.* 257:811–15

111. Page, I. H. 1981. Antihypertensive drugs. Our debt to industrial chemists. *New Eng. J. Med.* 304:615–18

Ann. Rev. Pharmacol. Toxicol. 1985. 25:325–47

THE TOXICITY OF SMOKE FROM POLYMERIC MATERIALS DURING THERMAL DECOMPOSITION

Yves Alarie

Department of Industrial Environmental Health, University of Pittsburgh School of Public Health, Pittsburgh, Pennsylvania 15261

INTRODUCTION

Synthetic polymers, because of their chemical composition, release smoke that is qualitatively different from the smoke of commonly used natural polymers such as cotton and wood (1, 2). In addition, the rate of release of smoke from synthetic polymers can be much faster than that for cotton or wood and the yield of principal toxicants may be higher (1, 2). For these reasons, we need to develop methods to evaluate the acute toxicity of smoke from both synthetic and natural materials.

Ideally, we should be able to make a complete qualitative and quantitative analysis of the smoke from each polymer, but such data cannot be obtained easily. As a result, researchers in this area have relied on animal exposures to rapidly evaluate possible differences in the potency of smoke from various materials. Most have measured key toxic gases such as carbon monoxide, hydrogen cyanide, formaldehyde, and hydrogen chloride while exposing animals to these substances. In addition, a large number of studies have been made on over 300 other polymeric materials by investigators in many countries. Several summaries of these investigations have recently appeared (1–4). In May of 1984, the Secretary of State of New York recommended that toxicity data on smoke from polymeric materials be filed at the Department of State as determined by the Uniform Fire Prevention and Building Code Council (5). The implementation of this recommendation is now under way.

325

0362-1642/85/0415-0325$02.00

MEASURING THE ACUTE TOXICITY OF SMOKE

Researchers have used two different approaches to evaluate acute lethality during exposure to smoke.

Type I or Time to an Effect Approach

The time to an effect approach consists of thermally decomposing a given amount of material and exposing animals until a particular effect is observed. Many investigations have been conducted using this method. Among others, Hilado (6) has investigated more than 200 polymers and the Federal Aviation Administration has investigated 75 aircraft cabin materials with this approach (7). Its major drawback is that all the exposed animals die and taking the average time to death as a measure of toxicity is invalid. Furthermore, ranking acute lethality with this method is impossible for the following reasons:

1. By definition, toxicity is based on the amount of chemical or physical agent necessary to produce a given level of effect (8, 9). Therefore, if smoke from material A is to be declared more toxic than smoke from material B, it is necessary to demonstrate that less material A is needed to cause death.

2. The time element in these experiments is related to the rapidity of action of the toxicants released and their concentration in the exposure chamber in addition to the time it takes for the samples to decompose. In general, it has been demonstrated that as the concentration of toxicants increases the time for a given level of effect to occur is shorter. In addition, the proportion of animals exhibiting the effect increases (10–12).

The Type I approach yields only descriptive data on the time it takes to kill all the animals, i.e. onset of the effect, when the same amount (one gram) of each material is used. This is illustrated by the data in Table 1. Three materials produced 100% mortality within a planned 30-minute exposure period when one gram of each material was thermally decomposed. Because mortality in every case was 100%, we have no idea of how toxic the smoke from each material really was. Perhaps only 0.1 gram would have been sufficient to cause death.

The results in another test using the same approach with other polymers are presented in Table 2. When one gram of polymer was decomposed, a factor of 3.5 existed between the fastest and slowest times required for 100% mortality, being six minutes for wool and 21 minutes for Nylon 6. Also presented in Table 2 are the smallest amounts of each polymer that when thermally decomposed still induced 100% mortality, as well as the time it took for this to occur. It can be seen that reducing one gram by a factor of ten still killed all the animals, but the time for this effect to occur approximately only doubled. The most rapid effect occurred with red oak, 15 minutes, and the slowest with wool, 23

Table 1 Toxicity of thermal decomposition products from various polymers decomposed at 600°C

Polymers	Weight charged in furnace	% mortality	Time to death	References
Polytetrafluoroethylene	1 gram	100	22.9 minutes	13
Polypropylene	1 gram	100	21.7 minutes	14
Polyether sulfone	1 gram	100	6.05 minutes	15

minutes. From the data observed in this experiment (16), it was also possible to calculate the amount of material needed to kill 50% of the animals (LC_{50}) and the time needed to kill 50% of the animals (LT_{50}) when this amount was used. These data are also given in Table 2. They permit a valid comparison of toxicity and show that red oak is almost eight times less toxic than Nylon 6. They also show that the differences between LT_{50} values are small. If the LT_{50} is taken as a measure of toxicity, red oak seems more toxic than Nylon 6. This is obviously wrong, since it takes eight times less Nylon 6 than red oak to produce 50% mortality. Thus, the time required for a given level of effect to occur is secondary; it is an important measurement, but it cannot replace quantity as a measure for ranking toxicity.

Type II or Amount for an Effect for a Given Duration of Exposure Approach

The Type II approach consists of determining the amount of material necessary to produce sufficient smoke to kill 50% of the animals (LC_{50}) following exposure of all groups and all animals in each group to the exact same duration of exposure. The only laboratory adhering strictly to this protocol is the National Bureau of Standards (17).

With this protocol, each material was thermally decomposed and all animals were exposed to the smoke for 30 minutes. Lethality was then observed over a period of 14 days. A concentration-response relationship was obtained from a series of experiments that varied the amount of material being decomposed to yield between 0 and 100% mortality. The LC_{50} was calculated by using an appropriate statistical method. While it sometimes occurred that a few animals died close to the end of the exposure period rather than following exposure, such a small deviation is of minor consequence. Results obtained with this method using a variety of polymers are presented in Table 3. Valid conclusions about the toxicity of smoke from these materials in comparison with Douglas fir were possible, since the protocol followed basic toxicological principles with proper statistical analysis.

Table 2 Lethality data obtained for thermal decomposition products of various polymers decomposed under the same conditions[a]

Samples	Amount of material used (grams)	% mortality	Exposure time for 100% mortality (minutes)	Amount to kill 50% of the animals (grams)[b]	Time to kill 50% of the animals at the LC_{50} (minutes)[c]
Polyphenylene sulfide	1	100	11	0.135	27
	0.2	100	20		
Polyaryl sulfone	1.0	100	11	0.092	29
	0.15	100	26		
Nylon 6	1	100	21	0.04	30
	0.047	100	30		
Douglas fir	1	100	13	0.09	23
	0.11	100	22		
Wool	1.0	100	6	0.10	29
	0.12	100	23		
Red oak	1.0	100	12	0.31	23
	0.4	100	15		

[a] Taken from (16).
[b] This would be described as the LC_{50}.
[c] Not reported by these authors but approximated from their tables. This is described as the LT_{50}.

Table 3 Comparison of toxicity of thermal decomposition products (non-flaming mode) obtained at the National Bureau of Standards for 30 minutes of exposure and 14 days observation period[a]

Material	LC_{50} material LC_{50} Douglas fir
Red oak flooring boards	1.45
Flexible polyurethane foam	1.31
Acrylonitrile-butadiene-styrene pellets	1.27
Wool: unbleached, unwoven fibers	1.07
Douglas fir	1.00
Poly (vinylchloride) pellets	0.74
Polyphenylsulfone pellets	0.71
Poly (vinylchloride) with zinc Ferrocyanide	0.48
Modacrylic knit fabric	0.26
Polytetrafluoroethylene	0.006

[a] Taken from (17)

Type III or Amount for an Effect Within a Planned Duration of Exposure Approach

The Type III approach combines the methodology of both Type I and Type II. In a strict sense, the 50% mortality calculation (LC_{50}) should be based on a similar exposure period for all animals at all concentrations of smoke, as in the Type II approach. A variation on this method is to allow deaths to occur within a given, or planned, duration of exposure rather than merely observing deaths following a given exposure period. One advantage of this variation is that it is less costly, but delayed toxicity cannot be as accurately measured as with the Type II approach unless a larger number of animals are exposed. The second advantage is that deaths are observed with a time frame more appropriate to fire situations than during a 14-day observation period following exposure.

Several investigators have used this approach and have sometimes made post-exposure observations on the surviving animals (16, 18–22). Data from these investigators are presented in Tables 4–7 and the last two columns of Table 2. These tables make it very easy to see the toxicity of the thermal decomposition of polymeric materials. However, the thermal decomposition methods used and durations of exposure varies widely. Therefore, it is impossible to compare the results obtained from these methods.

With the Type III approach, the amount of toxicant necessary to kill 50% (LC_{50}) of the animals can be combined with the time necessary to kill 50% (LT_{50}) of the animals in order to make a comparison among materials for both potency (LC_{50}) and rapidity of action (LT_{50}). This can be done by plotting both variables, as shown in Figure 1, for a wide variety of materials (see also Table

Table 4 Amount of material decomposed at 800°C necessary to kill 50% of the animals (mice) in 10 minutes[a]

Materials	Amount of material (grams)
Polyacrylonitrile	0.16
Polyamide 6	0.023
Polypropylene	0.030
Acrylonitrile-butadiene-styrene	0.034
Polyurethane A	0.038
Polyethylene	0.052
Macrolon	0.095
Polystyrene	0.12
Polyvinylchloride	0.14

[a] Taken from (18)

Table 5 Amount of materials decomposed up to 1000° necessary to kill 50% of the animals within an exposure period of two hours but also including death within a two-week post-exposure observation period[a]

Materials	Amount of materials (grams)
Y-2000: Aromatic polyamide	0.15
Y-1797: Aromatic-type nylon with flame retardant	0.205
Y-1796: Aromatic type nylon without flame retardant	0.36
Y-4959: Polyarelene rigit material	2.20
Y-4397: Polyimide resin on fiberglass	4.71

[a] Taken from (19)

Table 6 Amount of material decomposed to kill 50% of the animals (LC_{50}) within a planned 30-minute exposure period. Heating rate at 20°C/minute[a]

	Materials	LC_{50} (gram)	Time to kill 50% of the animals (minutes)
GM-21:	Flexible urethane foam	12.9	13
GM-47:	Expanded polystyrene	5.8	11
PTFE:	Polytetrafluoroethylene	0.64	8
PVC:	Polyvinylchloride (92% homopolymer)	7.0	10
MOD:	Modacrylic	4.9	18
UF:	Urea formaldehyde foam	2.5	22
D. fir:	Douglas fir	63.8	22
Wool:	Wool fiber, undyed	3.0	27

[a] Taken from (20)

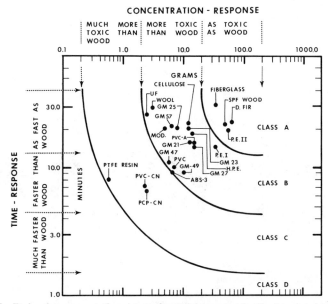

Figure 1   Each point represents the amount of material (gram on the X axis) needed to produced sufficient smoke to kill 50% of the animals tested (LC$_{50}$) and the time (minutes on the Y axis) necessary for this effect to occur (LT$_{50}$) using this amount of material. Vertically each material is classified in terms of potency, horizontally each material is classified in terms of onset of action, always in comparison to Douglas fir, the wood standard. To combine both potency and onset of action, parallel quadrants separate class A, B, C, and D materials. A description of the materials presented is given in Table 8. Taken from (21).

8) in order to compare them with Douglas fir, which is used as the standard (21).

It should be understood that with Type II and III approaches the investigators predetermined the exposure period or planned for an exposure period relevant to a fire survival situation. With the Type II protocol, the investigators were trying to find out the maximum amount of smoke tolerable for a particular period of time without producing a lethal effect afterward. With the Type III

Table 7   Amount of material decomposed to kill 50% of the animals within a period of two hours with decomposition of samples at 822°C[a]

Materials	Amount (grams)
FR-polycarbonate	8.6
High-impact polystyrene	8.9
Wool	9.4
Red oak	16.8
Phenolic general purpose	47.5

[a] Taken from (22)

Table 8 Samples tested and summary of the results presented in Figure 1

Abbreviation	Sample name and description	LC_{50} (grams)	LT_{50} (minutes)	Class[a]
PRC materials[b]				
GM 21	Flexible polyurethane foam	12.9	13	B
GM 23	Same as GM 21, with fire retardant	10.4	18	B
GM 25	High-resilience flexible polyurethane foam	8.3	19	B
GM 27	Same as GM 25, with fire retardant	14.4	15	B
GM 29	Rigid polyurethane foam	10.4	28	B
GM 31	Same as GM 29, with fire retardant	8.2	23	B
GM 35	Rigid polyurethane foam, fluorocarbon blown	7.5	17	B
GM 37	Same as GM 35, CO_2 blown	8.0	15	B
GM 41	Rigid isocyanurate foam	6.4	18	B
GM 43	Same as GM 41, contains some polyurethane	6.1	16	B
GM 47	Polystyrene expanded	5.8	11	B
GM 49	Same as GM 47, with fire retardant	10.0	9	B
GM 57	Phenol formaldehyde-phenol resin, expanded with blowing agent	6.3	20	B
Non-PRC materials				
PTFE	Polytetrafluoroethylene resin	0.64	8	C
PVC	Polyvinylchloride (92% homopolymer)	7.0	10	B
PVC-A	Polyvinylchloride (46% homopolymer)	15.2	15	B
PVC-CN	Polyvinylchloride (46% homopolymer + 5% zinc ferrocyanide)	2.3	7	C
PCP-CN	Polyvinylchloride (92% homopolymer + 5% zinc ferrocyanide)	2.5	6	C
ABS-3	Standard acrylonitrile/butadiene/styrene	6.3	9	B
Mod.	Modacrylic	4.9	18	B
Wool	Wool fibers — undyed	3.0	27	B
UF	Urea formaldehyde foam	2.5	22	B
Cellulose	Blowing type cellulose fiber insulation	11.9	21	B
D. fir	Douglas fir	63.8	22	A
Fiberglass	Fiberglass building insulation, 3.5 in. thick with paper and vapor barrier	35.7	25	A
PE I	Polyester resin — commercial acrylic modified unsaturated	34.8	14	B
PE II	Polyester resin — experimental acrylic modified unsaturated	57.4	18	A
HPE	Polyester resin, styrenated halogen modified	14.4	16	B
SPF wood	Compressed spruce, pine, fir slab	48.7	19	A

[a] From Figure 1
[b] From the Product Research Committee (PRC) sample bank at the National Bureau of Standards and (21)

protocol, a standard was used first and attempts were made to obtain 50% mortality at exactly a specified duration of exposure, such as 30 minutes, as in (20). This was impossible to achieve and the investigators had to settle for a time close to it. For example, when Douglas fir was used as the standard, 50% mortality occurred at 22 minutes instead of the desired 30 minutes (20, 21). However, once the results for the standard are obtained, all other materials can be rated against it for both LC_{50} and LT_{50}.

UNDERSTANDING THE LIMITATIONS OF THE DATA IN TERMS OF REDUCING FIRE FATALITIES DUE TO SMOKE INHALATION

Toxicity Data

Fire is one of the most serious problems affecting modern life and our ability to minimize its effects has improved little over the past 50 years (1). Cullis & Hirshcler (1) placed things in perspective when they pointed out that during the period from 1961 to 1972 fires killed over three times more Americans (143, 550) in the United States than died in the Vietnam War. The US has the worse fire-fatality record of the industrialized nations (1). Only motor vehicle accidents and falls rank higher as a cause of death (23). Recently, most attention has focused on the toxicity of smoke, since approximately 80% of fire victims die from smoke inhalation rather than burns (24). Three major recent examples where this was the case are the fire at the MGM Hotel in Las Vegas, when 85 persons died, most from smoke inhalation (25); the fire at a jail in Biloxi, Mississippi, where 29 prisoners died, all from inhaling the smoke from the wall padding of a single cell (26); and the fire at the Westchase Hilton Hotel in Houston, Texas (27).

The main reason for undertaking the toxicological testing of materials under thermal stress is to provide information on how to select those that will reduce fatalities due to smoke inhalation. Obviously, materials releasing smoke of low toxicity are preferable to materials whose smoke contains potent toxicants.

However, one must also consider that during an actual fire, so much toxicant can be released that nobody survives a 30-minute exposure regardless of the burning materials. Another time, the amount of smoke can be so small or the dilution so great that everyone is likely to survive no matter what materials are involved. For this reason, it makes no sense to regard toxicological data alone, or to think that small differences in LC_{50} or LT_{50} will be important in reducing fire fatalities (20, 21). Developing classifications and rankings for materials on the basis of potency, as presented in Figure 1, can cover only orders of magnitude. Toxicologists have generally recognized a factor of ten as separating different classes of toxic level (8, 9).

Table 9   Amount of materials loaded in the furnace and heated at 20°C/minute resulting in 50% lethality (LC_{50}) within a planned 30-minute exposure period[a]

Foam samples	LC_{50} (grams)	LT_{50} (minutes)	Volume of material at LC_{50} (in^3)
A	34.3	19.5	17
B	7.2	19.3	20
C	10.6	20.5	20

[a] Taken from (29)

A second point to consider is the toxicity of smoke from wood. Although wood is taken as a standard in toxicological testing, smoke from wood is toxic. For example, in one thermal decomposition system a maximum 100 ppm of CO per gram of Douglas fir was easily reached (20), while in another 88 ppm of CO per gram was observed (17). Thus, wood can produce acute lethal effects. If we intend to reduce fire fatalities due to smoke inhalation, it is not enough to use materials whose smoke is less toxic than wood. We must also insist on better fire prevention with measures such as the installation of smoke alarms and sprinkler systems. Some important new developments in synthetic polymeric materials are also worth noting. For example, new inorganic polymers are being developed that do not burn or release toxic gases (28).

The final point to consider is that materials used in building are not used on a weight basis but rather on a volume, surface area, or length basis. For example, three different types of synthetic foam for mattresses have been tested with the Type III method previously described (20); the results are presented in Table 9. A factor of five was found between the most and the least toxic foams when the LC_{50} was given in grams. However, on a volume basis there was no difference among these materials. In order to make the best selection, it is necessary to know how much of each sample is required to obtain the same comfortable mattress on a volume basis. Unless the difference is rather large (i.e. by a factor of ten or so), the choice is difficult. We must consider that smoke's capacity to impair visibility and heat release, which will influence the impact of the fire, are determined by the weight of material, not by its volume. Ease of ignition and flame spread are two other important characteristics of burning material, and these unfortunately are not related to weight or volume. Thus, toxicity is only one of many factors to be considered in the selection of materials.

In some cases, the toxicological data on synthetic polymers used on a weight, volume, surface area, or length basis is of such a nature that we must question their employment in large quantities or in areas likely to be exposed to high heat without proper fire prevention systems. The use of polymers showing extremely high toxicity of their thermal decomposition products will probably be the exception rather than the rule. Indeed, during the past ten years, only two types of materials were found, both at the University of Pittsburgh (10, 20, 21) and at the National Bureau of Standards (17), to fit this category: fluoropolymers and polyvinyl chloride. During recent testing at Arthur D. Little (R. C. Anderson, personal communication), a third material was found with a toxicity at least ten times higher than that of the fluoropolymers.

A recent series of tests on the decomposition of communication cables using the Type III method of testing indicated the toxicity of fluoropolymers. The results of these tests are presented in Table 10. The LC_{50} values (in grams or inches) given there are only good approximations of the LC_{50}, since it was not technically possible to cut these wires into smaller quantities, permitting a full series of experiments to statistically calculate the LC_{50}. Nevertheless, these cable amounts and lengths are extremely small. The tests showed that carbon monoxide clearly was not the toxicant produced by the burning cables, nor can hydrogen cyanide be involved, since these polymers contain no nitrogen. As in the case of another fluoropolymer, polytetrafluoroethylene (20), the extremely toxic gas released during the tests was probably perfluoroisobutylene (30), whose acute inhalation toxicity (31) is of the same level as the nerve agent Soman (32). We do not know the mechanism of action of this toxic gas nor do we know an effective treatment for it. These polymers have been attractive as

Table 10   Amount of materials loaded in the furnace and heated at 20°C/minute resulting in 50% lethality (LC_{50}) within a planned 30-minute exposure period[a]

Observations	High-temperature coaxial cable covered with Teflon®-FEP[b]	High-temperature telephone cable with 25 pairs of wire covered with Teflon®-FEP
LC_{50} (grams)	0.29	1.96
LC_{50} (inches)	0.25	0.5
LT_{50} (minutes)	28	28
Temperature at initial decomposition and exposure of animals (°C)	325	325
Temperatures between which major decomposition occurred	400–500	400–500
Maximum CO reached in exposure chamber during decomposition (ppm)	< 50	< 50
Residue after burning (mostly wire) (mg)	42	760

[a] Taken from (29)
[b] ®Registered trademark of E.I. DuPont de Nemours for fluoropolymers

building materials because their flame spread (if any) is extremely low, their heat release is 25% that of wood, and they release no smoke to impair visibility (1). Nevertheless, the toxicity of their thermal decomposition products is so high that it must be a primary factor in determining their use.

Extrapolation from Animals to Humans

Two factors must be considered in extrapolating test data to real conditions. The first one is that laboratory animals, mice or rats, are used for testing. The second one is that the principal toxicants in the decomposition products of various materials are not always the same. These factors greatly complicate our task in extrapolating toxicity test results to humans.

When wood burns, carbon monoxide is the main toxicant (17, 20), and carbon monoxide is the main toxicant in other polymeric materials as well. The relative toxicity ranking established for carbon monoxide in laboratory animals can justifiably be extrapolated to humans because the mechanism of toxicity in both is the same. This gas is absorbed in mice or rats in the same manner as it is in humans; the only difference is that it is absorbed faster, and thus acts more quickly, in animals due to their higher minute ventilation/body weight (33). The same is true with hydrogen cyanide. However, if material A, in which the principle toxicant is hydrogen cyanide, is found to be ten times more toxic in mice than material B, whose principal toxicant is carbon monoxide, can we then extrapolate that material A is also ten times more toxic than material B if humans are exposed? From the data on the relative acute toxicity of hydrogen cyanide and carbon monoxide in mice (12) and the best approximations of their lethal levels for humans (34), such an extrapolation is justified, since the potency ratio between CO and HCN is similar for mice and humans.

When the principal toxicant is hydrogen chloride, as in polyvinyl chloride (35, 36), 58% of the polymer is chlorine and almost all of it is released as hydrogen chloride (1). In this case a correction factor must be applied in order to extrapolate to humans the results obtained in mice. This is because such gases as hydrogen chloride, hydrogen fluoride, and hydrogen bromide are highly soluble in water and react at the surface of the nasal mucosa. Mice and rats breathe exclusively through the nose; thus, such gases are readily scrubbed by the upper airways and are prevented from reaching the lungs and systemic circulation, reducing their toxic action (37–39). In an actual fire, humans breathe exclusively through the mouth, since smoke is irritating to the nose (40). In order to prevent the nasal mucosa from removing these gases, mice and rats can be exposed to the toxicant via tracheal cannula (37–39).

As shown in Table 11, the toxicity of smoke from polyvinylchloride and from hydrogen chloride differed by a factor of seven to ten between mice breathing through a tracheal cannula and normal mice breathing through the nose. In contrast, carbon monoxide and hydrogen cyanide were equally toxic

Table 11 Acute lethality in mice exposed to thermal decomposition products of various polymers or exposed to hydrogen chloride, carbon monoxide, or hydrogen cyanide. LC_{50} is given in grams loaded in the furnace for the polymers and in ppm for the gases.

	LC_{50} values	
Samples	Cannulated mice	Normal, non-cannulated mice
Polyvinyl chloride A[a,b]	2.2	15.2
GM-41 isocyanurate foam[c]	11.7	6.4
GM-57 phenol formaldehyde foam[b]	2.9	6.3
Hydrogen chloride[d]	1,095	10,157
Hydrogen cyanide[e]	166	166
Carbon monoxide[e]	3,500	3,500

[a] This sample contained 46% polyvinylchloride and inorganic inert filler.
[b] Taken from (20, 37)
[c] Taken from (20)
[d] Taken from (37)
[e] Taken from (12)

no matter which way they were inhaled. The difference in toxicity was small between GM-41 and GM-57, which release hydrogen cyanide and carbon monoxide respectively as the main toxicants during thermal decomposition (20). The LC_{50} of hydrogen chloride in cannulated mice (1095 ppm) is comparable to the predicted lethal concentration (1000–2000 ppm) in humans for a short exposure duration (34). This further reinforces the theory that a factor of seven to ten must be applied in extrapolating the acute lethal effect of this gas, or of smoke where the principal toxicant is hydrogen chloride, from experiments conducted with normal mice.

There may be other instances where such a correction factor is needed. For example, when perfluoroisobutylene is released from fluoropolymers and is the main toxicant in smoke (30), humans may be more or less susceptible to this gas than mice or rats. There are no data in the literature on the acute lethal level of this gas in humans and no correction factor can be applied at this time.

SMALL-SCALE FIRE MODELS AND EXPOSURE SYSTEMS

Criteria for Small-Scale Fires

Various apparatus have been used to evaluate smoke from polymers in a manner comparable to what can happen in an actual fire, and a list of combustion devices and their limitations has been presented (1–4). None of them is perfectly adequate. Testing methods must follow general criteria and investigators must make a variety of measurements to establish general relationships to real fires. Among the criteria and measurements required for adequate testing we can list the following:

1. The temperature should be high enough to decompose all samples being tested.
2. Sufficient air (oxygen) should surround the samples at all times during decomposition.
3. The temperature or radiant energy used should not be higher than average developing fires, i.e. around 400–800°C, since we do not want to incinerate the samples nor do we want to supply energy greatly in excess of what would occur in an actual fire.
4. Both non-flaming and flaming decomposition products should be investigated, simultaneously or as they follow each other in a fire.
5. The combustion-exposure chamber system should minimize the deposition of gases and particulates on the walls and the reaction of decomposition products with the walls.
6. The residence time of decomposition products at elevated temperature is an important variable. If residence time is very long, the larger molecular-weight organic constituents of the smoke will further decompose to gases such as CO_2, CO, H_2O, HCN, and HCl. Little work has been done on this subject.
7. The combustion system should be large enough to accomodate low-density materials, layered materials, and composite materials in a configuration, horizontal or vertical, appropriate to their intended use.
8. The rate at which the samples decompose must be monitored. This is a most important measurement, since the size of a fire is proportional to the burning rate of the material. Few studies have included this information.
9. Monitoring of at least carbon monoxide, carbon dioxide, and oxygen is necessary; they relate to the size and intensity of the fire. Tests of polymers containing nitrogen may require monitoring the hydrogen cyanide. In halogen-containing polymers, the halogens should also be measured if carbon monoxide or hydrogen cyanide are not the principal toxicants in the smoke.
10. The combustion system must permit the investigation of concentration-response relationships in order that acute lethal effects or other toxic effects can be quantitatively evaluated. This can be accomplished in two ways: (a) increase or decrease the size of the sample while keeping the dilution air constant or (b) keep the size of the sample constant while changing the dilution air.
11. Two major types of decomposition systems have been used. The first type is a fixed-temperature system. As long as the temperature is high enough to

decompose the sample, this testing method is valid (17). The second type is a system in which the temperature increases linearly, from 5 to 35°C per minute, until the sample decomposes. This method is equally valid.

12. The latter system requires that particular care be taken in determining the rate of heat increase. During tests of thermoplastic polymeric materials such as polystyrene foam or polymethylmethacrylate, a heating rate of 35°C per minute can cause explosions and flash-overs if these materials are burned in quantities of ten grams or more. A rate of 5°C per minute is probably too low for the adequate testing of thermosetting plastics such as urea-formaldehyde foam. A good working temperature rate for most heat-increase tests is probably around 20°C per minute (20). The criteria listed above reflect personal experience. I offer them as a guide to researchers interested in initiating research work in this field.

Exposure Systems

Investigators testing for toxicity in burning polymeric materials have used both static and dynamic exposure systems. Either is adequate for recreating the conditions of an actual fire. However, the advantages, disadvantages, and results of testing with these systems vary. Given below are the most important differences between the two exposure systems.

STATIC EXPOSURE SYSTEM   The static exposure system is most commonly used by the National Bureau of Standards (NBS) (17), which employs a cup furnace to decompose materials, and by Hilado (6), who uses a tube furnace. The NBS uses two temperature settings to test polymeric materials. The first setting produces thermal decomposition products at a temperature just below the ignition temperature of each material; the second setting produces thermal decomposition products in the flaming mode. One weakness of NBS tests done in the past has been their failure to measure the rate of material decomposition. Simple modifications of these exposure systems could allow for this measurement. The decomposition temperature required by NBS protocol seems reasonable. However, a low-oxygen condition has prevailed in the cup furnace during tests of large volumes of low-density samples. This can be rectified by increasing the cup size. The NBS tests have shown sufficiently rapid mixing and minimal deposition of thermal decomposition products on the walls of the exposure system.

By changing the sample size, the NBS investigators obtained concentration-response relationships for acute lethality (11), as did Hilado (16) in later experiments. NBS protocol requires determining the autoignition temperature of the materials being tested prior to establishing the temperatures at which they decompose. This could present problems during the testing of composite or layered materials; carpets, for example, can have different layers with a wide range of autoignition temperatures.

DYNAMIC EXPOSURE SYSTEMS   Two different dynamic exposure systems have been used to test the toxicity of polymeric materials and both yield valid concentration-response relationships for evaluating the acute lethal effects of a variety of polymers. The first system is a standardized method designated DIN53-436 by the German Standards Institution and commonly referred to as the DIN method (41); Herpol has also used this system (42). In the DIN system, samples are placed in a quartz tube. A furnace, set at 300–600°C, moves over the samples at a given rate for a fixed period of time, such as 30 minutes, and gradually decomposes the samples. Smoke escaping from the tube is then directed into the exposure chamber and diluted with room air to vary the toxicity level. A temperature of 600°C is high enough to decompose almost entirely all common polymeric materials. However, this decomposition system does not permit direct measurement of the rate of decomposition. In addition, Herpol reports (42) that tests of a large number of samples in multiple experiments show considerable differences in the behavior of the same samples as they decompose. Because of this drawback a comparison of toxicity between materials has been impossible. Nevertheless, it seems that with some modifications this approach should work. Indeed, LeMoan & Chaigneau (18) have obtained valid concentration-response relationships for several polymers, as listed in Table 4, using a similar decomposition system that changes the sample size rather than the dilution air to produce different levels of toxic effects.

The second dynamic-exposure system was originally developed by Barrow et al (43) and adapted to test a wide variety of polymers (20, 21, 44). This method is now known as the University of Pittsburgh protocol. In this method, the sample is placed in a furnace and heated, beginning at room temperature, at an established rate of 20°C per minute. Air flowing through the furnace at a rate of 11 liters per minute carries the smoke toward the exposure chamber. Cool air is also added to prevent excessive oxygen depletion and temperature increase. A schematic of this system is presented in Figure 2. The system generates smoke that continuously changes in chemical composition as the temperature increases. Animals are exposed to the smoke when 0.2 or 1% weight loss is recorded and continue to be exposed for 30 minutes, less if they all die prior to this time. Since initial polymer decomposition temperatures are seldom less than 200°C, the final temperature reached is 800°C, high enough to decompose all materials. Thus, the animals are first exposed to thermal decomposition products produced during pyrolysis at low temperature and then to products occurring during flaming conditions, if flaming ignition occurs. During exposure, CO, CO_2, and O_2 are monitored continuously. Depending on the nature of

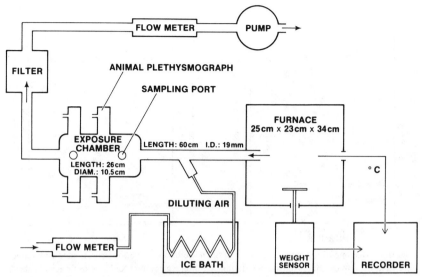

Figure 2 Experimental method to study the toxicity of thermal decomposition products from synthetic and natural polymers decomposed by increasing heat from room temperature at a rate of 20°C per minute. Taken from (20).

the polymer, formaldehyde, hydrogen cyanide and hydrogen chloride are also measured.

Some examples of the results obtained with this method are presented in Figures 3 and 4. Figure 3 illustrates the differences in toxicity observed between two cellulosic materials, Douglas fir and a heavily flame-retarded cellulose insulation fiber sample. The variation between these two cellulosic substances is clear. When the Douglas fir was heated, release of CO occurred at the point of flaming ignition and was responsible for the deaths of the animals. The flame retardant prevented flaming ignition of the cellulose fibers, but decomposition released a much larger amount of CO. Thus, although both samples were mainly cellulose, one was six times more toxic because it produced much more CO. Figure 4 illustrates the difference between two thermosetting plastics so difficult to ignite that they did not do so under experimental conditions. Urea-formaldehyde foam insulation released large amounts of HCN, but only above 450°C. Moreover, less than 20% of the 2.49 grams of urea-formaldehyde loaded in the furnace produced toxic smoke. The principal toxicant of phenol formaldehyde is carbon monoxide, which is released at temperatures above 300°C. Both samples released formaldehyde at fairly low temperatures. However, the amount of formaldehyde released was considerably lower than the lethal level for this chemical (45).

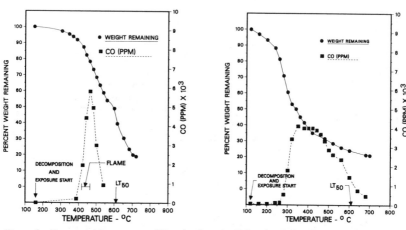

DOUGLAS FIR - DECOMPOSITION AT THE LC_{50} 63.8 GRAMS

CELLULOSE FIBER - DECOMPOSITON AT THE LC_{50} 11.9 GRAMS

Figure 3   Decomposition patterns of Douglas fir and cellulose insulation fibers treated with flame retardant. Carbon monoxide release and flaming ignition temperature for Douglas fir as indicated. Beginning of exposure and temperature at which 50% lethality occurred as indicated. Both samples were heated at 20°C per minute, beginning at room temperature. Modified from (20).

With the dynamic exposure method of toxicity testing, the measurement of time for 50% mortality (LT_{50}) was calculated from the start of decomposition. This is dependent on the thermal stability of the polymers as well as on the rapidity of action of the toxicant released.

REPRODUCIBILITY OF TOXICITY MEASUREMENTS

The reproducibility of test results is an important aspect to consider when proposing protocols for the evaluation of toxicity. In 1982 the National Bureau of Standards organized a round-robin discussion of protocol among several laboratories. The group judged very good the results of experiments using the National Bureau of Standards testing method (17). More recently, the protocol used by the University of Pittsburgh was tested in three laboratories: the results are presented in Table 12. Considering that the Pittsburgh method contains two sources of variability, i.e. decomposition of the samples and biological variation, the results presented in Table 12 indicate good repeatability. The results obtained within the same laboratory were comparable and reproduced well and the results obtained by other different laboratories were also comparable. In fact, the results presented in Table 12 are well within the variation obtained in one laboratory performing oral LD_{50} tests (46).

PHENOL FORMALDEHYDE - DECOMPOSITION AT THE LC$_{50}$ 8.26 GRAMS   UREA FORMALDEHYDE - DECOMPOSITION AT THE LC$_{50}$ 2.49 GRAMS

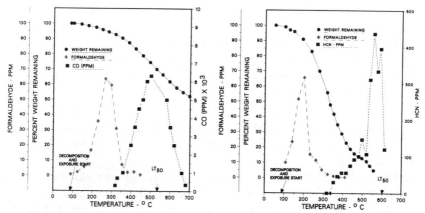

Figure 4   Decomposition patterns of phenol-formaldehyde foam and urea formaldehyde foam insulation with formaldehyde, carbon monoxide, and hydrogen cyanide release. Beginning of exposure and temperature at which 50% lethality occurred as indicated. Both samples were heated at 20°C per minute, beginning at room temperature. Modified from (20).

Table 12   Repeatability and reproducibility of the acute lethality measurement (LC_{50}) using the University of Pittsburgh experimental protocol described in (4, 20)

Materials	University of Pittsburgh	Biotecs Laboratory[b]	Arthur D. Little[c]
Douglas fir[a]	64	57	50
	78	61	
	56	64	
		59	
Average for Douglas fir ± (SD) = 61.1 (8.2) (n = 8)			
Phenol formaldehyde foam (GM-57)[a]	6.3	7.4	4.8
Polyester-fiberglass PEI[a]	35	36	
Polyester-fiberglass PE II[a]	57	58	
Vinyl coated wire[a]	15		15
Polyurethane foam flexible	13		9
Polyester-fiberglass halogen retardant HPE[a]	14	15	

[a] Samples furnished by the University of Pittsburgh
[b] Data supplied by C. P. Carpenter of Biotecs Laboratory, Mellon Institute, Pittsburgh
[c] Taken from (4)

CONCLUSION

During the past ten years, major advances have been made in the study of the toxicity of smoke from polymeric materials. Such advances have been possible because of the collaboration among toxicologists, analytical chemists, fire technology experts, and polymer chemists. We now recognize that smoke from different polymers will produce acute lethal effects different from the smoke of wood. Below is a summary of our basic findings:

1. Some synthetic polymers will release a much larger amount of carbon monoxide than wood does (17, 20, 21). In these cases the principal toxicant is the same as with wood or cotton, the difference being the yield of carbon monoxide per gram of polymer.
2. Because of their nitrogen content, some synthetic polymers release substantial amounts of hydrogen cyanide. Hydrogen cyanide is much more potent and faster acting than carbon monoxide; this is the reason why the smoke from these polymers is classified as more toxic and faster acting than wood smoke (20, 21). The results of Clark et al (47) indicate that high levels of cyanide are now being found in victims of smoke inhalation. Treatment of this condition will require much more involved procedures than the simple administration of oxygen.
3. Some synthetic polymers release large amounts of hydrogen chloride. This gas is more toxic to humans than carbon monoxide (34) and victims surviving exposure to this gas suffer very serious pulmonary complications (36, 48, 49). As a result, emergency room physicians must try to anticipate this type of toxic effect, which is quite different from intoxication by carbon monoxide or hydrogen cyanide. This is particularly important since polyvinylchloride is a very widely used polymer (1) and is likely to be involved in most fires. Unfortunately, there is no adequate treatment for intoxication by this gas, and recovery from pulmonary injury is extremely slow (36, 49).
4. Some synthetic polymers release CO or HCN at a very fast rate, much higher than the rate at which CO is released from wood or cotton (50). Because of this higher rate of emission, there is less chance for dilution. As a result, the overall exposure concentration will be higher (50), making these polymers more hazardous than wood or cotton in a fire.
5. Some synthetic polymers, the fluoropolymers, release toxicants, probably perfluoroisobutylene and other fluorinated hydrocarbons, that have been shown to be extremely toxic (30, 31). This explains why they fall in the category labeled much more toxic than wood (20, 21). We do not know the mechanism of their toxic action nor what kind of treatment should be used for their victims.

These five reasons explain why, in general, smoke from decomposing synthetic polymers is faster acting and more toxic than smoke from wood. This can also be seen from the data presented in Figure 2.

Synthetic polymers were introduced into the US in large quantities only about thirty years ago (1). They have been instrumental in raising the American standard of living and their applications in science are useful and widespread. They also present serious problems when they decompose under heat. We must discover how best to use toxicity data in combination with the other properties of these materials to reduce deaths due to smoke inhalation. Clearly we have passed the point of questioning whether smoke from synthetic polymers is more toxic than smoke from wood. The answer obviously is yes. Now our task is to make sure that those who use large quantities of synthetic materials understand the toxicity of their thermal decomposition products and choose substances no more potentially toxic than wood. Combustible building materials, synthetic or natural, should be used with extreme care as replacements for noncombustible materials such as concrete, metals, glass, and ceramics. Finally, only synthetic polymers whose smoke is no more toxic than wood should be used in place of wood; smoke from wood is already toxic enough (20, 21). Only a better selection of building materials, combined with more effective fire prevention, will help improve our record on fire fatalities.

ACKNOWLEDGEMENT

Figures 1–4 reprinted with permission from Academic Press. Written under Grant 60NANB4D001 from the National Bureau of Standards. The conclusions are those of the author.

Literature Cited

1. Cullis, C. F., Hirschler, M. M. 1981. *The Combustion of Organic Polymers.* Oxford: Clarendon. 420 pp.
2. Landrock, A. H. 1983. *Handbook of Plastics Flammability and Combustion Toxicology. Principles, Materials, Testing, Safety and Smoke Inhalation Effects.* Park Ridge, NJ: Noyes. 308 pp.
3. Kaplan, H. L., Grand, A. F., Hartzell, G. E. 1983. *Combustion Toxicology, Principles and Test Methods.* Lancaster, PA: Technomic. 174 pp.
4. Anderson, R. C., Daring, K. M., Long, M. 1983. Study to assess the feasibility of incorporating combustion toxicity requirements into building material and furnishing codes of New York State. *Final Rep. Dep. State, Off. Fire Prevention and Control, Albany, NY.* Cambridge, MA: Arthur D. Little, Ref. 88712
5. Shaffer, G. S. 1984. Fire gas toxicity. Recommendations of the Secretary of State to the Uniform Fire Prevention and Building Code Council. Albany, NY: State of New York, Dept. State, 12231
6. Hilado, J. C., Cumming, H. J., Casey, C. J. 1978. Relative toxicity of materials in fire situations. *Modern Plastics* April: 92–96
7. Crane, C. R., Sanders, D. C., Endecott, B. R., Abbott, J. K., Smith, P. W. 1977. *Inhalation Toxicology: I. Design of a Small-Animal Test System. II. Determination of the Relative Toxic Hazards of 75 Aircraft Cabin Materials.* Washington, DC: Rep. FAA-AM-77-9, Dept. Transport., Fed. Aviation Admin., Office of Aviation Med.
8. Hodge, H. C., Sterner, J. H. 1949. Tabulation of toxicity classes. *Am. Ind. Hyg. Assoc. J.* 10:93–96
9. Klaassen, C. D., Doull, J. 1980. Evaluation of safety: Toxicologic evaluation. In *Casarett and Doull's Toxicology: The Basic Science of Poisons* ed. J. Doull, C.

D. Klaassen, M. O. Amdur, pp. 93–96. New York: Macmillan. 2nd ed.

10. Anderson, R. C., Alarie, Y. 1978. Screening procedure to recognize "supertoxic" decomposition products from polymeric materials under thermal stress. *J. Combust. Toxicol.* 5:54–63

11. Anderson, R. C., Alarie, Y. 1978. Approaches to the evaluation of the toxicity of decomposition products of polymeric materials under thermal stress. *J. Combust. Toxicol.* 5:214–21

12. Matijak-Schaper, M., Alarie, Y. 1982. Toxicity of carbon monoxide, hydrogen cyanide and low oxygen. *J. Combust. Toxicol.* 9:21–61

13. Hilado, C. J., Schneider, J. E. 1982. Toxicity of pyrolysis gases from polytetrafluoroethylene. *J. Combust. Toxicol.* 6:91–93

14. Hilado, C. J., Schneider, J. E., Brauer, D. P. 1979. Toxicity of pyrolysis gases from polypropylene. *J. Combust. Toxicol.* 6:109–111

15. Hilado, C. J., Olcomendy, E. M. 1979. Toxicity of pyrolysis gases from polyether sulfone. *J. Combust. Toxicol.* 6:117–20

16. Hilado, C. J., Huttlinger, N. V. 1978. Concentration-response data on toxicity of pyrolysis gases from some natural and synthetic polymers. *J. Combust. Toxicol.* 5:196–213

17. Levin, B. C., Fowell, A. J., Birky, M. M., Paabo, M., Stolte, A., Malek, D. 1982. *Further Development of a Test Method for the Assessment of the Acute Inhalation Toxicity of Combustion Products*. Washington, DC: US Dept. Commerce, Natl. Bur. Stand., Rep. NBSIR-82-2532

18. LeMoan, G., Chaigneau, M. 1977. Toxicite des produits de combustion des matieres plastiques. III. Methode rapide d'evaluation par la determination de la DL_{50} chez la souris. *Ann. Pharmaceut. France* 35:461–64

19. Lawrence, W. H., Raje, R. R., Singh, A. R., Autian, J. 1978. Toxicity of pyrolysis products: Influence of experimental conditions. The MSTL/UT and NASA/JCS procedures. *J. Combust. Toxicol.* 5:39–53

20. Alarie, Y., Anderson, R. C. 1979. Toxicologic and acute lethal hazard evaluation of thermal decomposition products of synthetic and natural polymers. *Toxicol. Appl. Pharmacol.* 51:341–62

21. Alarie, Y., Anderson, R. C. 1981. Toxicologic classification of thermal decomposition products of synthetic and natural

polymers. *Toxicol. Appl. Pharmacol.* 57:181–88

22. Nelson, G. L., Hixson, E. J., Denine, E. P. 1978. Combustion product toxicity studies of engineering plastics. *J. Combust. Toxicol.* 5:222–38

23. Einhorn, I. N. 1983. Toxicity of combustion products. *Intl. Fire Chief* 49:13–15

24. Berl, W., Halpin, B. 1979. *Human Fatalities from Unwanted Fires*. Washington, DC: Natl. Bur. Stand., Contract Rep. NBS-GCR-168. 57 pp.

25. Birky, M., Malek, D., Paabo, M. 1983. Study of biological samples obtained from victims of MGM Grand Hotel fire. *J. Analyt. Toxicol.* 7:265–71

26. Bell, J. R. 1983. Twenty-nine die in Biloxi, Mississippi jail fire. *Fire J.* 77:44–55

27. Bell, J. R., Klen, T. J., Willey, A. E. 1982. Investigative report on the Westchase Hilton Hotel, Houston, Texas, March 6, 1982, 12 fatalities. National Fire Protection Association report. *Fire J.* 77:11–22

28. Birchall, J. D., Kelly, A. 1983. New inorganic materials. *Sci. Am.* 248:104–15

29. Matijak-Schaper, M., Stock, M. F., Alarie, Y. 1982. Toxicity of thermal decomposition products from commonly used synthetic polymers. *Fire Sci. Technol.* Vol. 1, No. 1, microfiche card 1 of 1. New York: Comtex Scientific

30. Arito, H., Soda, R. 1977. Pyrolysis products of polytetrafluoroethylene and polyfluoroethylene propylene with reference to inhalation toxicity. *Ann. Occupat. Hyg.* 20:247–55

31. Smith, L. W., Gardner, R. J., Kennedy, G. L. 1982. Short-term inhalation toxicity of perfluoroisobutylene. *Drug Chem. Toxicol.* 5:295–303

32. Fonnum, F., Aas, P., Sterri, S., Helle, K. B. 1984. Modulation of the cholinergic activity of bronchial muscle during inhalation of Soman. *Fund. Appl. Toxicol.* 4:S52–S57

33. Haldane, J. 1895. The action of carbonic oxide on man. *J. Physiol.* 18:430–62

34. Henderson, Y., Haggard, H. W. 1943. *Noxious Gases and the Principles of Respiration Influencing Their Action*. New York: Reinhold. 294 pp. 2nd ed.

35. Barrow, C. S., Lucia, H., Alarie, Y. 1978. A comparison of the acute inhalation toxicity of hydrogen chloride versus the thermal decomposition products of polyvinylchloride. *J. Combust. Toxicol.* 6:3–12

36. Wong, K. L., Stock, M. F., Alarie, Y.

C. 1983. Evaluation of the pulmonary toxicity of plasticized polyvinylchloride thermal decomposition products in guinea pigs by repeated CO_2 challenges. *Toxicol Appl. Toxicol.* 70:236–48

37. Anderson, R. C., Alarie, Y. 1980. Acute lethal effects of polyvinylchloride thermal decomposition products in normal and cannulated mice. Washington, DC: *Soc. Toxicol. Meet.*, p. A–2 (Abstr.)

38. Morris, J. B., Smith, F. A. 1980. Regional deposition and absorption of inhaled hydrogen fluoride. Washington, DC: *Soc. Toxicol. Meet.* p. A–4 (Abstr.)

39. Morris, J. B., Smith, F. A. 1982. Regional deposition and absorption of inhaled hydrogen fluoride in the rat. *Toxicol. Appl. Pharmacol.* 62:81–89

40. Alarie, Y., Kane, L., Barrow, C. S. 1980. Sensory irritation: The use of an animal model to establish acceptable exposure to airborne chemical irritants. In *Toxicology: Principles and Practice,* ed. A. L. Reeves pp. 48–92. New York: Wiley

41. Klimisch, H. J., Hollander, H. W. M., Thyssen, J. 1980. Comparative measurements of the toxicity to laboratory animals of products of thermal composition generated by the method of DIN-53-436. *J. Combust. Toxicol.* 7:209–30

42. Herpol, C. 1980. Biological evaluation of toxicity caused by combustion of building materials. *Fire Mater.* 4:127–43

43. Barrow, C. S., Lucia, H., Stock, M. F., Alarie, Y. 1979. Development of methodologies to assess the relative hazards from thermal decomposition products of polymeric materials. *Am. Ind. Hyg. Assoc. J.* 40:408–23

44. Sangha, G. K., Matijak, M., Alarie, Y. 1981. Toxicologic evaluation of thermoplastic resins at and above processing temperatures. *Am. Ind. Hyg. Assoc. J.* 42:481–85

45. Alarie, Y. 1981. Toxicological evaluation of airborne chemical irritants and allergens using respiratory reflex reactions. *Proc. Inhalation Toxicol. Technol. Symp.* ed. B. K. J. Leong, pp. 207–231. Ann Arbor: Ann Arbor Science

46. Weil, C. S., Carpenter, C. P., Est, J. S., Smyth, H. F. Jr. 1966. Reproducibility of single oral dose toxicity testing. *Am. Ind. Hyg. Assoc. J.* 27:483–87

47. Clark, C. J., Campbell, D., Reid, W. H. 1981. Blood carboxyhemoglobin and cyanide levels in fire survivors. *Lancet* 1:1332–35

48. Dyer, R. F., Esch, V. H. 1976. Polyvinyl chloride toxicity in fires. Hydrogen chloride toxicity in fire fighters. *J. Am. Med. Assoc.* 235:393–97

49. Colardyn, F., Van er Straeten, M., Lamont, H., Van Peteghem, T. 1976. Acute inhalation-intoxication by combustion of polyvinylchloride. *Intl. Arch. Occupat. Environ. Health* 38:121–27

50. Alarie, Y., Stock, M. F., Matijak-Schaper, M., Birky, M. M. 1983. Toxicity of smoke during chair smoldering tests and small scale tests using the same materials. *Fund. Appl. Toxicol.* 3:619–26

Ann. Rev. Pharmacol. Toxicol. 1985. 25:349–80

ANTIBIOTIC TOLERANCE AMONG CLINICAL ISOLATES OF BACTERIA

Sandra Handwerger and Alexander Tomasz

The Rockefeller University, 1230 York Avenue, New York, New York 10021

INTRODUCTION

One of the unique features of β lactam antibiotics and other cell-wall inhibitors like vancomycin and bacitracin is that they can rapidly kill and in many cases lyse susceptible bacteria. Many other types of antibacterial agents (e.g. trimethoprim or chloramphenicol) are primarily bacteriostatic: they inhibit multiplication but do not cause an irreversible inactivation of the cell. In 1970 the characterization of a novel type of pneumococcal mutant was reported in the literature (1). This mutant grows in normal generation times and is as sensitive to growth inhibition by penicillin as the wild-type parent strain. However, while cultures of the parent strain are rapidly lysed and killed during exposure to penicillin, mutant cultures undergo only a very slow loss of viability and do not lyse at all. In other words, in these mutants penicillin and other cell-wall inhibitors act primarily as bacteriostatic agents. The term *antibiotic tolerance* has been coined to describe this novel type of bacterial response to antibiotic treatment.

Since the publication of the report on the pneumococcal mutant, tolerant strains have been isolated in the laboratory from mutagen-treated cultures of a number of other bacterial species (see Table 1). Subsequent reports have established that tolerance is not only a laboratory phenomenon. In 1974, Best and his colleagues tested 60 clinical isolates of *Staphylococcus* and found that one of these (strain Evans) is tolerant to oxacillin (2). Strain Evans has an oxacillin minimum inhibitory concentration (MIC) of 0.8 μg/ml, a value close to that of the majority of oxacillin-sensitive staphylococci. Upon addition of 6 μg/ml of oxacillin to a culture of the Evans strain, though, the bacteria only stop growing; under similar conditions other strains undergo rapid lysis. In

349

Table 1 Tolerant mutants isolated in the laboratory

Method of selection	Parent strain	Defective component		References
		Autolysin	Other	
Autolysin defect	Streptococcus pneumoniae R36A	N-acetylmuramic acid–L-alanine amidase (amidase)		1
	Streptococcus faecium ATCC9790	Muramidase		9
	Bacillus subtilis 168	Amidase?		10
	Bacillus licheniformis	Amidase or muramidase		11
	Bacillus subtilis 168	Amidase and glucosaminidase		12
Antibiotic survival	Escherichia coli K12	Transglycosylase?		8
	Escherichia coli K1776	Transglycosylase and endopeptidase		7
	Escherichia coli K2452 (temperature sensitive)	Normal level	Trigger pathway?	6
	Streptococcus pneumoniae R36A	Normal level	Trigger pathway?	13
	Staphylococcus aureus Evans	?	?	14
	Streptococcus pyogenes T4-56	?	?	16
Protease production	Bacillus subtilis 168	Normal level	Autolysin inactivation by protease	15

1976, a similar screening by Mayhall et al noted a high prevalence of tolerant cells among clinical isolates of staphylococci (3). Another naturally occurring tolerant strain, *Streptococcus sanguis* Wicky, was described in 1977 (4). Again, this strain is exquisitely sensitive to penicillin inhibition but does not lyse and loses viability only very slowly during treatment with any concentration of penicillin, even up to 10,000 times its MIC value.

A publication of major impact was the report by Sabath and colleagues in 1977 in *Lancet* that described the unsuspected frequency with which tolerant strains of staphylococci can be isolated from clinical specimens originating in deep-seated infections (5). Since then, reports of tolerance among isolates of gram-positive organisms have increased in frequency. A computer-library search (MEDLINE) indicates that five reports about tolerant isolates were published between 1970 and 1977; there were over 35 reports of tolerant clinical isolates between 1977 and 1984, and strains exhibiting the tolerant response now include more than 20 species. Most of these are gram-positive bacteria. The only gram-negative tolerant isolates so far described appear to be laboratory mutants of *Escherichia coli* (6–8).

The better-characterized tolerant laboratory mutants have already been used extensively as experimental tools for the analysis of the mechanism of action of penicillin and other wall inhibitors. The apparently widespread occurrence of tolerant bacteria among natural isolates poses a number of additional questions and moves the phenomenon of antibiotic tolerance into the realm of clinical medicine. Do the naturally occurring tolerant bacteria isolated on the basis of criteria from the clinical diagnostic laboratory have a biochemical basis of tolerance similar to that of the laboratory isolates? Do tolerant bacteria found among clinical isolates arise through antibiotic selection? Do infections with tolerant strains pose any problems in chemotherapy with β lactams or other cell–wall inhibitory antibiotics? The purpose of this review is to attempt a critical evaluation of reports on natural tolerant isolates of bacteria with these three questions in mind.

Antibiotic Tolerance and Antibiotic Resistance

Since tolerance can improve the chances of bacterial survival quite dramatically during antibiotic treatment, the phenomenon is often referred to as a novel form of antibiotic resistance. This terminology can be confusing, since in the mechanistic sense tolerance may actually be contrasted with resistance.

Resistance results in the need for a higher concentration of antibiotic to prevent growth; that is, the MIC is increased. Although higher concentrations are required for growth inhibition of resistant organisms, once exposed to this concentration, the organisms will cease growing and killing (and in some bacteria lysis) will begin. Tolerant organisms, on the other hand, show only small or no change in MIC, but upon exposure to this concentration lysis is blocked and viability is lost only very slowly. Figure 1 illustrates the contrast-

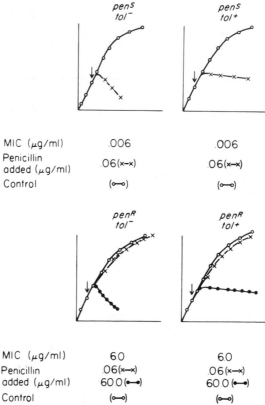

MIC (μg/ml)	.006	.006
Penicillin added (μg/ml)	.06(x—x)	.06(x—x)
Control	(o—o)	(o—o)

MIC (μg/ml)	6.0	6.0
Penicillin added (μg/ml)	.06(x—x)	.06(x—x)
	60.0(•—•)	60.0(•—•)
Control	(o—o)	(o—o)

Figure 1   Response of antibiotic-tolerant and antibiotic-resistant strains to penicillin treatment. Viable titer of bacterial cultures (ordinate) is plotted against time (abscissa). Cultures receive penicillin at the times indicated by the arrows. In the upper panel, a penicillin–sensitive nontolerant (pen^{S}tol$^-$) and a penicillin–sensitive tolerant (pen^{S}tol$^+$) culture receives 0.06 μg per ml penicillin [corresponding to 10 times the MIC equivalent concentration (x–x–x–x)]. Loss of viability in the pen^{S}tol$^-$ culture may be contrasted with the primarily bacteriostatic response of the pen^{S}tol$^+$ bacteria.

In the lower panel, a pair of penicillin-resistant nontolerant (pen^{R}tol$^-$) and penicillin-resistant tolerant (pen^{R}tol$^+$) bacteria receive penicillin at two concentration: 0.06 μg (x–x–x–x) and 60.0 μg (———) per ml. The lower concentration of antibiotic, below the MIC value of these resistant strains (MIC = 6.0 μg/ml), has no effect on growth. The higher concentration of penicillin (concentration to 10 times the MIC value) causes loss of viability in the tol$^-$ strain and bacteriostasis in the tol$^+$ strain.

ing features and possible combinations of the tolerance and resistance traits. A specific example of the combination of high-level penicillin resistance with tolerance recently has been described in the case of South African pneumococci (17).

Another example of confusing terminology arises when authors refer to erythromycin or chloramphenicol tolerance. From what has been outlined above, it should be clear that the term *tolerance* refers to bacteria in which a typically bactericidal-bacteriolytic response to antibiotics is changed in the direction of bacteriostasis. There is little use in referring to the response of bacteria to a typically bacteriostatic drug as tolerance.

THE MECHANISM OF THE IRREVERSIBLE EFFECTS OF β LACTAM ANTIBIOTICS

The tolerant phenotype presumably results from some block in the sequence of events between antibiotic exposure and bacterial killing. It is critical, therefore, to understand current models of the mechanism of action of cell–wall active antibiotics, in particular β lactams, in order to comprehend what has gone awry in the tolerant cell. In current models, all the antibacterial effects of β lactam antibiotics, whether inhibition of growth, killing, or lysis of the cells, are initiated by the inhibition of a set of bacterial enzymes that catalyze the terminal stages of cell-wall assembly. These enzymes (penicillin-binding proteins or PBPs) are anchored in the bacterial plasma membrane. Penicillin covalently binds (acylates) the active sites of PBPs, causing inactivation of these enzymes. How then does inhibition of these enzymes cause eventual lysis and death? It appears that antibiotic-induced lysis, and to some extent killing, depends on the activity of a group of ubiquitous bacterial enzymes, called autolysins or murein hydrolases, that can hydrolyze covalent bonds in the cell wall surrounding the bacterial cell (see Figure 2).

The Role of Autolysins in Antibiotic-Induced Bacterial Killing

Mutants defective in autolysins have been isolated in a number of bacterial species. Such mutants have a common phenotype: they do not undergo lysis and lose viability with reduced rates during treatment with β-lactam antibiotics and other cell-wall inhibitors. In other words, these mutants exhibit antibiotic tolerance.

Biochemical and physiological analysis of an antibiotic-tolerant mutant of the pneumococcus was first described in 1970. The tolerant phenotype appeared to be associated with the low specific activity of a cell wall–hydrolyzing enzyme activity, an N-acetylmuramic acid-L-alanine amidase (amidase) (1). This finding has been confirmed by the demonstration that DNA isolated from the mutants can introduce (via genetic transformation) the autolytic defect into lysis-prone recipient cells and the transformants all show a tolerant response to all cell-wall inhibitors. In tolerant mutants subsequently isolated from laboratory mutants of other species, tolerance is also associated with defective autolytic activities.

Tolerant mutants differ in their degrees of tolerance: i.e. in the residual rates

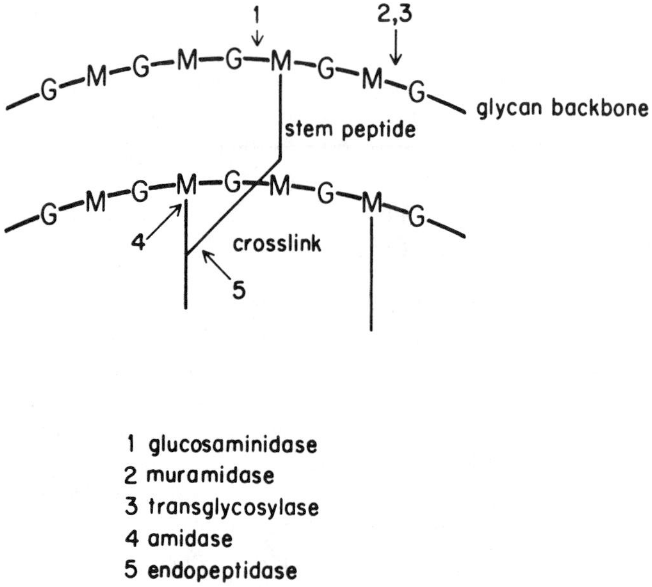

1 glucosaminidase
2 muramidase
3 transglycosylase
4 amidase
5 endopeptidase

Figure 2   Sites of action of autolytic enzymes; a cartoon of the types of covalent bonds in the cell-wall peptidogylcan: two glycan strands with a pair of cross-linked stem peptides and one uncross-linked stem peptide. Letters M and G represent N-acetylmuramic acid and N-acetylglucosamine residues respectively. Numbers with arrows indicate the sites of action of various autolytic enzymes.

of lysis and viability loss during antibiotic treatment. Whether or not the extent of the defect in autolysin activity determines the degree of resistance to lysis (and killing) is not yet clear. In *E. coli,* which produces several autolytic enzymes, mutants defective in one or two of these enzyme activities have been obtained. The degree of tolerance appears to be related both to the residual enzyme level and to the number of defective autolytic activities (7).

What is the normal role of these hydrolytic enzymes required for antibiotic-induced killing? The type and number of autolytic enzymes differ among bacterial species: e.g. amidase has been described in pneumococci (18); muramidase has been described in lactobacilli; and transglycosylase, peptidase, and amidase activity has been described in *E. coli* (19). None of the mutants shows poor growth or abnormality in functions essential for growth in test-tube cultures, implying that the enzyme activity lost in the mutants does not perform an essential physiological role. The mutants described thus far are not totally devoid of autolysin, however: in each 0.1%–10% of activity remains, and it is possible that this small amount of autolysin activity is sufficient for some essential aspect of cell-wall growth. In several bacteria, autolysins appear to be required for normal cell separation. Autolysin-defective (Lyt⁻) mutants show defective cell separation as manifested by chaining in pneumococci (1) and *Bacillus* species (12) and packet or clump formation in staphylococci (20). Autolysin activity has also been implicated in competence, flagellar extrusion, cell-wall turnover, and sporulation (19).

The major conclusion emerging from the analysis of the autolysin-defective mutants is that interference with cell-wall synthesis in bacteria can rapidly upset the cellular control of autolytic enzymes, triggering their activity on a level that is suicidal for the cell. It is intriguing to consider that the unsurpassed antibacterial power of β-lactam antibiotics may be linked to an enzyme activity that, under in vitro conditions at least, is not essential for the growth of the target bacteria.

The Pleiotropy of Tolerance

Although the great majority of tolerant mutants isolated in the laboratory have defective autolytic systems, one should recall that the majority of these mutants have been selected for an autolytic defect. If selection is for *survival* during antibiotic treatment, as is likely to be the case in the tolerant clinical isolates, then in theory at least any number of complex factors that play a role in bactericidal activity may be altered by mutation and provide antibiotic tolerance. Experience in the laboratory supports this idea (see Table 1 and mechanism 2 below).

It may be worth describing in some detail the types of mutational changes that conceivably could cause the tolerant phenotype. This could also serve to illustrate the variety of factors that can modulate the irreversible effects of β-lactam antibiotics. Figure 3 shows schematically the presumed pathway between β-lactam binding and eventual cell death. Briefly, in this model inhibition of one or more PBPs by β-lactam antibiotics results in inhibition of cell-wall synthesis, generating some regulatory signal in the cell that can trigger the uncontrolled activity of autolytic enzyme(s). These enzymes inflict various degrees of irreparable structural damage on the cell wall, possibly by first cleaving a limited number of covalent bonds in the cell wall, which produces focal nicks too small to be resolved by electron microscopy. Exposure of the underlying plasma membrane would then cause cell death. More extensive damage to the wall would lead to actual wall degradation and anatomical-sized gaps in the wall, followed by rupture of the plasma membrane and escape of the cytoplasmic contents (lysis). [For a more detailed view of the pathways by which cell-wall inhibitors result in bacterial killing, see (19, 21–23).] In Figure 3, sites at which alterations in this pathway might result in tolerance are numbered to correspond to the mechanisms discussed below.

1. It has been shown that β-lactam antibiotics that bind to the penicillin-binding proteins (PBP) 1a and 1b of *E. coli* are those most effective in triggering rapid viability loss and lysis. Preferential binding to other PBPs may

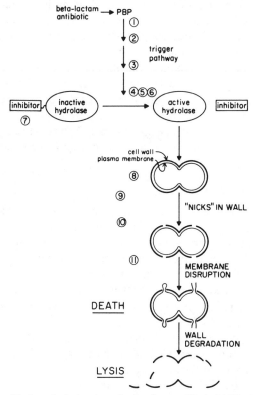

Figure 3   Scheme of the hypothetical pathway leading from antibiotic-inhibited PBPs to cell lysis. See text.

cause only a slow loss of viability, while the rate of killing and lysis by other cell-wall inhibitors would remain unaltered. While such mutants have not yet been reported, drug-specific tolerance (e.g. tolerance to β-lactam antibiotics but not to vancomycin) has been described in both laboratory mutants and clinical isolates (5, 13, 24, 25).

2. A second type of tolerance mutation with normal levels of autolysin activity but without the capacity to induce lytic activity has been described (6, 13). When mutagen-treated pneumococci are exposed to several cycles of treatment with bactericidal doses of ampicillin, among 100 isolates sharing the tolerant phenotype 80 have defective autolysin; the rest have a normally functioning autolytic system. Despite the presence of normal autolytic activity, these mutants are tolerant, i.e. they show slow lysis and death during antibiotic treatment. Williamson & Tomasz have suggested that tolerance may be due to a defect in some signal needed to trigger autolytic activity (13). A similar isolate

has been characterized in *E. coli* (7). Several isolates of resistant South African pneumococci are also highly tolerant but contain only moderately reduced levels of autolysin. These may also contain a defect in the triggering pathway (17).

3. It is well known that non-growing bacteria or bacteria with inhibited protein synthesis are tolerant to cell-wall active antibiotics (26, 27). Normally, the addition of penicillin to growing bacteria results first in interference with cell-wall synthesis and next in inhibition of protein synthesis. In some mutants, the time needed to shut down protein synthesis after penicillin addition may be shortened so that the bacterium in effect assumes the phenotype of a non-growing cell (28).

4. Since the destructive activity of autolysins is provoked by inhibition of cell-wall synthesis, it is conceivable that in some tolerant mutant this suicidal coupling between the halt in wall synthesis and autolysin activity is somehow circumvented.

5. Some autolytic enzymes are sensitive to proteolysis. *Bacillus subtilis* mutants that overproduce extracellular proteases appear resistant to the lytic action of β-lactam antibiotics (15).

6. A lower specific activity of autolytic enzymes seems to be the basis of tolerance in numerous strains of bacteria, as described in the original tolerant laboratory mutants (1, 9, 10, 11, 12). *Streptococcus sanguis* strain Wicky may also represent this type of tolerance (4).

7. If autolysin activity is negatively controlled in vivo, as was first suggested for pneumococci (29, 30), then overproduction of an inhibitor may result in the tolerant phenotype. Lipoteichoic acids appear to inhibit autolysin activity in several bacterial species (29–33). Some tolerant *Staphylococcus aureus* strains produce greater quantities of lipoteichoic acids and secrete greater amounts upon exposure to oxacillin than nontolerant strains (34). Extracts of these cultures added to nontolerant cultures inhibit lytic activity (5). Thus, tolerant staphylococcal strains might represent regulatory mutants that produce increased quantities of autolysin inhibitor.

8. In pneumococci, biosynthetic replacement of choline with ethanolamine results in the formation of cell walls resistant to the effects of autolysin (35). Such bacteria are tolerant to cell-wall antibiotics. An analogous mutational defect resulting in alteration of the autolysin substrate (cell wall) represents still another possible mechanism of tolerance.

9. Persistence, a phenomenon most frequently reported in *S. aureus,* is the survival of a small fraction (less than 0.1%) of cultures despite prolonged antibiotic exposure (36). Subcultures of these survivors yield cultures with the same response, i.e. less than 0.1% survival. This phenomenon may be related to the existence of a stage in the cell-divisional cycle in which autolytic activity is low. Mutants may exist in which the probability of an average cell being in

this low autolytic (tolerant) phase is increased (38). This would raise the percentage of persisters, resulting in apparent tolerance.

Indeed, several authors have suggested that only a fraction of *S. aureus* cultures are actually tolerant in a fashion analogous to the heterogeneity of methicillin-resistant staphylococci (37, 39). While this represents a possible mechanism of tolerance, examination of time-kill studies by these and other investigators indicate that tolerant *S. aureus* show a decreased rate of killing for the culture population as a whole (2, 14, 24, 40). Although survival after 24 hours may differ from strain to strain and reflect a relative degree of tolerance, this situation is not different from that of other tolerant organisms. All tolerant strains, including laboratory autolysin-defective mutants, undergo some loss of viability, albeit slowly, and thus demonstrate variable numbers of survivors after 24 hours (1, 2, 9). This should not be construed to imply that only a portion of the population is tolerant.

10. Bacteria growing at acidic pH values are known to shift to the synthesis of different phospholipids (41) and the plasma membrane of such cells appears to have increased resistance to stress (42). Bacteria growing at low pH values also become tolerant to the killing effect of cell-wall inhibitors (43, 44). Such a membrane alteration conceivably is the basis of tolerance in certain types of bacterial fermentation mutants that overproduce acidic catabolites.

11. Bacterial mutants that produce plasma membranes with altered chemical composition and increased resistance to osmotic lysis may also show the tolerant phenotype.

The main purpose of Figure 3 is to emphasize the complexity of the processes that contribute to the irreversibility of the action of β-lactam antibiotics. Most of the mutational blocks listed are hypothetical. Specific selection processes will have to be designed to test whether or not they actually exist among the numerous tolerant strains described from clinical sources.

THE DETECTION OF TOLERANT BACTERIA: METHODOLOGY

Although tolerance was originally defined as a decreased rate of killing or slow loss of viability upon exposure to bactericidal antibiotics, for clinical purposes tolerance more recently has been considered present when the minimal bactericidal concentration (MBC) is significantly higher (generally 32-fold) than the minimum inhibitory concentration, where the MBC is defined as the concentration of antibiotic yielding 99.9% killing of the inoculum. Notwithstanding the obvious practical values of this assay, one should realize that this method is at best a very insensitive end-point titration and can produce serious artifacts.

A critical review of the literature describing reports of clinical isolates tentatively identified as tolerant makes it apparent that technical problems in these studies frequently make it difficult to accept their claims. It seems worthwhile to spell out types of problems that contribute to this situation.

Technical Problems with the MBC Determination

Cultures of penicillin-sensitive nontolerant bacteria contaminated with a minority population of either β–lactamase producing or intrinsically resistant cells of the same species may fortuitously produce false tolerance. Subculture and retesting of survivors should eliminate this problem (45). On the other hand, the incidence of tolerance may be falsely decreased due to antibiotic carryover. When a loop full of bacteria from the drug-containing MIC tube is transferred to the surface of drug-free agar, dilution of the drug by the volume of the agar medium does not necessarily occur. Adding penicillinase to cultures prior to agar plating for viability or MBC determinations may be necessary to reliably determine tolerance in some strains (46). However, not all investigators have begun to take this precaution.

Comparison of the rates of viability loss between cultures exhibiting different degrees of chaining can cause obvious problems: longer chains may appear more resisant to killing because of the larger numbers of viable units per chains.

Gwynn and colleagues (47) have observed that bacteria may escape the cidal effect of antibiotics during MIC determination by adhering to test-tube walls above the meniscus of the antibiotic-containing medium. While the factors that can actually contribute to the ability of such bacteria to survive are not completely clear, it is obvious that these cells are reintroduced into the body of the culture fluid during stirring, which many investigators do just prior to testing the viable titers of cells in the MIC tubes. This effect can produce falsely high survival rates and misleadingly indicate tolerance. Taylor et al evaluated the influence of this effect on MBC determinations on 40 strains of *S. aureus,* including several that previously had been described as tolerant. Using the simple technical precaution of mixing the cultures after overnight incubation four hours prior to plating for MBC determination, they found no strains with MBC exceeding the MIC by fourfold or more (48). Presumably organisms adhering to the test tube walls above the meniscus were mixed into the antibiotic-containing broth, eliminating the falsely elevated MBCs (49).

Phenotypic Tolerance

Studies on the mechanism of the cidal and lytic effects of cell-wall inhibitors have revealed that the rate and degree of these irreversible antibacterial effects can be dramatically modulated by factors in the bacterial environment (44, 58). Table 2 is a compilation of some of the factors that can cause phenotypic tolerance in genetically nontolerant bacteria. The biochemical mechanism of these effects is not well understood and discussion of these is outside the scope of this review. Phenotypic tolerance has importance for our discussion in two

Table 2 Environmental factors causing phenotypic tolerance

Factor	Species	Proposed mechanism	References
Low pH	Group B streptococci, B. subtilis, E. coli, S. aureus, S. pneumoniae	Suboptimal pH for autolysin and/or membrane stabilization	43, 44
Serum	S. faecalis	Diminished autolysin activity or decreased growth rate	50
High Ca or Mg concentration	N. gonorrhoeae	Outer membrane stabilization	51, 52
Inhibition of growth (e.g. stationary phase or bacteriostatic antibiotics)	All bacteria	Decreased autolysin activity?	26, 27, 53
High inoculum size	S. viridans, Listeria monocytogenes, Group G streptococci	?	60, 62, 63, 74
Composition of growth medium	Group B and D streptococci, S. aureus	May be due to pH effect	24, 57, 61, 87
Protease	B. subtilis	Protease sensitive autolysin	15
Forssman antigen	S. pneumoniae	Inhibition of autolysin	29, 30
Lipoteichoic acids	S. aureus, S. faecalis, Lactobacillus spp.	Inhibition of autolysin	2, 31, 32
Cardiolipin	S. faecalis	Inhibition of autolysin	32

respects. First, conditions may arise during the screening of isolates that result in the appearance of tolerance (see Table 3) and, second, conditions may occur at the sites of infection that promote a decreased rate of killing of (genotypically) nontolerant organisms. Probably the most frequent technical pitfall is the use of stationary-phase cultures in the MBC and viability determinations. It has long been known that β-lactam antibiotics are active against growing cells and that conditions that prevent growth, such as chloramphenicol treatment or amino-acid deprivation, will diminish effective bacterial killing (26, 27, 53). Clearly, then, growing rather than stationary-phase cultures must be used to assess tolerance accurately. The American Society for Microbiology suggests that inocula be prepared by either dilution of overnight cultures or use of growing cultures (54, 55), and many clinical laboratories use overnight cultures to directly inoculate MIC and MBC tubes. Using such stationary cultures will necessarily result in diminished killing rates. Overnight cultures of bacteria that have been in the stationary phase for an unknown length of time cannot be assumed to resume growth instantly upon dilution into fresh medium, particularly not if that medium contains antibiotics. Thus, bacteria reported to be tolerant only after tests using stationary-phase cultures (39, 56) should not be considered truly tolerant unless cultures of growing cells (log phase) demonstrate similar findings.

Additional major variables affecting the rate of killing include media composition, pH, and inoculum size (24, 57–60). Autolysin activity in nontolerant organisms may be decreased with exposure to low pH, causing cultures to appear tolerant (43, 50, 52). Venglarcik et al (61) attempted to correlate the effects of media and growth phase with pH. *S. aureus* cultures showed lowest final inoculum pH after overnight incubation in tryptic soy broth (TSB); highest final pH was obtained after a three-hour incubation in Mueller-Hinton broth (MHB). Those conditions resulting in low-inoculum pH were associated with the highest MBCs, so that 10 of 20 strains appeared tolerant. Under conditions promoting higher final pH, no strains appeared tolerant. Tryptose phosphate and tryptic soy broth seem to allow the lowest pH values and thus the least degree of killing.

The significance of the inoculum effect noted in several species is unclear. Tolerance appears to increase when large inocula are used and to decrease with small inocula (60, 62). Since most authors do not specify whether organisms were diluted to the appropriate concentrations or grown to a given density, it is not apparent whether this is related to growth phase rather than inoculum alone. Best noted no difference in killing rate between staphylococcal cultures with inocula of 10^5 and 10^8 when both cultures were logarithmic phase (14). In group G streptococci, however, inoculum size and growth phase may independently increase the appearance of tolerance. Organisms are killed rapidly when log or stationary-phase cultures are diluted to low inocula (10^4), but log-phase

Table 3 Tolerant clinical isolates

Species/group	Source[a]	Phase of inoculum[b]	Media[c]	$\dfrac{MBC \geq}{MIC}$[d]	Incidence of tolerance[e]	Comments	References
Streptococcus							
S. viridans	gingivae/blood	NS	NS	10	15/58	patients receiving pen. prophylaxis	85
S. viridans	blood	NS	NS	10	16/80		107
S. viridans	blood	log	THB	32	0/10		87
S. viridans	mult	stat	THB	32	5/9	penicillinase added	75
S. sanguis	gingivae/blood	NS	NS	10	4/21	patients receiving pen. prophylaxis	85
S. sanguis	mult	log	THB	32 killing curves	4/5	penicillinase added	46
S. mitior	gingivae/blood	NS	NS	10	19/94	patients receiving pen. prophylaxis	85
S. mitior (nutritional variants)	blood	log	THB	16	9/11	penicillinase added	74
S. mutans	gingivae/blood	NS	NS	10	4/15	patients receiving pen. prophylaxis	85
S. milleri	gingivae/blood	NS	NS	10	1/9	pen. prophylaxis	85
S. salivarius	gingivae/blood	NS	NS	10	0/17	pen. prophylaxis	85
S. pneumoniae	mult	stat	THB	32	0/11	penicillinase added	75
S. pneumoniae	blood/CSF	log	C + y	killing curves	5 (only report of tolerant isolates)	also highly resistant	17
Group A	mult	stat	THB	16	11/12		90
Group A	mult	stat	THB	32	1/16		75
Group B	blood/CSF	log	MHB	32 killing curves	4/100	penicillinase added	
Group B	mult	stat	THB	32	13/33		
Group B	mult	stat	THB	32	1/16	penicillinase added	
Group C	mult	log	nutrient broth and serum	32	16/17	penicillinase added serum may increase tolerance	

Group D	mult	stat	THB	32	17/18	penicillinase added	
S. faecalis, S. faecium	blood	log	MHB	32	majority of 34	only mean MBC/MIC data shown	
S. bovis	blood	log	MBH	32	4/4	patients responding poorly to treatment	63
Group G	mult	log	THB	32 killing curves	0/9, 0/9 vanco		
Group G	mult	log	THB	32	0/19, 1/19 vanco		93
Group G	mult	NS	NS	32	1/9, 8/9 vanco		92
Lactobacillus							
Lactobacillus spp.	mult	stat	MHB	achievable serum level	31/40		96
Lactobacillus spp.	mult	stat	MHB	killing curves	16/17		72, 124
Listeria							
L. monocytogenes	mult	NS	dextrose phosphate	killing curves	most of 20	only mean MBC data shown	95
L. monocytogenes	mult	log	TSB	16 killing curves	50/50		62
Clostridium							
C. perfingens	feces	stat	MHB	8	most of 50 tol to vanco	only mean MBC data shown	125
Staphylococcus							
S. aureus	mult	stat	MHB	50 killing curves	33/60 oxa	fewer tolerant using 48-hour MBC	3
S. aureus	blood	log	MHB	32	28/63 naf		5
S. aureus	mult	stat	MHB	100	8/30 cloxa		126
S. aureus	blood	stat	MHB	16 killing curves	16/35 meth, 17/35 oxa, 23/35 ceph		56
S. aureus	blood	stat	MHB	100	34/34 meth		81
S. aureus	blood	log	TSB	10	16/45 oxa		79

	Source[a]	Phase[b]	Medium[c]		Tolerance[d,e]	Comments[f]	Ref.
S. aureus	bovine mastitis	log	MHB	32	7/24 cloxa	penicillinase added	82
S. aureus	blood	stat	BHI	16	6/13 naf, 5/13 vanco		24
S. aureus	blood	stat	MHB	16	5/13 naf, 7/13 vanco		127
S. aureus	mult	NS	MHB	32	2/20 moxalactam		25
S. aureus	mult	NS	BHI	32	9/15 oxa, 4/10 vanco		40
S. aureus	mult	stat	MHB	killing curves	19/30 oxa, 19/30 ceph		106
S. aureus	blood	stat, log	MHB	32	12/15 ceph, 12/15 oxa	penicillinase added	80
S. aureus	blood/endo-carditis	stat	TSB	32	32/50 oxa, naf or ceph		
S. aureus	blood/bac-teremia	stat	TSB	32	35/54 oxa, naf or ceph		59
S. aureus	mult	stat	MHB	16	25/40 oxa, 20/40 ceph		48
S. aureus	mult	log	MHB	16	0/9 oxa, 0/9 ceph	mixed cultures 4 hours prior to plating (see text)	
S. aureus	mult	log	MHB	8	0/40 oxa	penicillinase added	

[a] Mult = multiple sources, CSF = cerebrospinal fluid

[b] NS = not specified, log = logarithmic phase, stat = stationary phase

[c] MHB = Mueller Hinton broth, THB = Todd Hewitt broth, C + y = casein hydrolysate medium with yeast extract, TSB = tryptic soy broth, BHI = brain heart infusion

[d] Criterion for determination of tolerance; if only numeral given, refers to ratio of MBC to MIC greater than which isolates considered tolerant; killing curves not used unless specified.

[e] Number of tolerant isolates/total number of strains evaluated; refers to penicillin tolerance unless otherwise indicated.

[f] Penicillinase was not added unless specified.

cultures concentrated to high inocula (10^7–10^8) are killed more rapidly than stationary-phase cultures (63).

A more important consequence of phenotypic tolerance concerns its effects on the bactericidal action of antibiotics in vivo. Diminished killing by antibiotics may occur at sites of infection due to changes in the local environment. Low pH, which results in phenotypic tolerance in vitro, may be encountered in phagosomes of polymorphonuclear neutrophils (64), in synovial fluid during septic arthritis (65), in cerebrospinal fluid during meningitis (66), in the endobronchium during pneumonia (67), and in abcesses and empyemas (68). Slow bacterial growth occurs in osteomyelitis (O. Zak, personal communication) and within endocarditic vegetations (69). Additionally, high inocula and stationary-phase growth are associated with phenotypic tolerance, and these conditions may exist in endocarditis, septic arthritis, and other deep-seated infections. Phenotypic tolerance may be superimposed on genotypic tolerance in the laboratory with an additive effect: autolysin-defective pneumococcal mutants show even slower killing by penicillin when growth is inhibited by amino-acid deprivation (S. Handwerger, A. Tomasz, unpublished observations). Such effects may also occur in vivo under conditions disposing to phenotypic tolerance.

Nontechnical Problems with the MBC Determination

Even if standardized, the MBC determination yields only viability at an arbitrary endpoint, with no information about the rate of killing during the preceding 24 hours (see Figure 4). Since tolerance is defined as a slow rate of killing, lysis or viability (time kill) curves that examine multiple time points will necessarily yield more information. In the quantitation of tolerance by the MBC determination, it is assumed that higher concentrations of the drug will cause higher rates of viability loss. This need not be the case. For example, cultures of tolerant *S. sanguis* strains exposed to a wide range of concentrations of penicillin (1–10,000 times the MIC value) lose their viability with the same very slow rate (46). Several investigators have noted that tolerant strains may have an infinite MBC value (37). In nontolerant cells, the rate of cidal action of penicillin increases only up to a certain concentration, above which the rate either stabilizes or actually decreases. In many species of bacteria, it has been shown that the use of increased penicillin concentrations does not increase the rate of killing in either tolerant or nontolerant strains (14, 26, 70, 71). In fact, use of very high concentrations of antibiotic may give precisely the opposite effect. This phenomenon, known as the paradoxical or Eagle effect, was described by Eagle in 1948: in some species of bacteria, the rate of antibiotic killing is diminished at very large multiples of the MIC (70). For this reason, use of a single very high concentration, such as 50–100 times the MIC, for determining tolerance should be avoided.

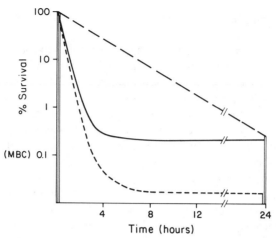

Figure 4 Relationship between killing rates and the MBC value. Curves show three possible types of kinetics for the loss of viability during treatment with penicillin at a concentration of one time the MIC value. The vertical bar at 0 minutes indicates the inoculum; bars at 24 hours represent percent of survival as determined by the MBC value. The lower bar represents less than 0.1% survival reached along the rapidly declining killing curve of the nontolerant bacterium (- - - - -). The higher bars indicate survival of more than 0.1% of the cells, which indicates tolerance by the MBC test. However, rates (and mechanisms) of killing in the two "tolerant" cultures are completely different. The truly tolerant mutant undergoes slow loss of viability (———), while the other culture (————) has an initial rapid rate of killing typical of nontolerant cells but a higher survival rate, which may be due to physiologically heterogeneous inoculum (e.g. higher percentage of dormant cells that are phenotypically tolerant). Alternatively, these cells may represent increased persisters or a subpopulation of resistant cells.

In some strains of bacteria, additional problems may hamper the characterization of tolerant isolates. Instability of the tolerant trait (loss during storage of frozen cultures) has been reported in staphylococci (5, 36, 59), and an extreme cell concentration dependence of tolerance has been noted among *S. sanguis* isolates (60). The mechanism of these effects is not understood.

Improved Methods of Detection

Time-kill studies remain the most reliable means of determining tolerance. In many bacterial species, including *E. coli, N. gonorrhoeae, S. pneumoniae,* group A streptococci, lactobacilli, and *S. aureus,* treatment of growing cultures (generation time 30–90 minutes) with 5–10 × the MIC of penicillin results in a 2–3 log decrease in viability within four hours. Treatment with 1–2 times the MIC equivalent causes a similar degree of killing within 6–8 hours (1, 5, 6, 7, 14, 16, 52, 72). In contrast, tolerant mutants of *E. coli,* pneumococci, group A streptococci, lactobacilli, and *S. aureus,* as well as tolerant strains of *Listeria monocytogenes* and *Streptococcus sanguis,* show no decrease in viable titer or, at maximum, a one-log fall (1, 4, 5, 6, 7, 14, 16, 72, 73). [Watanakunakorn

(56) found no difference between rates of killing of staphylococci determined to be tolerant or nontolerant on the basis of high MBC–MIC ratios. However, only stationary-phase cultures were used, and the "nontolerant" strains showed no loss of viability after six hours of incubation with oxacillin.] Thus, within 2–6 hours after the addition of antibiotic, tolerant and nontolerant strains can be differentiated by their relative rates of killing. A reliable and relatively simple method for clinical laboratories might use viability plating just prior to antibiotic addition and, four hours later, at a single antibiotic concentration. This method would not represent a significant increase in workload compared to MBC determinations and would reliably differentiate between rates of antibiotic killing. The same precautions regarding technique outlined for MBC determinations are required for this type of testing.

Recently, more rapid methods have been suggested for the detection of tolerance in the clinical laboratory. A disk-diffusion test substituting a penicillinase disk for a penicillin-susceptibility disk was successful for a small number of *S. viridans* initially screened (74), but use of high inocula caused false-positive results, and further testing with other streptococcal species yielded sensitivities as low as 57% (75). Similar methods have been used for screening a number of other gram-positive isolates (76, 77). A more recently proposed method incorporating penicillin gradient plates and replica plating appears promising but requires further testing (78). Plating technique results have been most frequently compared to MBC–MIC ratios to verify their sensitivity and specificity (75). More detailed analyses comparing test results to viability curves are needed to determine the reliability of these newer techniques.

THE INCIDENCE OF TOLERANCE AMONG CLINICAL ISOLATES

Given the number of possible variables, it is not surprising that estimates of the incidence of tolerance range widely (see Table 2). Estimates of tolerance to β–lactamase resistant penicillins among strains of *S. aureus* generally vary from 30–70% (5, 40, 79, 80), although one report cites 100% of isolates (81) and another no tolerant isolates (48). Tolerant isolates have also been reported in the veterinary literature (82). Staphylococcal isolates generally show cross-tolerance among the β lactams: i.e. strains tolerant to one β lactam show the same response to others. Vancomycin tolerance has also been reported, although the incidence appears lower. Tolerance to vancomycin may accompany β-lactam tolerance or appear independently (5, 83, 84). The mechanism of this phenomenon is unknown. One isolate of *S. epidermidis* has been reported as tolerant to vancomycin, but was only "tolerant" in the stationary phase (39).

Among the streptococcal species, the viridans group shows a high incidence of penicillin tolerance, with the possible exception of *S. salivarius* (85). A small study of nutritionally variant *S. mitior* found most strains tested to be tolerant (74). A significant fraction of *S. viridans* species may also show tolerance to vancomycin (86). Krogstad et al (87) did not find any tolerance among ten viridans streptococci; however, their methodology differed from that of the former study.

Group D streptococci of both enterococcal *(S. faecalis, S. faecium)* and nonenterococcal *(S. bovis)* groups show a high incidence of tolerance (50, 87, 88, 89). Incidence was reported to be high in Group A strains by one group, but only stationary-phase cultures were used for testing (90). The pediatric literature of the past ten years has noted that in vitro killing of Group B streptococci by penicillin is slow (71); the occurrence of tolerance in clinical isolates (by the MBC–MIC ratio) has been reported as 4% (91), 30% (90), and over 80% (57), depending on the media used for culture. Isolates of Group G streptococci tolerant to penicillin and vancomycin have been reported, but the single report showing a high incidence of tolerance to vancomycin does not specify methodology (92), and other investigators, using time-kill curves and log-phase cultures, have found a low incidence of tolerance (less than 5%) (63, 93). Tolerant isolates also have been reported among group C streptococci (94), but these were tested in medium containing serum, which appears to decrease the activity of autolysin in other streptococcal strains (87).

Listeria monocytogenes strains also show tolerance to penicillin and ampicillin (73, 95). A survey of 50 strains showed that all had MBCs greater than eightfold the MIC, and many were not killed at concentrations one thousand-fold greater (62). These findings are confirmed by time-kill studies, which show that viability decreases less than one log after 24 hours over a range of penicillin or ampicillin concentrations. Among 40 strains of *Lactobacillus* spp., 95% were tolerant to ampicillin, 78% to penicillin, and 85% to cephalo-thin (96).

Will tolerance become an increasingly frequent finding, possibly forcing alterations in standard therapeutic regimens? The effect of environmental pressures on possible selection for tolerance has not yet been investigated. Penicillin-resistant *S. viridans* species arise in the mouth and pharyngeal flora during penicillin therapy. Such strains may appear within the first 48 hours of therapy and persist for several months after treatment is complete (97, 98). They may cause endocarditis in susceptible patients (99, 100). Tolerance similarly might emerge and, in cases where only inhibitory sensitivity testing was done, may have been previously unnoticed. In the laboratory, tolerant mutants may be isolated by repeated passage on penicillin-containing media; such selection might occur in vivo, just as selection of resistant clones has been documented. Holloway et al (85) found a high percentage of tolerant viridans streptococci in patients receiving penicillin prophylaxis. The incidence in patients receiving no treatment is unknown. In a small study of children with *S. aureus* bacteremia, Hilty and colleagues (79) found a higher incidence of tolerant isolates in patients with prolonged hospital stays, suggesting that tolerant organisms might be a significant source of nosocomial infections. Several of the highly resistant South African pneumococci isolated from hospitalized children also showed a high degree of tolerance (17). Most of the patients had chronic illnesses and had received repeated exposure to antibiotics, and in some children the organisms appeared nosocomially acquired (101). Thus, the antibiotic pressure of the hospital environment might encourage selection of tolerant organisms just as it does highly resistant strains.

A related avenue requiring further investigation is the means of transfer of tolerance among bacteria. In the laboratory, tolerance can be conferred by transformation with relative ease (1, 12). Transduction (102) by bacteriophage may be another means by which tolerance can be transferred. If tolerant organisms can be selected by antibiotic pressure, this trait could then easily spread, increasing the incidence of clinically significant isolates that demonstrate tolerance.

TOLERANT BACTERIA IN VIVO

There is general agreement that the effective cure of bacterial infections at sites of impaired host defense requires the use of bactericidal antibiotics such as β lactams (103, 104). One thus would expect that tolerant bacterial strains with their selective resistance to the irreversible effects of β lactam antibiotics would pose serious problems to chemotherapy in immunocompromised patients or in deep-seated infections such as endocarditis, meningitis, and osteomyelitis. On the other hand, the presence of host factors may make tolerant pathogens more sensitive to the irreversible effects of antibiotics in vivo than in vitro. In tolerant *S. sanguis,* for example, treatment with human lysozyme plus penicillin results in loss of viability, although neither alone has this effect (46). This emphasizes the importance of in vivo investigations of tolerant bacteria.

Animal Studies

The rabbit endocarditis model has been used in several studies attempting to determine the effect of tolerance on the establishment and outcome of infection during antibiotic treatment and prophylaxis. The bacterial pathogens in which tolerance has been most frequently noted, i.e. staphylococci, viridans streptococci, and group D streptococci, are those most frequently causing infective endocarditis. In a Mayo Clinic study of 150 cases of infective endocarditis, 38% were caused by viridans streptococci, 20% by staphylococci, and 18% by group D streptococci (105). Reports on the incidence of tolerant strains among these species indicate high frequencies: up to 50% among *S. sanguis* and other viridans strains (74, 75, 85), 30–70% among staphylococci (40, 106), and over 90% among group D streptococci (75, 87). Why tolerant strains appear so frequently at this infection site is not clear. Nevertheless, this association makes the use of the endocarditis model particularly suited for testing the in vivo role of tolerance.

While the endocarditis model is presumed to be most useful for the reasons cited above, it is also possible that nontolerant organisms manifest a phenotypically tolerant response while growing on the heart valve due to the high bacterial density, diminished metabolic activity, and slow growth rate that occurs within vegetations (69); thus, differences between tolerant and nontolerant organisms might be less apparent than in a setting where inoculum is lower or growth rate more rapid.

A number of studies with viridans streptococci have noted the relative difficulty of eliminating tolerant over nontolerant isolates from valvular vegetations in experimental endocarditis. A preliminary report comparing a tolerant *S. sanguis I* with a nontolerant *S. sanguis II* in rabbit endocarditis suggested that tolerant organisms are less responsive to killing by penicillin (107). Lowy et al (108) compared the efficacy of treatment regimens on infection with a tolerant *S. sanguis* and a nontolerant *S. mitis*. The high-dose regimen (80,000 U/kg every eight hours) achieved serum concentrations comparable to those in patients treated for endocarditis. Unfortunately, these two viridans strains seem to differ in their virulence properties, since one day after inoculation rabbits receiving *S. mitis* showed greater bacteremia and, left untreated, died sooner than those receiving *S. sanguis*. In animals treated with low-dose penicillin (5,000 U/kg every eight hours), rabbits infected with the *sanguis* strain developed vegetations with significantly higher bacterial counts than those infected with *S. mitis,* despite the apparent greater virulence of the *mitis* strain. However, there was no difference noted between the bacterial counts of *sanguis* and *mitis* vegetations in animals receiving the high-dose penicillin regimen. These authors concluded that, while tolerant pathogens clearly survive better during a lower-dose penicillin regimen, increasing the dosage (i.e. penicillin concentration and length of treatment) successfully eliminates the tolerant bacteria also. This presumably is achieved by the slow rate of killing of *S. sanguis,* which is clearly demonstrable in the test tube during prolonged (several days) exposure to the antibiotic (4).

Brennan & Durack (60) also compared tolerant and nontolerant *S. sanguis* in the rabbit model of endocarditis, using an inoculum and a dose regimen similar to those of the high-dose regimen of Lowy et al. Vegetations excised from untreated animals showed the same number of organisms, suggesting that virulence for the two strains is equal. In rabbits treated with intramuscular (IM) procaine penicillin, the number of organisms surviving five days is significantly greater after inoculation with tolerant than with nontolerant *S. sanguis;* the addition of streptomycin in a small number of animals results in sterilization of all vegetations by day five. This study suggests that the presence of tolerance may indeed affect the outcome of treatment of viridans endocarditis. The detection of tolerant colonies from vegetations may have been significantly improved in this study with the use of penicillinase in plates for viability counting.

Several studies have used the endocarditis model to test the sensitivity of tolerant versus nontolerant pathogens to prophylaxis with β-lactam antibiotics. While it is generally agreed that treatment of established disease requires bactericidal antibiotics, the issue is less clear regarding prophylaxis. Originally, it was assumed that antibiotic prophylaxis prevents endocarditis by eradicating organisms already lodged on the valve (109). Were this the case, tolerant organisms would evade prophylaxis, as they would grow after the antibiotic is withdrawn. More recently, it has been shown that penicillin also decreases adherence to fibrin-platelet matrices in vitro and to cardiac valves during bacteremia (86, 110, 111). If prevention of adherence is an equally important factor in preventing disease, then tolerance might have less effect on the efficacy of prophylaxis. Experimental tests of these questions have yielded information that suggests that both the cidal effect of the antibiotics and the suppression of adherence play a role in successful prophylaxis and that tolerant bacteria potentially pose problems in chemoprophylaxis.

Hess et al (112) tested four *S. sanguis* strains of relatively similar MIC values (.006–0.1 μg/ml) but vastly different in vitro MBC values (.02 μg/ml–32 mg/ml). The strains appeared to have comparable virulence, i.e. similar abilities to adhere to the traumatized valvular surfaces and give rise to dense populations in untreated rabbits. Rabbits received single intramuscular injection of procaine penicillin 30 minutes prior to inoculation with 10^8 bacteria. Two days later, 44 of 70 (70%) animals infected with a highly tolerant strain had developed endocarditis, while only two of 22 (9%) animals infected with nontolerant strains had detectable bacterial vegetations. The results of this experiment suggest that tolerant bacteria can evade prophylaxis by virtue of their relative resistance to the killing action of penicillin.

However, other studies indicate that penicillin can suppress the ability of both tolerant and nontolerant bacteria to adhere to heart valves during the initial phase of effective contact and colonization, before clearance removes most bacteria from the circulation. Lowy et al (110) briefly exposed tolerant *S. sanguis* to penicillin in vitro. Under the conditions used, bacteria underwent no loss of viability but did secrete over 90% of the acylated lipoteichoic acids, which have been postulated to function as adhesins (113). After removal of penicillin, pretreated bacteria were mixed with an equal number of untreated cells of an isogenic strain distinguishable by genetic markers and the mixed cultures were introduced into rabbits with previously traumatized heart valves.

Animals were sacrificed 15 minutes and two hours after inoculation. Differential counting (using the genetic markers) of bacteria in vegetations at both times revealed ten to one-hundredfold greater numbers of untreated compared to pretreated bacteria. This finding confirms the notion that penicillin treatment interferes with bacterial adherence by a process that does not depend on the cidal activity of the antibiotic. The interplay of cidal activity, which should be relatively ineffective against tolerant cells, and anti-adherence activity, which affects tolerant as well as nontolerant cells, is well demonstrated in the studies of Glauser et al (86, 111). They have shown that antibiotics for which *S. viridans* is tolerant may adequately prevent endocarditis (111) in the rat. Glauser and colleagues (86) further compared amoxicillin prophylaxis of tolerant *S. intermedius* and *S. sanguis* with nontolerant *S. mitior*. Their observations suggest that amoxicillin prevents endocarditis by two mechanisms: (*a*) bactericidal action, a process to which tolerant cells are less sensitive, and (*b*) decreased adherence, which affects tolerant and nontolerant strains equally.

The studies with tolerant viridans streptococci briefly reviewed above outline the types of problems tolerant pathogens may cause in the chemotherapy and chemoprophylaxis of endocarditis. The results with tolerant strains of *Staphylococcus aureus* are less clear. One reason may be the apparent instability of the tolerance trait in staphylococci (5, 59). Using the rabbit endocarditis model, Goldman & Petersdorf (114) found no difference in survival during methicillin treatment after inoculation of 10^4 logarithmic-phase organisms of a tolerant versus nontolerant *S. aureus* strain. (However, the tolerant strain showed a high MBC–MIC ratio at only 24 and not 48 hours.) Survival of the nontolerant strain in vegetations of untreated animals was significantly greater than that of the tolerant, however, suggesting diminished virulence of the tolerant strain. When stationary-phase organisms were used to inoculate the animals, those receiving the tolerant strains survived longer. It is unclear whether these findings are related to tolerance or represent only differences in virulence. In a recent study of bacteremic *S. aureus,* pyelonephritis inoculation with tolerant organisms resulted in a larger renal microbial population after eight weeks than did inoculation with nontolerant organisms. However, animals treated with methicillin showed no difference in clinical outcome between groups (115). These widely disparate results suggest that virulence factors unrelated to antibiotic response may alter the outcome of in vivo studies. Further studies with isogenic strains that show similar virulence are needed before conclusions about the effect of tolerance upon *S. aureus* infections can be drawn.

Clinical Studies

In 1976, Mayhall, Medoff, & Marr (3) described three patients with staphylococcal bacteremia who responded poorly to treatment with oxacillin; the three strains were subsequently shown to be tolerant. Sabath's report (5) of tolerance in clinical isolates of *S. aureus* described seven patients who had responded poorly to treatment. Since then, there have been multiple case reports of treatment failures and recurrence of infection ascribed to tolerant organisms, including staphylococci and groups A, B, and D streptococci (71, 83, 84, 89, 90, 116–119). The significance of such reports is unclear, since a large proportion of common pathogens, such as staphylococci and streptococci, are tolerant. Multiple other causes, including occult septic foci, exist for treatment failure in invasive bacterial disease, and persistent bacteremia or treatment failure may occur without apparent cause in patients infected with nontolerant organisms (63, 93, 120–122).

In 1979, a retrospective chart review of 20 patients with a variety of *S. aureus* infections first suggested that those with organisms tolerant to the antibiotics received (nafcillin, vancomycin, or cefazolin) have a longer duration of bacteremia and a poorer prognosis, but the two groups were not exactly matched for type of infection or underlying disease (123). A small study of staphylococcal bacteremia in children showed no difference in mortality rate between those with tolerant and those with nontolerant organisms. Duration of fever or positive blood cultures was not reported (79). In 1980, Rajashekaraiah et al (80) evaluated 50 patients with *S. aureus* endocarditis and 54 with *S. aureus* bacteremia. Over 60% of the patients in each group were infected with organisms tolerant by their criterion, an MBC–MIC ratio greater than or equal to 16. Inocula for these determinations were obtained from overnight cultures grown in TSB, conditions likely to overestimate the incidence of tolerance (61). Endocarditis patients infected with tolerant staphylococci had more prolonged fever, more complications, and were more frequently admitted to the intensive care unit than those with nontolerant organisms; mortality was greater in the tolerant group but the difference was not statistically significant. No difference in outcome was detected between groups for patients with bacteremia alone. In a collaborative study of *S. aureus* endocarditis among Veterans Administration hospitals, patients infected with tolerant organisms also had more prolonged fever, although the rate of bacteriologic cure was the same (J. Rahal, personal communication). These studies strongly suggest that infection with tolerant organisms adversely affects the course of treatment of endocarditis. That persistent fever and complications in endocarditis patients do not produce a difference in ultimate mortality is not surprising in light of the laboratory finding that tolerant organisms lose viability more slowly than nontolerant organisms but are ultimately killed by cell-wall antibiotics.

Clearly, more study is needed to further define the effects of infection by tolerant organisms, staphylococci as well as other species, upon the course and outcome of treatment. Investigation is also necessary to determine which antibiotic regimens hasten eradication of infection and whether this prevents increased early morbidity. A randomized study of a large number of patients with strict definitions of tolerance and prescribed antibiotic therapy is needed. At present, it seems reasonable to suggest that, in patients infected with tolerant organisms, persistent bacteremia or a poor response to antibiotics should prompt a change in therapy to include bactericidal antibiotics.

CONCLUSIONS

We have attempted to evaluate the body of information on tolerance in clinical isolates that has accumulated over the fifteen years since tolerance was first described. The phenomenon of antibiotic tolerance, initially reported as the unique response of lysis-defective pneumococci to penicillin treatment, is clearly not restricted to laboratory mutants. Clinical isolates in which the penicillin-induced loss of viability is substantially slower than in other isolates of the same species have been detected during the last fifteen years among a number of human pathogens, including Listeria, *Staphylococcus aureus, Streptococcus pneumoniae,* and group D and viridans streptococcal species.

It is difficult to compare the mechanistic basis of the tolerance of clinical isolates to those of the autolysin-defective laboratory strains. Most laboratory tolerant strains have been selected for an autolysin defect and clearly demonstrate both diminished lysis and killing upon exposure to cell–wall active antibiotics. Although no mutants show a complete lack of killing, in each autolysin-defective strain the cell population as a whole undergoes loss of viability very slowly. While some natural isolates exist that may demonstrate this type of tolerance, e.g. *S. sanguis,* enterococci, and Listeria, multiple other types of tolerance appear to exist in nature that differ in degree and probably in mechanism. Additionally, the mechanism of killing itself is not clear for all species: although the model of penicillin-induced lysis and death explains the observed phenomena in pneumococci and several other species, cell death may also occur by other routes not accompanied by lysis, as it was first described, e.g. in Group A streptococci. Other possible mechanisms for the production of tolerance have been described in the laboratory and still a further number have been proposed. Many of these are likely to occur in nature and remain to be discovered.

It is also difficult to evaluate the frequency of tolerance among natural isolates since in many cases the sole criterion used for the identification of tolerance has been the elevated MBC–MIC ratio. The insensitivity of this method and the numerous experimental variables that can influence MBC determination, causing unrealistic estimations of tolerance, have been discussed briefly and a more reliable method suggested. Although elevated ratios may serve as a first hint of tolerance in a clinical specimen, such claims should be confirmed by more detailed studies in the microbiology laboratory, using genetically and physiologically homogeneous cultures of the isolate.

The physiological state of the target bacterium and factors in the bacterial environment can profoundly modulate the irreversible effects of β-lactam antibiotics. Phenotypic tolerance due to such factors is likely to be a major variable influencing both the detection of tolerance in vitro and the efficacy of such antibiotics in vivo. Another important question is whether such tolerant bacteria are selected in the natural environment under antibiotic pressure in a fashion similar to antibiotic-resistant mutants.

Tolerant isolates appear to be unusually frequent among bacterial pathogens causing valvular endocarditis in man. The reason for this propensity is not clear. Studies with the rabbit endocarditis model strongly suggest that infections with tolerant isolates of viridans streptococci require more prolonged treatment for cure during penicillin therapy than do infections with nontolerant strains. Sensitivity to the cidal effect of penicillin also appears to be one of the factors influencing the success of prophylaxis in this experimental model. Strain-to-strain differences in virulence complicate the intrepretation of many animal studies. A critical evaluation of the role of tolerance in such models of infection will have to wait until isogenic pairs of tolerant and nontolerant isolates of the same strain of bacteria and of identical virulence properties become available.

Clinical studies thus far suggest that the outcome of treatment of staphylococcal endocarditis with tolerant organisms may not differ but that during the course of treatment prolonged fever and other complications may occur. Based on the present evidence, it seems unwise to change existing successful therapeutic regimens that have shown high therapeutic-to-toxic ratios. However, it seems appropriate to suggest that MBC determinations be routinely done on pathogens isolated from the blood of endocarditis patients. If the presence of tolerant organisms is confirmed (by repeating viability determinations at an earlier time point also, e.g. after four hours incubation of the MIC tubes), then a change to a bactericidal antibiotic regimen should be considered.

Both animals studies and clinical investigations to date have focused on the role of tolerance in endocarditis. The implications of tolerance at other sites of infection remain to be evaluated.

ACKNOWLEDGMENTS

We would like to acknowledge comments and helpful discussions by several colleagues: Drs. Wilfredo Talavera, Elaine Tuomanen, Richard B. Roberts, Warren Johnson, Fritz D. Schoenknecht, John C. Sherris, and James J. Rahal. Sandra Handwerger was supported in part by a training fellowship from the American Lung Association.

Literature Cited

1. Tomasz, A., Albino, A., Zanati, E. 1970. Multiple antibiotic resistance in a bacterium with suppressed autolytic system. *Nature* 227:138–40
2. Best, G. K., Best, N. H., Koval, A. V. 1974. Evidence of participation of autolysins in bactericidal action of oxacillin of *Staphylococcus aureus*. *Antimicrob. Agents Chemother.* 6:825–30
3. Mayhall, C. G., Medoff, G., Marr, J. J. 1976. Variation in the susceptibility of strains of *Staphylococcus aureus* to oxacillin, cephalothin, and gentamicin. *Antimicrob. Agents Chemother.* 10:707–12
4. Horne, D., Tomasz, A. 1977. Tolerant response of *Streptococcus sanguis* to beta lactams and other cell wall inhibitors. *Antimicrob. Agents Chemother.* 11:888–96
5. Sabath, L. D., Lavadiere, M. Wheeler, N., Blazevic, D., Wilkinson, B. J. 1977. A new type of penicillin resistance in *Staphylococcus aureus*. *Lancet* 1:443–47
6. Kitano, K., Tomasz, A. 1979. *Escherichia coli* mutants tolerant to beta-lactam antibiotics. *J. Bacteriol.* 140:955–62
7. Kitano, K., Williamson, R., Tomasz, A. 1980. Murein hydrolase defect in the beta lactam tolerant mutants of *Escherichia coli*. *FEMS Microbiol. Letts.* 7:133–36
8. Harkness, R. E., Ishiguro, E. E. 1983. Temperature sensitive autolysis defective mutants of *Escherichia coli*. *J. Bacteriol.* 155:15–21
9. Shungu, D. L., Cornett, J. B., Shockman, G. D. 1979. Morphological and physiological study of autolytic defective *Streptococcus faecium* strains. *J. Bacteriol.* 136:598–608
10. Ayusawa, D., Yoneda, Y., Yanane, K., Maruo, B. 1975. Pleiotropic phenomena in autolytic enzyme content, flagellation and simultaneous hyperproduction of extracellular amylase and protease in a *Bacillus subtilis* mutant. *J. Bacteriol* 124:459–69
11. Rogers, H. J., Forsberg, C. W. 1971. Autolysins in the killing of bacteria by some bactericidal antibiotics. *J. Bacteriol.* 108:1235–43
12. Fein, J. E., Rogers, H. J. 1976. Autolytic enzyme deficient mutants of *B. subtilis* 168. *J. Bacteriol* 127:1427–42
13. Williamson, R., Tomasz, A. 1980. Antibiotic tolerant mutants of *Streptococcus pneumoniae* that are not deficient in autolytic activity. *J. Bacteriol.* 144:105–13
14. Best, G. K., Koval, A. V., Best, N. H. 1975. Susceptibility of clinical isolates of *Staphylococcus aureus* to killing by oxacillin. *Can. J. Microbiol.* 21:1692–97
15. Jolliffe, L. K., Doyle, R. J., Streips, U. N. 1982. Extracellular proteases increase tolerance of *Bacillus subtilis* to nafcillin. *Antimicrob. Agents Chemother.* 22:83–89
16. Gutmann, L., Tomasz, A. 1982. Penicillin resistant and penicillin tolerant mutants of group A streptococci. *Antimicrob. Agents Chemother.* 22:128–36
17. Liu, H., Zighelboim, S., Tomasz, A. 1981. Penicillin tolerance in multiply-resistant natural isolates of *S. pneumoniae 21st Intersci. Conf. Antimicrob. Agents Chemother., Am. Soc. Microbiol., Chicago, 1981* (Abstr.)
18. Holtje, J. V., Tomasz, A. 1976. Purification of the pneumococcal N-acetyl-muramyl-L-alanine amidase to biochemical homogeneity. *J. Biol. Chem.* 251:4199–207
19. Rogers, H. J., Forsberg, C. W. 1980. *Microbial Cell Walls and Membranes.* London: Chapman & Hall
20. Chaterjee, A. N., Wong, W., Young, F. E., Gilpin, R. W. 1976. Isolation and characterization of a mutant of *Staphylococcus aureus* deficient in autolytic activity. *J. Bacteriol.* 125:961–67
21. Tomasz, A. 1983. Murein hydrolases. In *The Target of Penicillin*, ed. R. Hakenbeck, pp. 155–64. Berlin: Walter de Gruyter
22. Tomasz, A. 1981. Penicillin tolerance and the control of murein hydrolases. In *Beta Lactam Antibiotics*, ed. M. R. J. Salton, G. D. Shockman, pp. 227–48. New York: Academic
23. Tomasz, A. 1979. From penicillin binding proteins to the lysis and death of bacteria: A 1979 view. *Rev. Infect. Dis.* 1:434–67
24. Norden, C. W., Keleti, E. 1981. Antibiotic tolerance in strains of *Staphylococcus aureus*. *J. Antimicrob. Chemother.* 7:599–605
25. Peterson, L. R., Gerding, D. N., Hall, W. H., Schierl, E. A. 1978. Medium dependent variation in bactericidal activity of antibiotics against susceptible *Staphylococcus aureus*. *Antimicrob. Agents Chemother.* 13:665–68
26. Hobby, G. L., Meyer, K., Chaffee, E. 1942. Observations on the mechanism of action of penicillin. *Proc. Soc. Exp. Biol.* 50:281–85
27. Lederberg, J., Zinder, N. 1948. Concentration of biochemical mutants of bacteria

with penicillin. *J. Am. Chem. Soc.* 70:4267–68

28. Mychajlonka, M., McDowell, T. D., Shockman, G. D. 1980. Inhibition of peptidoglycan, ribonucleic acid and protein sythesis in tolerant strains of *Streptococcus mutans. Antimicrob. Agents Chemother.* 17:572

29. Holtje, J. V., Tomasz, A. 1975. Lipoteichoic acid: A specific inhibitor of autolysin activity in pneumococcus. *Proc. Natl. Acad. Sci. USA* 72:1690–94

30. Holtje, J. V., Tomasz, A. 1975. Biological effects of lipoteichoic acids. *J. Bacteriol.* 124:1023–27

31. Cleveland, R. F., Holtje, J. V., Wicken, A. J., Tomasz, A., Daneo-Moore, L., Shockman, G. D. 1975. Inhibition of bacterial wall lysins by lipoteichoic acids and related compounds. *Biochem. Biophys. Res. Commun.* 67:1128–35

32. Cleveland, R. F., Wicken, A. J., Daneo-Moore, L., Shockman, G. D. 1976. Inhibition of wall autolysis in *Streptococcus faecalis* by lipoteichoic acids and lipids. *J. Bacteriol.* 126:192–97

33. Tomasz, A., Waks, S. 1975. Mechanism of action of penicillin: Triggering of the pneumococcal autolytic enzyme by inhibitors of cell wall synthesis. *Proc. Natl. Acad. Sci. USA* 72:4162–65

34. Raynor, R. H., Scott, D. F., Best, G. K. 1979. Oxacillin induced lysis of *Staphylococcus aureus. Antimicrob. Agents Chemother.* 16:134–40

35. Mosser, J. L., Tomasz, 1970. Choline containing teichoic acid as a structural component of pneumococcal cell wall and its role in sensitivity to lysis by an autolytic enzyme. *J. Biol. Chem.* 245: 287–98

36. Sabath, L. D. 1982. Mechanisms of resistance to beta-lactam antibiotics in strains of *Staphylococcus aureus. Ann. Int. Med.* 97:339–44

37. Goessens, W. H. F., Fontijne, P., van Raffe, M., Michel, M. F. 1984. Tolerance percentage as a criterion for the detection of tolerant *Staphylococcus aureus* strains. *Antimicrob. Agents Chemother.* 25:575–78

38. Moyed, H. S., Bertrand, K. P. 1983. *hip A,* A newly recognized gene of *Escherichia coli* K12 that affects frequency of persistence after inhibition of murein synthesis. *J. Bacteriol.* 155:768–75

39. Traub, W. H. 1981. Variable tolerance of a clinical isolate of *Staphylococcus epidermidis. Chemotherapy* 27:432–43

40. Bradley, J. J., Mayhall, C. G., Dalton, H. P. 1978. Incidence and characteristics of antibiotic tolerant strains of *Staphylococcus aureus. Antimicrob. Agents Chemother.* 13:1052–57

41. Carson, D., Pieringer, R. A., Daneo-Moore, L. 1979. Effect of growth rate on lipid and lipoteichoic acid composition in *Streptococcus faecium. Biochim. Biophys. Acta* 575:225–33

42. Op den Kamp, J. A. F., van Iterson, W., van Deenen, L. L. M. 1967. Studies on the phospholipids and morphology of protoplasts of *Bacillus megaterium. Biochim. Biophys. Acta* 135:862–84

43. Horne, D., Tomasz, A. 1981. pH Dependent penicillin tolerance of group B streptococci. *Antimicrob. Agents Chemother.* 20:128–35

44. Goodell, W., Lopez, R., Tomasz, A. 1976. Suppression of lytic effect of beta lactams on *Escherichia coli* and other bacteria. *Proc. Natl. Acad. Sci. USA* 73:3293–329

45. De Repentigny, L., Turgeon, P. L. 1981. Screening of *Neisseria gonorrhoeae* for tolerant response to beta lactam antibiotics. *Antimicrob. Agents Chemother.* 19:645–48

46. Horne, D., Tomasz, A. 1980. Lethal effect of a heterologous murein hydrolase on penicillin treated *Streptococcus sanguis. Antimicrob. Agents Chemother.* 17:235–46

47. Gwynn, M. N., Webb, L. T., Rolison. G. N. 1981. Regrowth of *Pseudomonas aeruginosa* and other bacteria after the bactericidal action of carbenicillin and other beta lactam antibiotics. *J. Infect. Dis.* 144:263–69

48. Taylor, P. C., Schoenknecht, F. D., Sherris, J. C., Linner, E. C. 1983. Determination of minimum bactericidal concentrations of oxacillin for *Staphylococcus aureus. Antimicrob. Agents Chemother.* 23:142–50

49. Ishida, K. P., Guze, A., Kalmanson, G. M., Albrandt, K., Guze, L. B. 1982. Variables in demonstrating methcillin tolerance in *Staphylococcus aureus* strains. *Antimicrob. Agents Chemother.* 21:688–90

50. Storch, G. A., Krogstad, D. J., Parquette, A. 1981. Antibiotic induced lysis of enterococci. *J. Clin. Invest.* 68:639–45

51. Wegener, W. S., Hebeler, B. H., Morse, S. A. 1977. Cell envelope of *Neisseria gonorrhoeae:* Penicillin enhancement of peptidoglycan hydrolysis. *Infect. Immun.* 18:717–25

52. Goodell, E. W., Fazio, M., Tomasz, A. 1978. Effect of benzylpenicillin on the synthesis and structure of the cell envelope of *N. gonorrhoeae. Antimicrob. Agents Chemother.* 13:514–26

53. Jawetz, E., Gunnison, J. B., Speck, R. S., Coleman, V. R. 1951. Studies on antibiotic synergism and antagonism. *Arch. Int. Med.* 87:349–59

54. Anhalt, J. P., Sabath, L. D., Barry, A. L. 1980. Special tests: Bactericidal activity, activity of antimicrobics in combination, and detection of beta lactamase production. In *Manual of Clinical Microbiology*, ed. E. H. Lenette, pp. 478–83. Washington: Am. Soc. Microbiol. 3rd ed.

55. Washingon, J. A., Sutter, V. L. 1980. Dilution susceptibility tests: Agar and macro-broth dilution procedures. See Ref. 54, pp. 453–58

56. Watanakunakorn, C. 1978. Antibiotic tolerant *Staphylococcus aureus*. *J. Antimicrob. Chemother.* 4:561–68

57. Kim, K. S., Yoshimori, R. N., Imagawa, D. T., Anthony, B. F. 1979. Importance of medium in demonstrating penicillin tolerance by group B streptococci. *Antimicrob. Agents Chemother.* 16:214–16

58. Lopez, R., Ronda-Lain, C., Tapia, A., Waks, S. B., Tomasz, A. 1976. Suppression of the lytic and bactericidal effects of cell wall inhibitory antibiotics. *Antimicrob. Agents Chemother.* 10:697–706

59. Mayhall, C. G., Apollo, E. 1980. Effect of storage and changes in bacterial growth phase and antibiotic concentrations on antimicrobial tolerance in *Staphylococcus aureus*. *Antimicrob. Agents Chemother.* 18:784–88

60. Brennan, R. O., Durack, D. T. 1983. Therapeutic significance of penicillin tolerance in experimental streptococcal endocarditis. *Antimicrob. Agents Chemother.* 23:273–77

61. Venglarcik, J. S., Blair, L. L., Dunkle, L. M. 1983. pH Dependent oxacillin tolerance of *Staphylococcus aureus*. *Antimicrob. Agents Chemother.* 23:232–35

62. Wiggins, G. L., Albritton, W. L., Feeley, J. C. 1978. Antibiotic susceptibility of clinical isolates of *Listeria monocytogenes*. *Antimicrob. Agents Chemother.* 13:854–60

63. Lam, K., Bayer, A. S. 1983. Serious infections due to group G streptocci. *Am. J. Med.* 75:561–70

64. Mandell, G. L. 1970. Intraphagosomal pH of human polymorphonuclear neutrophils. *Proc. Soc. Exp. Med.* 134:447–49

65. Ward, T. T., Steigbigel, R. T. 1978. Acidosis of synovial fluid correlates with synovial fluid leukocytosis. *Am. J. Med.* 64:933–36

66. Bland, R. D., Lister, R. C., Ries, J. P. 1974. Cerebrospinal fluid lactic acid level and pH in meningitis. *Am. J. Dis. Child.* 128:151–56

67. Bodem, C. R., Lampton, L. M., Miller, D. P., Tarka, E. F., Everett, E. D. 1983. Endobronchial pH: Relevance to aminoglycoside activity in gram negative bacillary pneumonia. *Am. Rev. Resp. Dis.* 127:39–41

68. Light, R. W., Girard, W. M., Jenkinson, S. G., George, R. B. 1980. Parapneumonic effusions. *Am. J. Med.* 69:507–12

69. Durack, D. T., Beeson, P. B. 1972. Experimental bacterial endocarditis II: Survival of bacteria in endocardial vegetations. *Br. J. Exp. Path* 53:50–53

70. Eagle, H., Musselman, A. D. 1948. The rate of bactericidal action of penicillin in vitro as a function of its concentration and its paradoxically reduced activity at high concentrations against certain organisms. *J. Exp. Med.* 88:99–131

71. Schauf, V., Devekis, A., Riff, L., Serota, A. 1976. Antibiotic killing kinetics of group B streptococci. *J. Pediatr.* 89:194–98

72. Bayer, A. S., Chow, A. W., Morrison, J. O., Guze, L. B. 1980. Bactericidal synergy between penicillin or ampicillin and aminoglycosides against antibiotic tolerant lactobacilli. *Antimicrob. Agents Chemother.* 17:359–63

73. Gordon, R. C., Barrett, F. F., Clark, D. J. 1972. Influence of several antibiotics, singly and in combination on the growth of *Listeria monocytogenes*. *J. Pediatr.* 80:667–70

74. Holloway, Y., Dankert, J. 1981. Penicillin tolerance in nutritionally variant streptococci. *Antimicrob. Agents Chemother.* 22:1073–75

75. Slater, G. J., Greenwood, D. 1983. Detection of penicillin tolerance in streptococci. *J. Clin. Pathol.* 36:1353–56

76. Peterson, L. R., Denny, A. E., Gerding, D. N., Hall, W. H. 1980. Determination of tolerance to antibiotic bactericidal activity on Kirby-Bauer susceptibility plates. *Am. J. Clin. Pathol.* 74:645–50

77. Traub, W. H. 1982. Simple screening method for gram positive beta lactam antibiotic tolerance on routine laboratory Bauer Kirby plates. *Chemotherapy* 28:110–18

78. Kim, K. S., Anthony, B. F. 1983. Use of penicillin gradient and replicate plates for the demonstration of tolerance to penicillin in streptococci. *J. Infect. Dis.* 148:488–91

79. Hilty, M. D., Venglarcik, J. S., Best, G.

K. 1980. Oxacillin-tolerant staphylococcal bacteremia in children. *J. Pediatr.* 96:1035–37

80. Rajashekaraiah, K. R., Rice, T., Rao, V. S., Marsh, D., Ramakrishna, B., Kallick, C. A. 1980. Clinical significance of tolerant strains of *Staphylococcus aureus* in patients with endocarditis. *Ann. Int. Med.* 93:796–82

81. Bradley, H. E., Weldy, P. L., Hodes, D. S. 1979. Tolerance in *Staphylococcus aureus. Lancet* 2:150

82. Craven, N., Anderson, J. C. 1983. Penicillin (cloxacillin)-tolerant *Staphylococcus aureus* from bovine mastitis: Identification and lack of correlation between tolerance in vitro and response to therapy in vivo. *Res. Vet. Sci.* 34:266–71

83. Faville, R. J., Zaske, D. E., Kaplan, E. L., Crossley, K., Sabath, L. D., Quie, P. G. 1978. *Staphylococcus aureus* endocarditis: Combined therapy with vancomycin and rifampin. *J. Am. Med. Assoc.* 240:1963–65

84. Gopal, V., Bisno, A. L., Silverblatt, F. J. 1976. Failure of vancomycin treatment in *Staphylococcus aureus* encocarditis. *J. Am. Med. Assoc.* 236:1604–6

85. Holloway, Y., Dankert, J., Hess, J. 1980. Penicillin tolerance and bacterial endocarditis. *Lancet* 1:589

86. Glauser, M. P., Bernard, J. P., Moreillon, P., Francoli, P. 1983. Successful single dose amoxicillin prophylaxis against experimental endocarditis. *J. Infect. Dis.* 147:568–75

87. Krogstad, D. J., Parquette, A. R. 1980. Defective killing of enterococci: A common property of antimicrobial agents acting on the cell wall. *Antimicrob. Agents Chemother.* 17:965–68

88. Kaye, D. 1982. Enterococci—Biologic and epidemiologic characteristics and in vitro susceptibility. *Arch. Int. Med.* 142:2006–9

89. Savitch, C. B., Barry, A. L., Hoeprich, P. D. 1978. Infective endocarditis caused by *Streptococcus bovis* resistant to the lethal effect of penicillin G. *Arch. Int. Med.* 138:931–34

90. Allen, J. L., Sprunt, K. 1978. Discrepancy between minimum inhibitory and minimum bactericidal concentration of penicillin for group A and group B betahemolytic streptococci, *J. Pediatr.* 93:69–71

91. Kim, K. S., Anthony, B. F. 1981. Penicillin tolerance in group B streptococci isolated from infected neonates. *J. Infect. Dis.* 144:411–19

92. Noble, J. T., Tyburski, M. B., Berman, M., Greenspan, J., Tenenbaum, M. J.

1980. Antimicrobial tolerance in group G streptococci. *Lancet* 2:982–83

93. Rolston, K. V. I., LeFrock, J. L., Schell, R. F. 1982. Activity of 9 antimicrobial agents against Lancefield group C and group G streptococci. *Antimicrob. Agents Chemother.* 22:930–32

94. Portnoy, C., Prentis, J., Richards, G. K. 1981. Penicillin tolerance of human isolates of group C streptococci. *Antimicrob. Agents Chemother.* 20:235

95. Moellering, R. C., Medoff, G., Leech, I., Wennerstein, C., Kunz, L. J. 1972. Antibiotic synergism against *Listeria monocytogenes. Antimicrob. Agents Chemother.* 1:30–34

96. Bayer, A. S., Chow, A. W., Concepcion, N., Guze, L. B. 1978. Susceptibility of 40 lactobacilli to six antimicrobial agents with broad gram positive spectra. *Antimicrob. Agents Chemother.* 14:720–22

97. Garrod, L. P., Waterworth, P. M. 1962. The risks of dental extraction during penicillin treatment. *Br. Heart J.* 24:39–46

98. Sprunt, K., Redman, W., Leidy, G. 1968. Penicillin resistant alpha streptococci in pharynx of patients given oral penicillin. *Pediatrics* 42:957–68

99. Parrillo, J. E., Borst, G. C., Mazur, M. H., Iannini, P., Klempner, M. S., et al. 1979. Endocarditis due to resistant viridans streptococci during oral penicillin chemoprophylaxis. *New Engl. J. Med.* 300:296–300

100. Doyle, E. F., Spaguolo, M., Taranta, A., Kuttner, A. G., Markowitz, M. 1967. The risk of bacterial endocarditis during antirheumatic prophylaxis. *J. Am. Med. Assoc.* 201:807–12

101. Ward, J. B. 1981. Antibiotic resistant *Streptococcus pneumoniae:* Clinical and epidemiologic aspects. *Rev. Infect. Dis.* 3:254–66

102. Bradley, H. E., Wetmur, J. G., Hodes, D. S. 1980. Tolerance in *Staphylococcus aureus:* Evidence for bacteriophage role. *J. Infect. Dis.* 141:233–37

103. Bayer, A. S. 1982. Staphylococcal bacteremia and endocarditis. *Arch. Int. Med.* 142:1169–77

104. Drake, T. A., Sande, M. A. 1983. Studies of the chemotherapy of endocarditis. *Rev. Infect. Dis.* 5(Suppl. 2):S345–55

105. Wilson, W. R., Giuliani, E. R., Danielson, G. K., Geraci, J. E. 1982. General considerations in the diagnosis and treatment of infective endocarditis. *Mayo Clinic Proc.* 57:31–40

106. Goessens, W. H. F., Fontijne, P., Michel, M. F. 1982. Factors influencing

detection of tolerance in *Staphylococcus aureus*. *Antimicrob. Agents Chemother.* 22:364–68

107. Pulliam, L., Inokuchi, S., Hadley, W. K., Mills, J. 1979. Penicillin tolerance in experimental streptococcal endocarditis. *Lancet* 1:957

108. Lowy, F. D., Neuhaus, E. G., Chang, D. S., Steigbigel, N. H. 1983. Penicillin therapy of experimental endocarditis induced by tolerant *Streptococcus sanguis* and nontolerant *Streptococcus mitis*. *Antimicrob. Agents Chemother.* 23:67–73

109. Durack, D. T., Petersdorf, R. G. 1973. Chemotherapy of experimental streptococcal endocarditis. *J. Clin. Invest.* 52:592–98

110. Lowy, F. D., Chang, D. S., Neuhaus, E. G., Horne, D. S., Tomasz, A., Steigbigel, N. H. 1983. Effect of penicillin on the adherence of *Streptococcus sanguis* in vitro and in the rabbit model of endocarditis. *J. Clin. Invest.* 71:668–75

111. Glauser, M. P., Francoli, P. 1982. Successful prophylaxis against experimental streptococcal endocarditis with bacteriostatic antibiotics. *J. Infect. Dis.* 146:806–10

112. Hess, J., Dankert, J., Durack, D. 1983. Significance of penicillin tolerance *in vivo:* Prevention of experimental *Streptococcus sanguis* endocarditis. *J. Antimicrob. Chemother.* 11:555–64

113. Horne, D., Tomasz, A. 1979. Release of lipoteichoic acid from *Streptococcus sanguis:* Stimulation of release during penicillin treatment. *J. Bacteriol.* 137:1180–84

114. Goldman, P. L., Petersdorf, R. G. 1979. Significance of methicillin tolerance in experimental staphylcoccal endocarditis. *Antimicrob. Agents Chemother.* 15:802–6

115. Guze, P. A., Kalmanson, G. M., Guze, L. B. 1982. The role of antibiotic tolerance in the response to treatment of pyelonephritis due to *Staphylococcus aureus* in rats. *J. Infect. Dis.* 145:169–73

116. Steinbrecher, U. P. 1981. Serious infection in an adult due to penicillin tolerant group B streptococcus. *Arch. Int. Med.* 141:1714

117. Svenungsson, B., Kalin, M., Lindgren, L. G. 1982. Therapeutic failure in pneumonia caused by a tolerant strain of *Staphylococcus aureus*. *Scand. J. Infect. Dis.* 14:309–11

118. Broughton, D. D., Mitchell, W. G., Grossman, M., Hadley, W. K., Cohen, M. S. 1976. Recurrence of group B streptococcal infection. *J. Pediatr.* 89:183–85

119. Musher, D. M., Fletcher, T. 1982. Tolerant *Staphylococcus aureus* causing vertebral osteomyelitis. *Arch. Int. Med.* 142:632–34

120. Sheagren, J. N. 1984. *Staphylococcus aureus:* The persistent pathogen, part II. *New Engl. J. Med.* 310:1437–42

121. Reymann, M. T., Holley, H. P., Cobbs, C. G. 1978. Persistent bacteremia in staphylococcal endocarditis. *Am. J. Med.* 65:729–37

122. Kaye, D. 1980. Editorial: The clinical significance of tolerance of *Staphylococcus aureus*. *Ann. Int. Med.* 93:924–25

123. Denny, A. E., Peterson, L. R., Gerding, D. N., Hall, W. H. 1979. Serious staphylococcal infections with strains tolerant to bactericidal antibiotics. *Arch. Int. Med.* 139:1026–103

124. Kim, K. S., Morrison, J., Bayer, A. S. 1982. Deficient autolytic enzyme activity in antibiotic tolerant lactobacilli. *Infect. Immun.* 36:582–85

125. Jung, W. K. 1983. Susceptibility of 50 isolates of *Clostridium perfringens* to cefotaxime, fosfonomycin, penicillin G and vancomycin; Variable tolerance for vancomycin. *Chemotherapy* 29:99–103

126. Rozenberg-Arska, M., Fabius, G. T. J., Beens-Dekkers, M. A. A. J., Duursma, A., Sabath, L. D., Verhoef, J. 1970. Antibiotic sensitivity and synergism of penicillin tolerant *Staphylococcus aureus*. *Chemotherapy* 25:352–55

127. Nelson, R. E., Washington, J. A. 1981. Paradoxic and tolerant effects of moxalactam on *Staphylococcus aureus*. *J. Infect. Dis.* 144:178

Ann. Rev. Pharmacol. Toxicol. 1985. 25:381–412

THE MECHANISMS OF ANTIINFLAMMATORY STERIOD ACTION IN ALLERGIC DISEASES

Robert P. Schleimer

Department of Medicine, Division of Clinical Immunology, The Johns Hopkins University School of Medicine, Baltimore, Maryland 21239

INTRODUCTION

Since the recognition of the antiinflammatory actions of adrenal extracts, the adrenal glucocorticosteroids (hereinafter referred to as steroids) have been the mainstay in the therapy of severe allergic diseases of the skin, the nasal airways, and the lungs. In fact, if their use was not accompanied by undesirable side effects, steroids easily might be the only drugs used. A great deal of progress has been made in our efforts to understand the mechanisms of antiinflammatory steroid action; the purpose of this review is to discuss our present state of knowledge, with an emphasis on steroid actions in the allergic, IgE-mediated diseases. The review has been divided into three major parts: the in vivo actions of steroids, in the clinical setting and in experimental model systems; the in vitro actions of steroids, in particular the effects of steroids on inflammatory cell types likely to be important effectors of allergic disease; and the theories of steroid action, again from the perspective of their antiallergic effects.

THE EFFECTS OF STEROIDS ON IN VIVO MANIFESTATIONS OF ALLERGIC DISEASE

Clinical Findings

This section discusses the antiallergic actions of steroids. The diseases under consideration are broken down into those of the lung, the skin, and the nasal

381

0362-1642/85/415-0381$02.00

airways. I have attempted to discuss the etiology of these diseases in order to put the discussion of steroid action in context.

BRONCHIAL ASTHMA   Bronchial asthma is a disease characterized by increased bronchial reactivity, hypertrophy of bronchial smooth muscle, inflammatory cell infiltrate, hypersecretion of mucus, and narrowing of the airways. Its causes are not yet clear. In about one-third of the cases in North America, the disease is clearly IgE/allergen-mediated (extrinsic asthma); in one-third of the cases it has an allergic component; and in one-third (intrinsic asthma) the etiology is not known. Studies done in the early 1950s by Carryer, Cooke, and others demonstrated the effectiveness of ACTH and cortisone against both intrinsic and extrinsic forms of asthma (1–3). The steroid effect required between several hours and several days to be fully expressed (2, 4) (Figure 1). The airway obstruction in chronic asthma is also associated with a loss of elastic recoil, resulting in hyperinflation of the chest; all of these symptoms are reversed with steroid therapy (5). The relatively recent introduction of inhaled steroid preparations, such as beclomethasone dipropionate aerosol, has provided an effective alternative to systemic steroids, with fewer systemic side effects (6).

One characteristic that sets asthmatic patients apart from normal people is a hyperreactivity of the airways to irritant chemicals such as ozone and sulphur dioxide, as well as to exogenously applied mediators such as histamine, methacholine, and prostaglandin F_2. Thus, while these agents cause little or no decrease in airway function in normals, even at high concentrations, asthmatic

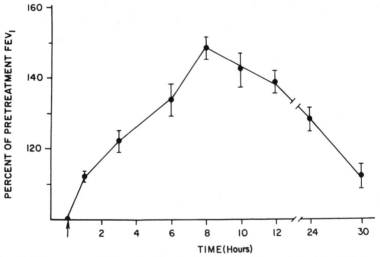

Figure 1   Improvement of airway function in asthmatics receiving a single 40 mg injection of prednisone phosphate [taken from (4)].

subjects experience a marked decrease in airflow following inhalation or parenteral challenge (7, 8). Hargreave and his colleagues have suggested that the sensitivity of asthmatic patients to the airway-constricting effects of methacholine and histamine parallels the severity of their disease (8). It is not yet clear whether this bronchial hyperreactivity is a cause, or merely a symptom, of the disease. Studies indicate that hyperreactivity may be the result of prior exposure to antigen (9), to increased permeability of bronchial epithelium (10), or to local inflammation involving influx of neutrophils (11). Although Arkins et al have claimed that steroid therapy does not reduce asthmatic bronchial hyperreactivity (12), the increase of hyperreactivity following antigen challenge appears to be blocked by steroids (9).

In many severe asthmatic patients, strenuous exercise produces what has been called exercise-induced asthma by an as-yet undetermined mechanism. In contrast to the cases of allergic or intrinsic asthma, steroid therapy, either by inhalation or orally, is only marginally effective against exercise-induced asthma (13–15).

Allergic asthma has been thought for many years to be due to the union of the inhaled allergen with specific IgE on the surface of the pulmonary mast cells, followed by the release of mast-cell inflammatory mediators such as histamine and leukotrienes. The bronchospasm and hypersecretion seen are thought to be due to the action of these mediators. Recent work by Hogg and his associates reconciles this concept with the fact that the bulk of the pulmonary mast cells reside beneath the epithelial barrier, which is impermeable to most allergens. They have proposed that the release of mediators by the small number of superepithelial and interepithelial mast cells is sufficient to increase epithelial permeability so as to allow the allergen access to the large number of subepithelial mast cells (Figure 2)(10). Pare & Hogg have proposed that steroid therapy may block this permeability increase (10).

ALLERGIC DISEASES OF THE SKIN   At the same time that steroids were found to be effective antiasthmatic drugs, researchers were establishing their effectiveness against many other immunologically based diseases, including diseases of the skin such as atopic dermatitis, pemphigus vulgaris, and cutaneous-contact hypersensitivity (16–18). Although the etiology of atopic dermatitis is unclear, an IgE-dependent mechanism is suspected. There is a strong correlation between the severity of the disease and serum IgE levels (19). Furthermore, a marked (approximately sevenfold) elevation of Fc_ϵ receptor–positive lymphocytes is seen in these patients. Steroid therapy reduces the number of Fc_ϵ receptor–positive lymphocytes in these patients to the normal range (approximately 1%) (20). Although steroids are effective in the therapy of atopic skin diseases, they do not affect the immediate allergic skin test wheal and flare

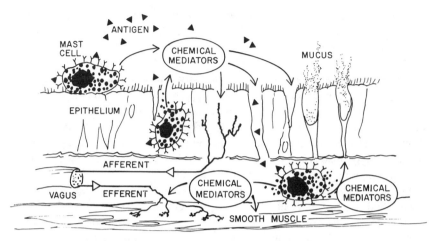

Figure 2 Immediate response to antigen inhalation. Mast cells on the epithelial surface release mediators that increase epithelial permeability and allow the access of antigen to subepithelial mast cells. Degranulation of subepithelial mast cells stimulates smooth muscle contraction and mucus secretion [modified from (10)].

response (2, 3, 21, 22). These paradoxical findings may be reconciled by recognition of the importance of the late cutaneous response (see below).

ALLERGIC RHINITIS   Steroid therapy effectively alleviates the symptoms of allergic rhinitis, commonly known as hay fever (21, 23). However, the disease is rarely severe enough to justify systemic steroid therapy and its associated side effects. While the early success of intranasally applied steroids may have been related to systemic absorption of the drugs (24–26), steroids are now available that clearly act locally, without causing any of the systemic side effects, such as adrenal suppression (Figure 3) (27).

Clinical Research

The administration of antigens, or inflammation-provoking substances, can produce reactions that in many ways resemble the naturally occurring allergic diseases. In this section, discussion will focus on such in vivo experimental models, their relevance to particular allergic diseases, and their use as models for the study of steroid action.

THE LATE-PHASE REACTION   In atopic subjects, the administration of allergen produces an immediate, vigorous, IgE-dependent response that varies according to the site of administration (bronchospasm in the lungs, wheal and flare in the skin, and sneezing and rhinorrhea in the nose). In a subset of these subjects, the response reappears four to ten hours after the administration of the

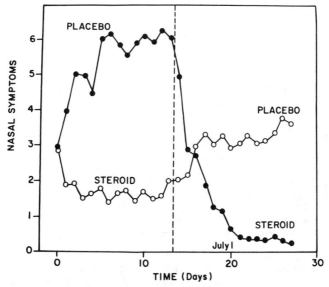

Figure 3   Double-blind cross-over trial of intranasal beclomethasone dipropionate aerosol in hay fever. Placebo and steroid (400 μg daily) groups were switched at the time indicated by the dashed line [adapted from (22)].

allergen in what has been termed the late-phase reaction [elegantly reviewed by Gleich in (28)]. This reaction can also be produced by compound 48/80, a polyamine that causes mast-cell degranulation, and in the rat by a 1400 molecular–weight (MW) component of mast-cell granules (29–31). There is additional evidence that the late-phase reaction (LPR) occurs as a consequence of mast-cell degranulation. The size of the LPR correlates with the size of the preceding immediate reaction to antigen (31, 32). Furthermore, the LPR is clearly IgE-mediated, based on studies that show that it can be produced by specific anti-IgE antibody (22, 33), and it can be passively transferred in skin with purified, antigen-specific IgE antibody (34). While mast-cell degranulation may be necessary to produce an LPR, it may not be sufficient. This hypothesis is based on the studies of Dolovich et al, who showed a minimal LPR in the skin following challenge with codeine (35).

The LPR reflects to a large extent the significant infiltration of inflammatory cells from the blood into the site of allergen administration (see below). Treatment of subjects with steroids prevents the occurrence of the LPR in the lungs, the skin, and the nose (Figure 4) (22, 36–38). Owing to the lack of effect of steroids in inhibiting the immediate response in these models, their effectiveness against the LPR, and their effectiveness in allergic disease, Gleich has suggested that the LPR may be a better model of allergic diseases than the immediate allergic response (28).

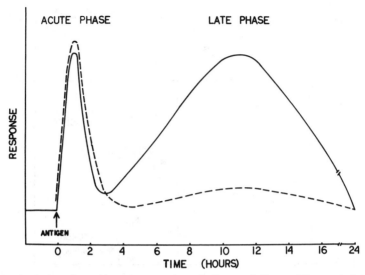

Figure 4   Action of steroids against experimental allergen challenge. Allergen challenge is characterized by an immediate and late-phase response in the skin, the nose, and the airway (solid line). Steroid treatment selectively blocks the late response (dashed line).

BRONCHIAL PROVOCATION   As mentioned above, challenging allergic subjects produces a biphasic response characterized by a reduction in lung function (e.g. decreased peak expiratory flow and forced-expiratory volume). Most (33, 36, 39–42), but not all (43–45), investigators find no effect of steroid therapy on the immediate response; the LPR is consistently inhibited by steroid treatment in these studies. Bronchial biopsies of asthma patients have shown that, during a naturally occurring episode of asthma, the number of pulmonary mast cells falls approximately 70%, perhaps indicating in vivo degranulation (46). Salvato claimed that therapy with 3–5 mg of dexamethasone per day reduces the number of mast cells in the bronchial biopsies (46). However, in autopsies of patients who died of acute asthma, Connell demonstrated a marked reduction of tissue mast cells (47). Of the twelve patients in Connell's study, the three who had been on steroid therapy had higher numbers of tissue mast cells than the remaining nine.

During an asthmatic episode, marked changes in the mucociliary apparatus occur. Challenge with ragweed allergen produces a significant decrease in the velocity of tracheal mucociliary transport, which may result from the release of leukotrienes in the airways (see below) (48). Large exudation of mucus into the airways is a marked pathological feature of asthma (47). In vitro studies with human airway tissue by Marom and coworkers indicate that mucus secretion is stimulated by sulfidopeptide leukotrienes and that treatment with dexamethasone in vitro can inhibit the secretion of mucus (Figure 2) (49, 50).

Much emphasis has been placed on identifying the chemical mediator(s) responsible for constricting the airways following bronchial challenge. Unfortunately, many of the likely mediators (histamine, leukotrienes, platelet-activating factor) have such a rapid half-life that their detection in the blood following challenge in the lungs is difficult. Thus far, bronchial-challenge studies have demonstrated a rise in blood histamine and platelet factor four and a high molecular–weight factor chemotactic for neutrophils that is presumably mast cell–derived (44, 51, 52). Serum neutrophil chemotactic factor levels have been seen to rise during both the immediate and the late-phase responses (52).

Leukotrienes Leukotrienes C_4, D_4, and E_4 are sulfidopeptide derivatives of arachidonic acid that are potent constrictors of bronchiolar smooth muscle, both in vitro and in vivo (53–56). These compounds, formerly known as slow-reacting substance of anaphylaxis (SRS-A), are from 600–10,000 times as potent as histamine in causing contraction of isolated human bronchi and in reducing lung function (peak expiratory flow) in normal subjects (55, 56). Since large quantities of leukotrienes are produced by mast cells, basophils, and other inflammatory cells, as well as by isolated lung tissue challenged with antigen, the leukotrienes figure prominently as important potential mediators of asthma (see below). Leukotriene B_4, a dihydroxy derivative of arachidonic acid that lacks the sulfidopeptide moiety, has been found in elevated concentrations in the sputa of asthmatic patients (57). The effects of steroids on leukotriene formation are discussed below.

THE ALLERGEN CHALLENGE OF THE SKIN   Studies of the skin have mostly employed one of three techniques: allergen challenge followed by tissue biopsy; denudement of a surface of skin, followed by challenge and then a coverslip cover (the skin window) that is later removed in order to classify and enumerate the cells adhering to it; and skin blister techniques, in which a blister provides an in vivo chamber for the study of mediators and cells. Challenge with allergen produces a cellular infiltrate that is similar in all of these model systems. Polymorphonuclear leukocyte (PMN) infiltration (approximately 4–8 hours) is followed by the influx of eosinophils and basophils; after approximately 24 hours the infiltrate becomes largely mononuclear (lymphocytes, monocytes, and macrophages) (58–61). During the first four hours following allergen, the number of identifiable mast cells decreases, suggesting that mast-cell degranulation has occurred (62). This conclusion is supported by the finding that the mast-cell mediators histamine and PgD_2 appear in skin-blister fluid following allergen challenge (63). The chemotaxis of PMN, eosinophils, basophils, and other agents into the tissue may be stimulated by mast cell–derived, large molecular–weight, specific chemotactic factors that remain to be

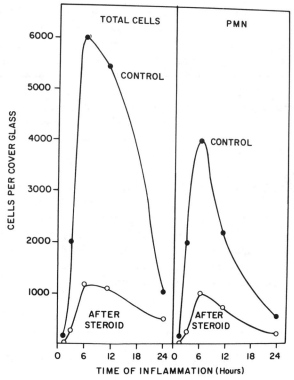

Figure 5   Steroid inhibition of the cellular infiltrate during inflammation, using the skin-window technique [taken from (75a)].

fully characterized, as well as by compounds such as LTB_4 and PgD_2, which can, especially in combination, cause an intense PMN infiltrate in human skin (64) (see below).

As noted earlier, the induration and erythema of the cutaneous late-phase reaction to antigen are inhibited by prior steriod therapy. Most (2, 3, 16, 21, 22, 65–70), but not all (71), investigators find no effect of steroid therapy on the immediate cutaneous (wheal and flare) reaction. A prominent histological feature of steroid action on the late cutaneous response to antigen is an inhibition of the influx of all leukocyte types (PMN, eosinophils, basophils, mononuclear cells, lymphocytes) into the tissue (70, 72–75) (Figure 5). This is one of the most important antiinflammatory actions of the steroids, and it probably occurs by an interference with the adherence of the cells to vascular endothelium prior to their emigration from the circulation into the tissue (see below).

NASAL CHALLENGE   Studies of nasal challenge have been hampered by the lack of a reliable, objective criterion by which to judge the action of the allergen. The major physiological changes are sneezing and the obstruction of nasal airways. The latter can be measured as an increase in nasal-airway resistance (NAR); however, NAR changes occur on a cyclical basis in unchallenged subjects, making baseline values somewhat unreliable. Topical steroid therapy has been reported to cause either a reduction (76, 77) or no change (37, 78) in the allergen-induced increase in nasal-airway resistance. Pipkorn has reported a decrease in the histamine content of nasal mucosa following topical steroids and has concluded that this is due to a reduction in mast-cell histamine content rather than to a decrease in mast-cell numbers (79, 80). Steroid therapy has been reported to reduce the number of eosinophils in nasal smears and the number of mast cells in nasal scrapings (81, 82). Okuda & Mygind have suggested that steroids may reduce the allergen-induced increases in endothelial/epithelial permeability that occur in rhinitis patients (83). Recently, Naclerio et al have developed a nasal-challenge model that allows for the measurement of chemical mediators following allergen challenge (84, 85). Following allergen challenge, histamine, PgD_2, kinins, leukotrienes, and other mediators have been demonstrated in the nasal secretions (84–87). This model system should allow for an objective study of the action of steroids in vivo against experimental allergic rhinitis.

STEROID EFFECTS ON WHITE BLOOD CELLS   The administration of steroid orally or parenterally causes significant changes in the circulating white blood–cell profile. Data in Figure 6 summarize the reported effects of a medium dose (e.g. 50 mg prednisone or 350 mg hydrocortisone) of steroid on leukocyte numbers. About 4–8 hours (depending on route of administration) following steroid administration, PMN levels rise to roughly twice resting levels, while the numbers of lymphocytes, monocytes, eosinophils, and basophils fall by approximately 80% (88–92) (Figure 6). Since PMN are the predominant white blood–cell type, total white counts rise slightly or do not change.

The increase in PMN counts reflects an increase of the half-life of the PMN from 7–10 hours, as well as an increase in the circulating, marginal, and therefore total blood-granulocyte pool (93). Studies with radiolabeled lymphocytes by Fauci & Dale indicate that the steroid selectively depletes the recirculating lymphocyte population (94). Further, lymphocyte marker studies indicate that T_μ and not T_γ lymphocytes are susceptible to the steroid effect (95). The decrease in lymphocyte numbers in man is due to redistribution of the circulating lymphocytes rather than to a lysis of lymphocytes, as occurs in the rat and mouse (96). Radiolabeled cell studies in the rat indicate that the fall in eosinophil numbers is due to reversible sequestration of the cells rather than to death (97). The numbers of lymphocytes, monocytes, and basophils in the circulation display a diurnal variation that is inversely related to diurnal levels of cortisol (98–100).

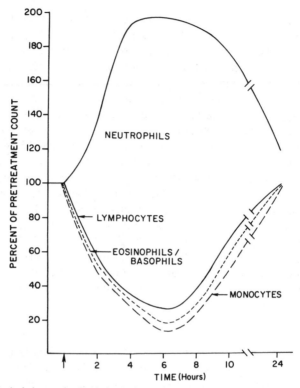

Figure 6   Typical changes in circulating leukocyte numbers following administration of steroid [taken from (88, 90–92)].

VASCULAR EFFECTS OF STEROIDS   The vascular endothelium plays a gate-keeper role in the inflammatory response, since it controls the entry of plasma proteins as well as circulating leukocytes into a localized tissue site. Increased permeability of vascular endothelium can occur directly as a result of stimulation with histamine or with the combination of bradykinin and PgE_2 or PgI_2 (101, 102). However, the increase in permeability caused by LTB_4, the complement fragment C_{5a}, and the bacterial peptide FMLP requires PMN (and probably Pg derived from either the PMN, the vascular endothelium, or both) (64, 101–104). In vivo microscopic studies in animals clearly show that steroids reduce the sticking of leukocytes to vascular endothelium following the administration of an inflammatory stimulus (105–109). Thus, some of the effects of steroids in reducing edema may be related to an inhibition of the interaction between PMN and vascular endothelium required to increase vascular permeability.

In addition to the inhibition of inflammatory-cell adherence to endothelium, steroids are effective vasoconstrictors (110–113). This action is the basis of a widely used test of topical steroid action (called the McKenzie test) (113) and may in part be related to the so-called permissive effects of steroids on adrenergic activity (111) (see below).

MAST CELLS, BASOPHILS, ANAPHYLAXIS   The union of allergen and IgE on the surface of mast cells and basophils produces degranulation and the release of chemical mediators of inflammation [for review, see (114)]. The most dramatic result of this reaction in vivo is anaphylaxis; chronic elicitation of this response is an important component of most, if not all, allergic diseases. It is for this reason that much research into steroid mechanisms of action has been focused on the mast cell and basophil. A considerable amount of this work has been carried out in vitro and will be discussed in another section.

Skin mast cells   Studies on the effect of steroid treatment on the number of mast cells in the skin of rats and human subjects have shown either no effect (115–118), a decrease (119–121), or, in some cases, a mild cytotoxic effect (122–123). Recent studies have shown that topical application of a potent steroid to human volunteers produces a reduction of tissue mast cells only after the production of cutaneous atrophy (124).

Basophils   One of the cell types that infiltrates a skin-test site during experimental allergen challenge is the basophil. Significant numbers of basophils have been observed in skin windows, skin blisters, and skin biopsies following allergic challenge (125–128). Of particular interest is the observation of Dvorak and coworkers, who note a profound basophil infiltrate at the site of allergic-contact dermatitis involving delayed-type hypersensitivity reactions (129, 130). This basophil influx may be caused by a lymphocyte-derived basophil chemotactic factor (131). As I discussed above, steroid treatment inhibits the local influx of basophils to a tissue site (132, 133).

Anaphylaxis   Naturally, it has not been possible to study the effect of steroids on experimental anaphylaxis in man, although the clinical evidence clearly suggests that they are not effective. There is some indication that treatment with steroid reduces the incidence and severity of radiocontrast dye reactions, a response that may be due to mediator release from basophils/mast cells. (134). Steroid treatment clearly protects against lethal anaphylaxis in the mouse and rabbit (135, 136), but not the guinea pig (137).

PMN   Steroids clearly reduce the adherence of PMN to vessel walls and their subsequent efflux into LPR tissue sites in animals and man (see above). Some interesting, but as yet unresolved, questions are: what are the biochemical changes responsible for adherence and which cell type expresses them, the leukocyte or the endothelial cell? Which cell type is the target cell for this most important action of steroids, the leukocyte or the endothelium? Recent studies indicate that the attachment of human PMN to bovine endothelial-cell monolayers is increased by prior exposure of the endothelial cells, but not the PMN, to LTB_4 (138), suggesting that the endothelial cell is the cell in which the adherence event is modulated. Several studies indicate that steroid treatment in vivo and in vitro can impair the adherence of PMN to nylon fibers (139–141). Therapeutically achievable concentrations of steroids in vivo and in vitro do not limit the chemotactic activity of PMN in vitro (141; R. P. Schleimer, D. W. MacGlashan, Jr., M. R. Mogowski, R. Daiuta, unpublished observations), nor do they inhibit the phagocytic activity of PMN (142). Low concentrations of dexamethasone have been reported to inhibit the release of plasminogen activator by PMN (143).

EOSINOPHILS   The eosinophil has long been an enigmatic cell; however, recent studies strongly implicate the eosinophil as an active killer of parasites and a central causative cell type in allergic diseases. Eosinophils arrive, sometimes in great numbers, at tissue sites following mast-cell degranulation and the appearance of eosinophil chemotactic factors (144, 145). Several lines of evidence implicate the eosinophil in asthma: (a) the circulating eosinophil count correlates well with the severity of asthma (146); (b) patients who die of asthma show a marked eosinophilic infiltrate in airway tissue, especially at sites of pronounced epithelial damage (47, 147); (c) the eosinophil's major basic protein (MBP) is a potent cytotoxin for bronchiolar epithelium (148); and (d) levels of MBP found in the sputa of asthmatics are sufficient to cause damage to epithelial cells (148).

Steroid therapy prevents the entry of eosinophils into a site of inflammation (149)(see above). This may be related in part to the pronounced reduction in circulating eosinophil levels. Gleich and associates have shown that steroid therapy of asthmatics improves lung function [peak expiratory flow rate (PEFR)], at the same time reducing blood eosinophil numbers and serum and sputum levels of MBP (150).

MONONUCLEAR PHAGOCYTES   The role of monocytes and macrophage in allergic diseases is not well characterized. Since antigen presentation is probably required for IgE production as well as for IgG production, macrophages (or perhaps dendritic cells) presumably are involved in the inductive phase of the allergic response. Recent studies demonstrating receptors for IgE on monocytes and macrophages, coupled with the appearance of these cells in the LPR and the recognition that under some circumstances they can release leukotrienes, leaves open the possibility of a significant role for these cells in allergic reactions (151, 152). The number of Fc_ϵ receptor–positive cells is elevated in patients with severe allergic disease and is reduced to normal levels or lower by steroid therapy (151).

Steroid treatment reduces the numbers of circulating monocytes and tissue macrophages. The reduction of tissue-macrophage numbers is largely the result of a decrease in the precursor (monocyte) number (153, 154), which in turn is the result of reduced production in the bone marrow (155). As is the case with PMN, steroids do not inhibit monocyte phagocytosis, but they do interfere with intracellular killing of microorganisms (156).

Immunoglobulins   The effects of steroids on specific IgE synthesis remain to be determined. Available information indicates that 2–4 weeks of steroid therapy have little or no effect on total IgE levels (157–159). While IgG antibody levels may be reduced slightly by similar steroid therapy (158–160), no evidence has been obtained for an inhibition of the specific IgG antibody response (161–163).

THE EFFECTS OF STEROIDS ON IN VITRO MODELS OF ALLERGIC DISEASE

Introduction

There is considerable uncertainty as to which cell types and chemical mediators are the most influential in causing allergic disease. By necessity, therefore, in vitro model systems employing a given cell type are only useful insofar as that cell is an important effector in the disease process. This section emphasizes the cells that have been strongly implicated in this role [i.e. mast cells, basophils, and mononuclear phagocytes (very little data are available on PMN and eosinophils)]. Although lymphocytes certainly play a part in the inductive phases of allergic processes and a wealth of knowledge on steroid effects on lymphocytes is available, less attention is given to these cells here, since their effector role is likely to be relatively small.

Steroid action in general requires the binding of steroids to an intracytoplasmic receptor, alteration of the ligand-receptor complex, translocation to the nucleus, and induction of RNA and then protein synthesis to produce an effector protein [for review, see (164, 165)]. Because of this, steroid effects in most in vitro systems require incubations of several hours to occur. Unfortunately, many studies were performed before this fact was known; these studies, in which steroid effects were usually demonstrated only at very high concentrations of drug, have been omitted from the present discussion.

Mast Cells and Basophils

Exposure of human basophils to steroids in culture for 24 hours leads to an inhibition of the subsequent histamine release induced by an IgE-dependent

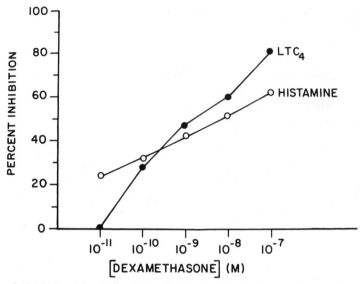

Figure 7   Inhibition of the release of histamine (o—o) and leukotriene C_4 (●—●) from anti-IgE–stimulated human basophils by dexamethasone.

stimulus but not of the release induced by a calcium ionophore, the chemotactic peptide Fmet-leu-phe, or phorbol diesters (166–68). This steroid effect is not caused by a modulation of the number of cell-surface IgE or IgE Fc receptors (167). Recent studies have shown that low concentrations of steroid inhibit the anti-IgE–induced release of leukotriene C_4 from basophils (169) (Figure 7).

Administration of steroid in vivo does not lead to an inhibition of basophil histamine release tested subsequently in vitro (92; K. L. Lampl, L. M. Lichtenstein, R. P. Schleimer, unpublished observations). Furthermore, basophils taken from asthmatics on continuous steroid therapy respond normally to anti-IgE (170). Lampl and coworkers have shown, however, that basophils derived from steroid-treated subjects are resistant to the in vitro action of dexamethasone, suggesting that steroid treatment in vivo has altered their in vitro responsiveness and perhaps their functions other than histamine release as well (171).

Although the IgE-dependent release of histamine and arachidonic acid in vitro is inhibited by steroids in murine mast cells (172, 173), this is not the case in human pulmonary mast cells (174). Incubation with dexamethasone does not inhibit the release of histamine, PgD_2, or leukotriene C_4 from human lung mast cells, whether they are in situ in lung fragments or in a highly purified state (174). This finding is consistent with the lack of effect of steroids in vivo against the immediate response to antigen (see above). In contrast, in the mouse and rat the protective effects of steroids in anaphylactic models may be related to an inhibition of the immediate mast-cell degranulation response.

Lung Tissue

Challenge of perfused lung tissue or lung fragments in vitro with antigen or anti-IgE leads to the release of mediators derived from mast cells (histamine, leukotriene C_4, prostaglandin D_2, and others) and other sources (6-keto-prostaglandin $F_{1\alpha}$, prostaglandin E_2, and $F_{2\alpha}$) (174–178). Overnight incubation of human lung fragments with relevant concentrations of steroids does not inhibit the subsequent release of the mast cell-derived mediators histamine, SRS (leukotriene C_4), PgD_2, or TxB_2, but it does produce a pronounced inhibition of the release of other arachidonate metabolites, including 6-keto-prostaglandin $F_{1\alpha}$ (174, 179). As is discussed below, inhibition of the release of arachidonic acid metabolites is likely to be an important mechanism of antiinflammatory steroid action.

Mononuclear Phagocytes

The in vivo studies discussed above indicate that steroids inhibit the entry of monocytes into tissue and their subsequent differentiation to become macrophages. In vitro studies support this concept, showing that steroids inhibit monocyte chemotaxis and differentiation (180–182). Other in vitro studies indicate that steroids inhibit the mononuclear-cell antigen-presenting function for T lymphocyte proliferation (183). Monocyte HLA DR surface antigen is increased by steroid treatment, and antigen presentation is normal if steroid-treated monocytes are washed free of steroid before being pulsed with antigen (183).

Because of the difficulty in obtaining human macrophages, most of the studies discussed below have been carried out using murine peritoneal macrophages. The mechanism by which steroids interfere with antigen presentation is not clear. Several studies indicate that macrophage phagocytic activity and phagosome-lysosome fusion is unaffected by steroids (184–86). Perhaps an important mechanism by which steroids inhibit macrophage activity in presenting antigen and inducing T-cell proliferation is the inhibition of Ia antigen induction and the synthesis of interleukin-1 (187, 188).

Steroids inhibit the in vitro release of some macrophage-derived mediators but not of others. Steroids inhibit the mediators released at cell activation and not the constitutively produced mediators (or the constitutive functions, such as phagocytosis) (Table 1). In addition to inhibiting macrophage plasminogen–activator release, steroids have been reported to induce a plasminogen-activator inhibitor in hepatoma cells, possibly potentiating the antifibrinolytic actions of steroids (192). Finally, human pulmonary macrophages produce a mucus secretagogue (193). It is possible that some of the action of steroids in inhibiting mucus release in vivo and in vitro is in inhibiting the release of this secretagogue from macrophages (193, 194).

Table 1   Effects of steroids in vitro on the release of macrophage-derived mediators

Mediator	Release		Inhibited by steroids	Reference
	Activation-dependent	Constitutive		
Interleukin-1	+		+	187, 188
Plasminogen activator	+		+	189, 190
Elastase	+		+	190
Collagenase	+		+	190
Lysozyme		+	−	190
Colony-stimulating factor	+		+	191
Fibronectin		+	−	191a
Macrophage-derived growth factor		+	−	191a

Lymphocytes

The suppressive effects of steroids against lymphocyte-mediated reactions (e.g. delayed hypersensitivity, graft rejection) are probably in large part due to an inhibition of lymphocyte proliferation (195). Proliferation is inhibited by the combined effects of a reduction in both antigen presentation and the synthesis of interleukin 1 and interleukin 2 (195–198) (see above). Steroids inhibit the generation of cytotoxic lymphocytes but not their action (199–201). T lymphocytes in mouse and rat are lysed by the steroid-induced activation of an endogenous endonuclease that destroys the DNA; human T lymphocytes are resistant to the lytic actions of steroids (202, 203).

MOLECULAR THEORIES OF STEROID ACTION

Introduction

In the late sixties and early seventies, a unified concept for all steroid action emerged (164, 165). Thus far, all cells that show a response to steroids (whether they be sex steroids, mineralocorticoids, or glucocorticoids) contain a specific intracytoplasmic steroid receptor. The unified concept states that steroid action is mediated through receptor binding and eventual alteration in the synthesis of proteins. Recent work indicates that steroids also can alter posttranslational processing of protein synthesis (e.g. glycosylation, cleavage, and compartmentalization). This presumably also occurs via steroid-receptor action at the level of gene expression (204, 204a).

For many years before the emergence of this unified concept, antiinflammatory steroid action was thought to be the result of lysosomal stabilization, since high concentrations of steroids acutely prevent the emptying of isolated lysosomes caused by irradiation and other agents (205). Lysosomal stabilization is no longer a tenable hypothesis, however, because it occurs in the absence of a nucleus and functioning protein-synthetic apparatus, high concentration of steroids are required, the time course of action (immediate) is not consistent with the in vivo time course, and for other reasons (206).

Phospholipase Inhibition

Appreciation of the critical importance of arachidonic-acid metabolites in inflammation is increasing. Just a little over a decade ago, Vane and Smith & Willis demonstrated that a major mechanism of action of non-steroidal antiin-flammatory drugs such as aspirin is an inhibition of the synthesis of prostaglandins (207, 208). At about the same time, Kunze & Vogt pointed out that the rate-limiting step in the production of arachidonic acid metabolites (cyclooxygenase metabolites as well as lipoxygenase metabolites such as leukotrienes and HETES) is the phospholipase A_2 enzyme that liberates arachidonic acid from phospholipid stores (209).

Gryglewski and coworkers, Lewis & Piper, and Levine and associates demonstrated that prolonged exposure to steroids leads to inhibition of prostaglandin release in several different tissues (210–212). It rapidly became clear that this steroid action was due to inhibition of the release of arachidonic acid rather than to inhibition of the cyclooxygenase enzyme (213, 214). Inhibitors of protein or RNA synthesis block the steroid effect, suggesting that steroids induce the synthesis of an inhibitor of arachidonic-acid release (215, 216). Subsequent studies by Flower & Blackwell, Hirata and coworkers, and others have uncovered several steroid-induced proteins that inhibit the liberation of arachidonic acid in many different tissues (217–223). One of these proteins, termed macrocortin, was first identified in the perfusate of steroid-treated guinea pig lungs and subsequently in rat leukocytes (217, 219). This polypeptide (MW 16,000, from guinea-pig lung) is stored by rat peritoneal leukocytes and rapidly released following exposure to steroids (219). Macrocortin has been shown to act directly in inhibiting the release of radiolabeled fatty acid from phosphatidylcholine.

Characterization of phospholipase inhibitory proteins from rabbit PMN and rat leukocytes reveals a protein of 40k MW (termed lipomodulin), as well as proteins of 200k, 30k, and 16k (218, 224, 225). Collaborative studies suggest that macrocortin (16k) as well as the 30k-protein are split products of lipomodulin (224). The phospholipase inhibitors are inactivated by phosphorylation and are often phosphorylated during their generation; they can be activated in vitro with alkaline phosphatase and apparently in vivo by target cells (221, 224, 226, 227). Lipomodulin is active in vivo in preventing carrageenan pleurisy in rats (227).

The applicability to humans of this data on phospholipase-inhibitory proteins is not yet entirely clear. Steroids have been shown to inhibit arachidonic acid–metabolite release by both pathways in several human cell and tissue types (169, 212, 228, 229). Furthermore, Hirata et al have demonstrated the presence of antilipomodulin antibodies in patients with rheumatic disease (230). Their finding in mice that antilipomodulin binds to I-J determinants and causes selective loss of suppressor cells raises the intriguing possibility that this may also be occurring in the patients with circulating antilipomodulin (230, 231).

Another function of phospholipase-inhibiting proteins may be in the regulation of IgE biosynthesis. Rat and allergic human lymphocytes produce IgE binding factors (232–236). In the nonglycosylated state, the rat IgE binding factor inhibits the formation of IgE-producing cells (232, 234, 237). Steroids, or a 16k fragment of lipomodulin, prevent glycosylation of the IgE binding factor, thus yielding the suppressive form of the factor. Antilipomodulin has the opposite effect (226, 233). The regulation of glycosylation by glucocorticoids is not without precedent (204). Thus far, the effects of steroid therapy on specific IgE synthesis in man have not been determined. However, owing to the apparent lack of effect on IgG synthesis and the rapid therapeutic action of steroids in allergic diseases (hours to days), it seems unlikely that regulation of IgE synthesis in vivo is a critical mechanism of steroid antiallergic actions.

The β-Adrenergic Theory of Asthma

An interaction between steroids and the β-adrenergic arm of the autonomic nervous system may explain some of the steroids' antiasthmatic effects. Researchers have known for some time that asthmatic patients show a reduced response to the effects of β-agonists, whether or not they have been receiving adrenergic drugs (228, 239). Steroid therapy restores the effects of β-agonists in asthmatics (240–242) (Figure 8). Based on these and other observations, Szentivanyi proposed that asthma is due to reduced β-adrenergic tone and that the efficacy of steroids is due to their permissive, or restorative, effects on the β-adrenergic system (243, 244).

A reduced response (desensitization) can be induced in vivo or in vitro by continued exposure to β-agonists. When normal subjects are desensitized in such a fashion, a single dose of intravenously administered steroid restores their response to inhaled β-agonists (245, 246).

Although the most important antiasthmatic action of β-agonists may be their dilating effects on smooth muscle, β-agonists also inhibit the function of inflammatory cells such as mast cells, basophils, PMN, and lymphocytes by elevating intracellular cyclic AMP levels [for review, see (247)]. Lymphocytes and PMN from asthmatics show a lower cyclic AMP response to β-agonists than do normals; the response is restored by previous in vivo steroid therapy (248–250). Steroids increase the number of β receptors on lung tissue in vitro

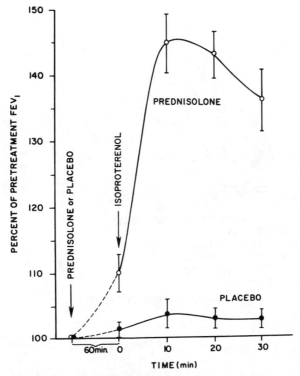

Figure 8 Permissive effect of steroid therapy on the β-adrenergic response in asthmatics. Isoproterenol response is weak in untreated patients (placebo), while one-hour pretreatment with 40 mg prednisolone allowed a brisk bronchodilatory response to isoproterenol [taken from (245)].

and cause some β_1 receptors to become β_2 receptors in 3T3 cells (251–253). However, in PMN, steroid prevents the desensitization-induced uncoupling of receptors from adenylate cyclase rather than altering receptor numbers (254). Thus, the so-called permissive effects of steroids on the β-adrenergic response in asthmatics may be related to steroid modulation of β receptor number, receptor subtype, or β-receptor coupling to the adenylate cyclase.

SUMMARY AND CONCLUSIONS

The beneficial actions of steroids for patients with allergic diseases cannot be explained by any single mechanism. A graphic summary of the most important antiallergic actions of steroids is shown in Figure 9. In this case, steroid action against asthma is discussed—the mechanisms may be the same or very similar in allergic disease of the skin and nasal airways. The immediate reaction, involving mast cell–mediator release, constriction of airways smooth muscle,

LATE PHASE — UNTREATED

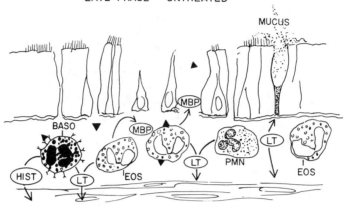

1. INFLAMMATORY CELL INFILTRATE
2. BRONCHOCONSTRICTION
3. HYPERSECRETION OF MUCUS
4. EPITHELIAL PERMEABILITY
5. EPITHELIAL DESTRUCTION
6. EDEMA

LATE PHASE — STEROID TREATED

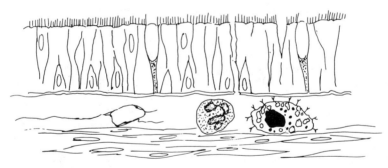

1. NO INFLAMMATORY CELL INFILTRATE
2. NO BRONCHOCONSTRICTION
3. NO HYPERSECRETION OF MUCUS
4. NO EPITHELIAL PERMEABILITY
5. NO EPITHELIAL DESTRUCTION
6. NO EDEMA
7. REDUCED ARACHIDONATE METABOLITES
8. INCREASED β-ADRENERGIC TONE

Figure 9 Model of steroid action on the late-phase response to bronchial-inhalation challenge with allergen (see Figure 2 for acute-response model). In the absence of steroid treatment (top), an inflammatory-cell infiltrate occurs, leading to bronchoconstriction, mucus secretion, edema, and epithelial destruction. Steroid therapy (bottom) prevents the inflammatory cell infiltrate and the concomitant sequelae.

increase of epithelial permeability, and mucus secretion (see Figure 2), is relatively unaffected by steroids. In the untreated subject, this immediate reaction is followed by the late-phase reaction (top panel, Figure 9). In this reaction, an inflammatory-cell infiltrate occurs (neutrophils, eosinophils, basophils, and monocytes are attracted by chemotactic factors). Eosinophil-derived MBP produces widespread focal destruction of airway epithelium, cell-derived mediators maintain mucus hypersecretion and epithelial hyper-meability, and bronchial hyperractivity and reduced β-adrenergic tone are manifest by mechanisms not yet understood.

In the steroid-treated subject, the inflammatory-cell infiltrate is profoundly reduced, and the usual consequences of that infiltrate, i.e. epithelial cell destruction and increased permeability, mucus hypersecretion, bronchocon-striction, and edema, therefore do not occur (Figure 9, bottom). In addition to this, the function of those cells that do enter the tissue (e.g. basophils, monocytes) is reduced. Furthermore, many of the target tissue responses themselves (e.g. mucus secretions and epithelial-cell permeability) appear to be inhibited directly by steroids. Finally, the smooth-muscle and perhaps the inflammatory-cell response to adrenergic tone (both neural and circulating catecholamines) is potentiated by the steroids.

It is somewhat difficult to factor out the relative importance of the inhibition of arachidonic acid–metabolite release in this picture. Since the vascular-permeability response leading to edema often requires a chemotactic stimulus and cyclooxygenase metabolites, or neutrophils, steroid effects on vascular permeability may be mediated in part via inhibition of arachidonic acid–metabolite formation. The lack of effect of aspirin in patients with asthma limits the potential importance of this mechanism to lipoxygenase products. However, the inhibition of phospholipase has as a consequence more than just the inhibition of arachidonic acid–metabolite release; many cells are activated by phospholipase-dependent mechanisms. Such may be the case with vascular endothelial cells, mucus-producing goblet cells, epithelial cells, and others. If that is the case, then steroids may exert many of their actions (e.g. inhibition of inflammatory cell adherence to vascular endothelium, inhibition of mucus secretion, etc) by way of a phospholipase-inhibiting intermediate.

ACKNOWLEDGMENTS

I would like to thank Drs. Lawrence M. Lichtenstein and Marshall Plaut for critical review of the manuscript and Mrs. Carol Dankelman for expert assis-tance in preparation of the manuscript. The author is supported by grants AI20136 and AM31891 from the National Institutes of Health.

Literature Cited

1. Carryer, H. M., Koelsche, G. A., Prickman, L. E., Maytum, C. K., Lake, C. F., et al. 1950. The effect of cortisone on bronchial asthma and hay fever, occurring in subjects sensitive to ragweed pollen. *J. Allergy* 21:282–87
2. Feinberg, S. M., Dannenberg, T. B., Malkiel, S. 1951. ACTH and cortisone in allergic manifestations. *J. Allergy* 22: 195–210
3. Cooke, R. A., Sherman, W. B., Mentel, A. E. O., Chapin, H. B., Howell, C. M., et al. 1951. ACTH and cortisone in allergic diseases. *J. Allergy* 22:211–36
4. Ellul-Micallef, R., Fenech, F. F. 1975. Intravenous prednisone in chronic bronchial asthma. *Thorax* 30:312–15
5. Gold, W. M., Kaufman, H. S., Nadel, J. A. 1967. Elastic recoil of the lungs in chronic asthmatic patients before and after therapy. *J. Appl. Physiol.* 23:433–38
6. Brown, M., Storey, G., George, W. H. S. 1972. Beclomethasone dipropionate: A new steroid aerosol for the treatment of allergic asthma. *Br. Med. J.* 1:585–90
7. Curry, J. J. 1946. The action of histamine on the respiratory tract in normal and asthmatic subjects. *J. Clin. Invest.* 25:-785–91
8. Hargreave, F. E., Ryan, G., Thomson, N. C., O'Byrne, P. M., Latimer, K., et al. 1980. Bronchial responsiveness to histamine or methacholine in asthma: Measurement and clinical significance. *J. Allergy Clin. Immunol.* 68:347–55
9. Cockroft, D. W., Ruffin, R. E., Dolovich, J., Hargreave, F. E. 1977. Allergen-induced increase in nonallergic bronchial reactivity. *Clin. Allergy* 7:503–13
10. Pare, P. O., Hogg, J. C. 1980. *Topical Steroid Treatment for Asthma and Rhinitis*, pp. 12–21. London: Bailliere Tindall
11. Holtzman, M. J., Fabbri, L. M., O'Byrne, P. M., Gold, B. D., Aizawa, E. H., et al. 1983. Importance of airway inflammation for hyperresponsiveness induced by ozone. *Am. Rev. Respir. Dis.* 127:686–90
12. Arkins, J. A., Schlerter, D. P., Fink, J. N. 1968. The effect of corticosteroids on methacholine inhalation in symptomatic bronchial asthma. *J. Allergy* 41:209–16
13. Konig, P., Jaffe, P., Godfrey, S. 1974. Effect of corticosteroids on exercise-induced asthma. *J. Allergy* 54:14–19
14. Hills, E. A., Davies, S., Geary, M. 1974. The effect of betamethasone valer-ate aerosol in exercise-induced asthma. *Postgrad. Med. J.* 67–68 (Suppl.)
15. Hartley, J. P. R., Charles, T. J., Seaton, A. 1977. Betamethasone valerate inhalation and exercise-induced asthma in adults. *Br. J. Dis. Chest* 71:253–58
16. Sulzberger, M. B., Sauer, G. C., Herrmann, F., Baer, R. L., Milberg, I. L. 1951. Effects of ACTH and cortisone on certain diseases and physiological functions of the skin: 1. Effects of ACTH. *J. Invest. Dermatol.* 16:323–37
17. MacGregor, R. R., Sheagren, J. N., Lipsett, M. B., Wolff, S. M. 1969. Alternate-day prednisone therapy. Evaluation of delayed hypersensitivity responses, control of disease and steroid side effects. *New Engl. J. Med.* 280:1429–34
18. Rabhan, N. B., Kopf, A. W. 1971. Alternate-day prednisone therapy for *pemphigus vulgaris*. *Arch. Dermatol.* 103:615–22
19. Ogawa, M., Berger, P. A., McIntyre, O. R., Clendenning, W. E., Ishizaka, K. 1971. IgE in atopic dermatitis. *Arch Dermatol.* 103:575–80
20. Spiegelberg, H. L., O'Connor, R. D., Simon, R. A., Mathison, D. A. 1979. Lymphocytes with immunoglobulin E Fc receptors in patients with atopic disorders. *J. Clin. Invest.* 64:714–20
21. Leith, W., Graham, M. J., Burrage, W. S. 1951. The effect of ACTH on the immediate skin reaction and passive transfer test in man. *J. Allergy* 22:99–105
22. Poothullil, J., Umemoto, L., Dolovich, J., Hargreave, F. E., Day, R. P. 1976. Inhibition by prednisone of late cutaneous allergic responses induced by antiserum to human IgE. *J. Allergy Clin. Immunol.* 57:114–17
23. Schwartz, E. 1954. Oral hydrocortisone therapy in bronchial asthma and hay fever. *J. Allergy* 25:112–19
24. Herxheimer, H., McAllen, M. 1956. Treatment of hay-fever with hydrocortisone snuff. *Lancet* 1:537–39
25. Godfrey, M. P., Maunsell, K., Pearson, R. S. 1957. Prednisone snuff in hay-fever. A controlled trial. *Lancet* 1:767–69
26. Norman, P. S., Winkenwerder, W. C., Murgatroyd, G. W., Parsons, J. W. 1966. Evidence for the local action of intranasal dexamethasone aerosols in the suppression of hay fever symptoms. *J. Allergy* 38:93–99
27. Mygind, N. 1973. Local effect of intra-nasal beclomethasone dipropionate aerosol in hay fever. *Br. Med. J.* 4:464–66

28. Gleich, G. J. 1982. The late phase of the immunoglobulin IgE-mediated reaction: A link between anaphylaxis and common allergic disease? *J. Allergy Clin. Immunol.* 70:160–69

29. Oertel, H., Kaliner, M. 1981. The biologic activity of mast cell granules in rat skin: Effects of adrenocorticosteroids on late-phase inflammatory responses induced by mast cell granules. *J. Allergy Clin. Immunol.* 68:238–45

30. Oertel, H. L., Kaliner, M. 1981. The biologic activity of mast cell granules. III. Purification of inflammatory factors of anaphylaxis (IF-A) responsible for causing late-phase reactions. *J. Immunol.* 127:1398–402

31. DeShazo, R., Levinson, A. I., Dvorak, H. F., Davis, R. W. 1979. The late phase skin reaction: Evidence for activation of the coagulation system in an IgE-dependent reaction in man. *J. Immunol.* 122:692–98

32. Robertson, D. G., Kerigan, A. T., Hargreave, F. E., Chalmers, R., Dolovich, J. 1974. Late asthmatic responses induced by ragweed pollen allergen. *J. Allergy* 54:244–54

33. Dolovich, J., Hargreave, F. E., Chalmers, R., Shier, K. J., Gauldie, J., et al. 1973. Late cutaneous allergic responses in isolated IgE-dependent reactions. *J. Allergy* 52:38–76

34. Solley, G. O., Gleich, G. J., Jordon, R. E., Schroeter, A. L. 1976. The late phase of the immediate wheal and flare skin reaction. Its dependence upon IgE antibodies. *J. Clin. Invest.* 58:408–20

35. Dolovich, J., Denberg, J., Kwee, Y. N., Belda, T., Blajchman, M., et al. 1983. Does non-immunologic mast cell mediator release/activation elicit a late cutaneous response? *Ann. Allergy* 50:241–45

36. McCarthy, D. S., Pepys, J. 1971. Allergic bronchopulmonary aspergillosis. *Clin. Allergy* 1:415–32

37. Mygind, N., Johnsen, N. J., Thomsen, J. 1977. Intranasal allergen challenge during corticosteroid treatment. *Clin. Allergy* 7:69–74

38. Gronneberg, R., Strandberg, K., Stalenheim, G., Zetterstrom, O. 1981. Effect in man of antiallergic drugs on the immediate and late phase cutaneous allergic reactions induced by anti-IgE. *Allergy* 36:201–8

39. Booij-Noord, H., Orie, N. G. M., deVries, K. 1971. Immediate and late bronchial obstructive reactions to inhalation of house dust and protective effects of disodium cromoglycate and predni-

sone. *J. Allergy Clin. Immunol.* 48:344–54

40. Booij-Noord, H., deVries, K., Sluiter, H. J., Orie, N. G. M. 1972. Late bronchial obstructive reaction to experimental inhalation of house dust extract. *Clin. Allergy* 2:43–61

41. Pepys, J., Davies, R. J., Breslin, A. B. X., Hendrick, D. B., Hutchcroft, B. J. 1974. The effects of inhaled beclomethasone diproprionate (Becotide) and sodium cromoglycate on asthmatic reactions to provocation tests. *Clin. Allergy* 4:13–24

42. Nakazawa, T., Yoyoda, T., Furukawa, M., Taya, T., Kobayashi, S. 1976. Inhibitory effects of various drugs on dual asthmatic responses in wheat-flour sensitive subjects. *J. Allergy Clin. Immunol.* 58:1–9

43. Herxheimer, H. 1954. Influence of cortisone on induced asthma and bronchial hyposensitization. *Br. Med. J.* 1:184–88

44. Martin, G. L., Atkins, P. C., Dunsky, E. H., Zweiman, B. 1980. Effects of theophylline, terbutaline and prednisone on antigen-induced bronchospasm and mediator release. *J. Allergy Clin. Immunol.* 66:204–12

45. Burge, P. S. 1982. The effects of corticosteroids on the immediate asthmatic reaction. *Eur. J. Resp. Dis.* 122:163–66 (Suppl.)

46. Salvato, G. 1959. Mast cells in bronchial connective tissue of man. Importance of such cells in allergic tissue injury. *Experientia* 15:308–9

47. Connell, J. T. 1971. Asthmatic deaths. Role of the mast cell. *J. Am. Med. Assoc.* 215:769–76

48. Ahmed, T., Greenblatt, D. W., Birch, S., Marchette, B., Wanner, A. 1981. Abnormal mucociliary transport in allergic patients with antigen-induced bronchospasm: Role of slow reacting substance of anaphylaxis. *Am. Rev. Respir. Dis.* 124:110–14

49. Marom, Z., Shelhamer, J. H., Bach, M. K., Morton, D. R., Kaliner, M. 1982. Slow-reacting substances, leukotrienes C_4 and D_4, increase the release of mucus from human airways in vitro. *Am. Rev. Respir. Dis.* 126:449–51

50. Marom, Z., Shelhamer, J., Alling, D., Kaliner, M. 1984. The effects of corticosteroids on mucous glycoprotein secretion from human airways in vitro. *Am. Rev. Respir. Dis.* 129:62–65

51. Knauer, K. A., Lichtenstein, L. M., Adkinson, N. F. Jr., Fish, J. E. 1981. Platelet activation during antigen-

induced airway reactions in asthmatic subjects. *New Engl. J. Med.* 304:1404–7

52. Nagy, L., Lee, T. H., Kay, A. B. 1982. Neutrophil chemotactic activity in antigen-induced late asthmatic reactions. *New Engl. J. Med.* 306:497–501

53. Samuelsson, B., Borgeat, P., Hammarstrom, S., Murphy, R. C. 1979. Introduction of a nomenclature: Leukotrienes. *Prostaglandins* 17:785–87

54. Lewis, R. A., Austen, K. F., Drazen, J. M., Clark, D. A., Marfat, A., et al. 1980. Slow reacting substances of anaphylaxis: Identification of leukotrienes C and D from human and rat sources. *Proc. Natl. Acad. Sci. USA* 77:3710–14

55. Dahlen, S. E., Hedqvist, P., Hammarstrom, S., Samuelsson, B. 1980. Leukotrienes are potent constrictors of human bronchi. *Nature* 288:484–86

56. Weiss, J. W., Drazen, J. M., Coles, N., McFadden, E. R., Weller, P. F., et al. 1982. Bronchoconstrictor effects of leukotriene C in humans. *Science* 216:196–98

57. O'Driscoll, B. R. C., Cromwell, O., Kay, A. B. 1984. Sputum leukotrienes in obstructive airways diseases. *Clin. Exp. Immunol.* 55:397–404

58. Kline, B. S., Cohen, M. B., Rudolph, J. A. 1932. Histologic changes in allergic and nonallergic wheals. *J. Allergy* 3:531–41

59. Rebuck, J. W., Hodsoon, J. M., Priest, R. J., Barth, C. L. 1963. Basophilic granulocytes in inflammatory tissues of man. *Ann. NY Acad. Sci.* 103:409–26

60. Eidinger, D., Raff, M., Rose, B. 1962. Tissue eosinophils in hypersensitivity reactions as revealed by the human skin window. *Nature* 196:683–84

61. Kimura, I., Tanizaki, Y., Takahashi, K., Saito, K., Veda, N., Sato, S. 1974. Emergence of basophils at sites of local allergic reactions using a skin vesicle test. *Clin. Allergy* 4:281–90

62. Atkins, P., Green, G. R., Zweiman, B. 1973. Histologic studies of human skin test responses to ragweed, compound 48/80, and histamine. *J. Allergy Clin. Immunol.* 51:263–73

63. Pienkowski, M., Adkinson, N. F. Jr., Norman, P. S., Lichtenstein, L. M. 1984. Mediators during cutaneous allergic immediate and late-phase reactions. *J. Allergy Clin. Immunol.* 73:147

64. Soter, N. A., Lewis, R. A., Corey, E. J., Austen, K. F. 1983. Local effects of synthetic leukotrienes (LTC$_4$, LTD$_4$, LTE$_4$ and LTB$_4$) in human skin. *J. Invest. Dermatol.* 80:115–19

65. Stollermann, G. H., Rubin, S. J., Plotz, C. M. 1951. Effect of cortisone on passively induced skin hypersensitivity in man. *Proc. Soc. Exp. Biol. Med.* 76:261–65

66. Mancini, R. E., Colombi, P. A., Galli, H., Orcivoli, L. 1961. Effect of glucocorticoid hormones on experimentally induced allergic reactions on human skin. *J. Allergy* 32:471–82

67. Nyfors, A. 1970. The influence of cortico-steroids on the allergic skin wheal reaction and the delayed type reaction (mantoux). *Acta Allergol.* 25:53–62

68. Gallant, S. P., Bullock, J., Wong, D., Maibach, H. I. 1973. The inhibitory effect of antiallergy drugs on allergen and histamine induced wheal and flare response. *J. Allergy Clin. Immunol.* 51:11–21

69. Slott, R. I., Zweiman, B. 1979. A controlled study of the effect of corticosteroids on immediate skin test reactivity. *J. Allergy Clin. Immunol.* 54:229–34

70. Zwieman, B., Slott, R. I., Atkins, P. C. 1976. Histologic studies of human skin test responses to ragweed and compound 48/80. *J. Allergy Clin. Immunol.* 58:657–63

71. Hauge, H. E., Vale, J. R. 1965. The influence of triamcinolone on the allergic skin wheal reaction. *Acta Allergol.* 20:496–502

72. Rebuck, J. W., Smith, R. W., Margulis, R. R. 1951. The modification of leukocytic function in human windows by ACTH. *Gastroenterology* 19:644–57

73. Rebuck, J. W., Mellinger, R. C. 1953. Interruption by topical cortisone of leukocytic cycles in acute inflammation in man. *Ann. NY Acad. Sci.* 56:715–32

74. Eidinger, D., Wilkinson, R., Bose, B. 1964. A study of cellular responses in immune reactions utilizing the skin window technique. I. Immediate hypersensitivity reactions. *J. Allergy* 35:77–85

75. Slott, R. I., Zweiman, B. 1975. Histologic studies of human skin test responses to ragweed and compound 48/80. *J. Allergy Clin. Immunol.* 55:232–40

75a. Bishop, C. R., Athens, J. W., Boggs, D. R., Warner, H. R., Cartwright, G. E., et al. 1968. Leukokinetic studies. XIII. A non-steady-state kinetic evaluation of the mechanism of cortisone-induced granulocytosis. *J. Clin. Invest.* 47:249–60

76. Vilsvik, J. S., Jenssen, A. O., Walstad, R. 1975. The effect of beclomethasone dipropionate aerosol on allergen induced nasal stenosis. *Clin. Allergy* 5:291–94

77. Pipkorn, U. 1982. Budesonide and nasal

allergen challenge testing in man. *Allergy* 37:129–34

78. Pelikan, Z., DeVries, K. 1974. Effects of some drugs applied topically to the nasal mucosa before nasal provocation tests with allegen. *Acta Allergol.* 29:337–53

79. Pipkorn, U. 1982. Budesonide and nasal mucosal histamine content and anti-IgE induced histamine release. *Allergy* 37:591–95

80. Pipkorn, U. 1983. Effect of topical glucocorticoid treatment on nasal mucosal mast cells in allergic rhinitis. *Allergy* 38:125–29

81. Sorenson, H., Mygind, N., Pedersen, C. B., Prytz, S. 1976. Long term treatment of nasal polyps with beclomethasone dipropionate aerosol. *Acta Oto-Laryngol.* 82:260–62

82. Hastie, R., Chir, B., Heroy, J. H., Levy, D. A. 1979. Basophil leukocytes and mast cells in human nasal secretions and scrapings studied by light microscopy. *Lab. Invest.* 40:554–61

83. Okuda, M., Mygind, N. 1980. See Ref. 10, pp. 22–33

84. Naclerio, R. M., Meier, H. L., Sobotka, A. K., Norman, P. S., Lichtenstein, L. M. 1984. In vivo model for the evaluation of topical antiallergic medications. *Arch. Oto-Laryngol.* 110:25–27

85. Naclerio, R. M., Meier, H. C., Adkinson, N. F. Jr., Kagey-Sobotka, A., Meyers, D. A., et al. 1983. In vivo demonstration of inflammatory mediator release following nasal challenge with antigen. *Eur. J. Respir. Dis.* 64(Suppl. 128):26–32

86. Proud, D., Togias, A., Naclerio, R. M., Crush, S. A., Norman, P. S., et al. 1983. Kinins are generated in vivo following nasal airway challenge of allergic individuals with allergen. *J. Clin. Invest.* 72:1678–85

87. Creticos, P. S., Peters, S. P., Adkinson, N. F. Jr., Naclerio, R. M., Hayes, E. C., et al. 1984. Peptide leukotriene release after antigen challenge in patients sensitive to ragweed. *New Engl. J. Med.* 310:1626–30

88. Herbert, P. H., DeVries, J. A. 1949. The administration of adrenocorticotropic hormone to normal human subjects. The effect of the leukocytes in the blood and on circulating antibody levels. *Endocrinology* 44:259–73

89. Saunders, R. H., Adams, E. 1950. Changes in circulating leukocytes following the administration of adrenal cortex extract (ACE) and adrenocorticotropic hormone (ACTH) in infectious mono-

nucleosis and chronic lymphatic leukemia. *Blood* 5:732–41

90. Fauci, A. S., Dale, D. C. 1974. The effect of in vivo hydrocortisone on subpopulations of human lymphocytes. *J. Clin. Invest.* 53:240–46

91. Fauci, A. S. 1976. Mechanisms of corticosteroid action on lymphocyte subpopulations. II. Differential effects of in vivo hydrocortisone, prednisone and dexamethasone on in vitro expression of lymphocyte function. *Clin. Exp. Immunol.* 24:54–62

92. Dunsky, E. H., Zweiman, B., Fischler, E., Levy, D. A. 1979. Early effects of corticosteroids on basophiles, leukocyte histamine, and tissue histamine. *J. Allergy Clin. Immunol.* 63:426–32

93. Athens, J. W., Haab, O. P., Raab, S. O., Mauer, A. M., Ashenbrucker, H., et al. 1961. Leukokinetic studies. IV. The total blood, circulating and marginal granulocyte pools and the granulocyte turnover rate in normal subjects. *J. Clin. Invest.* 40:989–95

94. Fauci, A. S., Dale, D. C. 1975. The effect of hydrocortisone on the kinetics of normal human lymphocytes. *Blood* 46:235–43

95. Haynes, B. F., Fauci, A. S. 1978. The differential effect of *in vivo* hydrocortisone on the kinetics of subpopulations of human peripheral blood thymus-derived lymphocytes. *J. Clin. Invest.* 61:703–7

96. Cupps, T. R., Fauci, A. S. 1982. Corticosteroid-mediated immunoregulation in man. *Immunolog. Rev.* 65:133–55

97. Andersen, V., Bro-Rasmussen, F., Hougaard, K. 1969. Autoradiographic studies of eosinophil kinetics: Effects of cortisol. *Cell Tissue Kinet.* 2:139–46

98. Osada, Y. 1956. Diurnal rhythms of the numbers in circulating basophils and eosinophils in healthy adults. *Bull. Inst. Publ. Health Tokyo* 5:5–9

99. Thomson, S. P., MaMahon, L. J., Nugent, C. A. 1980. Endogenous cortisol: A regulator of the number of lymphocytes in peripheral blood. *Clin. Immunol. Immunopath.* 17:506–14

100. Abo, T., Kawate, T., Itoh, K., Kumagai, K. 1981. Studies on the biperiodicity of the immune response. 1. Circadian rhythms of human T, B and K cell traffic in the peripheral blood. *J. Immunol.* 126:1360–63

101. Wedmore, C. V., Williams, T. J. 1981. Control of vascular permeability by polymorphonuclear leukocytes in inflammation. *Nature* 289:646–50

102. Bjork, J., Hedqvist, P., Arfors, K. E.

1982. Increase in vascular permeability induced by leukotriene B$_4$ and the role of polymorphonuclear leukocytes. *Inflammation* 6:189–96

103. Issekutz, A. C. 1981. Vascular responses during acute neutrophilic inflammation. Their relationship to in vivo neutrophil emigration. *Lab. Invest.* 45:435–41

104. Hedqvist, P., Dahlen, S. E. 1983. Pulmonary and vascular effects of leukotrienes imply involvement in asthma and inflammation. *Adv. Prostgland. Thromb. Leukotriene Res.* 1:27–32

105. Michael, N., Whorton, C. M. 1951. Delay of the early inflammatory response by cortisone. *Proc. Soc. Exp. Biol. Med.* 76:754–57

106. Moon, V. H., Tershakovec, G. A. 1952. Influence of cortisone upon acute inflammation. *Proc. Soc. Exp. Biol. Med.* 79:63–65

107. Ebert, R. H., Barclay, W. R. 1952. Changes in connective tissue reaction induced by cortisone. *Ann. Intern. Med.* 37:506–18

108. Barclay, W. R., Ebert, R. H., 1953. The effect of cortisone on the vascular reactions to serum sickness and tuberculosis. *Ann. NY Acad. Sci.* 56:634–36

109. Allison, F. Jr., Smith, M. R., Wood, W. B. Jr. 1955. Studies on the pathogenesis of acute inflammation. II. The action of cortisone on the inflammatory response to thermal injury. *J. Exp. Med.* 102:669–79

110. Ashton, N., Cook, C. 1952. In vivo observations of the effects of cortisone upon the blood vessels in rabbit ear chambers. *Br. J. Exp. Pathol.* 33:445–50

111. Zweifach, B. W., Shorr, E., Black, M. M. 1953. The influence of the adrenal cortex on behavior of terminal vascular bed. *Ann. NY Acad. Sci.* 56:626–33

112. Shulman, M. H., Fultin, G. P., Moront, G. P. 1954. Effect of cortisone on the healing of localized burns in the hamster cheek pouch. *New Engl. J. Med.* 251:257–61

113. McKenzie, A. W. 1962. Percutaneous absorption of steroids. *Arch. Dermatol.* 86:91–94

114. Wasserman, S. 1983. Mediators of immediate hypersensitivity. *J. Allergy Clin. Immunol.* 72:101–15

115. Baker, B. L. 1952. Mast cells of the omentum in relation to states of adrenocortical deficiency and excess. *Ann. NY Acad. Sci.* 56:684–92

116. Schoch, E. P., Glick, D. 1952. The effect of cold stress, ACTH, cortisone, pyrogen, and nitrogen mustard on tissue mast cells in the skin and subcutaneous tissues of the rat. *J. Invest. Dermatol.* 18:119–32

117. Baker, B. L. 1952. Mast cells of the omentum in relation to states of adrenocortical deficiency and excess. *Ann. NY Acad. Sci.* 56:684–90

118. Devitt, J. E., Pirozynski, W. J., Samuels, P. B. 1953. Mast cell resistance to hormonal influence. *Proc. Soc. Exp. Biol. Med.* 83:335–37

119. Asboe-Hansen, G. 1950. Effect of the adrenocorticotropic hormone of pituitary on mesenchymal tissues. *Scand. J. Clin. Lab. Invest.* 2:271–75

120. Cavallero, C., Braccini, C. 1951. Effect of cortisone on the mast cells of the rat. *Proc. Soc. Exp. Biol. Med.* 78:141–43

121. Asboe-Hansen, G. 1952. The mast cell. Cortisone action on connective tissues. *Proc. Soc. Exp. Biol. Med.* 80:677–79

122. Smith, D. E., Lewis, Y. S. 1954. Influence of hypophysis and adrenal cortex upon tissue mast cells of the rat. *Proc. Soc. Exp. Biol. Med.* 87:515–18

123. Wegelius, D., Asboe-Hansen, G. 1956. Hormonal effects on mast cells. Studies on living connective tissue in the hamster cheek pouch. *Acta Endocrinol.* 22:157–65

124. Lavker, R. M., Schechter, N. M. 1984. Cutaneous mast cell depletion results from topical corticosteroid usage. *Fed. Proc.* 43:1900 (Abstr.)

125. Aspegren, N., Fregert, S., Rorsman, H. 1963. Basophil leukocytes in allergic eczematous contact dermatitis. *Int. Arch. Allergy Appl. Immunol.* 23:150–56

126. Juhlin, L. 1963. Basophil leukocytes in blood and inflammatory exudate. *Acta Derm. Venereol.* 43:528–43

127. Felarca, A. B., Lowell, F. C. 1971. The accumulation of eosinophils and basophils at skin sites as related to intensity of skin reactivity and symptoms in atopic disease. *J. Allergy Clin. Immunol.* 48:125–33

128. Mitchell, E. B., Crow, J., Chapman, M. D., Jouchal, S. S., Pope, F. M., et al. 1982. Basophils in allergen-induced patch test sites in atopic dermatitis. *Lancet* 1:127–31

129. Dvorak, H. F., Mihm, M. C. 1972. Basophilic leukocytes in allergic contact dermatitis. *J. Exp. Med.* 135:235–54

130. Dvorak, H. F., Mihm, M. C., Dvorak, A. M., Johnson, R. A., Mansen, E. J., et al. 1974. Morphology of delayed type hypersensitivity reactions in man. *Lab. Invest.* 31:111–30

131. Kay, A. B., Austen, K. F. 1972. Chemotaxis of human basophil leukocytes. *Clin. Exp. Immunol.* 11:557–63

132. Juhlin, L. 1964. Effect of fluocinolone on basophil and eosinophil leukocytes in inflammatory exudate. *Acta Derm. Venereol.* 44:327–29

133. Okuda, M., Sakaguchi, K., Ohtsuka, H. 1983. Intranasal beclomethasone: Mode of action in nasal allergy. *Ann. Allergy* 50:116–20

134. Greenberger, P. A., Patterson, R., Simon, R., Lieberman, P., Wallace, W. 1981. Pretreatment of high-risk patients requiring radiographic contrast media studies. *J. Allergy Clin. Immunol.* 67:185–87

135. Nelson, C. T., Fox, C. L., Freeman, E. B. 1950. Inhibitory effect of cortisone on anaphylaxis in the mouse. *Proc. Soc. Exp. Biol. Med.* 75:181–83

136. Berthrong, M., Rich, A. R., Griffith, P. C. 1950. A study of the effect of adreno-corticotropic hormone (ACTH) upon the experimental cardiovascular lesions produced by anaphylactic hypersensitivity. *Bull. Johns Hopkins Univ.* 86:131–40

137. Dworetzky, M., Code, C. F., Higgins, G. M. 1950. Effect of cortisone and ACTH on eosinophils and anaphylactic shock in guinea pigs. *Proc. Soc. Exp. Biol. Med.* 75:201–6

138. Hoover, R. L., Karnovsky, M. J., Austen, K. F., Corey, E. J., Lewis, R. A. 1984. Leukotriene B_4 action on endothelium mediates augmented neutrophil/endothelial adhesion. *Proc. Natl. Acad. Sci. USA* 81:2191–93

139. MacGregor, R. R., Spagnuolo, P. J., Lentnek, A. L. 1974. Inhibition of granulocyte adherence by ethanol, prednisone and aspirin, measured with an assay system. *New Engl. J. Med.* 291:642–46

140. MacGregor, R. R. 1976. The effect of antiinflammatory agents and inflammation on granulocyte adherence. *Am. J. Med.* 61:597–607

141. Clark, R. A. F., Gallin, J. I., Fauci, A. S. 1979. Effects of in vivo prednisone on in vitro eosinophil and neutrophil adherence and chemotaxis. *Blood* 53:633–41

142. Allison, F., Adcock, M. H. 1965. Failure of pretreatment with glucocorticoids to modify the phagocytic and bactericidal capacity of human leukocytes for encapsulated type 1 pneumococcus. *J. Bacteriol.* 89:1256–61

143. Granelli-Piperno, A., Vassalli, J. D., Reich, E. 1977. Secretion of plasminogen activator by human polymorphonuclear leukocytes. *J. Exp. Med.* 146:1693–706

144. Kay, A. B., Stechschulte, D. J., Austen, K. F. 1971. An eosinophil leukocyte chemotactic factor of anaphylaxis. *J. Exp. Med.* 133:602–8

145. Paterson, N. A. M., Wasserman, S. I., Said, J. W., Austen, K. F. 1976. Release of chemical mediators from partially purified human lung mast cells. *J. Immunol.* 117:1356–62

146. Horn, B. R., Robin, E. D., Theodore, J., Kessel, A. V. 1975. Total eosinophil counts in the management of bronchial asthma. *New Engl. J. Med.* 292:1152–55

147. Fitten, W. V., Holley, K. E., Kephart, G. M., Gleich, G. J. 1982. Identification by immunofluorescence of eosinophil granule major basic protein in lung tissues of patients with bronchial asthma. *Lancet* 2:11–15

148. Gleich, G. J., Frigas, E., Filley, W. V., Loegering, D. A. 1984. Eosinophils and bronchial inflammation. In *Asthma III. Pathophysiology, Immunopharmacology, Treatment*, ed. A. B. Kay, K. F. Austen, L. M. Lichtenstein, pp. 195–210 New York: Academic

149. Dunsky, E. H., Atkins, P. C., Zweiman, B. 1977. Histologic responses in human skin test reactions to ragweed. IV. Effects of a single intravenous injection of steroids. *J. Allergy Clin. Immunol.* 59:142–46

150. Frigas, E., Loegering, D. A., Solley, G. O., Farrow, G. M., Gleich, G. J. 1981. Elevated levels of the eosinophil granule major basic protein in the sputum of patients with bronchial asthma. *Mayo Clinic Proc.* 56:345–53

151. Melewicz, F. M., Zeiger, R. S., Mellon, M. H., O'Connor, R. D., Speigelberg, H. L. 1981. Increased peripheral blood monocytes with Fc receptors for IgE in patients with severe allergic disorders. *J. Immunol.* 126:1592–95

152. Joseph, M., Jonnel, A. B., Torpier, G., Capron, A., Arnoux, B., et al. 1983. Involvement of immunoglobulin E in the secretory process of alveolar macrophages from asthmatic patients. *J. Clin. Invest.* 71:221–30

153. Thompson, J., VanFurth, R. 1970. The effect of glucocorticosteroids on the kinetics of mononuclear phagocytes. *J. Exp. Med.* 131:429–42

154. Belsito, D. V., Flotte, T. J., Lim, H. W., Baer, R. C., Thorbecke, G. J., et al. 1982. Effect of glucocorticosteroids on epidermal langerhans cells. *J. Exp. Med.* 155:291–302

155. Thompson, J., VanFurth, R. 1973. The effect of glucocorticosteroids on the proliferation and kinetics of promonocytes

and monocytes of the bone marrow. *J. Exp. Med.* 137:10–21

156. Rinehart, J. J., Sagone, A. I., Balcerzak, S. P., Ackerman, G. A., LoBuglio, A. F. 1975. Effects of corticosteroid therapy on human monocyte function. *New Engl. J. Med.* 292:236–41

157. Kumar, L., Hornbrook, M., Newcomb, R. W., 1971. A year-round study of serum IgE levels in asthmatic children. *J. Allergy Clin. Immunol.* 48:305–12

158. Settipane, G. A., Pudupakkam, R. K., McGowan, J. H. 1978. Corticosteroid effect on immunoglobulins. *J. Allergy Clin. Immunol.* 62:162–66

159. Posey, W. C., Nelson, H. S., Branch, B., Pearlman, D. S. 1978. The effects of acute corticosteroid therapy for asthma on serum immunoglobulin levels. *J. Allergy Clin. Immunol.* 62:340–48

160. Butler, W. T., Rossen, R. D. 1977. Effects of corticosteroids on immunity in man. 1. Decreased serum IgG concentration caused by 3 or 5 days of high doses of methylprednisolone. *J. Clin. Invest.* 52:2629–40

161. Larson, D. L., Tomlinson, L. J. 1951. Quantitative antibody studies in man. I. The effect of adrenal insufficiency and of cortisone on the level of circulating antibodies. *J. Clin. Invest.* 30:1451–55

162. Hahn, E. O., Houser, H. B., Rammelkamp, C. H., Denny, F. W., Wannamaker, L. W. 1951. Effect of cortisone on acute streptococcal infections and poststreptococcal complications. *J. Clin. Invest.* 30:274–81

163. Friedman, H. T. 1953. The influence of cortisone and hydrocortisone on the production of circulating antibody in human beings. *J. Allergy* 24:342–47

164. Baxter, J. D., Funder, J. W. 1979. Hormone receptors. *New Engl. J. Med.* 301:1149–61

165. Schmidt, T. J., Litwack, G. L. 1982. Activation of the glucocorticoid receptor complex. *Physiol. Rev.* 62:1131–92

166. Schleimer, R. P., Lichtenstein, L. M., Gillespie, E. 1981. Inhibition of basophil histamine release by antiinflammatory steroids. *Nature* 292:454–55

167. Schleimer, R. P., MacGlashan, D. W. Jr., Gillespie, E., Lichtenstein, L. M., 1982. Inhibition of basophil histamine release by antiinflammatory steroids. II Studies on the mechanism of action. *J. Immunol.* 129:1632–36

168. Bergstrand, H., Bjornesson, A., Lundquist, B., Nilsson, A., Brattsand, R. 1984. Inhibitory effect of glucocorticosteroids on anti-IgE-induced histamine release from human basophilic leuko-

cytes: Evidence for a dual mechanism of action. *Allergy* 39:217–30

169. Schleimer, R. P., Peters, S. P., Lichtenstein, L. M. 1984. Inhibition of basophil leukotriene release by antiinflammatory steroids. *Proc. Coll. Int. Allergol.* In press (Abstr.)

170. Findlay, S. R., Lichtenstein, L. M. 1980. Basophil "releasability" in patients with asthma. *Am. Rev. Respir. Dis.* 122:53–59

171. Lampl, K. L., Lichtenstein, L. M., Schleimer, R. P. 1984. In vitro resistance to dexamethasone (DEX) of basophils from steroid-dependent asthmatics. *J. Allergy Clin. Immunol.* 73:166 (Abstr.)

172. Daeron, M., Sterk, A. R., Hirata, F., Ishizaka, T. 1982. Biochemical analysis of glucocorticoid-induced inhibition of IgE-mediated histamine release from mouse mast cells. *J. Immunol.* 129:1212–18

173. Heiman, A. S., Crews, F. T. 1984. Hydrocortisone selectively inhibits IgE-dependent arachidonic acid release from rat peritoneal mast cells. *Prostaglandins* 27:335–43

174. Schleimer, R. P., Schulman, E. S., MacGlashan, D. W. Jr., Peters, S. P., Hayes, E. C., et al. 1983. Effects of dexamethasone on mediator release from human lung fragments and purified human lung mast cells. *J. Clin. Invest.* 71:1830–35

175. Brocklehurst, W. E. 1960. The release of histamine and formation of a slow reacting substance (SRS-A) during anaphylactic shock. *J. Physiol.* 151:416–23

176. Sheard, P., Killingback, R. G., Blair, A. M. J. N. 1967. Antigen induced release of histamine and SRS-A from human lung passively sensitized with reaginic serum. *Nature* 216:283–84

177. Piper, P. J., Walker, J. L. 1973. The release of spasmogenic substances from human chopped lung tissue and its inhibition. *Br. J. Pharmacol.* 47:291–304

178. Schulman, E. S., Newball, H. H., Demers, L. M., Fitzpatrick, P. A., Adkinson, N. F. Jr. 1981. Anaphylactic release of thromboxane A$_2$, prostaglandin D$_2$ and prostacylin from human lung parenchyma. *Am. Rev. Respir. Dis.* 124:402–6

179. Hammond, C. B., Hammond, M. D., Taylor, W. A. 1982. Selective inhibition by betamethasone of allergen-induced release of SRS-A from human lung. *Int. Arch. Allergy Appl. Immunol.* 67:284–86

180. Rinehart, J. J., Balcerzak, S. P., Sagone, A. L., LoBuglio, A. F. 1974. Effects of corticosteroids on human monocyte function. *J. Clin. Invest.* 54:1337–43

181. Tanner, A. R., Halliday, J. W., Powell, L. W. 1980. Effect of long-term corticosteroid therapy on monocyte chemotaxis in man. *Scand. J. Immunol.* 11:335–40

182. Rinehart, J. J., Wuest, D., Ackerman, G. A. 1982. Corticosteroid alteration of human monocyte to macrophage differentiation. *J. Immunol.* 129:1436–40

183. Gerrard, T. L., Cupps, T. R., Jurgensen, C. H., Fauci, A. S. 1984. Hydrocortisone-mediated inhibition of monocyte antigen presentation: Dissociation of inhibitory effect and expression of DR antigens. *Cell Immunol.* 85:330–39

184. Bell, P. G. H., Hinde, I. J. 1953. The effect of cortisone on macrophage activity in mice. *Br. J. Exp. Pathol.* 34:273–75

185. VanFurth, R., Jones, T. C. 1975. Effect of glucocorticosteroids on phagosome-lysosome interaction. *Infect. Immun.* 12:888–90

186. VanZwet, T. L., Thompson, J., VanFurth, R. 1975. Effect of glucocorticosteroids on the phagocytosis and intracellular killing by peritoneal macrophages. *Infect Immun.* 12:699–705

187. Smith, K. A. 1980. T cell growth factor. *Immunolog. Rev.* 51:337–57

188. Snyder, D. S., Unanue, E. R. 1982. Corticosteroids inhibit murine macrophage Ia expression and interleukin 1 production. *J. Immunol.* 129:1803–5

189. Vassalli, J. D., Hamilton, J., Reich, E. 1977. Macrophage plasminogen activator: Induction by concanavalin A and phorbol myristate acetate. *Cell* 11:695–705

190. Werb, Z. 1978. Biochemical actions of glucocorticoids on macrophages in culture. Specific inhibition of elastase, collagenase and plasminogen activator secretion and effects on other metabolic functions. *J. Exp. Med.* 147:1695–712

191. Ralph, P., Ito, M., Broxmeyer, H. E., Nakoinz, I. 1978. Corticosteroids block newly induced but not constitutive functions of macrophage cell lines: Myeloid colony-stimulating activity, production, latex phagocytosis and antibody-dependent lysis of RBC and tumor targets. *J. Immunol.* 121:300–3

191a. Lacronique, J. G., Rennard, S. I., Bitterman, P. B., Ozaki, T., Crystal, R. G. 1984. Alveolar macrophages in idiopathic pulmonary fibrosis have glucocorticoid receptors, but glucocorticoid therapy does not suppress alveolar macrophage release of fibronectin and alveolar macrophage derived growth factor. *Am. Rev. Resp. Dis.* 130:450–56

192. Coleman, P. L., Barouski, P. A., Gelehrter, J. D. 1982. The dexamethasone-induced inhibitor of fibrinolytic activity in hepatoma cells. A cellular product which specifically inhibits plasminogen activator. *J. Biol. Chem.* 257:4260–64

193. Marom, Z., Shelhamer, J. H., Kaliner, M. 1984. Human pulmonary macrophage-derived mucus secretagogue. *J. Exp. Med.* 159:844–60

194. Marom, Z., Shelhamer, J., Alling, D., Kaliner, M. 1984. The effects of corticosteroids on mucous glycoprotein secretion from human airways in vitro. *Am. Rev. Respir. Dis.* 129:62–65

195. Nowell, P. C. 1961. Inhibition of human leukocyte mitosis by prednisone in vitro. *Cancer Res.* 21:1518–21

196. Gillis, S., Crabtree, G. R., Smith, K. A. 1979. Glucocorticoid-induced inhibition of T cell growth factor production. II. The effect on the in vitro generation of cytolytic T cells. *J. Immunol.* 123:1632–38

197. Larsson, E. L., Iscove, N. N., Coutinho, A. 1980. Two distinct factors are required for induction of T cell growth. *Nature* 283:664–67

198. Larsson, E. L. 1980. Cyclosporin A and dexamethasone suppress T cell responses by selectively acting at distinct sites of the triggering process. *J. Immunol.* 124:2828–33

199. Williams, T. W., Granger, G. A. 1969. Lymphocyte in vitro cytotoxicity: Correlation of derepression with release of lymphotoxin from human lymphocytes. *J. Immunol.* 103:170–78

200. Balow, J. E., Hunninghake, G. W., Fauci, A. S. 1977. Corticosteroids in human lymphocyte-mediated cytotoxic reactions. *Transplantation* 23:322–28

201. Gillis, S., Crabtree, G. R., Smith, K. A. 1979. Glucocorticoid-induced inhibition of T cell growth factor production. I. The effect on mitogen-induced lymphocyte proliferation. *J. Immunol.* 123:1624–31

202. Claman, H. N., Moorhead, J. W., Benner, W. H. 1974. Corticosteroids and lymphoid cells in vitro. I. Hydrocortisone lysis of human, guinea pig, and mouse thymus cells. *J. Lab. Clin. Med.* 78:499–507

203. Cohen, J. J., Duke, R. C. 1984. Glucocorticoid activation of a calcium-dependent endonuclease in thymocyte nuclei leads to cell death. *J. Immunol.* 132:38–42

204. Firestone, G. L., Payvar, F., Yamamoto, K. R. 1982. Glucocorticoid regulation of

protein processing and compartmentalization. *Nature* 300:221–25

204a. Ringold, G. M. 1985. Steroid-hormone regulation of gene expression. *Ann. Rev. Pharmacol. Toxicol.* 25: In press

205. Weissman, G., Thomas, L. 1962. Studies on lysosomes. I. The effects of endotoxin, endotoxin tolerance, and cortisone on the release of acid hydrolases from a granular fraction of rabbit liver. *J. Exp. Med.* 116:433–50

206. Persellin, R. H., Ku, L. C. 1974. Effects of steroid hormones on human polymorphonuclear leukocyte lysosomes. *J. Clin. Invest.* 54:919–25

207. Vane, J. R. 1971. Inhibition of prostaglandin synthesis as a mechanism of action for aspirin-like drugs. *Nature New Biol.* 231:232–35

208. Smith, J. B., Willis, A. L. 1971. Aspirin selectively inhibits prostaglandin production in human platelets. *Nature New Biol.* 231:235–37

209. Kunze, H., Vogt, W. 1971. Significance of phospholipase A for prostaglandin formation. *Ann. NY Acad. Sci.* 180:123–25

210. Gryglewski, R. J., Panczenko, B., Korbut, R., Grodzinsky, L., Ocetkiewicz, A. 1975. Corticosteroids inhibit prostaglandin release from perfused mesenteric blood vessels of rabbit and from perfused lungs of sensitized guinea pigs. *Prostaglandins* 10:343–55

211. Lewis, G. P., Piper, P. J. 1975. Inhibition of release of prostaglandins as an explanation of some of the actions of antiinflammatory corticosteroids. *Nature* 254:308–11

212. Kantrowitz, F., Robinson, D. R., McGuire, M. B., Levine, L. 1975. Corticosteroids inhibit prostaglandin produced by rheumatoid synovia. *Nature* 258:737–39

213. Hong, S. L., Levine, C. 1976. Inhibition of arachidonic acid release from cells as the biochemical action of antiinflammatory corticosteroids. *Proc. Natl. Acad. Sci. USA* 73:1730–34

214. Nijkamp, F. P., Flower, R. J., Moncada, S., Vane, J. R. 1976. Partial purification of rabbit aorta contracting substance-releasing factor without inhibition of its activity by antiinflammatory steroids. *Nature* 263:479–82

215. Tam, S., Hong, S. L., Levine, L. 1977. Relationships among the steroids of antiinflammatory properties and inhibition of prostaglandin production and arachidonic acid release by transformed mouse fibroblasts. *J. Pharm. Exp. Ther.* 203:162–68

216. Danon, A., Assouline, G. 1978. Inhibition of prostaglandin biosynthesis by corticosteroids requires RNA and protein synthesis. *Nature* 273:552–54

217. Flower, R. J., Blackwell, G. J. 1979. Antiinflammatory steroids induce biosynthesis of a phospholipase A_2 inhibitor which prevents prostaglandin generation. *Nature* 278:456–59

218. Hirata, F., Schiffmann, E., Venkatasubramanian, K., Salomon, D., Axelrod, J. 1980. A phospholipase A_2 inhibiting protein in rabbit neutrophil induced by glucocorticoids. *Proc. Natl. Acad. Sci. USA* 77:2533–36

219. Blackwell, G. J., Carnuccio, R., DiRosa, M., Flower, R. J., Parente, L., et al. 1980. Macrocortin: A polypeptide causing the antiphospholipase effect of glucocorticoids. *Nature* 287:147–49

220. Carnuccio, R., DiRosa, M., Persico, P. 1980. Hydrocortisone-induced inhibitor of prostaglandin biosynthesis in rat leukocytes. *Br. J. Pharmacol.* 68:14–16

221. Hirata, F. 1981. The regulation of lipomodulin, a phospholipase inhibitory protein in rabbit neutrophils by phosphorylation. *J. Biol. Chem.* 256:7730–33

222. Russo-Marie, F., Duval, D. 1982. Dexamethasone-induced inhibition of prostaglandin production does not result from a direct action on phospholipase activities but is mediated through a steroid-inducible factor. *Biochim. Biophys. Acta* 712:177–85

223. Gupta, C., Katsumata, M., Goldman, A. S., Herold, R., Piddington, R. 1984. Glucocorticoid-induced phospholipase A_2-inhibitory proteins mediate glucocorticoid teratogenicity in vitro. *Proc. Natl. Acad. Sci. USA* 81:1140–43

224. Hirata, F., Notsu, Y., Iwata, M., Parente, L., DiRosa, M., et al. 1982. Identification of several species of phospholipase inhibitory protein(s) by radioimmunoassay for lipomodulin. *Biochem. Biophys. Res. Commun.* 109:223–30

225. Coote, P. R., DiRosa, M., Flower, R. J., Parente, L., Merrett, M., et al. 1983. Detection and isolation of a steroid-induced antiphospholipase protein of high molecular weight. *Proc. Br. Pharm. Soc.* Sept.: C3 (Abstr.)

226. Uede, T., Hirata, F., Hirashima, M., Ishizaka, K. 1983. Modulation of the biologic activities of IgE-binding factors. 1. Identification of glycosylation-inhibiting factor as a fragment of lipomodulin. *J. Immunol.* 130:878–84

227. Blackwell, G. J., Carnuccio, R., DiRosa, M., Flower, R. J., Langham, C. S. J.,

et al. 1982. Glucocorticoids induce the formation and release of antiinflammatory and antiphospholipase proteins into the peritoneal cavity of the rat. *Br. J. Pharmacol.* 76:185–94

228. Mitchell, M. D., Carr, B. R., Mason, J. I., Simpson, E. R. 1982. Prostaglandin biosynthesis in the human fetal adrenal gland: Regulation by glucocorticosteroids. *Proc. Natl. Acad. Sci. USA* 79: 7547–51

229. Hammarstrom, S., Hamberg, M., Duell, E. A., Stawiski, M. A., Anderson, T. P., et al. 1977. Glucocorticoid in inflammatory proliferative skin disease reduces arachidonic and hydroxyeicosatetraenoic acids. *Science* 197:994–96

230. Hirata, F., Carmine, R. D., Nelson, C. A., Axelrod, J., Schiffmann, E., et al. 1981. Presence of autoantibody for phospholipase inhibitory protein lipomodulin in patients with rheumatic diseases. *Proc. Natl. Acad. Sci. USA* 78:3190–94

231. Hirata, F., Iwata, M. 1983. Role of lipomodulin, a phospholipase inhibitory protein, in immunoregulation by thymocytes. *J. Immunol.* 130:1930–36

232. Hirashima, M., Yodoi, J., Ishizaka, K. 1980. Regulatory role of IgE-binding factors from rat T lymphocytes. III. IgE-specific suppressive factor with IgE-binding activity. *J. Immunol.* 125:1442–48

233. Yodoi, J., Hirashima, M., Hirata, F., DeBlas, A. L., Ishizaka, K. 1981. Lymphocytes bearing Fc receptors for IgE. VII. Possible participation of phospholipase A_2 in the glycosylation of IgE-binding factors. *J. Immunol.* 127:476–80

234. Hirashima, M., Uede, T., Huff, T., Ishizaka, K. 1982. Formation of IgE-binding factors by rat T lymphocytes. IV. Mechanisms for the formation of IgE-suppressive factors by antigen stimulation of BCG-primed spleen cells. *J. Immunol.* 128:1909–16

235. Deguchi, H., Suemura, M., Ishizaka, A., Osaki, Y., Kishimoto, S., et al. 1983. IgE class-specific suppressor T cells and factors in humans. *J. Immunol.* 131:2751–56

236. Ishizaka, K., Sandberg, K. 1981. Formation of IgE binding factors by human T lymphocytes. *J. Immunol.* 126:1692–96

237. Yodoi, J., Hirashima, M., Ishizaka, K. 1981. Lymphocyte-bearing Fc receptors for IgE. VI. Suppressive effect of glucocorticoids on the expression of Fc_ϵ receptors and glycosylation of IgE binding factors. *J. Immunol.* 127:471–76

238. Cookson, D. V., Reed, C. E. 1963. A comparison of the effects of isoproterenol in the normal and asthmatic subject. *Am. Rev. Respir. Dis.* 88:636–43

239. Lockey, S. D., Glennon, J. A., Reed, C. E. 1967. Comparison of some metabolic responses in normal and asthmatic subjects to epinephrine and glucagon. *J. Allergy* 40:349–59

240. Logsdon, P. J., Middleton, E., Coffey, R. G. 1972. Stimulation of leukocyte adenylcyclase by hydrocortisone and isoproterenol in asthmatic and nonasthmatic subjects. *J. Allergy* 50:45–56

241. Pun, L. Q., McCulloch, M. W., Rand, M. J. 1973. The effect of hydrocortisone on the bronchodilator activity of sympathomimetic amines and on the uptake of isoprenaline in the isolated guinea pig trachea. *Eur. J. Pharmacol.* 22:162–68

242. Ellul-Micallef, R., Fenech, F. F. 1975. Effect of intravenous prednisone in asthmatics with diminished adrenergic responsiveness. *Lancet* 2:7948

243. Szentivanyi, A. 1968. The beta adrenergic theory of the atopic abnormality in bronchial asthma. *J. Allergy* 42:203–32

244. Brodie, B. B., Davies, J. I., Hynie, S. Krishna, G., Weiss, B. 1966. Interrelationships of catecholamines with other endocrine systems. *Pharmacol. Rev.* 18:273–89

245. Tashkin, D. P., Conolly, M. E., Deutsch, R. I., Hui, K. K., Littner, M., et al. 1982. Subsensitization of beta-adrenoceptors in airways and lymphocytes of healthy and asthmatic subjects. *Am. Rev. Respir. Dis.* 125:185–93

246. Holgate, S. T., Baldwin, C. J., Tattersfield, A. E. 1977. β-adrenergic agonist resistance in normal human airways. *Lancet* 2:375–77

247. Bourne, H. R., Lichtenstein, L. M., Melmon, K. L., Henney, C. S., Weinstein, Y., et al. 1974. Modulation of inflammation and immunity by cyclic AMP. *Science* 184:19–28

248. Parker, C. W., Smith, J. W. 1973. Alterations in cyclic adenosine monophosphate metabolism in human bronchial asthma. 1. Leukocyte responsiveness to β-adrenergic agents. *J. Clin. Invest.* 52: 48–59

249. Parker, C. W., Huber, M. G., Baumann, M. L. 1973. Alterations in cyclic AMP metabolism in human bronchial asthma. III. Leukoctye and lymphocyte responses to steroids. *J. Clin. Invest.* 52:1342–48

250. Busse, W. W., Anderson, C. L., Cooper, W. 1981. Cortisol protection of the granulocyte response to isoproterenol

during an in vitro influenza virus incubation. *J. Allergy. Clin. Immunol.* 67:178–84

251. Mano, K., Akbarzadeh, A., Townley, R. G. 1979. Effect of hydrocortisone on beta-adrenergic receptors in lung membrane. *Life Sci.* 25:1925–30

252. Fraser, C. M., Venter, J. C. 1980. The synthesis of β-adrenergic receptors in cultured human lung cells: Induction by glucocorticoids. *Biochem. Biophys. Res.*

Commun. 94:390–97

253. Lai, E., Rosen, O. M., Rubin, C. S. 1982. Dexamethasone regulates the β-adrenergic receptor subtype expressed by 3T3-L1 preadipocytes and adipocytes. *J. Biol. Chem.* 257:6691–96

254. Davies, A. O., Lefkowitz, R.. J. 1983. In vitro desensitization of beta adrenergic receptors in human neutrophils. Attenuation by corticosteroids. *J. Clin. Invest.* 71:565–71

Ann. Rev. Pharmacol. Toxicol. 1985. 25:413–31

THE CURRENT AND FUTURE USE OF THROMBOLYTIC THERAPY

Sol Sherry and Ellen Gustafson

Department of Medicine and Thrombosis Research Center, Temple University School of Medicine, Philadelphia, Pennsylvania 19140

INTRODUCTION

In 1977, the Food and Drug Administration (FDA) approved streptokinase (SK) for the treatment of deep-vein thrombosis and pulmonary embolism and urokinase (UK) for the treatment of pulmonary embolism. Three years later, the FDA, in conjunction with the National Institutes of Health (NIH), sponsored a consensus development conference on these thrombolytic agents (1). After reviewing the data, the panel issued a strong positive statement encouraging physicians to employ these plasminogen activators in the management of proximal deep-vein thrombosis and the more severe forms of pulmonary embolism. This recommendation has resulted in a surge of interest in thrombolytic therapy with the following result: (*a*) increased acceptance of streptokinase and urokinase therapy for the indications previously noted; (*b*) expanded indications for their use; (*c*) application of new techniques and dosage schedules for their administration; and (*d*) development of new thrombolytic agents.

This review provides an update on the current state of the clinical use of thrombolytic agents and their future expectations.

GENERAL ASPECTS

Primary Mechanism for Thrombolysis

The rationale for using plasminogen activators for therapeutic thrombolysis is based on the evidence that the most sensitive mechanism for thrombolysis is the activation of fibrin-bound plasminogen to fibrin-bound plasmin, the latter then acting on its substrate in a relatively inhibitor-free environment (2, 3). Fun-

413

damental to an understanding of the special fibrinolytic properties of the plasminogen-plasmin system is that in vivo plasminogen exists in two phases, plasma or soluble-phase plasminogen and fibrin-bound or gel-phase plasminogen, with the plasminogen-plasmin system operating differently in each phase.

Plasminogen, the inactive precursor of the proteolytic enzyme plasmin, is a normal circulating constituent in plasma (its concentration in plasma is analogous to that of prothrombin) and possesses several binding sites for fibrin, the primary one having a very high affinity constant (3, 4); during clotting, approximately 5% of the surrounding plasma plasminogen becomes bound to fibrin and at a site that also serves as the major binding site for α_2-antiplasmin, the immediate, stoichiometric, and irreversible inhibitor of plasmin. In addition, evidence exists that fibrin enhances the rate of activation of plasminogen by plasminogen activators and that there are specific receptor sites on fibrin for plasminogen activators (4). Thus, when a plasminogen activator is in circulation and comes in contact with fibrin, activation of fibrin-bound or gel-phase plasminogen occurs; this produces selective fibrinolysis. Here there are no competing substrates for the action of fibrin-bound plasmin; the latter's action is carried out in a relatively inhibitor-free environment (the affinity of the fibrin-bound plasmin cannot be overcome by its affinity for α_2-antiplasmin); and fibrinolysis proceeds without any evidences of systemic proteolysis. These molecular events provide the rationale for the use of plasminogen activators rather than plasmin (or other proteolytic enzymes) for therapeutic thrombolysis and, more recently, for the development of plasminogen activators more specific for fibrin.

During streptokinase or urokinase therapy, there is also activation of plasma or soluble-phase plasminogen in the circulating blood and this leads to the appearance of free plasmin; the latter degrades fibrinogen, blood-clotting factors V and VIII, and some components of complement. While this action is controlled and dampened by various checks and balances, primarily through the action of such major inhibitors as α_2-antiplasmin and α_2-macroglobulin (slow and non-stoichiometric), there is evidence of considerable fibrinogen proteolysis, with the appearance of significant amounts of breakdown products. The resulting hypofibrinogenemia, impairment of platelet function (fibrinogen is necessary for normal platelet function) and the anticoagulant properties of fibrinogen breakdown products lead to an impaired hemostatic mechanism; this increases the risk of a bleeding episode, the major complication of thrombolytic therapy.

Plasminogen Activators in Clinical Practice

STREPTOKINASE   Streptokinase (SK) is the first of the plasminogen activators introduced into clinical medicine, originally for the lysis of extravascular deposits of fibrin and fibrin coagula, and later for intravascular thrombolysis (5, 6). At present, its approved indications are for the treatment of deep-vein thrombosis, pulmonary embolism, arterial thrombosis and embolism, coronary thrombosis (by intracoronary perfusion), and for the lysis of clotted arteriovenous cannulae (dialysis shunts, for example).

SK is produced from cultures of Lancefield Group C β hemolytic streptococci and has a molecular weight of 47,000 daltons. SK does not directly cleave plasminogen but activates plasminogen indirectly via the formation of an intermediate. The intermediate, a stoichiometric 1:1 complex of human plasminogen or plasmin and SK, then converts plasminogen into active plasmin (7).

In the utilization of streptokinase for therapeutic purposes, variable amounts of circulating antistreptokinase antibody, the consequence of previous streptococcal infections, must be overcome. The cumbersome dose titrations employed in the past to determine the amount of streptokinase required to neutralize such antibodies are no longer performed. Clinical experience with large numbers of patients has shown that a loading dose of 250,000 units given intravenously is sufficient to overcome the antibody level in 90–95% of patients and to initiate a thrombolytic state (8). The exceptions are those patients who have been treated recently with streptokinase, who have had a hemolytic streptococcal infection within the previous six months, or who have maintained a high antibody level.

The antigenic response to SK has been well studied. Antibody titers may rise even during the first day and peak in very high titers from day 7–10. High titers persist for three months and then slowly decline. By seven months after a course of therapy, an initial loading dose of 250,000 units is generally sufficient for initiating another course of therapy. In vivo, SK has two half lives: a rapid one of 16 minutes, which represents antibody complexing and its removal, and a slower one of about 83 minutes, which represents the biologic half life of this protein, its complex with plasminogen or plasmin, and their degradation products (9). However, the half life of the active moieties (free streptokinase and the activator complex) is shorter than the latter, although its duration has not yet been defined.

As noted previously, the administration of streptokinase results in the activation of both plasma plasminogen and thrombus plasminogen; the latter action is primarily responsible for thrombolysis, while the former, which also occurs rapidly and extensively, results in a transient state of hyperplasminemia. The level of this hyperplasminemia and its duration depends upon the rate of plasminogen activation, the concentration of α_2-antiplasmin (normally there is sufficient α_2-antiplasmin to inactivate about half of all the plasmin that can be formed from plasma plasminogen), the rate of inactivation of plasmin by the slower nonstoichiometric and progressive but reversible inhibitor complex formed with α_2-macroglobuin, and the rate of clearance of plasmin by the reticuloendothelial system. Thus, the state of hyperplasminemia and its effects vary considerably among patients and are primarily observed early during the therapy, when plasminogen is being rapidly activated (first few hours). Subsequently, when plasma plasminogen has been reduced to near zero levels, plasmin activity progressively declines and disappears, despite the continuation of the streptokinase infusion.

During the period of brisk hyperplasminemia, which is usually well tolerated by the patient, most of the fibrinogen is partially degraded; fragment X (a poorly clottable fibrinogen derivative with strong antithrombin activity) appears early, but later there is a progressive appearance of such incoagulable fragments as Y, D, and E, which, with the exception of the latter, are inhibitors of fibrin polymerization. In addition to the effects of fibrinogenolysis on both the coagulation mechanism and the ability of platelets to aggregate normally, there is also a partial degradation of factors V and VIII; all these changes induce a hemostatic defect that resolves slowly as the therapy is continued. This aberration, and the dissolution of fibrin previously laid down at sites of invasive procedures, are responsible for the increased risk of bleeding.

While the activation of plasma plasminogen is a hazard of therapy, it probably also contributes to its success: the induced hemostatic defect inhibits new fibrin formation at the thrombotic site and circulating plasmin may augment the process of thrombolysis; activation of plasma plasminogen perfusing a clot could also contribute to this phenomenon.

UROKINASE   Urokinase (UK), currently approved for the treatment of pulmonary embolism and coronary thrombosis (by intracoronary perfusion) and for intravenous catheter clearance (central venous lines, for example), is presently isolated and purified either from human fetal kidney cultures or from human urine; it exists in two forms whose molecular weights are 54,000 and 31,600 daltons. The former is believed to be the native form, the latter an active fragment. UK, an active protease, directly cleaves plasminogen to plasmin. Of the two forms of plasminogen (10), activation of lys-plasminogen proceeds more rapidly than with glu-plasminogen. Interestingly, while it is a native human plasminogen activator, UK is different from the activator(s) appearing in plasma following stimulation of the intrinsic or extrinsic mechanisms of fibrinolysis (11); this suggests that the urinary source of urokinase is in local production in the kidney rather than in excretion from plasma. Although there are no antibodies to overcome with urokinase as there are with streptokinase, nevertheless plasma inhibitors to urokinase and a rapid rate of clearance require that a loading dose be given when the agent is infused systemically; the most frequently used loading dose to initiate a thrombolytic state with urokinase, comparable to that achieved with SK, is 2,000 units per pound of body weight. Since the methods of standardizing urokinase and streptokinase are different, their units are not the same; in practice, the in vivo activity of approximately three units of UK is comparable to one unit of SK. The half-life of UK in vivo has been estimated at 14 ± 6 minutes (12).

UK has several theoretical advantages as a thrombolytic agent in clinical practice: (a) it is non-antigenic and its use is free of allergic reactions; (b) no anti-UK antibodies are present to interfere with drug action, although a variability exists in its rates of inactivation and clearance; and (c) compared to SK it has a greater affinity for fibrin-bound plasminogen than for plasma plasminogen. This increased affinity for fibrin-bound plasminogen allows clot lysis to occur with a milder hemostatic defect (13). Nevertheless, in studies comparing UK with SK that were designed to produce approximately equivalent levels of circulating plasminogen activator activity (14) and are currently being used in practice, no significant differences in clinical efficacy were observed, nor were there significant differences in the incidence of hemorrhagic complications (the initiation of a bleeding complication is most frequently due to the lysis of a hemostatic plug at the site of a recent invasive procedure and not to the hematologic changes, while the latter is more responsible for the duration and severity of the bleeding episode). Considering these observations, the much lower cost of SK has made it the more favored therapeutic agent in clinical medicine.

Factors Regulating In Vivo Thrombolysis

Once a thrombolytic state is established in vivo with either UK or SK, there is little correlation between the level of circulating plasma clot–dissolving activity and the rate or extent of thrombolysis (13). The latter appears to be dependent primarily on local factors in and around the thrombus rather than on measurable changes in the circulation. These factors include: (a) the accessibility of the activator to the thrombus; (b) the surface area of the clot exposed to the plasminogen activator; (c) the concentration of fibrin-bound plasminogen within the clot; (d) the activator concentration surrounding the thrombus; and (e) the age of the clot [fresh clots dissolve more readily than older ones (15)]. As a result, at present there are no useful tests for regulating dosage of the agents or rates of administration so as to maximize the speed of resolution of a thrombus; modifications of commonly employed regimens (see below) have been empirical, including attempts to reinforce the plasminogen content of thrombi (16). No evidence exists that any of these modifications has improved the therapeutic results.

Monitoring of Therapy

With the accumulation of evidence that the hematologic findings associated with thrombolytic therapy correlate poorly with either the clinical result or in predicting bleeding complications (13), monitoring of these changes during therapy no longer appears necessary or useful. Rather, during treatment one seeks only evidence that sufficient plasminogen activator is present in the circulation to activate plasminogen. At present, when SK or UK are administered systemically, it is recommended that three to four hours following the onset of the infusion a blood sample be obtained that demonstrates a prolongation of the partial thromboplastin time, a reduction in plasma fibrinogen, the appearance of increased levels of fibrinogen-fibrin degradation products, or a shortening of the euglobulin lysis time. If these do not occur, the patient is probably resistant to the activator; under these circumstances, one either switches to another activator or discontinues the treatment and initiates anticoagulant therapy instead.

With local perfusions, where lower doses of SK or UK are administered, the systemic hematological changes are milder, but one can usually demonstrate a reduction in plasma fibrinogen even though the partial thromboplastin time may remain unaffected. (The commonly employed clinical laboratory determination of fibrinogen is the most sensitive test for demonstrating plasma-plasminogen activation because it measures the totality of normal and slowly clottable fibrinogen as well as the antithrombin and antipolymerizing action of fibrinogen degradation products.)

Adverse Reactions

ALLERGIC REACTIONS   Allergic reactions have been observed in 1–2% of patients receiving streptokinase. These may include rash, urticaria, angioneurotic edema, bronchospasm, and anaphylactoid reaction. Most of these can be prevented by premedicating the patient with intravenously administered hydrocortisone (repeatable at 12-hour intervals during prolonged infusions). In the unusual instance of an anaphylactoid reaction, therapy should be stopped and the patient treated in the usual manner for such reactions.

FEVER   A febrile episode is not uncommon following streptokinase administration. The incidence of such febrile episodes (usually mild) can be reduced to less than 5% by hydrocortisone premedication. With urokinase, fevers may also occur in 1–2% of patients, although the mechanism is obscure. Allergic reactions are not seen with urokinase.

BLEEDING COMPLICATIONS   Bleeding is the major and most serious complication associated with thrombolytic therapy. The incidence has been variable and is dependent upon the investigator's definition of bleeding; some have reported all bleeding episodes, including minor cutdown or venipuncture oozing, others only transfusion-dependent episodes, and some only life-threatening episodes.

Attention to proper techniques and patient selection are critical factors in determining the incidence of bleeding. Bleeding can be expected to be initiated in a large percentage of patients with a recent invasive procedure; this is due to the lysis of a fibrin-stabilized hemostatic plug. However, this bleeding usually can be prevented by careful planning or controlled by pressure dressings. Severe bleeds requiring systemic therapy (cryoprecipitate, fresh-frozen plasma, or whole blood) occur in about 5% of cases. While most of these are at sites of known vascular injury, others are not (gastrointestinal, retroperitoneal or cerebral). The lowest incidence of severe bleeds, less than 1%, has been reported in patients receiving a single bolus injection of SK (high-dose, brief-duration therapy) for the lysis of a coronary thrombus (17).

Contraindications

Patient selection is very important if one is to minimize bleeding complications. Absolute contraindications include: (*a*) active bleeding lesions; (*b*) the presence of vascular intracranial disorders, such as cerebrovascular accident or a transient cerebral ischemic episode within the previous two months, cerebral tumors, or a cerebral arterio-venous malformation; and (*c*) cardio-pulmonary resuscitation because of underlying chest trauma.

Relative contraindications include: (*a*) age over 70; (*b*) large abrasive wounds, fractures, major surgery, or deep-closed biopsies within the previous ten-day period; (*c*) severe or accelerated hypertension (diastolic pressures greater than 110 mm Hg); and (*d*) any known increased bleeding risk, such as the presence of a constitutional or acquired coagulation or platelet defect, severe liver failure, or advanced uremia.

Not sufficiently stressed in the literature is the apparent synergistic action of heparin anticoagulation in increasing the bleeding incidence in patients receiving SK or UK therapy. In one study, the incidence of bleeding with low-dose SK (approximately one-tenth the usual dose) plus full-dose heparin therapy was as great as that observed with high-dose SK alone (18); in another study, the combination of low-dose SK with low-dose heparin was worse than high-dose SK alone (19). And while a low incidence of bleeding complications (0.8%) has been reported for patients receiving high-dose, short-duration intravenously administered SK (1.0–1.5 million units) for acute myocardial infarction (17), a recent study involving a smaller dose of SK (750,000 units) combined with high-dose heparin therapy had a 12.3% incidence of serious bleeding complications, including two intracerebral bleeds (20). The simultaneous use of heparin with SK or UK therapy should be avoided whenever possible.

THROMBOLYTIC THERAPY FOR SPECIFIC CLINICAL STATES

Deep-Vein Thrombosis

RATIONALE   While anticoagulation is the mainstay of therapy for a deep-vein thrombosis, it serves only as a secondary preventive measure; it slows or stops the underlying thrombotic process and in so doing inhibits extension of the venous thrombosis and decreases the likelihood of pulmonary embolism or its recurrence. However, anticoagulation has no acute demonstrable effect on the original thrombus. The natural history of such thrombi is to undergo organization and subsequent recanalization but with loss of normal venous valvular function. Serial venographic studies carried out during the first week in patients treated with heparin following an attack of proximal deep-vein thrombophlebitis have shown that complete resolution of the venous thrombosis can be expected to occur in only 10% or less of patients and some resolution may be evident in approximately another 15%, but the remainder (75%) show either no resolution or some progression of the underlying process (21). Pathologic and radiologic studies have shown that large venous thrombi that do not undergo rapid resolution are organized and recanalized, but the new channel contains no valves or, where valves remain, they are functionally inadequate because of cicatricial changes and anatomic disfiguration. Thus, most patients are left with persistent venous hypertension in the affected extremity (22, 23), remain symptomatic (pain, swelling), and are at permanent high risk for recurrent thrombophlebitis and a disabling post-phlebitic insufficiency syndrome. In a study by Elliott et al (22), 21 of 25 patients treated with adequate anticoagulation alone for proximal thrombophlebitis were available for two-year follow-up studies; 19 were still symptomatic, with four having developed venous claudication and one suffering from venous ulcers. In Arnesen's study, which followed patients for an average of 6.5 years, similar results were obtained (23). Of the 18 patients in the heparin group available for follow-up, none had a normal venogram, only six were asymptomatic, and three of the 12 symptomatic patients had developed a full-blown post-phlebitic insufficiency syndrome.

RESULTS   The consequences described above can be avoided if blood flow is restored to normal before venous valvular function is seriously impaired, and this can be accomplished by thrombolytic therapy in a majority of cases (15), particularly when the lesion is less than 72 hours old. Not only has this therapy avoided many of the late complications observed when anticoagulation is used as the only form of therapy (21), but the immediate effect has been a more rapid improvement in the clinical picture (24). Thus, thrombolytic therapy, when used properly in appropriately selected cases (25, 26) and in tandem with anticoagulation, offers the physician a significant advance in the therapy of proximal deep-vein thrombosis, including socioeconomic considerations (27).

INDICATIONS   At present thrombolytic therapy is recommended for all cases of adequately documented (usually by venography) proximal deep-vein thrombosis of the upper and lower extremities, provided that the benefit-risk ratio favors its use.

RECOMMENDED METHOD OF ADMINISTRATION AND DOSAGE   Thrombolytic therapy for deep-vein thrombosis is most commonly carried out by a sustained intravenous infusion via an infusion pump into an antecubital vein. The recommended dosage for streptokinase is a loading dose of 250,000 units given over a 30-minute period, followed by a sustaining infusion of 100,000 units per hour. The therapy is continued for periods of up to 72 hours depending on the clinical result. The objective is to restore blood flow to normal as gauged by non-invasive techniques and to discontinue therapy when this is achieved. Heparinization is then instituted to prevent recurrence. Guidelines for this form of therapy have been published (25, 26).

As yet, urokinase has not been approved for deep-vein thrombosis, but it has been used successfully for this purpose with currently recommended dosages, i.e. a loading dose of 2,000 units per pound of body weight given intravenously over a 10-minute period, followed by a sustaining infusion of 2000 units per pound of body weight per hour until blood flow has been restored (28, 29).

Acute Pulmonary Embolism

RATIONALE   The natural history of pulmonary embolism in anticoagulated patients is not very dissimilar from that of the venous thrombi from which they arise (21). This is based on the following evidence: (a) heparin does not acutely affect the pulmonary hypertension that frequently occurs with a large embolic episode and, although the hypertension moderates with time, increased pulmonary vascular resistance and pulmonary hypertension persist, along with a reduction in the total pulmonary capillary blood volume; (b) perfusion defects are still present in a significant percentage of cases (25–30%) when studied serially over several years; and (c) pathological observations reveal that pulmonary emboli frequently undergo organization and recanalization, ultimately leaving fibrous webs and bands as hallmarks of previous emboli. To prevent these late consequences, which can affect the long-term prognosis, rapid restoration of blood flow following a large embolic episode is required.

RESULTS   Successful lysis of acute pulmonary emboli can be achieved in the majority of cases (13, 14), and the acute clinical effects are considerably better than those observed with anticoagulation alone (30, 31), as are the late consequences (32).

INDICATIONS   Barring significant contraindications, thrombolytic therapy is recommended for any of the following conditions: (a) pulmonary embolism with evidence of acute pulmonary hypertension; (b) pulmonary embolism associated with protracted shock; and (c) pulmonary embolism with a perfusion defect (single or multiple) equivalent to one lobe or more.

RECOMMENDED METHOD OF ADMINISTRATION AND DOSAGE   Once the diagnosis is established by objective methods, treatment is carried out by an intravenous infusion as for deep-vein thrombosis except that the duration of therapy with streptokinase is 24 hours; with urokinase it is 12 hours. However, if the pulmonary artery pressure is being monitored or a pulmonary angiogram is performed, the infusion can be administered directly into the pulmonary artery; under these circumstances, a loading dose of SK or UK is unnecessary. While the results of direct perfusion into the pulmonary artery are very impressive (33), they are not very different from those achieved using the intravenous route.

Arterial Thrombosis and Embolism

RATIONALE   Rapid removal of an acute thrombotic or embolic arterial obstruction, if feasible, has always been considered a primary objective of therapy so as to avoid tissue necrosis or permanent impairment of the circulation. Thrombolytic therapy provides either an alternative or an adjunct to surgery.

RESULTS AND INDICATIONS   When used in the same manner as for venous thrombosis or pulmonary embolism, thrombolytic therapy produces results on the arterial side similar to those achieved in the lesser circulation (15, 34). Also, as on the venous side, emboli are more readily lysed than thrombi (34). Nevertheless, because many immediate successful surgical techniques are available for managing acute arterial thrombo-embolic problems, especially in the extremities, the indications for the use of systemic thrombolytic therapy as currently practiced is usually restricted to situations where an operative procedure is refused or is not likely to be tolerated or where the lesion is not accessible, e.g. in more distal vessels of the extremities.

Recently, however, a number of investigators (35–39) have extended the indications and usefulness of thrombolytic therapy by passing catheters to the immediate proximity of an acute thrombus or embolus and locally perfusing the vessel with a thrombolytic agent. The advantages of such an approach are: (a) delivery of the agent to the intended site is assured; (b) higher local concentrations of these activators are achieved with lower dosage schedules, thus maximizing rates of clot lysis while minimizing systemic effects and bleeding complications; and (c) the duration of therapy can be shortened and effectively tailored to the desired therapeutic objective with the aid of serial angiographic studies or suitable alternatives (oscillometry, for example). This approach is now being used for all lesions accessible to local perfusion; it has allowed the vascular surgeon to employ both surgical techniques and lytic therapy to best advantage in the total management of complex problems (40), and has allowed the interventional radiologist to employ both thrombolysis and percutaneous transluminal balloon angioplasty for the total management of a thrombosed atherosclerotic vessel (41).

As with venous thrombo-emboli, the age of the clot is an important determinant in the success of lysis. While several investigators (34, 42) have reported lysing older peripheral arterial thrombotic occlusions (several weeks to several months in duration) with relief of ischemic symptoms (intermittent claudication, etc), the success rate progressively declines with age of the thrombus; the duration of therapy to achieve reperfusion is also lengthened, and bleeding complications are increased. Consequently, the value of thrombolytic therapy for chronic peripheral arterial occlusions by local perfusion of the affected vessel remains controversial.

RECOMMENDED DOSAGE FOR LOCAL PERFUSION   Many dosage regimens have been used; they range from 5,000–50,000 units per hour for streptokinase and from 15,000–200,000 units per hour for urokinase. Since there are no reports of studies with dosage as the only variable, the superiority of one dosage schedule over another has not been established. Higher dosages may be expected to produce more rapid rates of lysis but with more extensive hematological changes; lower doses are usually given with larger amounts of heparin and may be subject to a higher incidence of bleeding.

Acute Myocardial Infarction

RATIONALE   The amount of myocardium that becomes necrotic with acute myocardial infarction determines the acute outcome and long-term prognosis. Major efforts in the past to develop methods for substantially reducing the size of myocardial infarction have not been very successful (43). Coronary thrombolysis is a promising treatment for this purpose, since an actue thrombus at the proximal border of an atherosclerotic obstruction usually underlies myocardial infarction (44, 45). While the use of fibrinolytic therapy is predicated on its potential for lysing an acutely obstructing thrombus and restoring blood flow, other actions may play a salutory role in this condition, as follows: (a) reduction in plasma viscosity consequent to the degradation of fibrinogen, and (b) improved flow through the lysis of platelet-fibrin thrombo-emboli in the microcirculation of the ischemic area (46). The latter effect could salvage myocardium otherwise destined to infarct and/or reduce the electrical instability of the marginal zone of ischemia.

METHODS OF ADMINISTRATION AND RESULTS   Three forms of therapy with plasminogen activators have been investigated for salvaging myocardium in patients undergoing a myocardial infarction: (a) sustained intravenous infusion for 24 hours, (b) intracoronary perfusion, and (c) high-dose, brief-duration (one hour) intravenous infusion.

Sustained 24-hour intravenous infusion   Sustained 24-hour intravenous infusion is the original form of therapy introduced for the treatment of acute myocardial infarction with streptokinase (6) and was employed in a series of trials begun in the mid-sixties and continued throughout the seventies (47). While the dosage and the duration of therapy varied, most of the studies used a regimen similar to that described for pulmonary embolism.

Many of these trials, including the well-designed European Cooperative Study (48), claimed a significant reduction in mortality compared to untreated controls. A recent review of the total data (47) suggests that the therapy probably was associated with a reduction in mortality of approximately 20%. However, the cardiological community in the United States either never took these studies seriously or expressed only passing interest (49). The reasons for this were:

1. The importance of coronary thrombosis as the precipitating factor in acute myocardial infarction, even when the latter was transmural, was minimized on the basis of a study (50) that was readily accepted by leading academic cardiologists, even though most of the information on this subject still indicated a high association (51). And when coronary thrombosis was present at autopsy, it was relegated to a secondary event of little or no pathogenic significance (50).
2. To satisfy the biometricians and cardiologists, trials had to be conducted in patients with a proven myocardial infarction (evolutionary changes in the electrocardiogram and elevated enzyme levels). Thus, many studies were undertaken only in patients whose zone of infarction was already completed or almost so. Under these circumstances, successful lysis of a coronary thrombus could only be expected to have limited goals, i.e. to prevent further extension of an already fairly fully developed infarct or to reduce the myocardial irritability arising from the marginal zone of ischemia.
3. The advent of coronary care units, with their constant monitoring of patients and their aggressive management of early rhythm or hemodynamic disturbances, not only reduced mortality to a point where trial numbers would have to be expanded greatly to prove a significant reduction in mortality, but also could have salvaged the same patients likely to be helped by the lysis of a thrombus.
4. The multiple invasive procedures carried out in coronary care units significantly enhanced the risk of bleeding associated with thrombolytic therapy, and it became increasing dangerous to treat patients by protracted systemic infusions (52).
5. Studies on infarct size reduction, which could have served as an alternative to mortality trials and allowed for an answer using much fewer patients, could not be carried out because of the lack of an acceptable method for measuring infarct size in the living patients.

Local intracoronary perfusion   With the demonstration that (*a*) coronary catheterization, angiography, and ventriculography could be carried out relatively safely in patients during the first few hours of an evolving myocardial infarction, and (*b*) an occluding thrombus was responsible for the lack of perfusion of the jeopardized mycardium, the opportunity was provided to treat such patients by direct local perfusion of the obstructed vessel before extensive infarction had taken place, and to evaluate the results.

Since the initial encouraging report by Rentrop (53), many investigators, as noted in a recent review (54), have substantiated his findings. On the average, in 75% (range 62–95%) of the patients studied, the obstructed coronary vessel was successfully recanalized by local streptokinase perfusion, usually within 20–30 minutes of the introduction of the agent into the obstructed artery. While the proven benefits of such therapy are still being debated, considerable evidence has accumulated that this therapy, when successful, does reduce infarct size (55–58); a recent trial also has claimed a significant reduction in mortality (59).

The dosages employed by cardiologists for perfusion of the obstructed coronary artery have ranged from 2,000–8,000 units per minute, usually given over a one-hour period (total dosage has varied between 100,000–500,000 units). Because of the insertion of a catheter (femoral artery approach), the patients have received heparin along with the streptokinase. Based on a survey of the current literature (54), the bleeding complication rate using this form of therapy has been 4.8%. The other significant problem encountered has been a 16% incidence [range 5–25% (54)] of recurrent thrombosis in the previously affected artery. Consequently, following thrombosis, a number of institutions employ coronary by-pass surgery or transluminal balloon angioplasty when a high degree of stenosis underlies the site of previous thrombosis (60).

Almost all studies on intracoronary perfusion have been conducted with SK, but in a recent trial the local perfusion of UK produced equivalent results to those observed with SK (61).

High-dose, brief-duration intravenous infusion of SK   In order to make streptokinase therapy for acute evolving myocardial infarction available to a much larger number of patients (many hospitals do not have catherization laboratories or trained personnel available at all times) without the morbidity associated with coronary catherization and without the delays in initiating treatment (coronary catheterization and angiography may take up to two hours), attempts are now underway to reproduce the results of intracoronary thrombolysis by high-dose, brief-duration intravenously administered streptokinase. The objective of the high dose is to flood the circulation with sufficient streptokinase to produce rapid thrombolysis of a coronary thrombus. Thus, doses of 500,000–1,500,000 units of SK have been infused over an hour's time, with the latter dose being the most popular. The rationale for the brief duration is to allow for early recovery of the hemostatic mechanism, thus minimizing the likelihood of a serious or protracted bleeding episode.

The initial results have been very encouraging (62–66): angiographic studies have demonstrated a reperfusion rate of 44–60% (average 51%), a bleeding complication rate of only 0.8%, and an average reocclusion rate of 18% (range 9–29%) (54).

More recent studies have reported higher rates of reperfusion (67, 68); however, these regimens are sufficiently different in design [duration of therapy (67) or simultaneous use of high-dose heparin therapy with a very significant increase in bleeding episodes (68)] to consider these studies independently of the others.

As with intracoronary perfusion, evidence is accumulating that high-dose, brief-duration, intravenously administered SK reduces infarct size (54), while the first major randomized trial evaluating mortality with this form of therapy will be completed soon (R. Schroder, personal communication).

Clotted Intravenous Catheters and Shunts

Streptokinase has been approved and has been used successfully for the treatment of arteriovenous cannula occlusion. After failure of other methods to relieve the thrombotic occlusion, 250,000 units of SK in 2 ml of an intravenous solution are injected into each occluded limb of the cannula; the cannula limbs are clamped off for two hours, the lysed contents are then aspirated, the cannula limbs are flushed, and the clamps are removed.

Urokinase has been approved and both UK (69) and SK (70) have been used successfully for clearing various types (intravenous alimentation catheters and Hickman catheters, for example) of occluded central venous lines. In this situation, small amounts of UK or SK are injected into the catheter in an amount equal to the volume of the catheter and the catheter is clamped distally. After a period of time (between five minutes and an hour), the catheter is aspirated of its contents and flushed.

Miscellaneous Uses of Thrombolytic Therapy

UNSTABLE ANGINA   Since a fair percentage of patients with unstable angina reveal evidence of partially obstructing thrombi during coronary catheterization, several investigators have reported on the potential value of SK therapy either intravenously (71) or by intracoronary perfusion (72) for this condition. Further investigation of thrombolytic therapy for this entity is indicated.

CEREBRAL VENOUS SINUS THROMBOSIS   Because of the high mortality rate of cerebral venous sinus thrombosis and the lack of any effective therapy for this condition, attempts have been made by several investigators to treat such patients with thrombolytic therapy (73, 74). While the reports are encouraging, the numbers of patients are small and the investigation still in an early stage.

PROSTHETIC VALVES   Thrombotic occlusion of a prosthetic valve is an acute catastrophe that could lend itself to thrombolytic therapy as an alternative to emergency surgery. There are several reports on the successful use of SK and UK for this condition (75, 76).

NEW THROMBOLYTIC AGENTS CURRENTLY UNDER CLINICAL INVESTIGATION

Tissue Plasminogen Activator

As previously noted, the activation of plasma plasminogen by streptokinase or urokinase in the circulating blood usually leads to a significant hemostatic defect (fibrinogen reduced, fibrinogen breakdown products increased, impaired platelet function, and other conditions). In contrast, the activator made by endothelial cells, fibroblasts, tumor cells, etc, utilizes fibrin as a co-factor for the activation of plasminogen. Thus, when this type of human activator, referred to as tissue-type plasminogn activator (TPA), is introduced into the blood stream, minor hemostatic abnormalities ensue; its activity is restricted primarily to activation of the fibrin-bound plasminogen, the most sensitive mechanism for thrombolysis. The theoretical advantage of TPA and TPA-like agents is that they could greatly increase the safety of thrombolytic therapy and ultimately change the practice habits of all physicians, i.e. to use thrombolytic therapy initially for all acute thrombo-embolic events followed by anticoagulation to prevent a recurrence. Currently, an extensive investigation is underway to evaluate TPA. Originally the material was obtained in tissue culture from a human melanoma cell line; preliminary studies on the lysis of venous and coronary thrombi with this preparation have been encouraging (77, 78). The agent is now being made in tissue culture by recombinant DNA techniques (rTPA) utilizing a mammalian cell line, and this material is undergoing clinical study (79).

Acylated Streptokinase-Plasminogen Activator Complex

Another development in the use of thrombolytic therapy involves the acylation of the streptokinase-plasminogen activator complex; this inactivates the SK activator so that, when the acylated streptokinase-plasminogen activator complex is introduced into the blood stream, no hemostatic abnormalities are produced. However, after the acylated compound binds to fibrin, deacylation takes place; this releases the original activator complex so as to activate the plasminogen bound to fibrin. Although animal studies with such preparations have been very encouraging (80), recent observations in man indicate that the presently used substances are deacylating in the general circulation and induce a hemostatic defect (81, 82).

Literature Cited

1. Sherry, S., Bell, W. R., Duckert, F. H., Fletcher, A. P., Gurewich, V., et al. 1980. Thrombolytic therapy in thrombosis: A National Institutes of Heatlh consensus development conference. *Ann. Intern. Med.* 93:141–44
2. Alkjaersig, N., Fletcher, A. P., Sherry, S. 1959. The mechanism of clot dissolution by plasmin. *J. Clin. Invest.* 38:1086–95
3. Collen, D. 1981. On the regulation and control of fibrinolysis. *Thromb. Haemostasis* 45:77–89
4. Wiman, W., Wallen, P. 1977. The specific interaction between plasminogen and fibrin. A physiological role of the lysine binding site in plasminogen. *Thromb. Res.* 10:213–22
5. Johnson, A. J., McCarty, W. R. 1959. The lysis of artificially induced intravascular clots in man by intravenous infusion of streptokinase. *J. Clin. Invest.* 38:1627–43
6. Fletcher, A. P., Sherry, S., Alkjaersig, N., Smyrniotis, F. E., Jick, S. 1959. The maintenance of a sustained thrombolytic state in man. II: Clinical observations in patients suffering from early myocardial infarction and other thromboembolic disorders. *J. Clin. Invest.* 38:1096–111
7. Castellino, F. J., Violand, B. N. 1979. The fibrinolytic system—Basic considerations. *Prog. Cardiovas. Dis.* 21:241–54
8. Verstraete, M., Tytgat, G., Amery, A., Vermylen, J. 1966. Thrombolytic therapy with streptokinase using a standard dosage. *Thromb. Diath. Haemorrh.* 16(Suppl. 21):494–500
9. Fletcher, A. P., Alkjaersig, N., Sherry S. 1958. The clearance of heterologous proteins from the circulation of normal and immunized man. *J. Clin. Invest.* 37:1306–15
10. Robbins, K. C. 1982. The plasminogen-plasmin enzyme system. In *Hemostasis and Thrombosis*, ed. R. Colman, J. Hirsh, V. J. Marder, E. W. Salzman, pp. 623–39. Philadelphia/Toronto: Lippincott. 1135 pp.
11. Aoki, N., von Kaulla, K. N. 1971. Dissimilarity of human vascular plasminogen activator and human urokinase. *J. Lab. Clin. Med.* 78:354–62

12. Fletcher, A. P., Alkjaersig, N., Sherry, S., Genton, E., Hirsh, J., et al. 1965. The development of urokinase as a thrombolytic agent. Maintenance of a sustained thrombolytic state in man by its intravenous infusion. *J. Lab. Clin. Med.* 65:713–38
13. Urokinase-Pulmonary Embolism Trial Study Group. 1973. The urokinase pulmonary embolism trial. *Circulation* 47(Suppl. 2):1–108
14. Urokinase-Streptokinase Pulmonary Embolism Trial. 1974. Phase II results. A national cooperative trial. *J. Am. Med. Assoc.* 229:1606
15. Marder, V. J., Bell, W. R. 1982. Fibrinolytic therapy. See Ref. 10, pp. 1037–57
16. Kakkar, V. V., Sagan, S., Scully, M. F., Lane, D. A. 1978. Intermittent plasminogen-streptokinase treatment of deep vein thrombosis. In *New Concepts of Streptokinase Dosimetry*, ed. M. Martin, W. Schoop, J. Hirsh, pp. 142–58. Bern/Stuttgart/Vienna: Huber. 246 pp.
17. Schroder, R. 1983. Systemic versus intracoronary streptokinase infusion in the treatment of acute myocardial infarction. *J. Am. Coll. Cardiol* 1:1254–61
18. Hirsh, J. 1978. The use of anticoagulants in patients treated with streptokinase. See Ref. 16, pp. 135–40
19. Schulman, S., Lockner, D., Granqvist, S., Bratt, G., Paul, G., et al. 1984. A comparative randomized trial of low-dose versus high-dose streptokinase in deep vein thrombosis of the thigh. *Thromb. Haemostasis* 51:261–65
20. Ganz, W., Geft, I., Shah, P. K., Lew, A. S., Rodriguez, L., et al. 1984. Intravenous streptokinase in evolving acute myocardial infarction. *Am. J. Cardiol.* 53:1209–16
21. Sherry, S. 1982. Clinical management of the thrombosed vessel: An overview. *Angiology* 33:6–10
22. Elliott, M. S., Immelman, E. J., Jeffery, P., Benatar, S. R., Funston, M. R., et al. 1979. A comparative randomized trial of heparin versus streptokinase in the treatment of acute proximal venous thrombosis; an interim report of a prospective trial. *Br. J. Surg.* 66:838–43
23. Arnesen, H., Hoiseth, A., Ly, B. 1982.

Streptokinase or heparin in the treatment of deep vein thrombosis. Follow-up results of a prospective study. *Acta Med. Scand.* 211:65–68

24. Robertson, B. R., Nilsson, I. M., Nylander, G. 1968. Value of streptokinase and heparin in treatment of acute deep vein thrombosis. *Acta Chir. Scand.* 134:203–8

25. Bell, W. R., Meek, A. G. 1979. Guidelines for the use of thrombolytic agents. *N. Engl. J. Med.* 301:1266–70

26. Marder, V. J. 1979. The use of thrombolytic agents: Choice of patient, drug administration, laboratory monitoring. *Ann. Intern. Med.* 90:802–8

27. O'Donnell, T. F., Browse, N. L., Burnand, K. G., Leathomas, M. 1977. The socioeconomic effects of an ileo-femoral thrombosis. *J. Surg. Res.* 22:483–88

28. Vande Loo, J. C. W., Kriessmann, A., Trubestein, G., Knoch, K., de Swart, C. A. M., et al. 1983. Controlled multicenter pilot study of urokinase-heparin and streptokinase in deep vein thrombosis. *Thromb. Haemostasis* 50:660–63

29. D'Angelo, A., Mannucci, P. M. 1984. Outcome of treatment of deep-vein thrombosis with urokinase: Relationship to dosage, duration of therapy, age of the thrombus and laboratory changes. *Thromb. Haemostasis* 51:236–39

30. Miller, G. A. H., Hall, R. J. C., Paneth, M. 1977. Pulmonary embolectomy, heparin and streptokinase: Their place in the treatment of acute massive embolism. *Am. Heart J.* 93:568–74

31. Ly, B., Arnesen, H., Eie, H., Hol, R. 1978. A controlled trial of streptokinase and heparin in the treatment of major pulmonary embolism. *Acta Med. Scand.* 203:465–70

32. Sharma, G. V. R. K., Burleson, V. A., Sasahara, A. A. 1980. Effect of thrombolytic therapy on pulmonary capillary blood volume in patients with pulmonary embolism. *N. Engl. J. Med.* 303:842–45

33. Demeter, S. L., Fuenning, C. 1983. Intra-pulmonary artery streptokinase. *Angiology* 34:70–77

34. Martin, M. 1979. Thrombolytic therapy in arterial thromboembolism. *Prog. Cardiovas. Dis.* 21:351–74

35. Dotter, C. T., Rosch, J., Seaman, A. J. 1974. Selective clot lysis with low-dose streptokinase. *Radiology* 111:31–37

36. Fiessinger, J. N., Vayssairat, M., Juillet, Y., Aiach, M., Janneau, D., et al. 1980. Local urokinase in arterial thromboembolism. *Angiology* 31:715–20

37. Katzen, B. T., van Breda, A. 1981. Low dose streptokinase in the treatment of arterial occlusions. *Am. J. Roentgenol.* 136:1171–78

38. Hargrove, W. C. III, Barker, C. F., Berkowitz, H. D., Perloff, L. J., McLean, G., et al. 1982. Treatment of acute peripheral arterial and graft thromboses with low-dose streptokinase. *Surgery* 92:981–93

39. Chaise, L. S., Comerota, A. J., Soulen, R. L., Rubin, R. N. 1982. Selective intra-arterial streptokinase therapy in the immediate postoperative period. *J. Am. Med. Assoc.* 247:2397–400

40. von Ryll Gryska, P., Raker, E. J. 1983. Post-embolectomy thrombosis treated with intra-arterial streptokinase. *Angiology* 34:620–25

41. Troop, B., Peterson, G. J., Pilla, T. 1983. Treatment of advanced vascular disease with intra-arterial thrombolytic therapy followed by arterial dilatation. *Angiology* 34:527–34

42. Hess, H., Ingrisch, H., Mietaschk, A., Rath, H. 1982. Local low-dose thrombolytic therapy of peripheral arterial occlusions. *N. Engl. J. Med.* 307:1627–30

43. Rude, R. E., Muller, J. E., Braunwald, E. 1981. Efforts to limit the size of myocardial infarcts. *Ann. Intern. Med.* 95:736–61

44. Phillips, S. J., Kongtahworn, C., Zeff, R., Benson, M., Iannone, L., et al. 1979. Emergency coronary artery revascularization: A possible therapy for acute myocardial infarction. *Circulation* 60:241–46

45. DeWood, M. A., Spores, J., Notske, R., Mouser, L. T., Burroughs, R., et al. 1980. Prevalence of total coronary occlusion during the early hours of transmural myocardial infarction. *N. Engl. J. Med.* 303:897–902

46. Nydick, I., Ruegsegger, P., Bouvier, C., Hutter, R. V., Abarquez, R., et al. 1961. Salvage of heart muscle by fibrinolytic therapy after experimental coronary occlusion. *Am. Heart J.* 61:93–100

47. Stampfer, M. J., Goldhaber, S. Z., Yusuf, S., Peto, R., Hennekens, C. H. 1982. Effect of intravenous streptokinase on acute myocardial infarction. *N. Engl. J. Med.* 307:1180–82

48. European Cooperative Study Group for Streptokinase Treatment in Acute Myocardial Infarction. 1979. Streptokinase in acute myocardial infarction. *N. Engl. J. Med.* 301:797–802

49. Sullivan, J. M. 1979. Streptokinase in myocardial infarction. *N. Engl. J. Med.* 301:836–37

50. Roberts, W. C., Buja, L. M. 1972. The

frequency and significance of coronary arterial thrombi and other observations in acute myocardial infarction. *Am. J. Med.* 52:425–43

51. Chandler, A. B., Chapman, I., Erhardt, L., Roberts, W. C., Schwartz, C. J. et al. 1974. Coronary thrombosis in myocardial infarction. *Am. J. Cardiol.* 34:823–32

52. Ness, P. M., Simon, T. L., Cole, C., Walston, A. 1974. A pilot study of streptokinase therapy in acute myocardial infarction: Observations on complications and relation to trial design. *Am. Heart J.* 88:705–12

53. Rentrop, P., Blanke, H., Wiegand, V., Karsch, K. R. 1979. Acute myocardial infarction: Intracoronary application of nitroglycerin and streptokinase in combination with transluminal catheterization. *Clin. Cardiol.* 5:354–63

54. Spann, J. F., Sherry, S. 1984. Coronary thrombolysis for evolving myocardial infarction. *Drugs* 28:465–83

55. Stack, R. S., Phillips, H. R., Grierson, D. S., Behar, V. S., Kong, Y., et al. 1983. Functional improvement of jeopardized myocardium following intracoronary streptokinase infusion in acute myocardial infarction. *J. Clin. Invest.* 72:84–95

56. Sheehan, F. H., Mathey, D. G., Schofer, J., Krebber, H. J., Dodge, H. T. 1982. Effects of interventions in salvaging left ventricular function in acute myocardial infarction: A study of intracoronary streptokinase. *Am. J. Cardiol.* 52:431–38

57. Schwarz, F., Schuler, G., Katus, H., Miehmel, H., van Olshausen, K., et al. 1982. Intracoronary thrombolysis in acute myocardial infarction: Correlations among serum enzymes, scintigraphic and hemodynamic findings. *Am. J. Cardiol.* 50:32–38

58. Cribier, A., Berland, J., Champoud, O., Moore, N., Behar, P. et al. 1983. Intracoronary thrombolysis in acute evolving myocardial infarction. Sequential angiographic analysis of left ventricular performance. *Br. Heart J.* 50:401–10

59. Kennedy, J. W., Ritchie, J. L., Davis, K. B., Fritz, J. K. 1983. Western Washington randomized trial of intracoronary streptokinase in acute myocardial infarction. *N. Engl. J. Med.* 309:1477–82

60. Serruys, P. W., Wyns, W., Van den Brand, M., Ribeiro, V., Fioretti, P., et al. 1983. Is transluminal coronary angioplasty mandatory after successful thrombolysis? Quantitative coronary angiographic study. *Br. Heart J.* 50:257–65

61. Tennant, S. N., Dixon, J., Venable, T. C., Page, H. L. Jr., Roach, A., et al. 1984. Intracoronary thrombolysis in patients with acute myocardial infarction: Comparison of efficacy of urokinase with streptokinase. *Circulation* 69:756–60

62. Schroder, R., Biamino, G., Enz-Rudiger, L., Linderer, T., Bruggemann, T., et al. 1983. Intravenous short-term infusion of streptokinase in acute myocardial infarction. *Circulation* 67:536–48

63. Rogers, W. J., Mantle, J. A., Hood, W. P., Baxley, W. A., Whitlow, P. L., et al. 1983. Prospective randomized trial of intravenous and intracoronary streptokinase in acute myocardial infarction. *Circulation* 68:1051–61

64. Schwarz, F., Hoffman, M., Schuler, G., Kubler, W. 1983. Combined intravenous and intracoronary streptokinase therapy in acute myocardial infarction. *J. Am. Coll. Cardiol.* 1:615

65. Spann, J. F., Sherry, S., Carabello, B. A., Denenberg, B. S., Mann, R. H., et al. 1984. Coronary thrombolysis by intravenous streptokinase in acute myocardial infarction: Acute and follow-up studies. *Am. J. Cardiol.* 53:655–61

66. Neuhaus, K. L., Teble, U., Sauer, G., Kreuzer, H., Kostering, H. 1983. High dose intravenous streptokinase in acute myocardial infarction. *Clin. Cardiol.* 6:426–34

67. Taylor, G. J., Mikell, F. L., Moses, H. W., Dove, J. J., Batchelder, J. E. 1984. Intravenous versus intracoronary streptokinase therapy for acute myocardial infarction. *Am. J. Cardiol.* 54:256–60

68. Alderman, E. L., Jutzy, K. R., Berts, L. E., Miller, R. G., Friedman, J. P., et al. 1984. Randomized comparison of intravenous versus intracoronary streptokinase for myocardial infarction. *Am. J. Cardiol.* 54:14–19

69. Lawson, M. 1982. The use of urokinase to restore the patency of occluded central venous catheters. *Am. J. Intraven. Ther. Clin. Nutr.* 9:29–32

70. Rubin, R. N. 1983. Local installation of small doses of streptokinase for treatment of thrombotic occlusion of long-term access catheters. *J. Clin. Oncology* 1:572–73

71. Lawrence, J. R., Shepard, J. T., Bone, T., Rogen, A. S., Fulton, W. F. M. 1980. Fibrinolytic therapy in unstable angina pectoris. A controlled clinical trial. *Thromb. Res.* 17:767–77

72. Vetrovec, G. W., Leinbach, R. C.,

Gold, H. K., Cowley, M. J. 1982. Intracoronary thrombolysis in syndromes of unstable ischemia: Angiographic and clinical results. *Am. Heart J.* 104:946–52

73. Bogdahrn, U., Fuhrmeister, U., Dominasch, D. 1983. Treatment of cerebral venous thrombosis: Thrombolytic agents versus heparin. In *Fibrinolytic Therapy,* ed. G. Trubestein, F. Etzel, pp. 299–303. Stuttgart/New York: Shattauer. 583 pp.

74. Leone, G., Laghi, F., Accorra, F., Catumaccio, R., Bizzi, B. 1983. Heparin-urokinase treatment in massive cerebral sinuses venous thrombosis. See Ref. 73, pp. 311–14

75. Peterffy, A., Henze, A., Savidge, G. F., Landou, C., Bjork, V. O. 1980. Late thrombotic malfunction of the Bjork-Shiley tilting disc valve in the tricuspid position. *Scand. J. Thorac. Cardiovasc. Surg.* 14:33–41

76. Witchitz, S., Veyrat, C., Moisson, P., Scheinman, N., Rozenstajn, L. 1980. Fibrinolytic treatment of thrombus on prosthetic heart valve. *Br. Heart J.* 44:545–51

77. Weimar, W., Stibbe, J., van Seyen, A. J., Billau, A., DeSomer, P., et al. 1981. Specific lysis of an ileofemoral thrombus by administration of extrinsic (tissue-type) plasminogen activator. *Lancet* 2: 1018–20

78. Sobel, B. E., Geltman, E. M., Tiefenbrunn, A. J., Jaffee, A. S., Spadaro, J. J., Jr. et al. 1984. Improvement of regional myocardial metabolism after coronary thrombolysis induced with tissue-type plasminogen activator or streptokinase. *Circulation* 69:983–90

79. Van de Werf, F., Bergmann, S. R., Fox, K. A. A., de Geest, H., Hoyng, C. F., et al. 1984. Coronary thrombolysis with intravenously administered human-type plasminogen activator produced by recombinant-DNA technology. *Circulation* 69:605–10

80. Dupe, R. J., English, P. D., Smith, R. A. G., Green, J. 1984. Acylenzymes as thrombolytic agents in dog models of venous thrombosis and pulmonary embolism. *Thromb. Haemostasis* 51: 248–53

81. Prowse, C. V., Hornsey, V., Ruckley, C. V., Boulton, F. E. 1982. A comparison of acylated streptokinase-plasminogen complex and streptokinase in healthy volunteers. *Thromb. Haemostasis* 47: 132–35

82. Walker, E. D., Davidson, J. F., Rae, A. P., Hutton, I., Lawrie, T. D. V. 1984. Acylated streptokinase-plasminogen complex in patients with acute myocardial infarction. *Thromb. Haemostasis* 51: 204–6

Ann. Rev. Pharmacol. Toxicol. 1985. 25:433–62

THE PHYSIOLOGY AND PHARMACOLOGY OF SPINAL OPIATES

T. L. Yaksh and R. Noueihed

Section of Neurosurgical Research, Mayo Clinic, Rochester, Minnesota 55905

INTRODUCTION

Opioid agonists with an action limited to the spinal cord produce powerful changes in an organism's response to otherwise painful stimuli. The effect is mediated by an action on opioid receptors located, we believe, on specific spinal elements that mediate the local processing of nociceptive information and its subsequent transmission to supraspinal centers. An extensive literature, reviewed elsewhere (1–2a), has made it abundantly clear that several classes of opioid receptors exist, including those with pharmacological profiles designated μ, δ, κ, σ and ϵ. In the following section we consider current thinking on the mechanism underlying the spinal action of opioids, the characteristics of the analgesia, and the characteristics of the receptor populations that mediate effect. Recently, it has become clear that spinal opioid receptors are also associated with a variety of systems in addition to those pertaining to sensory modulation. Thus, the spinal administration of opiates in the intact and unanesthetized animal has revealed powerful receptor-mediated effects on motor, cardiovascular, gastrointestinal, and bladder function. These subjects will also be briefly addressed.

OPIATES AND SPINAL FUNCTION

Several observations clearly demonstrate that opiates can exert a direct effect on spinal sensory and motor processing. The systemic administration of opiates in spinal-transected animals will at low doses selectively reduce the A-δ and C fiber and the thermally evoked ventral root reflex (3). Recording in the

433

0362-1642/85/415-0433$02.00

spinal-transected animal from wide dynamic-range neurons, a variety of systemically administered opiates have been shown to preferentially suppress the A-δ/C-evoked activity (4–7) as well as activity induced by a variety of somatic stimuli that evoke pain behavior in the unanesthetized animal [thermal >42°C (8, 9); cutaneous pinch, pressure (5)]. Although the effects are preferential for nociceptive input, less profound but measurable effects on receptive field size and the response to non-noxious stimuli have also been described (5, 8). An important question is whether the cells whose activity is affected by opiates project suprasegmentally or represent a population of local interneurons. Jurna & Grossmann (10) have demonstrated that lumbar neurons suppressed by systemically administered opiates can be antidromically fired from more rostral cord segments and thus do indeed represent "projection" neurons. These results on spinal nociceptors obtained with systemically administered opiates are probably mediated via an opioid receptor because: (a) the rank ordering of activity (the structure-activity relationship) bears a close correlation with the efficacy of these agents in opiate receptor bioassays: etorphine > fentanyl > levorphanol ≥ morphine ≥ d-1-methadone >> U-50488H ≥ meperidine >> dextrorphan = naloxone = 0 (4–13; T. L. Yaksh, unpublished data), and (b) their effects are antagonized by naloxone (see above) in a dose-dependent fashion (13).

The focal application of opiate alkaloids (morphine, levorphanol) and opioid peptides (e.g. met-enkephalin, leu-enkephalin, met-enkephalin amide) onto dorsal-horn neurons suppresses the activity evoked by noxious thermal or mechanical stimuli applied to the cutaneous receptive field (14–19). In the majority of these studies, naloxone given either systemically or iontophoretically can antagonize the suppression [but see (17)]. These results, suggesting that opiates act within the dorsal gray matter to suppress nociceptive activity, are supported by the observation that the effects of systemic opiates are reversed by naloxone iontophoresed into the dorsal gray (20).

Considerable skill and effort have been directed at understanding the mechanism whereby opiates in the spinal cord produce their particular effects. The ability of opiates to produce a powerful inhibition of small afferent fiber input with little effect on large afferent-evoked activity early led to speculation that opiates may act presynaptically. Alternately, the ability to suppress non-noxious activity in dorsal-horn neurons by high doses suggested that the selectivity is relative and depends on the temporal characteristics of the afferent input to the second-order neurons. This permits a postsynaptic effect to explain the observed events. The question of the substrate upon which opiates act to produce their physiological effects may be approached anatomically by noting the distribution of opioid ligand–binding sites and electrophysiologically by noting the spinal systems affected by opiates.

Binding Studies

Significant levels of μ, δ, and κ ligand binding have been demonstrated in the spinal cord, with the highest levels in the dorsal gray matter [see (2, 21)]. Ganglionectomies or rhizotomies result in a significant but clearly subtotal reduction in binding (22), suggesting that a proportion of these binding sites may be on primary afferents. The demonstration of binding in dorsal root ganglion cells (DRG) and in dorsal roots supports this association (23, 24). In fetal mouse spinal cord–ganglion preparations, opioid binding appears in the ganglion initially but does not appear in the cord until invasion by the ganglion cell neurites (25). Capsaicin, a neurotoxin that destroys small afferents (26), produces a significant reduction in the levels of markers for small primary afferents (27) and produces a reduction in ^{3}H-dihydromorphine binding in rat spinal cord comparable to that seen with rhizotomy (28). These observations jointly suggest that opiate binding sites may be found in primary afferents. Nevertheless, the subtotal loss of binding after neurotoxic and anatomical lesions argues that residual opioid binding exists on non-afferent elements.

The Primary Afferent Effects of Spinal Opiates

Evidence suggesting a presynaptic action for spinal opiates derives from studies examining the spinal release of neurotransmitters, the effects of opiates on primary afferent excitability, and the effects on dorsal root ganglion cell culture systems.

1. Substance P, a putative neurotransmitter found in small primary afferents, is released in vivo by A-δ/C fiber activity from spinal cord (29, 30). This evoked release is attenuated in vitro (31, 32) and in vivo (29, 30) by the local superfusion of opiates; the inhibition is antagonized by naloxone.

2. When current is applied by microelectrode in the dorsal-horn terminal field of a single primary afferent, the amount of change required to antidromically activate that axon permits assessment of the excitability of these terminals. Primary afferent depolarization, classically assumed to result in a decrease in neurotransmitter release, is reflected by a decrease in the threshold current required to evoke an antidromic discharge. Systemically administered opioid alkaloids in doses that result in behaviorally defined changes in pain in cats produce a significant decrease in terminal excitability (33). These effects of opiates appear to be mediated by an action on afferent terminals, because the focal iontophoretic delivery of morphine and met-enkephalin into the dorsal spinal gray also evokes a reliable decrease in the excitability of A-δ and C fiber but not of A-β terminals, which are naloxone antagonized (34).

3. Studies in chicken and mouse dorsal-root ganglion cultures have revealed that opiate alkaloids [morphine (32), etorphine (35)] and peptides [leu-

enkephalin (36), dynorphin (37), D-ala^2-met-enkephalin (32), morphiceptin (36)] have no effect on resting membrane potential or input resistance but do produce a shortening of the duration of the action potential antagonized by naloxone (32, 38, 39). This appears to occur by the attenuation of a voltage-dependent inward calcium current or by the enhancement of a voltage-dependent outward current. It must be stressed that all DRG cells do not respond to opiates, and those that do appear to have several populations of receptors (36, 40). This rather surprising finding has potential relevance for interpreting the physiological effects of opiates. In a cell culture system in which DRG cells synaptically drive spinal neurons, MacDonald & Nelson (35) demonstrated that etorphine iontophoretically applied to the spinal explant abolishes the EPSP evoked by stimulating the ganglion cell. This occurs in the absence of any change in either the membrane potential or the resistance of the second-order neuron. These data jointly suggest that opiates can diminish the depolarization-evoked release of a putative primary afferent neurotransmitter, perhaps by a local affect on the afferent terminals in the dorsal horn.

The Postsynaptic Effects of Spinal Opiates

To determine whether the observed effects of opiates on spinal nociceptive processing are pre- or postsynaptic, two ploys have been used: (a) to examine the ability of iontophoretically applied opioid to antagonize excitation evoked by glutamate, and (b) to apply the opiate near the terminals (in the substantia gelatinosa) and record from the cell body in the underlying nucleus proprious. Zieglgansberger and colleagues (15, 16) have noted that iontophoretic opiates applied in the vicinity of the cell body lead to a reduction in the rate of rise of the EPSP recorded intracellularly. This occurs in the absence of any evidence of hyperpolarization. Since spike initiation secondary to rapidly rising EPSP (generated, for example, by a synchronously arriving volley from rapidly conducting fibers) is less affected than the spike generated by slowly rising EPSP's (as generated by a dysynchronously arriving volley from small, slowly conducting afferents), the selective effects of opiates could be accounted for by this differential sensitivity to membrane conductance [but see (41) for a perceptive critique].

The majority of the studies that thus far have examined the response of neurons in the spinal cord to opiates have examined the neurons thought to lie within the nucleus proprious and whose dendrites lie more dorsally in the substantia gelatinosa. Duggan and colleagues, using multiple pipettes, examined the effect of opioids applied into the dorsal gray while recording from the vicinity of the more ventral cell body (42–44). In this work, morphine was observed to depress the responses evoked by thermal stimuli only when applied in the dorsal lamina; it was relatively inactive when given near the cell body. Peptides, in contrast, uniformly produce depression when administered along the dorsal-ventral axis of the neuron. Importantly, naloxone reverses the depressive effects of both the alkaloids and the peptides.

Sastry & Goh (45) have observed that morphine and met-enkephalin amide excite gelatinosa neurons but suppress underlying cells. Such actions are not inconsistent with the effects of opiates on afferents, given the possible role of gelatinosa neurons in presynaptic inhibition.

The mechanism of the action of opiates on cell function has been investigated in in vitro studies. Zieglgansberger & Sutor (46) have observed slices in which activity evoked by stimulating an attached rootlet as well as by iontophoretically applied glutamate is suppressed by focally applied D-Ala^2-D-Leu^5-enkephalin (DADL); this effect is reversed by naloxone. Recording intracellularly, the application of morphine, met-enkephalin, and DADL (47, 48) results in hyperpolarization concentration dependent over ranges of 30 nmol–100 μmol. Naloxone results in a significant antagonism of the observed hyperpolarization. Importantly, this hyperpolarization has been observed in the presence of calcium-free, high-magnesium solutions and is associated with an increase in membrane conductance. The results of manipulating extracellular potassium suggest that this conductance increase is largely related to the potassium ion.

In short, persuasive anatomical and electrophysiological data argue that exogenously administered opiates can act in the dorsal horn at sites that are both pre- and postsynaptic to the primary afferent to suppress nociceptive processing.

THE BEHAVIORAL EFFECTS OF SPINAL OPIATES

The powerful selective effects of systemically administered opiates on dorsal-horn neurons and nociceptive reflexes in spinal-transected animals and the pharmacological characteristics of these effects clearly demonstrate beyond question the existence of spinal opioid receptors that regulate the spinal processing of A-δ/C fiber input. Such studies, however, provide no information about the relevance of these opiate–receptor linked systems to behavior.

The Spinal-Injection Preparation

The early studies (49) on the functional role of these spinal receptor systems in the intact and unanesthetized preparation were facilitated by the demonstration that a chronic spinal catheter could be passed to various levels of the intrathecal space in the spinal cord of the rat (50), rabbit (50), cat (51), and primate (52). After the initial description of this phenomenon in rats, several modifications have been presented (53, 54). This simple approach has found use in the majority of studies published thus far on this topic. Recently, a variation in the approach in the rodent has been described that incorporates a cervical (55) or a lumbar penetration (56, 57). The direct-puncture technique described by Hylden & Wilcox (58) for the mouse must be considered an important contribution in view of the widespread use of this species. The use of osmotic minipumps to deliver opiates chronically through an intrathecal catheter in rats has been described (59).

Epidural animal preparations have been described for rat (56), cat (60), and primate (52). The present discussion will not deal with the results obtained using the epidural route, since these results are qualitatively comparable, although equipotent epidural doses generally exceed those observed after intrathecal administration and some drugs are comparatively inactive by the former route because it lies outside of the blood-brain barrier.

The question of the anatomical specificity of the intrathecal injection procedure has been discussed elsewhere (50, 61). The likelihood of a supraspinal redistribution of the drug can never be excluded and in fact increases with injection volumes, dose, lipid partition coefficient of drug (leading to increased blood levels), and time after injection. Failure to observe the effect associated with intrathecal action of the agent after intracisternal administration of an equal dose, or if such an injection produces a different behavioral syndrome, and if the effective intrathecal dose of the agent is inactive after intravenous injection, then the probability that the intrathecally administered drug is acting supraspinally is minimized. The intrathecal or epidural catheter preparation may cease functioning after an unpredictable period due to the formation of a fibrotic sheath that can prevent the drug from moving freely. A rightward shift in the dose response curve for intrathecal dynorphin has been reported in rats implanted more than a few days (62, 63). Durant & Yaksh (unpublished data) similarly have found a significant rightward shift in the dose response curve for morphine after epidural injection in rats, and this is associated with histologically defined fibrosis. Long-term studies must therefore build in controls to minimize the likelihood that loss of response to a particular agent is not simply due to a change in spinal drug distribution.

The Antinociceptive Effects of Spinal Opiates

Analgesia may be loosely considered the absence of an organized pain response in the presence of an otherwise adequate stimulus. Although complex, the central issue in assessing the effects of analgesic drugs is that somatic/visceral information must reach supraspinal centers to evoke the pain state. In animal models, the endpoint that signifies analgesia is the behavioral state in which the animal fails to respond with an organized behavioral response (hind paw lick, bar press) to escape an unconditioned stimulus that would otherwise evoke that behavior. Reliance on a task, the response components of which are spinally organized (e.g. the tail flick or skin twitch), makes it possible that drug effects that alter extensor/flexor tone (as with the Straub tail in the rat after morphine), or that postsynaptically alter the ability of flexor-reflex afferents to excite motoneurons, can yield results that are reflective of motor dysfunction and not sensory processing. While supraspinally organized responses are not devoid of interpretational difficulty, if the spinally administered drug blocks the ability of a somatic stimulus to evoke an organized escape response and the animal has the demonstrated ability to make the response (i.e. ambulation, vocalization, bar press) one can be certain to some degree that the spinal drug has altered the text of the ascending message. Thus, while spinally mediated reflexes are convenient and reliable, the need to examine measures that require supraspinally organized responses cannot be underestimated.

Table 1 summarizes the activity of spinally administered opiates on a number of spinally or supraspinally organized pain models in man and animals. It also presents the dose of intrathecal (animal) or epidural morphine (man) that represents the ED_{50} or is the dose that significantly increases the response baseline. As shown, spinal morphine produces: (a) an increase in the latency to respond in spinally mediated reflexes (tail flick, skin twitch) and supraspinally mediated responses (hot plate) evoked by strong cutaneous thermal stimuli; (b) an increase in the shock intensity applied to the tail or the hind paws (but not the ear) required to evoke squeak or bar press response; (c) a decrease in the likelihood of an agitation response to pinches applied to the paws; and (d) a reduction in the incidence of behavioral sequelia secondary to the intraperitoneal injection of an irritant. In terms of relative activity, the approximate rank ordering of the efficacy of intrathecal morphine in the mouse is writhing > tail flick = hot plate, and in the rat is pinch = hot plate = tail flick > tail shock = shock titration. We want to stress that the comparison of efficacy across different tests is in part artifactual, because the apparent ED_{50} values can be shifted radically by altering the endpoints on the criteria for failure to respond. Nevertheless, comparability of doses in the several thermal nociceptive tests reflecting the ability to block the two end-points suggests comparable substrates. In dogs, spinal morphine blocks the rise in blood pressure secondary to exercise ischaemia induced by reversible ligation of the iliac artery during mild activity on a treadmill (88).

In man, experimental pain models have proven less useful than in animals; nevertheless, measurable effects on the ability to tolerate cold water immersion and a pressure tourniquet to the lower limbs (but not upper limbs) are significantly increased in volunteers receiving clinically useful doses of epidural morphine. The majority of work on the antinociceptive effects of spinal opiates in man has been carried out in postoperative pain patients and patients suffering from terminal malignancies. As shown in Table 1, following thoracic and/or abdominal surgery, epidural morphine produces a powerful analgesia, as measured by a variety of behavioral endpoints, such as the visual analogue scale, the McGill pain questionnaire, and the mobilization scale (indicating the relative activity of the patient during the postoperative course). One powerful

Table 1 Pain models in mouse, rat, cat, primate, and human sensitive to spinal morphine

Pain Model	Species	Spinal morphine dose (nmol)[a]	References
EXPERIMENTAL			
Temperature			
Thermal-spinal reflex			
Tail flick	Mouse	0.9–2.4[b]	64
	Rat	1.3–11.9	65
Skin twitch	Cat	120[b]	51
Thermal-supraspinal			
Hot plate	Mouse	1.5–5.7[b]	66
	Rat	0.9–12.7[b]	64
Cold-supraspinal			
Limb immersion	Human	~ 30,000[c]	67
Electrical			
Shock vocalization	Rat	90[c]	68
Shock titration	Rat	135[c]	69
	Primate	3000[d]	70
Pressure			
Pinch	Rat	0.8–3.5[b]	71
Tourniquet pressure	Human	~ 10,500[c]	72
Inflammatory			
Writhing	Mice	0.08–0.21[b]	77
	Rat	0.3–12.1[b]	65
CLINICAL			
Postoperative: Thoracic/upper abdominal		2–8 mg	
Visual analogue scale			74–76
Modified McGill pain questionnaire			74
Mobilization scale			77
Duration or time to first analgesic (> 10 hours)			78–80
Cumulative consumption of additional analgesics			78, 80
Respiratory function			
Peak expiratory flow rate			76, 77
Vital capacity			76, 81
Forced expiratory volume at 1 second			77, 80, 81
CO_2 response curves			82
Pulmonary X-ray changes			77, 81
Terminal Cancer			
Visual analogue			83, 84
McGill pain questionnaire			84
Consumption of additional analgesics			84–86
Time between doses			84, 85, 87

[a] Intrathecal in animals; epidural in man.
[b] 95% CI of ED_{50}.
[c] Dose that produces a significant increase over baseline.
[d] Dose that just produces the maximum increase in the shock titration response.

method of quantification is an examination of the pattern of analgesic consumption during the postoperative course, since this represents a clearly quantifiable operant response on the part of the patient during the occurrence of pain. Thus, among groups receiving spinal opiates, the time to administration of the first alternative analgesic is significantly increased and the cumulative consumption of alternative analgesics is reduced. A variety of physiological, particularly respiratory, indices generally compromised after thoracic or abdominal information have also been studied with spinal opiates. In all cases, there is a significant improvement in performance, which indicates a reduction in the pain stimulus evoked by the expansion of the chest wall.

In terminal cancer pain, difficulties arise by virtue of (a) possible day-to-day variation in pain, and (b) problems of tolerance associated with long-term use of systemic or spinal opiates. Nevertheless, spinal opiates have been shown to acutely produce pain relief as assessed by behavioral measures such as the visual analogue scale and the McGill pain questionnaire. During long-term administration, the adequacy of spinal drug therapy is reflected in the time between doses (or, in the case of chronic infusion, in the stability over time of the dose required to produce reports of analgesia) and the level of consumption of additional pain medication; long-term administration of spinal opiates, either by percutaneous catheters [see, for example, (85, 87)] or by chronic infusion [see, for example, (84, 86)], has indeed been reported to result in adequate analgesia, with minimum alternative drug consumption, without a need for significant spinal drug–dose escalation for periods of between three and six months.

In short, spinally administered opiates can produce a powerful increase in the tolerance to thermal, mechanical, and chemical stimuli, as well as postoperative states that otherwise evoke verbal and behavioral manifestations of pain.

The Locus of Action of Spinally Administered Opiates

What corollaries can be drawn between the effects of intrathecally administered opiates on behavior and the effects on single-unit activity in spinal cord? In view of the presence of opioid binding in the DRG and dorsal roots, and the observation that in vitro opiates can produce a significant effect on the activity of subpopulations of DRG cells in culture, it is reasonable to speculate that the spinally administered opiates may exert a direct effect on the afferents. This effect appears limited to the culture preparation, however, because in adult animals recording in situ from rat dorsal root ganglion cells and from vagus nerve opiates have failed to produce any effect on measured membrane properties (89, 90). Alternately, failure to observe opiate effects on adult ganglion cells may be due to limited sampling. As noted (36, 40), opiate sensitivity is found in a limited population of neurons.

To examine the correlation between intrathecally administered agents and the effect on similar activity, drugs have been applied directly to the surface of the cat cord and the effect on the resting and evoked activity in the underlying neuronal pool has been examined. Doi & Jurna (91), in an outstanding series of experiments in the rat, observed that doses of intrathecal morphine that produce analgesia (69) result in a dose-dependent, naloxone-reversible suppression of activity in ascending axons evoked by A-δ and C, but not A-β, afferent stimulation. In other work, fentanyl (92), alftenanil (93), and morphine (94, 95) have been shown to produce a dose-dependent suppression of both resting activity and the activity evoked by the application of noxious thermal stimuli to the receptive field in anesthestized cats. These effects are also reversed by relatively low doses of intravenous naloxone. Importantly, the time course of the onset of the inhibition is shortest for fentanyl, longest for morphine. These time courses correspond closely with the time course reported for the onset of the block of the skin twitch response for these three agents in the cat (96) and the rat (69). Also of importance is that this ordering of the onset of activity corresponds closely with the lipid partition coefficient of these agents, which is known to correlate with the rate at which the material diffuses into the tissue (97). This close correspondence between time of onset of action in both single unit and behavioral studies, with lipid partition coefficients and the rate of drug diffusion, therefore is consistent with, but does not necessarily prove, that the effects on behavior are mediated by this particular population of wide dynamic-range neurons. As noted above, the possibility of a supraspinal movement of the drug cannot be discounted. The small amount of drug that does redistribute may account in part for the potent effects of spinally administered opiates. This is consistent with earlier speculations that there is a synergistic interaction between spinal and supraspinal opiate receptor–linked systems (98, 99). Nevertheless, the somatotopy of the antinociceptive effects of spinal opiates (51, 52, 69) in several species indicates that, at least acutely, the physiological effects of spinally administered opiates are mediated by an action on spinal receptors.

The Pharmacology of the Antinociceptive Effects of Spinal Opiates

As indicated in the preceding section, intrathecally or epidurally administered opiates will produce a significant attenuation in both experimental and clinical measures of assessing somatic or visceral pain in all species thus far examined, from mouse to man. What are the characteristics of the spinal receptor(s) through which these effects are mediated? An extensive literature based on in vivo and in vitro bioassays subsequently supported by ligand binding studies indicates the likelihood of discriminable populations of opioid receptors. Based on different structure-activity relationships viz different physiological measures, different affinities of the antagonists for the receptor acted upon by the several agents in a given preparation, and differential cross tolerance, five distinguishable pharmacological profiles have been identified and named as μ, κ, σ (100), δ (101), and ε (102) receptors. A comparable analysis carried out with intrathecally administered drugs permits one to assess the characteristics of the spinal receptor systems that mediate the unconditioned response of the intact and unanesthetized animal to otherwise noxious stimuli. Such an approach has several inherent advantages: (a) it permits the use of agents that do not cross the blood-brain barrier or are otherwise inactivated by a peripheral route (metabolism or protein binding); (b) spinal application allows assessment of the characteristics of the *spinal* receptors in the intact animal, and as such permits one to determine whether those spinal receptors can alter a supraspinally mediated escape response, i.e. alter the rostrad transmission of nociceptive information.

THE STRUCTURE-ACTIVITY RELATIONSHIP OF INTRATHECALLY ADMINIS-TERED OPIOIDS   Table 2 presents the structure-activity relationship for a series of opioid alkaloids and peptides given intrathecally in mice (tail flick, writhing), rat (hot plate, tail flick, writhing), and primate (shock titration). Where possible, the table is based on work from a single laboratory to permit examination of a variety of agents in comparable preparations. Where the full range of the dose response curves has been examined, it has been possible to produce a monotonic dose-dependent inhibition of the several endpoints, with maximum suppression achieved at doses that have no discriminable effect on the ability of the animal to make the response.

We want to emphasize several points made by the data presented in Tables 2 and 3.

1. In the rat, in spinal and/or supraspinally mediated responses to cutaneous thermal stimuli and in the primate in the shock titration test, μ and δ ligands produce a monotonic dose-dependent increase in the response latency or level of shock tolerated by the animal. Examination of the rank order of potency, in the rat in the two thermal response measures and between rat and primate, of opioids reported to have some degree of μ or δ selectivity indicates remarkable parallels between tests and between species. d-Stereoisomers of active agents are between 100–1,000 times less active than the l-isomer.

Examination of the rank order of potency in the rat and primate on thermal nociceptive measures and the shock titration indicates that among the more efficacious agents are those generally thought to possess significant mixed μ and δ affinity (e.g. β-endorphin, metkephamid). The spinal potency of β-endorphin has been noted by others (71). This observation is consistent with the finding that coactivation by intrathecal injection of μ and δ receptors results in an evident synergy (128). Whether this reflects the possibility that μ and δ receptors are allosterically coupled (129) is not known. In the mouse, intrathe-

Table 2 Potencies relative to morphine of intrathecally administered mu, delta, kappa, and sigma agonists in the mouse and primate

Ligand/putative receptor selectivity	Mouse		Rat[c]			Primate[d]
	Tail flick[a]	Writhing[b]	Tail flick	Hot plate	Writhing	Shock titration
Mu						
Morphine	1.0	1.0	1.0	1.0	1.0	1.0
Sufentanyl	—[e]	—	15.0	27.7	—	—
Levorphanol	—	—	8.1	10.2	7.8	—
Fentanyl	—	—	2.0	1.7	—	—
Alfentanil	—	—	0.9	0.76	—	—
D/L-methadone	—	—	0.1	0.6	—	1.0
Meperidine	—	—	0.07	0.05	—	0.2
Codeine	—	—	<0.01	<0.01	—	—
Delta						
DADL	150	2.5	1.5	1.0	<0.1	—
DPE$_2$	—	8.7	1.3	1.0	<0.06	—
Met-enkephalin	0.07	—	0.03	0.02	<0.01	—
Leu-enkephalin	0.03	—	<0.01	<0.01	<0.01	—
DSTLE	—	—	—	—	<0.1	—
Mu/delta						
D-ala^2-MEA	17	—	42.0	33.0	0.04	2.3
Beta-endorphin	—	—	33.0	25.0	2.6	27.0
Metkephamid	—	—	21.0	21.0	1.4	35.0
Etorphine	—	—	18.1	22.3	—	—
D-ala^2-met-enkephalin	—	—	0.7	0.9	—	—

Kappa				
U-50488H	32	<0.01	<0.01	0.03
Bremazocine	—	<0.01	0.05	0.09
EKC	1.1	<0.01	0.03	0.18
Dynorphin$_{1-10}$	38	<0.1	<0.1	1.1
Sigma				
SKF10047	—	<0.01	<0.01	<0.01
Partial agonists				
Nalbuphine	—	<0.01	<0.01	0.03
Buprenorphine	—	0.2	—	0.2
Nallorphine	—	<0.01	<0.01	—
Pentazocine	—	<0.01	<0.01	0.1
D-isomer				
D-methadone	—	<0.01	<0.01	<0.01
Dextrorphan	—	<0.01	<0.01	—

[a] Taken from (103): morphine, DADL, met/leu-enkephalin, D-ala^2-MEA, EKC; taken from (66): dynorphin, U-50488H.
[b] Taken from (73)
[c] Taken from (65, 69, 104-111); T. L. Yaksh, unpublished observations
[d] Taken from (52, 70); T. L. Yaksh, unpublished observations
[e] (—) not tested

Table 3 Range of doses of epidurally administered opioids required to produce clinically acceptable analgesia in postoperative or terminal cancer patients

Drug	Clinical situation	Dose range (mg)	Reference
Morphine	Upper abdominal; thoracic	4–10	76, 78[b], 80, 112[b]
	C-section; gynecologic	4–8	75[b], 113, 114, 115[b]
	lower abdominal; orthopedic	2–4	116, 117[b]
	terminal cancer[a]		83, 84, 85, 87
Methadone	Upper abdominal; thoracic	9	80
Diamorphine	Lumbar laminectomy; major abdominal vascular surgery	5	118, 119
β-Endorphin	Terminal cancer pain	3	120
Meperidine	Upper abdominal; thoracic	50–60	79, 121
Alfentanil	Orthopedic; abdominal	0.015–0.3	122
Pentazocine	Gynecologic; abdominal	10–15	123, 124
Fentanyl	Upper abdominal; thoracic	0.06	125
Bupenorphine	Major abdominal; orthopedic	0.06–0.3	126

[a] Doses required are variable, depending upon state of tolerance. Doses as high as 175 mg have been reported (127).
[b] Dose response curves were generated.

cal μ and δ ligands block the tail-flick response. Hylden & Wilcox (130) have shown that the hindlimb scratching response evoked by intrathecal substance P (sP) is suppressed in a dose-dependent fashion by intrathecally administered μ and δ ligands.

2. Putative κ agonists (ethylketocyclazocine, bremazocine, and U-50488H), partial agonists (buprenorphine), and partial agonists/antagonists (nalbuphine) show limited activity in the cutaneous thermal tests when given spinally or systemically. Ethylketocyclazocine, which is weakly active on the hot plate and tail flick [(73, 105, 110), but see (131)], is known to possess μ receptor activity as defined by in vitro binding and bioassay analysis, indicating that some of its activity during these tests may be discriminable from its κ agonist activity [see (1, 2)]. Agents having reportedly high levels of κ specificity, such as U-50488H, show little if any effect on hot plate and tail flick in the rat when given intrathecally (65), although significant antireflexive activity has been reported after systemic and intrathecal administration in the mouse (66).

Recently, dynorphin-like peptides, endogenous peptides with putative κ receptor affinity, have been shown to be equal to (62, 63, 73, 77, 132) or considerably less potent than morphine (C. Stevens, G. Harty, T. L. Yaksh, unpublished observations) (Table 2) in blocking thermally evoked reflexes. Comparable results with dynorphin$_{1-13}$ have been reported after spinal administration in the mouse on the thermally evoked tail flick (see Table 2) (66).

3. In the rat, intrathecally administered μ and κ ligands, or agents classified as partial agonists and mixed agonist-antagonist, produce a monotonic dose-dependent reduction in the writing response with no signs of an efficacy plateau. In the work summarized in Table 2, μ agonists displayed comparable activity on the visceral chemical and the two thermal response measures (see morphine ED_{50} values in Table 1). We want to stress that the quantitative similarity of the ED_{50} values on the writhing and thermal tests is a fortuitous function of the endpoint chosen in either class of test. In contrast, agents designated on the basis of in vitro bioassay and binding studies as being δ ligands (e.g. D-ala^2-D-leu^5-enkephalin, D-ser^2-thr^6-leu-enkephalin, leu-enkephalin-CH$_2$-leu-enkephalin) and that when given intrathecally in the rat display a rank order potency equal to or greater than morphine on the cutaneous thermal tests show little or no efficacy in the visceral chemical writhing measure at doses that (a) block the hot plate and tail flick responses or (b) do not produce evidence of motor dysfunction.

K ligands (U-50488H, dynorphin$_{1-13}$), which are minimally active on cutaneous thermal measures when given intrathecally in the rat, show an increase in activity on the writhing test. Consistent with the diminished efficacy of δ ligands in the rat writhing test, agents with significant μ and δ affinity, such as metkephamid and β-endorphin, display a marked reduction in their apparent potency in the writhing compared to the relatively selective μ agonist morphine, which shows little or no change in apparent efficacy. Przewlocki et al (73) reported that DADL produces a dose-dependent decrease in the writhing score but relative to morphine is less active than on the tail flick. With regard to dynorphin, these investigators observed blockade of the tail flick at doses above those that suppressed the writhing and in a range at which motor impairment could play a role (see below).

4. The low efficacy of met- and leu-enkephalin, putative δ receptor ligands, on the cutaneous thermal tests could be due to their lack of activity at the relevant receptor and/or to metabolism (133–136). Based on the half life of these peptides in brain tissue (134) and evidence suggesting that the magnitude of antinociceptive activity and metabolic stability do not appear to covary (135), it has been argued that the lack of activity is not related to their rapid turnover. Nevertheless, protecting an appropriate enkephalin from hydrolysis by the inhibition of enkephalinase A, by co-spinal administration of thiorphan, or by aminopeptidase inhibitors such as amastatin or bestatin (135) results in significant increases in the antinociceptive activity of intrathecally administered D-ala^2-met-enkephalin, met-, and leu-enkephalin (137, 138). When both terminals of the enkephalin molecule are protected either by the D-amino acid substitution and amidization (D-ala^2-D-met^5-enkephalin amide) or by D-alanine substitution along with enkephalinase A inhibition, the apparent potency after intrathecal injection or cutaneous thermal measures in the rat is in

excess of that observed with morphine (137). Significantly, neither met- nor leu-enkephalin in the presence of peptidase inhibitors in doses that block the tail flick had any detectable effect on the visceral chemical writhing responses (138). These observations are consistent with the previous findings that δ ligands have little effect on the visceral chemical response in the absence of motor deficit.

Recent studies have demonstrated that intrathecal opiates in the frog suppress the scratching response to acid applied to the skin. The phenomenon is characterized by a monotonic dose dependency, the rank ordering of potency being levorphanol > dynorphin > β-endorphin > morphine > met-enkephalin > naloxone = 0. The observed effects are antagonized by naloxone (139, 140). These results suggest the biological relevance of μ, δ and κ opioid binding sites previously described in amphibian brain (141).

NALOXONE ANTAGONISM   The effects of intrathecally administered opiates that result in a significant elevation in the nociceptive thresholds with no detectable effect on motor function have uniformly been reversed by naloxone. Systematic studies on the ability of naloxone to reverse opioid effects have demonstrated (a) that the antagonism produced by either systemic or intrathecal administration of naloxone is dose-dependent, with the magnitude of the antagonism proportional to the log of the dose (69), (b) that the order of sensitivity to naloxone antagonism on the tail flick and hot plate is by ranking: morphine ≃ β-endorphin ≃ D-ala^2-met-enkephalin amide ≃ alfentanil ≃ sufentanil ≃ ethylketocyclazocine > DADL (69, 96, 105, 106, 107, 142). This calculation of the apparent pA$_2$ [see (143)] has provided values of around seven for the former and six for the latter group of intrathecally administered agents [see (2)]. These results indicate that on these behavioral endpoints the agents in the spinal cord may be grouped according to two classes of sites distinguishable on the basis of the efficacy of naloxone. Han and colleagues (132), examining the antagonistic potency of naloxone on a thermal tail withdrawal response, observed that the rank order of sensitivity to naloxone is: [N-Me-Phe^3, D-Pro^4]morphiceptin, dihydroetorphine, morphine, D-ala^2-leu-enkephalin, D-ala^2-D-leu^5-enkephalin, ethylketocyclazocine, dynorphin B, dynorphin A.

Results comparable to those in the rat have been observed in the primate on the shock titration task (70). Thus, the pA$_2$ for morphine and β-endorphin is around 6.7–6.8, while that for DADL and metkephamid is around 6.0–6.3. The congruency of this line of investigation in two species on two different classes of measures provides a validating consistency for this complex analysis.

In the visceral chemical test, the naloxone pA$_2$ measured in the presence of spinal morphine is comparable to that obtained in the cutaneous thermal measures, indicating that in the rat spinal cord the receptor intrathecal morphine acts on to block the cutaneous thermal and visceral chemical cannot be distinguished. K ligands show lower sensitivity to naloxone antagonism (e.g. pA_2 values on the order of six) (65). Intrathecal ethylketocyclazocine thus displays complex characteristics such that, on cutaneous thermal tests, it behaves as if it is acting on a receptor acted on by morphine in the guinea pig ileum, for which naloxone has a relatively high affinity, while in the writhing model, at lower doses, the drug exerts its effects by a receptor in the ileum for which naloxone has a lower affinity [see (1, 2)].

TOLERANCE AND CROSS TOLERANCE   Rats rendered tolerant to morphine by intrathecal or systemic injections show cross tolerance between the two routes, suggesting that at analgesic doses intrathecal morphine exerts its effects on receptors acted on by systemic opiates (144). Withdrawal phenomena secondary to systemic morphine can be induced by intrathecal opiate antagonists (144, 145). Intrathecal D-chlornaltrexamine, an irreversible opiate antagonist, antagonizes the effects of systemic morphine and attenuates the development of dependence, as evidenced by signs of precipitated withdrawal (145).

With regard to cross tolerance between intrathecally administered opioid ligands, rats and primates rendered tolerant to intrathecal morphine show a relative loss of activity such that morphine $\geq$ β-endorphin $>>$ metkephamid $\geq$ DADL $= 0$ (69, 70, 104, 146). In animals desensitized by intrathecal injections of morphine or ethylketocyclazocine given at short intervals, dynorphin B shows a significant loss of activity in animals receiving the former but not the latter alkaloid (132). Thus, agents that have a relative selectivity for the δ or κ receptor show little loss of effect in animals rendered tolerant to morphine, whereas animals desensitized to intrathecal ethylketocyclazocine show a significant reduction of the effect of dynorphin.

Several inconsistencies preclude any simple interpretation of cross tolerance experiments, however. First, β-endorphin is thought to have mixed μ/δ receptor activity, yet a loss of activity in morphine-tolerant rats and primates has been reported (104, 146). In contrast, metkephamid is relatively resistant to the loss of activity in morphine-tolerant animals (70), yet, according to the loss of intrathecal activity in the writhing test (Table 2), a significant proportion of its activity may originate from a synergistic interaction with μ and δ receptors. Second, animals rendered tolerant to intrathecal D-ala^2-D-leu^5-enkephalin (147; A. Tung, T. L. Yaksh, unpublished observations) or metkephamid (70) show a significant loss of response to intrathecal morphine. Cross-tolerance studies can provide information on whether two agents interact at comparable sites, but such studies are subject to variables such as the dose, the time of exposure to the tolerance-producing agents, and the selectivity of the respective agonists. Moreover, it is not clear, for example, that the tolerance observed after acute or chronic administration reflects the same phenomenon. High doses may give rise to actions not specific to the receptor under investigation. The asymmetric cross-tolerance data, for example, may reflect this difficulty. The considerations of Rothman & Westfall (129, 148) regarding the allosteric coupling of the μ and δ receptors may also play a role in this observed asymmetry between μ and δ agonists.

The Pharmacology of Spinal Opioid Receptors in Man

Although adequate data do not exist to fully define the characteristics of the spinal receptors that modulate pain transmission in man, there is ample data to support distinct receptor interaction. First, patients tolerant to systemic morphine show cross-tolerance to spinally administered morphine (85). Second, although systematic studies have not been carried out, these effects of spinally administered opiates are antagonized by naloxone (149–151). Third, spinally administered agents produce analgesia with a structure-activity profile (see Tables 2 and 3) that can be roughly assessed. Although no systematic comparison is possible because of varying paradigms, the approximate rank order of potency seen in man resembles that observed after spinal injection in rat and primate animal models, i.e. on a molar basis: β-endorphin > fentanyl > morphine > pentazocine > meperidine (see Tables 2 and 3). Importantly, D-ala^2-D-leu^5-enkephalin given intrathecally in terminal cancer patients produces a powerful analgesia (152, 153). The reported activity of buprenorphine and pentazocine appears also to implicate a receptor-type interaction that resembles that displayed by the visceral chemical tests. Significantly, κ binding sites have been reported to predominate in human spinal cord (154), and some investigators have argued that κ binding sites predominate in other species as well [see (155)].

In summary, in the spinal cord, the different structure-activity profiles on different tests, the similarity of the profiles across species, the distinguishable pA$_2$ values, and the different degrees of cross-tolerance argue strongly for distinguishable populations of spinal opioid receptors that modulate spinal nociceptive processing. The particular pharmacological profiles observed in these models appear characteristic of the profiles observed in in vitro bioassay and binding studies designated μ, δ, and κ. Moreover, these observations suggest the likelihood that several classes of opioid receptors may be functionally associated with discrete sensory processing systems. Importantly, although limited data currently exist, the characteristics of the structure-activity relationship in man seem to resemble closely those obtained in rats and primates, suggesting parallels between these systems.

SPINAL OPIATES AND MOTOR FUNCTION

Early studies demonstrated that opiates in spinal-transected dogs did not influence monosynaptic stretch reflexes but suppressed crossed extensor reflexes and flexion reflexes [see (156)]. Such findings have been corroborated in part by electrophysiological studies, which indicate that opiates suppress polysynaptic and to a lesser degree monosynaptic flexion reflexes (157–160) and the firing of α-motoneurons evoked by muscle stretch (159). Importantly, this inhibition, particularly on the monosynaptic reflexes, is most manifest on those reflexes evoked by high- but not low-frequency stimulation (158, 159). In rats, morphine has been reported to enhance firing of populations of extensors (161, 162). In paraplegic man, morphine in a naloxone-reversible fashion blocks the polysynaptic reflex evoked by sural nerve stimulation of the tibially anterior muscle but has little effect on the monosynaptic "H"-reflex (163).

The mechanisms of these effects are not clear. As discussed above, opiates can exert demonstrated presynaptic effects, although apparently not on large afferents. Opiates have been shown to have a direct effect on glutamate-evoked excitation of motoneurons (15, 16, 164). Both recurrent (mediated by Renshaw cells and activated by motoneuron collaterals) and to a lesser extent direct (mediated by interneurons activated by large primary afferents) inhibition is suppressed by opiates (165, 166). The complexity of opiate effects on motor function is illustrated by the clear excitatory effect opiates have on Renshaw cell activity. This phenomenon is stereospecific and antagonized by naloxone (167, 168). Comparable results have been observed with iontophoretically applied enkephalins (17).

In unanesthetized animals and man, spinal opiates at analgesic doses do not show any measurable effect on behaviorally assessed monosynaptic reflexes [see (61)]. In primates, systematic studies have shown that intrathecal morphine at analgesic doses has no effect on muscle strength (52). At high doses (> 100 nmol) intrathecally administered morphine in rats has been shown to produce two syndromes: (a) conclusive seizures of the hindquarters coupled with hyperreflexia secondary to cutaneous stimuli, and (b) intense motor rigidity. Neither phenomenon is antagonized by naloxone (68). The mechanism of these effects is not clear but may result from the ability of morphine to block the action of glycine (166). Intrathecal strychnine or bicuculline produces a comparable syndrome (T. L. Yaksh, unpublished observations). The rigidity may reflect the paradoxical effect in which morphine in rat has been shown to excite extensor motor neurons (161). Intrathecal δ-ligands, such as D-ala^2-D-leu^5-enkephalin at high doses (> 40 nmol), result in a loss of hindlimb placing and stepping reflexes, with the limb showing some degree of motor tone but no voluntary movement. This phenomenon is not antagonized by naloxone (109). In doses greater than 3–5 nmol, intrathecal dynorphin (dyn $_{1–13}$) has been observed to produce a comparable syndrome also not antagonized by high doses of naloxone (62, 169; C. Stevens, G. Harty, T. L. Yaksh, unpublished observations). Motor dysfunctions observed with high doses in animal models after intrathecal injection have not been reported in man after either intrathecal μ or δ agonists.

Several points should be stressed. First, detectable motor dysfunctions for μ agonists occur at doses generally at or above those classified as analgesic in all response measures. δ ligands block the cutaneous thermal responses and K ligands (dynorphin) readily block the visceral chemical at doses less than those that produce signs of motor dysfunction. If the dose of spinal drug required to block a response such as a tail withdrawal approaches that where evidence of motor impairment is observed, the likelihood of a nonspecific effect on spinal function must be considered before a selective inhibition of the pain response can be ascribed. Thus, intrathecal DADL has been reported not to block the writhing response and intrathecal dynorphin does not appear to totally block the tail flick in rats at doses that do not produce evidence of motor dysfunction (65, 169). After spinal injections, care must therefore be taken to carefully separate a motor dysfunction from a sensory inhibition. In the case of work utilizing only a tail response, this appears difficult at best. Second, several motor phenomena appear to have a pharmacology different from that associated with analgesia. The failure of naloxone to antagonize is the principle example of this hypothesis. Third, because after intrathecal injection these phenomena are often observed at higher doses, the possibility of supraspinal redistribution represents a very real concern. Thus, the syndrome observed after high intrathecal doses of morphine in which the rat shows extreme truncal rigidity (the banana rat syndrome) can be readily induced by injections into supraspinal structures.

At subtoxic doses, the reported effects of opiates on spinal motor function and the presence of opioid binding in the ventral horn suggest that the failure to see any detectable effect on motor function may simply reflect the role of spinal opioid systems not normally active or too subtle for the gross analysis to which they have been thus far subjected [see, for example, (170a)]. Struppler and colleagues (149) have noted that epidural morphine and fentanyl at analgesic doses diminish in a naloxone-reversible manner flexor-reflex spasm observed in a patient suffering from multiple sclerosis. This occurs in the absence of any change in oligosynaptic or voluntary motor functions or changes in the perception of touch or vibration.

Spinal Opiates and Cardiovascular Function

Spinal morphine given in the unanesthetized rat, cat (170), dog (172) and man (171) has no effect on resting heart rate or blood pressure. In dogs either anesthetized with halothane or unanesthetized, intrathecal morphine and DADL have no effect on cardiac output or peripheral resistance (172; R. Noueihed, T. L. Yaksh, unpublished observations). In man, spinal opiates have no effect on skin temperature and sudomotor activity and, unlike spinal anesthetic, do not diminish the magnitude of the Valsalva maneuver (171). In rats, spinal morphine has been shown to produce an elevation in body temperature associated with peripheral vasoconstriction (173). This, however, has been interpreted as the activation of coordinated thermoregulatory responses perhaps secondary to a reduction in warm receptor input.

During high-intensity stimuli of a visceral or somatic nature in anesthetized man and animals, there is a significant increase in autonomic outflow measured by markers of pituitary (e.g. prolactin, ADH, ACTH, ß-endorphin), adrenomedullary, and sympathetic (catecholamines, methionine enkephalin) activity. Similarly, physiologial measures such as heart rate, blood pressure, and cardiac output are elevated. In anesthetized preparations, spinal morphine [in man (174–178); in dogs (R. Noueihed, T. L. Yaksh, unpublished observations)] or intrathecal DADL [in dogs (R. Noueihed, T. L. Yaksh, unpublished observations)] produces a significant, but variable, reduction in the release evoked by high-intensity stimulation (intraoperative in man or stimulation of the sciatic nerve in dogs).

SPINAL OPIATES AND THEIR EFFECTS ON GASTROINTESTINAL FUNCTION

Systemic opiates are known to alter gastrointestinal (GI) motility. Intrathecally administered morphine in mice produces a dose-dependent slowing of the transit of a radioactive stomach load (179). δ receptor ligands (D-ala^2-D-leu^5-enkephalin, D-ser^2-leu-enkephalin-thr^6, and D-leu^2-L-cys^2-enkephalin) are also active. The suppressive effects of both intrathecal μ and δ agents remain in the presence of spinal transaction (179, 180). K ligands (ethylketocyclazocine, dynorphin$_{1-7}$, or dynorphin$_{1-13}$) are uniformly inactive (181). Intrathecal morphine does not suppress the migrating motor complex in unanesthetized dogs (G. Telford, M. Hashmonai, J. Szurzewski, T. L. Yaksh, unpublished observations), but does induce propagated bursts of motor activity in the small bowel during the fed state and suppress the fed pattern otherwise observed after a meal (J. Malagalada, M. Camilliera, T. L. Yaksh, unpublished observations). In man, no systematic studies have been carried out with spinal opiates on gastric motility, but ileus, a not-uncommon finding with local anesthetics, and constipation have not been reported.

SPINAL OPIATES AND BLADDER FUNCTION

Spinally administered morphine produces a naloxone-reversible inhibition of the volume-evoked micturition reflex in unanesthetized man (182) and animals (183, 184). Cystometrograms in man show an increase in bladder capacity with unchanged urethral pressures (185). Sphincter EMGs indicate that external sphincter tone is slightly increased (186). Intrathecal morphine in unanesthetized dogs increases the threshold pressure required to evoke the micturition reflex (187). Dose-response curves carried out in unanesthetized rats with chronic indwelling bladder catheters reveal a clear structure-activity relationship: ß-endorphin ≥ DADL ≥ morphine > ethylketocyclazocine >> SKF10047. The effects of intrathecal agents on bladder function in man and animals are antagonized by naloxone. Animals rendered tolerant to the micturition-suppressing effects of intrathecal morphine show no change in the ED_{50} of intrathecal DADL (183). Comparable results have been observed in the anesthetized rat (187a), the unanesthetized cat, and the primate (T. L. Yaksh, unpublished observations). Intrathecal met-enkephalin, leu-enkephalin, and D-ala^2-met-enkephalin amide given in anesthetized cats reduce spontaneous bladder contractions (184). Although the mechanisms of this effect of opiates on bladder function are not clear, the observations suggest a vesico-sphincter dysynergia and are consistent with the inhibition of firing in vesico-postganglionic nerves (184). These findings represent a significant advance in understanding the central pharmacology of vesicle function. Although inhibition of micturition by spinal opiates is considered an undesirable side effect in their therapeutic use in pain management, it is likely that such observations may presage advances in the management of bladder disorders. Thus, the depressant effect of spinal morphine on spontaneous bladder tone has been used successfully to manage bladder spasm (188), while naloxone has been observed to augment the micturition reflex in spinal-transected animals (189).

SUMMARY

The use of the spinal-catheterized, unanesthetized animal in conjunction with systematic studies on the pharmacology of spinal drug action has provided a powerful tool by which complex functions mediated by spinal systems can be studied. The majority of work to date has focused on the spinal opioid–sensitive substrate that processes high-intensity stimulation. We want to emphasize two points, however. First, these methodological approaches have provided significant insights into the fact that non-opioid spinal receptor systems also play a role in pain modulation. Second, not only do the spinal systems modulate pain processing, they also play a precise role in the mediation of a variety of somatomotor and autonomic functions that are also amenable to investigation and manipulation using this methodology in the unanesthetized animal. The very complexity of the anatomy and biochemistry of the spinal gray emphasizes that the spinal cord substrates are not simply hard-wired systems and that spinal processing may be subject to very subtle alterations by the application of receptor-selective agents. Such insights clearly suggest the likelihood that such insights into spinal functioning possess significant clinical applicability. As indicated, such studies on basic spinal mechanisms have already led to certain fundamental advances in the clinical management of pain. The likelihood of comparable advances having clinical relevance in other aspects of spinal autonomic and motor dysfunction make this an exciting area of investigation.

In summary, examination of the pharmacology of the effects produced by intrathecally administered opioids in the unanesthetized and intact animal has revealed the relevance of diverse spinal opioid–receptor systems. The combination of this in vivo methodology with single-unit recording and ligand-binding techniques has begun to provide insights into the subtle actions of exogenous opioids on spinal sensory, autonomic, and somatomotor function. This information clearly yields insight into the natural role played by the endogenous opioid systems and potential advances in the management of clinical problems dependent on spinal processing.

ACKNOWLEDGEMENTS

We thank those investigators who shared recent data, apologize to those we failed to cite, and give our appreciation to Ms. Ann Rockafellow, who prepared the manuscript. This manuscript was written during support by DA02110, NS16541, NS19650 (TLY), and TW03188 (RN).

Literature Cited

1. Martin, W. R. 1983. Pharmacology of opioids. *Pharmacol. Rev.* 35:283–323
2. Yaksh, T. L. 1984. Multiple opiate receptor systems in brain and spinal cord. Part I. *Eur. J. Anaesthesiol.* 1:171–99
2a. Yaksh, T. L. 1984. Multiple opiate receptor systems in brain and spinal cord. Part II. *Eur. J. Anaesthesiol.* 1:201–25
3. Bell, J. A., Martin, W. R. 1977. The effect of narcotic antagonists naloxone, naltrexone and nalorphine on spinal cord C-fiber reflexes evoked by electrical stimulation or radiant heat. *Eur. J. Pharmacol.* 42:147–54
4. Le Bars, D., Menetrey, D., Conseiller, C., Besson, J. M. 1975. Depressive effects of morphine upon lamina V cell activities in the dorsal horn of the spinal cat. *Brain Res.* 93:261–77
5. Yaksh, T. L. 1978. Inhibition by etorphine of the discharge of dorsal horn neurons: Effects upon the neuronal response to both high- and low-threshold sensory input in the decerebrate spinal cat. *Exp. Neurol.* 60:23–40
6. Jurna, I., Heinz, G. 1979. Differential effects of morphine and opioid analgesics on A and C fiber-evoked activity in ascending axons of the rat spinal cord. *Brain Res.* 171:573–76
7. Woolf, C. J., Fitzgerald, M. 1981. Lamina-specific alteration of C-fibre evoked activity by morphine in the dorsal horn of

the rat spinal cord. *Neurosci. Lett.* 25:37–41
8. Einspahr, F. J., Piercey, M. F. 1980. Morphine depresses dorsal horn neuron responses to controlled noxious and non-noxious cutaneous stimulation. *J. Pharmacol. Exp. Ther.* 213:456–61
9. Toyyoka, H., Kitahata, L. M., Dohi, S., Ohtani, M., Hanaoka, K., et al. 1978. Effect of morphine on the Rexed lamina VII spinal neuronal response to graded radiant heat stimulation. *Exp. Neurol.* 62:146–58
10. Jurna, I., Grossmann, W. 1976. The effect of the activity evoked in ventrolateral tract axons of the cat spinal cord. *Exp. Brain Res.* 24:473–84
11. Iwata, N., Sakai, Y. 1971. Effects of fentanyl upon the spinal interneurons activated by Ad afferent fibers of the cutaneous nerve of the cat. *Jpn. J. Pharmacol.* 21:413–26
12. Piercey, M. F., Lahti, R. A., Schroeder, L. A., Einspahr, F. J., Barsahn, C. 1982. U-50488H, a pure kappa receptor agonist with spinal analgesic loci in the mouse. *Life Sci.* 31:1197–200
13. Yaksh, T. L. 1978. Opiate receptors for behavioral analgesia resemble those related to the depression of spinal nociceptive neurons. *Science* 199:1231–33
14. Calvillo, O., Henry, J. L., Neuman, R. S. 1979. Actions of narcotic analgesics

and antagonists on spinal units responding to natural stimulation in the cat. *Can. J. Physiol. Pharmacol.* 51:652–63

15. Zieglgansberger, W., Bayerl, H. 1976. The mechanisms of inhibition of neuronal activity by opiates in the spinal cord of the cat. *Brain Res.* 115:111–28

16. Zieglgansberger, W., Tulloch, I. F. 1979. The effects of methionine and leucine enkephalin on spinal neurones of the cat. *Brain Res.* 167:53–64

17. Davies, J., Dray, A. 1978. Pharmacological and electrophysiological studies of morphine and enkephalin on rat supraspinal neurones and cat spinal neurones. *Br. J. Pharmacol.* 63:87–96

18. Randic, M., Miletic, V. 1978. Depressant actions of methionine-enkephalin and somatostatin in cat dorsal horn neurones activated by noxious stimuli. *Brain Res.* 152:196–202

19. Satoh, M., Kawajiri, S.-I., Ukai, Y., Yamamoto, M. 1979. Selective and nonselective inhibition by enkephalins and noradrenaline of nociceptive responses of lamina V type neurons in the spinal dorsal horn of the rabbit. *Brain Res.* 177:384–87

20. Johnson, S. M., Duggan, A. W. 1981. Evidence that opiate receptors of the substantia gelatinosa contribute to the depression by intravenous morphine of the spinal transmission of impulses in unmyelinated primary afferents. *Brain Res.* 207:223–28

21. Wamsley, J. K. 1983. Opioid receptors: Autoradiography. *Pharmacol. Rev.* 35:69–83

22. LaMotte, C., Pert, C. B., Snyder, S. H. 1976. Opiate receptor binding in primate spinal cord: Distribution and changes after dorsal root section. *Brain Res.* 112:407–12

23. Fields, H. L., Emson, P. C., Leigh, B. K., Gilbert, R. F. T., Iversen, L. L. 1980. Multiple opiate receptor sites on primary afferent fibres. *Nature* 284:351–53

24. Ninkovic, M., Hunt, S. P., Gleave, J. R. W. 1982. Localization of opiate and histamine H_1-receptors in the primate sensory ganglia and spinal cord. *Brain Res.* 241:197–206

25. Hiller, J. M., Simon, E. J., Crain, S. M., Peterson, E. R. 1978. Opiate receptors in cultures of fetal mouse dorsal root ganglia (DRG) and spinal cord: Predominance in DRG neurites. *Brain Res.* 145:396–400

26. Scadding, J. W. 1980. The permanent anatomical effects of neonatal capsaicin

on somatosensory nerves. *J. Anat.* 132:473–84

27. Jessell, T. M., Iversen, L. L., Cuello, A. C. 1978. Capsaicin-induced depletion of substance P from primary sensory neurones. *Brain Res.* 152:183–88

28. Gamse, R., Holzer, P., Lembeck, F. 1979. Indirect evidence for presynaptic location of opiate receptors in chemosensitive primary sensory neurones. *Naunyn-Schmiedberg's Arch. Pharmacol.* 308:281–85

29. Yaksh, T. L., Jessell, T. M., Gamse, R., Mudge, A. W., Leeman, S. E. 1980. Intrathecal morphine inhibits substance P release from mammalian spinal cord *in vivo. Nature* 286:155–56

30. Kuraishi, Y., Hirota, N., Sugimoto, M., Satoh, M., Takagi, H. 1983. Effects of morphine on noxious stimuli-induced release of substance P from rabbit dorsal horn *in vivo. Life Sci.* 33:693–96

31. Jessell, T. M., Iversen, L. L. 1977. Opiate analgesics inhibit substance P release from rat trigeminal nucleus. *Nature* 268:549–51

32. Mudge, A. W., Leeman, S. E., Fischbach, G. D. 1979. Enkephalin inhibits release of substance P from sensory neurons in culture and decreases action potential duration. *Proc. Natl. Acad. Sci. USA* 76:526–30

33. Carstens, E., Tulloch, I., Zieglgansberger, W., Zimmerman, M. 1979. Presynaptic excitability changes induced by morphine in single cutaneous afferent C- and A-fibers. *Pflügers Arch.* 379:143–47

34. Sastry, B. R. 1980. Potentiation of presynaptic inhibition of nociceptive pathways as a mechanism for analgesia. *Can J. Physiol. Pharmacol.* 58:97–100

35. MacDonald, R. L., Nelson, P. G. 1978. Specific opiate-induced depression of transmitter release from dorsal root ganglion cells in culture. *Science* 199:1449–51

36. Werz, M. A., MacDonald, R. L. 1983. Opioid peptides with differential affinity for mu and delta receptors decrease sensory neuron calcium-dependent action potentials. *J. Pharmacol. Exp. Ther.* 227:394–402

37. Werz, M. A., MacDonald, R. L. 1984. Dynorphin reduces calcium-dependent action potential duration by decreased voltage-dependent calcium conductance. *Neurosci. Lett.* 46:185–90

38. Werz, M. A., MacDonald, R. L. 1982. Opioid peptides decrease calcium-dependent action potential duration of

mouse dorsal root ganglion neurons in cell culture. *Brain Res.* 239:315–21

39. Werz, M. A., MacDonald, R. L. 1982. Heterogeneous sensitivity of cultured dorsal root ganglion neurones to opioid peptides selective for μ- and δ-opiate receptors. *Nature* 299:730–33

40. Egan, T. M., North, R. A. 1981. Both μ and δ opiate receptors exist on the same neuron. *Science* 214:923–24

41. Duggan, A. W., North, R. A. 1984. Electrophysiology of opioids. *Pharmacol. Rev.* 35:219–81

42. Duggan, A. W., Hall, J. G., Headley, P. M. 1977. Suppression of transmission of nociceptive impulses by morphine: Selective effects of morphine administered in the region of the substantia gelatinosa. *Br. J. Pharmacol.* 61:65–76

43. Duggan, A. W., Hall, J. G., Headley, P. M. 1977. Enkephalins and dorsal horn neurones of the cat: Effects on responses to noxious and innocuous skin stimuli. *Br. J. Pharmacol.* 61:399–408

44. Duggan, A. W., Johnson, S. M., Morton, C. R. 1981. Differing distributions of receptors for morphine and Met[5]-enkephalinamide in the dorsal horn of the cat. *Brain Res.* 229:379–87

45. Sastry, B. R., Goh, J. W. 1983. Actions of morphine and met-enkephalin-amide on nociceptor driven neurones in substantia gelatinosa and deeper dorsal horn. *Neuropharmacology* 22:119–22

46. Zieglgansberger, W., Sutor, B. 1983. Responses of substantia gelatinosa neurons to putative neurotransmitters in an in vitro preparation of the adult rat spinal cord. *Brain Res.* 279:316–20

47. Yoshimura, M., North, R. A. 1983. Substantia gelatinosa neurones in vitro hyperpolarized by enkephalin. *Nature* 305:529–30

48. Murase, K., Nedeljkov, V., Randic, M. 1982. The actions of neuropeptides on dorsal horn neurons in the rat spinal cord preparation: An intracellular study. *Brain Res.* 234:170–76

49. Yaksh, T. L., Rudy, T. A. 1976. Analgesia mediated by a direct spinal action of narcotics. *Science* 192:1357–58

50. Yaksh, T. L., Rudy, T. A. 1976. Chronic catheterization of the spinal subarachnoid space. *Physiol. Behav.* 17:1031–36

51. Yaksh, T. L. 1978. Analgetic actions of intrathecal opiates in cat and primate. *Brain Res.* 153:205–10

52. Yaksh, T. L., Reddy, S. V. R. 1981. Studies in the primate on the analgetic effects associated with intrathecal actions

of opiate, α-adrenergic agonists and baclofen. *Anesthesiology* 54:451–67

53. LoPachin, R. M., Rudy, T. A., Yaksh, T. L. 1981. An improved method for chronic catheterization of the rat spinal subarachnoid space. *Physiol. Behav.* 27:559–61

54. Reddy, S. V. R., Maderdrut, J. L., Yaksh, T. L. 1980. Spinal cord pharmacology of adrenergic agonist-mediated antinociception. *J. Pharmacol. Exp. Ther.* 213:525–33

55. Dib, B. 1984. Intrathecal catheterization in the rat. *Pharmacol. Biochem. Behav.* 20:45–48

56. Bahar, M., Rosen, M., Vickers, M. D. 1984. Chronic cannulation of the intradural or extradural space in the rat. *Br. J. Anaesth.* 56:405–10

57. Satoh, M., Kubota, A., Iwama, T., Wada, T., Yasui, M., et al. 1983. Comparison of analgesic potencies of mu, delta and kappa agonists locally applied to various CNS regions relevant to analgesia in rats. *Life Sci.* 33:689–92

58. Hylden, J. L. K., Wilcox, G. L. 1980. Intrathecal morphine in mice: A new technique. *Eur. J. Pharmacol.* 67:313–16

59. Wiesenfeld, Z., Gustafsson, L. L. 1982. Continuous intrathecal administration of morphine via an osmotic minipump in the rat. *Brain Res.* 247:195–97

60. Tung, A. S., Yaksh, T. L. 1982. The antinociceptive effects of epidural opiates in the cat: Studies on the pharmacology and the effects of lipophilicity in spinal analgesia. *Pain* 12:343–56

61. Yaksh, T. L. 1981. Spinal opiate analgesia: Characteristics and principles of action. *Pain* 11:293–346

62. Herman, B., Goldstein, A. 1984. Antinociception and paralysis induced by intrathecal dynorphin A. *J. Pharmacol. Exp. Ther.* In press

63. Przewlocki, B., Shearman, G. T., Herz, A. 1983. Mixed opioid/non-opioid effects of dynorphin related peptides after intrathecal injection in the rat. *Neuropeptides* 3:233–40

64. Piercey, M. F., Varner, K., Schroeder, L. A. 1982. Analgesic activity of intraspinally administered dynorphin and ethylketocyclazocine. *Eur. J. Pharmacol.* 80:283–384

65. Schmauss, C., Yaksh, T. L. 1983. *In vivo* studies on spinal opiate receptor systems mediating antinociception. II. Pharmacological profiles suggesting a differential association of mu, delta and kappa receptors with visceral chemical

and cutaneous thermal stimuli in the rat. *J. Pharmacol. Exp. Ther.* 228:1–12

66. Piercey, M. F., Varner, K., Schroeder, L. A. 1982. Analgesic activity of intraspinally administered dynorphin and ethylketocyclazocine. *Eur. J. Pharmacol.* 80:283–384

67. Bromage, P. R., Camporesi, E., Leslie, J. 1980. Epidural narcotics in volunteers: Sensitivity to pain and carbon dioxide. *Pain* 9:145–60

68. Tang, A. H., Schoenfeld, M. J. 1978. Comparison of subcutaneous and spinal subarachnoid injections of morphine and naloxone in analgesic tests in the rat. *Eur. J. Pharmacol.* 52:215–23

69. Yaksh, T. L., Rudy, T. A. 1977. Studies on the direct spinal action of narcotics in the production of analgesia in the rat. *J. Pharmacol. Exp. Ther.* 202:411–28

70. Yaksh, T. L. 1983. *In vivo* studies on spinal opiate receptor systems mediating antinociception. I. Mu and delta receptor profiles in the primate. *J. Pharmacol. Exp. Ther.* 226:303–16

71. Kuraishi, Y., Satoh, M., Harada, Y., Akaike, A., Shibata, T., et al. 1980. Analgesic action of intrathecal and intracerebral ß-endorphin in rats: Comparison with morphine. *Eur. J. Pharmacol.* 67:143–46

72. Thompson, W. R., Smith, P. T., Hirst, M., Varkey, G. P., Knill, R. L. 1981. Regional analgesic effects of epidural morphine in volunteers. *Can. Anaesth. Soc. J.* 28:530–36

73. Przewlocki, R., Stala, L., Greczek, M., Shearman, G. T., Przewlocka, B., et al. 1983. Analgesic effects of μ-, δ- and κ-opiate agonists and, in particular, dynorphin at the spinal level. *Life Sci.* 33:649–52

74. Anderson, I., Thompson, W. R., Varkey, G. P., Knill, R. L. 1981. Lumbar epidural morphine as an effective analgesic following cholecystectomy. *Can. Anesth. Soc. J.* 28:523–29

75. Cahill, J., Murphy, D., O'Brien, D., Mulhrall, J., Fitzpatrick, G. 1983. Epidural buprenorphine for pain relief after major abdominal surgery: A controlled comparison with epidural morphine. *Anaesthesia* 38:760–64

76. Torda, T. A., Pybus, D. A. 1984. Extradural administration of morphine and bupivacaine: A controlled comparison. *Br. J. Anesth.* 56:141–46

77. Rawal, N., Sjöstrand, U., Christoffersson, E., Dahlström, B., Arvill, A., et al. 1984. Comparison of intramuscular and epidural morphine for postoperative analgesia in the grossly obese: Influence on postoperative ambulation and pulmonary function. *Anesth. Analg.* 63: 583–92

78. Nordberg, G. 1984. Pharmacokinetic aspects of spinal morphin analgesia. *Acta Anesth. Scand.* 79:7–37 (Suppl.)

79. Torda, T. A., Pybus, D. A. 1982. Comparison of four narcotic analgesics for extradural analgesia. *Br. J. Anesth.* 54: 291–95

80. Bromage, P., Camporesi, E. M., Chestnut, D. 1980. Epidural narcotics for postoperative analgesia. *Anesth. Analg.* 59: 473–80

81. Rybro, L., Schurizek, A., Petersen, T. K., Wernberger, M. 1982. Postoperative analgesia and lung function: A comparison of intramuscular with epidural morphine. *Acta Anaesth. Scand.* 26:514–18

82. Holland, R. B. 1982. Carbon dioxide response after epidural morphine. *Anaesthesia* 37:753–57

83. Coombs, D. W., Saunders, R. L., Gaylor, M. S., Block, A. R., Colton, T., et al. 1983. Relief of continuous chronic pain by intraspinal narcotic infusion via an implanted reservoir. *J. Am. Med. Assoc.* 250:2336–39

84. Coombs, D. W., Maurer, L. H., Saunder, R. L., Gaylor, M. 1984. Outcomes and complications of continuous intraspinal narcotic analgesia for cancer pain control. *Anesth. Intern. Care.* In press

85. Müller, H., Stoyanov, M., Börner, U., Hempelman, G. 1982. Epidural opiates for relief of cancer pain. In *Spinal Opiate Analgesia,* ed. T. L. Yaksh, H. Müller, 144:125–37. Berlin/Heidelberg/New York: Springer-Verlag. 147 pp.

86. Onofrio, B. M., Yaksh, T. L., Arnold, L. E. 1981. Continuous low dose intrathecal morphine administration in the treatment of chronic pain of malignant origin. *Mayo Clin. Proc.* 56:516–20

87. Zenz, M. 1984. Epidural opiates for the treatment of cancer pain. In *Recent Advances in Pain Therapy,* ed. M. Zimmerman. Berlin/Heidelberg/New York: Springer-Verlag. In press

88. Pomeroy, G., Ardell, J. F., Wurster, R. P. 1983. Role of spinal opiate receptors on the afferent component of the somatoautonomic reflexes in the exercising dog. *Soc. Neurosci.* 9:547 (Abstr.)

89. Williams, J., Zieglgansberger, W. 1981. Mature spinal ganglion cells are not sensitive to opiate receptor mediated actions. *Neurosci. Lett.* 21:211–16

90. Shefner, S. A., North, R. A., Zukin, R. S. 1981. Opiate effects on rabbit vagus nerve: Electrophysiology and radioligand binding. *Brain Res.* 221:109–16

91. Doi, T., Jurna, I. 1982. Analgesic effect of intrathecal morphine demonstrated in ascending nociceptive activity in the rat spinal cord and ineffectiveness of caerulein and cholecystokinin octapeptide. *Brain Res.* 234:399–407

92. Suzukawa, M., Matsumoto, M., Collins, J. G., Kitahata, L. M., Yuge, O. 1983. Dose-response suppression of noxiously evoked activity of WDR neurons by spinally administered fentanyl. *Anesthesiology* 58:510–13

93. Collins, J. G., Matsumoto, M., Kitahata, L. M., Yuge, O., Tanaka, A. 1983. Do pharmacokinetic parameters derived from systemic administration adequately describe spinal drug actions. *Anesthesiology* 59:A381 (Abstr.)

94. Homma, E., Collins, J. G., Kitahata, L. M., Kawahara, M. 1983. Suppression of noxiously evoked WDR dorsal horn neuronal activity by spinally administered morphine. *Anesthesiology* 58:232–36

95. Hanaoka, K., Tagami, M., Toyooka, H., Yamamura, H. 1982. Mechanism of intrathecally administered morphine analgesia. In *Anaesthesia and Intensive Care*, ed. T. L. Yaksh and H. Müller, pp. 24–29. Berlin: Springer-Verlag

96. Noueihed, R., Durant, P., Yaksh, T. L. 1984. Studies on the effects of intrathecal sufentanil, fentanyl and alfentanil in rats and cats. *Anesthesiology* 60:A218 (Suppl.)

97. Herz, A., Teschemacher, H.-J. 1971. Activities and sites of antinociceptive action of morphine-like analgesics and kinetics of distribution following intravenous, intracerebral and intraventricular application. *Adv. Drug Res.* 6:79–119

98. Yaksh, T. L., Rudy, T. A. 1978. Narcotic analgesics: CNS sites and mechanisms of action as revealed by intracerebral injection techniques. *Pain* 4:299–359

99. Yeung, J. C., Rudy, T. A. 1980. Multiplicative interaction between narcotic agonisms expressed at spinal and supraspinal sites of antinociceptive action as revealed by concurrent intrathecal and intracerebroventricular injections of morphine. *J. Pharmacol. Exp. Ther.* 215:633–42

100. Martin, W. R., Eades, C. G., Thompson, J. A., Huppler, R. E., Gilbert, P. E. 1976. The effects of morphine and nalorphine-like drugs in the nondependent and morphine-dependent chronic spinal dog. *J. Pharmacol. Exp. Ther.* 197:517–32

101. Lord, J. A. H., Waterfield, A. A., Hughes, J., Kosterlitz, H. W. 1977. Endogenous opioid peptides: Multiple agonists and receptors. *Nature* 267:495–99

102. Schulz, R., Faase, E., Wuster, M., Herz, A. 1979. Selective receptors for ß-endorphin on the rat vas deferens. *Life Sci.* 24:843–50

103. Hylden, J. L. K., Wilcox, G. L. 1982. Intrathecal opioids block a spinal action of substance P in mice: Functional importance of both µ and receptors. *Eur. J. Pharmacol.* 86:95–98

104. Yaksh, T. L., Gross, K. E., Li, C. H. 1982. Studies on the intrathecal effect of ß-endorphin in primate. *Brain Res.* 241:261–69

105. Tung, A. S., Yaksh, T. L. 1982. *In vivo* evidence for multiple opiate receptors mediating analgesia in the rat spinal cord. *Brain Res.* 247:75–83

106. Yaksh, T. L., Frederickson, R. C. A., Huang, S. P., Rudy, T. A. 1978. *In vivo* comparison of the receptor populations acted upon in the spinal cord by morphine and pentapeptides in the production of analgesia. *Brain Res.* 148:516–20

107. Yaksh, T. L., Henry, J. L. 1978. Antinociceptive effects of intrathecally administered human ß-endorphin in the rat and cat. *Can. J. Physiol. Pharmacol.* 56:754–60

108. Yaksh, T. L., Huang, S. P., Rudy, T. A., Frederickson, R. C. A. 1977. The direct and specific opiate-like effect of met^5-enkephalin and analogues on the spinal cord. *Neuroscience* 2:593–96

109. Schmauss, C., Shimohigashi, Y., Jensen, T. S., Rodbard, D., Yaksh, T. L. 1984. Studies on spinal opiate receptor pharmacology. III. Analgetic effects of enkephalin dimers as measured by cutaneous thermal and visceral chemical evoked responses. *Brain Res.* In press

110. Schmauss, C., Doherty, C., Yaksh, T. L. 1983. The analgetic effects of an intrathecally administered partial opiate agonist, nalbuphine hydrochloride. *Eur. J. Pharmacol.* 86:1–7

111. Russell, B., Yaksh, T. L. 1981. Antagonism by phenoxybenzamine and pentazocine of the antinociceptive effects of morphine in the spinal cord. *Neuropharmacology* 20:575–79

112. Pybus, D. A., Torda, T. A. 1982. Dose-effect relationships of extradural morphine. *Br. J. Anaesth.* 54:1259–62

113. Carmichael, F. J., Rolbiu, S. H., Hew, E. M. 1982. Epidural morphine for analgesia after caesarean section. *Can. Anaesth. Soc. J.* 29:359–63

114. Kotelko, D. M., Dailey, P. A., Shnider, S. M., Rosen, M. A., Hughes, S. C., et

al. 1984. Epidural morphine analgesia after caesarean delivery. *Obst. Gyn.* 63: 409–13

115. Rosen, M. A., Hughes, S. C., Shnider, S. M., Abboud, T. K., Norton, M., et al. 1983. Epidural morphine for the relief of postoperative pain after caesarean delivery. *Anesth. Analg.* 62:666–72

116. Gustafsson, L. L., Friberg-Nielsen, S., Garle, M., Mohall, A., Rane, A., et al. 1982. Extradural and parenteral morphine kinetics and effects in postoperative pain. A controlled clinical study. *Br. J. Anesth.* 54:1167–74

117. Martin, R., Salbaing, J., Blaise, G., Tetrault, J. P., Tetreault, L. 1982. Epidural morphine for postoperative pain relief: A dose response curve. *Anesthesiology* 56:423–26

118. Cowen, M. J., Bullingham, R. E. S., Paterson, G. M. C., McQuay, H. J., Turner, M., et al. 1982. A controlled comparison of the effects of extradural diamorphine and bupivacaine on plasma glucose and plasma cortisol in postoperative patients. *Anesth. Analg.* 61:15–18

119. Malins, A. F., Goodman, N. W., Cooper, G. M., Prys-Roberts, C., Baird, R. N. 1984. Ventilatory effects of pre- and postoperative diamorphine. A comparison of extradural with intramuscular administration. *Anaesthesia* 39:118–25

120. Oyama, T., Fukushi, S., Jin, T. 1982. Epidural ß-endorphin in treatment of pain. *Can. Anaesth. Soc. J.* 29:24–26

121. Rutter, D. V., Skewes, D. G., Morgan, M. 1981. Extradural opioids for postoperative analgesia. *Br. J. Anesth.* 53:915–20

122. Chauvin, M., Salbaing, J., Perrin, D., Levon, J. C., Viars, P. 1983. Comparison between intramuscular and epidural administration of alfentanil for pain relief and plasma kinetics. *Anesthesiology* 59: A197

123. Mori, T. 1982. Studies on comparison of the postoperative analgesic method between epidural morphine HC1 and pentazocine. *Acta Obstet. Gynaecol. Jpn.* 34:1819–26

124. Kalsa, P., Madan, R., Sabsena, R., Batra, R., Gode, G. 1983. Epidural pentazocine for postoperative pain relief. *Anesth. Analg.* 52:949–50

125. Welchew, E. A. 1983. The optimum concentration for epidural fentanyl. A randomized double-blind comparison with and without 1:200000 adrenalin. *Anaesthesia* 38:1037–41

126. Rondomanska, M., deCastro, J., Lecron, L. 1982. The use of epidural bu-

prenorphine for the treatment of postoperative pain. See Ref. 85, pp. 147–52

127. Coombs, D. 1983. Mechanism of epidural lidocaine reversal of tachyphylaxis to epidural morphine analgesia. *Anesthesiology* 59:486–87

128. Larson, A. A., Vaught, J. L., Takemori, A. E. 1980. The potentiation of spinal analgesia by leucine enkephalin. *Eur. J. Pharmacol.* 61:381–83

129. Vaught, J. L., Rothman, R. B., Westfall, T. C. 1982. Mu and delta receptors: Their role in analgesia and in the differential effects of opioid peptides on analgesia. *Life Sci.* 30:1443–55

130. Hylden, J. L. K., Wilcox, G. L. 1983. Pharmacological characterization of substance P-induced nociception in mice: Modulation by opioid and noradrenergic agonists at the spinal level. *J. Pharmacol. Exp. Ther.* 226:398–404

131. Wood, P. L., Rackham, A., Richard, J. 1981. Spinal analgesia: Comparison of the mu agonist morphine and the kappa agonist ethylketocyclazocine. *Life Sci.* 28:2119–25

132. Han, J.-S., Xie, G.-X., Goldstein, A. 1984. Analgesia induced by intrathecal injection of dynorphin B in the rat. *Life Sci.* 34:1573–79

133. Morley, J. S. 1980. Structure-activity relationships of enkephalin-like peptides. *Ann. Rev. Pharmacol. Toxicol.* 20:81–110

134. Craves, F. B., Law, P.-Y., Hunt, C. A., Loh, H. H. 1978. The metabolic disposition of radiolabeled enkephalins in vitro and in situ. *J. Pharmacol. Exp. Ther.* 206:492–506

135. Bajusz, S., Patthy, A., Kenessey, A., Graf, L., Szekely, J. I., Ronai, A. Z. 1978. Is there a correlation between analgesic potency and biodegradation. *Biochem. Biophys. Res. Commun.* 84: 1045–53

136. Barclay, R. K., Phillipps, M. A. 1980. Inhibition of enkephalin-degrading aminopeptidase activity by certain peptides. *Biochem. Biophys. Res. Commun.* 96: 1732–38

137. Yaksh, T. L., Harty, G. J. 1982. Effects of thiorphan on the antinociceptive effects of intrathecal D-ala²-met⁵-enkephalin. *Eur. J. Pharmacol.* 79:293–300

138. Noueihed, R., Umezawa, H., Yaksh, T. L. 1985. Potentiation of the effects of intrathecal methionine enkephalin by aminopeptidase inhibition. *Adv. Pain Res.* In press

139. Stevens, C. W., Pezalla, P. D. 1983. A

spinal site mediates opiate analgesia in frogs. *Life Sci.* 33:2097–103

140. Stevens, C. W., Pezalla, P. D. 1984. Naloxone blocks the analgesic action of levorphanol, but not of dextrorphan in the leopard frog. *Brain Res.* In press

141. Simon, E. J., Hiller, J. M., Groth, J., Itzhak, Y., Holland, M. J., et al. 1982. The nature of opiate receptors in the toad brain. *Life Sci.* 31:1367–70

142. Tseng, L.-F., Cheng, S. S., Fujimoto, J. M. 1983. Inhibition of tail-flick and shaking responses by intrathecal and intraventricular d-Ala^2-d-Leu^5-enkephalin and ß-endorphin in anesthetized rats. *J. Pharmacol. Exp. Ther.* 224:51–54

143. Tallarida, R. J., Cowan, A., Adler, M. W. 1979. pA$_2$ and receptor differentiation: A statistical analysis of competitive antagonism. *Life Sci.* 25:637–54

144. Yaksh, T. L., Kohl, R. L., Rudy, T. A. 1977. Induction of tolerance and withdrawal in rats receiving morphine in the spinal subarachnoid space. *Eur. J. Pharmacol.* 42:275–84

145. Delander, G. E., Takemori, A. E. 1983. Spinal antagonism of tolerance and dependence induced by systemically administered morphine. *Eur. J. Pharmacol.* 94:35–42

146. Yaksh, T. L., Howe, J. R., Harty, G. J. 1984. Pharmacology of spinal pain modulatory systems. In *Advances in Pain Research and Therapy,* ed. C. Benedetti, 7:57–70. New York: Raven

147. Tseng, L.-F. 1982. Tolerance and cross tolerance to morphine after chronic spinal D-Ala^2-D-Leu^5-enkephalin infusion. *Life Sci.* 31:987–92

148. Rothman, R. B., Westfall, T. C. 1982. Allosteric coupling between morphine and enkephalin receptors in vitro. *Mol. Pharmacol.* 21:548–57

149. Struppler, A., Burgmayer, B., Ochs, G. B., Pfeiffer, H. G. 1983. The effect of epidural application of opioids on spasticity of spinal origin. *Life Sci.* 33:607–10

150. Brookshire, G. L., Shnider, S. M., Abboud, T. K., Kotelko, D. M., Noueihed, R., et al. 1983. Effects of naloxone on the mother and neonate after intrathecal morphine for labor analgesia. *Anesthesiology* 59:A417

151. Abboud, T. K., Shnider, S. M., Dailey, P. A., Raya, J. A., Sarkis, F., et al. 1984. Intrathecal administration of hyperbaric morphine for relief of labour pain. *Br. J. Anesth.* In press

152. Onofrio, B. M., Yaksh, T. L. 1983. Intrathecal delta-receptor ligand produces analgesia in man. *Lancet* 1:1386–87

153. Moulin, D., Max, M., Kaiko, R., Inturrisi, C., Maggard, J., Foley, K. 1984. Analgesic efficacy of IT d-ala^2-d-leu^5-enkephalin (DADL) in cancer patients with chronic pain. *Pain* 2:511 (Suppl.)

154. Czlonkowski, A., Costa, T., Przewlocki, R., Pasi, A., Herz, A. 1983. Opiate receptor binding sites in human spinal cord. *Brain Res.* 267:392–96

155. Gouarderes, C., Audigier, Y., Cros, J. 1982. Benzomorphan binding sites in rat lumbo-sacral spinal cord. *Eur. J. Pharmacol.* 78:483–86

156. Wikler, A. 1950. Sites and mechanisms of action of morphine and related drugs in the central nervous system. *Pharmacol. Rev.* 2:435–506

157. Goldfarb, J., Kaplan, E. I., Jenkins, H. R. 1978. Interaction of morphine and naloxone in acute spinal cats. *Neuropharmacology* 17:569–75

158. Jurna, I., Schafer, H. 1965. Depression of post tetanic potentiation in the spinal cord by morphine and pethidine. *Experientia* (Basel) 21:226–27

159. Krivoy, W., Kroeger, D., Zimmermann, E. 1973. Actions of morphine on the segmental reflex of the decerebrate spinal cat. *Br. J. Pharmacol.* 47:457–64

160. Jurna, I. 1966. Inhibition of the effect of repetitive stimulation on spinal motoneurones of the cat by morphine and pethidine. *Intl. J. Neuropharmacol.* 5:117–23

161. Kuschinsky, K., Seeber, U., Langer, J., Sontag, K. H. 1978. Effects of opiates and of neuroleptics on alpha-motoneurones in rat spinal cord: Possible correlations with muscular rigidity and akinesia. In *Characteristics and Function of Opioids,* ed. J. M. Van Ree, L. Terenius, pp. 431–35. Amsterdam: Elsevier-North Holland

162. Jurna, I., Heinz, G., Blinn, S., Nell, T. 1978. The effect of substantia nigra stimulation and morphine on motoneurones and the tail flick response. *Eur. J. Pharmacol.* 51:239–50

163. Willer, J. C., Bussel, B. 1980. Evidence for a direct spinal mechanism in morphine-induced inhibition of nociceptive reflexes in humans. *Brain Res.* 287:212–15

164. Duggan, A. W., Davies, J., Hall, J. G. 1976. Effects of opiate agonists and antagonists on central neurons of the cat. *J. Pharmacol. Exp. Ther.* 196:107–20

165. Kruglov, N. A. 1964. Effect of morphine group analgesics on the central inhibitory mechanisms. *Intl. J. Neuropharmacol.* 3:197–203

166. Curtis, D. R., Duggan, A. W. 1969. The

depression of spinal inhibition by morphine. *Agents Act.* 1:14–19

167. Davies, J. 1976. Effects of morphine and naloxone on Renshaw cells and spinal interneurones in morphine dependent and non-dependent rats. *Brain Res.* 113:311–26

168. Davies, J., Duggan, A. W. 1974. Opiate agonist-antagonist effects on Renshaw cells and spinal interneurones. *Nature* 250:70–71

169. Kaneko, T., Nakazawa, T., Ikeda, M., Yamatsu, K., Iwama, T., et al. 1983. Sites of analgesic action of dynorphin. *Life Sci.* 33:661–64

170. Yasuoka, S., Yaksh, T. L. 1983. Effects on nociceptive threshold and blood pressure of intrathecally administered morphine and α-adrenergic agonists. *Neuropharmacology* 22:309–15

170a. Duggan, A. W., Morton, C. R., Johnson, S. M., Zhao, Z. Q. 1984. Opioid antagonists and spinal reflexes in the anaesthetized cat. *Brain Res.* 297:33–40

171. Bromage, P. R., Camporesi, E., Leslie, J. 1980. Epidural narcotics in volunteers: Sensitivity to pain and to carbon dioxide. *Pain* 9:145–60

172. Atchison, S. R., Yaksh, T. L., Durant, P. 1984. Cardiovascular and respiratory effects of intrathecal DADL in awake dogs. *Anesthesiology* 60: In press

173. Rudy, T. A., Yaksh, T. L. 1977. Hyperthermic effects of morphine: Set point manipulation by a direct spinal action. *Br. J. Pharmacol.* 61:91–96

174. Bormann, B., Weidler, B., Dermhardt, R., et al. 1983. Influence of epidural fentanyl on stress-induced elevation of plasma vasopressin (ADH) after surgery. *Anesth. Analg.* 62:727–32

175. Cowen, M. J., Bullingham, R. E. S., Paterson, G. M. C., McQuay, H. J., Turner, M., et al. 1982. A controlled comparison of the effects of extradural diamorphine and bupivacaine on plasma glucose and plasma cortisol in postoperative patients. *Anesth. Analg.* 61:15–18

176. El-Baz, N., Goldin, M. D. 1983. Continuous epidural morphine infusion for pain relief after open heart surgery. *Anesthesiology* 59:A193

177. Mori, T. 1982. Studies on changes of the plasma prolactin, growth hormone and ACTH levels following surgical stress and epidural microinjections of morphine hydrochloride for the postoperative

analgesic method. *Acta Obstet. Gynaecol. Jpn.* 34:1707–16

178. Rutberg, H., Hakanson, E., Anderberg, B., Jorfeldt, L., Martensson, J., et al. 1984. Effects of the extradural administration of morphine, or bupivacaine on the endocrine response to upper abdominal surgery. *Br. J. Anesth.* 56:233–38

179. Porrecca, F., Filla, A., Burks, T. F. 1982. Spinal cord-mediated opiate effects on gastrointestinal transit in mice. *Eur. J. Pharmacol.* 86:135–36

180. Porrecca, F., Burks, T. F. 1983. The spinal cord as a site of opioid effects on gastrointestinal transit in the mouse. *J. Pharmacol. Exp. Ther.* 227:22–27

181. Porrecca, F., Filla, A., Birks, T. F. 1983. Studies *in vivo* with dynorphin (1–9): Analgesia but not gastrointestinal effects following intrathecal administration to mice. *Eur. J. Pharmacol.* In press

182. Reiz, S., Westberg, M. 1980. Side effects of epidural morphine. *Lancet* 2:203–4

183. Brent, C. R., Harty, G., Yaksh, T. L. 1983. The effects of spinal opiates on micturition in unanesthetized animals. *Soc. Neurosci.* 9:743

184. De Groat, W. C., Kawatani, M., Hisamitsu, T., Lowe, I., Morgan, C., et al. 1983. The role of neuropeptides in the sacral autonomic reflex pathways of the cat. *J. Auton. Nerv. Sys.* 7:339–50

185. Rawal, N., Möllefors, K., Axelsson, K., Lingardh, G., Widman, B. 1983. An experimental study of urodynamic effects of epidural morphine and of naloxone reversal. *Anesth. Analg.* 62:641–47

186. Aoki, M., Watanabe, H., Namiki, A., Takahashi, T., Yokoyama, E., et al. 1982. Mechanism of urinary retention following intrathecal administration of morphine. *Masui* 31:939–43

187. Bolam, J. M., Robinson, C. J., Wurster, R. D. 1984. Micturition in conscious dogs following spinal opiate administration. *Soc. Neurosci.* 10:1108

187a. Dray, A. 1984. In vivo assessment of spinal and supraspinal opioid activity using the rat urinary bladder preparation. *Soc. Neurosci. Abstr.* 10:586

188. Baxter, A. D., Kiruluta, G. 1984. Detrusor tone after epidural morphine. *Anesth. Analg.* 63:464

189. Thor, K. B., Roppolo, J. R., deGroat, W. C. 1983. Naloxone induced micturition in unanesthetized paraplegic cats. *J. Urol.* In press

Ann. Rev. Pharmacol. Toxicol. 1985. 25:463–83

PHYSIOLOGICAL STUDIES WITH SOMATOCRININ, A GROWTH HORMONE–RELEASING FACTOR

William B. Wehrenberg, Andrew Baird, Fusun Zeytin, Fred Esch, Peter Böhlen, Nick Ling, Shao Y. Ying, and Roger Guillemin

Laboratories for Neuroendocrinology, The Salk Institute for Biological Studies, San Diego, California 92037

INTRODUCTION

Our knowledge of how hormones affect normal growth and development has derived from observing the pathophysiological effects of hormonal deficiency or excess in clinical and experimental studies. These observations have led to the identification of numerous hormones that exert significant effects on somatic growth, including growth hormone (GH), insulin, thyroid hormones, glucocorticoids, and androgens. As implied by its name, GH is the fundamental factor regulating growth. Moreover, it is of particular interest since it is the hormonal link between somatic development and its regulation by the central nervous system.

GH release by the anterior pituitary is controlled by hypothalamic releasing and inhibiting factors. The recognition (1) and characterization (2) of hypothalamic growth hormone release–inhibiting factor, somatostatin, in 1973 extended our knowledge of the regulation of GH secretion. The structural elucidation of growth hormone–releasing factor (GRF) was not accomplished until almost ten years later. In November 1982, Guillemin and associates (3) reported the isolation and characterization of a 44 amino acid peptide from a pancreatic tumor causing acromegaly with potent GH-releasing activity. These investigators also described two additional GH-releasing peptides consisting of

463

0362-1642/85/415-0463$02.00

the first 37 and 40 amino acids of the 44 amino acid peptide. The structure of the 40 amino acid GRF was confirmed shortly thereafter by Rivier et al (4) and Esch et al (5). This information has led to the successful characterization of human hypothalamic GRF (5a) as well as murine (6), porcine (7), bovine (8), and ovine and caprine GRF (8a).

The availability of synthetic GRF has opened a new era in our investigations of the regulation of GH secretion by the anterior pituitary. The purpose of this article is to review the literature concerning the in vivo actions of growth hormone–releasing factor.

THE ONTOGENY AND DISTRIBUTION OF GRF WITHIN THE CENTRAL NERVOUS SYSTEM

Based on its hypophysiotropic function, the distribution of GRF within the central nervous system had been hypothesized as being concentrated in the hypothalamus. Immunohistochemical studies conducted to evaluate this hypothesis show that the localization of this peptidergic system within the central nervous system is highly consistent with its physiological function of releasing GH from the anterior pituitary.

GRF immunoreactivity is not observed in the hypothalami of human fetuses younger than 29 weeks of age (9). Between 29 and 31 weeks of intrauterine life, numerous immunoreactive cells are found in the infundibular (arcuate) nucleus, showing typical neuroblastic aspects such as small diameter and no processes. No immunoreactive fibers can be found in the median eminence of the hypothalamus at these ages. The hypothalamic distribution of GRF neurons is similar in older fetuses and neonates; however, cell bodies appear more immunoreactive and short, immature processes are observed. GRF immunoreactive fibers first appear in the hypothalamus after the thirty-first week of fetal life and are numerous at birth. These fibers also appear in the median eminence, with endings in contact with the hypothalamic-hypophyseal portal vessels, at about the same time.

The ontogeny of the GRF system does not parallel the development of the other hypophysiotropic factors. Neurons staining for luteinizing hormone-releasing factor (LRF) are detectable by the eleventh week of fetal life (10), for somatostatin by the fourteenth week (11), and for corticotropin-releasing factor (CRF) by the sixteenth week (12). The appearance of somatotropic cells within the pituitary occurs as early as the eighth week of gestation. Thus, it appears that the initial stages of the development and differentiation of pituitary somatotrophs are independent of hypothalamic GRF input.

Numerous cell bodies containing GRF immunoreactivity are observed in the adult human and monkey hypothalami (13, 14); the vast majority of these cell bodies are in the medial basal hypothalamus, especially in the arcuate nucleus.

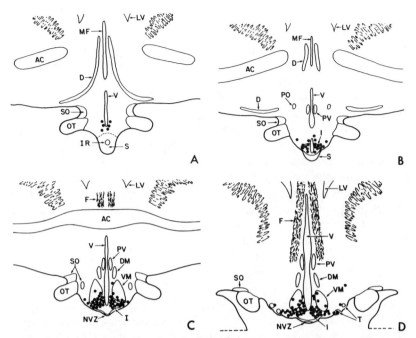

Figure 1 Diagrams of the frontal sections of the adult human hypothalamus showing the localization of GRF immunoreactive cell bodies. A–D are from anterior to posterior planes. Abbreviations: AC = anterior commissure; D = nucleus of diagonal band; DM = dorsomedial nucleus; F = fornix; I = infundibular nucleus; IR = infundibular recess; LV = lateral ventricle; MF = midline fissure; NVZ = neurovascular zone; OT = optic tract; PO = preoptic nucleus; PV = paraventricular nucleus; S = pituitary stalk; SO = supraoptic nucleus; T = lateral tuber nucleus; V = third ventricle; VM = ventromedial nucleus (taken from 9).

Some cell clusters extend into the lateral hypothalamus, and others extend dorsally near the ventromedial nucleus and along the wall of the third ventricle. Cell bodies are found as far anterior as the optic chiasm and as far posterior as the mamillary bodies (Figure 1). GRF immunoreactive fibers are present in the median eminence, arcuate nucleus, and ventromedial nuclei. Within the median eminence, the fibers appear grouped in bundles that terminate on the primary capillary plexus of the hypothalamic-hypophyseal portal system, an expected observation based on the functions of GRF.

The distribution of GRF immunoreactive structures within the rat hypothalamus is similar to that found in primate brains. The majority of cell bodies are found in the arcuate nucleus and in the medial perifornical region of the lateral hypothalamus (15–17, 22). Scattered cell bodies are also seen in the ventral and dorsal lateral hypothalamus. Of interest is the apparent absence of GRF-containing neurons in the ventromedial hypothalamus in the rat (16). Electrical stimulation (18) and lesion experiments (19–21) have strongly implicated the ventromedial hypothalamus as an important neural locus with regard to GRF. Since GRF cell bodies are located in areas contiguous to this region, it is likely that the effects observed by destruction or stimulation of the ventromedial nucleus are due to extension of the lesions or to diffusion of the stimulation to adjacent areas. Nevertheless, neurons within the ventromedial nucleus might exert an effect on GRF neurons in the arcuate nucleus.

Dense GRF immunoreactive processes and terminals are observed in the median eminence. Bloch et al (22) have demonstrated that neonatal treatment of rats with monosodium glutamate, a procedure that selectively destroys the neurons of the arcuate nucleus, results in the almost complete and selective loss of GRF staining in the median eminence. These results demonstrate that the arcuate nucleus is the main source of GRF in the median eminence. Fibers from GRF-staining neurons in the perifornical region run perpendicular to the basal surface of the hypothalamus. They then turn medially and run parallel to it until they terminate in the median eminence.

The ontogeny and distribution of GRF immunoreactivity has also been studied in the cat (23). As in other species, cell bodies are most abundant in the arcuate nucleus, with additional staining observed in the paraventricular, supraoptic, and dorsomedial nuclei and anterior periventricular areas. Again, little or no immunoreactivity is observed in the ventromedial nucleus. Consistent with what is observed in humans, the development of the GRF pathways in the cat is much later than that of the other hypothalamic releasing and inhibiting factors. Although the GRF cell bodies are developed by 15 days of age, only scarce GRF immunoreactive fibers in the median eminence can be observed. By 30 days of age nerve fibers are abundant and well developed, and terminals can be seen in close proximity to the primary capillary bed of the hypothalamic-hypophyseal portal system. GRF perikarya have also been observed outside the hypothalamus in the cat; however, questions concerning the specificity of the GRF antiserum in relation to feline GRF leave these observations open to interpretation.

GRF REGULATION OF GH RELEASE

Extensive studies on the in vivo action of GRF were initiated as soon as the synthetic replicate of GRF became available. Initial experiments were designed to establish the dose-response relationship and the specificity of GRF in stimulating GH release in a variety of animal models. Likewise, studies were conducted to evaluate whether the various GRFs characterized possess different biological activity. Since the 44 amino–acid peptide isolated from human tissue has in vivo biological activity similar to the 40 and 37 amino–acid peptides (Figure 2) and since human and murine GRF are equipotent in vivo

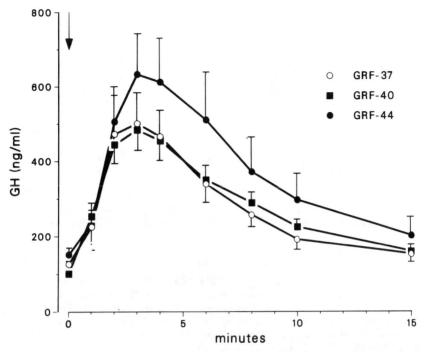

Figure 2   The relative potency of 0.02 nmole human GRF (1-44), (1-40), and (1-37) (see 3) in anesthetized male rats. Animals were treated with 60 mg/kg sodium pentobarbital administered intraperitoneally 15 minutes prior to the initiation of blood sampling. The peptides were administered intravenously immediately after time 0 in 0.5 ml saline. Data points represent the mean of results obtained in 19 rats; vertical bars represent the SEM (W. Wehrenberg, N. Ling, unpublished observations).

(23a), little distinction will be given here to which specific molecule of GRF was used in a given study.

Doses

HUMAN AND SUBHUMAN PRIMATES   The identification of a substance with direct and potent GH releasing activity has stimulated substantial clinical interest. Intravenous administration of GRF into normal adults in doses of 0.1–10 μg/kg body weight results in a significant increase in plasma GH concentrations (24–29). Peak concentrations of GH are reached 15–30 minutes post-injection and concentrations return to baseline values in between one and two hours (Figure 3). The pituitary GH response to GRF is specific; the secretion of no other anterior pituitary hormone is altered by GRF administration (24). Thorner et al (30) have reported that GRF is also effective in stimulating GH release following subcutaneous and intranasal administration.

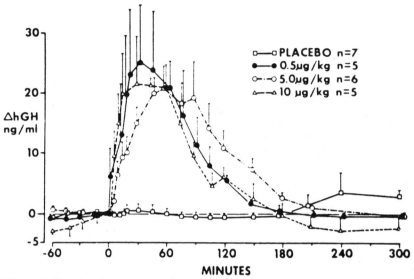

Figure 3 Elevation of plasma GH concentrations in response to GRF in normal adult human volunteers. Response to the 0.5, 5, and 10 μg/kg doses of GRF were all significantly higher than the placebo. GH concentrations rose within five minutes and reached a maximum at 30–45 minutes (0.5 μg/kg), 45–90 minutes (5 μg/kg), and 30–120 minutes (10 μg/kg). Results are expressed in ng hGH/ml (mean ± SEM) (taken from 25).

The minimum effective doses of GRF required for subcutaneous administration are approximately 30 times greater than those required for intravenous administration (30). Intranasal administration of GRF requires doses about 100 times greater than those required for intravenous administration (30, 31).

The specific pituitary GH response to GRF and its dose-response relationship has also been confirmed in subhuman primates (32). Increases in GH are observed in normal female monkeys following the intravenous administration of 5–100 μg GRF/kg. Maximum GH concentrations are measured approximately 30 minutes following injection; concentrations return to baseline within one hour following lower doses of GRF, but they remain elevated for up to two hours following higher doses.

The reports published thus far on the effects of GRF on GH secretion in humans and monkeys demonstrate a marked heterogeneity of the GH response to a given dose of GRF. This applies to the response observed within an individual given repeated doses of GRF and to the response observed between individuals. It is unclear what factors are involved in modulating the GH response to GRF. It is possible that somatostatin is actively involved, since this neuropeptide plays a major role in regulating GH secretion and it has already been shown to modulate the GH response to GRF in laboratory animals (33,

43). Regardless of the variability in the GH response to GRF, this peptide is already of immense importance in the clinical diagnosis of GH disorders.

OTHER SPECIES   Extensive research has been conducted on the biological relationships between GRF and GH in the laboratory rat. Initial studies were conducted in rats anesthetized with sodium pentobarbital. This animal model has proven very useful for the study of GRF, since pentobarbital anesthesia appears to inhibit the release of both endogenous somatostatin and GRF (34). Studies with GRF have demonstrated that the maximum GH response occurs within 3–5 minutes post-intravenous injection; concentrations begin to decline within 15 minutes and return to baseline by 30 minutes. The dose-response relationship for GRF has been clearly demonstrated in the rat, in contrast to results obtained in the human. The minimum effective dose of GRF to elicit a GH response is approximately 100 ng/kg and the maximum dose is in the range of 5 μg/kg (Figure 4). The subcutaneous administration of GRF is also effective, the minimum effective dose being approximately 25 μg/kg (35). Rats anesthetized with urethane also appear to be a useful model (35, 36). However, urethane anesthesia is known to increase somatostatin concentrations in hypothalamic-hypophyseal portal blood compared to sodium pentobarbital anesthesia (37), and thus it is not unexpected that the amount of GRF needed to stimulate GH secretion is greater in the urethane-anesthetized rat.

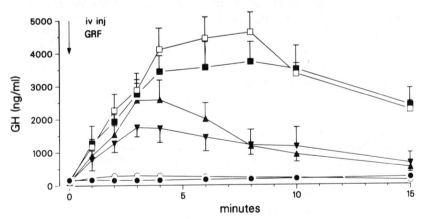

Figure 4   The increase in plasma GH concentrations following the intravenous administration of saline (●), 0.15 (○), 0.5 (◄), 1.5 (▲), 15 (□), and 25 μg/kg (■) of GRF in anesthetized male rats three months of age. Animals were treated immediately after the time 0 sample, data points represent the mean response in six rats, and vertical bars represent the SEM. Note that the increase in GH concentrations following the 0.15 μg/kg dose is significant (p <0.05), although it is difficult to illustrate this increase here because of the tremendous responses observed at the higher doses (taken from 90).

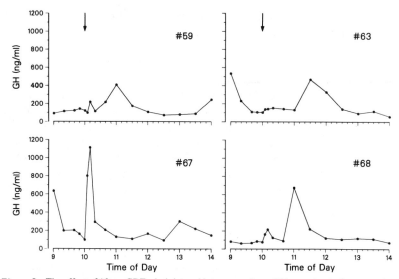

Figure 5   The effect of 10 μg GRF administered intravenously on GH secretion in four conscious, freely moving male rats. Injections (indicated by arrows) were made at a time known to be between spontaneous GH pulses. Note the absence of response in rat #63 and the partial response in rats #59 and #68 compared to the response in rat #67 (taken from 33).

While anesthetized animals are a very useful model for numerous studies, it is apparent that they are not the best model for studies designed to investigate some of the physiological interactions between GRF and GH. Ideally, such studies should be carried out in conscious, freely moving animals. Initial studies using this animal model yielded very perplexing results (33). The intravenous administration of GRF, which is unequivocally bioactive in vitro (3, 4) and in vivo in anesthetized rats (3, 4), only induces an increase in plasma GH concentrations in 30% of the rats tested (Figure 5). This inconsistency in response, which to some degree appears similar to the heterogeneity of responses observed in humans, can be completely eliminated by pretreating the rats with antibodies raised against somatostatin (Figure 6). An additional study was conducted to further establish the role of somatostatin in modulating the pituitary GH response to GRF. Following a 72-hour fast, a treatment reported to increase endogenous somatostatin release (38), rats were injected with GRF. The administration of GRF did not elicit a significant GH response in fasted rats, a result that can be reversed by pretreatment of the animals with somatostatin antibodies (33). These results demonstrate the dynamic and opposite roles exerted by GRF and somatostatin in regulating GH secretion (see further discussion below).

An additional fact that can complicate the interpretation of results obtained from studies involving the administration of GRF to conscious, freely moving

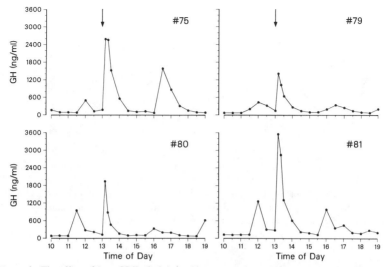

Figure 6   The effect of 1 μg GRF administered intravenously on GH secretion in four conscious, freely moving male rats pretreated with antiserum against somatostatin. Injections (indicated by arrows) were made at a time known to be between spontaneous GH pulses. Note the change in dose of GRF administered and scale of GH concentrations compared to Figure 5 (taken from 33).

animals is that the endogenous release of GH by the pituitary is pulsatile in nature (39). Using a monoclonal antibody raised against rat GRF (40), Wehrenberg et al (41) have shown that these spontaneous GH pulses are GRF dependent. The fact that plasma GH concentrations during spontaneous pulses can approach those observed in response to exogenously administered GRF make it difficult to delineate spontaneous and induced changes in plasma GH concentrations. To circumvent the problems created by endogenous somatostatin and GRF, Wehrenberg et al (42) treated conscious, freely moving animals with antiserum against somatostatin and with a monoclonal antibody against rat GRF that does not recognize GRF isolated from human tissue. This animal model is ideal in that it represents an immediate, noninvasive, yet reversible, functional lesion of the hypothalamo-pituitary axis that is specific only for endogenous somatostatin and rat GRF. Using this model, these investigators have shown that the pituitary GH response to repeated doses of human GRF is virtually unchanged over time (Figure 7). In addition, dose-response studies conducted in this animal model confirm studies performed in anesthetized rats. The minimum effective dose of GRF required to elicit a GH response is 100–200 ng/kg and the maximum GH response is observed with approximately 5 μg/kg (Figure 8).

GRF has been shown to be biologically active in all of the animal species tested thus far. Intravenous injection of 1–10 μg GRF in rabbits causes a

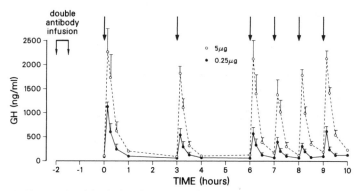

Figure 7   The capacity of the pituitary in conscious, freely moving male rats (n = 6) to secrete GH in response to repeated intravenous injections of a moderate (0.25 μg; ●) and maximal (5 μg; ○) dose of human GRF. Two hours before the first injection, the rats were treated with an antiserum against somatostatin and a monoclonal antibody against rat GRF that does not recognize human GRF. Arrows indicate the injection of human GRF. Data points represent the mean GH concentration and the vertical bars represent the SEM (taken from 42).

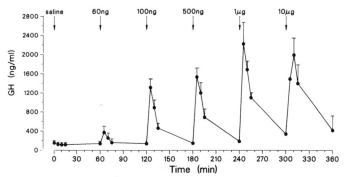

Figure 8   The dose-dependent response of the pituitary in conscious, freely moving male rats (n = 6) to secrete GH in response to human GRF administered intravenously. Two hours before the saline injection, the rats were treated with an antiserum against somatostatin and a monoclonal antibody against rat GRF that does not recognize human GRF. The dose and time of injection of human GRF are indicated, data points represent the mean GH concentration, and the vertical bars represent the SEM (taken from 42).

significant and dose-related increase in plasma GH concentrations (43). As in the rat, the GH response is significantly greater in rabbits pretreated with somatostatin antiserum than in rabbits pretreated with control serum. The GH response to repeated doses of GRF is also unaltered over time in rabbits, again illustrating the capacity of the pituitary to secrete GH. GRF is effective in releasing GH in dogs (3). In domestic animals, GRF stimulates GH secretion in ovine (44, 45), porcine (46), and bovine species (47). It is also active in chickens (48, 49) and turkeys (50). GRF releases GH in at least one lower vertebrate species, the goldfish (51). It is our opinion that, as further research is conducted, GRF will continue to be shown as a potent and specific releaser of GH across all species.

Animal Models for the Study of GRF Regulation of GH Release

As already discussed, the stimulation of GH secretion by GRF can be clearly illustrated in normal animals following various routes of administration. However, the GH response to GRF is quite variable due to the interaction of endogenous somatostatin and the pulsatile nature of spontaneous GH secretion. For this reason, various animal models have been investigated for their potential use in studying the GH response to GRF. Rats with electrolytic lesions of the ventromedial-arcuate region of the hypothalamus have a marked suppression of the GH release (52) that is not due to increased somatostatin release (21). Using such lesioned animals, Tannenbaum et al (54) and Wehrenberg et al (55) have reported a potent effect of GRF on GH secretion. Pretreatment of these animals with somatostatin antibodies results in an enhancement of the GH response to GRF. Other animal models in which spontaneous GH secretion can be modified have also been evaluated. Chemical lesion of the arcuate nucleus by neonatal treatment with monosodium glutamate and the pharmacological interruption of catecholamine synthesis and storage by α-methyl-p-tyrosine and reserpine respectively are all known to inhibit spontaneous GH release. In each of these animal models, the GH response to GRF is enhanced by prior treatment of the animals with somatostatin antiserum (55).

CENTRAL NERVOUS SYSTEM PATHWAYS INVOLVED IN GRF SECRETION

Numerous stimuli are known to release GH in vivo. Their actions are indirect, since they are unable to stimulate GH release in vitro. Initial reports are now appearing in the literature that indicate that these indirect pathways for releasing GH ultimately involve GRF. Opiates and opioid peptides are potent releasers of pituitary GH in vivo, yet are devoid of any GH releasing activity in vitro. Wehrenberg et al (42) reported that the GH response to morphine sulfate administration in rats can be completely blocked by the prior administration of GRF antibodies. These results have been expanded by the recent report by Miki et al (58) that shows that passive immunization of rats with an antibody raised against human GRF that recognizes rat GRF completely abolishes the GH response to FK 33–824, an enkephalin analogue. We have also observed that such passive immunization inhibits the GH-releasing activity of β-endorphin when administered into the lateral cerebral ventricles (57). Miki et al (58) have also shown that the α–adrenergic stimulating pathways involved in GH secretion require the active involvement of GRF. These initial observations indicate that GRF is the final common pathway for the ultimate regulation of GH secretion.

FACTORS MODULATING GRF REGULATION OF GH RELEASE

Other Hypothalamic Releasing Factors

The specificity of previously characterized hypothalamic releasing factors in releasing their respective pituitary target hormones is well established. Thyrotropin-releasing factor (TRF) stimulates the release of thyrotropin (TSH) and prolactin; luteinizing hormone–releasing factor (LRF) stimulates the release of luteinizing hormone (LH) and follicle-stimulating hormone (FSH); corticotropin-releasing factor (CRF) stimulates the release of adrenocorticotropin (ACTH) and β-endorphin. Likewise, GRF is specific for the release of GH (3, 4, 24, 34). Under numerous pathophysiological conditions, the secretion of anterior pituitary hormones is altered. For example, stress increases the secretion of ACTH and decreases the secretion of gonadotropins and TSH (60, 61). This change in pituitary secretion may be due to a variety of mechanisms, one of which might be changes in the pituitary response to the releasing factors in the presence or absence of other releasing factors (i.e. interactions). To investigate the possibility of interactions between the four hypothalamic releasing factors on anterior pituitary secretion, Wehrenberg et al (62) conducted in vitro and in vivo experiments using a $2 \times 2 \times 2 \times 2$ factorial design. This design allows for the evaluation of both main effects of the releasing factors as well as of all possible interactions between them. The results obtained confirm the specificity of each of the releasing factors on their respective target cells in the anterior pituitary under normal physiological conditions. There were no significant interactions between any of the releasing factors on anterior pituitary hormone secretion. These results suggest that changes in the pituitary secretion observed under pathophysiological conditions are not due to interactions of the releasing factors at the level of the pituitary, but rather to other secondary interactions that modify the hypothalamic release of the releasing factors or the pituitary response to the stimuli. An important implication of these results is that the clinical pituitary reserve test conducted in humans to evaluate pituitary response to the hypothalamic releasing factors can be expanded to include all four releasing factors, since any lack of response will reflect pituitary dysfunction and not an interaction of the releasing factors.

Hypothalamic Inhibiting Factor: Somatostatin

As discussed earlier, somatostatin plays an active role in modulating the GH response to GRF. One of the most perplexing observations made thus far is the apparent randomness of the GH response to GRF in conscious, freely moving animals (33, 43). When normal animals are pretreated with somatostatin antiserum, the GH response is normalized. These observations suggest that somatostatin is released in a pulsatile or episodic fashion. Arancibia et al (63) and Kasting et al (64) have reported that the concentrations of somatostatin released from the median eminence is pulsatile, with a period interval of approximately 60–120 minutes. Evidence thus suggests that both GRF and somatostatin are released in a pulsatile fashion. Apparently, somatostatin predominates in this system, since administration of somatostatin always reduces plasma GH concentrations (65) and the administration of GRF does not always increase GH (33). For the exogenous administration of GRF to be effective, hypothalamic somatostatin secretion must be at a nadir. Much work is needed in this area to further delineate the relationship between GRF and somatostatin in regulating GH secretion.

Pituitary Hormones

To date, only the effects of reduced or excess GH on the pituitary response to GRF have been reported. These reports have centered primarily on clinical studies in patients suffering from acromegaly or hypopituitarisms. Shibasaki et al (66) have observed that the time of peak GH concentrations, as well as the magnitude of the pituitary response to GRF, was highly variable in ten acromegalic patients. In light of the clinical history of these individuals, the significance of the results is unclear. A preliminary report has appeared that suggests that the exogenous administration of GH to normal subjects reduces the GH response to GRF (67).

The effects of GRF administration under conditions of GH deficiency can be summarized by stating that GRF is very useful in distinguishing pituitary dysfunction from hypothalamic dysfunction (68–71). The significance of this as a clinical tool is apparent. Pintor et al (72) have also observed that GRF has a prolactin-lowering effect in GH-deficient children. This observation will need further confirmation.

Other Endocrine Effects

Glucocorticoids enhance GH production by somatotrophs in in vitro systems (73–75). Yet in vivo, the exogenous administration of these steroids results in an inhibition of somatic growth. To study this apparent dichotomy in the actions of glucocorticoids, the pituitary response to GRF has been evaluated in intact and adrenalectomized rats receiving glucocorticoid replacement therapy. Administration of the glucocorticoid dexamethasone significantly enhanced the GH response to GRF in intact as well as in adrenalectomized rats (76). These observations demonstrate that these steroids enhance the pituitary GH response to GRF in vivo. This fact, coupled with the fact that glucocorticoids inhibit somatic growth, leads to the hypothesis that adrenocortical steroids are positive modulators of the GH response at the pituitary level but negative modulators at peripheral sites. Thyroid hormone also enhances GH production by somatotrophs in vitro (74, 75). Preliminary observations in vivo are consistent with these observations in that thyroid hormone appears to enhance the GH response to GRF (77). These results are in agreement with in vitro data (78).

Males of most vertebrate species, including humans and laboratory rodents, are much larger than their female counterparts. Sex differences in weight are known to be due to direct and potent anabolic effects of androgens on metabolic processes in target tissues. In addition, some evidence suggests that gonadal steroids mediate their effects on growth by regulating GH synthesis and release (79–84). Wehrenberg et al (85) have reported that testosterone replacement therapy in gonadectomized male rats causes a significant enhancement of the GH response to GRF, but estradiol replacement therapy in gonadectomized female rats does not alter the response. Other results in pre- and post-pubescent rats suggest that the enhanced response observed in male rats is not observed until after puberty.

Other Factors

The amino acid sequence of GRF shows considerable homology with peptides in the secretin-glucagon family of gut peptides and suggests that peptides within this family might interact. Glucagon, gastric inhibitory peptide (GIP), and secretin cause a slight inhibition of plasma GH concentrations when administered to anesthetized rats (86). When GIP is administered in combination with GRF, the pituitary GH response is significantly augmented. In contrast, when secretin is administered in combination with GRF, the pituitary response is significantly reduced. It is unclear whether these results reflect a direct interaction of these peptides with GRF receptors on the somatotrophs or are due to extrapituitary mechanisms.

One of the standard clinical tests to elicit pituitary GH secretion in man is insulin-induced hypoglycemia. The fact that hyperglycemia suppresses GH secretion is well known. In light of this relationship, the effects of blood glucose on the response of GH to GRF have been evaluated in humans (87, 88). Under conditions of hyperglycemia, the GH response to GRF is significantly suppressed.

Significant age-related variations in the spontaneous secretion of GH exist in man and experimental animals. At or near the time of puberty, GH secretion is near a maximum for both the frequency of spontaneous GH pulses and the magnitude of plasma GH concentrations. With advancing age, both of these parameters are significantly reduced. The cause of these age-related changes is unknown; however, a possible mechanism could be changes in pituitary response to GRF. The data reported in humans are unequivocal: the pituitary GH response to GRF in men in their twenties and thirties is significantly greater than the response observed in men in their forties or older (89). It is not known whether this change in response reflects decreased pituitary sensitivity to GRF or increased involvement of somatostatin.

Studies conducted in rats show an absence of any age-related change in GH response to GRF. Wehrenberg et al (90) have reported no age-related change in the pituitary response to either submaximal or maximal doses of GRF when administered to anesthetized male rats. Using a similar experimental design, Sonntag et al (91) have reported a decreased response to GRF in old rats as compared to young rats. In vitro data published by these investigators show that there is no change in the somatotrophs' response to GRF when these cells are isolated from hypothalamic influences. In light of these in vitro results, Sonntag et al (91) have suggested that the reduced response to GRF in vivo may be due to increased release of or enhanced sensitivity to somatostatin rather than to a decrease in the pituitary response to GRF.

There is no doubt that the somatomedins play a significant role in mediating the actions of GH. To date, we have little information on what role somatomedins have in the feedback regulation of GRF or how they might modify the GH response to GRF. Motilin is another peptide that might be involved, since it has been reported to have a direct effect on pituitary GH secretion in vitro (92), and passive immunization of animals with antiserum raised against motilin suppress plasma GH concentrations (93). An additional factor that may be involved is an enkephalin analog with growth hormone–releasing activity in vitro and in vivo (94–96). How these factors integrate into the regulation of GH secretion remains to be determined.

CHRONIC ADMINISTRATION OF GRF AND ITS EFFECTS ON SOMATIC GROWTH

The GH content of the anterior pituitary is very high compared to that of other anterior pituitary hormones. This suggests that the pituitary may have a large capacity to secrete GH after repeated or chronic administration of GRF. As previously discussed, the pituitary GH response to GRF does not change after repeated doses of GRF in the rat (Figure 7) (42). In contrast, earlier observations indicated that the pituitary becomes refractory to the continuous administration of GRF in less than one hour (34). In a more extensive study, Wehrenberg et al (97) have shown that the capacity of the pituitary to respond to GRF can be exhausted after a 12–24 hour administration of a relatively high dose of GRF in rats pretreated with somatostatin antiserum. The loss of response is due at least in part to depletion of pituitary GH content. The possible involvement of GRF receptor desensitization or down-regulation has not been evaluated and therefore can not be ruled out.

One of the most obvious applications for the chronic use of GRF is to enhance somatic growth. There is no doubt that GRF is critical in this process. Indeed, passively immunizing rats with GRF antibodies for as short a time as eight days causes a significant inhibition of somatic growth (98). The absence of any published reports indicating the successful use of GRF to enhance growth undoubtedly reflects the complex nature of the hypothalamic regulation of GH secretion by GRF and somatostatin.

TOXICOLOGICAL AND PHARMACOLOGICAL EFFECTS

The potential toxic effects of GRF have been evaluated in various animal models (28; W. Wehrenberg, N. Ling, P. Brazeau, R. Guillemin, unpublished observations). The gross and microscopic pathology of tissues obtained from animals receiving over 1,000 times the maximum effect dose of GRF are normal. No morbidity or mortality of animals was noted in studies in which large doses of GRF were administered for extended periods (more than seven days). Administration of GRF to humans does cause a transient flushing of the face and upper torso (24–29). These effects occur during the first few minutes following GRF administration, and no long-term effects have been observed.

CONCLUSIONS

Since the isolation and characterization of GRF, initially from tumor tissue but subsequently from normal hypothalamic tissue, most of the fundamental studies of the in vivo actions of GRF have been performed. Immunohistochemical mapping of GRF neurons in the central nervous system has been completed, the dose-response relationships between GRF and GH have been established, and the clinical use of the peptide has been initiated. Our present knowledge of the actions of GRF will serve as a solid foundation for the numerous additional studies that must be conducted before we will be able to completely understand the physiology of GRF. It is easiest to illustrate the immense amount of research that is currently being conducted and that remains to be performed by stating that in the week prior to the submission of this manuscript, over 100 abstracts on the actions of GRF were presented at the seventh international congress on endocrinology held in Quebec City, Canada.

ACKNOWLEDGEMENTS

W. B. Wehrenberg thanks the Andrew W. Mellon Foundation for its continued support. We thank C. Wong, B. Phillips, J. Wehrenberg, and the secretarial staff of the Laboratories for Neuroendocrinology for assistance in preparing this manuscript.

Literature Cited

1. Krulich, L., Dhariwal, A. P. S., McCann, S. M. 1968. Stimulatory and inhibitory effects of purified hypothalamic extracts on growth hormone release from rat pituitary in vitro. *Endocrinology* 83:783–90

2. Brazeau, P., Vale, W., Burgus, R., Ling, N., Butcher, M., et al. 1973. Hypothalamic polypeptide that inhibits the secretion of immunoreactive pituitary growth hormone. *Science* 179:77–79

3. Guillemin, R., Brazeau, P., Bohlen, P., Esch, F., Ling, N., Wehrenberg, W. B. 1982. Growth hormone-releasing factor from a human pancreatic tumor that caused acromegaly. *Science* 218:585–87

4. Rivier, J., Spiess, J., Thorner, M., Vale, W. 1982. Characterization of a growth hormone-releasing factor from a human pancreatic islet tumour. *Nature* 300:276–78

5. Esch, F. S., Bohlen, P., Ling, N. C., Brazeau, P. E., Wehrenberg, W. B., et al. 1982. Characterization of a 40 residue peptide from a human pancreatic tumor with growth hormone releasing activity. *Biochem. Biophys. Res. Commun.* 109: 152–58

5a. Ling, N., Esch, F., Bohlen, P., Brazeau, P., Wehrenberg, W. B., et al. 1984. Isolation, primary structure and synthesis of human hypothalamic somatocrinin: Growth hormone-releasing factor. *Proc. Natl. Acad. Sci. USA.* 81: 4302–6

6. Spiess, J., Rivier, J., Vale, W. 1983. Characterization of rat hypothalamic growth hormone-releasing factor. *Nature* 303:532–35

7. Bohlen, P., Esch, F., Brazeau, P., Ling, N., Guillemin, R. 1983. Isolation and characterization of the porcine hypothalamic growth hormone releasing factor. *Biochem. Biophys. Res. Commun.* 116: 726–34

8. Esch, F., Bohlen, P., Ling, N., Brazeau, P., Guillemin, R. 1983. Isolation and characterization of the bovine hypothalamic growth hormone releasing factor. *Biochem. Biophys. Res. Commun.* 117: 772–79

8a. Brazeau, P., Böhlen, P., Esch, F., Ling, N., Wehrenberg, W. B., Guillemin, R. 1984. Growth hormone–releasing factor from ovine and caprine hypothalamus: Isolation, sequence analysis and total synthesis. *Biochem. Biophys. Res. Commun.* In press

9. Bloch, B., Gaillard, R. C., Brazeau, P., Lin, H. D., Ling, N. 1984. Topographical and ontogenetic study of the neurons producing growth hormone-releasing factor in human hypothalamus. *Reg. Peptides* 8:21–31

10. Bugnon, C., Bloch, B., Lenys, D., Fellmann, D. 1978. Cytoimmunological study of the LH-RH neurons in humans during fetal life. In *Brain Endocrine Interaction. 3rd Int. Symp. Wurzburg, 1977. III. Neural Hormones and Reproduction,* ed. D. E. Scott, G. P. Kozlowski, A. Weindl, pp. 183–96. Basel: Karger

11. Bugnon, C., Fellmann, D., Bloch, B. 1977. Immunocytochemical study of the ontogenesis of the hypothalamic somatostatin-containing neurons in the human fetus. *Cell Tissue Res.* 183:319–28

12. Bugnon, C., Fellmann, D., Bresson, J. L., Clavequin, M. C. 1982. Etude immunocytochimique de l'ontogenese du systeme neuroglandulaire a CRF chez l'homme. *C.R. Acad. Sci.* 294:491–94

13. Bloch, B., Brazeau, P., Ling, N., Bohlen, P., Esch, F., et al. 1983. Immunohistochemical detection of growth hormone-releasing factor in brain. *Nature* 301:607–8

14. Bloch, B., Brazeau, P., Bloom, F., Ling, N. 1983. Topographical study of the neurons containing hpGRF immunoreactivity in monkey hypothalamus. *Neurosci. Lett.* 37:23–28

15. Jacobowitz, D. M., Schulte, H., Chrousos, G. P., Loriaux, D. L. 1983. Localization of GRF-like immunoreactive neurons in the rat brain. *Peptides* 4:521–24

16. Sawchenko, P. E., Swanson, L. W., Rivier, J., Vale, W. W. 1984. The distribution of growth hormone-releasing factor (GRF)-immunoreactivity in the central nervous system of the rat: An immunohistochemical study using antisera directed against rat hypothalamic GRF. *J. Comp. Neurol.* In press

17. Merchenthaler, I., Vigh, S., Schally, A. V., Petrusz, P. 1984. Immunocytochemical localization of growth hormone-releasing factor in the rat hypothalamus. *Endocrinology* 114:1082–85

18. Martin, J. B. 1972. Plasma growth hormone (GH) response to hypothalamic or extrahypothalamic electrical stimulation. *Endocrinology* 91:107–15

19. Frohman, L. A., Bernardis, L. L. 1968. Growth hormone and insulin levels in weanling rats with ventromedial hypothalamic lesions. *Endocrinology* 82: 1125–32

20. Frohman, L. A., Bernardis, L. L., Kant, K. J. 1968. Hypothalamic stimulation of growth hormone secretion. *Science* 162: 580–82
21. Eikelboom, R., Tannenbaum, G. S. 1983. Effects of obesity-inducing ventromedial hypothalamic lesions on pulsatile growth hormone and insulin secretion: Evidence for the existence of a growth hormone-releasing factor. *Endocrinology* 112:212–19
22. Bloch, B., Ling, N., Benoit, R., Wehrenberg, W. B., Guillemin, R. 1984. Specific depletion of immunoreactive growth hormone–releasing factor by monosodium glutamate in rat median eminence. *Nature* 307:272–73
23. Bugnon, C., Gouget, A., Fellmann, D., Clavequin, M. C. 1983. Immunocytochemical demonstration of a novel peptidergic neurone system in the cat brain with an anti-growth hormone-releasing factor serum. *Neurosci. Lett.* 38:131–37
23a. Wehrenberg, W. B., Ling, N. 1983. *In vivo* biological potency of rat and human growth hormone–releasing factor and fragments of human growth hormone-releasing factor. *Biochem. Biophys. Res. Commun.* 115:525–53
24. Thorner, M. O., Spiess, J., Vance, M. L., Rogol, A. D., Kaiser, D. L., et al. 1983. Human pancreatic growth-hormone-releasing factor selectively stimulates growth-hormone secretion in man. *Lancet* 1:24–28
25. Rosenthal, S. M., Schriock, E. A., Kaplan, S. L., Guillemin, R., Grumbach, M. M. 1983. Synthetic human pancreas growth hormone–releasing factor (hpGRF 1–44–NH2) stimulates growth hormone secretion in normal men. *J. Clin. Endocrinol. Metab.* 57:677–79
26. Chatelain, P., Cohen, H., Sassolas, G., Exclerc, J. L., Ruitton, A., et al. 1983. Somathormone plasmatique induite par la somatocrinine: Formes circulantes et active biologique. *Ann. Endocrinol.* 44: 159
27. Wood, S. M., Ch'ng, J. L. C., Adams, E. F., Webster, J. D., Joplin, G. F., et al. 1983. Abnormalities of growth hormone release in response to human pancreatic growth hormone releasing factor [GRF (1–44)] in acromegaly and hypopituitarism. *Br. Med. J.* 286:1687–91
28. Gelato, M. C., Pescovitz, O., Cassorla, F., Loriaux, D. L., Merriam, G. R. 1983. Effects of a growth hormone releasing factor in man. *J. Clin. Endocrinol. Metab.* 57:674–76
29. Losa, M., Stalla, G. K., Muller, O. A., von Werder, K. 1983. Human pancreatic

growth hormone-releasing factor (hpGRF): Dose-response of GRF- and GH- levels. *Klin. Wochenschr.* 61:1249–53
30. Thorner, M. O., Vance, M. L., Kaiser, D. L., Chitwood, J., Evans, W. S. 1984. Intravenous, subcutaneous, and intranasal administration of hpGRF-40 in normal men. *7th Int. Congress of Endocrinology, Quebec City,* p. 1415. Amsterdam: Excerpta Medica
31. Evans, W. S., Borges, J. L. C., Kaiser, D. L., Vance, M. L., Sellers, R. P., et al. 1983. Intranasal administration of human pancreatic tumor GH-releasing factor-40 stimulates GH release in normal men. *J. Clin. Endocrinol. Metab.* 57:1081–83
32. Almeida, O. F. X., Schulte, H. M., Rittmaster, R. S., Chrousos, G. P., Loriaux, D. L., et al. 1984. Potency and specificity of a growth hormone-releasing factor in a primate and *in vitro. J. Clin. Endocrinol. Metab.* 58:309–12
33. Wehrenberg, W. B., Ling, N., Bohlen, P., Esch, F., Brazeau, P., et al. 1982. Physiological roles of somatocrinin and somatostatin in the regulation of growth hormone secretion. *Biochem. Biophys. Res. Commun.* 109:562–67
34. Wehrenberg, W. B., Ling, N., Brazeau, P., Esch, F., Bohlen, P., et al. 1982. Somatocrinin, growth hormone releasing factor, stimulates secretion of growth hormone in anesthetized rats. *Biochem. Biophys, Res. Commun.* 109:382–87
35. Murphy, W. A., Lance, V. A., Sueiras-Diaz, J., Coy, G. H. 1983. Effects of secretin and gastric inhibitory polypeptide on human pancreatic growth hormone-releasing factor(1–40)–stimulated growth hormone levels in the rat. *Biochem. Biophys. Res. Commun.* 112: 469–74
36. Szabo, M., Dudlak, D., Thominet, J. L., Frohman, L. A. 1983. Ectopic growth hormone-releasing factor stimulates growth hormone secretion in the urethane-anesthetized rat in vivo. *Neuroendocrinology* 37:328–31
37. Chihara, K., Arimura, A., Schally, A. V. 1979. Immunoreactive somatostatin in rat hypophyseal portal blood: Effects of anesthetics. *Endocrinology* 104:1434–41
38. Tannenbaum, G. S., Epelbaum, J., Colle, E., Brazeau, P., Martin, J. B. 1978. Antiserum to somatostatin reverses starvation-induced inhibition of growth hormone but not insulin secretion. *Endocrinology* 102:1909–14
39. Tannenbaum, G. S., Martin, J. B. 1976. Evidence for an endogenous ultradian

rhythm governing growth hormone secretion in the rat. *Endocrinology* 98:562–70

40. Luben, R. A., Brazeau, P., Bohlen, P., Guillemin, R. 1982. Monoclonal antibodies to hypothalamic growth hormone–releasing factor with picomoles of antigen. *Science* 218:887–89

41. Wehrenberg, W. B., Brazeau, P., Luben, R., Bohlen, P., Guillemin, R. 1982. Inhibition of the pulsatile secretion of growth hormone by monoclonal antibodies to the hypothalamic growth releasing factor (GRF). *Endocrinology* 111:2147–48

42. Wehrenberg, W. B., Brazeau, P., Luben, R., Ling, N., Guillemin, R. 1983. A noninvasive functional lesion of the hypothalamo-pituitary axis for the study of growth hormone-releasing factor. *Neuroendocrinology* 36:489–91

43. Chihara, K., Minamitani, N., Kaji, H., Kodama, H., Kita, T., et al. 1983. Human pancreatic growth hormone-releasing factor stimulates release of growth hormone in conscious unrestrained male rabbits. *Endocrinology* 113:2081–85

44. Ohmura, E., Jansen, A., Chernick, V., Winter, J., Friesen, H. G., et al. 1984. Human pancreatic growth hormone releasing factor (hpGRF-1-40) stimulates GH release in the ovine fetus. *Endocrinology* 114:299–301

45. Baile, C. A., Della-Fera, M. A. 1984. An update on the roles for brain peptides in controlling behavior and metabolism. *Monsanto Techn. Symp. Fresno, Calif.*, pp. 13–34. St. Louis: Nutr. Chem. Div., Monsanto

46. Lance, V. A., Murphy, W. A., Sueiras-Diaz, J., Coy, D. H. 1984. Super-active analogs of growth hormone-releasing factor (1-29)-amide. *Biochem. Biophys. Res. Commun.* 119:265–72

47. Moseley, W. M., Krabill, L. F., Friedman, A. R., Olsen, R. F. 1984. Growth hormone response of steers injected with synthetic human pancreatic growth hormone-releasing factors. *J. Anim. Sci.* 58:430–35

48. Scanes, C. G., Carsia, R. V., Lauterio, T. J., Huybrechts, L., Rivier, J., et al. 1984. Synthetic human pancreatic growth hormone releasing factor (GRF) stimulates growth hormone secretion in the domestic fowl (*Gallus domesticus*). *Life Sci.* 34:1127–34

49. Leung, F. C., Taylor, J. E. 1983. In vivo and in vitro stimulation of growth hormone release in chickens by synthetic human pancreatic growth hormone releasing factor (hpGRFs). *Endocrinology* 113:1913–15

50. Proudman, J. A. 1984. Growth hormone and prolactin response to thyrotropin releasing hormone and growth hormone releasing factor in the immature turkey (41770). *Proc. Soc. Exp. Biol. Med.* 175:79–83

51. Peter, R. E., Nahorniak, C. S., Vale, W., Rivier, J. 1984. Human pancreatic growth hormone-releasing factor stimulates growth hormone release in goldfish. *J. Exp. Zool.* In press

52. Martin, J. B., Renaud, L. P., Brazeau, P. 1974. Pulsatile growth hormone secretion: Suppression by hypothalamic ventromedial lesions and by long-acting somatostatin. *Science* 186:538–40

53. Deleted in proof

54. Tannenbaum, G. S., Eikelboom, R., Ling, N. 1983. Human pancreas GH-releasing factor analog restores high-amplitude GH pulses in CNS lesion-induced GH deficiency. *Endocrinology* 113:1173–75

55. Wehrenberg, W. B., Bloch, B., Chong-Li, Z., Brazeau, P., Ling, N., et al. 1984. Pituitary response to growth hormone-releasing factor in rats with functional or anatomical lesions of the central nervous system that inhibit endogenous growth hormone secretion. *Reg. Peptides* 8:1–8

56. Deleted in proof

57. Wehrenberg, W. B., Bloch, B., Ling, N. 1985. Pituitary secretion of growth hormone in response to opioid peptides and opiates is mediated through growth hormone-releasing factor. *Neuroendocrinology* In press

58. Miki, N., Ono, M., Shizume, K. 1984. Evidence that opiatergic and α-adrenergic mechanisms stimulate rat growth hormone release via growth hormone-releasing factor (GRF). *Endocrinology* 114:1950–52

59. Deleted in proof

60. Sachar, E. J. 1975. Neuroendocrine abnormalities in depressive illness. In *Topics in Neuroendocrinology*, ed. E. J. Sachar, pp. 135–58. New York: Grune & Stratton.

61. Ducommun, P., Vale, W., Sakiz, E., Guillemin, R. 1967. Reversal of the inhibition of TSH secretion due to acute stress. *Endocrinology* 80:953–56

62. Wehrenberg, W. B., Baird, A., Ying, S. Y., Rivier, C., Ling, N., et al. 1984. Multiple stimulation of the adenohypophysis by combinations of hypothalamic releasing factors. *Endocrinology* 114:1995–2001

63. Arancibia, S., Epelbaum, J., Alonso, G., Assenmacher, I. 1983. Pulsatile secretion of somatostatin (SRIF) into the 3rd ventricle of unanesthetized rats. *C.R. Acad. Sci.* 296:47–52
64. Kasting, N. W., Martin, J. B., Arnold, M. A. 1981. Pulsatile somatostatin release from the median eminence of the unanesthetized rat and its relationship to plasma growth hormone levels. *Endocrinology* 109:1739–45
65. Brazeau, P., Rivier, W., Vale, W., Guillemin, R. 1974. Inhibition of growth hormone secretion in the rat by synthetic somatostatin. *Endocrinology* 94:184–87
66. Shibasaki, T., Shizume, K., Masuda, A., Nakahara, M., Hizuka, N., et al. 1984. Plasma growth hormone response to growth hormone-releasing factor in acromegalic patients. *J. Clin. Endocrinol. Metab.* 58:215–17
67. Rosenthal, S. M., Hulse, J. A., Kaplan, S. L., Grumbach, M. M. 1984. Exogenous growth hormone (GH) inhibits growth hormone releasing factor (GRF-44-NH)-induced GH secretion in normal men: Further evidence for GH autoregulation. See Ref. 30, p. 1144
68. Borges, J. L. C., Gelato, M. C., Rogol, A. D., Vance, M. L., MacLeod, R. M., et al. 1983. Effects of human pancreatic tumour growth hormone releasing factor on growth hormone and somatomedin C levels in patients with idiopathic growth hormone deficiency. *Lancet* 1:119–24
69. Grossman, A., Wass, J. A. H., Sueiras-Diaz, J., Savage, M. O., Lytras, N., et al. 1983. Growth-hormone-releasing factor in growth hormone deficiency: Demonstration of a hypothalamic defect in growth hormone release. *Lancet* 1:137–38
70. Takano, K., Hizuka, N., Shizume, K., Asakawa, K., Miyakawa, M., et al. 1984. Plasma growth hormone (GH) response to GH-releasing factor in normal children with short stature and patients with pituitary dwarfism. *J. Clin. Endocrinol. Metab.* 58:236–41
71. Pintor, C., Fanni, V., Loche, S., Locatelli, V., Cella, S. G., et al. 1983. Synthetic hpGRF 1-40 stimulates growth hormone and inhibits prolactin secretion in normal children and children with isolated growth hormone deficiency. *Peptides* 4:929–33
72. Pintor, C., Corda, R., Puggioni, R., Locatelli, V., Cella, S. G., et al. 1983. Prolactin-lowering effect of growth-hormone-releasing factor in children with growth-hormone deficiency. *Lancet* 1:1088–89

73. Bancroft, F. C., Levine, L., Tashjian, A. H. 1969. Control of growth hormone production by a clonal strain of rat pituitary cells: Stimulation by hydrocortisone. *J. Cell Biol.* 43:432
74. Shapiro, L., Samuels, H., Yaffee, B. 1979. Modulation of thyroid hormone nuclear receptor levels by 3'5' triiodo-L-thyronine in GH cell. *J. Biol. Chem.* 252:6052
75. Spindler, S., Mellon, S., Baxter, J. 1982. Growth hormone gene transcription is regulated by thyroid and glucocorticoid hormones in cultured rat pituitary tumor cells. *J. Biol. Chem.* 257:11627–32
76. Wehrenberg, W. B., Baird, A., Ling, N. 1983. Potent interaction between glucocorticoids and growth hormone–releasing factor in vivo. *Science* 221:556–58
77. Ruestow, P. C., Kramer, D. E., Szabo, M. 1984. Growth hormone (GH) response to systemic thyrotropin-releasing hormone (TRH) and GH-releasing factor (GRF) administration in rats: Effect of hypothyroidism and thyroid hormone replacement. See Ref. 30, p. 1145
78. Vale, W., Vaughan, J., Yamamoto, G., Spiess, J., Rivier, J. 1983. Effects of synthetic human pancreatic (tumor) GH releasing factor and somatostatin, triiodothyronine and dexamethasone on GH secretion *in vitro*. *Endocrinology* 112:1553–55
79. Somana, R., Visessuwan, S., Samridtong, A., Holland, R. C. 1978. Effect of neonatal androgen treatment and orchidectomy on pituitary levels of growth hormone in the rat. *J. Endocrinol.* 79:399–400
80. Eastman, C. J., Lazarus, L., Stuart, M. C., Casey, J. H. 1971. The effect of puberty on growth hormone secretion in boys with short stature and delayed adolescence. *Austr. NZ J. Med.* 1:154–59
81. Illig, R., Prader, A. 1970. Effect of testosterone on growth hormone secretion in patients with anorchia and delayed puberty. *J. Clin. Endocrinol. Metab.* 30:615–18
82. Jansson, J. O., Eriksson, E., Eden, S., Modigh, K. 1982. Effects of gonadectomy and testosterone replacement on growth hormone response to alpha-2 adrenergic stimulation in the male rat. *Psychoneuroendocrinology* 7:245–48
83. Shupnik, M. A., Baxter, L. A., French, L. R., Gorski, J. 1979. In vivo effects of estrogen on ovine pituitaries: Prolactin and growth hormone biosynthesis and

messenger ribonucleic acid translation. *Endocrinology* 104:729–35

84. Negro-Vilar, A., Ojeda, S. R., Advis, J. P., McCann, S. M. 1979. Evidence for noradrenergic involvement in episodic prolactin and growth hormone release in ovariectomized rats. *Endocrinology* 105:86–91

85. Wehrenberg, W. B., Baird, A., Ying, S. Y., Ling, N. 1985. The effects of testosterone and estrogen on the pituitary growth hormone response to growth hormone-releasing factor in rats. *Biol. Reprod.* In press

86. Murphy, W. A., Lance, V. A., Sueiras-Diaz, J., Coy, D. H. 1983. Effects of secretin and gastric inhibitory polypeptide on human pancreatic growth hormone-releasing factor (1-40)-stimulated growth hormone levels in the rat. *Biochem. Biophys, Res. Commun.* 112:469–74

87. Sharp, P. S., Foley, K., Chahal, P., Kohner, E. M. 1984. The effect of plasma glucose on the growth hormone response to human pancreatic growth hormone releasing factor in normal subjects. *Clin. Endocrinol.* 20:497–501

88. Masuda, A., Shibasaki, T., Shizume, K., Nakahara, M., Imaki, T., et al. 1985. The effect of glucose on growth hormone releasing factor-mediated GH secretion in man. *J. Clin. Endocrinol. Metab.* In press

89. Shibasaki, T., Shizume, K., Nakahara, M., Masuda, A., Jibiki, K., et al. 1984. Age-related changes in plasma growth hormone response to growth hormone-releasing factor in man. *J. Clin. Endocrinol. Metab.* 58:212–14

90. Wehrenberg, W. B., Ling, N. 1983. The absence of an age-related change in the pituitary response to growth hormone-

releasing factor in rats. *Neuroendocrinology* 37:463–66

91. Sonntag, W. E., Hylka, V. W., Meites, J. 1983. Impaired ability of old male rats to secrete growth hormone *in vivo* but not *in vitro* in response to hpGRF (1-44). *Endocrinology* 113:2305–7

92. Samson, W. K., Lumpkin, M. D., McCann, S. M. 1982. Motilin stimulates growth hormone release in vitro. *Brain Res. Bull.* 8:117–21

93. Samson, W. K., Lumpkin, M. D., Nilaver, G., McCann, S. M. 1984. Motilin: A novel growth hormone releasing agent. *Brain Res. Bull.* 12:57–62

94. Momany, F. A., Bowers, C. Y., Reynolds, G. A., Chang, D., Hong, A., et al. 1981. Design, synthesis and biological activity of peptides which release growth hormone *in vitro*. *Endocrinology* 108:31–39

95. Momany, F. A., Bowers, C. Y., Reynolds, G. A., Hong, A., Newlander, K. 1984. Conformational energy studies and *in vitro* and *in vivo* activity data on growth hormone-releasing peptides. *Endocrinology* 114:1531–36

96. Bowers, C. Y., Momany, F. A., Reynolds, G. A., Hong, A. 1984. On the *in vitro* and *in vivo* activity of a new synthetic hexapeptide that acts on the pituitary to specifically release growth hormone. *Endocrinology* 114:1537–45

97. Wehrenberg, W. B., Brazeau, P., Ling, N., Textor, G., Guillemin, R. 1984. Pituitary growth hormone response in rats during a 24-hour infusion of growth hormone-releasing factor. *Endocrinology* 114:1613–16

98. Wehrenberg, W. B., Bloch, B., Phillips, B. J. 1984. Antibodies to growth hormone-releasing factor inhibit somatic growth. *Endocrinology* 115:1218–20

Ann. Rev. Pharmacol. Toxicol. 1985. 25:485–508

THE CHEMOTHERAPY OF SCHISTOSOMIASIS

Sydney Archer

Cogswell Laboratory, Department of Chemistry, Rensselaer Polytechnic Institute, Troy, New York 12180

INTRODUCTION

Several major developments have occurred in the chemotherapy of schistosomiasis since Archer & Yarinsky reviewed the subject in 1972 (1). Perhaps the outstanding discovery has been the broad-spectrum, well-tolerated drug praziquantel, which is rapidly becoming the drug of choice in the treatment of schistosomiasis. Two other new broad-spectrum, clinically effective drugs that have made their appearance in recent years are oltipraz and amoscanate. We have also made some progress in understanding the mode of action of some of the older antischistosomal drugs such as hycanthone, oxamniquine, niridazole, and metrifonate, but little is known about the mechanism of action of the newer drugs. In order to focus attention on this problem, the Steering Committee of the Scientific Working Group on Schistosomiasis sponsored a symposium in Geneva January 30–February 1, 1984 (2) that was devoted exclusively to the biochemistry and chemotherapy of this disease. Wherever possible, this chapter devotes particular attention to the mode of action of clinically active agents and some of their relevant analogues.

HYCANTHONE

Hycanthone $\underline{2}$ has been shown to be a bioactive metabolite of lucanthone, $\underline{1}$. It is a potent antischistosomal drug when given orally, but it is more potent when administered parenterally. It is more active in hamsters than in mice against experimental *Schistosoma mansoni* infections (3, 4). It is clinically effective against *S. mansoni* and *S. haemotobium* infections when given in single intramuscular doses of about 3 mg/kg (1). Hycanthone is an antitumor agent in

485

0362-1642/85/415-0485$02.00

mice (5) and is a frameshift mutagen (6). It has been reported to be teratogenic (7) and possibly carcinogenic (8, 9).

The effects of lucanthone and hycanthone on nucleic acid and protein biosynthesis have been studied in bacterial and mammalian systems (10–12). The primary effect of both drugs is a pronounced but reversible inhibition of RNA synthesis; DNA and protein synthesis are affected to a lesser extent. Such effects are to be expected of intercalating drugs. It has been demonstrated that lucanthone and hycanthone intercalate into DNA (4, 13). Both drugs interfere with DNA-dependent RNA polymerase.

Hycanthone and lucanthone show delayed effects on schistosomes. Hepatic shifts with both drugs do not commence until about 72 hours after administration (14–16), yet almost all of the drugs disappear from the blood of the host 24 hours post-administration (17, 18). Despite indications that hycanthone and lucanthone have a similar mode of action, it is not clear why lucanthone has to be oxidatively metabolized before it exerts its schistosomicidal effects. The evidence that supports such a hypothesis has been summarized (1).

Recently, Cioli and his co-workers found that hycanthone inhibits the uptake of ^{3}H-uridine by adult hycanthone-sensitive *S. mansoni* worms (19), whereas under comparable experimental conditions lucanthone is ineffective in inhibiting uptake of this pyrimidine base by the schistosomes. These observations confirm the previously stated hypothesis concerning the bioconversion of 1 to 2. Cioli & Knopf (20) have studied the action of hycanthone both in vivo and in vitro using a new technique based on the transfer of schistosomes into the mesenteric veins of hamsters. They concluded that the action of 2 against *S. mansoni* is not due to a host-derived metabolite of hycanthone.

Cioli, Pica-Mattoccia, Rosenberg, & Archer (19) have proposed that the manifold effects of hycanthone can be accounted for on the basis of the mechanism of action shown in Figure 1.

Lucanthone, 1, is bio-oxidized to hycanthone, 2, as proposed earlier (5). The latter is converted enzymically to the ester, 3, presumably by either a kinase that results in the formation of a phosphate or by a sulfotransferase that affords a sulfate ester. The formation of the acetate ester from acetylCoA cannot be ruled out. Miller & Hulbert (21) suggest that under certain conditions hycanthone and hycanthone acetate may act as alkylating agents. In either case, 3 possesses a good leaving group that allows a non-enzymic dissociation to the ion 4-4a to occur. This ion intercalates into DNA and then monoalkylates this macromolecule to give the covalently bound drug-DNA complex, 5. In the case of hycanthone, these reactions occur in the mammalian host as well as in the schistosome. A similar mechanism has been proposed without supporting evidence to account for the mutagenic action of hycanthone (22). The mechanism shown in Figure 1 is compatible with the findings of Cioli & Knopf (20),

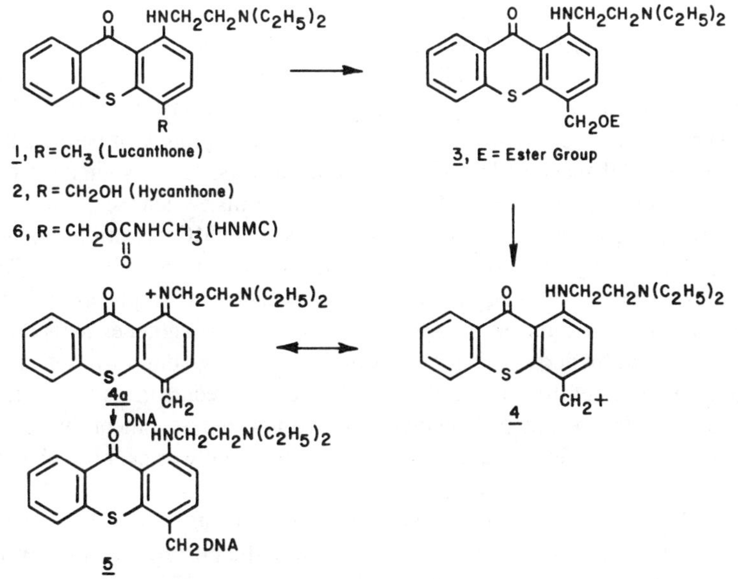

Figure 1   The mode of action of hycanthone

who concluded that the schistosomicidal activity of hycanthone does not depend on host bioactivation of the compound.

It has been known for some time that hycanthone and some of its congeners are antitumor agents (23, 24), but it is difficult to account for this property on the basis of intercalation alone. However, the mode of action shown in Figure 1 can also serve as the molecular basis for the antitumor activity of hycanthone.

In order to test this hypothesis, a surrogate, 6, of the ester, 3, was prepared because it was believed that sulfate or phosphate esters of 2 would be difficult to synthesize and use because of their high instability and reactivity. The N-methylcarbamate, 6 (HNMC), was readily prepared by treating hycanthone with methyl isocyanate (19).

The apparent association constant (Kapp) of the HNMC-calf thymus DNA complex is approximately fifteen times greater than that of the hycanthone-DNA complex, yet the ΔTm values of these complexes are nearly identical. Such observations can be rationalized on the basis of single-stranded DNA monoalkylation, as shown in Figure 1. Comparative dialysis experiments of these complexes showed that, in the time required for half of the hycanthone to dialyze away, only 2% of the HNMC dialyzes. The antitumor activities of 2 and HNMC in leukemic mice are almost identical, but HNMC exerts its action at one-tenth the dose of 2 and is also far more toxic. Such an increase in potency and toxicity could result from alkylation of DNA.

Cioli and coworkers have shown (25) that in adult hycanthone-sensitive *S*.

mansoni, hycanthone-induced inhibition of ^{3}H-uridine uptake is not reversed after removal of the drug from adult schistosomes but, in the case of hycanthone-resistant worms, ^{3}H-uridine uptake is restored after removal of the drug. According to the scheme outlined in Figure 1, hycanthone resistance is due to the absence of the enzyme that converts $\underline{2}$ to $\underline{3}$. Accordingly, it predicts that a surrogate of $\underline{3}$ that can undergo non-enzymic conversion to $\underline{4}$-$\underline{4a}$ in the schistosome should be active in hycanthone-resistant worms. When the above experiment is repeated with equimolar concentrations of HNMC, ^{3}H-uridine uptake is blocked in both hycanthone-sensitive and hycanthone-resistant worms. The in vitro experiments utilizing ^{3}H-uridine incorporation are duplicatible in vivo (26). *S. mansoni*–infected mice were treated with hycanthone; schistosomes were obtained by perfusion at various times after drug administration and the worms were tested for their ability to incorporate precursors of DNA, RNA, and protein. In hycanthone-sensitive adult worms precursor incorporation was inhibited, whereas in the case of immature or resistant worms, no such inhibition was noted. There was a close correlation between inhibition of macromolecule biosynthesis and parasite death. These results are also compatible with the mechanism shown in Figure 1, where the postulated lethal event is monoalkylation of schistosomal DNA.

When HNMC was administered in low doses (owing to the high toxicity of the drug) over a period of several days to mice infected with hycanthone-resistant *S. mansoni* worms, the mice were cured of their infection. Thus, HNMC is effective in vivo as well as in vitro.

It is well known that hycanthone has no effect on either immature *S. mansoni* or on adult *S. japonicum.* Recent experiments (27) on interbreeding between hycanthone-sensitive and hycanthone-resistant schistosomes have led to the conclusion that hycanthone resistance behaves like an autosomal recessive trait, which in turn suggests that hycanthone-resistant schistosomes are deficient in some factor(s). According to Figure 1, the missing factor is the enzyme that converts $\underline{2}$ to $\underline{3}$. A similar deficiency can account for the ineffectiveness of $\underline{2}$ in the immature *S. mansoni* and *S. japonicum.* Cioli and co-workers found that HNMC, $\underline{6}$, blocks ^{3}H-uridine uptake in both the immature forms of *S. mansoni* and the adult forms of *S. japonicum* (19). These results are compatible with the mechanism shown in Figure 1.

Thus far, the molecular mechanism of the mode of action of hycanthone as shown in Figure 1 can account for the manifold activities of the drug. Furthermore, the same mechanism can account for the cross-resistance with oxamniquine and IA-IV (16). Hillman and colleagues have suggested (28, 29) that hycanthone acts by binding irreversibly to the acetylcholine receptors of *S. mansoni.* This in turn leads to the paralysis of the digestive tract of the worm and eventual death by starvation. Although the evidence discussed above does not directly rule out such a hypothesis, it does not easily account for the many actions of hycanthone in mammalian and bacterial systems as well as in schistosomes by acetylcholine receptor blockade.

OXAMNIQUINE

A series of tetrahydroquinolines containing an aromatic methyl group adjacent to an electronegative substituent of the general formula 7 has been prepared in the laboratories of Pfizer Ltd. (30, 31). This group of compounds is closely related to the Mirasan analogue, Bayer 1593A, 8, (32).

7, X = NO$_2$, CN or Cl

R$_1$, R$_2$ = H or lower alkyl

8, Bayer 1593A

1.

The Pfizer compounds were active in *S. mansoni* infected mice; the most active member of the series was UK 3883 (7, X = NO$_2$, R$_1$ = H, R$_2$ = isopropyl). Armed with the knowledge that hycanthone is a metabolite of lucanthone and can be prepared by microbiological oxidation of 1 with *Aspergillus sclerotiorum* (1), the Pfizer group carried out a similar experiment on UK 3883 (33). They found that a similar conversion occurs that results in the formation of the hydroxymethyl analogue, oxamniquine, 9, which has proved to be a potent schistosomicide against experimental *S. mansoni* infections (34, 35). The drug is ineffective against *S. haemotobium* and *S. japonicum* infections (36, 37) but is a drug of choice in the treatment of *S. mansoni* infections in man (38). In South America, the recommended single oral dose is 12.5 mg/kg for patients weighing more than 40 kg and about 15 mg/kg for lighter individuals (39). In Zimbabwe, the dose necessary to achieve acceptable cure rates is 60 mg/kg given in four equal portions over a period of two days (40). This discrepancy in therapeutic regimens is probably a reflection of the differences in strain sensitivity to the drug. A large number of patients have been treated in Brazil with uniformly good cure rates at an acceptable level of mild side effects (41).

The genetic and mutagenic effects of oxamniquine are considerably weaker than those of hycanthone (42–44), but they are not entirely absent. Despite the fact that hycanthone and oxamniquine differ widely in their mutagenic potential, they are cross-resistant. In every case where hycanthone-resistant *S. mansoni* worms have been isolated from either man or animals, they have been found to be resistant to oxamniquine also (45–48). These observations suggest that the two drugs have a common mode of action with regard to their effect on

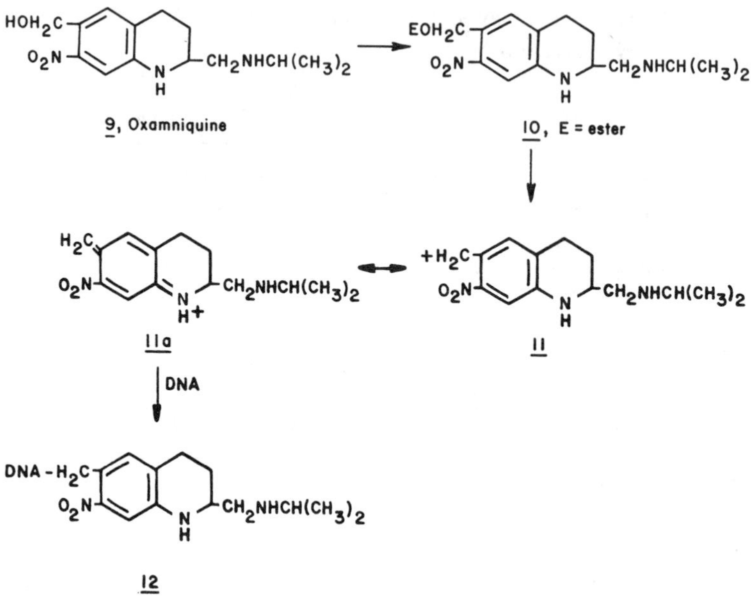

Figure 2 Proposed mode of action of oxamniquine

schistosomes. Accordingly, the scheme shown in Figure 2 has been proposed to account for the antischistosomal activity of oxamniquine.

As in the case of hycanthone, oxamniquine is enzymically converted, presumably by the same enzyme, to the ester, 10, where E is either a phosphate or a sulfate function. This species now possesses a good leaving group and may dissociate non-enzymically to give the ion 11-11a, which can alkylate DNA. The major difference between the mechanisms shown in Figures 1 and 4 is that in the latter case it is postulated that the ion 11-11a does not intercalate because oxamniquine does not possess a multiplanar ring system, which is a structural requirement for intercalation (49). Cioli (unpublished observations) has found that oxamniquine does not affect the Tm of calf thymus DNA, an observation that strongly supports the view that the drug is not an intercalating agent. Gale et al have remarked, "The most potent frameshift mutagens do seem to be intercalating agents, but whether intercalation is necessary for drug-induced mutagenesis (it is clearly not sufficient) or merely incidental remains to be established" (50). The lower mutagenic action of oxamniquine may be attributable to the fact that it is not an intercalating agent.

Recently, Cioli (51) has studied the effect of in vitro exposure of schistosomes to oxamniquine, hycanthone, and some related drugs on the in vivo survival of these worms. Adult hycanthone-sensitive *S. mansoni* worms were exposed for one hour at 37°C to concentrations of the drugs listed in Table 1. At

Table 1 Survival of *S. mansoni* transplanted into Nile rats after in vitro exposure to drugs

Drug	Concentration	Worm recovery relative to untreated controls (%)		Egg counts relative to untreated controls (%)	
		Total	Males only	Liver	Intestine
Oxamniquine	10 μg/ml	70	67	66	98
	20 μg/ml	37	26	52	36
	50 μg/ml	30	3	23	4
UK-3883	50 μg/ml	121	120	98	133
Hycanthone	0.5 μg/ml	23	0	11	0.1
Lucanthone	10 μg/ml	113	116	97	129

the end of 21–30 days, live worms were recovered and the schistosome eggs were counted.

At concentrations of 50 μg/ml oxamniquine causes a marked reduction in both worm recovery and egg counts but is far less potent than hycanthone. The corresponding methyl precursors, UK-3883, $\underline{7}$(X = NO$_2$, R$_1$ = H, R$_2$ = isopropyl), and lucanthone $\underline{1}$ are inactive. However, when UK-3883 and lucanthone are administered orally to *S. mansoni*–infected mice and the synthesis of macromolecules measured in vitro in worms obtained 1–3 days posttreatment, both drugs inhibit uptake of ^{3}H-thymidine. These results support the previous conclusion that both UK-3883 and lucanthone must be bio-oxidized to furnish the active metabolites, oxamniquine and hycanthone. The uptake of ^{3}H-uridine by hycanthone-resistant schistosomes is inhibited in the presence of oxamniquine, but the inhibition disappears when the worms are thoroughly washed prior to measurement of the uptake of the pyrimidine base. When *S. japonicum* worms are exposed to oxamniquine, similar results are obtained. The lack of activity of oxamniquine is due to a deficiency in these particular species of the enzyme necessary to convert oxamniquine to the ester $\underline{10}$ (Figure 2).

1A-IV

A series of benzothiopyrano (4.3.2-cd) indazoles has been prepared by Elslager and his associates according to the scheme shown in Figure 3 (52–55). Treatment of the dichlorothioxanthenone, $\underline{13}$, with the dialkylaminoalkyl hydrazines $\underline{14}$ furnishes the benothiopyranoindazoles $\underline{15}$. Microbiological conversion with *A. sclerotiorum* gives the desired analogues of hycanthone, $\underline{16}$. This procedure is identical to the one used in the original preparation of

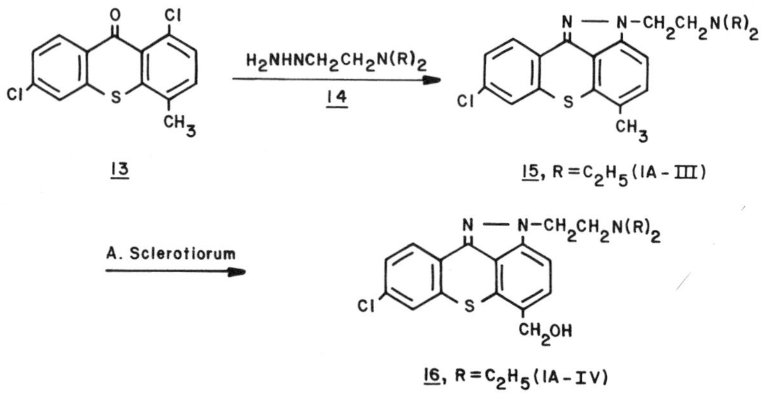

Figure 3   Synthesis of 1A-IV and analogues

hycanthone (1) except that, in the present instance, the hydrazines, 14, have been substituted for diethylaminoethylamine.

According to Elslager (55), 1A-IV and hycanthone are approximately equiactive when given intramuscularly, in the diet, or by gavage to mice infected with a Puerto Rican strain of *S. mansoni*. Single intramuscular injections of lucanthone or its analogue 1A-III (15, R = C_2H_5) have been ineffective in reducing the worm burden in hamsters, but hycanthone and 1A-IV have been curative in doses of 25–200 mg/kg. What is surprising is the observation that 1A-III, 1A-IV, and hycanthone are equally effective in mice when given in single intramuscular doses. Nevertheless, it has been concluded that 1A-IV is a bioactive metabolite of 1A-III.

Waring (56) has shown that 1A-III and 1A-IV reverse the supercoiling of closed circular duplex DNA and has concluded that these drugs are intercalating agents similar to lucanthone and hycanthone. The resemblance between hycanthone and 1A-IV is further strengthened by the finding that this pair of drugs is cross-resistant (57). Although the data on which to base a mechanism of action of 1A-IV are limited, it is tempting to postulate that 1A-IV and hycanthone act in a similar fashion, as shown in Figure 1.

The major difference between these drugs is that 1A-IV is claimed to be far less mutagenic than hycanthone (58, 59). Their mutagenic activity has been studied using the *S. typhimurium* strains TA-98 and TA-100 under in vitro and in vivo conditions. Waring (56) has commented that there does not appear to be a simple correlation between the ability of a drug to interact with DNA in the test tube and to induce mutagenesis in vivo. These observations can be rationalized on a molecular basis if we assume that 1A-IV is a poor substrate for the mammalian esterifying enzyme but a good one for the analogous enzyme in schistosomes. Investigations are in progress in the reviewer's laboratory to test this hypothesis.

PRAZIQUANTEL

A joint program sponsored by E. Merck, Darmstadt, and Bayer, A. G., on schistosomiasis chemotherapy has resulted in the discovery of the broad-spectrum schistosomicide, praziquantel, 18 (60). A vast literature of over 400 papers has appeared since the first publication on this drug, including a comprehensive review published in 1983 (61). Praziquantel is effective in mice, Syrian hamsters, and the multimammate rat, *mastomys natalenisis,* experimentally infected with *S. mansoni, S. haemotobium, S. japonicum, S. intercalatum,* and *S. matthei.* The drug is effective against young and adult *S. mansoni.* Praziquantel is active in monkeys and baboons infected with *S. haemotobium, S. mansoni,* and *S. japonicum* (62).

Extensive structure-activity studies have been carried out with a series of congeners of 18. The two most critical structural features of praziquantel are position -4 and position -2. An oxo group must be present at C-4; compounds with different substituents at this position are inactive in vivo and in vitro. Maximum activity has been observed when a cyclohexylcarbonyl group is present at position -2, but the p-aminobenzoyl and benzoyl analogues are also quite active. It should be noted that praziquantel possesses a chiral center at position $C-11b$. A precursor of 18 has been resolved and the optical isomers converted to $(+)$ and $(-)$ -praziquantel. Only the latter is biologically active (60, 61).

Praziquantel itself has a rapid onset of action both in vivo and in vitro. The drug appears to be less potent in mice than in larger animals, but this difference has been attributed to the relatively rapid drug elimination in mice (63).

A multi-center clinical trial of praziquantel was carried out using patients infected with *S. haemotobium, S. japonicum,* and *S. mansoni* in such countries as Brazil, Japan, the Philippines, and Zambia (64, 65). The initial double blind study used doses of 1×20 mg/kg, 2×20 mg/kg, and 3×20 mg/kg. This was followed by a single blind trial in Zambia using two different regimens; one employed a dose schedule of 3×20 mg/kg given at four-hour intervals and the other was a single oral dose of 50 mg/kg. Regardless of the dose regimen, there was only one failure in the 73 patients, who were followed for six months. Tolerance to the drug was very good. Since the initial clinical trials a number of other studies have been performed. The cure rates were uniformly excellent in all, regardless of the nature of the schistosome infection. The most common side effects are abdominal pain, headache, dizziness, and skin involvement, such as urticaria, which may be an allergic response to dying parasites. The currently recommended dosing schedules are: a single oral dose of 40 mg/kg for *S. haemotobium* and *S. mansoni* infections and 2×30 mg/kg given in divided doses in one day for *S. japonicum* (63). Praziquantel is well absorbed when given orally to man or animals. When ^{14}C-labelled drug is administered orally

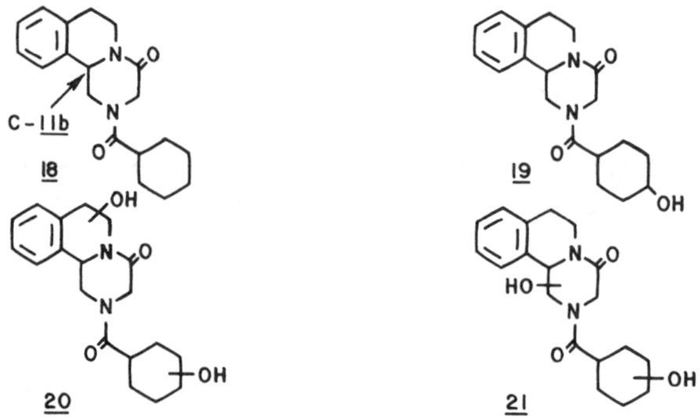

Figure 4   Metabolites of praziquantel

to volunteers in doses of either 20 mg/kg or 50 mg/kg, the maximum serum concentrations of unchanged praziquantel vary between 0.2 µg/ml and 1.0 µg/ml reached one to two hours post-administration. It was demonstrated earlier that at concentrations of 1 µg/ml the drug is lethal to adult *S. mansoni* worms (63). Praziquantel appears to be extensively metabolized, since only 5 to 7% of the total radioactivity present in the serum is unchanged drug. The half life of unchanged drug is about 1.5 hours. Between 80–85% of the ^{14}C-label is excreted via the kidney within four days. Thus, the drug and its metabolites are rapidly absorbed, rapidly metabolized, and rapidly eliminated. The major metabolite of 18 in man is the monohydroxylated compound 19, whose structure is secure. Two minor metabolites, probably derived by further oxidation of 19, are dihydroxylated derivatives, which on the basis of mass spectroscopic studies have been provisionally assigned structures 20 and 21 (see Figure 4) (63). In all likelihood, the position of the hydroxyl group in the cyclohexane ring of 20 and 21 is the same as it is in 19. The other hydroxyl in 21 is probably located at C−11b, because this is a benzylic carbon adjacent to a nitrogen atom.

Praziquantel is effective in patients infected with hycanthone- and oxamniquine-resistant *S. mansoni* (66). It is not mutagenic in a number of different species, including bacteria, yeasts, insects, and mammalian cells (67). The drug has no effect on DNA or protein synthesis and does not affect the uptake of nucleic acid precursors (63). On the basis of these observations, the mode of action of praziquantel clearly differs from those of hycanthone and oxamniquine.

Direct exposure of adult schistosomes to praziquantel results in immediate tetanic contraction of the musculature followed by a rapid vacuolization of the syncytial tegument. These effects occur at drug concentrations in the same range as therapeutic serum levels. In vitro, ^{14}C-praziquantel is rapidly taken up by schistosomes, but after transfer to a drug-free medium 93% of the radioactivity disappears from the worms. Although praziquantel is not an ionophor, the rapid contraction of the worms has been attributed to a change in calcium flux. In male schistosomes, praziquantel causes a rapid uptake of calcium ion with a concomitant loss of potassium. The muscle contractions can be abolished by lowering the ambient calcium ion levels or by increasing the concentration of magnesium ion (68). Vacuolization of the tegument is reversible and thus is not a lethal event (69). Death of the schistosome occurs when tegumental damage becomes severe and irreversible. Despite the body of evidence that points to the tegument as the locus of the schistosomicidal action of praziquantel, the exact mechanism whereby lethality is produced is not yet understood.

The general consensus at present is that praziquantel is effective orally in treating all human forms of schistosomiasis, is relatively well-tolerated, and thus far has produced no known cases of drug resistance. It is rapidly becoming the drug of choice for treating schistosomiasis.

OLTIPRAZ

Barreau and his colleagues synthesized oltipraz [4-methyl-5-(2-pyrazinyl)-1,2-dithiole-3-thione] 22 in 1976 (70). The drug is an effective schistosomicidal agent against experimental S. mansoni infections in mice and monkeys. In animals, oltipraz has little or no effect on the cardiovascular, respiratory, or central nervous systems. It responds negatively in the usual laboratory tests for mutagenic and immunosuppressant activity (71). In human S. mansoni infections, 3.0–4.5 g of the drug given in three divided doses in one day proved to be curative (72). Similar results have been reported from the Sudan. Two groups of young males were given 25 mg/kg and 35 mg/kg in two divided doses in one day. Cure rates of greater than 90% were observed. The most frequent side effects were vomiting and mild abdominal pain (73). Oltipraz is also effective in treating S. haemotobium and S. intercalatum infections. The most frequent side effects, in addition to those observed in other studies (73), are headache and paresthesias of the extremities, which appear to increase after exposure to sunlight. The cure rate in the S. haemotobium patients was 90% in those receiving a total dose of 25 mg/kg given in one or two days, and 87% in the S. intercalatum-infected patients, who received total doses ranging from 1.25 g –4.50 g over a three-day period. These clinical results suggest that oltipraz is a broad-spectrum, orally effective antischistosomal drug (74).

In contrast to praziquantel, oltripraz is a very slow-acting drug; approximately two months are required before the full schistosomicidal effects become manifest. One of the first signs of schistosomicidal activity of a drug in laboratory S. mansoni infections is the shift of the worms from their usual habitat in the mesenteric veins to the liver. This effect was first reported by Bang & Hairston in 1946 (75). In the case of oltipraz, the hepatic shift does not

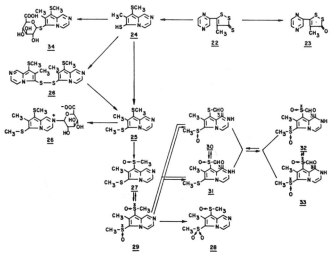

Figure 5 Metabolites of oltipraz

occur until nine days after drug administration (76). The first major effect of oltipraz observed is a reduction of schistosomal glutathione (GSH) levels. For example, two days after administration of 150 mg/kg of the drug to *S. mansoni*-infected mice, the GSH levels in the worm isolated from the mesenteric veins fall from 2.36 μM/g in untreated mice to 1.42 μM/g in those receiving the drug. This is a transient effect, since over the course of the next 15 days GSH levels return to control levels and then fall again. At higher doses, the GSH levels are depressed for several days before returning to normal, and at 250 mg/kg there does not appear to be any significant early reduction in GSH levels. However, at the higher doses, the initial control values are lower than normal. Despite these variable results, there does seem to be a distinct trend toward initial lowering of GSH levels in the schistosomes. In a series of oltipraz congeners, there seems to be a correlation between antischistosomal activity and lowering of GSH levels (Table 2).

Bieder and his associates have performed a thorough study of the metabolism of ^{14}C-oltipraz in rodents, monkeys, and man (77). Thirteen metabolites were isolated, purified, and identified. Their structures and interrelationships are shown in Figure 5.

With the exception of 23, which is the direct hydrolysis product of 27, all of the other metabolites result from a deep-seated rearrangement of oltripraz that this reviewer postulates to proceed via the unstable intermediate 24. The rest of the metabolites can be derived from 24, as shown in Figure 5. The percent distribution of the metabolites in rodents and monkeys is given in Table 3.

One possible mechanism that accounts for the formation of metabolites 25

Table 2 Antischistosomal activity and the effect on GSH of oltipraz congeners

Number	Structure	Antischis-tosomal activities	Single oral dose (mg/kg)	GSH levels[a]
35972 RP Oltipraz		+	250	1.42
36,642 RP		−	250	2.39
36,731 RP		−	250	2.42
37,528 RP		−	250	2.39
36,733 RP		+	50	1.70
38,650 RP		+	50	1.70
40,863 RP		−	200	2.37

[a]GSH content of worms two days after drug administration (μM/g). Control values were in the range 2.19–2.63 μM/g.

and 34 is shown in Figure 6. This differs from the scheme suggested by Bieder et al (77) in that GSH rather than CH_3S^- initiates the rearrangement. The methylation of the thiols can take place via well-known methyl transfer reactions. This scheme requires the intervention of mammalian glutathione, even though Bueding has been unable to show any reduced GSH levels in the host (76).

Very little is known about the mode of action of oltipraz. As far as this

Table 3   Percent distribution of the principal metabolites of ^{14}C-oltipraz in non-hydrolyzed urine[a]

Metabolites	Species		
	Mouse	Rat	Monkey
22, 23, 25, 26	9.4	14.4	7.9
27, 28	15.6	12.1	3.4
29	35.8	16.9	2.8
30	<1.0	2.0	8.1
31	8.2	26.1	15.2
32, 33	5.5	5.3	25.0
34, 35	20.5	23.2	47.6

[a]A possible mechanism to account for the formation of metabolites 25 and 34 is shown in Figure 6. This differs from the scheme suggested by Bieder et al (77) in that GSH rather than CH_3S^- initiates the rearrangement.

reviewer is aware, no studies have been reported on either the interaction of oltipraz with or the effect on the biosynthesis of macromolecules. Any proposed mechanism must account for the very slow onset of the drug and its effect on schistosomal GSH levels. It is tempting to suggest that a scheme slightly modified from that shown in Figure 6 can be used to account for the mode of action of oltipraz. As shown in this scheme, ring closure of 36 occurs by a nucleophilic attack of a pyrazine nitrogen atom on the carbon in the dithio ester, 36. In the schistosome this electrophilic carbon atom reacts with a macromolecule to give a covalently bound drug complex. If the macromolecule is an essential enzyme, then such a reaction could result in the slow death of the parasite. An investigation into the question of whether oltipraz does bind covalently in the schistosome would be a welcome test of the plausibility of this suggestion.

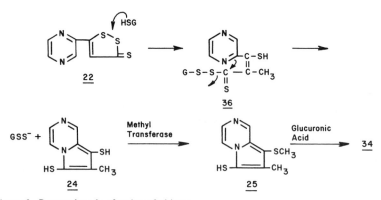

Figure 6   Proposed mode of action of oltipraz

NIRIDAZOLE

Niridazole, 39, a nitrothiazole, was first reported to have schistosomicidal activity over 20 years ago (78). The early studies were reviewed in 1972 (1); thus, this review deals with more recent developments.

The drug is an effective schistosomicide against *S. mansoni, S. haemotobium,* and *S. japonicum* infections in man (78, 79). The usual dose is 25–30 mg/kg given over a period of five to ten days. Factors other than the need for multiple dosing and the occurrence of occasional severe CNS side effects, which militate against the clinical acceptability of niridazole, are immunosuppression (80), mutagenicity, and carcinogenicity (81–81b). Recent studies support the hypothesis that some of the side effects of niridazole, in addition to its effectiveness as an antischistosomal compound, are related to the metabolism of the drug (82).

Faigle & Kebule showed that schistosomes absorb ^{14}C-niridazole and convert it to unidentified metabolites (83). Tracy, Catto, & Webster found that the radio label is bound covalently to schistosomal macromolecules (84). For example, when adult *S. mansoni* worm pairs are incubated with 70 μM of ^{14}C-niridazole for sixteen hours, about 30% of the total radioactivity that the parasites incorporate is precipitable with trichloroacetic acid (TCA). Vigorous attempts to dissociate the radiolabel from the TCA-precipitated material have been unsuccessful. About 85–90% of the radioactivity is associated with the protein fractions, 3–5% with RNA, and 4–7% with DNA. When this experiment is carried out in *S. mansoni*-infected mice, about 43% of the total parasite radio label is covalently bound to the macromolecular fraction, showing that covalent drug binding occurs under therapeutic conditions as well as in vitro.

| 39 | 40 | 41 | 2. |

Covalent drug binding has been demonstrated using cell-free schistosome preparations. Under these conditions, it has been found that the initial step in the metabolism of niridazole involves an NADPH-dependent enzymatic reduction of the nitro group. Such a reduction may lead to an as yet unidentified drug metabolite that can bind covalently to schistosomal macromolecules. 4'-Methylniridazole, 40, is inactive as a schistosomicide (84). The compound is taken up by adult worms but, in contrast to niridazole, 40, is recovered unchanged. Thus, 40 is not a substrate for schistosomal nitro-reductase. Blumer et al (85) found that the antibiotic and mutagenic activities of niridazole toward auxotrophs of *S. typhimurium* are linked to the levels of bacterial nitro

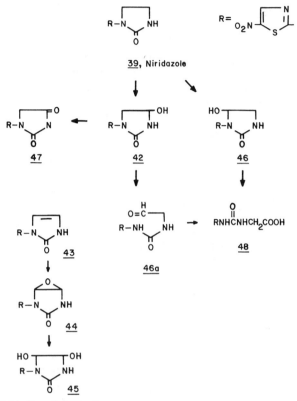

Figure 7   Metabolism of niridazole

reductase. Resistant strains are less sensitive to the mutagenic effects of the drug and have lower levels of nitro reductase.

An immunosuppressive metabolite was isolated from the urine of rats and of a patient treated with niridazole (86). The compound was subsequently shown to be 41 (87, 88). The compound is not formed in the liver but is produced by intestinal flora (89). Most, if not all, of the immunosuppressant action of 39 is due to this metabolite (90).

In contrast to the reductive metabolism of niridazole that is the predominant pathway in the schistosome, mammalian metabolism of the drug is oxidative in nature (82, 87). Hepatic microsomes obtained from DBA/2J mice were incubated with either niridazole or its metabolites in the presence of NADPH. Ethyl acetate extracts of the mixtures were analyzed by high-performance liquid chromatography (hplc). The oxidative metabolic pathway is shown in Figure 7.

Niridazole is hydroxylated to give 4- and 5-hydroxyniridazole (42 and 46 respectively). The former is dehydrated to afford 4,5-dehydroniridazole, 43, which is oxidized to the epoxide, 44. Finally, 44 is hydrated to give the diol, 45. 4-Ketoniridazole, 47, is formed from 4-hydroxyniridazole and not from either the dehydro derivative, 43, or the epoxide 44. 4-Hydroxyniridazole, 46, exists in tautomeric equilibrium with the open-chain form 46a, which is oxidized to the hydantoic acid, 48, by means of a NAD^+-dependent aldehyde dehydrogenase.

The delayed CNS toxicity that is an occasional toxic manifestation of niridazole therapy may be due to a metabolite rather than to the drug itself (87). 4-Ketoniridazole, 47, is more potent than niridazole in producing CNS toxicity, but the overt signs are different (91). On the other hand, the delayed onset of CNS toxicity has been correlated with oxidative metabolism of the drug.

The microsomal oxidative metabolism of ^{14}C-niridazole leads to covalent drug binding, and the requirements for such binding are the same as those necessary for oxidative metabolism. The 4,5-diol, 45, is the only stable end product of the microsomal oxidation of 4,5-dehydroniridazole, 43. Blumer et al have suggested that the reactive epoxide, 44, may be responsible for niridazole-induced tumor formation (85). The recent investigations of Webster and his colleagues (82) have established in part the molecular basis both for the antischistosomal action of niridazole and for the toxic effects of the drug. Although the proximate active metabolites remain to be identified, it is clear that the pathways leading to the antischistosomal action are different from those leading to the toxic effects of the drug.

AMOSCANATE

In 1976, Striebel (92) reported that 4'-isothiocyanato-4'-nitrodiphenylamine, amoscanate, 49, was an anthelmintic, active against intestinal nematodes, filariae, and schistosomes.

O_2N—⟨ ⟩—NH—⟨ ⟩—NCS

49, Amoscanate   3.

The yellow crystalline compound is insoluble in water and common organic solvents. This lack of solubility has created problems from the beginning with respect to proper dosage forms of the drug. The first experimental studies were carried out with material having a particle size of 30–50 μm. The curative single oral dose against *S. mansoni* in mice was 300 mg/kg. When micronized material was used, this dose dropped to 120 mg/kg. Ball mill treatment for 14 days in a suspension of 1% Cremophor EL (BASF) and 25% glycerol reduced the particle size to 0.5 μm. With particles of this size, the curative dose was 5–7.5 mg/kg (94). Amoscanate is active against hycanthone-resistant strains of

S. mansoni. Bueding also has reported that amoscanate is not mutagenic when tested against Salmonella strains TA-98 and TA-100 in either the presence or absence of liver microsomes (93). However, six species of mammals receiving 49 excreted an unidentified mutagenic metabolite probably produced by intestinal flora rather than by the metabolic action of the hosts (94).

Amoscanate has proved effective in experimental *S. haemotobium* and *S. japonicum* infections in mice (92) and is active in monkeys against the three common human forms of schistosomiasis. It does not produce any major organ toxicity (95). The drug is also active in humans (96).

Little is known about either the metabolic fate or the mode of action of amoscanate. Striebel (96a) has reported that the compound binds irreversibly to the amino groups of amino acids and proteins in vitro and in vivo by reaction with the isothiocyanate to form thiourea derivatives. About 80% of the drug in plasma is precipitated by perchloric acid and is not extractable with acetone. Presumably, the drug is covalently linked to plasma proteins.

Voge & Bueding have studied the tegumental alterations in *S. mansoni* induced by subcurative doses of amoscanate by means of scanning electron microscopy (97). The changes noted include swelling, constriction, and erosion of large surface areas. Most of the lesions were completely repaired 62 days after exposure to the drug. The authors raise the question of whether these surface changes are the result of drug-induced functional damage regardless of the type of drug used.

METRIFONATE

Metrifonate (trichlorfon, bilarcil) is an organophosphorous compound that by virtue of its inhibitory affect on cholinesterases has been used as an insecticide under the names Dipterex and Dylox. The compound is an effective schistosomicide in animals (98–100).

$$CCl_3CHONP(OCH_3)_2 \longrightarrow Cl_2C=CHOP(OCH_3)_2$$

50, Metrifonate   51, Dichlorvos   4.

Whatever side effects are produced result from the expected depression of plasma cholinesterase levels. The drug shows moderately high host-mediated mutagenic activity in *S. typhimurium* strain TA-100 (11) but is neither teratogenic nor carcinogenic in healthy rats and dogs (101).

It is generally believed that the schistosomicidal activity of metrifonate is not mediated via the drug itself but by its metabolite, dichlorvos, 51, which is a far more potent inhibitor of cholinesterase (102–104). The potency of metrifonate increases with pH and time, factors that do not affect the activity of 51. After metrifonate administration to patients, the plasma levels of 50 and 51 were 31 μM and 0.3 μM respectively. This level of dichlorvos is sufficient to cause a substantial inhibition of cholinesterase within fifteen minutes.

The most surprising aspect of the therapeutic profile of metrifonate is that the drug does not appear to be effective against human *S. mansoni* infections but it is quite active against *S. haemotobium* in man despite the fact that both species of schistosomes are susceptible to the drug in vitro (102, 105). The reasons for this discrepancy are not clear.

CONCLUDING COMMENTS

During the past fifteen years, major advances have occurred in the chemotherapy of schistosomiasis. Three new broad-spectrum compounds, amoscanate, oltipraz, and praziquantel, have appeared on the therapeutic horizon. Praziquantel has had extensive clinical use and has established itself as a drug of choice for the treatment of all human forms of the disease. These drugs emerged from routine screening of compounds: the serendipitous method of drug discovery has again produced active compounds. Unfortunately, the mechanisms by which these drugs exert their effects are not known. Considerable progress has been made with regard to the molecular basis for the action of two drugs that have fallen out of clinical favor in recent years, namely, hycanthone and niridazole. Insights into the modes of action of these drugs can be exploited to design new molecules free of the undesirable effects of the parent drugs. This has been accomplished inadvertantly in the case of oxamniquine. Its mechanism of action in schistosomes is thought to be almost identical with that of hycanthone but, because of highly significant structural differences, its mammalian effects are far more benign.

Investigators have begun to apply rational design to the chemotherapy of schistosomiasis. elKouni and his colleagues (106) have shown that the pathways in de novo pyrimidine biosynthesis in *S. mansoni* differ from the mammalian pathway. This difference, as well as some others, can be exploited by offering the chemist targets for new synthetic enzyme inhibitors.

Finally, from the clinical standpoint, the future looks brighter than ever for the more than 200 million individuals who suffer from schistosomiasis. The newer drugs can be given in one or two doses and are reasonably well-tolerated. As a result, widespread clinical therapy is now possible for the first time.

ACKNOWLEDGMENTS

I wish to thank Dr. Leslie Webster Jr. and Dr. James Tracy for supplying me with pre-prints of their papers and permission to quote from them, and the

World Health Organization for financial support. I am greatly indebted to Dr. Donato Cioli not only for allowing me to quote from papers in press, but also for many stimulating conversations.

Literature Cited

1. Archer, S., Yarinsky, A. 1972. Recent developments in the chemotherapy of schistosomiasis. In *Progress in Drug Research*, ed. E. Jucker, 16:11–67. Basel/Stuttgart: Birkhauser. 472 pp.
2. Steering Committee, Scientific Working Group in Schistosomiasis, sponsored by the UN Develop. Prog.; World Bank; World Health Organization, Special Programme for Research and Training in Tropical Diseases. 1984. *Symp. Biochem. Chemother. Schistosomiasis, Geneva, Jan. 1984*
3. Rosi, D., Peruzzotti, G., Dennis, E. W., Berberian, D. A., Freele, H., Archer, S. 1965. A new, active metabolite of Miracil D. *Nature* 208:1005–6
4. Rosi, D., Peruzzotti, G., Dennis, E. W., Berberian, D. A., Freele, H., et al. 1967. Hycanthone, a new, active metabolite of lucanthone. *J. Med. Chem.* 10:867–76
5. Hirschberg, E. 1975. Thioxanthenones: Miracil D and hycanthone. In *Mechanism of Action of Antimicrobial and Antitumor Agents*, ed. J. W. Corcoran, F. E. Hahn, 3:274–303. Berlin/Heidelberg: Springer-Verlag. 742 pp.
6. Hartman, P. E., Levine, E., Hartman, Z., Berger, H. 1971. Hycanthone: A frameshift mutagen. *Science* 172:1058–60
7. Moore, J. A. 1972. Teratogenicity of hycanthone in mice. *Nature* 239:107–9
8. Haese, W. H., Smith, D. L., Bueding, E. 1973. Hycanthone-induced hepatic changes in mice infected with *Schistosoma mansoni*. *J. Pharmacol. Exp. Ther.* 186:430–38
9. Yarinsky, A., Drobeck, H. P., Freele, H., Wiland, J., Gumaer, K. L. 1974. An 18-month study of parasitologenic and tumorigenic effects of hycanthone in *Schistosoma mansoni*-infected and non-infected mice. *Toxicol. Appl. Pharmacol.* 27:169–87
10. Bases, R., Mendez, F. 1969. Reversible inhibition of ribosomal RNA synthesis in Hela by lucanthone (Miracil D) with continued synthesis of DNA-like RNA. *J. Cell Physiol.* 74:283–94
11. Weinstein, I. B., Carchman, R., Marner, E., Hirschberg, E. 1967. Miracil D: Effects on nucleic acid synthesis, protein synthesis and enzyme induction in

Escherichia coli. Biochim. Biophys. Acta 142:440–49
12. Wittner, M., Tanowitz, H., Rosenbaum, M. 1971. Studies with the schistosomicide hycanthone. Inhibition of macromolecular synthesis and its reversal. *Exp. Mol. Pathol.* 14:124–33
13. Waring, M. 1971. Binding of drugs to supercoiled circular DNA; Evidence for and against intercalation. In *Progress in Molecular and Subcellular Biology*, ed. F. E. Hahn, 2:216–31. New York: Springer-Verlag
14. Khayyal, M. T., Girgis, N. L., Henry, W. 1969. Effectiveness of a single dose of hycanthone orally in experimental schistosomiasis in hamsters. *Bull. WHO* 40:963–65
15. Jewsburg, J. M., Homewood, C. A., Gibson, J. 1974. The effect of hycanthone on the distribution of *Schistosoma mansoni* in the mouse. *Ann. Trop. Med. Parasitol.* 65:365–66
16. Senft, A. W., Senft, D. G., Hillman, G. R., Polk, D., Kryger, S. 1976. Influence of hycanthone on morphology and serotonin uptake of *Schistosoma mansoni*. *Trop. Med. Hyg.* 25:832–40
17. Yarinsky, A., Hernandez, P., Dennis, E. W. 1970. The uptake of tritiated hycanthone by male and female *Schistosoma mansoni* worms and distribution of the drug in plasma and whole blood of mice following a single intramuscular injection. *Bull. WHO* 42:445–49
18. Hernandez, P. E., Dennis, E. W., Farah, A. 1971. Metabolism of the schistosomicidal agent hycanthone by rat and rhesus monkeys. *Bull. WHO* 48:27–34
19. Cioli, D., Pica-Mattoccia, L., Rosenberg, S., Archer, S. 1984. Hypothesis on the mode of action of the schistosomicidal drug, hycanthone. *Life Sci.* In press
20. Cioli, D., Knopf, P. M. 1980. A study of the mode of action of hycanthone against *Schistosoma mansoni in vivo* and *in vitro*. *Am. J. Trop. Med. Hyg.* 29:220–26
21. Miller, J. L., Hulbert, P. B. 1976. Hycanthone an alkylating agent. *J. Pharm. Pharmacol.* 28:18 (Suppl.)
22. Hartman, P. E., Hulbert, P. B. 1975. Genetic activity spectra of some antischistosomal compounds with particular emphasis on thioxanthenones and ben-

zothiopyranoindazoles. *J. Toxicol. Environ. Health* 2:243–70

23. Archer, S., Miller, K. J., Rej, R., Periana, C., Fricker, L. 1982. Ring hydroxylated analogues of lucanthone as antitumor agents. *J. Med. Chem.* 25: 220–27

24. Archer, S., Zayed, A.-H., Rej, R., Rugino, T. A. 1983. Analogues of hycanthone and lucanthone as antitumor agents. *J. Med. Chem.* 26:1240–46

25. Pica-Mattoccia, L., Lelli, A., Cioli, D. 1981. Effect of hycanthone on *Schistosoma mansoni* macromolecular synthesis *in vitro*. *Mol. Biochem. Parasitol.* 2: 295–307

26. Pica-Mattoccia, L., Cioli, D. 1983. Effect of hycanthone administered *in vivo* upon the incorporation of radioactive precursors into macromolecules of *Schistosoma mansoni*. *Mol. Biochem. Parasitol.* 8:99–107

27. Cioli, D., Pica-Mattoccia, L. 1984. Genetic analysis of hycanthone resistance in *Schistosoma mansoni*. *Am. J. Trop. Med. Hyg.* 33:80–88

28. Hillman, G. R., Senft, A. W. 1975. Anticholinergic properties of the antischistosomal drug hycanthone. *Am. J. Trop. Med. Hyg.* 24:827–34

29. Hillman, G. R., Senft, A. W., Gibler, W. B. 1978. The mode of action of hycanthone revisited. *J. Parasitol.* 64: 754–56

30. Baxter, C. A. R., Richards, H. C. 1971. Schistosomicides. 1. Derivatives of 2-aminomethyl - 1,2,3,4 - tetrahydroquinoline. *J. Med. Chem.* 14:1033–42

31. Richards, H. C., Foster, R. 1969. New series of 2-aminomethyl-tetrahydroquinoline derivatives displaying schistosomicidal activity in rodents and primates. *Nature* 222:581–82

32. Gonnert, R. 1961. The structure-activity relationship in several schistosomicidal compounds. *Bull. WHO* 25:702–6

33. Kaye, B., Woolhouse, N. M. 1972. The metabolism of a new schistosomicide 2 - isopropylamino - 6 - methyl - 7 - nitro-1,2,3,4-tetrahydroquinoline (UK-3883). *Xenobiotica* 2:169–78

34. Foster, R., Cheetam, B. L., King, B. L. 1973. Schistosomicide oxamniquine (UK-4271)II. Activity in primates. *Trans. R. Soc. Trop. Med. Hyg.* 67: 685

35. Foster, R., Cheetam, B. L. 1973. Studies with the schistosomicide oxamniquine (UK-4271). I. Activity in rodents and *in vitro*. *Trans. R. Soc. Trop. Med. Hyg.* 67:674–82

36. Pica-Mattoccia, L., Cioli, D. 1984. Studies on the mode of action of oxamniquine and related schistosomicidal drugs. *Am. J. Trop. Med. Hyg.* In press

37. Yarinsky, A., Hernandez, P., Ferrari, R. A., Freele, H. W. 1972. Effects of hycanthone against two strains of S. japonicum in mice. *Jpn. J. Parasitol.* 21: 101–8

38. Nash, T. G., Cheever, A. W., Ottensen, E. A., Cook, J. A. 1982. Schistosomal infections in humans: Perspective and recent findings. *Ann. Int. Med.* 97:740–54

39. Miller, M. J. 1976. Protozoan and helminth parasites; a review of current treatment. *Prog. Drug Res.* 20:433–64

40. Clarke, V. deV., Blair, D. M., Weber, M. C., Garneth, P. A. 1976. Dose finding trials of oral oxamniquine in Rhodesia. *S. Afr. Med. J.* 50:1867–71

41. Almeida Machado, P. 1982. The Brazilian program for schistosomiasis control, 1975–79. *Am. J. Trop. Med. Hyg.* 31:76–86

42. Ray, V. A., Holden, N. E., Ellis, J. H., Hynech, M. 1975. A comparative study on the genetic effects of hycanthone and oxamniquine. *J. Toxicol. Environ. Health* 1:211–27

43. Haese, W. H., Bueding, E. 1976. Long term hepatocellular effects of hycanthone and of two other antischistosomal drugs in mice infected with S. mansoni. *J. Pharmacol. Exp. Ther.* 197:703–12

44. Batzinger, R. P., Bueding, E. 1977. Mutagenic activities *in vitro* and *in vivo* of five antischistosomal compounds. *J. Pharmacol. Exp. Ther.* 200:1–9

45. Rogers, S. H., Bueding, E. 1971. Hycanthone resistance: Development in S. mansoni. *Science* 172:1057–58

46. Jansma, W. B., Rogers, S. W., Lire, C. L., Bueding, E. 1977. Experimentally produced resistance of S. mansoni to hycanthone. *Am. J. Trop. Med. Hyg.* 26:926–30

47. Katz, N., Dias, E. P., Aranjo, N., Souza, C. P. 1973. Estudo de uma cepa memana de S. mansoni resistente a agentes esquistosomicidas. *Rev. Soc. Brasil Med. Trop.* 7:381–87

48. Dias, L. C. S., Pedro, R. J., Debelardini, R. 1982. Use of praziquantel in patients with *schistosomiasis mansoni* previously treated with oxamniquine or hycanthone. *Trans. R. Soc. Trop. Med. Hyg.* 76:652–59

49. Deleted in proof

50. Waring, M., E. F. Gale, E. Cundliffe, D. E. Reynolds, M. H. Richmond, M. Waring. 1980. *The Molecular Basis for Antibiotic Action*. London/New York: Wiley. 646 pp. 2nd ed.

51. Pica-Mattoccia, P., Cioli D. 1984. Studies on the mode of action of oxamniquine and related schistosomicidal drugs. *Am. J. Trop. Med. Hyg.* In press

52. Elslager, E. F. 1970. Chemotherapy of schistosomiasis: Progress at a snail's pace. *Jpn. J. Trop. Med. Hyg.* 11:34–37

53. Elslager, E. F. 1970. 2H-[1]Benzothiopyrano[4,3,2-cd]indazole compounds. *US Patent 3,505,341*. April 7

54. Elslager, E. F. 1976. Benzo and benzothiopyranoindazole N-oxides. *US Patent 3,963,740*. June 15

55. Elslager, E. F. 1977. Benzo and benzothiopyranoindazole N-oxides. *US Patent 4,026,899*. May 31

56. Waring, M. 1973. Interaction of indazole analogs of lucanthone and hycanthone with closed circular duplex deoxyribonucleic acid. *J. Pharmacol. Exp. Ther.* 186:385–89

57. Werbel, L. M. 1975. Progress and prospects in the conquest of schistosomiasis. *Isr. J. Chem.* 14:185–92

58. Hulbert, P. B., Bueding, E., Hartman, P. E. 1976. Hycanthone analogs: Dissociation of mutagenic effects from antischistosomal effects. *Science* 186:647–48

59. Bueding, E. 1975. Dissociation of mutagenic and other toxic properties from schistosomicides. *J. Toxicol. Environ. Health* 1:329–34

60. Seubert, J., Pohlke, R., Loebich, F. 1977. Synthesis and properties of praziquantel, a novel broad-spectrum anthelmintic with excellent activity against schistosomes and cestodes. *Experientia* 33:1036–37

61. Andrews, P., Thomas, H., Pohlke, R., Seubert, J. 1983. Praziquantel. *Med. Res. Rev.* 3:147–200

62. Webbe, G., Janeus, E., Nelson, G. S., Sturock, R. F. 1981. The effect of praziquantel on *Schistosoma haemotobium, S. japonicum* and *S. mansoni* in primates. *Arzneimit. Forsch.* 31:542–44

63. Andrews, P. 1981. A summary of the efficacy of praziquantel against schistosomes in animal experiments and notes on its mode of action. *Arzneitmit. Forsch.* 31:538–41

64. Davis, A., Wagner, D. H. G. 1979. Multicentre trails of praziquantel in human schistosomiasis: Design and techniques. *Bull. WHO* 57:767–71

65. Davis, A., Biles, J. E., Ulrich, A.-M. 1979. Initial experiences with praziquantel in the treatment of human infections due to *Schistosoma haemotobium*. *Bull. WHO* 57:773–79

66. Dias, L. E. de S., Pedro, R. de J., Deberaldini, E. R. 1982. Use of prazequantil in patients with *Schistosomiasis mansoni* previously treated with oxamniquine and/or hycanthone: Resistance of *Schistosoma mansoni* to schistosomicidal agents. *Trans. R. Soc. Trop. Med. Hyg.* 76:652–59

67. Bartsch, H., Kuroki, T., Malaveille, C., Loprieno, N., Barale, R., et al. 1978. Absence of mutagenicity of praziquantel, a new, effective antischistosomal drug, in bacteria, yeasts, insects, and mammalian cells. *Mutation Res.* 58:133–42

68. Pax, R., Bennett, J. L., Fetterer, R. 1978. A benzodiazepine derivative and praziquantel: Effects on musculature of *Schistosoma mansoni* and *Schistosoma japonicum*. *Naunyn Schmiedebergs Arch. Exp. Pharmakol.* 304:309–15

69. Mehlhorn, H., Becker, B., Andrews, P., Thomas, H., Frenkel, J. K. 1981. *In vivo* and *in vitro* experiments on the effects of praziquantel on Schistosoma mansoni. *Arzneimit. Forsch.* 31:544–54

70. Barreau, M., Cotrel, C., Jeanmart, C. 1977. 1,2-Dithiolethiones. *Chem. Abstr.* 87:593, *152171r*

71. LeRoy, J. P., Barreau, M., Cotrel, C., Jeanmart, C., Messer, M., Benazet, F. 1978. Laboratory studies of 35972 R. P. A new schistosomicidal compound. In *Current Chemotherapy—Proc. 10th Intl. Congr. Chemother.* ed. W. Siegenthaler, R. Luthy, 1:148–50. Washington, DC: Am. Soc. Microbiol.

72. Pieron, R., Lesobre, B., Mafart, Y., Lancastre, F. 1980. Effaits de l'oltipraz en traitment bref dans la bilharziose. *Med. Trop.* 40:302–11

73. Bella, H., Rahim, A. G. A., Mustafa, M. D., Ahmed, M. A. M., Wasfi, S., Bennett, J. L. 1982. Oltipraz-antischistosomal efficacy in Sudanese infected with *Schistosoma mansoni*. *Am. J. Trop. Med. Hyg.* 31:775–78

74. Gentilini, M., Duflo, B., Richard-Lenoble, D., Brucker, G., Danis, M., et al. 1980. Assessment of 35972 RP (oltipraz), a new antischistosomal drug against *Schistosoma haemotobium, Schistosoma mansoni* and *Schistosoma intercalatum*. *Acta Tropica* 37:271–74

75. Bang, F. B., Hairston, N. G. 1946. Chemotherapy of experimental *Schistosomiasis japonica*. *Am. J. Hyg.* 44:349–66

76. Bueding, E., Dolan, P., LeRoy, J. P. 1982. The antischistosomal activity of oltipraz. *Res. Commun. Chem. Pathol. Pharmacol.* 37:293–303

77. Bieder, A., Decouvelaere, B., Gaillard, C., Depaire, H., Heusse, D., et al. 1983. Comparison of the metabolism of oltipraz

in the mouse, rat, monkey and in man. *Arzneimit. Forsch.* 33:1289–97

78. Lambert, C. R., Wilhelm, M., Stroebel, H., Kradolfer, F., Schmidt, P. 1964. A new compound active against bilharziasis and amebiasis. *Experimentia* 20:452

79. Katz, N. 1977. Chemotherapy of *Schistosomiasis mansoni. Adv. Pharmacol. Chemother.* 14:1–70

80. Webster, L. T. Jr., Butterworth, A. E., Mahmoud, A. A. F., Mingola, E. N., Warren, K. W. 1975. Suppression of delayed hypersensitivity in schistosome-infected patients by niridazole. *New Engl. J. Med.* 292:1144–47

81. Urman, H. K., Bulay, O., Clayson, D. B., Shubik, P. 1975. Carcinogenic effects of niridazole. *Cancer Lett.* 1:69–74

81a. Bulay, O., Clayson, D. B., Shubik, P. 1978. Carcinogenetic effects of niridazole in rats. *Cancer Lett.* 4:305–10

81b. Bulay, O., Patail, K., Wilson, R., Shubik, P. 1979. Kidney tumors induced in rats by the antischistosomal drug niridazole. *Cancer Res.* 39:4996–5002

82. Webster, L. T. Jr., Tracy, J. W., Blumer, J. L., Catto, B. A., Sissors, D. L. 1984. Relationships of niridazole metabolism to antiparasitic efficacy and host toxicity. In *Proc. 9th Intl. Congr. Pharmacol., Vol. 2.* London: Macmillan. In press

83. Faigle, J. W., Kebule, H. 1966. The metabolic fate of CIBA 32644-Ba. *Acta Tropica* 9:8–22 (Suppl.)

84. Tracy, J. W., Catto, B. A., Webster, L. T. Jr. 1982. Reductive metabolism of niridazole by adult schistosoma: Correlation with covalent drug binding to parasite macromolecules. *Mol. Pharmacol.* 24:291–99

85. Blumer, J. L., Novak, R. F., Lucas, S. V., Simpson, J. M., Webster, L. T. Jr. 1979. Aerobic metabolism of niridazole by rat liver microsomes. *Mol. Pharmacol.* 16:1019–30

86. Lucas, S. V., Daniels, J. C., Schubert, R. D., Simpson, J. M., Mahamoud, A. A. F., et al. 1977. Identification and purification of immunosuppressive activity in the urine of rats and a human patient treated with niridazole. *J. Immunol.* 118:418–22

87. Blumer, J. L., Simpson, J. M., Lucas, S. V., Webster, L. T. Jr. 1980. Toxicogenetics of niridazole in inbred mice. *J. Pharmacol. Exp. Ther.* 212:509–13

88. Tracy, J. W., Fairchild, E. H., Lucas, S. V., Webster, L. T. Jr. 1980. Isolation, characterization and synthesis of an im-

munoregulatory metabolite of niridazole: 1 - Thiocarbamyl - 2 - imidazolidinone. *Mol. Pharmacol.* 18:313–19

89. Tracy, J. W., Webster, L. T. Jr. 1981. The formation of 1-thiocarbamyl-2-imidazolidinone from niridazole in mouse intestine. *J. Pharmacol. Exp. Ther.* 217:363–68

90. Tracy, J. W., Kazura, J. W., Webster, L. T. Jr. 1982. Suppression of cell-mediated immune responses *in vivo* and *in vitro* by 1-thiocarbamyl-2-imidazolidinone. *Immunoharm.* 4:187–200

91. Catto, B. A., Valencia, C. I., Hafiz, K., Fairfield, E. H., Webster, L. T. Jr. 1984. 4-Ketoniridazole: A major metabolite with central nervous system toxicity different than niridazole. *J. Pharmacol. Exp. Ther.* 228:662–68

92. Striebel, H. P. 1976. 4'-Isothiocyanato-4'-nitrodiphenylamine (C-9333-GO/CGP 4540), an anhelmintic with an unusual spectrum of activity against intestinal nematodes, filariae and schistosomes. *Experientia* 32:457–58

93. Bueding, E., Batzinger, R., Petterson, G. 1976. Antischistosomal and some toxicological properties of a nitrodiphenylaminothiocyanate (C9333-GO/CGP 4540). *Experientia* 32:604–6

94. Batzinger, R. P., Bueding, E., Reddy, B. S., Weisburger, J. H. 1978. Formation of a mutagenic drug metabolite by intestinal microorganisms. *Cancer Res.* 38:608–12

95. Crawford, K. A., Asch, H. L., Bruce, J. L., Bueding, E., Smith, E. R. 1983. Efficacy of amoscanate against experimental schistosoma infections in monkeys. *Am. J. Trop. Med. Hyg.* 32:1055–64

96. Hupei. Cooperative study of nithiocyamine. 1980. Observations of 4,022 schistosomiasis cases treated with nithiocyamine in a three-day regimen. *Natl. Med. J. China* 60:679–82

96a. Striebel, H. P. 1984. Paper presented at WHO Symp. Biochem. Chemother. Schistosomiasis. See Ref. 2

97. Voge, M., Bueding, E. 1980. *Schistosoma mansoni* tegumental surface alterations induced by subcurative doses of the schistosomicide amoscanate. *Exp. Parasitol.* 50:251–59

98. James, C., Webbe, G. 1974. Treatment of *Schistosoma haemotobium* in the baboon with metrifonate. *Trans. R. Soc. Med. Hyg.* 63:413

99. James, C., Webbe, G. 1974. The susceptibility of *Schistosoma japonicum* in hamsters to metrifonate. *Ann. Trop. Med. Parasitol.* 68:487

100. James, C., Webbe, G., Preston, J. M. 1972. A comparison of the susceptibility to metrifonate of *Schistosoma haemotobium, S. matthei* and *S. mansoni* in hamsters. *Ann. Trop. Med. Parasitol.* 66: 467–74

101. Davis, A. 1975. Clinically available antischistosomal drugs. *J. Toxicol. Environ. Health* 1:191–201

102. Nordgren, I., Bengtsson, E., Holmstedt, B., Petterson, B.-M. 1981. Levels of metrifonate and dichlorvos in plasma and erythrocytes during treatment of schistosomiasis with bilarcil. *Acta Pharmacol. Toxicol.* 49:79–86

103. Reiner, E. 1981. Esterases in schistosomes. Reaction with substrates and inhibitors. *Acta Pharmacol. Toxicol.* 49: 72–78

104. Reiner, E., Krauthacker, B., Simeon, V., Skrinjaric-Spoljar, M. 1975. Mechanism of inhibition in vitro of mammalian acetylcholinesterase and cholinesterase in solutions of 0,0-dimethyl-2,2-2-trichloro-1-hydroxyethyl phosphonate. *Biochem. Pharmacol.* 24:717–22

105. Katz, N., Pellegrino, J., Pereira, J. P. 1968. Experimental chemotherapy of schistosomiasis. III. Laboratory and clinical trials with trichlorophone, an organophosphorus compound. *Rev. Soc. Brasil. Med. Trop.* 4:237–45

106. elKouni, M. H., Niedzwicki, J. G., Lee, K.-Y., Iltzsch, M. H., Senft, A. W., Cha, S. 1983. Enzymes of pyrimidine metabolism in *Schistosoma mansoni. Fed. Proc.* 42:2207

Ann. Rev. Pharmacol. Toxicol. 1985. 25:509–28

THE ROLE OF OXYGEN RADICALS AS A POSSIBLE MECHANISM OF TUMOR PROMOTION

W. Troll and R. Wiesner

Department of Environmental Medicine, New York University Medical Center, New York, New York 10016

INTRODUCTION

In recent years, considerable progress has been made in our understanding of the basic concepts of carcinogenesis. Epidemiological and experimental animal studies indicate that cancer can develop in tissues in a multistep process. The concept of two-stage carcinogenesis was first described by Berenblum (1) in mouse skin and this description has been the primary model for investigating the mechanism of tumor promotion. Tumor induction can be divided into two distinct treatment stages: initiation and promotion. The initiation phase requires a single application of either a direct or an indirect carcinogen at a subthreshold dose and is essentially irreversible; the promotion stage requires repeated treatments *after* initiation and is initially reversible, later becoming irreversible (2). The initiation step in this process probably involves a heritable modification in the genetic material of the cells, as evidenced by the good correlation between the mutagenicity and the carcinogenicity of many chemical agents (3). Most tumor-initiating agents are electrophilic reactants or must be converted metabolically into a chemically reactive electrophilic form that then binds covalently to cellular DNA and other macromolecules (4). Initiation is produced after a single exposure to an initiating carcinogen that presumably converts a small proportion of the target cell population to cells that are competent to be transformed into tumors (5). On the other hand, promoters are not mutagenic and do not bind covalently to DNA. Many promoters, like phorbol esters, are almost exclusively membrane-active agents. The cell mem-

509

0362-1642/85/415-0509$02.00

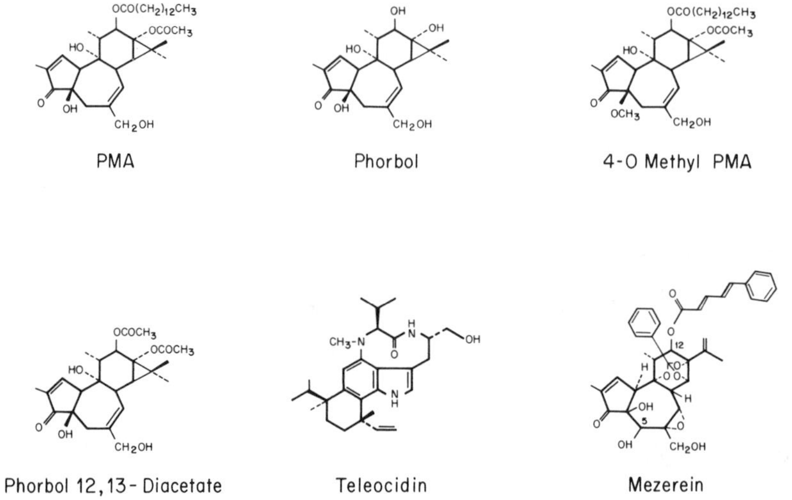

Figure 1   Structures of PMA, phorbol, 4-O-methyl PMA, phorbol 12,13-diacetate, teleocidin, and mezerein.

branes of many tissues contain high-affinity, specific receptors that interact with biologically active phorbol esters in a reversible and saturable manner (6, 7). Promotion requires multiple or prolonged exposure to the promoting agent before tumor growth becomes inevitable. Promotion has been further divided into at least two phases (8, 9). An additional step different from promotion has also been described, i.e. the progression of a benign lesion to a malignant neoplasm (10).

Evidence for the existence of two-stage carcinogenesis has been shown in a number of other species and tissues and with other promoting agents (11).

The most potent tumor promoter is phorbol-myristate-acetate (PMA), which has been isolated from croton oil (12, 13). In addition to the phorbol esters, a wide variety of other compounds [teleocidin (14), mezerein (15), and various organic peroxides (16) (Figure 1)] have been shown to have skin tumor–promoting activity. Although tumor promoters cause many cellular and biochemical changes in mouse skin, it is difficult to determine which of the many effects associated with tumor promotion are in fact essential components of the promotion process.

PROTEASE ACTION IN TUMOR PROMOTION

The observation that the inflammatory tumor promoter PMA induces proteases in mouse skin led to the suggestion that proteases play a role in tumor promotion. Further studies have shown that the action of proteases in tumor promotion and neoplastic transformation can be modified by protease inhibitors when these inhibitors are applied directly to tissues or when fed to animals or man.

The first indication that proteases affect tumor promotion was the observation that protease inhibitors suppress tumor induction by PMA in mouse skin. Low doses (1–10 μg) of tosyl-L-lysine chloromethyl ketone (TLCK), tosyl-phenylalanine-chloromethyl ketone (TPCK), and tosyl-L-arginine methyl ester (TAME) counteract the effect of PMA on mouse skin in two-stage carcinogenesis (17). The number and incidence of tumors are decreased and the latent period is increased. The most effective agent is TPCK. This inhibition by protease inhibitors has been confirmed by Hozumi et al, who used the protease inhibitor leupeptin (18), one of the small inhibitors isolated from streptomycetes (19), to suppress tumorigenesis in the mouse-skin model. The importance of proteases in the tumorigenic process was further kindled by the discovery of Reich and his associates that tumor cells contain more plasminogen activator than their normal counterparts (20). Plasminogen activators are trypsin-like serine proteases. Furthermore, the level of plasminogen activator is increased when fibroblasts are transformed by viruses or promoters (21). Intracellular plasminogen activator appears to be associated with the membrane fraction (22).

In the early studies, the inhibitors were applied percutaneously. Later experiments have shown that feeding a raw soybean diet rich in protease inhibitors suppresses the appearance of tumors in mouse skin treated with nitroquinoline oxide and PMA (23), of breast tumors induced by X-ray irradiation in Sprague-Dawley rats (24), and of spontaneous liver cancer in C_3H mice (25). Similarly, feeding leupeptin (26) or N,N-dimethylamino-[p-p'-(guanidinobenzyloxy)]-benzilcarbonyloxyglycolate, an effective trypsin inhibitor, also delays and suppresses rat mammary tumors induced by 7,12-dimethyl benz(a)anthracene (DMBA) (27).

Additional evidence for the reduction of tumor formation by protease inhibitors has been obtained with the oral administration of ε-aminocaproic acid, which inhibits 1,2,dimethyl-hydrazine-induced mouse colorectal tumors (28). Furthermore, the feeding of a synthetic protease inhibitor [N,N-dimethylcarbamoylmethyl 4-(4 guanidinobenzoyloxy)-phenylace-tate]methanesulfate (FOY-305) suppresses the incidence of carcinomas in mouse skin induced by repeated applications of the carcinogen 3-methylcholanthrene, which presumably has both initiating and promoting capabilities (29). FOY-305 is a strong inhibitor of trypsin, thrombin, and kallikrein.

Ingested protease inhibitors may play a direct role in blocking tumor promotion in mouse skin, or they may act in an indirect manner by limiting the digestion of proteins (30).

Two major inhibitors purified from soybeans are the Kunitz inhibitor and the Bowman-Birk inhibitor (31). When the Bowman-Birk inhibitor is fed to rodents, a large part of the inhibitor is excreted in the feces as a protease: protease inhibitor complex that retains its antiprotease activity. We have proposed that the anticarcinogenic activity of Bowman–Birk like inhibitors may be an indirect one resulting from the consequent inhibition of protein digestion (32).

In addition to protease inhibitors, other agents that block the induction of tumors by PMA in mouse skin are the anti-inflammatory steroids, dexamethasone (33) and fluocinolone acetonide (34); certain retinoids (35); a combination of retinoids and anti-inflammatory agents (36); and certain antioxidants (16).

The finding that these agents block tumor promotion has raised new questions about how tumor promotion is derailed by these agents.

OXYGEN RADICALS IN TUMOR PROMOTION

Recent developments have stimulated a growing interest in the possible role of free oxygen radicals in tumor promotion. More and more, the data support the view that these radicals are important in promotion in vivo as well as in vitro.

Tumor induction by PMA in mouse skin is accompanied by an inflammatory response; within 24 hours after promotion treatment, polymorphonuclear leukocytes (PMNs) infiltrate the dermis (37). Protease inhibitors applied directly to mouse skin block this response (17). When phagocytes (PMNs and macrophages) are exposed to appropriate stimuli, a series of metabolic events takes place known as the respiratory burst (38, 39). Many agents, both particulate and soluble, are able to evoke this response, which is accompanied by the production of superoxide anions ($O_2^-\cdot$), hydrogen peroxide (H_2O_2), hydroxy radical ($\cdot OH$), and singlet oxygen. The production of reactive oxygen species by phagocytic cells contributes to the antimicrobial and antitumor activity of these cells (38–40).

Evidence from our laboratory suggests that tumor promoters such as PMA may enhance tumor formation by stimulating superoxide anion production through the action of an NADPH-dependent oxidase. Very small amounts of PMA (5–10 ng) stimulate the formation of superoxide anions, H_2O_2 (41), and chemiluminescence (42) in PMNs. Mezerein, a diterpene related to the phorbol esters, also stimulates $O_2^-\cdot$ production (43) as well as that of chemiluminescence (42). Indole alkaloids such as teleocidin, lyngbyatoxin, debromoaplysiatoxin, and aplysiatoxin (14), which are chemically distinct from the phorbol esters, are another class of tumor promoters that stimulates $O_2^-\cdot$ production in human PMNs (44). The degree of stimulation of PMNs by various phorbol esters correlates with their promoting activity in mouse skin. PMA is greater than phorbol dibutyrate, which is greater than phorbolol myristate acetate (45).

On the other hand, phorbol, phorbol diacetate, and 4-0-methyl phorbol myristate acetate, which are inactive in tumor promotion, are also inactive in stimulating $O_2^- \cdot$ production (42, 45). PMA, but not 4-0-methyl-PMA, also stimulates the release of $O_2^- \cdot$ and H_2O_2 in guinea pig macrophages (46). No superoxide anion production has been observed in either human or Chinese hamster fibroblast cultures (47). These oxygen radicals induced by the promoter may contribute to tumor promotion by being released at an inappropriate time.

One might expect protease inhibitors capable of inhibiting tumor promotion in mouse skin to be able to antagonize the stimulation by PMA in human leukocytes. Such is indeed the case; a number of protease inhibitors (soybean trypsin inhibitor, lima bean trypsin inhibitor, benzamidine, and antipain) suppress the production of $O_2^- \cdot$ in PMNs stimulated by PMA. Soybean trypsin inhibitor antagonizes the stimulatory effect of a variety of other stimulating agents and inhibits $O_2^- \cdot$ production in rat PMNs as well as in alveolar macrophages (41). TLCK and TPCK suppress oxygen consumption and superoxide production in PMA-stimulated rat pulmonary macrophages (48). Crude extracts of canned legumes, as well as protease inhibitors purified from these legumes, have been effective in blocking the effect of PMA on the $O_2^- \cdot$ response of PMNs (49).

Derivatives of Vitamin A have also been shown to inhibit tumor promotion (35). Thus, it is not surprising that retinol and Vitamin A analogs (retinyl acetate and retinoic acid) effectively inhibit $O_2^- \cdot$ production in PMA-stimulated PMNs in a dose-dependent manner (42, 50). Similar to PMNs, rat alveolar macrophages also show a decrease in $O_2^- \cdot$ formation when stimulated by PMA in the presence of retinol. Stimulation of $O_2^- \cdot$ production by mezerein and teleocidin B is also inhibited by retinol. The mechanism of action of retinol in this system could be explained by its alteration of cell membrane fluidity. Retinoic acid has been shown to alter membrane fluidity in red cell membranes (51). Thus, the inhibition of PMA stimulation of PMNs observed with retinoids may involve a general effect such as an alteration in the dynamic properties of plasma membranes (50).

The anti-inflammatory corticosteroid dexamethasone, which can strongly inhibit tumor promotion (33), also inhibits the PMA-stimulated PMNs. The anti-inflammatory property of the steroids may in part be due to their antioxidant properties (52). An alternative explanation is that the inhibitory action of dexamethasone is due to the elaboration of a protease inhibitor. Dexamethasone has been shown to induce an inhibitor of plasminogen activator (53, 54).

Superoxide production probably is initiated on the cell surface by the interaction of the cell surface with appropriate stimuli. Surface-active agents such as cytochalasin E and Concanavalin A generate $O_2^- \cdot$ formation in PMNs and monocytes (55). In addition, anti-IgE induces production of $O_2^- \cdot$ in human basophils (56). The $O_2^- \cdot$ production in all of these cells is inhibited by potent inactivators of serine proteases in a dose-dependent fashion. The inhibitory effect of inactivators of chymotrypsin-like proteases is more effective than that of inhibitors of trypsin-like proteases, suggesting that a chymotrypsin-like protease is involved in $O_2^- \cdot$ production by PMNs and basophils. $O_2^- \cdot$ produced by the xanthine-xanthine oxidase superoxide anion–generating system is not impaired by protease inhibitors, indicating that these inhibitors do not themselves react with superoxide.

More direct evidence for the involvement of free radicals in tumor promotion comes from the work of Slaga et al (2), who have shown that a number of free radical–generating compounds (benzoyl peroxide, chloroperbenzoic acid, lauroyl peroxide) are effective skin tumor promoters in Sencar mice after initiation with DMBA. A significant number of papillomas and squamous cell carcinomas are produced by benzoyl peroxide, which is not effective as a complete carcinogen or as an initiator.

One expected effect of PMA stimulation is an increase in lipid peroxidation. However, Logani et al observed that lipid peroxidation in mouse skin is decreased by PMA treatment and that TPCK has no effect on this response (57). In contrast, Belman & Garte (58) found that mouse epidermal lipid peroxidation is unchanged after one treatment with PMA but is markedly suppressed after six treatments.

Stimulation of superoxide release by PMA has been observed only in phagocytes. Recently, Fisher & Adams (59; S. M. Fischer, unpublished data) presented evidence that treatment of isolated mouse epidermal cells with PMA results in increased production of chemiluminescence, an index of the generation of superoxide anions and singlet oxygen. The PMA-mediated chemiluminescence is dose-dependent and peaks within 15 minutes. The extent of the response correlates with the tumor-promoting ability of the phorbol esters tested. This response can be suppressed by superoxide dismutase (SOD) and Cu(II)-3,5,diisopropylsalicylate (CuDIPS) as well as by retinoic acid. Inhibitors of the arachidonic acid cascade, such as benoxaprofen and phenidone, also suppress the response. The data suggest that the metabolism of arachidonic acid is responsible for the PMA-stimulated response in mouse epidermal cells. Thus, free radicals may be generated by tumor promoters without the intervention of PMNs.

DEFENSE MECHANISMS AGAINST FREE OXYGEN RADICALS

The reduction of molecular oxygen in all aerobic eukaryotic cells results in intermediates ($O_2^- \cdot$, H_2O_2, and $\cdot OH$) that are highly toxic. As a result, organisms have developed an elaborate system of defenses against these intermediates (60). The primary defense is provided by enzymes that catalytically scavenge the intermediates of oxygen reduction. Superoxide anions are eliminated by SOD, which catalyzes a dismutation reaction leading to the formation of $O_2^- \cdot$ plus H_2O_2. The latter can be destroyed by the action of catalases and glutathione peroxidase (61). Although $O_2^- \cdot$ and H_2O_2 individually may not be particularly damaging in aqueous solution, it has been postulated that their combined action leads to the formation of a highly reactive product, the hydroxy radical via the Haber-Weiss reaction (62), according to the following equation:

$$O_2^- \cdot + H_2O_2 \rightarrow \cdot OH + OH^- + O_2$$

This reaction is very slow; however, there is substantial evidence that, when catalyzed by metal ions present in all biological systems, this reaction can proceed at a pace that would make it biologically relevant (63). Hydroxy radicals will attack and destroy most molecules in living cells (39, 40); hence, efficient methods of removing $O_2^- \cdot$ and H_2O_2 are necessary to prevent the damage that can result from these radicals.

Treatment of adult mouse skin with 2 μg PMA results in decreased levels of both SOD and catalase activities in the epidermis. A fairly good correlation has been found between the tumor-promoting ability of various promoters and their ability to decrease the activity of these enzymes. The effect of PMA is selective for SOD and catalase, since general protein synthesis is not inhibited by PMA (64). Mezerein, a resiniferonal derivative with weak promoting activity that nevertheless acts as a strong stage II promoter, is more potent than PMA in lowering the levels of SOD and catalase. Therefore, lowered SOD and catalase levels may be characteristic of stage II promotion.

Reduced levels of SOD have been found in human lymphoblast and fibroblast cultures after PMA treatment (47). Such treatment also lower levels of both SOD and catalase in $C_3H/10T\frac{1}{2}$ cells (J. Yavelow, personal communication).

Two types of superoxide dismutases are found in all eukaryotic cells: a copper and zinc-containing SOD (CuZnSOD) and a manganese-containing SOD (MnSOD) (61). Lowered levels of CuZnSOD and especially of MnSOD are characteristic of many of the tumor systems studied so far (65). CuZnSOD activity is significantly decreased in the liver of rabbits bearing the VX-2 carcinoma in the maxillary sinus, whereas MnSOD is not affected. However, in the VX-2 carcinoma itself no MnSOD activity and only low levels of CuZnSOD have been found (66). In a separate study, solid tumors were induced in CBA/J mice by implantation of Ehrlich carcinoma cells. Depressed levels of SOD activity were seen in a number of the organs of these tumor-bearing mice. In liver, spleen, and kidneys, the MnSOD activity was lowered some time after implantation, even though there was no evidence of metastases in these organs (67). An earlier study showed that Ehrlich carcinomas in inbred

CBA mice contain reduced amounts of SOD activity when compared to the activity of control mice. Furthermore, when CuDIPS was administered at various doses, reduction in tumor size, delay of metastases, and a significant increase in survival of the hosts were observed (68). CuDIPS is a lipid-soluble, low molecular–weight compound that exhibits superoxide dismutase activity and therefore can act as an intracellular $O_2^- \cdot$ scavenger. CuDIPS also reduces the frequency of PMA-induced mouse papillomas and inhibits the induction of ornithine decarboxylase (ODC) (69), the enzyme shown by Boutwell to be characteristic of tumor promotion (70).

An excess of free radicals, in conjunction with a deficiency in protective enzymes such as SOD and catalase, could lead to adverse effects that may contribute to the cancer phenotype.

THE ROLE OF TUMOR PROMOTERS IN MUTAGENESIS

Free oxygen radicals generated during phagocytosis can be harmful or beneficial with respect to neoplasia. Products of phagocytosis such as $O_2^- \cdot$, H_2O_2, and $\cdot OH$ are part of the killing mechanism of neutrophils and macrophages (40). On the other hand, these products can peroxidize lipids and form cytotoxic metabolites such as malondialdehyde, which is capable of interacting with DNA and producing mutations (71). Additional evidence for the genotoxic effects of the products of phagocytosis has been furnished by the observation that mutagenic activity could be associated with human PMNs stimulated by phagocytosis. When histidine-requiring mutants of *Salmonella typhimurium* strain TA 100 are incubated with PMNs, these bacteria revert to histidine independence (72). The mutagenicity of PMNs from patients with chronic granulomatous disease (CGD) is markedly diminished compared to that of normal cells. Neutrophils from a patient with CGD have a defect in the NADPH oxidase-superoxide generating system and are thus unable to generate $O_2^- \cdot$ and H_2O_2. Further support for the idea that phagocytosis induces mutations comes from work with luminous bacteria. In this case, dark mutants of luminous bacteria incubated with human neutrophils activated by opsonized zymosan revert to hereditary stable luminescent forms. Heat-killed phagocytes are not mutagenic. Scavengers of oxygen radicals, such as β carotene, mannitol, and benzoate, as well as SOD, prevent these mutations (73). Moreover, $O_2^- \cdot$ generated from potassium superoxide induces mutagenic and cytotoxic effects in Chinese hamster ovary (CHO) cells. These effects are reversed by SOD (74).

PMA-stimulated PMNs cause other types of cytotoxic changes in CHO cells, resulting in a concentration-dependent increase in sister-chromatid exchanges. PMA alone and PMNs from a patient with CGD did not increase sister-chromatid exchanges. A significant increase in sister-chromatid exchanges is induced when the cells are exposed to a cell-free superoxide-generating system (75).

The production of reactive oxygen species could explain how leukocytes induce mutation and generate sister-chromatid exchanges and suggests that PMA may participate in tumor promotion in vivo by stimulating toxic oxygen radical production in PMNs.

IN VITRO TUMOR PROMOTION SYSTEMS

PMA can enhance the level of transformation induced by chemical carcinogens (76), ultraviolet light (77), and X-ray in $C_3H/10T\frac{1}{2}$ cells (78) just as it enhances promotion in vivo. Protease inhibitors have been shown to prevent tumor promotion in vivo and they also have the ability to inhibit malignant transformation in vitro. Protease inhibitors that have the ability to suppress X-ray transformation in $C_3H/10T\frac{1}{2}$ cells include antipain, leupeptin, and the Bowman-Birk inhibitor, whereas antipain and soybean trypsin inhibitor suppress PMA enhancement of transformation (79). Similar results have been obtained by Borek et al (80). Antipain, elastatinal, chymostatin, and leupeptin also block chemical transformation of $C_3H/10T\frac{1}{2}$ cells (81).

Mouse erythroleukemia cells respond to PMA by an increase in cell adhesiveness. This response is associated with activation of protease activity. TLCK prevents cell adhesiveness. Pentamide isethionate, a trypsin-like inhibitor, decreases cell adhesiveness as well as PMA-induced proteolytic activity (82).

The enhancement of X–ray induced sister-chromatid exchanges by PMA in $C_3H/10T\frac{1}{2}$ cells is also suppressed by antipain and leupeptin (83).

Induction of skin tumors and ornithine decarboxylase by PMA is inhibited by retinoids (35). Thus, the ability of retinoids (β-all trans retinoic acid and the trimethyl methoxyphenyl analog of N-ethyl retinamide) to inhibit not only X–ray induced transformation but also the enhancement of this transformation by PMA in both $10T\frac{1}{2}$ and hamster embryo cells is to be expected. The effectiveness of the retinoids in preventing promotion takes place a short time after their addition to the media and their action is irreversible (84).

Zimmerman & Cerutti (85) have shown that active oxygen species act directly as a promoter in $C_3H/10T\frac{1}{2}$ cells. Extracellular superoxide produced by xanthine-xanthine oxidase has the capacity to promote $C_3H/10T\frac{1}{2}$ fibroblasts. Cell cultures initiated with [137]Cs γ-rays or benzo[a]pyrene diol epoxide I transform three to 30 times more effectively when subsequently treated with xanthine-xanthine oxidase for three weeks. SOD or SOD together with catalase reduces the number of transformed foci.

The effect of SOD and catalase on bleomycin and X–ray induced transformation has been examined in hamster embryo cells. SOD, but not catalase, inhibits the transformation induced by X-rays and bleomycin and the enhancement by PMA of X–ray induced transformation (86). These results support the idea that oncogenic transformation is mediated in part by free radicals and that SOD is most effective in inhibiting events associated with promotion.

Mouse epidermal cells (JB6) have been shown to respond to late-stage tumor promoters with an irreversible induction of anchorage-independent growth. Mezerein, a strong stage-II promoter, stimulates promotion of anchorage-independent growth of JB6 cells without accompanying induction of DNA double- or single-strand scissions. On the other hand, both benzoyl peroxide, a complete tumor promoter, and H_2O_2, an efficient stage-I tumor promoter, produce single-strand DNA scission under conditions that do not induce anchorage-independent growth. These data lead one to believe that strand scission in DNA may not be involved in late-stage promotion in JB6 cell lines (87).

However, PMA and mezerein induce DNA single-strand breaks in primary mouse epidermal cells when incubated in the presence of macrophages. PMA or macrophages alone do not induce strand breaks. One concludes from this data that active phorbol ester tumor promoters cause the release of a clastogenic factor from macrophages that can then exert its effect on a known target cell, the epidermal cell (88). Induction of anchorage independence by PMA in JB6 mouse epidermal cell lines is inhibited by antioxidants, CuZnSOD, and CuDIPS, but not by catalase. Scavengers of ·OH (benzoate, mannitol) are moderately active, suggesting that O_2^-· and possibly ·OH, but not H_2O_2, play a role as mediators of promotion of neoplastic transformation by PMA in JB6 mouse epidermal cells (89).

The addition of fresh medium to mouse mammary tumor cells (Mm 5 mt/C1) induces ornithine decarboxylase. Further, PMA enhances this induction. SOD, catalase, SOD plus catalase, and mannitol (a scavenger of hydroxy radicals) partially inhibit ODC induction, supporting the notion that active oxygen species O_2^-·, H_2O_2 and ·OH participate in the induction of ODC (90).

DNA DAMAGE BY FREE RADICALS

At the biochemical level, the major difference between initiators and promoters is their site of action. Whereas initiators (or their metabolites) bind covalently to DNA, the primary site of action of the phorbol ester tumor promoters appears to be the cell membrane through their interaction with specific cell receptors (6, 7). It usually has been assumed that tumor promoters (in particular PMA) exert their pleotropic effects entirely by interaction with epigenetic targets. However, recent observations have provided evidence that the phorbol ester tumor promoters may act directly or indirectly to produce DNA damage and chromosomal aberrations via activated forms of oxygen.

Very low levels of PMA induce extensive DNA strand break damage (DSBD) in human PMNs. Just as in the case of mouse skin, nonpromoting analogues are inactive. Damage is decreased by the addition of either catalase or SOD, providing evidence that the damage is caused by products of the respiratory burst (91). The damage to DNA involves both superoxide anion and H_2O_2, but the precise radical has not been determined. A likely candidate is the highly reactive $\cdot OH$ radical, which can be formed from $O_2^- \cdot$ and H_2O_2 in the presence of certain trace metals (63). However, the use of $\cdot OH$ scavengers does not provide any definite proof of $\cdot OH$ involvement (92). The following observations provide strong evidence that PMA-induced DNA damage is related to the respiratory burst: (a) DSBD is prevented by the inhibitor 2-deoxyglucose, which blocks superoxide production by interfering with the hexose monophosphate shunt responsible for generating NADPH. (b) The PMNs from patients with CGD have a defect in the NADPH-oxidase superoxide-generating system and are thus unable to generate $O_2^- \cdot$ and H_2O_2. Exposure of PMNs from patients with CGD to PMA induces no detectable DSBD. (c) PMA-stimulated PMNs induce DSBD in mouse erythroleukemia cells. DSBD is blocked by catalase but not be SOD. Complete inhibition by catalase but not by SOD is also obtained when DSBD is induced in PMNs by xanthine-xanthine oxidase, which enzymatically generates superoxide anions. Other promoters that produce DSBD in leukocytes are benzoyl peroxide and teleocidin B (93).

The action of oxygen radicals may also exert its effect through the formation of a clastogenic factor, a diffusible cellular product that induces chromosomal damage. PMA, but not its weakly or nonpromoting derivatives, induces chromosomal aberrations with high efficiency in phytohaemogglutinin-stimulated lymphocytes (94). The clastogenic activity of the compounds tested (PMA, 4-O-methyl PMA, and phorbol) parallels their effectiveness as promoters in the mouse skin system. This clastogenic activity of PMA is indirect because it can be suppressed by SOD, which catalyzes the breakdown of $O_2^- \cdot$. It is mediated by secondary products formed by the cell in response to the interaction with PMA. Active oxygen species, as well as metabolites of arachidonic acid, are intermediates in the formation and action of the clastogenic factor because CuZnSOD, certain antioxidants, and inhibitors of the cyclooxygenase and lipooxygenase pathways are anticlastogenic (95, 96). PMA also induces the formation of a diffusable clastogenic factor in human leukocytes (97).

Clastogenic activity also can be detected in concentrated ultrafiltrates of media from cultures of fibroblasts of patients with Bloom's syndrome (98). No activity has been found in the media of normal fibroblasts. Because bovine SOD strongly suppresses the clastogenic potency of the ultrafiltrates, the authors speculate that the primary genetic defect in Bloom's syndrome may be a deficiency in the detoxification of active oxygen species that cause the formation of a clastogenic factor. Preliminary evidence suggests that the clastogenic factor consists of free arachidonic acid plus lipid hydroperoxides and aldehydic compounds. Cerutti et al have proposed a model for "membrane-mediated chromosomal damage," i.e. membrane-active agents such as PMA stimulate the arachidonic acid cascade, elicit an oxidative burst, and perturb membrane integrity so that phospholipids become more susceptible to auto-oxidation and induce chromosomal damage (99).

Radiation causes strand breaks (100) and modification of bases in DNA (101, 102). It is well established that hydroxy radicals are responsible for this damage (62). Modification of thymine in cellular DNA through the action of γ-irradiation results in formation of 5-hydroxymethyl-2'-deoxyuridine (HMdU) (102). If PMA is similar to ionizing radiation in generating ·OH radicals, one would expect the same type of modification of the thymine moiety in DNA as has been shown to occur with γ-irradiation. Preliminary results indeed show that PMA-stimulated neutrophils cause formation of HMdU in DNA coincubated with PMNs in the presence of ferrous ions or autologous serum (103). H_2O_2 also modifies thymine, forming ring-saturated products such as thymine glycol (104). Therefore, it appears that at least some of the properties of tumor promoters, expressed through the PMN-mediated generation of oxygen radicals, are similar to initiating carcinogens in causing modification of DNA constituents.

TUMOR PROMOTION IN OTHER SYSTEMS

The significance of the concept of tumor promotion has been questioned because initially mouse skin was the only vehicle in which induction of tumors by PMA could be demonstrated. Recent developments, however, show that two-stage carcinogenesis is not limited to mouse skin, and the importance of promotion in the development of several other cancers has been confirmed.

In addition to the phorbol esters, several other substances exhibit promoting activity. Phenobarbital appears to act as a tumor promoter by increasing the incidence of tumors in the liver when its administration is preceded by initiation with 2-acetylaminofluorene (105). Similarly, the incidence of bladder cancer in animals has been enhanced after a single dose of a carcinogen followed by consumption of diets containing saccharin or sodium cyclamate (106, 107). Bile acids promote colon cancer initiated by N-methyl-N-nitro-N-nitrosoguanidine (108).

Although tobacco smoke contains a number of known carcinogens, the incidence of cancer associated with smoking could just as well be related to the tumor promoters in smoke. The risk of cancer occurrence in heavy smokers who have given up the habit for 15 years is only slightly higher than that of individuals who have never smoked. This reduction in risk is more consistent with the view that promoters rather than initiators are the major agents of cigarette smoke that cause cancer (109).

Prolonged inhalation of asbestos produces two types of lung cancer. Asbestos has a promoting effect on tumor development in rodent trachael grafts previously exposed to subcarcinogenic doses of 7,12-dimethylbenz(a)-anthracene. Increased DNA synthesis and the induction of ornithine decarboxylase accompany the morphological changes induced by asbestos in tracheal epithelium cells. The addition of exogenous SOD, but not catalase, to these cultures prevents the cytotoxicity induced by asbestos, suggesting that $O_2^-\cdot$ may be important in mediating asbestos cytotoxicity (110).

Production of duodenal adenocarcinomas in mice initiated by methyl-azoxy-methanol acetate is enhanced when hydrogen peroxide is given in the drinking water (111). This effect, which is larger in mice with low levels of catalase (112), has been ascribed to the promoting action of oxygen radicals, probably $\cdot OH$ radicals generated from H_2O_2.

The decisive action of an initiating carcinogen is to cause formation of a cancer-initiated cell that differs from normal cells in having an increased risk of tumor formation on subsequent exposure to carcinogens or promoting agents. A possible model for a cancer-initiated cell is one that has lowered repair capacity, as do cells of individuals with genetic diseases such as *Xeroderma pigmentosum* or *Ataxia telangectasia*. For example, an initial insult to cells by viral infection or chemical carcinogens (e.g. N-acetyl-N-amino-fluorene) results in the loss of their ability to repair carcinogen-induced damage (113). This is also true of lung explants exposed to cigarette smoke (114).

The effect of one agent (promoter) increasing the effect of another (initiator) has been noted in some epidemiological studies (115, 116). Ionizing radiation, which experimentally is used as an initiator in cell culture (78) or to induce breast cancer in rats (23), may act as an initiator in man. Asbestos workers who are smokers have a ten-fold higher lung cancer mortality than asbestos workers who do not smoke (11). Cigarette-smoking uranium miners occupationally exposed to radon have radiation-induced lung cancer rates about five times higher than those of miners who do not smoke (115). Here, we have a choice of whether to assign the role of initiator to the radiation or to the tobacco smoke.

A clearer human case for ionizing radiation acting as an initiator is the description of a 15-fold increase in risk for cutaneous cancer in psoriatic patients undergoing PUVA treatment (8-methoxypsoralen plus long-wave ultraviolet light) if they had been previously treated with ionizing radiation (116). A possible mechanism suggested for these findings is the lowering of DNA repair capacity by the ionizing radiation (116). The phenomenon described here has some relevance to multistage carcinogenesis, where a single dose of one agent (X-rays) predisposes cells to the action of subsequent exposure to a second agent (PUVA). A single X-ray treatment of V79 cells acts in a manner expected from an initiator. PUVA-induced mutability of the hypoxanthine guanine-phosphoribosyl locus of V79 cells increases for at least 108 days after the initial insult by X-ray treatment (117).

A second possible mechanism for increased vulnerability to promoter-induced damage after the primary damage by the initiating agent has occurred is a diminution in the capacity of the cells to detoxify active oxygen species. This might lead to increased amounts of DNA damage and the release of clastogenic factors. It has been postulated that clastogenic factors contribute to the chromosomal fragility of Bloom's syndrome and *Ataxia telangectasia* (96). The agents that detoxify active oxygen species include protective enzymes such as SOD that inhibit transformation when added to tissue culture systems (86).

POINTS TO PONDER

A number of problems concerning the role of free oxygen radicals in tumor promotion remain to be solved. How does the tumor promoter recognize the initiated cell and convert it to a tumor? What are the ultimate reactive species producing promotional or clastogenic changes in cellular DNA? What is the relationship between DNA damage induced by active oxygen and tumor promotion? How does one relate tumor induction in mouse skin with the phenomenon of oxygen radical production in neutrophils? In what way do protease inhibitors, retinoids, and antioxidants work to inhibit tumorigenesis? These and other questions still remain to be answered before the underlying mechanism of tumor promotion can be fully understood.

SUMMARY

In this chapter we have reviewed the evidence that free oxygen radicals play a role in tumor promotion. We have emphasized the fact that protease as well as other inhibitors exert their action by modulating the oxygen radical response. The finding that chemical agents are capable of blocking the carcinogenic process offers some hope that cancer may be prevented by diets rich in these agents.

Nutrition is an important modifying factor in chemical carcinogenesis. A relationship between diet and cancer incidence has been demonstrated by studies that show a wide variation in cancer incidence from country to country and even within the same country, depending on the dietary habits of the populations (118). Even more convincing is the fact that in migrant populations the incidence of cancer changes from the level characteristic of the mother country to that of the new country as the immigrants adapt to the dietary preferences of their new home (119, 120).

The Western diet, which is rich in fat content but low in vegetables, appears to contribute to a higher occurrence of breast, colon, and prostatic cancers (121, 122). The incidence of these cancers is lower in populations eating vegetarian diets (123–125).

We have shown that protease inhibitors interfere with tumor promotion by modulating the oxygen radical response. Protease inhibitors are widely distributed in plants, especially soybeans, which are a major source of protein in vegetarian diets. Therefore, the finding that protease inhibitors interfere with tumor promotion, taken together with the lower incidence of cancer in populations eating vegetarian diets, offers hope for the future that protease inhibitors may play an important role in preventing cancer.

ACKNOWLEDGMENTS

We wish to thank Drs. Thomas W. Kensler, Michael A. Trush, and Susan Fisher for reprints and preprints of publications. We express our warm thanks to Susan Benninghoff for her helpful secretarial assistance. This investigation was supported by PHS grant number CA 16060, awarded by the National Cancer Institute, DHHS.

Literature Cited

1. Berenblum, I. 1941. The cocarcinogenic action of croton resin. *Cancer Res.* 1:44–48

2. Slaga, T. J., Klein-Szanto, A. J. P., Triplett, L. L., Yotti, L. P., Trosko, J. E. 1981. Skin tumor promoting activity of benzoyl peroxide, a widely used free radical-generating compound. *Science* 213:1023–25

3. McCann, J., Choi, E., Yamasaki, E., Ames, B. N. 1975. Detection of carcinogens as mutagens in the *Salmonella/* microsome test: Assay of 300 chemicals. *Proc. Natl. Acad. Sci. USA* 72:5135–39

4. Miller, E. C., Miller, J. A. 1976. The metabolism of chemical carcinogens to reactive electrophiles and their possible mechanisms of action in carcinogenesis. In *Chemical Carcinogens,* ed. C. E. Searle, pp. 737–62. Washington, DC: Am. Chem. Soc.

5. Hicks, R. M. 1983. Pathological and biochemical aspects of tumor promotion. *Carcinogenesis* 4:1209–14

6. Driedger, P. E., Blumberg, P. M. 1980. Specific binding of phorbol ester tumor promoters. *Proc. Natl. Acad. Sci. USA* 77:567–71

7. Shoyab, M., Todaro, G. J. 1980. Specific high affinity cell membrane receptors for biologically active phorbol and ingenol esters. *Nature* 288:451–55

8. Boutwell, R. K. 1964. Some biological aspects of skin carcinogenesis. *Prog. Exp. Tumor Res.* 4:207–50

9. Slaga, T. J., Fischer, S. M., Nelson, K., Gleason, G. L. 1980. Studies on mechanism of action of anti-tumor-promoting agents: Evidence for several stages in promotion. *Proc. Natl. Acad. Sci. USA* 77:3659–63

10. Boutwell, R. K. 1983. Diet and anticarcinogenesis in the mouse skin two-stage model. *Cancer Res.* 43:2465s–68s (Suppl.)

11. Diamond, L., O'Brien, T. G., Baird, W. M. 1980. Tumor promoters and the mechanism of tumor promotion. *Adv. Cancer Res.* 32:1–74

12. Van Duuren, B. L., Orris, L. 1965. The tumor-enhancing principles of *Croton tiglium. Cancer Res.* 25:1871–75

13. Hecker, E. 1968. Cocarcinogenic principles from the seed oil of *Croton tiglium* and from other euphorbiaceae. *Cancer Res.* 28:2338–49

14. Fujiki, H., Mori, M., Nakayasu, M., Terada, T., Sugimura, T., Moore, R. E. 1981. Indole alkaloids: Dihydroteleocidin B, teleocidin, and lyngbyatoxin A as members of a new class of tumor promoters. *Proc. Natl. Acad. Sci. USA* 78:3872–76

15. Mufson, R. A., Fischer, S. M., Verma,

A. K., Gleason, G. L., Slaga, T. J. 1979. Effects of 12-O-tetradecanoylphorbol-13-acetate and mezerein on epidermal ornithine decarboxylase activity, isoproterenol-stimulated levels of cyclic adenosine 3:5-monophosphate, and induction of mouse skin tumors. *Cancer Res.* 39:4791–95

16. Slaga, T. J., Solanki, V., Logani, M. 1983. Studies on the mechanism of action of antitumor promoting agents: Suggestive evidence for the involvement of free radicals in promotion. In *Radioprotectors and Anticarcinogens,* ed. O. F. Nygaard, M. G. Simic, pp. 471–85. New York: Liss

17. Troll, W., Klassen, A., Janoff, A. 1970. Tumorigenesis in mouse skin: Inhibition by synthetic inhibitors of proteases. *Science* 169:1211–13

18. Hozumi, M., Ogawa, M., Sugimura, T., Takeuchi, T., Umezawa, H. 1972. Inhibition of tumorigenesis in mouse skin by leupeptin, a protease inhibitor from *Actinomycetes. Cancer Res.* 32:1725–29

19. Umezawa, H. 1972. *Enzyme Inhibitors of Microbial Origin,* pp. 15–52. Baltimore: Univ. Park

20. Ossowski, L., Quigley, J. P., Kellerman, G. M., Reich, E. 1973. Fibrinolysis associated with oncogenic transformation. Requirement of plasminogen for correlated changes in cellular morphology, colony formation in agar and cell migration. *J. Exp. Med.* 138:1056–64

21. Reich, E. 1975. Plasminogen activator: Secretion by neoplastic cells and macrophages. In *Proteases and Biological Control,* ed. E. Reich, D. B. Rifkin, E. Shaw, pp. 333–42. Cold Spring Harbor, NY: Cold Spring Harbor Lab.

22. Quigley, J. P. 1976. Association of a protease (plasminogen activator) with a specific membrane fraction isolated from transformed cells. *J. Cell Biol.* 71:472–86

23. Troll, W., Belman, S., Wiesner, R., Shellabarger, C. J. 1979. Protease action in carcinogenesis. In *Biological Function of Proteinases,* ed. H. Holzer, H. Tschesche, pp. 165–70. Berlin: Springer-Verlag

24. Troll, W., Wiesner, R., Shellabarger, C. J., Holtzman, S., Stone, J. P. 1980. Soybean diet lowers breast incidence in irradiated rats. *Carcinogenesis* 1:469–72

25. Becker, F. F. 1981. Inhibition of spontaneous hepatocarcinogenesis in C3H/HEN mice by Edipro A, an isolated soy protein. *Carcinogenesis* 2:1213–14

26. Fukui, Y., Takamura, M., Yamamura, M., Yamamoto, M. 1975. Effect of leupeptin on carcinogenesis of rat mammary tumor induced by 7,12-dimethylbenz[a]-anthracene. *Proc. Jpn. Cancer Assoc. 34th Ann. Meet.,* p. 20 (Abstr.). Tokyo: Univ. of Tokyo Press

27. Yamamura, M., Nakamura, M., Fukui, Y., Takamura, C., Yamamoto, M., et al. 1978. Inhibition of 7,12-dimethylbenz[a]anthracene-induced mammary tumorigenesis in rats by a synthetic protease inhibitor, [N,N-dimethylamino-p-(p'-guanidinobenzoyloxy) benzilcarbonyloxy] glycolate. *Gann* 69:749–52

28. Corasanti, J. G., Hobika, G. H., Markus, G. 1982. Interference with dimethylhydrazine induction of colon tumors in mice by ε-aminocaproic acid. *Science* 216:1020–21

29. Ohkoshi, M., Fujii, S. 1983. Effect of the synthetic protease inhibitor [N,N-dimethylcarbamoyl-methyl-4-(4-guanidinobenzoyloxy) - phenylacetate] methanesulfate on carcinogenesis by 3-methylcholanthrene in mouse skin. *J. Natl. Cancer Inst.* 71:1053–57

30. Troll, W., Frenkel, K., Wiesner, R. 1984. Protease inhibitors as anticarcinogens. *J. Natl. Cancer Inst.* 73(6): In press

31. Birk, Y. 1976. Proteinase inhibitors. *Methods Enzymol.* 45(Pt. B):695–707

32. Yavelow, J., Finlay, T. H., Kennedy, A. R., Troll, W. 1983. Bowman-Birk soybean protease inhibitor as an anticarcinogen. *Cancer Res.* 43:2454s–59s (Suppl.)

33. Belman, S., Troll, W. 1972. The inhibition of croton oil-promoted mouse skin tumorigenesis by steroid hormones. *Cancer Res.* 32:450–54

34. Schwartz, J. A., Viaje, A., Slaga, T. J., Yuspa, S. H., Hennings, H., Lichti, U. 1977. Fluocinolone acetonide: A potent inhibitor of skin tumor promotion and epidermal DNA synthesis. *Chem. Biol. Interact.* 17:331–47

35. Verma, A. K., Shapas, B. G., Rice, H. M., Boutwell, R. K. 1979. Correlation of the inhibition by retinoids of tumor promoter-induced mouse epidermal ornithine decarboxylase activity and of skin tumor promotion. *Cancer Res.* 39:419–25

36. Week, C. E., Slaga, T. J., Hennings, H., Gleason, G. L., Bracken, W. M. 1979. Inhibition of phorbol-ester induced tumor promotion in mice by vitamin A analog and anti-inflammatory steroid. *J. Natl. Cancer Inst.* 63:401–6

37. Janoff, A., Klassen, A., Troll, W. 1970. Local vascular changes induced by the

cocarcinogen, phorbol myristate acetate. *Cancer Res.* 30:2568–71

38. Babior, B. M. 1978. Oxygen-dependent microbial killing of phagocytes. *N. Engl. J. Med.* 298:659–68, 721–25

39. Badwey, J. A., Karnovsky, M. L. 1980. Active oxygen species and the functions of phagocytic leukocytes. *Ann. Rev. Biochem.* 49:695–726

40. Klebanoff, S. J. 1980. Oxygen metabolism and the toxic properties of phagocytes. *Ann. Intern. Med.* 93:480–89

41. Goldstein, B. D., Witz, G., Amoruso, M., Troll, W. 1979. Protease inhibitors antagonize the activation of polymorphonuclear leukocyte oxygen consumption. *Biochem. Biophys. Res. Commun.* 88: 854–60

42. Kensler, T. W., Trush, M. A. 1981. Inhibition of phorbol ester-stimulated chemiluminescence in human polymorphonuclear leukocytes by retinoic acid and 5,6-epoxyretinoic acid. *Cancer Res.* 41:216–22

43. Troll, W., Witz, G., Goldstein, B., Stone, D., Sugimura, T. 1982. The role of free oxygen radicals in tumor promotion and carcinogenesis. In *Carcinogenesis. A Comprehensive Survey. Cocarcinogenesis and Biological Effects of Tumor Promoters,* ed. E. Hecker, N. E. Fusenig, W. Kunz, F. Marks, H. W. Thielmann, 7:593–97. New York: Raven

44. Formisano, J., Troll, W., Sugimura, T. 1983. Superoxide response induced by indole alkaloid tumor promoters. *Ann. NY Acad. Sci.* 407:429–31

45. Goldstein, B. D., Witz, G., Amoruso, M., Stone, D. S., Troll, W. 1981. Stimulation of human polymorphonuclear leukocyte superoxide anion radical by tumor promoters. *Cancer Lett.* 11:257–62

46. Pick, E., Keisari, Y. 1981. Superoxide anion and hydrogen peroxide production by chemically elicited peritoneal macrophages—induction by multiple nonphagocytic stimuli. *Cell Immunol.* 59: 301–18

47. Kinsella, A. R., Gainer, H. St. C., Butler, J. 1983. Investigation of a possible role for superoxide anion production in tumor promotion. *Carcinogenesis* 4: 717–19

48. Hoffman, M., Autor, A. P. 1982. Effect of cyclooxygenase inhibitors and protease inhibitors on phorbol-induced stimulation of oxygen consumption and superoxide production by rat pulmonary macrophages. *Biochem. Pharmacol.* 31:775–80

49. Yavelow, J., Gidlund, M., Troll, W.

1982. Protease inhibitors from processed legumes effectively inhibit superoxide generation in response to TPA. *Carcinogenesis* 3:135–38

50. Witz, G., Goldstein, B. D., Amoruso, M., Stone, D. S., Troll, W. 1980. Retinoid inhibition of superoxide anion radical production by human polymorphonuclear leukocytes stimulated with tumor promoters. *Biochem. Biophys. Res. Commun.* 97:883–88

51. Meeks, R. G., Chen, R. F. 1979. The effect of membrane detergents and retinoic acid on membrane microviscosity. *Fed. Proc.* 38:540 (Abstr.)

52. Demopoulos, H., Pietronigro, D., Seligman, M., Flamm, E. 1980. The possible role of free radical reactions in carcinogenesis. *J. Environ. Pathol. Toxicol.* 3:273–304

53. Troll, W. 1975. Blocking tumor promotion by protease inhibitors. In *Fundamentals in Cancer Prevention,* ed. P. N. Magee, S. Takayama, T. Sugimura, T. Matsushima, pp. 41–53. Tokyo: Univ. Tokyo Press

54. Cwikel, B. J., Barouski-Miller, P. A., Coleman, P. L., Gelehrter, T. D. 1984. Dexamethasone induction of an inhibitor of plasminogen activator in HTC hepatoma cells. *J. Biol. Chem.* 259:6847–51

55. Kitagawa, S., Takaku, F., Sakamoto, S. 1980. Evidence that proteases are involved in superoxide production by human polymorphonuclear leukocytes and monocytes. *J. Clin. Invest.* 65:74–81

56. Kitagawa, S., Takaku, F., Sakamoto, S. 1980. Serine protease inhibitors inhibit superoxide production by human basophils stimulated by anti-IgE. *Biochem. Biophys. Res. Commun.* 95:801–6

57. Logani, M. K., Solanki, V., Slaga, T. J. 1982. Effect of tumor promoters on lipid peroxidation in mouse skin. *Carcinogenesis* 3:1303–6

58. Belman, S., Garte, S. 1984. Proteases and cyclic nucleotides. In *Prostaglandins, Leukotrienes and Cancer,* ed. T. Slaga, S. Fisher. The Hague: Nijhoff. In press

59. Fischer, S. M., Adams, L. M. 1984. Inhibition of tumor promoter stimulated chemiluminescence in mouse epidermal cells by inhibitors of arachidonic acid metabolism. *Proc. Am. Assoc. Cancer Res.* 25:82

60. Fridovich, T. 1978. The biology of oxygen radicals. The superoxide radical is an agent of oxygen toxicity; superoxide dismutases provide an important defense. *Science* 201:875–80

61. Fridovich, T. 1983. Superoxide radical: An endogenous toxicant. *Ann. Rev. Pharmacol. Toxicol.* 23:239–57
62. McLennan, G., Oberley, L. W., Autor, A. P. 1980. The role of oxygen-derived free radicals in radiation-induced damage and death of nondividing eucaryotic cells. *Radiat. Res.* 84:122–32
63. Halliwell, B. 1978. Biochemical mechanisms accounting for the toxic action of oxygen on living organisms. The key role of superoxide dismutase. *Cell. Biol. Int. Rep.* 2:113–28
64. Solanki, V., Rana, R. S., Slaga, T. J. 1981. Diminution of mouse epidermal superoxide dismutase and catalase activities by tumor promoters. *Carcinogenesis* 2:1141–46
65. Oberley, L. W., Buettner, G. R. 1979. Role of superoxide dismutase in cancer: A review. *Cancer Res.* 39:1141–49
66. Takada, Y., Noguchi, T., Okabe, T., Kajiyama, M. 1982. Superoxide dismutase in various tissues from rabbits bearing the VX-2 carcinoma in the maxillary sinus. *Cancer Res.* 42:4233–35
67. Leuthauser, S. W. C., Oberley, L. W., Oberley, T. D., Loven, D. P. 1984. Lowered superoxide dismutase activity in distant organs of tumor-bearing mice. *J. Natl. Cancer Inst.* 72:1065–74
68. Leuthauser, S. W. C., Oberley, L. W., Oberley, T. D., Sorenson, J. R. J., Ramakrishna, K. 1981. Antitumor effect of a copper coordination compound with superoxide dismutase-like activity. *J. Natl. Cancer Inst.* 66:1077–81
69. Kensler, T. W., Bush, D. M., Kozumbo, W. J. 1983. Inhibition of tumor promotion by a biomimetic superoxide dismutase. *Science* 221:75–77
70. O'Brien, T. G., Simsiman, R. C., Boutwell, R. K. 1975. Induction of the polyamine-biosynthetic enzymes in the mouse epidermis and their specificity for tumor promotion. *Cancer Res.* 35:2426–33
71. Mukai, F. H., Goldstein, B. D. 1976. Mutagenicity of malonaldehyde, a decomposition product of peroxidized polyunsaturated fatty acids. *Science* 191:868–69
72. Weitzman, S. A., Stossel, T. P. 1981. Mutation caused by human phagocytes. *Science* 212:546–47
73. Barak, M., Ulitzur, S., Merzbach, D. 1983. Phagocytosis-induced mutagenesis in bacteria. *Mutat. Res.* 121:7–16
74. Cunningham, M. L., Lokesh, B. R. 1983. Superoxide anion generated by potassium superoxide is cytotoxic and mutagenic to Chinese hamster ovary cells. *Mutat. Res.* 121:299–304
75. Weitberg, A. B., Weitzman, S. A., Destrempes, M., Latt, S. A., Stossel, T. P. 1983. Stimulated human phagocytes produce cytogenic changes in cultured mammalian cells. *N. Engl. J. Med.* 308:26–30
76. Mondal, S., Brankow, D. W., Heidelberger, C. 1976. Two-stage chemical oncogenesis in cultures of C₃H/10T½ cells. *Cancer Res.* 36:2254–60
77. Mondal, S., Heidelberger, C. 1976. Transformation of 10T½/C18 mouse embryo fibroblasts by ultraviolet irradiation and a phorbol ester. *Nature* 260:710–11
78. Kennedy, A. R., Mondal, S., Heidelberger, C., Little, J. B. 1978. Enhancement of X-ray transformation by 12-O-tetradecanoyl-phorbol-13-acetate in a cloned line of C₃H mouse embryo cells. *Cancer Res.* 38:439–43
79. Kennedy, A. R., Little, J. B. 1981. Effects of protease inhibitors on radiation transformation *in vitro*. *Cancer Res.* 41:2103–8
80. Borek, C., Miller, R., Pain, D., Troll, W. 1979. Conditions for inhibiting and enhancing effects of the protease inhibitor antipain on X-ray induced neoplastic transformation in hamster and mouse cells. *Proc. Natl. Acad. Sci. USA* 74:1800–3
81. Kuroki, T., Drevon, C. 1979. Inhibition of chemical transformation in C₃H/10T½ cells by protease inhibitors. *Cancer Res.* 39:2755–61
82. Fibach, E., Kidron, M., Nachson, I., Mayer, H. 1983. Phorbol ester-induced adhesion of murine erythroleukemia cells: Possible involvement of cellular proteases. *Carcinogenesis* 4:1395–99
83. Nagasawa, H., Little, J. B. 1979. Effect of tumor promoters, protease inhibitors, and repair processes in X-ray-induced sister chromatid exchanges. *Proc. Natl. Acad. Sci. USA* 76:1943–47
84. Borek, C. 1982. Radiation oncogenesis in cell culture. *Adv. Cancer Res.* 37:159–232
85. Zimmerman, R., Cerutti, P. 1984. Active oxygen acts as a promoter of transformation in mouse embryo fibroblasts C3H10T1/2/C18. *Proc. Natl. Acad. Sci. USA* 81:2085–87
86. Borek, C., Troll, W. 1983. Modifiers of free radicals inhibit *in vitro* the oncogenic actions of X-rays, bleomycin, and the tumor promoter 12-O-tetradecanoylphorbol 13-acetate. *Proc. Natl. Acad. Sci. USA* 80:1304–7

87. Gensler, H. L., Bowden, G. T. 1983. Evidence suggesting a dissociation of DNA strand scissions and late-stage promotion of tumor cell phenotype. *Carcinogenesis* 4:1507–11
88. Dutton, D., Bowden, G. T. 1984. Clastogenic effects of tumor promoters in primary mouse epidermal cells coincubated with macrophages. *Proc. Am. Assoc. Cancer Res.* 25:151 (Abstr.)
89. Nakamura, Y., Gindhart, T. D., Colburn, N. H. 1984. Antioxidants, superoxide dismutase and Cu(II)DIPS inhibit promotion of neoplastic transformation by TPA in JB6 cells: Role of reactive oxygen in tumor promotion. *Proc. Am. Assoc. Cancer Res.* 25:139 (Abstr.)
90. Friedman, J., Cerutti, P. A. 1983. The induction of ornithine decarboxylase by phorbol-12-myristate 13-acetate or by serum is inhibited by antioxidants. *Carcinogenesis* 4:1425–27
91. Birnboim, H. C. 1982. DNA strand breakage in human leukocytes exposed to a tumor promoter, phorbol myristate acetate. *Science* 215:1247–49
92. Birnboim, H. C. 1982. Factors which affect DNA strand breakage in human leukocytes exposed to a tumor promoter, phorbol myristate acetate. *Can. J. Physiol. Pharmacol.* 60:1359–66
93. Birnboim, H. C. 1983. Importance of DNA strand-break damage in tumor promotion. See Ref. 16, pp. 539–56
94. Emerit, I., Cerutti, P. A. 1981. Tumor promoter phorbol-12-myristate-13-acetate induces chromosomal damage via indirect action. *Nature* 293:144–46
95. Emerit, I., Levy, A., Cerutti, P. 1983. Suppression of tumor promoter phorbolmyristate acetate-induced chromosome breakage by antioxidants and inhibitors of arachidonic acid metabolism. *Mutat. Res.* 110:327–35
96. Emerit, I., Cerutti, P. A. 1982. Tumor promoter phorbol 12-myristate 13-acetate induces a clastogenic factor in human lymphocytes. *Proc. Natl. Acad. Sci. USA* 79:7509–13
97. Emerit, I., Cerutti, P. A. 1983. Clastogenic action of tumor promoter phorbol-12-myristate-13-acetate in mixed human leukocyte cultures. *Carcinogenesis* 4:1313–16
98. Emerit, I., Cerutti, P. 1981. Clastogenic activity from Bloom syndrome fibroblast cultures. *Proc. Natl. Acad. Sci. USA* 78:1968–72
99. Cerutti, P. A., Amstad, P., Emerit, I. 1983. Tumor promoter phorbolmyristate-acetate induces membrane-

mediated chromosomal damage. See Ref. 16, pp. 527–38
100. Schulte-Frohlinde, D. 1983. Kinetics and mechanism of polynucleotide and DNA strand break formation. See Ref. 16, pp. 53–71
101. Teebor, G. W., Frenkel, K., Goldstein, M. S. 1982. Identification of radiation-induced thymine derivative in DNA. *Adv. Enzyme Regul.* 20:39–54
102. Teebor, G. W., Frenkel, K., Goldstein, M. S. 1984. Ionizing radiation and tritium transmutation both cause formation of 5-hydroxy-methyl 2'-deoxyuridine in cellular DNA. *Proc. Natl. Acad. Sci. USA* 81:318–21
103. Troll, W., Frenkel, K., Teebor, G. 1984. Free oxygen radicals: Necessary contributors to tumor promotion and cocarcinogenesis. In *Cellular Interactions by Environmental Tumor Promoters,* ed. H. Fujiki et al., 207–18 Tokyo: Jpn. Sci. Soc.
104. Demple, B., Linn, S. 1982. 5,6-Saturated thymine lesions in DNA: Production by ultraviolet light or hydrogen peroxide. *Nucleic Acids Res.* 10:3781–89
105. Peraino, C., Fry, R. J. M., Staffelt, E. 1971. Reduction and enhancement by phenobarbital of hepatocarcinogenesis induced in the rat by 2-acetylaminofluorene. *Cancer Res.* 31:1506–12
106. Hicks, R. M. 1982. Promotion in bladder cancer. See Ref. 43, 7:139–53
107. Cohen, S. M., Arai, M., Jacobs, J. B., Friedell, G. H. 1979. Promoting effect of saccharin and DL-tryptophan in urinary bladder carcinogenesis. *Cancer Res.* 39:1207–17
108. Reddy, B. S., Weisburger, J. H., Wynder, E. L. 1978. Colon cancer: Bile salts as tumor promoters. In *Carcinogenesis, Mechanisms of Tumor Promotion and Cocarcinogenesis,* ed. T. J. Slaga, A. Sivak, R. K. Boutwell, 2:453–74. New York: Raven
109. Marx, J. L. 1978. Tumor promoters: Carcinogenesis gets more complicated. *Science* 201:515–18
110. Mossman, B., Light, W., Wei, E. 1983. Asbestos: Mechanism of toxicity and carcinogenicity in the respiratory tract. *Ann. Rev. Pharmacol. Toxicol.* 23:595–615
111. Hirota, N., Yokoyama, T. 1981. Enhancing effect of hydrogen peroxide upon duodenal and upper jejunal carcinogenesis in rats. *Gann* 72:811–12
112. Ito, A., Watanabe, H., Naito, M., Naito, Y., Kawashima, K. 1984. Correlation between induction of duodenal tumor by

hydrogen peroxide and catalase activity in mice. *Gann* 75:17–21

113. Teebor, G. W., Frenkel, K. 1983. The initiation of DNA excision-repair. *Adv. Cancer Res.* 38:23–59

114. Rasmussen, R. E., Boyd, C. H., Dansie, D. R., Kouri, R. E., Henry, C. J. 1981. DNA replication and unscheduled DNA synthesis in lungs of mice exposed to cigarette smoke. *Cancer Res.* 41:2583–88

115. Whittemore, A., McMillan, A. 1983. Lung cancer mortality among U.S. uranium miners: A reappraisal. *J. Natl. Cancer Inst.* 71:489–99

116. Stern, R. S., Thibodeau, L. A., Kleinerman, R. A., Parrish, J. A., Fitzpatrick, T. B. 1979. Risk of cutaneous carcinoma in patients treated with oral methoxsalen photochemotherapy for psoriasis. *N. Engl. J. Med.,* 300:809–13

117. Frank, J. P., Williams, J. R. 1982. X-ray induction of persistent hypersensitivity to mutation. *Science* 216:307–8

118. Armstrong, B., Doll, R. 1975. Environmental factors and cancer incidence and mortality in different countries, with special reference to dietary factors. *Int. J. Cancer* 15:617–31

119. Haenszel, W., Kurihara, M. 1968. Studies of Japanese migrants. I. Mortality from cancer and other diseases among Japanese in the U.S. *J. Natl. Cancer Inst.* 40:43–68

120. Staszewski, J., Haenszel, W. 1965. Cancer mortality among the Polish-born in the United States. *J. Natl. Cancer Inst.* 35:291–97

121. Carroll, K. K. 1975. Experimental evidence of dietary factors and hormone-dependent cancers. *Cancer Res.* 35:3374–83

122. Wynder, F., Mabuchi, K., Whitmore, W. 1971. Epidemiology of cancer of the prostate. *Cancer* 28:344–60

123. Phillips, R. L. 1975. Role of life-style and dietary habits in risk of cancer among Seventh-Day Adventists. *Cancer Res.* 35:3513–22

124. Correa, P. 1981. Epidemiological correlations between diet and cancer frequency. *Cancer Res.* 41:3685–90

125. Winn, D. M., Ziegler, R. G., Pickle, L. W., Gridley, G., Blot, W. J., Hoover, R. N. 1984. Diet in the etiology of oral and pharyngeal cancer among women from the southern United States. *Cancer Res.* 44:1216–22

Ann. Rev. Pharmacol. Toxicol. 1985. 25:529–66

STEROID HORMONE REGULATION OF GENE EXPRESSION

Gordon M. Ringold

Department of Pharmacology, Stanford University School of Medicine, Stanford, California 94305

INTRODUCTION

The remarkable diversity in form and function of cells within a single organism stems not from intrinsic differences in genetic composition but from the selective and highly controlled expression of subsets of that genetic repertoire. A major focus of current biological research is the elucidation of the mechanisms by which gene expression can be regulated both during development and in response to environmental stimuli. It is the ability of steroid hormones to act as gene regulatory molecules that has focused tremendous attention on their mode of action.

Each class of steroid hormone appears to mediate its biological response by binding to an intracellular receptor protein that is confined to target tissues [reviewed in (1, 2)]. Interaction of the hormone with its cognate receptor leads to an alteration in the structure of the protein that is manifested by an increased affinity of the steroid-receptor (SR) complex for DNA [reviewed in (3)]. By analogy with other ligand-protein interactions, the role of the hormone itself can best be viewed as an allosteric modifier of receptor structure. One exception to this general model is the membrane receptor for progesterone found on *Xenopus* oocytes (4).

Although SR complexes bind to all DNAs, albeit with low binding constants, it is their high-affinity interactions with specific DNA sequences that seem to be important for the ensuing alterations in gene expression. As a result, only a small number of genes within the target cell become transcriptionally activated. It is my intent in this review to summarize key observations from the

529

0362-1642/85/415-0529$02.00

large body of work that has led to our current understanding of steroid receptor structure and function as it pertains to activation of gene transcription. In addition, I will briefly introduce novel modes by which steroids effect changes in gene expression. It is through a concerted interplay of gene regulatory events, in large part (if not completely) initiated by direct stimulation of transcription by SR complexes, that predictable and reproducible effects on cell function transpire. Particular attention will be paid to systems that have been and those that have promise of being especially useful in deciphering the intricacies of steroid receptor action. The reader will be directed to other sources for more detailed discussions of receptor structure, modification, and activation, as well as for additional information pertaining to specific systems.

THE EVOLUTION OF THE MODEL OF STEROID RECEPTOR ACTION

Although perhaps not generally appreciated, some of the earliest studies involving detection of receptors with radioactive ligands were performed by Jensen & DeSombre in the course of their studies on estrogen-responsive tissues (1). They observed that ^3H estradiol accumulated in tissues such as uterus that are known to exhibit marked physiological changes in response to hormone treatment. Based on these observations, Jensen postulated the existence of highly specific receptors for estradiol in these target tissues. Subsequent analysis of the estradiol receptor by Jensen's and Gorski's groups led to the observation that the unoccupied receptor resides primarily in the cytoplasm, whereas after hormone treatment the bulk of the receptor becomes tightly associated with the nucleus (5, 6). Similar data were later obtained for other classes of steroids (2). The proposed two-step model of steroid hormone action was widely accepted and as postulated suggested that the hormone causes net migration of receptor protein from the cytosolic to the nuclear compartment. Since it was clear that steroids cause alterations in the production of specific proteins in various systems (see below), the idea that the nuclear form of the SR complex regulates gene expression arose [for reviews see (7, 8)]. The observation that the receptor could bind to DNA in vitro, but only after binding to the hormone, added significantly to the model (9, 10).

Recent technological developments have provided powerful new approaches to the study of steroid receptors. As a result of such studies, the classical two-step model has had to undergo minor modifications. First, novel methods for fractionating cells into nuclear and cytoplasmic fractions led to the observation that unoccupied estrogen receptors reside primarily, if not completely, within the nucleus (11, 12). Second, immunocytochemistry with monoclonal antibodies against the human estrogen receptor also indicate that both the naive and ligand-bound forms of the receptor are localized within the nucleus (13).

Thus, the alteration of receptor structure and/or function associated with binding of hormone could reflect a redistribution of the receptor from a non–DNA containing nuclear compartment to the chromosomal DNA. The earlier studies on receptor localization were undoubtedly compromised by the fact that, upon lysing cells in large aqueous volumes, receptors appear to dissociate from nuclear components. Similar observations have been made for unrelated proteins such as α DNA polymerase (14) and the dioxin receptor (15). In the case of two steroid hormones, ecdysone and Vitamin D, as well as that of thyroxine, the unoccupied form of their corresponding receptors remains with the nuclear fraction even under harsh disruption conditions [reviewed in (16)]. The nature of the sites to which any or all of these receptors bind in the absence of hormone remains obscure. However, Barrack & Coffey (17) have suggested that estrogen receptors may be associated with a rather ill-defined but increasingly provocative structure composed of DNA and protein that they have called the nuclear matrix. Since both DNA replication and transcription machinery may be associated with this structure, Gorski (18) has raised the intriguing possibility that steroid receptors might remain immobilized on the nuclear matrix; the hormonal activation of the receptor would then be envisioned to expose a DNA binding site that would cause the SR complex to become tightly associated with DNA while remaining bound to other nuclear proteins.

In sum, although refinements continue to be made in our understanding of steroid receptor disposition within cells, the basic two-step model proposed in the late 1960s remains valid. To recapitulate, the interaction of the steroid hormone with its cognate receptor leads to an alteration in the physical state of the protein, resulting in its conversion to a form with increased affinity for DNA. Whether the receptor ever resides in the cytosol after its synthesis and whether the receptor ever exists in a soluble form within the nucleus are interesting issues, but ones that are perhaps ancillary to the mechanisms by which these proteins modulate gene activity.

REGULATION OF GENE EXPRESSION

Shortly after the discovery of steroid receptors, several groups postulated that physiological changes induced by steroid (and perhaps other classes of) hormones might be a result of alterations in gene expression [for reviews see (2, 3, 7)]. The then recent discoveries of messenger RNA and the elucidation of gene regulatory mechanisms in bacteria made this suggestion quite fashionable. Development of tools by which to analyze specific proteins in well-defined systems has allowed this prediction to be proven. Suggestive experiments also implied that specific messenger RNAs accumulated in response to treatment of cells with these hormones. Two noteworthy sets of experiments deserve mention. First, Sekeris (19) was ahead of his time in utilizing in vitro translation to document that ecdysone-stimulated increases in *dopa* decarboxylase are due to increased production of the corresponding mRNA. Second, Tomkins and his colleagues utilized metabolic inhibitors in novel ways to suggest that the induction of tyrosine aminotransferase (TAT) by glucocorticoids in HTC, rat hepatoma cells, is due to a direct action of the glucocorticoid-receptor complex on TAT mRNA production (20). Subsequent analyses in a large variety of systems confirmed these general notions. It was not, however, until the discovery of reverse transcriptase and the advent of nucleic acid hybridization and cloning techniques that detailed mechanistic studies on gene activation by steroid hormones became a reality. Since that time, tremendous advances have been made in characterizing the basic principles involved in steroid-mediated induction of gene expression. A general requirement for understanding the detailed mechanisms for gene activation by steroid hormones has been to obtain the DNA encoding the regulated gene product, in particular the region(s) of the DNA involved in the hormonal responsiveness of that gene. The development of recombinant DNA techniques has allowed investigators to obtain unlimited quantities of these important DNA sequences and to test whether, for example, SR complexes interact directly with the DNA adjacent to the coding region. The major focus of this review will be on systems in which the availability of the appropriate DNAs has facilitated a dissection of the molecular aspects of steroid-regulated gene expression.

RECEPTOR STRUCTURE

There is a paucity of data regarding the structure of steroid receptors as it pertains to their role as gene-regulatory molecules. Nevertheless, it is worthwhile at this juncture to briefly review some of the salient features of these proteins and to point out areas that remain to be explored. Until very recently, all data regarding these receptors were derived from their detection with radioactive ligands. The advent of affinity-labeling reagents and monoclonal antibodies for several of these receptors has facilitated the undertaking of more refined structural analyses.

Unactivated Receptors

The unactivated form of steroid receptors has generally been obtained by homogenizing cells at low temperatures in hypotonic buffers. If kept at low temperatures, the receptors remain in this state even when bound to hormone and acquire DNA-binding capabilities only when warmed, exposed to high salt, or subjected to a variety of other experimental conditions [reviewed in (3, 16)]. The recent observation that transition metal oxyanions (molybdate has been used most extensively) stabilize the unactivated form of receptors has facilitated their characterization (21, 22). Ion-exchange chromatography, isoelectric focusing, and aqueous two-phase partitioning have been used to assess receptor charge. The bulk of the experimental results indicates that the unactivated form of steroid receptors is acidic, with isoelectric points between 4 and 6. Sucrose gradient sedimentation and gel filtration have been the standard means by which to determine the size and shape of steroid receptors. Striking similarities are observed among receptors for various classes of steroids; in all cases studied to date, the unactivated receptor appears to exist as a multimer having a molecular weight of 200–300 Kd, with sedimentation values of 8–10S and Stokes radii of 7–10 nm. Furthermore, the receptors exist as prolate ellipsoids with axial ratios ranging from about 10–20. These and other properties of individual steroid receptors are summarized in recent reviews (16, 23, 24).

Activated Receptors

Most studies of the activated form of steroid receptors have utilized receptors that have been activated in vitro. Various experimental approaches support the notion that receptors lose net negative charge upon activation, resulting in proteins with isoelectric points of 5.5–7.0. Recent evidence indicates that glucocorticoid receptors exist as phosphoproteins in vivo (25), that progesterone receptors can be phosphorylated in vitro and may be phosphoproteins in vivo (26, 27), and that inhibitors of phosphatases such as molybdate and vanadate prevent activation whereas incubation with calf alkaline phosphatase activates receptors (see 24). The speculative hypothesis therefore exists that the activation of steroid receptors involves dephosphorylation of the receptor protein itself.

The activated forms of steroid receptors always have lower sedimentation (S) values than the unactivated forms. Conversion of the 8–10S form to a 3–4S form is characteristic and, since this alteration is associated with conditions that would dissociate oligomeric structures (e.g. high salt, elevated temperature, and dilution), it seems likely that the most stable activated form of steroid receptors is a monomeric structure. Preliminary evidence suggests, however, that a multimeric form may be involved in gene activation (28).

Except for the chick progesterone receptor, which appears to be composed of two dissimilar hormone-binding subunits of about 110 and 80 Kd (29), all the steroid receptors seem to contain a single species of protein ranging in molecular weight from about 60 Kd for the Vitamin D receptor to about 120 Kd for the androgen receptor [reviewed in (16)]. The chick progesterone receptor appears to consist of a small DNA-binding subunit (A) and a large non-DNA-binding subunit (B).

Extremely illuminating experiments relating to receptor structure have recently been performed using radioactively labeled covalent-affinity reagents for the glucocorticoid, progesterone, estrogen, and androgen receptors. Of particular note is the observation that under denaturing conditions of SDS-polyacrylamide gel electrophoresis, the unactivated and activated forms of the receptor are indistinguishable. Similar conclusions have been reached using monoclonal or polyclonal antibodies to, among others, the glucocorticoid (30, 31), progesterone (32), and Vitamin D (33) receptors. Lastly, purification of glucocorticoid (34) and estrogen (35) receptors in their activated state confirms the generality that, with the exception of the avian progesterone receptor, steroid receptors are composed of single hormone-binding polypeptides.

Functional Receptor Domains

Our knowledge of the functional domains inherent in the monomeric form of steroid receptors comes primarily from partial proteolysis studies of the rat and mouse glucocorticoid receptor. This receptor of 90–95 Kd appears to be composed of three distinct domains that can be resolved by judicious or in some cases accidental use of proteases (23, 26). A fragment of about 40 Kd that retains both hormone and DNA binding activities can be released from the receptor by mild treatment with chymotrypsin and occurs spontaneously in cell extracts (23, 36–38). Further digestion with trypsin-like proteases yields the so-called mero-receptor (23, 39) of approximately 23 Kd that contains only the hormone binding domain. The region of the receptor that has no obvious function contains the major antigenic determinants (36) and is likely to play a crucial role in modulating DNA binding activity, perhaps by serving as a binding domain for other nuclear proteins or by facilitating proper receptor-receptor interactions. The physiological importance of this region is indicated by the behavior of mutant forms of the glucocorticoid receptor that are ostensibly devoid of this "modulating" domain. In mouse S49 lymphoma cells carrying this mutated form of the receptor, the so-called nt^i receptor, the typical cytolytic response to glucocorticoids does not occur (40, 41). Furthermore, the nt^i receptor exhibits increased binding affinity for non-specific DNA sequences (42). Recently, receptor fragments devoid of the "modulating" domain have been prepared in vitro from purified receptor. These fragments retain the ability to recognize and bind to specific DNA sequences adjacent to glucocorticoid inducible genes, albeit with reduced affinity when compared to native gluco-corticoid-receptor complexes (28, 43). Thus, the role of this region of the receptor may be to aid in discriminating between specific and non-specific DNA binding sites. This will be discussed in more detail in a following section. Those readers who wish more detail on the characteristics of proteolytic fragments derived from the glucocorticoid receptor and the mutant forms of the receptors, as well as information on other steroid receptors, are directed to one or more of the following reviews (16, 23, 44, 45).

GLUCOCORTICOID INDUCIBLE GENES

Glucocorticoid Induction of MMTV (A Summary of the Viral Life-Cycle)

Viruses have played a leading role in deciphering the intricacies of biological regulatory mechanisms in both procaryotic and eukaryotic organisms. In the case of steroid hormone action, the fortuitous observation that glucocorticoids stimulate production of mouse mammary tumor virus (MMTV) in cultures of mouse mammary carcinoma cells (46) has led to what is now perhaps the best characterized model of how steroids regulate gene transcription. MMTV is a typical retrovirus containing a single-stranded RNA genome that replicates via a DNA intermediate called the provirus. Viral DNA is synthesized by the virion-associated reverse transcriptase and eventually becomes covalently integrated, apparently in a random fashion, into the host cell's chromosomes. At that point, the proviral DNA becomes a stable genetic element akin to any other cellular gene encoding a polypeptide sequence and can be viewed as being equivalent to the genes encoding TAT, globin, or albumin, for example. It is transcribed by RNA polymerase II (47) to yield a primary transcript of about 9,000 bases in length that is utilized both to produce some of the viral proteins and to encapsidate into progeny virions. In addition, smaller spliced RNAs are synthesized as templates for translation of the major viral glycoproteins (gp52 and gp36), as well as a protein of unknown function whose production is restricted to a subset of mammary cells [for recent reviews, see (48, 49)].

In order to appreciate the intricacies of this system, the reader should be aware of the general structure of the MMTV provirus (see Figure 1). As a consequence of the fascinating process by which reverse transcriptase generates the provirus (50, 51), sequences represented within the 3' and 5' ends of viral RNA are duplicated to generate a DNA molecule containing direct repeats at its termini. These so-called long terminal repeat (LTR) sequences contain most, if not all, of the regulatory signals involved in the control of viral gene transcription (50, 51). In the case of MMTV, the LTR is approximately 1,350 base pairs in length, with about 130 of these arising from the 5' end of viral RNA. Thus, it is convenient from the viruses' and the investigator's point of view that the LTR that contains the viral regulatory signals is encoded within the viral RNA itself.

INDUCTION OF MMTV RNA   The great interest in studying MMTV as a model system has been predicated on early studies showing that the glucocorticoid-mediated increase in production of virus by mammary tumor cells is a consequence of increased production of viral RNA (52, 53). More importantly, the induction of viral RNA is rapid, independent of ongoing protein synthesis, and

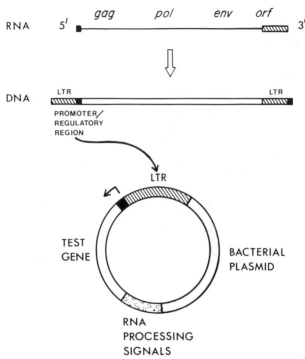

Figure 1   The structure of MMTV RNA, DNA, and a prototypical chimeric gene. The intact viral RNA (approximately 9000 bases) is illustrated with the coding regions indicated: *gag* = group-specific antigens or coat proteins; *pol* = viral polymerase or reverse transcriptase; *env* = envelope glycoproteins; *orf* = a protein of unknown function encoded within a 3' open reading frame. The linear form of double-stranded MMTV DNA contains long terminally repeated (LTR) sequences derived from both the 3' and 5' ends of viral RNA; these are indicated as the solid 5' region (130 base pairs) and the slashed 3' region (approximately 1200 base pairs). This structure is maintained when the viral DNA integrates into chromosomal DNA to form the provirus. A generic structure for chimeric recombinant plasmids is shown in which one of the MMTV LTR sequences (which contains the promoter and regulatory region) is placed adjacent to a marker or test gene whose activity can be easily measured after transfection of the DNA into recipient tissue culture cells. In addition to the LTR promoter/regulatory region and the test gene itself (clear), sequences required for RNA processing usually from the virus SV40, and all or a portion of a bacterial plasmid (stippled) that allows manipulation and propagation of the DNA in *E. coli,* are included in the recombinant molecule. [For a more detailed discussion, see (65).] Similar constructions have been utilized to characterize the promoter and regulatory regions of several steroid-inducible genes.

mediated by the cellular glucocorticoid receptor (54, 55). Particularly noteworthy was the observation that the accumulation of viral RNA is due to an increase in its rate of synthesis (56, 57); this was the first experimental demonstration that steroid hormones could directly affect the transcription of a specific gene. Lastly, infection of heterologous (i.e. non-mammary) cells by MMTV revealed two crucial points: (*a*) glucocorticoid inducibility is retained in a variety of cell types, including mink lung, cat kidney, and rat liver (58, 59), and (*b*) the sites of proviral integration in host-cell DNA are ostensibly random (60, 61). Thus, the signals that impart glucocorticoid sensitivity to MMTV must be encoded within the viral genome. An additional point borne out by these studies is that the functional region of the glucocorticoid receptor must be highly conserved, since the induction of MMTV RNA is retained in cells from widely divergent species.

TRANSFECTION OF MOLECULARLY CLONED MMTV DNA   The advent of molecular cloning has resulted in prodigious advances in our abilities to dissect the coding, non-coding, and regulatory components of specific DNA sequences. The first such experiments with MMTV entailed introduction of cloned proviral DNA into mouse fibroblasts (62, 63) by the newly developed methods of DNA-mediated gene transfer or transfection (64). These studies corroborated the information previously garnered by analysis of virally infected heterologous cells (see above) and strengthened the argument that the proviral DNA itself carries glucocorticoid regulatory sequences. The likely possibility that such sequences reside near the promoter region was tested by assessing the hormone responsiveness of chimeric genes in which an MMTV LTR is fused to heterologous coding sequences (see Figure 1). In all cases, the production of the fused gene product exhibits glucocorticoid inducibility in a variety of tissue-culture cell lines. Among the proteins that have been expressed in a hormone-dependent fashion are mouse dihydrofolate reductase (65), v-*ras* of the Harvey sarcoma virus (66), herpes simplex thymidine kinase (67–69), and the *E. coli* enzymes β-galactosidase and XGPRT (70, 71). These experiments provide convincing evidence that sequences within the MMTV LTR are sufficient to confer hormone sensitivity on the MMTV promoter.

In addition to studies employing chimeric genes, Fasel et al (72) and Yamamoto and colleagues (73) have introduced fragments of the MMTV genome into mouse L cells by co-transfection with the herpes virus TK gene. Again, production of MMTV RNA is hormone inducible. However, a surprising result was obtained by Yamamoto et al (73), who found that glucocorticoids also stimulate the production of MMTV RNA in cells transfected with non-LTR DNA fragments. As will be discussed below, specific binding sites for the glucocorticoid-receptor complex exist not only within the LTR but within internal viral DNA fragments as well (74). It is tempting to speculate that MMTV may harbor the vestiges of multiple glucocorticoid-regulated promoters that were once derived from cellular genes. This may reflect the possibility that, during the rapid evolution of the virus, the acquisition of multiple regulatory regions conferred upon it a selective advantage.

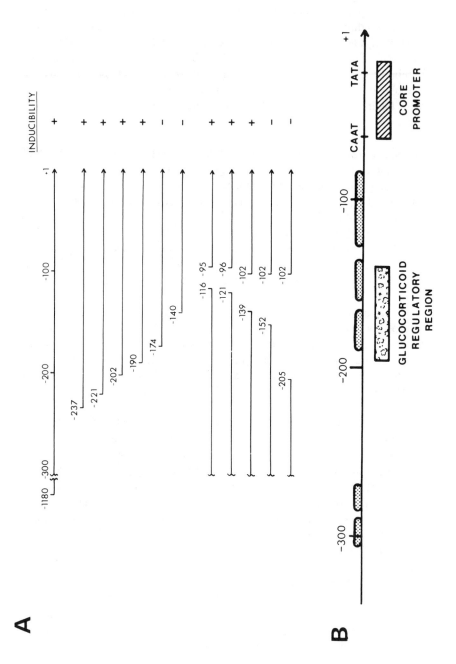

MAPPING THE GLUCOCORTICOID REGULATORY REGION WITHIN THE LTR By studying the behavior of chimeric genes that have had specific portions of the LTR removed, several groups have defined the region of DNA required for hormonal responsiveness (Figure 2A). The MMTV LTR contains a so-called TATA box and a CAAT sequence approximately 25 and 65 nucleotides respectively upstream from the start of transcription (Figure 2B). These short nucleotide sequences are thought to be important signals for the initiation of transcription by RNA polymerase II [for review see (75)]. By convention, nucleotides upstream of the transcription initiation site are denoted by negative numbers; thus, a deletion that removes all but 65 nucleotides upstream of this site is denoted as a −65 deletion.

Majors & Varmus (69) have reported that an LTR deleted to residue −190 retains hormone inducibility, whereas one deleted to residue −140 does not. Similar data from Hynes et al (76) and Buetti & Diggelmann (68) indicate that inducibility is retained in molecules containing about 200 residues upstream of the initiation site, whereas those retaining only 137 nucleotides lose hormone responsiveness. Lee and Ringold and their colleagues (77, 78) have also found that a −221 deletion is glucocorticoid responsive, whereas a −174 deletion is not. Consistent with these observations, Chandler et al (79) and Hager et al (80) have found that hormonal sensitivity is conferred by small regions of the LTR. The sum of these deletion analyses indicate that the 5' border of the regulatory region resides between residues −190 and −174.

Internal and 3' deletions have also been constructed that delimit the extent of the regulatory region. Hynes et al (76) showed that sequences downstream of −52 are not necessary for hormonal response. Majors & Varmus (67) and Lee and colleagues (77, 78) found that deletion of sequences between −98 and

←——

Figure 2 (A) Deletion mapping of the glucocorticoid regulatory region within the MMTV LTR. The top line represents the entire MMTV LTR; the arrow at residue +1 indicates the site at which transcription initiates; the position −100 indicates 100 base pairs upstream of that site. The portion of the LTR remaining in each deletion mutant is indicated by a solid line; the end points of the deletions have been determined by DNA sequence analysis. Inducibility (+) denotes positive stimulation of expression by the glucocorticoids of a test gene fused to the indicated LTR fragment. This figure is a composite of selected deletion mutants analyzed by several groups (68, 69, 76–78). (B) Summary of the functional regions and glucocorticoid-receptor (GR) complex binding sites within the MMTV LTR. The glucocorticoid regulatory region has been identified by analysis of deletion mutants, as shown above. The core promoter is the minimal region required for basal levels of transcription (76, 78, 80) and includes the characteristic TATA and CAAT boxes [see (75)]. Indicated as the stippled, hot-dog shaped regions are the sites protected from DNase digestion by purified GR complexes as reported by Payvar et al (28). The reader should note that the exact GR binding sites are somewhat different according to Scheidereit et al (111). Two major conclusions derived from this evidence are that the functional glucocorticoid regulatory region encompasses strong GR complex binding sites but that not all binding sites are functional as hormone-regulatory sequences.

-120 and between -97 and -138 respectively do not abrogate inducibility, whereas deletion of sequences between -103 and -151 does. Thus, it appears that the 3' border of the regulatory region resides between residues -138 and -151. A deletion that removes residues -103 to -158, however, retains full inducibility (78). The reason for the anomalous behavior of this mutant is not clear, but it is possible that a fortuitous reconstruction of a functional regulatory region has occurred. This is plausible since there appear to be multiple binding sites for the glucocorticoid-receptor complex within this region (see below).

In addition to delineating the sequences important in responsiveness to hormone, these deletion studies have also shown that the regulatory region is distinct and dissociable from the core promoter region (i.e. those sequences required for appropriate initiation by RNA polymerase at levels equivalent to those seen in the absence of hormone). Dobson et al (81) have reported that a -64 deletion retains the ability to produce RNA that initiates at the appropriate site within the LTR. The level of RNA produced (in the presence or absence of hormone) is comparable to that seen in non–hormone treated cells containing DNAs fused to the full-length LTR. Similar conclusions have been reached by Majors & Varmus (67), Hynes et al (76), and Chandler et al (79). In contrast to these results, Hager's and Khoury's laboratories (80, 82) have reported that, upon deletion of the hormone regulatory sequences, the uninduced level of transcription increases to that seen when the intact LTR is hormone stimulated. These researchers suggest, therefore, that the regulatory region functions as a negative control element and that hormone stimulation relieves its negative effect. Such results have not been seen by any other investigators, and it is difficult to ascertain what experimental details may account for these rather disparate results. The presence of a strong promoter-enhancing sequence (see below) in Hager's & Khoury's constructions may be responsible for this effect.

Several groups have recently reported that the glucocorticoid regulatory region can confer hormone inducibility on heterologous promoters. When the region upstream of residue -102 of the MMTV LTR, which lacks the MMTV core promoter, is fused to promoter fragments derived from the herpes virus TK gene (79), the Rous sarcoma virus LTR (69), the SV40 early promoter (83), and the adenovirus major late promoter (84), expression of the linked marker gene becomes glucocorticoid inducible. Thus, there is no obvious requirement for specific interactions between the regulatory region and the core promoter.

A revealing aspect of both the deletion analyses and the characterization of hybrid promoters is that the absolute spacing between the core promoter and the hormone regulatory region need not be constant. Molecules in which the two elements have been brought closer together by deletion of internal sequences function perfectly well, and several of the functional hybrid promoter constructs move the regulatory region further away from the site of transcription initiation. Chandler et al (79) have reported that the hormone regulatory region can even be placed 1,000 base pairs away and in the opposite orientation from the promoter and still retain at least partial ability to promote glucocorticoid-inducible expression of a linked TK gene. Hynes et al (76) have also reported that if the MMTV LTR is fused to the herpes TK gene with its own promoter intact, glucocorticoid-stimulated transcripts that initiate at each of the promoters can be detected in transfected cells. These observations have led to the proposal that the glucocorticoid regulatory region of MMTV acts as a hormone-dependent enhancer (79). Enhancers are rather remarkable DNA sequences first found in SV40 (85–87) that can activate promoters from hundreds or even thousands of base pairs away in an orientation-independent fashion. The mechanism(s) by which enhancers activate transcription remains obscure; however, since they exhibit both species and tissue specificity, they are most likely to be sites of protein-DNA interactions (88, 89). The fact that the glucocorticoid regulatory region and enhancers have some properties in common suggests that enhancer-binding proteins may share functional characteristics with steroid receptors. Intriguingly, however, the MMTV promoter is responsive to the SV40 enhancer in the presence or absence of glucocorticoids and to the MuLV enhancer in the presence of glucocorticoids (65, 89a); this suggests that the mechanisms by which enhancers and the SR-complex activate transcription are distinct.

Other Glucocorticoid Regulated Genes

Examples of glucocorticoid regulated genes abound in the literature. It is not my intent to chronicle all such examples, but rather to provide unifying themes from the most extensively studied genes. Human and rat growth hormone genes are induced two- to threefold by glucocorticoids after gene transfer into mouse fibroblasts (90, 91). In the case of the rat gene, this reflects a similar induction profile in rat pituitary-cell cultures (92). The sequences responsible for the glucocorticoid effect appear to reside within 500 base pairs of the transcription initiation site (93).

α2u-Globulin is a protein of about 19 Kd that is produced in the liver and secreted in the urine of male rats (94). In the animal, normal levels of this protein require a combination of hormones, including glucocorticoids, androgens, growth hormone, thyroxine, and insulin (95, 96). Androgens will induce production of this protein in females, but only after ovariectomy; thus, estrogens appear to play a dominant inhibitory role (97). In tissue culture, only the glucocorticoid response has been reproduced. Unlike MMTV, however, the induction of α2u RNA is dependent on on-going protein synthesis and therefore is probably not due to a direct activation of the gene by the glucocorticoid receptor complex (98). It is interesting, therefore, that a genomic clone of α2u globulin transfected into mouse L cells retains glucocorticoid sensitivity (99). Perhaps there is a general class of glucocorticoid-inducible proteins in cells as disparate as hepatocytes and fibroblasts that is capable of mediating the induction of this RNA. Further delineation of the molecular details involved in the complex response of this gene to other hormones awaits the development of appropriate hormone-responsive tissue-culture systems or the introduction of altered forms of the gene into mouse embryos and their subsequent analysis in transgenic mice.

Several other glucocorticoid-responsive genes have recently been cloned and sequences of the 5' flanking regions have been determined. Of particular interest is a short nucleotide sequence shared between the tyrosine amino-transferase (TAT) and tryptophan oxygenase (TO) genes, both of which are glucocorticoid-inducible in rat liver (100). This sequence is related to the consensus hexanucleotide T-G-T-T-C-T that is found in all of the high-affinity glucocorticoid-receptor binding sites in MMTV, hMT-IIa, and chick lysozyme (see below).

METALLOTHIONEIN   A cellular gene that has been extensively characterized and that responds to glucocorticoids in a fashion akin to that of MMTV is the human metallothionein-IIa gene (hMT-IIa). Metallothioneins (MT) constitute a family of small proteins that bind heavy metals. Their production can be induced by the heavy metals themselves and in some but not all cases by glucocorticoids (101). The hormonal induction of these genes is a primary effect and is at the level of transcription, as determined by direct measurement of RNA synthesis (102, 103). The mouse MT-I gene, when transfected into L cells, retains cadmium inducibility but not glucocorticoid sensitivity (104). Unlike this gene, the hMT-IIa gene retains both metal and hormone sensitivity when transfected into mouse cells (105). Deletion analysis of chimeric genes carrying the hMT-IIa promoter region fused to a TK coding region has shown that the 5' border of the region of DNA required for glucocorticoid responsive-ness lies between residues -268 and -236 (105). As in the case of MMTV, the core promoter can be dissociated from the hormone regulatory region. The hMT-IIa region also appears to have the capacity for promoting transcription when placed at a distance and either 3' or 5' to the promoter (M. Karin, personal communication). Thus, again, the glucocorticoid regulatory region may be acting in a fashion analogous to viral enhancer sequences. The MT genes, as mentioned above, also respond to metals; analysis of the deletion mutants clearly indicates that the sequences involved in this response are distinct from those involved in hormonal induction (105).

LYSOZYME   The chick lysozyme gene can be induced by estrogens, pro-gestins, androgens, and glucocorticoids each via its own receptor in the chick oviduct (106). The induction of ovalbumin in this system will be discussed below. Renkawitz et al (107) have recently constructed a chimeric gene in which the lysozyme promoter region is fused to the coding region for the SV 40 T antigen. No glucocorticoid or estrogen response could be detected by immunofluorescence assay for T-antigen after transfection of this DNA into HeLa or MCF-7 cells. These are both human cell lines that contain functional glucocorticoid receptors; MCF-7 also contains estrogen receptors. However, when the DNA is microinjected into chick oviduct cells but not into fibroblasts, the fusion gene retains responsiveness to glucocorticoids and progesterone (108). Analysis of 5' deletion mutants indicates that the 5' border of the regulatory region for both classes of steroids lies between residues −208 and −164 (108). Further fine mapping will be required to test whether exactly the same sequences are necessary for responsiveness to both progesterone and glucocorticoids.

GLUCOCORTICOID RECEPTOR BINDING TO SPECIFIC DNA SEQUENCES

As suggested by the observation that steroid receptors are DNA binding proteins (see above) and by analogy with known prokaryotic gene-regulatory proteins, the hypothesis has been put forth that stimulation of transcription requires high-affinity interactions with specific DNA sequences [reviewed in (3)]. The selective binding of the glucocorticoid-receptor (GR) complex to fragments of MMTV DNA was first reported by Payvar et al (74). Using a nitrocellulose filter binding assay, they found that DNA fragments derived from internal regions of MMTV are recognized preferentially by highly purified GR complexes compared to bacterial plasmid sequences. The significance of GR binding sites within the structural portions of the MMTV genome remains unclear; however, as mentioned earlier, vestiges of glucocorticoid-regulated promoters may exist within these regions of the viral genome. Although these first studies detailed what may be an unusual situation, subsequent efforts in several laboratories have focused on GR binding to LTR sequences. Both by filter binding assay and by direct visualization in the electron microscope, it has become clear that the LTR harbors multiple specific binding sites for the GR complex (28, 74, 109, 110). All of the binding sites reside upstream of the core promoter. By employing monoclonal antibodies to the GR, Schneidereit et al (111) have convincingly demonstrated that the binding is indeed due to the receptor protein itself. Using a DNA competition assay in which crude receptor preparations are used for detecting DNA binding sites, Pfahl has also found that sequences upstream of the promoter are efficient sites for GR binding (112).

More refined binding studies have been reported in which purified GR complexes are used to protect LTR fragments from degradation with DNAse I.

The results of these experiments, summarized in Figure 2B, indicate that there are several binding domains within the LTR; these are located between residues -305 and -289, -283 and -269, -189 and -166, -159 and -135, and -127 and -84, according to Payvar et al (28), and between residues -192 and -164 and -127 and -72, according to Schneidereit et al (111). The two domains furthest upstream appear to contain lower affinity sites, as determined by nitrocellulose and electron microscopic binding assays, whereas the highest affinity domains appear to be the ones between -189 and -135 (28). This is particularly gratifying, since this is exactly the region that functions as the gene regulatory region of the LTR as determined by the deletion analyses described earlier. It is noteworthy that each of the binding domains appears to be capable of binding GR complexes independently and that no evidence for cooperative interactions has been reported. As alluded to earlier, the binding form of the receptor, when viewed in the electron microscope, appears to exist as an oligomer of two or perhaps four subunits. Finally, alteration of one domain (i.e. by insertion of a short DNA fragment) affects only that binding site; in agreement with the deletion studies, the only such DNA insertions that affect inducibility lie within the -189 to -135 regions (113). It is interesting to note that the two most upstream regions between -305 and -269 and the large downstream region between -127 and -84 appear to be neither required nor sufficient to support hormone-stimulated transcription from the MMTV promoter. Deletions and alterations of these regions do not affect inducibility, in contrast to the sequences between -189 and -135, which appear to be highly susceptible to such alterations.

Nitrocellulose filter binding and DNAse I footprinting of partially purified GR complexes to the hMT-II promoter region have recently been reported (114). The results are consistent with those found for MMTV and are not confused by the presence of several ostensibly irrelevant binding regions. A single region that lies between residues -266 and -241 is protected from digestion with DNAse I by the GR complex. As summarized earlier, this is consistent with data indicating that the hormone regulatory region resides downstream of residue -268 (105).

In experiments virtually identical to those just described, the GR complex from rat liver has been found to bind specifically to sequences upstream of the chick lysozyme transcription initiation site (108). A strong binding site resides between nucleotides -74 and -39, whereas a weaker site exists between residues -208 and -161. The latter binding region coincides almost precisely with the sequences required for a functional glucocorticoid (and progesterone) response in chick oviduct cells (108). The specific binding of the rat liver GR complex to a chicken gene provides another example of the conserved function of this steroid receptor.

A Common DNA Sequence in the GR Binding Domains

The sequence T-G-T-T-C-T or derivatives of the degenerate octanucleotide ^T_ACTG^T_ATCT are present, sometimes in multiple copies, within all of the binding regions to which the GR complex binds in vitro (28, 111, 114). These include all of the binding regions in the MMTV LTR, the internal MMTV fragments, the hMT-IIa promoter, and the chick lysozyme promoter. In addition, this same hexanucleotide is present at approximately residue −100 in the promoter regions of TAT and TO, two rat liver genes that are glucocorticoid inducible (100).

That this hexanucleotide is important for GR receptor binding is corroborated by experiments in which the contacts between the receptor and MMTV DNA have been studied (115). In these studies, MMTV LTR sequences were subjected to methylation at the N−7 position of the G residues within the hexanucleotide. When methylated, the GR complex is unable to bind to that specific domain but not the others. Furthermore, all of the G residues within the hexanucleotide in four separate binding domains are protected from methylation by dimethyl sulfate when the GR complex is prebound. Similar data have been obtained in studies of GR binding to the hMT-IIa regulatory region (114).

It is important to point out that in both the MMTV LTR and the chick lysozyme promoter, not all bona fide binding sites are functional as hormone regulatory regions, at least as tested by transfection analysis. As an example, even though the binding sites between residues −127 and −84 are preserved in various deletion mutants of the LTR, such molecules are incapable of supporting a glucocorticoid response (69, 77, 78). What then are the crucial elements that constitute a functional regulatory region? Although there is no answer to this question at present, the methylation protection experiments of Schneidereit & Beato may provide a clue (115). They have noted that the protected G residues in the MMTV regulatory region are 10 base pairs (one turn of the helix in B-form DNA) apart and are therefore on the same face of the helix. The N−7 position of the G residue, which is the one susceptible to methylation, is in the major groove of the double helix. Inspection of the sequence in this region shows clearly that there are two pairs of G residues that could contact the receptor within the major groove between nucleotides −170 and −189. Thus, a dimer of GR complexes could bind to this region of DNA. In the case of the non-functional sites this paired arrangement of contacts does not exist, and thus dimer formation may not occur. I point out, however, that the available evidence from electron microscopy indicates that tetramers of GR complexes bind to all sites (28). Thus, it may be another aspect of the symmetry of the paired G residues (or more likely some other characteristic of the surrounding DNA sequence) that is important in allowing for a productive interaction of receptor. More detailed studies of the functional regions will be required to gain further insight into this problem.

Affinity of the Receptor for DNA Sequences: Is That All There Is?

Does the binding of GR complexes to naked DNA in vitro reflect the situation within a cell? Is the binding affinity of the GR complex for specific sequences relative to extraneous DNA sufficient to account for its ability to find limited number of sites in vivo? Although there have been no binding constants reported, the relative affinities between specific and non-specific sites appear to be several thousand–fold (112). These values seem to be insufficient to account for the high degree of selectivity inherent in steroid activation of genes; researchers have estimated that a minimum 10^5–10^6 fold difference in binding affinity between specific and non-specific sequences might be required for activation of a gene by steroid receptors (116). Thus, additional factors probably are required for biologically relevant binding to occur in vivo. Along these lines, Payvar et al (117) have recently identified a 72 Kd protein that copurifies with the GR complex; this protein is itself incapable of binding to DNA but increases the affinity of the GR complex for LTR sequences. Additional proteins, both chromosomal and non-chromosomal, are likely to be involved in the formation of a functional GR complex at specific sites. In addition, one must remember that other proteins associated with the chromatin may mask non-functional binding sites. In such a case, a feature of the authentic regulatory regions with which GR complexes interact might be that they are in an open configuration relative to the surrounding chromatin. Speculation on events subsequent to the binding interactions will be presented in a following section.

SEX STEROID REGULATION OF GENE EXPRESSION

The Chick Oviduct

The production of egg white proteins in the chick oviduct is dependent on its exposure to estrogen and progesterone (7). The tubular gland cells of the immature chick oviduct are stimulated to proliferate and differentiate by exogenous administration of estrogen; during this time, ovalbumin, conalbumin, ovomucoid, and lysozyme become major products of these cells. If the hormone is withdrawn, egg white protein synthesis decreases but can be restimulated by a second injection of estrogen. In a primed oviduct, this so-called secondary induction occurs more rapidly and is generally of greater magnitude than in the primary induction. Moreover, in a primed oviduct, not only estrogen but progesterone, glucocorticoids, and androgens are able to induce the production of several of the egg white proteins (106). Each of these hormones appears to act through its cognate receptor.

Nucleic acid hybridization and cloning technologies were first utilized in the steroid hormone field to assess the effects of estrogen and progesterone on ovalbumin RNA levels (118). The pioneering work of O'Malley and Schimke and their colleagues clearly documented that the hormones increase mRNA levels (119, 120). Although estrogen does have an effect on the turnover rate of ovalbumin mRNA (121), the major impact of the hormones is clearly at the level of transcription (122, 123). Extensive and excellent reviews of the early characterization of this system are available (124, 125).

THE OVALBUMIN GENE   The ovalbumin gene is one of three tandemly linked related genes (the others are the X and Y genes) that are induced in response to estrogen (125–127). Unlike the ovalbumin gene that responds to estrogen, progesterone, and glucocorticoids in a primed oviduct, the Y gene responds only to progesterone and estrogen, whereas the X gene responds solely to estrogen (126, 127). Furthermore, in a mature laying hen, the X and Y genes are expressed at levels approximately 10% and 1% that of ovalbumin. By far the most extensive characterization has been performed on the ovalbumin gene itself.

THE HORMONE CONTROL REGION(S) OF THE OVALBUMIN GENE   Chimeric genes containing the 5' flanking region of the ovalbumin gene fused to the coding region for chick β-globin have been constructed. When globin is introduced into most mammalian cell lines, its expression is directed by the ovalbumin promoter but is not hormone responsive (128). However, in chick oviduct cells the ovalglobin fusion retains estrogen inducibility (129).

More extensive analysis of the ovalbumin regulatory region has been performed by transfection of primary tubular gland cells derived from chick oviduct (129). Analysis of deletion mutants of the ovalbumin 5' flanking sequences indicates that: (a) the core promoter lies downstream of residue −95, and basal transcription is heavily dependent on sequences between residues −77 and −48 (128) as well as the TATA box (centered at residue −32), which is generally required for appropriate positioning of the transcription initiation site (75); (b) sequences required for the progesterone response are present between nucleotides −222 and −95 (129); the precise boundaries of the functional region have not been identified. As in the case of the glucocorticoid regulated genes already described, the core promoter and the hormone regulatory regions of the ovalbumin gene appear to be distinct and separable. Particularly intriguing are recent results indicating that the responsiveness of this gene to estrogen and glucocorticoids also requires sequences within the same -222 to -95 region (130). More precise mapping studies will have to be performed to ascertain whether the sequences responsible for each of these hormonal responses are clustered, overlapping, or perhaps even identical.

THE LYSOZYME GENE   The chick lysozyme gene is responsive to both progesterone and glucocorticoids. As described above, analysis of deletion mutants in microinjected chick oviduct cells indicates that the left-hand border of the regulatory region lies between residues -208 and -164 for both progesterone and glucocorticoids (107, 108). As in the other steroid-inducible genes, the core promoter and the hormone regulatory regions appear not to overlap.

Mammalian Genes Responsive to Sex Steroids

UTEROGLOBIN   The best characterized mammalian gene that responds to progesterone is that for uteroglobin, a protein secreted into the lumen of the uterus that itself has progesterone binding activity. Nucleic acid hybridization studies have documented that its induction in rabbit uteri is consequent to an increase in mRNA levels (131) and that this is due to an increase in the rate of uteroglobin RNA synthesis (132). Interestingly, estrogen is also capable of inducing mRNA levels, although not to the same degree as progesterone; when added together, the hormones appear to have an additive effect (131). Transfection studies with this gene have not yet been reported; however, binding studies with progesterone receptor indicate the presence of specific binding sites in the 5' flanking region (see below).

ANDROGEN-INDUCIBLE PROSTATIC C3 GENE   Prostatic steroid binding protein is a tetramer composed of three different polypeptides (C1, C2, C3) whose expression is under strict androgen control (133). The androgen induction of the three is due to alterations in the levels of the corresponding mRNAs and is accomplished at least in part by increased transcription of the genes. Transfection of a C3 genomic clone containing approximately 3.5Kb of 5' flanking DNA into the androgen-responsive S115 mammary carcinoma line results in androgen inducibility of C3 RNA sequences (134).

ESTROGEN-INDUCIBLE GENE PS2 FROM HUMAN MCF-7 CELLS   The human breast cancer cell line MCF-7 is estrogen dependent for growth, expresses several estrogen-inducible genes, and undergoes hormone-dependent morphological alterations. Recently, a cDNA encoding a specific estrogen-inducible mRNA (pS2) has been cloned and utilized to document that the induction by estrogens is primary (135). The experiments performed to date are analogous to those described earlier for the glucocorticoid-mediated induction of MMTV (54) and for the estrogen-mediated induction of vitellogenin in *Xenopus* oocytes (136).

Binding of Sex Steroid Receptors to Specific DNA Sequences

Initial observations that the chick oviduct progesterone receptor could bind to specific sites within the 5' flanking region of egg white genes utilized a DNA competition assay in which the receptor itself does not need to be purified. The results of such experiments indicate that fragments of DNA from the ovalbumin, X, Y, ovomucoid, and conalbumin genes contain high affinity sites for the progesterone receptor. More detailed mapping studies point to a region between residues -250 and -300 of the ovalbumin gene that contains a particularly efficient binding site (137). It is noteworthy that, based on functional studies described above, the region between -250 and -300 is dispensable for progesterone action in vivo (129). Thus, detection of receptor binding sites using a DNA competition assay by itself has not been useful for identifying authentic regulatory regions of the ovalbumin gene.

Nitrocellulose filter binding assays and nuclease protection experiments with chick progesterone receptor have also been reported (138, 139). In these studies, a highly purified A subunit of the chick oviduct receptor has been employed; note that the B subunit, which also binds progesterone, is not a DNA binding protein. The results indicate that the A subunit of the receptor exhibits preferential binding to 5' flanking regions of the ovalbumin and Y genes by a factor of 10 over other DNA sequences. A major binding site in the ovalbumin gene lies between residue -247 and -135, consistent with the region ostensibly required for progesterone responsiveness (137). It is important to recognize, however, that the ten-fold higher affinity of the A subunit for specific sites is probably too low to account for the high degree of selectivity observed in vivo. Thus, additional factors may be involved in the sequence-specific binding of the progesterone receptor to regulatory sites.

The mammalian, unlike the chick, progesterone receptor appears to consist of a single polypeptide chain of about 110 Kd (32). Such a receptor, purified to approximately 50% homogeneity, exhibits binding specificity toward the 5' flanking region of the rabbit uteroglobin gene (140). Two sites that appear to have higher affinities than others reside within nucleotides -394 to -251 and -193 to $+10$. The functional regulatory region associated with this gene remains to be determined.

Lastly, specific binding of the estrogen-receptor complex to a 5' flanking region of the chicken vitellogenin gene has been reported (141). Both DNA competition and DNAse protection assays indicate a prominent binding region between residues -550 and -660; multiple binding sites are present within this region. Of particular interest in this case, the estrogen receptor binding region corresponds to the location of a DNAse hypersensitive site that appears after estrogen treatment (142). Whether this region plays any role in estrogen inducibility per se remains to be determined; however, no functional regulatory region has yet been identified more than 250 nucleotides upstream of the transcription initiation site in any of the other steroid-inducible genes character-ized to date. Along these lines, it is worth pointing out that a striking sequence homology has been identified around position -140 in five estrogen-inducible genes of the chick (108); the derived consensus sequence $(AAA_A^TTGG_G^AC)$ bears little resemblance to the binding site identified in the vitellogenin gene; however, its role in estrogen inducibility is only speculative.

HOW DO STEROID-RECEPTOR COMPLEXES STIMULATE TRANSCRIPTION?

Prodigious advances have been made in our understanding of the mechanisms by which steroids regulate gene transcription. Moreover, the emerging data now allow us to focus our attention on a more precise definition of the molecular details involved. As a framework, I present the following possibili-ties as general mechanisms by which binding of the steroid-receptor (SR) complex to a regulatory region could facilitate increased transcription initia-tion.

1. SR complexes could relieve a negative effect of the regulatory region on promoter efficiency, perhaps by removing a repressor protein.
2. Direct protein-protein interactions between SR complexes and RNA polymerase may stimulate polymerase function.
3. Local unwinding of the DNA near the RNA polymerase binding site might increase the efficiency of polymerase binding to the core promoter.
4. SR complexes may alter the conformation of the DNA at the regulatory region in such a way as to facilitate the entry of transcription factors that can slide up or down the DNA (even over long distances) in search of poised polymerase molecules.
5. Binding of the SR complex could induce a change in the structure of the chromatin (i.e. by removing nuclear proteins) that could be propagated to the core promoter in such a way as to facilitate polymerase binding; such an alteration could occur over short or long distances.

It is of course difficult at this point to unequivocally discard or accept any of these possibilities. Nevertheless, some may be more likely than others. Since with only one exception, noted above, removing the hormone regulatory sequences from a core promoter does not lead to hormone-independent high-level expression, it seems highly unlikely that the function of the SR complex is to relieve a negative influence of that region on transcription.

Several studies have documented that the glucocorticoid regulatory region of

MMTV functions at various positions relative to the promoter (65, 69, 76, 79). Most of the changes in spacing have been over only 100–200 base pairs; however, in at least one case, partial function was retained even when the regulatory region was placed 1000 base pairs from the promoter. In addition, induction of a distal promoter is seen in some situations despite the presence of a functional intervening promoter. In view of these results, it is difficult to envision how direct interactions of the SR complex with polymerase could be of central importance in the facilitation of transcription initiation. Likewise, local unwinding of the DNA (i.e. over 1–3 turns of the helix), which is of importance in forming stable RNA polymerase complexes in *E. coli*, appears to be of little importance if the regulatory region can be moved over several hundred base pairs. A caveat to these arguments, of course, is the fact that we know little about the organization of these sequences in three-dimensional space. It is possible, therefore, that even when the regulatory region is moved relative to the promoter, additional DNA binding proteins help keep these regions in close apposition. The suggestion that the receptors themselves may be fixed on the nuclear matrix at all times (17, 18) could facilitate such interactions.

Bacterial Models

Positive transcriptional regulators in prokaryotic systems share several charac- teristics with steroid receptors. Foremost among these, they bind to specific DNA sequences near the corresponding promoters and in some cases (e.g. the cyclic AMP binding protein of *E. coli*, CRP) require a ligand to convert them to a DNA binding form. Whether the mechanisms by which steroid receptors and bacterial protein activate transcription are similar or not remains to be deter- mined.

In the case of the phage λ repressor, which also acts as a positive regulator at the Prm promoter, it appears that transcription is augmented by altering the isomerization rate at which functional (i.e. open) RNA polymerase complexes (143, 144) are formed rather than by altering the affinity of the RNA polymerase itself for the promoter (145). Ptashne and his colleagues have suggested that this stimulation occurs as a consequence of direct protein-protein interactions with the RNA polymerase (146). The data supporting this view are highly circumstantial; however, mutants that bind to the appropriate DNA sequence yet do not stimulate transcription support this hypothesis (145, 147).

Several *E. coli* promoters that are activated by cAMP have been intensively studied [for an excellent review see (148)]. In both the *lac* and *gal* promoters, the cAMP-CRP complex appears to stimulate transcription in two ways: (*a*) by shifting the RNA polymerase binding site by 20 and 5 nucleotides respectively, and (*b*) by increasing RNA polymerase open complex formation at the down- stream site (149). Augmented transcription initiation may be due to increasing the affinity of the RNA polymerase for promoter sites rather than to affecting the isomerization of polymerase from the closed to the open (active) state. Although binding of the cAMP-CRP complex alters the structure of the DNA to form a more compact molecule, evidence indicates that this change is not due to a transition from right-handed to left-handed DNA or from local unwinding of the DNA (148). Indirect evidence suggests that stimulation of transcription by cAMP-CRP may instead involve direct interactions with RNA polymerase (148–151). In the presence of cAMP, CRP appears to stabilize RNA polymerase binding to the upstream promoter, and the affinity of the cAMP-CRP complex for its binding site in the *lac* and *gal* promoters is increased by the addition of RNA polymerase (148–151). However, the distance between the CRP binding site and the start of transcription varies substantially among cAMP-regulated genes, ranging from 35 to 135 base pairs. Thus, one's notions concerning the nature of the putative interaction between the polymerase and CRP must take this into account.

Effects of Steroid Hormones on Chromatin Structure

Transcriptionally active genes in eukaryotes exhibit altered chromatin configurations as detected by their relative sensitivity to nucleases (152). The DNA within relatively large domains encompassing a gene or gene cluster are preferentially digested by DNAse I if the gene has been or is actively being transcribed. Within these domains, specific sites are more sensitive to digestion by 1–2 orders of magnitude (153). These so-called hypersensitive sites (HS) can generally be found within the 5' flanking region of active genes, often at the 3' end of the gene as well, and at times at internal sites in genes (153, 154). Interesting correlations suggest that the appearance of the HS sites is related to transcriptional activation. However, the basis for the appearance of HS sites is not at all clear, and to date no cause-effect relationship has been established between their appearance and the activation of transcription. With this as background, it is intriguing to note that steroid hormones can alter both the general pattern of DNAse sensitivity and HS sites in regulated genes.

GENERAL ALTERATIONS IN DNASE SENSITIVITY   Vitellogenin, the precursor of the major yolk proteins, is induced by estradiol in the livers of oviparous vertebrates (155). Four closely related genes encode vitellogenins in *Xenopus laevis,* and recent data from Gerber-Huber et al (156) have shown that at least two of these become generally more sensitive to DNAse in the livers of estrogen-treated males. Similarly, the chick ovalbumin gene is associated with a relatively DNAse-sensitive region of the chromatin that persists even after withdrawal of estrogen (157). Interestingly, the chromatin domain in which the ovalbumin, as well as X and Y genes, resides extends over approximately 100 kilobases and is flanked at the borders of the DNAse-sensitive region by a short middle repetitive sequence, CR1 (158). Thus, these genes probably are fixed in an open chromatin configuration during exposure of the tissue to hormone. This structure is maintained even after removal of the hormone when the gene is no longer active. This can be viewed as equivalent to a developmental alteration that is required but is itself insufficient for gene transcription. Similar long-lived and perhaps irreversible changes in chromatin structure surrounding the MMTV LTR are seen after glucocorticoid treatment (159).

ACQUISITION OF HYPERSENSITIVE SITES   Burch & Weintraub (142) have recently reported that there are three classes of HS sites detectable in the chick vitellogenin gene. Prior to estradiol-mediated activation of vitellogenin expression, HS sites exist within and 3' to the gene in liver and oviduct but not in erythrocytes, brain, or fibroblasts. These sites exist in embryonic liver even prior to development of estrogen receptors. Thus, this class of HS sites (HS-A) may reflect the potential for tissue-specific expression in an estrogen-responsive cell; note, however, that vitellogenin is not expressed in oviduct. A second class of sites (HS-B) are detected in the 5' flanking region of the gene in liver but not in the oviduct after estrogen treatment. These sites remain hypersensitive after removal of hormone and may therefore be involved in the memory phenomenon (i.e. the rapid secondary induction after hormone withdrawal) associated with estrogen induction of vitellogenin in liver (160) and several of the egg-white genes in the oviduct. Lastly, one HS site (HS-C) appears in response to estrogen approximately 700 base pairs upstream of the start of transcription. This site disappears after removal of the hormone and reappears upon re-induction. Such a site is likely to reflect directly an alteration in DNA structure associated with binding of the estrogen-receptor complex. Whether this site is part of the binding site itself remains to be determined. A similar analysis of HS sites in the MMTV LTR reveals the presence of a hormone-dependent and reversible site that indeed maps within the functional glucocorticoid regulatory region (159). It is noteworthy that the HS site seems to coincide with the binding region that is functional in stimulating transcription and not with all receptor binding domains. Mapping of HS sites in the rat TAT gene has revealed the presence of a glucocorticoid-inducible site approximately 2000 base pairs upstream of the start of transcription (161). Again, whether this reflects the presence of a receptor binding site or is the consequence of receptor binding at a distal site is as yet unknown. DNAse HS sites are also present in at least three locations in the 5' flanking region of the actively transcribed ovalbumin gene (162).

Chromatin Structure, DNA Supercoiling, and Transcriptional Activation

Are the observed steroid-induced alterations in chromatin structure responsible for increased transcriptional activity and if so how? Alternatively, are these changes a consequence of the process of gene activation by steroid-receptor complexes? Although there are no clear answers to these questions at the moment, there are interesting parallels to be drawn with other gene regulatory systems and with proteins that alter higher order structures of DNA.

Several lines of evidence point to the fact that supercoiling of DNA can profoundly affect gene expression [for review, see (163)]. Elegant genetic experiments have implicated the *E. coli* supX gene in the control of transcription, in some cases from promoters that can also be regulated by the cAMP-CRP complex (164). The supX gene encodes the enzyme topoisomerase I (165), one of a class of enzymes that change the degree of DNA supercoiling [for review, see (166)]. Promoters such as the *lac* promoter appear to be active only when the DNA is highly negatively supercoiled by the enzyme DNA gyrase; topoisomerase I relaxes negative supercoils and thus renders the promoter less active. Thus, mutations in supX, which inactivate topoisomerase I, would result in a higher degree of negative supercoiling and effect more efficient transcription from the promoter. Support for this idea comes from the observation that inhibitors of DNA gyrase such as nalidixic acid strongly inhibit the transcription from some promoters but not others (167, 168). The mechanism by which negative supercoiling stimulates transcription is unclear, but perhaps an alteration in the structure of the promoter region facilitates RNA polymerase binding or formation of open complexes (169). These, as we've already discussed, are the functions attributed to the λ repressor and the cAMP-CRP complex. Physical studies of naked DNA have also demonstrated that changes in superhelical density have profound effects on sequences that have the potential for existing in alternative secondary structures [for example, see (170)].

A remarkable example in eukaryotic cells in which supercoiling appears to have a central role in gene expression is that of the yeast mating type genes, which are transcribed from one chromosomal location but not another (171, 172). Using autonomously replicating plasmids in different strains of yeast, Nasmyth (173) has shown that the degree of supercoiling of the DNA seems to determine whether the mating type gene is expressed or not. The product of an unlinked gene, called SIR or MAR, appears to be responsible for controlling the structure of the DNA and may be analogous to the bacterial gyrase. It is noteworthy that the alterations of the mating type genes affect the chromatin structure surrounding the gene profoundly such that nucleosome (histone octamer) phasing may also be affected.

It is clearly premature to do so; nevertheless, it is tempting to speculate that steroid-receptor complexes may also alter DNA and chromatin structure by introducing negative supercoils into DNA. Since in chromatin negative supercoils are taken up by the nucleosome, such alterations may result in dramatic effects on the structure of the surrounding chromatin. As suggested by Yamamoto & Alberts (3), such an alteration may propagate over patches of chromatin, making the region more accessible to transcription factors or polymerase itself. Furthermore, the acquisition of DNase HS sites in the presence of hormone may reflect exposure of a specific DNA sequence that can serve as the recognition site for transcription factors. In each of these cases, the effect of the steroid-receptor complex could be propagated over quite large distances to effect alterations in promoter utilization. Evidence from several deletion and insertion mutants in the MMTV LTR indeed suggest that some property of activating the regulatory region must be propagated to the core promoter (69, 78). The effect could be manifested either by direct propagation of a physical alteration or by the movement of a transcriptional factor in search of a poised transcription complex. This latter hypothesis has also been put forth to explain how viral enhancer sequences can activate promoters from a distance (86).

A final speculation regarding the steroid-receptor complex is the possibility that specific interaction with another protein or set of proteins is responsible for gene activation. One can envision a scenario in which binding of the steroid-receptor complex to the regulatory region serves as the focus for the interaction of a gyrase-like protein that itself is responsible for altering the topology of the chromatin. In such a case, it might be that all steroid-receptor complexes interact with the same or a closely related protein.

DEVELOPMENTAL AND POST-TRANSCRIPTIONAL CONTROL OF GENE EXPRESSION

Steroid hormones have profound effects on cellular physiology, many of which are due to the direct activation of transcription by steroid-receptor complexes. However, the products of the genes activated by a given hormone may in themselves have dramatic effects on gene expression. The notion of such a cascade phenomenon is exemplified by the activation of genes in Drosophila polytene chromosomes by the moulting hormone ecdysone. Ashburner and colleagues (174) identified five gene loci (i.e. the early genes) activated in Drosophila salivary glands in the absence of protein synthesis. In a temporally defined order and incumbent on de novo protein synthesis, a large series of middle and late genes subsequently become activated. Coordinate with the activation of these genes, the early genes return to a quiescent state. This highly regulated developmental program is initiated by a single administration of ecdysone and, although this hypothesis is not yet proven, suggests that the products of the early genes (i.e. those directly activated by the hormone) themselves have profound gene regulatory activities. Also related to such a cascade are instances in which one steroid induces the production of the receptor for a different steroid. The best documented example is the estrogen-mediated induction of progesterone receptors in various tissues [for example, see (175)].

Another case in which a steroid hormone appears to regulate gene expression indirectly is the glucocorticoid-mediated induction of the acute phase reactant, α-1 acid glycoprotein (AGP). The RNA encoding this protein is induced several hundred–fold both in rat liver and in HTC cells, and at least in the latter case it requires ongoing protein synthesis (176–178). Most surprisingly, the induction of the RNA appears not to be at the level of gene transcription (179). One interpretation of these results is that the glucocorticoid-receptor complex directly activates a gene whose product is required for the production of stable AGP transcripts. This novel mechanism of gene regulation may be more general than previously believed; a thyroid hormone–inducible gene in rat liver also appears to be induced by a nontranscriptional mechanism (H. Towle, personal communication). Additional mechanisms may be involved in the ability of steroid (and other) hormones to alter the half-lives of existing mRNAs. For example, the induction of ovalbumin mRNA by estrogen in the chick oviduct is in part due to a stabilization of the RNA (121).

Glucocorticoids have also been implicated in inducing a glycoprotein-processing pathway for MMTV proteins in rat hepatoma cells that could in principle dramatically alter the pattern of cellular membrane and/or secreted proteins (180). Again, one presumes that the hormone-receptor complex activates a gene that encodes in this case a protein-processing factor.

Lastly, steroid hormones have dramatic effects on cell differentiation as exemplified by the estrogen-induced proliferation of tubular gland cells of the chick oviduct (119, 120), as well as the glucocorticoid-mediated conversion of myeloid precursors to macrophages (181) or preadipocytes to adipocytes (182). Similarly, sex steroids are often required for the proliferation and differentiation of tissues involved in the reproduction or maintenance of secondary sex characteristics. In these cases that require complex activation of a large set of coordinately regulated genes, it is indeed likely that products of the steroid-inducible genes have diverse functions in controlling the expression of the tissue-specific genes. Thus, an integrated physiological response to a steroid hormone will entail not only the primary activation of a few specific genes (as a consequence of receptor binding to regulatory DNA sequences) but the concerted interplay of other cellular regulatory factors that affect gene expression at both transcriptional and post-transcriptional levels.

QUESTIONS AND PROSPECTS FOR THE FUTURE

Many of the most pressing questions regarding steroid hormone action have been discussed throughout the text. Nevertheless, it may be useful to restate these more explicitly and to point out experimental approaches and obstacles that may arise.

1. What constitutes an SR complex binding site and what distinguishes a functional binding site from the others? These issues are central to understand-

ing the high degree of selectivity inherent in the cellular response to a particular hormone. For the moment, the most direct experimental approach to this problem will be to undertake fine mapping analysis of binding sites and functional regulatory regions using the powerful techniques of point mutagenesis and transfection. The possibility that two different steroid receptors may recognize the same DNA sequence can also be addressed in this fashion.

2. How does binding of an SR complex stimulate transcription? This, of course, is the central question not only for steroid hormones but for positive regulatory proteins in all organisms. It is sobering that the molecular details of how phage proteins or cAMP-CRP complexes activate transcription in *E. coli* remain hazy. Experimentally, it would be extremely useful if an in vitro, hormone-dependent transcription system could be developed. This will require both luck and a much better understanding of the requirements for polymerase II transcription of genes. Although limited success has recently been obtained in isolating a promoter-specific factor [for example see (183)], no one has yet reported an effect of SR complexes on transcription in a cell-free system. The physical state of the template, in particular with regard to its chromatin structure, may be a crucial aspect of this problem.

3. What is the role of chromatin structure in the control of transcription and how do SR complexes influence it? Although it is clear that chromosomal position profoundly influences the ability of a hormone-responsive gene to be transcribed (60, 184), isolating defined fragments of DNA that are packaged in a native chromatin state is an extremely difficult proposition. Our present understanding of the proteins involved in high-order chromatin structure is limited. Nevertheless, the utility of nucleases and chemical probes in detecting alterations in chromatin structure has been documented. Novel attempts to isolate minichromosomes in bovine papilloma virus vectors containing the glucocorticoid regulatory region of MMTV are underway (185) and have already provided the basis for future attempts to study this most difficult area. These minichromosomes may indeed be ideal substrates for attempts to obtain hormone-regulated transcription in vitro.

4. In several cases, steroid hormones appear to inhibit specific gene transcription (97, 186). Can SR complexes also act as direct transcriptional repressor molecules or do they induce the synthesis of such repressors?

5. What is the primary structure of the steroid receptors? Which domains are important in hormone binding, DNA binding, and transcriptional activation? Are there other proteins that interact specifically with each of the steroid receptors? The relative paucity of highly purified receptor protein has made these questions unapproachable; however, literally dozens of laboratories around the world are applying recombinant DNA technology to this problem. Undoubtedly by the time this review is published, the first reports of receptor cloning will be upon us. This will facilitate not only a detailed analysis of receptor structure and function but will provide insight into receptor evolution,

ontogeny of receptors, and issues related to the control of receptor gene expression.

6. It is striking that the hormone sensitivity of any particular gene is generally confined to one or at most a few tissues. This is true despite the presence of functional receptors in many tissues. An area of great interest, and at this time little insight, is how tissue-specific expression of genes may determine their hormone responsiveness. A point worth noting is that the activation of genes by SR complexes may be quite distinct from developmental activation of genes (unless, of course, the hormone itself influences the developmental program). The analysis of genes that undergo a change from hormone insensitivity to hormone sensitivity during a well-defined differentiative program may be of significant utility in approaching this problem.

7. As alluded to earlier, many of the effects of steroid hormones on gene expression are due to the products of the genes directly activated by SR complexes. A challenge for the future is to unravel the complex network of events that leads to a highly orchestrated cellular response such as steroid-induced differentiation. It is particularly exciting to entertain the possibility that steroid hormones may provide a key to understanding not only how genes are transcriptionally activated in eukaryotic cells but, in addition, to understanding the control of developmental transitions and tissue differentiation at a molecular level.

ACKNOWLEDGMENTS

I thank all of my colleagues who provided me with the innumerable reprints and preprints that made it possible to write this manuscript. The suggestions made by A. Chapman, M. Danielsen, D. Knight, R. Roth, H. Schulman, and F. Torti were invaluable in my attempt to make the review of use to a wide spectrum of scientists; if I have failed the blame is solely mine. Most importantly, the preparation of this manuscript was facilitated by the excellent assistance of Karen Benight. The work in my laboratory has been supported by grants from the NIH, the National Foundation March of Dimes, and by an Established Investigator Award from the American Heart Association.

Literature Cited

1. Jensen, E. V., DeSombre, E. R. 1972. Mechanism of action of the female sex hormones. *Ann. Rev. Biochem.* 41:203–30
2. Gorski, J., Gannon, F. 1976. Current models of steroid hormone action: A critique. *Ann. Rev. Physiol.* 38:425–50
3. Yamamoto, K. R., Alberts, B. M. 1976. Steroid receptors: Elements for modulation of eukaryotic transcription. *Ann. Rev. Biochem.* 45:721–46

4. Godeau, J. F., Schorderet-Slatkine, S., Hubert, P., Baulieu, E.-E. 1978. Induction of maturation in *Xenopus laevis* oocytes by a steroid linked to a polymer. *Proc. Natl. Acad. Sci. USA* 75:2353–57
5. Jensen, E. V., Suzuki, T., Kawashima, T., Stumpf, W. E., Jungblut, P. W., DeSombre, E. R. 1968. A two-step mechanism for the interaction of estradiol with rat uterus. *Proc. Natl. Acad. Sci. USA* 59:632–38

6. Gorski, J., Toft, D. O., Shyamala, G., Smith, D., Notides, A. 1968. Hormone receptors: Studies on the interaction of estrogen with the uterus. *Rec. Prog. Horm. Res.* 24:45–80

7. O'Malley, B. W., McGuire, W. L., Kohler, P. O., Korenman, S. G. 1969. Studies on the mechanism of steroid hormone regulation of synthesis of specific proteins. *Rec. Prog. Horm. Res.* 25:105–60

8. Tomkins, G. M., Martin, D. W. 1970. Hormones and gene expression. *Ann. Rev. Genet.* 4:91–106

9. Yamamoto, K., Alberts, B. M. 1972. *In vitro* conversion of estradiol-receptor protein to its nuclear form: Dependence on hormone and DNA. *Proc. Natl. Acad. Sci. USA* 69:2105–9

10. Baxter, J. D., Rousseau, G. G., Benson, M. C., Garcea, R. L., Ito, J., Tomkins, G. M. 1972. Role of DNA and specific cytoplasmic receptors in glucocorticoid action. *Proc. Natl. Acad. Sci. USA* 69:1892–96

11. Sheridan, P. J., Buchanan, J. M., Anselmo, V. C., Martin, P. M. 1979. Equilibrium: The intracellular distribution of steroid receptors. *Nature* 282:579–82

12. Welshons, W. V., Lieberman, M. E., Gorski, J. 1984. Nuclear localization of unoccupied estrogen receptors. *Nature* 307:747–49

13. King, W. J., Greene, G. L. 1984. Monoclonal antibodies localize estrogen receptor in the nuclei of target cells. *Nature* 307:745–47

14. Foster, D. N., Guney, T. 1976. Nuclear location of mammalian DNA polymerase activities. *J. Biol. Chem.* 251:7893–98

15. Whitlock, J. P. Jr., Galeazzi, D. 1984. TCDD receptors in wild type and variant mouse hepatoma cells: Nuclear location and strength of nuclear binding. *J. Biol. Chem.* 259:980–85

16. Vedeckis, W. V. 1984. Steroid hormone receptor structure in normal and neoplastic cells. In *Hormonally Sensitive Tumors,* ed. V. P. Hollander. New York: Academic. In press

17. Barrack, E. R., Coffey, D. S. 1983. The role of the nuclear matrix in steroid hormone action. In *Biochemical Actions of Hormones,* ed. G. Litwack, 10:23–90. New York: Academic

18. Gorski, J., Welshons, W., Sakai, D. 1984. Remodeling the estrogen receptor model. *Mol. Cell. Endocrinol.* 36:11–15

19. Sekeris, C. E. 1964. Action of ecdysone on RNA and protein metabolism in the Blowfly, Calliphora erythrocephola. In *Mechanisms of Hormone Action,* ed. P. Karlson, pp. 149–67. New York: Academic

20. Peterkofsky, B., Tomkins, G. 1968. Evidence for the steroid-induced accumulation of tyrosine-aminotransferase mRNA in the absence of protein synthesis. *Proc. Natl. Acad. Sci. USA* 60:222–28

21. Leach, K. L., Dahmer, M. K., Hammond, N. D., Sando, J. J., Pratt, W. B. 1979. Molybdate inhibition of glucocorticoid-receptor inactivation and transformation. *J. Biol. Chem.* 254:11884–90

22. Toft, D., Nishigori, H. 1979. Stabilization of the avian progesterone receptor by inhibitors. *J. Steroid Biochem.* 11:413–16

23. Sherman, M. R. 1984. Structure of mammalian steroid receptors: Evolving concepts and methodological developments. *Ann. Rev. Physiol.* 46:83–105

24. Dahmer, M. K., Housley, P. R., Pratt, W. B. 1984. Effects of molybdate and endogenous inhibitors on steroid-receptor inactivation, transformation, and translocation. *Ann. Rev. Physiol.* 46:67–81

25. Housley, P. R., Pratt, W. B. 1983. Direct demonstration of glucocorticoid-receptor phosphorylation by intact L cells. *J. Biol. Chem.* 258:4630–35

26. Weigel, N. L., Tash, J. S., Means, A. R., Schrader, W. T., O'Malley, B. W. 1981. Phosphorylation of hen progesterone receptor by cAMP dependent protein kinase. *Biochem. Biophys. Res. Commun.* 102:513–19

27. Dougherty, J. J., Puri, R. K., Toft, D. O. 1982. Phosphorylation *in vivo* of chicken oviduct progesterone receptor. *J. Biol. Chem.* 257:14226–30

28. Payvar, F., DeFranco, D., Firestone, G. L., Edgar, B., Wrange, O., et al. 1983. Sequence-specific binding of glucocorticoid receptor to MTV DNA at sites within and upstream of the transcribed region. *Cell* 35:381–92

29. Schrader, W. T., O'Malley, B. W. 1978. Molecular structure and analysis of progesterone receptors. In *Receptors and Hormone Action,* ed. B. W. O'Malley, L. Birnbaumer, pp. 189–225. New York: Academic

30. Westphal, H. M., Moldenhauer, G., Beato, M. 1982. Monoclonal antibodies to the rat liver glucocorticoid receptor. *EMBO J.* 1:1467–71

31. Gametchu, B., Harrison, R. W. 1984. Characterization of a monoclonal antibody to the rat liver glucocorticoid receptor. *Endocrinology* 114:274–85

32. Logeat, F., Hai, M. T. V., Fournier, A., Legrain, P., Buttin, G., Milgrom, E.

1983. Monoclonal antibodies to rabbit progesterone receptor: Cross-reaction with other mammalian progesterone receptors. *Proc. Natl. Acad. Sci. USA* 80:6456–59

33. Pike, J. W. 1984. Monoclonal antibodies to chick intestinal receptors for 1,25-dihydroxyvitamin D_3. *J. Biol. Chem.* 259:1167–73

34. Wrange, O., Carlstedt-Duke, J., Gustafsson, J.-A. 1979. Purification of the glucocorticoid receptor from rat liver cytosol. *J. Biol. Chem.* 254:9284–90

35. Bresciani, F., Sica, V., Weisz, A. 1979. Properties of estrogen receptor purified to homogeneity. See Ref. 17, 6:461–80

36. Carlstedt-Duke, J., Okret, S., Wrange, O., Gustafsson, J.-A. 1982. Immunochemical analysis of the glucocorticoid receptor: Identification of a third domain separate from the steroid-binding and DNA-binding domains. *Proc. Natl. Acad. Sci. USA* 79:4260–64

37. Westphal, H. M., Beato, M. 1980. The activated glucocorticoid receptor of rat liver. Purification and physical characterization. *Eur. J. Biochem.* 106:395–403

38. Govindan, M., Sekeris, C. 1978. Purification of two dexamethasone-binding proteins from rat liver cytosol. *Eur. J. Biochem.* 89:95–104

39. Sherman, M. R., Pickering, L. A., Rollwagen, F. M., Miller, L. K. 1978. Meroreceptors: Proteolytic fragments of receptors containing the steroid-binding site. *Fed. Proc.* 37:167–73

40. Sibley, C. H., Tomkins, G. M. 1974. Mechanisms of steroid resistance. *Cell* 2:221–27

41. Dellweg, H.-G., Hotz, A., Mugele, K., Gehring, U. 1982. Active domains in wild-type and mutant glucocorticoid receptors. *EMBO J.* 1:285–89

42. Yamamoto, K. R., Stampfer, M. R., Tomkins, G. M. 1974. Receptors from glucocorticoid-sensitive lymphoma cells and two classes of insensitive clones: Physical and DNA-binding properties. *Proc. Natl. Acad. Sci. USA* 71:3901–5

43. Scheidereit, C., Geisse, S., Westphal, H. M., Beato, M. 1983. The glucocorticoid receptor binds to defined nucleotide sequences near the promoter of mouse mammary tumor virus. *Nature* 304:749–52

44. Yamamoto, K. R., Gehring, U., Stampfer, M. R., Sibley, C. H. 1976. Genetic approaches to steroid hormone action. *Rec. Prog. Horm. Res.* 32:3–32

45. Bourgeois, S., Gasson, J. C. 1984. Genetic and epigenetic bases of glucocorticoid resistance in lymphoid cell lines. See Ref. 17, 12: In press

46. McGrath, C. M. 1971. Replication of mammary tumor virus in tumor cell cultures: Dependence on hormone-induced cellular organization. *J. Natl. Cancer Inst.* 47:455–67

47. Stallcup, M. R., Ring, J., Yamamoto, K. R. 1978. Synthesis of mouse mammary tumor virus ribonucleic acid in isolated nuclei from cultured mammary tumor cells. *Biochem.* 17:1515–21

48. Dickson, C., Peters, G. 1983. Proteins encoded by mouse mammary tumor virus. *Curr. Top. Microbiol. Immunol.* 106:1–34

49. Ringold, G. M. 1983. Regulation of mouse mammary tumor virus gene expression by glucocorticoid hormones. *Curr. Top. Microbiol. Immunol.* 106:79–103

50. Temin, H. M. 1981. Structure, variation and synthesis of retrovirus long terminal repeat. *Cell* 27:1–3

51. Varmus, H. E. 1982. Form and function of retroviral proviruses. *Science* 216:812–20

52. Parks, W. P., Scolnick, E. M., Kozikowski, E. H. 1974. Dexamethasone stimulation of murine mammary tumor virus expression. A tissue culture source of virus. *Science* 12:158–60

53. Ringold, G. M., Lasfargues, E. Y., Bishop, J. M., Varmus, H. E. 1975. Production of mouse mammary tumor virus by cultured cells in the absence and presence of hormones: Assay by molecular hybridization. *Virology* 65:135–47

54. Ringold, G. M., Yamamoto, K. R., Tomkins, G. M., Bishop, J. M., Varmus, H. E. 1975. Dexamethasone-mediated induction of mouse mammary tumor virus RNA: A system for studying glucocorticoid action. *Cell* 6:299–305

55. Scolnick, E. M., Young, H. A., Parks, W. P. 1976. Biochemical and physiological mechanisms in glucocorticoid hormone induction of mouse mammary tumor virus. *Virology* 69:148–56

56. Ringold, G. M., Yamamoto, K. R., Bishop, J. M., Varmus, H. E. 1977. Glucocorticoid-stimulated accumulation of mouse mammary tumor virus RNA: Increased rate of synthesis of viral RNA. *Proc. Natl. Acad. Sci. USA* 74:2879–83

57. Young, H. A., Shih, T. Y., Scolnick, E. M., Parks, W. P. 1977. Steroid induction of mouse mammary tumor virus: Effect upon synthesis and degradation of viral RNA. *J. Virol.* 21:139–46

58. Vaidya, A. B., Lasfargues, E. Y., Huebel, G., Lasfargues, J. C., Moore,

D. H. 1976. Murine mammary tumor virus: Characterization of infection of non-murine cells. *J. Virol.* 18:911–17

59. Ringold, G. M., Cardiff, R. D., Varmus, H. E., Yamamoto, K. R. 1977. Infection of cultured hepatoma cells by mouse mammary tumor virus. *Cell* 10:11–18

60. Ringold, G. M., Shank, P. R., Varmus, H. E., Ring, J., Yamamoto, K. R. 1979. Integration and transcription of mouse mammary tumor virus DNA in rat hepatoma cells. *Proc. Natl. Acad. Sci. USA* 76:665–69

61. Cohen, J. C., Shank, P. R., Morris, V. L., Cardiff, R. D., Varmus, H. E. 1979. Integration of the DNA of mouse mammary tumor virus in virus infected normal and neoplastic tissue of the mouse. *Cell* 16:333–45

62. Buetti, E., Diggelmann, H. 1981. Cloned mouse mammary tumor virus DNA is biologically active in transfected mouse cells and its expression is stimulated by glucocorticoid hormones. *Cell* 23:335–45

63. Hynes, N. E., Kennedy, N., Rahmsford, U., Groner, B. 1981. Hormone responsive expression of an endogenous proviral gene of mouse mammary tumor virus after molecular cloning and gene transfer into cultured cells. *Proc. Natl. Acad. Sci. USA* 78:2038–42

64. Wigler, M., Sweet, R., Sim, G. K., Wold, B., Pellicer, A., et al. 1979. Transformation of mammalian cells with genes from prokaryotes and eukaryotes. *Cell* 16:777–85

65. Lee, F., Mulligan, R., Berg, P., Ringold, G. 1981. Glucocorticoids regulate expression of dihydrofolate reductase cDNA in mouse mammary tumor virus chimeric plasmids. *Nature* 294:228–32

66. Huang, A. L., Ostrowski, M. C., Berard, D., Hager, G. L. 1981. Glucocorticoid regulation of the HaMuSV p21 gene conferred by sequences from mouse mammary tumor virus. *Cell* 27:245–55

67. Groner, B., Kennedy, N., Rahmsdorf, U., Herrlick, P., van Ooyen, A., Hynes, N. E. 1982. Introduction of a proviral mouse mammary tumor virus gene and a chimeric MMTV-thymidine kinase gene into L cells results in their glucocorticoid responsive expression. In *Hormones and Cell Regulation,* ed. J. E. Dumont, J. Nunez, G. Schultz, 6:217–28. Amsterdam: Elsevier North Holland

68. Buetti, E., Diggelmann, H. 1983. Glucocorticoid regulation of mouse mammary tumor virus: Identification of a short essential region. *EMBO J.* 2:1423–29

69. Majors, J., Varmus, H. 1983. A small

region of the mouse mammary tumor virus long terminal repeat confers glucocorticoid hormone regulation on a linked heterologous gene. *Proc. Natl. Acad. Sci. USA* 80:5866–70

70. Hall, C. V., Jacob, P. E., Ringold, G. M., Lee, F. 1983. Expression and regulation of *E. coli lac* Z gene fusions in mammalian cells. *J. Mol. Appl. Genet.* 2:101–10

71. Chapman, A. B., Costello, M. A., Lee, F., Ringold, G. M. 1983. Amplification and hormone-regulated expression of a MMTV-Eco gpt fusion plasmid in mouse 3T6 cells. *Mol. Cell. Biol.* 3:1421–29

72. Fasel, N., Pearson, K., Buetti, E., Diggelmann, H. 1982. The region of mouse mammary tumor virus DNA containing the long terminal repeat includes a long coding sequence and signals for hormonally regulated transcription. *EMBO J.* 1:3–7

73. Yamamoto, K. R., Payvar, F., Firestone, G. L., Maler, B. A., Wrange, O., et al. 1983. Biological activity of cloned mammary tumor virus DNA fragments that bind purified glucocorticoid receptor protein *in vitro. Cold Spring Harbor Symp. Quant. Biol.* 47:977–84

74. Payvar, F., Wrange, O., Carlstedt-Duke, J., Okret, S., Gustaffson, J. A., Yamamoto, K. R., 1981. Purified glucocorticoid receptors bind selectively *in vitro* to a cloned DNA fragment whose transcription is regulated by glucocorticoids *in vivo. Proc. Natl. Acad. Sci. USA* 78:6628–32

75. Nevins, J. R. 1983. The pathway of eukaryotic mRNA formation. *Ann. Rev. Biochem.* 52:441–66

76. Hynes, N., Van Ooyen, A. J. J., Kennedy, N., Herrlich, P., Ponta, H., Groner, B. 1983. Subfragments of the large terminal repeat cause glucocorticoid-responsive expression of mouse mammary tumor virus and of an adjacent gene. *Proc. Natl. Acad. Sci. USA* 80:3637–41

77. Ringold, G. M., Dobson, D. E., Grove, J. R., Hall, C. V., Lee, F., Vannice, J. L. 1983. Glucocorticoid regulation of gene expression: Mouse mammary tumor virus as a model system. *Rec. Prog. Horm. Res.* 39:387–424

78. Lee, F., Hall, C. V., Ringold, G. M., Dobson, D. E., Luh, J., Jacob, P. E. 1984. Functional analysis of the steroid hormone control region of mouse mammary tumor virus. *Nucleic Acids Res.* 12:4191–206

79. Chandler, V. L., Maler, B. A., Yamamoto, K. R. 1983. DNA sequences

bound specifically by glucocorticoid receptor *in vitro* render a heterologous promoter responsive *in vivo*. *Cell* 33:489–99

80. Hager, G. L., Lichtler, A. C., Ostrowski, M. C. 1983. The MMTV glucocorticoid regulatory sequence: A positive or negative element? In *Current Communications in Molecular Biology, Enhancers and Eukaryotic Gene Expression*, ed. Y. Gluzman, S. Shenk, pp. 161–64. Cold Spring Harbor, New York: Cold Spring Harbor Biol. Lab.

81. Dobson, D. E., Lee, F., Ringold, G. M. 1983. Separation of promoter and hormone regulatory sequences in MMTV. In *Gene Expression*, ed. D. Hamer, M. Rosenberg, pp. 87–94. New York: Liss

82. Kessel, M., Khoury, G. 1983. Induction of cloned genes after transfer into eukaryotic cells. In *Gene Amplification and Analysis*, ed. E. F. Papas, M. Rosenberg, I. G. Chirikjian, 3:234–60. New York: Elsevier

83. Ringold, G. M., Chapman, A., Costello, M., Dobson, D., Hall, C., et al. 1983. Glucocorticoid regulation of mouse mammary tumor virus gene expression. In *Mechanisms of Drug Action*, ed. T. Singer, T. E. Mansour, R. N. Ondarza, pp. 91–105. New York: Academic

84. Culpepper, J., Lee, F. 1984. A fragment of the MMTV LTR confers hormonal responsiveness on a heterologous promoter. *Mol. Cell. Biol.* In press

85. Banerji, J., Rusconi, S., Schaffner, W. 1981. Expression of a beta globin gene is enhanced by remote SV40 DNA sequences. *Cell* 27:299–308

86. Moreau, P., Hen, R., Wasylyk, B., Everrett, R., Gaub, M. P., Chambon, P. 1981. The SV40 72 base pair repeat has a striking effect on gene expression both in SV40 and other chimeric recombinants. *Nucleic Acids Res.* 9:6047–69

87. Fromm, M., Berg, P. 1982. Deletion mapping of DNA regions required for SV40 early region promotor function *in vivo*. *J. Mol. Appl. Gen.* 1:457–81

88. Laimins, L. A., Khoury, G., Gorman, C., Howard, B., Gruss, P. 1982. Host-specific activation of transcription by tandem repeats from Simian virus 40 and Moloney murine sarcoma virus. *Proc. Natl. Acad. Sci. USA* 79:6453–57

89. Khoury, G., Gruss, P. 1983. Enhancer elements. *Cell* 33:313–14

89a. Ostrowski, M. C., Huang, A. L., Kessel, M., Wolford, R. G., Hager, G. L. 1984. Modulation of enhancer activity by the hormone responsive regulatory element from mouse mammary tumor virus. *EMBO J.* 3:1891–99

90. Doehmer, J., Barinaga, M., Vale, W., Rosenfeld, M. G., Verma, I. M., Evans, R. M. 1982. Introduction of rat growth hormone gene into mouse fibroblasts via a retroviral DNA vector: Expression and regulation. *Proc. Natl. Acad. Sci. USA* 79:2268–72

91. Karin, M., Eberhardt, N. L., Mellon, S. H., Malich, N., Richards, R. I., et al. 1984. Expression and hormonal regulation of the rat growth hormone gene in transfected mouse L cells. *DNA* 3:147–55

92. Martial, J. A., Baxter, J. D., Goodman, H. M., Seeburg, P. H. 1977. Regulation of growth hormone messenger RNA by thyroid and glucocorticoid hormones. *Proc. Natl. Acad. Sci. USA* 74:1816–20

93. Robins, D. M., Paek, I., Seeburg, P. H., Axel, R. 1982. Regulated expression of human growth hormone genes in mouse cells. *Cell* 29:623–31

94. Roy, A. K., Neuhaus, O. W. 1966. Proof of the hepatic synthesis of a sex-dependent protein in the rat. *Biochim. Biophys. Acta* 127:82–87

95. Roy, A. K., Chatterjee, B., Demyan, W. F., Milin, B. S., Motwani, N. M., et al. 1983. Hormone and age-dependent regulation of α_{2u}-globulin gene expression. *Rec. Prog. Horm. Res.* 39:425–61

96. Kurtz, D. T., Feigelson, P. 1977. Multihormonal induction of hepatic α_{2u}-globulin mRNA as measured by hybridization to complementary DNA. *Proc. Natl. Acad. Sci. USA* 74:4791–95

97. Roy, A. K., McMinn, D. M., Biswas, N. M. 1975. Estrogenic inhibition of the hepatic synthesis α_{2u} globulin in the rat. *Endocrinology* 97:1501–8

98. Chen, C.-L. C., Feigelson, P. 1979. Cycloheximide inhibition of hormonal induction of α_{2u}-globulin mRNA. *Proc. Natl. Acad. Sci. USA* 76:2669–73

99. Kurtz, D. T. 1981. Hormonal inducibility of rat α-2μ globulin genes in transfected mouse cells. *Nature* 291:629–31

100. Shinomiya, T., Scherer, G., Schmid, W., Zentgraf, H., Schutz, G. 1984. Isolation and characterization of the rat tyrosine aminotransferase gene. *Proc. Natl. Acad. Sci. USA* 81:1346–50

101. Karin, M., Herschman, H. R. 1979. Dexamethasone stimulation of metallothionein synthesis in HeLa cell cultures. *Science* 204:176–77

102. Hager, L. J., Palmiter, R. D. 1981. Transcriptional regulation of mouse liver metallothionein-I gene by glucocorticoids. *Nature* 291:340–42

103. Karin, M., Andersen, R. D., Slater, E., Smith, K., Herschman, H. R. 1980. Metallothionein mRNA induction in HeLa cells in response to zinc or dexamethasone is a primary induction response. *Nature* 286:295–97

104. Mayo, K. E., Warren, R., Palmiter, R. D. 1982. The mouse metallothionein-I gene is transcriptionally regulated by cadmium following transfection into human or mouse cells. *Cell* 29:99–108

105. Karin, M., Haslinger, A., Holtgreve, H., Cathala, G., Slater, E., Baxter, J. D. 1984. Activation of a heterologous promoter in response to dexamethasone and cadmium by metallothionein gene 5'-flanking DNA. *Cell* 36:371–79

106. Moen, R. C., Palmiter, R. D. 1980. Changes in hormone responsiveness of chick oviduct during primary stimulation with estrogen. *Dev. Biol.* 78:450–63

107. Renkawitz, R., Beug, H., Graf, T., Matthias, P., Grez, M., Schutz, G. 1982. Expression of a chicken lysozyme recombinant gene is regulated by progesterone and dexamethasone after microinjection into oviduct cells. *Cell* 31:167–76

108. Renkawitz, R., Schutz, G., von der Ahe, D., Beato, M. 1984. Sequences in the promoter region of the chicken lysozyme gene required for steroid regulation and receptor binding. *Cell* 37:503–10

109. Geisse, S., Scheidereit, C., Westphal, H. M., Hynes, N. E., Groner, B., Beato, M. 1982. Glucocorticoid receptors recognize DNA sequences in and around murine mammary tumor virus DNA. *EMBO J.* 1:1613–19

110. Govindan, M. V., Spiess, E., Majors, J. 1982. Purified glucocorticoid-hormone complex from rat liver cytosol binds specifically to cloned mouse mammary tumor virus long terminal repeats *in vitro*. *Proc. Natl. Acad. Sci. USA* 79:5157–61

111. Scheidereit, C., Geisse, S., Westphal, H. M., Beato, M. 1983. The glucocorticoid receptor binds to defined nucleotide sequences near the promoter of mouse mammary tumor virus. *Nature* 304:749–52

112. Pfahl, M. 1982. Specific binding of the glucocorticoid-receptor complex to the mouse mammary tumor virus promoter region. *Cell* 31:475–82

113. DeFranco, D., Wrange, O., Merryweather, J., Yamamoto, K. R. 1984. Biological activity of a glucocorticoid regulated enhancer: DNA sequence requirements and interactions with other transcriptional enhancers. In *Genome Rearrangement*, ed. I. Herskowitz, M. Simon. New York: Academic. In press

114. Karin, M., Haslinger, A., Holtgreve, H., Richards, R. I., Krauter, P., et al. 1984. Characterization of DNA sequences through which cadmium and glucocorticoid hormones induce human metallothionein-II$_A$ gene. *Nature* 308:513–19

115. Scheidereit, C., Beato, M. 1984. Contacts between hormone receptor and DNA double helix within a glucocorticoid regulatory element of mouse mammary tumor virus. *Proc. Natl. Acad. Sci. USA* 81:3029–33

116. Yamamoto, K. R., Alberts, B. 1975. The interaction of estradiol-receptor protein with the genome: An argument for the existence of undetected specific sites. *Cell* 4:301–10

117. Payvar, F., Wrange, O. 1984. Relative selectivities and efficiencies of DNA binding by purified intact and protease-cleaved glucocorticoid receptor. In *Steroid Hormone Receptors: Structure and Function,* ed. H. Eriksson, J.-A. Gustafsson, pp. 267–82. Amsterdam: Elsevier/North-Holland Biomed.

118. Cox, R. F., Haines, M. E., Emtage, J. S. 1974. Quantitation of ovalbumin mRNA in hen and chick oviduct by hybridization to complementary DNA. *Eur. J. Biochem.* 49:225–36

119. Chan, L., Means, A. R., O'Malley, B. W. 1973. Rates of induction of specific translatable messenger RNAs for ovalbumin and avidin by steroid hormones. *Proc. Natl. Acad. Sci. USA* 70:1870–74

120. Rhoads, R. E., McKnight, G. S., Schimke, R. T. 1973. Quantitative measurement of ovalbumin messenger RNA activity. *J. Biol. Chem.* 248:2031

121. Palmiter, R. D., Carey, N. H. 1974. Rapid inactivation of ovalbumin messenger ribonucleic acid after acute withdrawal of estrogen. *Proc. Natl. Acad. Sci. USA* 71:2357–61

122. Schutz, G., Nguyen-Huu, M. C., Giesecke, K., Hynes, N. E., Groner, B., et al. 1978. Hormonal control of egg white protein messenger RNA synthesis in the chicken oviduct. *Cold Spring Harbor Symp. Quant. Biol.* 42:617–24

123. McKnight, G. S., Palmiter, R. D. 1979. Transcriptional regulation of the ovalbumin and conalbumin genes by steroid hormones in the chick oviduct. *J. Biol. Chem.* 254:9050–58

124. Schimke, R. T., McKnight, G. S., Shapiro, D. J. 1975. Nucleic acid probes and analysis of hormone action in oviduct. See Ref. 17, 3:245

125. Rosen, J., O'Malley, B. W. 1975. Hormonal regulation of specific gene ex-

pression in the chick oviduct. See Ref. 17, 3:271

126. Heilig, R., Muraskowsky, R., Mandel, J.-L. 1982. The ovalbumin gene family. *J. Mol. Biol.* 156:1–19

127. LeMeur, M., Glanville, N., Mandel, J. L., Gerlinger, P., Palmiter, R., Chambon, P. 1981. The ovalbumin gene family: Hormonal control of X and Y gene transcription and mRNA accumulation. *Cell* 23:561–71

128. Knoll, B. J., Zarucki-Schulz, T., Dean, D. C., O'Malley, B. W. 1983. Definition of the ovalbumin gene promoter by transfer of an ovalglobin fusion gene into cultured cells. *Nucleic Acids Res.* 11:6733–54

129. Dean, D. C., Knoll, B. J., Riser, M. E., O'Malley, B. W. 1983. A 5'-flanking sequence essential for progesterone regulation of an ovalbumin fusion gene. *Nature* 305:551–54

130. Dean, D. C., Gope, R., Knoll, B. J., Riser, M. E., O'Malley, B. W. 1984. A similar 5' flanking region is required for estrogen and progesterone induction of ovalbumin gene expression. *J. Biol. Chem.* 259:9967–70

131. Loosfelt, H., Fridlansky, F., Savouret, J.-F., Atger, M., Milgrom, E. 1981. Mechanism of action of progesterone in the rabbit endometrium. *J. Biol. Chem.* 256:3465–70

132. Kumar, N. M., Chandra, T., Woo, S. L. C., Bullock, D. W. 1982. Transcriptional activity of the uteroglobin gene in rabbit endometrial nuclei during early pregnancy. *Endocrinology* 111:1115–20

133. Parker, M. G., Scrace, G. T., Mainwaring, W. I. P. 1978. Testosterone regulates the synthesis of major proteins in rat ventral prostate. *Biochem. J.* 170:115–21

134. Page, M. J., Parker, M. G. 1983. Androgen-regulated expression of a cloned rat prostatic C3 gene transfected into mouse mammary tumor cells. *Cell* 32:495–502

135. Brown, A. M. C., Jeltsch, J.-M., Roberts, M., Chambon, P. 1984. Activation of pS2 gene transcription is a primary response to estrogen in the human breast cancer cell line MCF-7. *Proc. Natl. Acad. Sci. USA.* 81:6344-48

136. Hayward, M. A., Brock, M. L., Shapiro, D. J. 1982. Activation of vitellogenin gene transcription is a direct response to estrogen in *Xenopus laevis* liver. *Nucleic Acids Res.* 10:8273–84

137. Mulvihill, E. P., LePennec, J.-P., Chambon, P. 1982. Chicken oviduct progesterone receptor: Location of specific regions of high-affinity binding in cloned DNA fragments of hormone-responsive genes. *Cell* 28:621–32

138. Compton, J. G., Schrader, W. T., O'Malley, B. W. 1982. Selective binding of chicken progesterone receptor A subunit to a DNA fragment containing ovalbumin gene sequences. *Biochem. Biophys. Res. Commun.* 105:95–104

139. Compton, J. G., Schrader, W. T., O'Malley, B. W. 1983. DNA sequence preference of the progesterone receptor. *Proc. Natl. Acad. Sci. USA* 80:16–20

140. Bailly, A., Atger, M., Atger, P., Cerbon, M.-A., Alizon, M., et al. 1983. The rabbit uteroglobin gene: Structure and interaction with the progesterone receptor. *J. Biol. Chem.* 258:10384–89

141. Jost, J.-P., Seldran, M., Geiser, M. 1984. Preferential binding of estrogen-receptor complex to a region containing the estrogen-dependent hypomethylation site preceding the chicken vitellogenin II gene. *Proc. Natl. Acad. Sci. USA* 81:429–33

142. Burch, J. B. E., Weintraub, H. 1983. Temporal order of chromatin structural changes associated with activation of the major chicken vitellogenin gene. *Cell* 33:65–76

143. Chamberlin, M. J. 1974. The selectivity of transcription. *Ann. Rev. Biochem.* 43:721–75

144. McClure, W. R. 1980. Rate-limiting steps in RNA chain initiation. *Proc. Natl. Acad. Sci. USA* 77:5634–38

145. Hawley, D. K., McClure, W. R. 1983. The effect of a lambda repressor mutation on the activation of transcription initiation from the lambda P_{RM} promoter. *Cell* 32:327–33

146. Guarente, L., Nye, J. S., Hochschild, A., Ptashne, M. 1982. Mutant λ phage repressor with a specific defect in its positive control function. *Proc. Natl. Acad. Sci. USA* 79:2236–39

147. Hochschild, A., Irwin, N., Ptashne, M. 1983. Repressor structure and the mechanism of positive control. *Cell* 32:319–25

148. de Crombrugghe, B., Busby, S., Buc, H. 1984. Cyclic AMP receptor protein: Role in transcription activation. *Science* 224:831–38

149. Spassky, A., Busby, S., Buc, H. 1984. On the action of the cyclic AMP-cyclic AMP receptor protein complex at the *Escherichia coli* lactose and galactose promoter regions. *EMBO J.* 3:43–50

150. Taniguchi, T., de Crombrugghe, B. 1983. Interactions of RNA polymerase and the cyclic AMP receptor protein on

DNA of the *E. coli* galactose operon. *Nucleic Acids Res.* 11:5165–80

151. Shanblatt, S. H., Revzin, A. 1983. Two catabolite activator protein molecules bind to the galactose promoter region of *E. coli* in the presence of RNA polymerase. *Proc. Natl. Acad. Sci. USA* 80:1594–98

152. Weintraub, H., Groudine, M. 1976. Chromosomal subunits in active genes have an altered conformation. *Science* 193:848–56

153. Wu, C. 1980. The 5' ends of Drosophila heat shock genes in chromatin are hypersensitive to DNAse I. *Nature* 286:854–60

154. Elgin, S. C. R. 1981. DNAase I-hypersensitive sites of chromatin. *Cell* 27:413–15

155. Wilks, A. J., Cato, A. C. B., Cozens, P. J., Mattaj, I. W., Jost, J.-P. 1981. Isolation and fine structure organization of an avian vitellogenin gene coding for the major estrogen-inducible mRNA. *Gene* 16:249–59

156. Gerber-Huber, S., Felber, B. K., Weber, R., Ryffel, G. U. 1981. Estrogen induces tissue specific changes in the chromatin conformation of the vitellogenin genes in *Xenopus. Nucleic Acids Res.* 9:2475–94

157. Lawson, G. M., Knoll, B. J., March, C. J., Woo, S. L. C., Tsai, M.-J., O'Malley, B. W. 1982. Definition of 5' and 3' structural boundaries of the chromatin domain containing the ovalbumin multigene family. *J. Biol. Chem.* 257:1501–7

158. Stumph, W. E., Baez, M., Beattie, W. G., Tsai, M.-J., O'Malley, B. W. 1983. Characterization of deoxyribonucleic acid sequences at the 5' and 3' borders of the 100 kilobase pair ovalbumin gene domain. *Biochemistry* 22:306–15

159. Zaret, K. S., Yamamoto, K. R. 1984. Reversible and persistent changes in chromatin structure accompanying activation of a glucocorticoid-dependent enhancer element. *Cell* 38:29–38

160. Baker, H. J., Shapiro, D. J. 1978. Rapid accumulation of vitellogenin messenger RNA during secondary estrogen stimulation of *Xenopus laevis. J. Biol. Chem.* 253:4521–24

161. Becker, P., Renkawitz, R., Schutz, G. 1984. Tissue-specific DNaseI hypersensitive sites in the 5' flanking sequences of the tryptophan oxygenase and the tyrosine aminotransferase genes. *EMBO J.* 3:2015–20

162. Kaye, J. S., Bellard, M., Dretzen, G., Bellard, F., Chambon, P. 1984. A close association between sites of DNase I hypersensitivity and sites of enhanced cleavage by micrococcal nuclease in the 5'-flanking region of the actively transcribed ovalbumin gene. *EMBO J.* 3:1137–44

163. Smith, G. R. 1981. DNA supercoiling: Another level for regulating gene expression. *Cell* 24:599–600

164. Dubnau, E., Margolin, P. 1972. Suppression of promoter mutations by the pleiotropic *supX* mutation. *Mol. Gen. Genet.* 117:91–112

165. Sternglanz, R., DiNardo, S., Voelkel, K. A., Nishimura, Y., Hirota, Y., et al. 1981. Mutations in the gene coding for *Escherichia coli* DNA topoisomerase I affect transcription and transposition. *Proc. Natl. Acad. Sci. USA* 78:2747–51

166. Gellert, M. 1981. DNA topoisomerases. *Ann. Rev. Biochem.* 50:879–910

167. Shuman, H., Schwartz, M. 1975. The effect of nalidixic acid on the expression of some genes in *Escherichia coli* K-12. *Biochem. Biophys. Res. Commun.* 64:204–9

168. Sanzey, B. 1979. Modulation of gene expression by drugs affecting deoxyribonucleic acid gyrase. *J. Bacteriol.* 138:40–47

169. Yang, H.-L., Heller, K., Gellert, M., Zubay, G. 1979. Differential sensitivity of gene expression *in vitro* to inhibitors of DNA gyrase. *Proc. Natl. Acad. Sci. USA* 76:3304–8

170. Singleton, C. K., Wells, R. D. 1982. Relationship between superhelical density and cruciform formation in plasmid pVH51. *J. Biol. Chem.* 257:6292–95

171. Klar, A. J. S., Strathern, J. N., Broach, J. R., Hicks, J. B. 1981. Regulation of transcription in expressed and unexpressed mating type cassettes of yeast. *Nature* 289:239–44

172. Nasmyth, K. A., Tatchell, K., Hall, B. D., Astell, C., Smith, M. 1981. A position effect in the control of transcription at yeast mating type loci. *Nature* 289:244–50

173. Nasmyth, K. A. 1982. The regulation of yeast-mating-type chromatin structure by SIR: An action at a distance affecting both transcription and transposition. *Cell* 30:567–78

174. Ashburner, M., Chihara, C., Meltzer, P., Richards, G. 1973. Temporal control of puffing activity in polytene chromosomes. *Cold Spring Harbor Symp. Quant. Biol.* 38:655–62

175. Horwitz, K. B., Koseki, Y., McGuire, W. L. 1978. Estrogen control of progesterone receptor in human breast can-

cer: Role of estradiol and antiestrogens. *Endocrinology* 103:1742–51

176. Vannice, J. L., Ringold, G. M., McLean, J. W., Taylor, J. M. 1983. Induction of the acute-phase reactant, alpha-1-acid glycoprotein, by glucocorticoids in rat hepatoma cells. *DNA* 2:205–12

177. Baumann, H., Firestone, G. L., Burgess, T. L., Gross, K. W., Yamamoto, K. R., Held, W. A. 1983. Dexamethasone regulation of α_1-acid glycoprotein and other acute phase reactants in rat liver and hepatoma cells. *J. Biol. Chem.* 258:563–70

178. Feinberg, R. F., Sun, L.-H. K., Ordahl, C. P., Frankel, F. R. 1983. Identification of glucocorticoid-induced genes in rat hepatoma cells by isolation of cloned cDNA sequences. *Proc. Natl. Acad. Sci. USA* 80:5042–46

179. Vannice, J. L., Taylor, J. M., Ringold, G. M. 1984. Glucocorticoid-mediated induction of α_1-acid glycoprotein: Evidence for hormone-regulated RNA processing. *Proc. Natl. Acad. Sci. USA.* In press 81:4241–45

180. Firestone, G. L., Payvar, F., Yamamoto, K. 1982. Glucocorticoid regulation of protein processing and compartmentalization. *Nature* 300:221–25

181. Sachs, L. 1978. Control of normal cell differentiation and the phenotypic reversion of malignancy in myeloid leukaemia. *Nature* 274:535–39

182. Chapman, A. B., Knight, D. M., Dieckmann, B. S., Ringold, G. M. 1984. Analysis of gene expression during differentiation of adipogenic cells in culture and hormonal control of the developmental program. *J. Biol. Chem.* In press

183. Dynan, W. S., Tijan, R. 1983. Isolation of transcription factors that discriminate between different promoters recognized by RNA polymerase II. *Cell* 32:669–80

184. Feinstein, S. C., Ross, S. R., Yamamoto, K. R. 1982. Chromosomal position effects determine transcriptional potential of integrated mammary tumor virus DNA. *J. Mol. Biol.* 156:549–65

185. Ostrowski, M. C., Richard-Foy, H., Wolford, R. G., Berard, D. S., Hager, G. L. 1983. Glucocorticoid regulation of transcription at an amplified episomal promoter. *Mol. Cell. Biol.* 3:2045–57

186. Birnberg, N. C., Lissitzky, J.-C., Hinman, M., Herbert, E. 1983. Glucocorticoids regulate proopiomelanocortin gene expression *in vivo* at the levels of transcription and secretion. *Proc. Natl. Acad. Sci. USA* 80:6982–86

Ann. Rev. Pharmacol. Toxicol. 1985. 25:567–92

OCCUPATIONAL EXPOSURES ASSOCIATED WITH MALE REPRODUCTIVE DYSFUNCTION[1]

Susan Donn Schrag and Robert L. Dixon

Office of Health Research, US Environmental Protection Agency, Research Triangle Park, North Carolina 27711

INTRODUCTION

Dibromochloropropane (DBCP)-induced sterility in male workers who applied the nematocide has focused scientific, public, and regulatory attention on the potential nontherapeutic chemicals have to affect the human reproductive capacity. Questions are increasingly being asked about the effect of industrial and environmental chemicals on the relatively poor quality of human semen and on what some interpret as a general decline in mean sperm counts (1). Over the past decade, estimates of declining fertility have abounded. In the United States, nearly seven million couples are involuntarily infertile and three million couples contain at least one partner who is sterile; and in 1976, 25% of all married couples with the wife of child-bearing age (15–44 years old) had impaired fecundity (2). Even so, the relationships between occupational and environmental chemicals and reproductive failure remain poorly defined.

Occupational chemical exposure may be thought of as a model for many of the chemicals that contaminate our environment. Exposure levels are generally higher and more closely monitored in the workplace, and individual exposure can be more reliably estimated there. Because health surveillance programs often exist, cause-and-effect relationships may be established more convincingly. Yet many confounding factors complicate this task. Workers are rarely exposed to a single agent. Our total environment, including the work environment, is a multi-chemical world that makes it difficult to single out one reproductive toxin. Occupational settings provide the potential for both acute and chronic chemical exposure, with their resultant particular effects. This chapter focuses only on the effects of chronic exposure.

Chemicals, however, are not the only hazards that might affect human reproductive capacity. Physical agents such as altitude (3), temperature, and radiation (ionizing and non-ionizing) may also play a role (4). Elevated workplace temperatures might have not only a direct effect on the male gonads, but may also increase the absorption of toxic substances by increasing lung ventilation and circulatory rates. Absorption of pesticides increases in high-temperature work environments, perhaps because of the effect of the heat itself, because of the tendency of workers to remove protective clothing, or because of a combination of these two factors. Such potentially synergistic relationships between physical and chemical agents in the occupational environment rarely undergo rigorous scientific examination (5). Likewise, personal habits such as smoking (6), consuming alcoholic beverages, taking drugs either therapeutically or recreationally, or eating patterns and diet selection are each suspected to a greater or lesser degree of being confounding factors.

In the past, females have most often been the focus of studies of occupational exposures and reproductive effects, primarily because reproductive endpoints can be more easily determined in women than in men. A woman's menstrual cycle is established at puberty and continues throughout her reproductive life. Estrogens and progestins can be measured, and their effects are reflected in cellular changes in female accessory sex organs and in the regularity of the menstrual cycle. Women are particularly alert to delayed or missed periods, which may indicate spontaneous abortion or pregnancy wastage. Chemical agents may also appear in the secretory fluids of the accessory sex organs; certain ones are concentrated in breast milk. In many cases, the health of a child and the effects associated with nursing provide sensitive indicators of occupational toxicity.

In contrast, males lack an obvious and easily measurable reproductive cycle, and the primary clinical indicator, semen analysis, offers unsure clues to reproductive performance. Because only one sperm is required to fertilize the ovum, it is difficult to establish the probability of a pregnancy based on a reduction in the approximately 30 million sperm usually ejaculated (7). Normal mean semen parameters are 20 million sperm per milliliter of semen; only about 60% of the sperm is motile and about the same proportion is morphologically normal (8). Sperm density fluctuates daily in the same individual, and the predictability of the other variables has not been evaluated. Sperm density is an absolute predictor only when azoospermia is noted. Unless sperm are totally immobile, motility is difficult to quantify. And, although some investigators have reported a correlation between sperm morphology and chemical exposure, the link between changes in morphology and altered fertility has not been demonstrated convincingly (9).

Furthermore, no effects on sperm are yet confirmed to be associated with birth defects, and there is no male equivalent to nursing. Impotency is an unsure endpoint and decreased libido seldom causes a man to see a physician or to report to the factory's clinic. Likewise, with the exception of the sperm penetration assay, there are no good laboratory indicators of human sperm functionality [see (10)]. Because the scientist has fewer reliable clinical endpoints for men, the study of male reproductive toxicity is difficult and the drawing of conclusions is tenuous.

However, progress is being made in developing and evaluating tests to better identify chemical hazards and to estimate human health risks. Wyrobek (11, 12) has suggested that sperm morphology is a stable semen parameter and a reliable predictor of fertility and feels that careful longitudinal studies can reveal the selected changes in sperm morphology that accompany defined chemical exposures. A Y-body test, which scores the frequency of sperm with two florescent spots and is thought to represent sperm with two Y-chromosomes due to meiotic nondisjunction, has been used to evaluate human sperm; unfortunately, it has no direct counterpart in commonly used laboratory animals (13). The interspecies sperm penetration assay has recently been validated as a reliable predictor of fertility (14), and lack of sperm penetrating ability has been associated with chemical exposure (15). Post-testicular events such as sperm maturation, capacitation, acrosome reaction, cervical mucus penetrability, and fertilizing capacity are only occasionally assessed (16). Serum gonadotropins and androgen levels can be monitored, and size and weight of the testes can be easily derived. It is also possible to biopsy the testis, although this clinical procedure is rarely performed in investigations of the effects of industrial chemicals.

The study of occupational reproductive toxicology involves both the biological and the epidemiological sciences, and as a result the difficulties in designing a truly successful study are many (17). Surveillance of human reproductive capacity involves both prospective and retrospective studies, but they generally lack statistical power because of the unsure endpoints available and the generally low number of men observed (18, 19). Pregnancy loss and spontaneous abortion may also be important indicators of abnormal sperm function and have been included in surveillance programs (20, 21). The obvious need for better data collection on exposures and reproductive endpoints, as well as for greater coordination of these data and their analyses, has been discussed elsewhere (22–28).

OCCUPATIONAL EXPOSURE

While a large number and wide variety of therapeutic agents have been reported to affect male reproductive capacity based on laboratory and clinical reports (29), the list of industrial chemicals thought to affect the human male is much shorter. Because this is an area of increasing scientific interest and importance, various investigators have summarized existing knowledge and have offered their own lists of about a dozen potentially harmful industrial chemicals each (30, 31–33). However, except for length, agreement among these lists is far from perfect.

For some of these listed agents the mechanism of action is obvious, while for others the molecular interactions that account for their toxicity are generally unrecognized. Many are cytotoxic and generally toxic, and some also share carcinogenic, mutagenic, and/or teratogenic properties. Yet the reproductive hazard of greatest concern is probably the chemical that does not share mutagenic or carcinogenic potential, is not generally cytotoxic, acts by disrupting biological processes unique to the reproductive process, and is subtle in its onset.

This review focuses on those industrial chemicals thought to affect human male reproductive capacity for which published data are available (Table 1). Reports in the literature that associate industrial chemicals with male reproductive dysfunction are evaluated, laboratory approaches used in an attempt to identify hazards are examined, and the clinical signs indicating infertility are noted.

Agents with Confirmed Adverse Effects

For the following agents, whose adverse reproductive effects have been confirmed, there is a strong scientific concensus regarding a cause-and-effect relationship. Either a number of studies have shown toxicity or the effect of the chemical is predictable based on its known biological activity.

CARBON DISULFIDE   Carbon disulfide (CS_2) is a solvent used primarily in the production of viscose rayon, and chronic exposure is associated with apparent nervous system toxicity. European studies of the reproductive effects of occupational exposure reveal multiple statistically significant effects on endpoints of spermatogenesis (34, 35), on levels of serum FSH and LH (35–37), and on libido (34–36). These effects have been found to persist in 66% of the workers subject to follow-up examinations (35). However, dose-response relationships have not been statistically established for any of the parameters.

In a US study of low CS_2 exposure over considerably shorter periods of time (measured in months rather than years), Meyer (38) failed to demonstrate significant differences in semen parameters when exposed men were compared

Table 1 Occupational exposures associated with male reproductive dysfunction[a]

Agents with confirmed adverse effects	Agents with inconclusive effects	Agents with no observed adverse effects
Carbon disulfide	Anesthetic gases	Epichlorohydrin
Dibromochloropropane (DBCP)	Arsenic	Glycerine
Lead	Benzene	p-TBBA
Oral contraceptives	Boron	PBB
	Cadmium	PCB
	Carbaryl	
	Chlordecone	
	Chloroprene	
	DNT and TDA	
	Ethylene dibromide	
	Manganese	
	Mercury	
	Pesticides	
	PCP	
	Radiation-ionizing	
	Radiation-nonionizing	
	Solvents	
	TCDD (dioxin)	
	Vinyl chloride	

[a]Classification based upon analysis of currently available literature. Refer to text for specific comments.

to controls. Yet Romanian (34, 35), Italian (36), and Finnish (37) experiences seem to support the inclusion of CS_2 on any list of male reproductive hazards because of its multiple effects. The data also suggest that levels of occupational exposure should be well controlled.

DIBROMOCHLOROPROPANE   Dibromochloropropane (DBCP) originally was registered as a soil fumigant used to control nematodes. In 1979, the Environmental Protection Agency (EPA) banned the sale, distribution, and movement of DBCP in commerce, two years after suspending most end-use products. This was the first regulatory action taken by a US agency based on reproductive toxicity, and the literature is replete with references. The US Public Health Service reported that DBCP is mutagenic and "may reasonably be anticipated to be a human carcinogen" (39).

   Whorton et al (40) were the first to describe the reproductive effects of DBCP. They reported azoospermia and oligospermia, as well as increased serum levels of FSH and LH, in 14 of 25 men working in a pesticide factory. No other major abnormalities were detected, and testosterone levels were normal. Although exposure levels could not be quantified, the observed effects appeared to be related to duration of DBCP exposure. In recent years, reports of

DBCP testicular toxicity have been published by investigators throughout the world (41–48).

Glass et al (49) reported studies of male DBCP applicators and determined that the effects of the agent are limited to individuals in certain situations, such as applicators involved in irrigation set-up work and in the calibration of equipment. Once released from those situations, the sperm counts of these individuals return to normal. Statistical reanalysis of these data by Kahn & Whorton (50) showed that all applicator groups had reduced sperm counts in a dose-related manner and that reversibility was not a certainty. Glass (51) responded to these criticisms.

In studies of Y-chromosome nondisjunction, DBCP-exposed workers had a higher average YFF frequency compared to nonexposed individuals (13). An agent that increases Y-chromosomal nondisjunction (the frequency of YFF sperm) might be anticipated to result in increased pregnancy wastage.

International efforts have also been directed toward determining the reversibility of DBCP's effects (52–54). Wheater (55), responding to an inquiry in the *Journal of the American Medical Association,* rightly suggested that the DBCP effect appears reversible and that the more severe and potentially long-lasting reproductive effects, such as decreased testicular size, are probably restricted to production workers [see (43–45)] since farm workers and applicators are exposed only sporadically to diluted material.

Effects in chemical workers surveyed in Michigan were consistent with the known testicular effects of DBCP and again demonstrated the reversibility of the effect over time (47). Whorton & Milby (56) reexamined 21 men with DBCP-reduced sperm count after termination of exposure in 1977. When initially examined, 12 of the men were azoospermic and nine were oligospermic. Almost all of the oligospermic men improved considerably, while none of the 12 azoospermic men recovered.

Lipshultz et al (57) reported the gonadotoxic effects of DBCP on the largest group of workers to date. Semen analyses, serum hormonal determinations (LH, FSH, and testosterone), and genital examinations were completed on 228 workers at two chemical production sites. Their dose-response model suggested significant changes in sperm density after more than 100 adjusted hours of exposure. Broadening the focus of DBCP studies, Kharrazai et al (58) looked for effects on wives of DBCP-exposed field applicators and found an apparent increased risk of spontaneous abortion, although the health of the liveborn infants seemed unaffected.

A four-year reassessment of 20 Israeli workers with DBCP-induced testicular dysfunction, as well of the outcome of the pregnancies that accompanied their recovery process, demonstrated that the reversibility of the gonadotoxic effects was related to previous exposure time and was most likely to occur in patients with normal FSH levels (54). A delayed toxic effect of DBCP on

Sertoli and Leydig cell function was suggested to explain the lack of recovery. Pregnancies occurring after recovery from DBCP-induced spermatogenic impairment apparently are not associated with an increased risk of fetal congenital malformation.

Of all environmental agents, DBCP presents the clearest picture relating occupational exposure to testicular toxicity and human reproductive dysfunction [see (58a)]. Exposure levels have been estimated and dose-response relationships investigated. Studies have also focused on recovery from both mild and severe testicular effects. Thus, DBCP offers a valuable data base for assessing the reliability of laboratory test methods to predict the toxicity of similarly acting chemicals and for correlating human reproductive endpoints with chemically induced dusfunction and subsequent recovery.

LEAD   Lead exists in the environment in both inorganic and organic forms. People working as smelters, with batteries, as artisans such as stained-glass workers (59), and as painters may absorb inorganic lead. However, because organic or tetraethyl lead (TEL) is used as an additive to gasoline, it is the most common form of lead found in the environment. Although the literature includes two early reports showing reduced libido and increased impotency among TEL workers [see (30)], a study of US TEL workers found no detectable health differences between them and a group of matched controls (60).

Evidence of the deleterious effects of lead on human reproduction dates back to ancient Rome, where Gilfillan has suggested that lead in drinking vessels produced sufficient toxicity among the upper classes to result in declining populations (61). In addition, lead also has long been known as a spermicidal agent and an abortifacient (62).

Although most of the literature dealing with the effects of lead on reproduction relates to women and children (63), there is clear evidence that lead is also a male reproductive toxin. Lancranjan et al (63a) reported finding dose-related disturbances of spermatogenic endpoints, including asthenospermia, hypospermia, and teratospermia among the 150 lead workers studied. However, gonadotropin levels were unaffected. The results of their study suggest that lead may act directly on spermiogenesis.

Even more research has been directed toward the effects of lead on chromosomes. Thomas & Brogan (62) cite ten international studies that report an increased incidence of chromosomal damage in workers exposed to lead (e.g. 64–67) and six studies that fail to establish such an association (e.g. 68, 69). Interestingly, DeKnudt et al (64) examined the chromosomes of workers exposed to lead, zinc, and cadmium and found aberrations only among the lead workers. In addition, Nordenson et al (67) noted that, although the sperm effect for the groups in their study correlated in a dose-dependent manner with blood lead levels, individual blood lead levels were poor predictors of chromosome damage.

The evidence is convincing that lead affects spermatogenesis, results in abnormal sperm morphology, and is associated with infertility. Lead also appears to have a genotoxic potential. Thus, every effort should be made to reduce occupational and environmental lead exposure.

ORAL-CONTRACEPTIVE FORMULATION   Although this review could include the occupational hazards associated with a variety of therapeutic agents with known reproductive effects, it discusses only a single example because few well-designed studies are available. Harrington et al (70–71a) have described an investigation in a Puerto Rico factory that formulated oral contraceptives using synthetic estrogens and progestins. During a twelve-month period, 25 (20%) of the male employees experienced symptoms associated with hyperestrogenism. All of the affected males had gynecomastia, and three also reported a history of decreased libido or impotence. Elevated plasma ethinyl estradiol levels accounted for the effects observed. Hyperestrogenism among men, women, and children resulting from the adults' exposure to diethylstilbestrol (DES) and other estrogens while working in pharmaceutical plants has been a worldwide concern [see (70, 72, 73)]. Diaminostilbene, an optical brightener structurally similar to DES, has also been implicated as a male reproductive toxin. In 1981, the National Institute of Occupational Safety and Health (NIOSH) investigated a report of sexual impotence among male workers employed in the manufacture of diaminostilbene [see (74)]. This investigation indicated that more than one-third of the men in the affected area had a history of probable or possible impotency. The toxic effects of the oral contraceptives observed are predictable based on the pharmacological actions of the drugs involved.

Agents with Inconclusive Effects

The following agents are those whose reproductive effects are ir conclusive. Clinical studies of them have been performed or case studies reported, but the data lack the strength necessary to be convincing. Often their effects are chromosomal aberrations whose ultimate effect on male reproduction is unclear. The literature reviewed does not conclusively support the effects suggested in textbooks and reviews that may list a particular substance as harmful.

ANESTHETIC GASES   A 1967 report from Russia was one of the first to register concern about human health risks associated with the operating room environment. Vaisman [see (75)] noted a wide range of health complaints, including such adverse pregnancy outcomes as spontaneous abortion, premature delivery, and congenital malformations, among 21 of 31 reported pregnancies. Worldwide interest ensued, with initial reports focusing on the exposure of female nurses from Denmark (76), the United States (77–79), and Great Britain (80).

Among males occupationally exposed to anesthetic gases, infertility has been reported (76, 81). Their wives are reported to have an increased rate of spontaneous abortions (76, 81, 82), and among their children there apparently are greater numbers of congenital malformations (81, 83–88), low birth weights (81, 84), and a higher rate of female births (84, 89).

Wyrobek et al (90) analyzed semen samples from 46 male anesthesiologists who worked for at least one year in hospital operating rooms reventilated with modern gas-scavenging devices and observed no significant differences in the number and morphology of the sperm between the exposed group and controls. The outcome remained the same when the analysis was limited to men having no confounding factors such as varicocele, recent illness, medication, heavy smoking, or frequent sauna use. It is interesting to note, however, that the men who had one or more confounding factors (excluding anesthetic gases) showed significantly higher percentages of sperm abnormalities than did the group of men without such factors.

The study of the relationship between occupational exposure to anesthetic gases and reproductive toxicity is different from the study of exposure to other agents for two reasons. First, because of the educational level, socioeconomic status, and training of the veterinarians (91), dentists (82), and physicians exposed (80, 81, 83, 84), their responses to questionnaires appear to reflect an increased concern with and cognizance of health-related issues. This point is supported by the study results of Knill-Jones et al (86), who suspected bias in respondents reporting minor congenital abnormalities because there was no consistency in the type of abnormality reported and no increase in reports of major abnormalities. Second, the number of people exposed to anesthetics is large and is organized into professional associations that have sponsored large-scale epidemiological surveys (81–83). This is not true for any of the other occupational groups examined in this review.

Finally, although a causal relationship between anesthetic gases and male reproductive dysfunction has not been clearly established, it is obvious that waste gas concentrations should be maintained at a minimum and that other contributing factors should also be carefully controlled (88).

ARSENIC   This literature review identified only one major research effort devoted exclusively to the study of arsenic and its noncarcinogenic effects on human males (91a, 91b). The preliminary report (91a) described the detection of significantly higher numbers of chromosomal aberrations among nine Swedish smelter workers than among a control group. The follow-up report (91b) found similar results among the total cohort of 39 arsenic-exposed workers.

The researchers were very careful to point out that because of very large individual variations and the fact that the correlation between the frequency of all aberrations and arsenic exposure was not very good, it is nearly impossible to conclude that arsenic damages DNA structure. Arsenic appears to inhibit the repair of DNA damaged by the synergism of arsenic and smoking and/or by other agents such as lead and selenium. Arsenic is a known human carcinogen, but its effect, if any, on male reproduction remains unclear.

BENZENE   Reports published in the early 1970s supported the concern that exposure to high concentrations of benzene used as a solvent can cause chromosomal aberrations in male workers [see (92)]. A 1980 review of occupational benzene exposure reported that the results of tests showing weak toxic effects on the reproductive organs of male animals have prompted additional research supported by the American Petroleum Institute and the Chemical Manufacturers Association (93). The results of those studies are not yet available.

BORON   In the mid-1970s, Soviet scientists reported infertility associated with oligospermia and decreased libido among men working in factories in which boric acid is produced and among those living in communities where boron concentrations in artesian well water are high [see (94)]. In the US, much less concern surrounds the possible health hazards associated with boron compounds because laboratory tests suggest that inorganic boron compounds are not highly toxic (95).

CADMIUM   Despite the fact that the effects of cadmium on male reproduction have been studied throughout the world for two decades, the results are inconclusive and even confusing [see (96)]. Epidemiological and case study data suggest an association between the occupational inhalation of cadmium dusts and fumes and prostate cancer [see (97)]. Autopsy reports indicate no spermatids or sperm in the testes of a small group of men engaged in the manufacture of copper-cadmium alloy (98). There is one self-report of impotence in an alkaline storage battery worker (99), but no significant differences in urinary excretion of steroids were observed among the total of ten battery workers compared with a control group of lead-exposed workers. In addition, chromosomal aberrations have been associated with workers manufacturing cadmium pigments (100).

Cadmium is used in electroplating, in plastics manufacturing, in battery production, and in paint mixing. The Occupational Safety and Health Administration (OSHA) has estimated that 360,000 workers are exposed currently, and this number is expected to increase. Better scientific surveillance of cadmium workers and more carefully designed protocols are necessary to define clearly cadmium's reproductive effects.

CARBARYL   Carbaryl (Sevin) is one of the least acutely toxic of the carbamate insecticides. Whorton et al (101) and Wyrobek et al (102) used virtually the same cohort of exposed men to study the effects of carbaryl exposure on fertility by checking for infertile marriages and by measuring sperm counts and serum gonadotropins. Both groups have reported no significant differences between the cohort and a control group for any of the endpoints, although the carbaryl-exposed group included nearly three times as many oligospermic men as the control group. Because sperm counts are known to be statistically less sensitive to small changes, Wyrobek et al (102) analyzed sperm morphology and determined a non–dose related, significant elevation in sperm head abnormalities compared to controls, a condition that may not be reversible. Both studies had low participation rates, relied on self-reports of exposure levels, and used less-than-ideal control groups for comparisons. In a recent article discussing methods for evaluating the effects of environmental chemicals on human sperm production, Wyrobek et al (33) list carbaryl as an agent suggestive of adverse effects.

CHLORDECONE   Chlordecone (Kepone) is a chlorinated hydrocarbon insecticide that was produced in the US, added to other chemicals in West Germany, and then exported to Central and South America, where it was used to control banana borer weevils. From March 1974 through July 1975, the Life Science Products Company of Hopewell, Virginia, was the sole producer of Kepone and, because it is no longer produced, the exposures of the employees at that time have served as the basis for all published reports about the reproductive toxicity of Kepone (104–106).

The Center for Disease Control became aware of Kepone toxicity in 1975, but the scientific community was not alerted until a report by Cannon et al in 1978 (104) described a previously unrecognized clinical illness characterized by neurological symptoms (Kepone shakes) and oligospermia, with abnormal and immobile sperm predominating. Kepone appears to be a direct-acting male reproductive toxin. None of the reports attempt to analyze the data in terms of a dose-response relationship between Kepone levels in serum or fat and the degree of oligospermia, and none of the reports associate sterility with the altered semen parameters. However, the excretion of stored Kepone was hastened in 13 patients who received cholestyramine, an anion-exchange resin, in a controlled clinical trial (105). The researchers chose sperm counts as a dependent variable because neurological signs were more difficult to quantify and found that the number of mobile sperm increased as blood Kepone concentrations decreased in 12 of 13 patients.

CHLOROPRENE   Chloroprene is a pungent, colorless liquid used in the manufacture of synthetic rubber. Although it has been reported to affect male reproductive capacity (107–110), all reports quote the same obscure original Russian study (111). In summarizing that study, Sanotskii (109) writes, "Examinations of chloroprene workers revealed functional disturbances in spermatogenesis after six to ten years of work in chloroprene production, and morphological disturbances after 11 years or more. The questionnaire showed that cases of spontaneous abortion in the wives of chloroprene workers occurred more than three times as frequently as in the control group." Because of the inadequacy of the data, it is impossible to draw reliable conclusions regarding the male reproductive toxicity of chloroprene.

DINITROTOLUENE AND TOLUENE DIAMINE   A 1980 preliminary survey by NIOSH of the Olin Corporation plant in Kentucky detailed reduced sperm counts and higher miscarriage rates among 21 workers exposed to dinitrotoluene (DNT) and toluene diamine (TDA) (112). Olin disputed the report (113) and commissioned another. Subsequently, Hamill et al (114) found no differences between the 84 men in the exposed group and the 119 nonexposed workers in measures of sperm count, sperm morphology, FSH levels, testicular volume, reproductive histories, and urogenital function. These results, from Olin's Louisiana plant, differ considerably from those reported in Kentucky; thus, DNT and TDA should remain on the list of agents with inconclusive effects on male reproduction.

ETHYLENE DIBROMIDE   The use of ethylene dibromide (EDB) as a fumigant recently has received widespread public attention, even though its major, although declining, use is with lead as an anti-knock compound in leaded gasoline. Wong et al (115) assessed the reproductive performance of male workers in four plants exposed to EDB and in one plant found a statistically significant, non–dose related decrease in the expected number of children born to workers' wives. These investigators properly point out the drawbacks associated with their use of national fertility tables. A randomly chosen, in-plant control group would have been a more representative population; testing of such a group would be more likely to detect a decrease in fertility. Semen analysis of 44 occupationally exposed men in Florida, New Jersey, and Texas found no significant differences between the sperm counts of these men and two large statistical comparison groups (116). Ter Haar (117) concludes that neither sperm counts (116, 117) nor the incidence of live births among the workers' wives (115) indicates decreased fertility among exposed males. The data are meager, however, and the small number of workers with potential exposure (only about 1,000 worldwide) (117) is insufficient to draw firm conclusions about the reproductive toxicity of EDB.

MANGANESE   Workers can be exposed to manganese in the steel-manufacturing, chemical, and manganese-mining industries. Although specific studies of the reproductive effects of manganese are not available, reports of manganese poisoning among miners have included reproductive effects. Of fifteen manganese-poisoned Chilean miners, all of whom exhibited psychomotor and neurological disturbances, 27% experienced disturbances of libido and 20% had difficulty ejaculating (117a). This and similar reports [see (30)] were published decades ago. Manganese appears to be a rather weak reproductive toxin that, in cases of severe poisoning, affects both sexual desire and the ability to perform.

METHYLMERCURY   Chronic exposure to methylmercury results in severe central nervous system damage, particularly to the fetus. These effects were identified in the 1970s in Minamata, Japan, where pregnant women consumed fish contaminated with methylmercury. There also is some weak evidence that dental personnel suffer minor genetic damage as a result of mercury exposure (118).

Two case reports involving a total of nine men have outlined such reproductive effects of methylmercury as hypospermia, decreased libido, and impotence (119, 120), symptoms that persisted for at least five years. McFarland & Reigel (120) noted these chronic effects among six men who were exposed only briefly. A dose-related decrease in libido and significantly higher incidences of hypospermia, asthenospermia, and teratospermia have also been noted in 50 chronically exposed men who did not exhibit signs of poisoning (119).

As a possible reproductive toxin, methylmercury presents a unique methodological problem. First, because its primary effect is on the nervous system, symptoms may be classified as psychological in origin and remain unreported. When symptoms are reported, McFarland et al note that the physician often associates them with the depression that commonly occurs in methylmercury poisoning. Second, few males are occupationally exposed to methylmercury.

PESTICIDES   Spurred by the discovery of the toxic potential of DBCP, researchers have widened their search for additional reproductive toxins among the pesticides. Reports have been made of residual levels of DDE and BHC isomers in the semen (121), hexachlorobenzene in the fat, and DDT in the testicles and fat (122) of a randomly drawn sample of 50 fertile and infertile men.

Among occupationally exposed men, there are reports of disturbed spermatogenesis and increased chromosomal breakage (especially of the Y chromosome) (123) as well as impotence (124). In both of those reports, however, the number of workers was very small (five and four respectively). Moreover, the workers recovered potency after discontinuing exposure and receiving hormone therapy. A recent report cites no differences in the total number of pregnancies, sex ratios, spontaneous abortions, and birth defects in a sample of 314 agricultural pilots and 178 sibling families (125). Obviously, much more research is needed in this area before any conclusions about the reproductive consequences of pesticide accumulation can be determined.

PENTACHLOROPHENOL   Pentachlorophenol (PCP), a widely used wood preservative, has been found in the semen of exposed workers [see (126)], and a significantly increased incidence of chromosomal aberrations in their peripheral lymphocytes has been documented (127). Although reproductive dysfunction has not been reported, these findings suggest a higher priority for future investigations of this chemical.

RADIATION: IONIZING   Ionizing radiation has recognized cytotoxic and carcinogenic effects, and careful attempts have been made to establish clinical and occupational exposure levels that provide an adequate margin of safety. However, in recent years, exposure levels once thought to be safe have been questioned. The effects of ionizing radiation on male reproduction are much easier to predict than is the threshold for such effects. The clinical effects of ionizing radiation on the testes and other male reproductive endpoints have been well studied (128–130). The effects of chronic occupational exposure include significant decreases in serum gonadotropins (131) and significant changes in semen parameters (132). The effects of ionizing radiation on spermatogenesis are usually reversible and recovery of fertility has been observed within a few years (133–135).

RADIATION: NONIONIZING   In contrast to ionizing radiation, the biological effects of microwaves are much less apparent. Yet, the level of human exposure continues to increase annually, as does scientific and regulatory concern. The most obvious effects of nonionizing radiation observed in laboratory studies are those associated with thermal effects. Analyzing the human risk associated with nonthermal effects is of greater priority but is also more difficult. The 1975 report of a group of 31 men who experienced decreased libido and decreased semen parameters after long-term occupational exposure to microwaves from an unspecified source appears to be one of the only studies available on this subject (136).

SOLVENTS (HYDROCARBONS AND GLYCOL ETHERS)   A provocative study of the possible role of the father's occupation in the risk of malignant diseases among his offspring found a significant excess of fathers employed in hydrocarbon-related occupations in a group of 386 Quebec children who died before the age of five (137). One possibility suggested to explain this effect is a direct effect of some hydrocarbon contained in petroleum and oil on spermatogenesis that transmits the carcinogenic defect to the child. Of course, direct exposure is a more easily accepted possibility, assuming the association reported also shares a cause-and-effect relationship.

Other researchers have focused their concern on measuring spermatogenesis among workers exposed to the group of chemical solvents known as glycol ethers. Cook et al (138) reported no significant gross abnormalities or clinically meaningful differences in fertility indices among 15 of 97 men studied who submitted semen samples. The small number of participants and the fact that men in the exposed group had smaller testicles makes drawing realistic conclusions about this study impossible. Glycol ethers deserve further attention because they have been associated with male reproductive toxicity in laboratory animals [see (139)].

2,3,6,8-TETRACHLORODIBENZO-p-DIOXIN   2,3,6,8-Tetrachlorodibenzo-p-dioxin (dioxin, TCDD) is a toxic contaminant of trichlorophenol synthesis, of hexachlorophene manufacturing, and of the herbicide 2,4,5-trichlorophenoxy-acid (2,4,5-T). The acute effects of TCDD are associated primarily with the skin and the liver.

In July, 1976, an unfortunate explosion discharged products containing TCDD over an area of 700 acres in Seveso, Italy. The immediate health effect was chloracne, but concern about reproductive effects arose. Follow-up studies two years after the incident showed that the number of pregnancies, the incidence of spontaneous abortions, the rate of chromosomal aberrations, and the number of birth defects remained within expected rates for that area of Italy (140, 141). Similar results were obtained in an interviewer–administered questionnaire survey of a group of Michigan wives of men potentially exposed to dioxins as well as wives of in-plant controls (142). In addition, a recent comparison of 204 men exposed to TCDD in herbicide manufacturing and 163 not exposed to TCDD revealed no significant differences between the groups in pregnancies, live births, infant deaths, miscarriages, birth defects, and stillbirths (143). An unpublished study of railroad workers involved in cleaning up a dioxin spill found a 40% decrease in sperm count and plasma testosterone [see (144)], yet none of the data thus far have been able to confirm the reproductive effects of paternal exposure.

A group of major chemical-manufacturing companies recently settled a class-action lawsuit litigated on behalf of Vietnam veterans exposed to TCDD in the defoliant Agent Orange. A report that children fathered by veterans with symptoms of Agent Orange toxicity show twice the incidence of congenital anomalies as do children fathered by men without symptoms may have prompted that decision [see (144)]. However, Agent Orange exposure was not quantified, nor were other comparisons of the symptomatic and asymptomatic men published. Thus, the effects of paternal exposure to TCDD on reproductive function and the incidence of spontaneous abortions or stillbirths are unresolved, as is the more general question of the possibility that paternal exposure to chemicals can account for congenital abnormalities.

VINYL CHLORIDE   Vinyl chloride monomer (VCM), used in the manufacture or polymerization of polyvinylchloride (PVC), is a known human carcinogen that has been associated with an increased incidence of angiosarcoma, a rare liver tumor. Beginning in 1975, there were reports of increased incidences of chromosomal aberrations among small numbers of PVC manufacturers [see (4, 145, 146)]. As research in this area expanded, larger numbers of PVC workers were examined, and increased chromosomal abnormalities were related to the duration and extent of exposure (147).

Follow-up studies of workers who reduced their exposure showed concomitant decreases in chromosomal abnormalities (148, 149), and a Czech study (150) detected no chromosomal aberrations among men working in an environment where the VCM maximum allowable concentration (MAC) was 1 ppm. Comparisons of measurements of conventional chromosomal abberations with sister-chromatid exchanges demonstrated the former to be more sensitive in detecting changes (151, 152). However, differences among the various studies cited in the composition of the populations under study make direct comparisons difficult. Hatch et al (153) have proposed study guidelines that might solve some of the difficulties in drawing conclusions from inadequate study designs.

Wives of VCM-exposed workers have been reported to have a significant excess of fetal loss (154–157). However, these results must be assessed against the weakness inherent in interviews with fathers (157).

Among the symptoms experienced by men exposed to VCM in the workplace, impotence and loss of libido have been reported [see (30)]. However, there have been no reports of infertile men, and the true impact of chromosomal aberrations on male fertility cannot be assessed.

Agents With No Observed Adverse Effects

This category, agents with no observed adverse reproductive effects, is reserved for chemicals sometimes mentioned as affecting human male reproduction about which there are little or no published data. Also included in this category are chemicals that have been studied and that fail to show a toxic effect.

EPICHLOROHYDRIN   Epichlorohydrin (ECH) is a colorless liquid used in the manufacture of insecticides and many other products. It is an alkylating agent and is a suspected human carcinogen. Milby et al (158) have reported the results of an industry-supported study of the sperm counts of men from two

ECH production plants in which no significant differences among any of the groups were found, even after a variety of analyses. However, this study does not allow firm conclusions about ECH's toxic potential because the control group of "chemical plant workers unexposed to any agents known to be toxic to the testes" was inadequate at best, its participation rates were low, it did not examine such confounding factors as age or smoking, and, although it conducted a medical history and physical examination of "each of the participants," the only data analyzed were number of years worked and sperm density.

GLYCERINE   The manufacture of glycerine may result in exposure to allyl chloride, epichlorohydrin (see above), and 1,3-dichloropropene, agents that are structurally similar to DBCP (see above). This similarity to DBCP has prompted a fertility study of male manufacturers of glycerine (159). No statistically significant differences were demonstrated among the exposed and the control groups when serum gonadotropins, semen variables, and testicle size were analyzed. Thus, it appears that the manufacture of glycerine poses no obvious threat to male reproductive capacity.

PARA-TERTIARY BUTYL BENZOIC ACID   Para-tertiary butyl benzoic acid (p-TBBA) is an organic acid used in cutting oil and in paint that has adverse testicular effects in animals. Prompted by the results of animal studies, Whorton et al (160) studied the testicular function of 90 men occupationally exposed to p-TBBA. They concluded that the levels of p-TBBA exposure experienced at the selected chemical plant had no apparent clinical or epidemiological effect on sperm count, gonadotropin level, and fathering children. The design used in this study is based on studies of DBCP and serves as a prototype for similar investigations.

POLYBROMINATED BIPHENYLS   Polybrominated biphenyls (PBBs) are used as fire retardants in plastics. In 1973–1974, their accidental mixture with cattle feed in Michigan attracted a great deal of public attention because their presence later was detected both in breast milk and in blood serum. Yet Roseman et al (161) reported no effect on spermatogenesis among 52 PBB-exposed men who were studied four years after exposure, and no correlations were observed between serum PBB levels and sperm density or serum testosterone levels. However, because these studies were undertaken some time after the accident, it is not clear whether the lack of an apparent effect reflects recovery.

Interestingly, large surveys of the affected farmers and their customers have shown no relationship between serum PBB levels and the number of subjective symptoms reported (162). Stross (163) has concluded, "Present evidence suggests that people exposed to PBB have few objective findings at this time, and reactive depression may be responsible for the high prevalence of constitutional symptoms."

POLYCHLORINATED BIPHENYLS   Polychlorinated biphenyls (PCBs) have been broadly used in carbonless carbon paper, paints, and as fluids in capacitors and transformers. Because of their extensive use and their capacity to be stored in fat, PCBs are widely found in fish, birds, and animals, including humans. An accidental contamination of rice oil with PCBs and other impurities in 1968 was responsible for a variety of primarily skin ailments in Japanese men and women and their offspring. Its persistence in breast milk has been the focus of many studies, but the male reproductive effects of PCBs are virtually unexamined.

An extensive study of the health of 326 PCB-exposed US capacitor-manufacturing workers included the measurement of sex hormones and explored reproductive histories using a family history questionnaire (164). No abnormal values were reported; in fact, Fischbein et al (164) were surprised by the "striking paucity" of physical abnormalities other than frequent skin problems. However, semen analyses of the 168 males in the study were not performed, so definite conclusions about the reproductive effects of PCBs cannot be drawn.

Male-Mediated Reproductive Effects

The results of studies of men occupationally exposed to anesthetic gases and hydrocarbons have prompted many questions regarding the effect of such exposure on conception and the morphology and physiological functioning of offspring. Soyka et al (165) have reviewed this area, and the research of others points out the difficulty of determining effects. Following a comprehensive study of the pregnancy experiences of the wives of 764 workers in a Swedish copper smelter, Beckman & Nordstrom (166) reported no difference in the number of congenital malformations in offspring but noted a significantly increased rate of fetal death. They believe their results are consistent with the hypothesis that chemical exposure of males resulting in genetic damage will be reflected in an increased rate of fetal loss as the result of dominant lethal mutations.

Hemminki et al (167) recently analyzed spontaneous abortions in an industrialized Finnish community according to the occupation and workplace of both the woman and her husband. The abortion incidence among wives employed in a single factory whose husbands worked at a large metallurgical factory was more than three times higher than among women whose husbands worked elsewhere.

Some scientists have suggested that a seminal defect in the husband may be a cause of abortion (168). However, in a retrospective study of 534 pregnancies, Homonnai et al (169) found that the sperm quality of the men whose wives were repeated or habitual aborters was better than in the control group and found no evidence in routine semen analysis that sperm quality was predictive of abortions. These investigators conclude that the cause of the abortions seems to be either a female factor or chromosomal aberration. Kline and coworkers (170) have commented on the power of environmental monitoring of spontaneous abortions and have suggested an important role for such studies in defining reproductive hazards to both men and women.

Fabro (171) has recently summarized paternally induced adverse effects on pregnancy and has discussed the potential mechanisms of these effects.

PRIORITIES FOR THE FUTURE

Too little effort has been directed toward using semen as an indicator of chemical exposure and toward using sperm as a biological indicator of chemical effects. In addition, as a route of exposure, chemicals in semen might have significant effects on sperm motility and function or might act directly or indirectly on the uterus and accessory sex organs to affect fertilization or implantation. Mann (172) has reviewed the literature on the appearance of chemicals in semen, but greatly increased efforts should be undertaken to assess their presence and to document altered biological indicators such as sperm parameters or semen biochemical markers.

The structures and the biological activities of chemicals with either confirmed or suspected adverse effects on male reproduction range broadly, making it difficult to establish priorities for future human studies. Nonetheless, a few warning flags are too obvious to ignore. They indicate that future research should focus on: (a) chemicals that are reactive and capable of covalent interactions in biological systems; these chemicals often are cytotoxic and affect spermatogenesis as well; (b) chemicals defined as mutagens and/or carcinogens in short-term laboratory tests; (c) chemicals demonstrated to cause aneuploidy or other chromosomal aberrations; (d) chemicals that affect sperm motility in vitro or are positive in other short-term reproductive screening tests; (e) chemicals that share hormonal activity or affect hormone action; and (f) chemicals that act directly or indirectly to affect the hypothalamo-pituitary-gonadal axis.

CONCLUSION

Relatively unreliable laboratory tests, clinical endpoints, monitors of exposure, indicators of biological effects, and epidemiological studies each have contributed to the difficulties researchers are experiencing in their attempts to define the role of occupational and environmental chemicals in the etiology of male reproductive dysfunction. An increased effort should be undertaken to develop coordinated research to improve our ability to identify reproductive hazards in the laboratory, to detect reproductive dysfunction in exposed populations, to establish causal relationships, and to assess human risk. The current state of the scientific literature in this area documents the need for such a comprehensive effort.

ACKNOWLEDGEMENT

The authors gratefully acknowledge the patience and help Ms. Vickie Whitaker and Mrs. Myra Stewart provided during numerous revisions of this manuscript.

Literature Cited

1. Dougherty, R. C., Whitaker, M. J., Tang, S. Y., Bottcher, R., Keller, M., et al. 1981. Sperm density and toxic substances—A potential key to environmental health hazards. In *Environmental Health Chemistry*, ed. J. D. McKinney, pp. 263–78. Ann Arbor, MI: Ann Arbor Sci.

2. Mosher, W. D. 1980. Reproductive impairments among currently married couples: United States 1976. *Advancedata* 55:1–11

3. Donayre, J., Guerra-Garcia, R., Moncloa, F., Sobrevilla, L. A. 1968. Endocrine studies at high altitude. IV. Changes in the semen of men. *J. Reprod. Fertil.* 16:55–58

4. WHO. 1981. *Health Effects of Combined Exposures in the Work Environment.* Geneva: WHO Techn. Rep. Ser. 662

5. Waxweiler, R. J. 1981. Epidemiologic problems associated with exposure to several agents. *Environ. Health Persp.* 42:51–56

6. Evans, H. J., Fletcher, J., Torrance, M., Hargreave, T. B. 1981. Sperm abnormalities and cigarette smoking. *Lancet* 1:627–29

7. Macleod, J., Wang, Y. 1979. Male fertility potential in terms of semen quality: A review of the past, a study of the present. *Fertil. Steril.* 31:103–16

8. Eliasson, R. 1983. Morphological and chemical methods of semen analysis for quantitating damage to male reproductive function in man. See Ref. 17, pp. 263–75

9. James, W. H. 1982. Possible consequences of the hypothesized decline in sperm counts. In *Human Fertility Factors (with Emphasis on the Male),* ed. A. Spira, P. Jouannet, pp. 183–200. Paris: INSERM

10. Templeton, A., Aitken, J., Mortimer, D., Best, F. 1982. Sperm function in patients with unexplained infertility. *Br. J. Obstet. Gynaecol.* 89:550–54

11. Wyrobek, A. J. 1983. Methods for evaluating the effects of environmental chemicals on human sperm production. *Environ. Health Persp.* 48:53–59

12. Wyrobek, A. J., Gordon, L. A., Watchmaker, G., Moore, D. H. II. 1982. Human sperm morphology testing: Description of a reliable method and its statistical power. In *Indicators of Genotoxic Exposure,* ed. B. A. Bridges, B. E. Butterworth, I. B. Weinstein, Banbury Rep. 13, pp. 527–41. Cold Spring Harbor, NY: Cold Spring Harbor Biol. Lab.

13. Kapp, R. W. Jr., Picciano, D. J., Jacobson, C. B. 1979. Y-Chromosomal nondisjunction in dibromochloropropane-exposed workmen. *Mutat. Res.* 64:47–51

14. Hall, J. L. 1981. Relationship between semen quality and human sperm penetration of zona-free hamster ova. *Fertil. Steril.* 35:457–63

15. Stenchever, M. A., Williamson, R. A., Leonard, J., Karp, L. E., Ley, B., et al. 1981. Possible relationship between in utero diethylstilbestrol exposure and male fertility. *Am. J. Obstet. Gynecol.* 140:186–93

16. Vernon, R. B., Muller, C. H., Herr, J. C., Feuchter, F. A., Eddy, E. M. 1982. Epididymal secretion of a mouse sperm surface component recognized by a monoclonal antibody. *Biol. Reprod.* 26: 523–27

17. Vouk, V. B., Sheehan, P. J., eds. 1983. *Methods for Assessing the Effects of Chemicals on Reproductive Functions.* New York: Wiley. 541 pp.

18. Bloom, A. D., ed. 1981. *Guidelines for*

Studies of Human Populations Exposed to Mutagenic and Reproductive Hazards. White Plains, NY: March of Dimes Birth Defects Found. 163 pp.

19. Levine, R. J., Symons, M. J., Balogh, S. A., Arndt, D. M., Kaswandik, N. T., et al. 1980. A method for monitoring the fertility of workers: I. Method and pilot studies. *J. Occup. Med.* 22:781–91

20. Hemminki, K., Axelson, O., Niemi, M-L. 1983. Assessment of methods and results of reproductive occupational epidemiology: Spontaneous abortions and malformations in the offspring of working women. *Am. J. Ind. Med.* 4:293–307

21. Wilcox, A. J. 1983. Surveillance of pregnancy loss in human populations. *Am. J. Ind. Med.* 4:285–88

22. McDonald, J. C., Harrington, J. M. 1981. Early detection of occupational hazards. *J. Soc. Occup. Med.* 31:93–98

23. Sever, L. E. 1981. Reproductive hazards of the workplace. *J. Occup. Med.* 23:685–89

24. Whorton, M. D. 1983. Accurate occupational illness and injury data in the US: Can this enigmatic problem ever be solved? *Am. J. Publ. Health* 73:1031–32

25. Rutstein, D. D., Mullan, R. J., Frazier, T. M., Halperin, W. E., Melius, J. M., et al. 1983. Sentinel health events (occupational): A basis for physician recognition and public health surveillance. *Am. J. Publ. Health* 73:1054–61

26. Infante, P. F., Tsongas, T. A. 1983. Occupational reproductive hazards: Necessary steps to prevention. *Am. J. Ind. Med.* 4:383–90

27. Whorton, M. D. 1983. Adverse reproductive outcomes: The occupational health issue of the 1980s. *Am. J. Publ. Health* 73:15–16

28. Cordes, D. H. 1980. *Reproductive Hazards in the Workplace.* Tucson, AZ: Ctr. Occup. Safety Health. 19 pp.

29. Spira, A., Jouannet, P., eds. 1982. *Human Fertility Factors (with Emphasis on the Male).* Paris: INSERM

30. Barlow, S. M., Sullivan, F. M. 1982. *Reproductive Hazards of Industrial Chemicals.* New York: Academic. 610 pp.

31. Nisbet, I. C. T., Karch, N. J. 1983. *Chemical Hazards to Human Reproduction.* Park Ridge, NJ: Noyes Data. 245 pp.

32. Stellman, J. M. 1979. The effects of toxic agents on reproduction. *Occup. Health Safety* April:36–43

33. Wyrobek, A. J., Gordon, L. A., Burkhart, J. G., Francis, M. W., Kapp, R. W. Jr., et al. 1983. An evaluation of human sperm as indicators of chemically induced alterations of spermatogenic function. A report of the U.S. Environmental Protection Agency Gene-Tox Program. *Mutat. Res.* 115:73–148

34. Lancranjan, I., Popescu, H. I., Klepsch, I. 1969. Changes of the gonadic function in chronic carbon disulfide poisoning. *Med. Lav.* 60:566–71

35. Lancranjan, I. 1972. Alterations of spermatic liquid in patients chronically poisoned by carbon disulphide. *Med. Lav.* 63:29–33

36. Cirla, A. M., Bertazzi, P. A., Tomasini, M., Villa, A., Graziano, C., et al. 1978. Study of endocrinological functions and sexual behavior in carbon disulphide workers. *Med. Lav.* 69:118–29

37. Wagar, G., Tolonen, M., Stenman, U.-H., Helpio, E. 1981. Endocrinologic studies in men exposed occupationally to carbon disulfide. *J. Toxicol. Environ. Health* 7:363–71

38. Meyer, C. R. 1981. Semen quality in workers exposed to carbon disulfide compared to a control group from the same plant. *J. Occup. Med.* 23:435–39

39. Public Health Service. 1983. *Third Annual Report on Carcinogens.* Springfield, VA: Natl. Techn. Inf. Serv. 229 pp.

40. Whorton, D., Krauss, R. M., Marshall, S., Milby, T. H. 1977. Infertility in male pesticide workers. *Lancet* 2:1259–61

41. Biava, C. G., Smuckler, E. A., Whorton, D. 1978. The testicular morphology of individuals exposed to dibromochloropropane. *Exp. Mol. Pathol.* 29:448–58

42. Marquez Mayaudon, E. 1978. 1,2 Dibromo-3-chlor-propane (DBCP) nematocide with sterilizing action on man. *Salud Publica Mex.* 20:195–200

43. Potashnik, G., Ben-Aderet, N., Israeli, R., Yanai-Inbar, I., Sober, I. 1978. Suppressive effect of 1,2-dibromo-3-chloropropane on human spermatogenesis. *Fertil. Steril.* 30:444–47

44. Potashnik, G., Yanai-Inbar, I., Sacks, M. I., Israeli, R. 1979. Effect of dibromochloropropane on human testicular function. *Isr. J. Med. Sci.* 15:438–42

45. Whorton, D., Milby, T. H., Krauss, R. M., Stubbs, H. A. 1979. Testicular function in DBCP exposed pesticide workers. *J. Occup. Med.* 21:161–66

46. Sandifer, S. H., Wilkins, R. T., Loadholt, C. B., Lane, L. G., Eldridge, J. C. 1979. Spermatogenesis in agricultural workers exposed to dibromochloropropane (DBCP). *Bull. Environ. Contam. Toxicol.* 23:703–10

47. Egnatz, D. G., Ott, M. G., Townsend, J. C., Olson, R. D., Johns, D. B. 1980.

DBCP and testicular effects in chemical workers: An epidemiological survey in Midland, Michigan. *J. Occup. Med.* 22:727–32

48. Levine, R. J., Blunden, P. B., DalCorso, R. D., Starr, T. B., Ross, C. E. 1983. Superiority of reproductive histories to sperm counts in detecting infertility at a dibromochloropropane manufacturing plant. *J. Occup. Med.* 25:591–97

49. Glass, R. I., Lynness, R. N., Mengle, D. C., Powell, K. E., Kahn, E. 1979. Sperm count depression in pesticide applicators exposed to dibromochloropropane. *Am. J. Epidemiol.* 109:346–51

50. Kahn, E., Whorton, D. 1980. Re: "Sperm count depression in pesticide applicators exposed to dibromochloropropane." *Am. J. Epidemiol.* 112:161–65

51. Glass, R. I. 1980. Sperm count depression in pesticide applicators exposed to dibromochloropropane—The first author replies. *Am. J. Epidemiol.* 112:164

52. Ramirez, A. L., Ramirez, C. M. 1980. Esterilidad masculina causada por la exposicion laboral al nematicida 1, 2-dibromo-3-cloropropano. *Acta Med. Cost.* 23:219–22

53. Lantz, G. D., Cunningham, G. R., Huckins, C., Lipshultz, L. I. 1981. Recovery from severe oligospermia after exposure to dibromochloropropane. *Fertil. Steril.* 35:46–53

54. Potashnik, G. 1983. A four-year reassessment of workers with dibromochloropropane-induced testicular dysfunction. *Andrologia* 15:164–70

55. Wheater, R. H. 1978. Short-term exposures to pesticide (DBCP) and male sterility. *J. Am. Med. Assoc.* 239:2795

56. Whorton, M. D., Milby, T. H. 1980. Recovery of testicular function among DBCP workers. *J. Occup. Med.* 22:177–79

57. Lipshultz, L. I., Ross, C. E., Whorton, D., Milby, T., Smith, R., Joyner, R. E. 1980. Dibromochloropropane and its effect on testicular function in man. *J. Urol.* 124:464–68

58. Kharrazi, M., Potashnik, G., Goldsmith, J. R. 1980. Reproductive effects of dibromochloropropane. *Isr. J. Med. Sci.* 16:403–6

58a. Whorton, M. D., Foliart, D. E. 1983. Mutagenicity, carcinogenicity and reproductive effects of dibromochloropropane (DBCP). *Mutat. Res.* 123:13–30

59. Landrigan, P. J., Tamblyn, P. B., Nelson, M., Kerndt, P., Kronovetter, K. J., et al. 1980. Lead exposure in stained glass workers. *Am. J. Ind. Health* 1:177–80

60. Robinson, T. R. 1976. The health of long service tetraethyl lead workers. *J. Occup. Med.* 18:31–40

61. Gilfillan, S. C. 1965. Lead poisoning and the fall of Rome. *J. Occup. Med.* 7:53–60

62. Thomas, J. A., Brogan, W. C. III. 1983. Some actions of lead on the sperm and on the male reproductive system. *Am. J. Ind. Med.* 4:127–34

63. Rom, W. N. 1980. Effects of lead on reproduction. See Ref. 110, pp. 33–42

63a. Lancranjan, I., Popescu, H. I., Gavanescu, O., Klepsch, I., Serbanescu, M. 1975. Reproductive ability of workmen occupationally exposed to lead. *Arch. Environ. Health* 30:396–401

64. DeKnudt, G., Leonard, A., Ivanov, B. 1973. Chromosome aberrations observed in male workers occupationally exposed to lead. *Environ. Physiol. Biochem.* 3:132–38

65. Forni, A., Cambiaghi, G., Secchi, G. C. 1976. Initial occupational exposure to lead. *Arch. Environ. Health* 31:73–78

66. Sarto, F., Stella, M., Acqua, A. 1978. Cytogenetic studies in 20 workers occupationally exposed to lead. *Med. Lav.* 69:172–80

67. Nordenson, I., Beckman, G., Beckman, L., Nordstrom, S. 1978. Occupational and environmental risks in and around a smelter in northern Sweden. IV. Chromosomal aberrations in workers exposed to lead. *Hereditas* 88:263–67

68. O'Riordan, M. L., Evans, H. J. 1974. Absence of significant chromosome damage in males occupationally exposed to lead. *Nature* 247:50–53

69. Schmid, E., Bauchinger, M., Pietruck, S., Hall, G. 1972. Die cytogenetische Wirkung von Blei in menschlichen peripheren Lymphocyten in vitro und in vivo. *Mutat. Res.* 16:401–6

70. Harrington, J. M., Stein, G. F., Rivera, R. O., deMorales, A. V. 1978. The occupational hazards of formulating oral contraceptives—A survey of plant employees. *Arch. Environ. Health* 33:12–15

71. Harrington, J. M., Rivera, R. O., Lowry, L. K. 1978. Occupational exposure to synthetic estrogens—The need to establish safety standards. *Am. Ind. Hyg. Assoc. J.* 39:139–43

71a. Harrington, J. M. 1982. Occupational exposure to synthetic estrogens: Some methodological problems. *Scand. J. Work Environ. Health.* 8:167–71

72. Poller, L., Thomson, J. M., Otridge, B. W., Yee, K. F., Logan, S. H. M. 1979. Effects of manufacturing oral contracep-

tives on blood clotting. *Br. Med. J.* 1:1761–62

73. Burton, D. J., Shmunes, E. 1973. *Health Hazard Evaluation Report 71-9.* Cincinnati, OH: Haz. Eval. Serv. Br., Natl. Inst. Occup. Safety Health

74. Landrigan, P. J., Melius, J. M., Rosenberg, M. J., Coye, M. J., Binkin, N. J. 1983. Reproductive hazards in the workplace: Development of epidemiologic research. *Scand. J. Work Environ. Health* 9:83–88

75. Edling, C. 1980. Anesthetic gases as an occupational hazard. A review. *Scand. J. Work Environ. Health* 6:85–93

76. Askrog, V., Harvald, B. 1970. Teratogen effekt af inhalationsanestetika. *Nord. Med.* 83:498–500

77. Cohen, E. N., Belville, J. W., Brown, B. W. 1971. Anesthesia, pregnancy, and miscarriage: A study of operating room nurses and anesthetists. *Anesthesiology* 35:345–47

78. Corbett, T. H., Cornell, R. G., Lieding, K., Endres, J. L. 1973. Incidence of cancer among Michigan nurse-anesthetists. *Anesthesiology* 38:260–63

79. Corbett, T. H., Cornell, R. G., Endres, J. L., Lieding, K. 1974. Birth defects among children of nurse-anesthetists. *Anesthesiology* 41:341–44

80. Knill-Jones, R. P., Rodrigues, L. V., Moir, D. D., Spence, A. A. 1972. Anaesthetic practice and pregnancy: Controlled survey of women anaesthetists in the United Kingdom. *Lancet* 1:1326–28

81. Tomlin, P. J. 1979. Health problems of anaesthetists and their families in the West Midlands. *Br. Med. J.* 1:779–84

82. Cohen, E. N., Brown, B. W. Jr., Cascorbi, H. F., Corbett, T. H., Jones, T. W., et al. 1975. A survey of anesthetic health hazards among dentists. *J. Am. Dent. Assoc.* 90:1291–96

83. American Society of Anesthesiologists, Ad Hoc Committee. 1974. Occupational disease among operating room personnel: A national study. *Anesthesiology* 41: 321–40

84. Tomlin, P. J. 1978. Teratogenic effects of waste anaesthetic gases. *Br. Med. J.* 108:1046

85. Deleted in proof

86. Knill-Jones, R. P., Newman, B. J., Spence, A. A. 1975. Anaesthetic practice and pregnancy: Controlled survey of male anaesthetists in the United Kingdom. *Lancet* 2:807–9

87. Spence, A. A., Cohen, E. N., Brown, B. W. Jr., Knill-Jones, R. P., Himmelberger, D. U. 1977. Occupational hazards for operating room-based physicians: Analysis of data from the United States and the United Kingdom. *J. Am. Med. Assoc.* 238:955–59

88. Cohen, E. N. 1980. Waste anesthetic gases and reproductive health in operating room personnel. See Ref. 110, pp. 69–75

89. Mirakhur, R. K., Badve, A. V. 1975. Pregnancy and anaesthetic practice in India. *Anaesthesia* 30:18–22

90. Wyrobek, A. J., Brodsky, J., Gordon, L., Moore, D. H. II, Watchmaker, G., et al. 1981. Sperm studies in anesthesiologists. *Anesthesiology* 55:527–32

91. Manley, S. V., McDonell, W. N. 1980. Anesthetic pollution and disease. *J. Am. Vet. Med. Assoc.* 176:515–18

91a. Beckman, G., Beckman, L., Nordenson, I. 1977. Chromosome aberrations in workers exposed to arsenic. *Environ. Health Perspect.* 19:145–46

91b. Nordenson, I., Beckman, G., Beckman, L., Nordstrom, S. 1978. Occupational and environmental risks in and around a smelter in northern Sweden: II. Chromosomal aberrations in workers exposed to arsenic. *Hereditas* 88:47–50

92. Forni, A. 1978. Chromosome changes and benzene exposure. A review. *Rev. Environ. Health* 3:5–17

93. Brief, R. S., Lynch, J., Bernath, T., Scala, R. A. 1980. Benzene in the workplace. *Am. Ind. Hyg. Assoc. J.* 41:616–23

94. Krasovskii, G. N., Varshavskaya, S. P., Borisov, A. I. 1976. Toxic and gonadotropic effects of cadmium and boron relative to standards for these substances in drinking water. *Environ. Health Perspect.* 13:69–75

95. Lee, I. P., Sherins, R. J., Dixon, R. L. 1978. Evidence for induction of germinal aplasia in male rats by environmental exposure to boron. *Toxicol. Appl. Pharmacol.* 45:577–90

96. Pruett, J. G., Winslow, S. G. 1982. *Health Effects of Environmental Chemicals on the Adult Human Reproductive System.* Bethesda, MD: FASEB, Spec. Publ. 62 pp.

97. Owen, W. L. 1976. Cancer of the prostate: A literature review. *J. Chron. Dis.* 29:89–114

98. Smith, J. P., Smith, J. C., McCall, A. J. 1960. Chronic poisoning from cadmium fumes. *J. Pathol. Bacteriol.* 80:287–96

99. Favino, A., Candura, F., Chiappino, G., Cavalleri, A. 1968. Study on the androgen function of men exposed to cadmium. *Med. Lav.* 59:105–10

100. O'Riordan, M. L., Hughes, E. G., Evans, H. J. 1978. Chromosome studies on blood lymphocytes of men occupationally exposed to cadmium. *Mutat. Res.* 58:305–11
101. Whorton, M. D., Milby, T. H., Stubbs, H. A., Avashia, B. H., Hull, E. Q. 1979. Testicular function among carbaryl-exposed employees. *J. Toxicol. Environ. Health* 5:929–41
102. Wyrobek, A. J., Watchmaker, L., Gordon, L., Wong, K., Moore, D. II., et al. 1981. Sperm shape abnormalities in carbaryl-exposed employees. *Environ. Health Perspect.* 40:255–65
103. Deleted in proof
104. Cannon, S. B., Veazey, J. M. Jr., Jackson, R. S., Burse, V. W., Hayes, C., et al. 1978. Epidemic Kepone poisoning in chemical workers. *Am. J. Epidemiol.* 107:529–37
105. Cohn, W. J., Boylan, J. J., Blanke, R. V., Fariss, M. W., Howell, J. R., et al. 1978. Treatment of chlordecone (Kepone) toxicity with cholestyramine. *N. Engl. J. Med.* 298:243–48
106. Taylor, J. R., Selhorst, J. B., Houff, S. A., Martinez, A. J. 1978. Chlordecone intoxication in man: 1. Clinical observations. *Neurology* 28:626–30
107. Infante, P. F. 1980. Chloroprene: Adverse effects on reproduction. See Ref. 110, pp. 87–101
108. Infante, P. F., Wagoner, J. K., Young, R. J. 1977. Chloroprene: Observations of carcinogenesis and mutagenesis. In *Origins of Human Cancer, Book A: Incidences of Cancer in Humans,* ed. H. H. Hiatt, J. D. Watson, J. A. Winsten, 4:205–17. Cold Spring Harbor, NY: Cold Spring Harbor Biol. Lab. 1899 pp.
109. Sanotskii, I. V. 1976. Aspects of the toxicology of chloroprene: immediate and longterm effects. *Environ. Health Perspect.* 17:85–93
110. Infante, P. F., Legator, M. S., eds. 1980. *Proceedings of a Workshop on Methodology for Assessing Reproductive Hazards in the Workplace.* Washington, DC: US GPO
111. Fomenko, V. N., et al. 1974. The possibility of extrapolating animal data to man when studying the mutagenic and gonadotropic effect of chemical factors. *Vses. Nauchnaya Konf. Lab. Zzivotnie Med. Issled.,* Moscow pp. 44–46 (in Russian)
112. Ahrenholz, S. H., Meyer, C. R. 1980. *NIOSH Health Hazard Evaluation Rep. HE-79-113-728: Toulene Diamine.* Brandenburg, KY: Olin Chem. Co.
113. Cooper, C., ed. 1980. Reproductive hazards to workers at issue in Kentucky plant. *Pest. Tox. Chem. News.* 8:3–4
114. Hamill, P. V. V., Steinberger, E., Levine, R. J., Rodriguez-Rigau, L. J., Lemeshow, S., et al. 1982. The epidemiologic assessment of male reproductive hazard from occupational exposure to TDA and DNT. *J. Occup. Med.* 24:985–93
115. Wong, O., Utidjian, H. M. D., Karten, V. S. 1979. Retrospective evaluation of reproductive performance of workers exposed to ethylene dibromide (EDB). *J. Occup. Med.* 21:98–102
116. Griffiths, J., Heath, R., Davido, R. 1978. Spermatogenesis in agricultural workers potentially exposed to ethylene dibromide. *Interim Report. Health Effects Monitoring Branch, EPA* Research Triangle Park, NC: EPA. 25 pp.
117. Ter Haar, G. 1980. An investigation of possible sterility and health effects from exposure to ethylene dibromide. In *Ethylene Dichloride: A Potential Health Risk,* ed. B. Ames, P. Infante, R. Reitz, Banbury Rep. 5, pp. 167–88. Cold Spring Harbor, NY: Cold Spring Harbor Biol. Lab.
117a. Schuler, P., Oyanguren, H., Maturana, V., Valenzuela, A., Cruz, E., et al. 1957. Manganese poisoning: Environmental and medical study at a Chilean mine. *Ind. Med. Surg.* 26:167–73
118. Verschaeve, L., Susanne, C. 1979. Genetic hazards of mercury exposure in dental surgery. *Mutat. Res.* 64:149
119. Popescu, H. I. 1978. Poisoning with alkylmercury compounds. *Br. Med. J.* 1:1347
120. McFarland, R. B., Reigel, H. 1978. Chronic mercury poisoning from a single brief exposure. *J. Occup. Med.* 20:532–34
121. Szymczynski, G. A., Waliszewski, S. M. 1981. Content of chlorinated pesticides in human semen of a random population. *Intl. J. Androl.* 4:669–74
122. Szymczynski, G. A., Waliszewski, S. M. 1981. Comparison of the content of chlorinated pesticide residues in human semen, testicles and fat tissue. *Andrologia* 13:250–52
123. Shabtai, F., Bichacho, S., Halbrecht, I. 1978. Cytogenetic observations in infertile men working with insecticidal compounds. *Acta Genet. Med. Gemellol.* 27:51–56
124. Espir, M. L. E., Hall, J. W., Shirreffs, J. G., Stevens, D. L. 1970. Impotence in farm workers using toxic chemicals. *Br. Med. J.* 1:423–25
125. Roan, C. C., Matanoski, G. E., McIl-

nay, C. Q., Olds, K. L., Pylant, F., et al. 1984. Spontaneous abortions, stillbirths, and birth defects in families of agricultural pilots. *Arch. Environ. Health* 39:56–60

126. Mann, T., Lutwak-Mann, C. 1981. *Male Reproductive Function and Semen.* New York: Springer-Verlag. 495 pp.

127. Schmid, E., Bauchinger, M., Dresp, J. 1982. Chromosome analyses of workers from a pentachlorophenol plant. In *Mutagens in Our Environment,* ed. M. Sorsa, H. Vainio, pp. 471–77. New York: Liss

128. Rowley, M. J., Leach, D. R., Warner, G. A., Heller, C. G. 1974. Effect of graded doses of ionizing radiation on the human testis. *Radiat. Res.* 59:665–78

129. Lushbaugh, C. C., Casarett, G. W. 1976. The effects of gonadal irradiation in clinical radiation therapy: A review. *Cancer* 37:1111–20

130. Ash, P. 1980. The influence of radiation on fertility in man. *Br. J. Radiol.* 53:271–78

131. Popescu, H. I., Klepsch, I., Lancranjan, I. 1975. Eliminations of pituitary gonadotropic hormones in men with protracted irradiation during occupational exposure. *Health Phys.* 29:385–88

132. Popescu, H. I., Lancranjan, I. 1975. Spermatogenesis alteration during protracted irradiation in man. *Health Phys.* 28:567–73

133. Annamalai, M., Iyer, P. S., Panicker, T. M. R. 1978. Radiation injury from acute exposure to an Iridium-192 source: Case history. *Health Phys.* 35:387–89

134. MacLeod, J. 1974. Effects of environmental factors and of antispermatogenic compounds on the human testis as reflected in seminal cytology. In *Male Fertility and Sterility,* ed. R. E. Mancini, L. Martini, 5:123–48. New York: Academic

135. MacLeod, J., Hotchkiss, R. S., Sitterson, B. W. 1964. Recovery of male fertility after sterilization by nuclear radiation. *J. Am. Med. Assoc.* 187:637–41

136. Lancranjan, I., Maicanescu, M., Rafaila, E., Klepsch, I., Popescu, H. I. 1975. Gonadic function in workmen with long term exposure to microwaves. *Health Phys.* 29:381–83

137. Fabia, J., Thuy, T. D. 1974. Occupation of father at time of birth of children dying of malignant diseases. *Br. J. Prev. Soc. Med.* 28:98–100

138. Cook, R. R., Bodner, K. M., Kolesar, R. C., Uhlmann, C. S., VanPeenen, P. F., et al. 1982. A cross-sectional study of ethylene glycol monomethyl ether process employees. *Arch. Environ. Health* 37:346–51

139. Hardin, B. D. 1983. Reproductive toxicity of the glycol ethers. *Toxicology* 27:91–102

140. Reggiani, G. 1979. Estimation of the TCDD toxic potential in the light of the Seveso accident. *Arch. Toxicol. Suppl.* 2:291–302

141. Homberger, E., Reggiani, G., Sambeth, J., Wipf, H. K. 1979. The Seveso accident: Its nature, extent and consequences. *Ann. Occup. Hyg.* 22:327–67

142. Townsend, J. C., Bodner, K. M., VanPeenen, P. F. D., Olson, R. D., Cook, R. R. 1982. Survey of reproductive events of wives of employees exposed to chlorinated dioxins. *Am. J. Epidemiol.* 115:695–713

143. Suskind, R. R., Hertzberg, V. S. 1984. Human health effects of 2,4,5-T and its toxic contaminants. *J. Am. Med. Assoc.* 251:2372–80

144. Fabro, S., ed. 1984. Agent orange and dioxin. *Reprod. Tox.* 3:5–7

145. Purchase, I. F. H., Richardson, C. R., Anderson, D. 1975. Chromosomal and dominant lethal effects of vinyl chloride. *Lancet* 2:410–11

146. Heath, C. W. Jr., Dumont, C. R., Gamble, J., Waxweiler, R. J. 1977. Chromosomal damage in men occupationally exposed to vinyl chloride monomer and other chemicals. *Environ. Res.* 14:68–72

147. Purchase, I. F. H., Richardson, C. R., Anderson, D., Paddle, G. M., Adams, W. G. F. 1978. Chromosomal analyses in vinyl chloride-exposed workers. *Mutat. Res.* 57:325–34

148. Anderson, D., Richardson, C. R., Weight, T. M., Purchase, I. F. H., Adams, W. G. F. 1980. Chromosomal analyses in vinyl chloride exposed workers. Results from analysis 18 and 42 months after an initial sampling. *Mutat. Res.* 79:151–62

149. Hansteen, I.-L., Hillestad, L., Thiis-Evensen, E., Heldaas, S. S. 1978. Effects of vinyl chloride in man: A cytogenetic follow-up study. *Mutat. Res.* 51:271–78

150. Rossner, P., Sram, R. J., Novakova, J., Lambl, V. 1980. Cytogenetic analysis in workers occupationally exposed to vinyl chloride. *Mutat. Res.* 73:425–27

151. Anderson, D., Richardson, C. R., Purchase, I. F., Evans, H. J., O'Riordan, M. L. 1981. Chromosomal analysis in vinyl chloride exposed workers: Comparison of the standard technique with the sister-chromatid exchange technique. *Mutat. Res.* 83:137–44

152. Kucerova, M., Polivkova, Z., Batora, J. 1979. Comparative evaluation of the frequency of chromosomal aberrations and the SCE numbers in peripheral lymphocytes of workers occupationally exposed to vinyl chloride monomer. *Mutat. Res.* 67:97–100

153. Hatch, M., Kline, J., Stein, Z. 1981. Power considerations in studies of reproductive effects of vinyl chloride and some structural analogs. *Environ. Health Perspect.* 41:195–201

154. Infante, P. F., Wagoner, J. K., McMichael, A. J., Waxweiler, R. J., Falk, H. 1976. Genetic risks of vinyl chloride. *Lancet* 1:734–35

155. Infante, P. F., Wagoner, J. K., McMichael, A. J., Waxweiler, R. J., Falk, H. 1976. Genetic risks of vinyl chloride (letter). *Lancet* 1:1289–90

156. Infante, P. F., Wagoner, J. K., Waxweiler, R. J. 1976. Carcinogenic, mutagenic and teratogenic risks associated with vinyl chloride. *Mutat. Res.* 41:131–42

157. Waxweiler, R. J., Falk, H., McMichael, A., Mallov, J. S., Grivas, A. S., et al. 1977. *A Cross-Sectional Epidemiologic Survey of Vinyl Chloride Workers.* Cincinnati, OH: Natl. Inst. Occup. Safety and Health

158. Milby, T. H., Whorton, M. D., Stubbs, H. A., Ross, C. E., Joyner, R. E., et al. 1981. Testicular function among epichlorohydrin workers. *Br. J. Ind. Med.* 38:372–77

159. Venable, J. R., McClimans, C. D., Flake, R. E., Dimick, D. B. 1980. A fertility study of male employees engaged in the manufacture of glycerine. *J. Occup. Med.* 22:87–91

160. Whorton, M. D., Stubbs, H. A., Obrinsky, A., Milby, T. H. 1981. Testicular function of men occupationally exposed to para-tertiary butyl benzoic acid. *Scan. J. Work Environ. Health* 7:204–13

161. Rosenman, K. D., Anderson, H. A., Selikoff, I. J., Wolff, M. S., Holstein, E. 1979. Spermatogenesis in men exposed to polybrominated biphenyl (PBB). *Fertil. Steril.* 32:209–13

162. Landrigan, P. J., Wilcox, K. R. Jr., Silva, J. Jr., Humphrey, H. E. B., Kauffman, C., et al. 1979. Cohort study of Michigan residents exposed to polybrominated biphenyls: Epidemiologic and immunologic findings. *Ann. NY Acad. Sci.* 320:284–94

163. Stross, J. K., Smokler, I. A., Isbister, J., Wilcox, K. R. 1981. The human health effects of exposure to polybrominated biphenyls. *Toxicol. Appl. Pharmacol.* 58:145–50

164. Fischbein, A., Wolff, M. S., Lilis, R., Thornton, J., Selikoff, I. J. 1979. Clinical findings among PCB-exposed capacitor manufacturing workers. *Ann. NY Acad. Sci.* 320:703–15

165. Soyka, L.F., Joffe, J. M. 1980. Male mediated drug effects on offspring. In *Drug and Chemical Risks to the Fetus and Newborn,* ed. R. H. Schwarz, S. J. Yaffe, pp. 49–66. New York: Liss

166. Beckman, L., Nordstrom, S. 1982. Occupational and environmental risks in and around a smelter in northern Sweden. IX. Fetal mortality among wives of smelter workers. *Hereditas* 97:1–7

167. Hemminki, K., Kyyronen, P., Niemi, M.-L., Koskinen, K., Sallmen, M., et al. 1983. Spontaneous abortions in an industrialized community in Finland. *Am. J. Publ. Health* 73:32–37

168. Furuhjelm, M., Jonson, B., Lagergren, C.-G. 1962. The quality of human semen in spontaneous abortion. *Intl. J. Fertil.* 7:17–21

169. Homonnai, Z. T., Paz, G. F., Weiss, J. N., David, M. P. 1980. Relation between semen quality and fate of pregnancy: Retrospective study on 534 pregnancies. *Intl. J. Androl.* 3:574–84

170. Kline, J., Stein, Z., Susser, M., Warburton, D. 1980. Spontaneous abortion studies: Role in surveillance. See Ref. 110, pp. 279–89

171. Fabro, S., ed. 1984. Paternally-induced adverse pregnancy effects. *Reprod. Tox.* 3:13–16

172. Mann, T., Lutwak-Mann, C. 1982. Passage of chemicals into human and animal semen: Mechanisms and significance. *CRC Critical Rev. Toxicol.* 11:1–14

Ann. Rev. Pharmacol. Toxicol. 1985. 25:593–620

THE FUNCTION OF MYOSIN AND MYOSIN LIGHT CHAIN KINASE PHOSPHORYLATION IN SMOOTH MUSCLE

Kristine E. Kamm and James T. Stull

Department of Pharmacology and Moss Heart Center, University of Texas Health Science Center at Dallas, Dallas, Texas 75235

INTRODUCTION

An in-depth understanding of the regulation of contractile tone in smooth muscle takes its form from detailed biochemical descriptions of (*a*) specific effects unique to individual effector inputs at the membrane, (*b*) mechanisms of mediation of the effector signal (second messengers), and (*c*) modes and sites of action of second messengers both within the contractile protein regulatory system and within the membrane-associated homeostatic mechanisms. Most early physiological and pharmacological studies on smooth muscle preparations focused primarily on extracellular effectors and their interactions with the membrane components ultimately involved in the control of intracellular Ca^{2+} concentration. Evaluation of the steady-state contractile response has been interpreted as an index of sarcoplasmic Ca^{2+} concentration, with the underlying assumption that Ca^{2+} activates contractile proteins through a simple switch-like mechanism. The discoveries that the 20,000-dalton light chain of smooth muscle myosin could be phosphorylated [1], and that the phosphorylation of smooth muscle myosin is associated with an increase in its actin-activated Mg^{2+}-ATPase activity [2], have led to a number of biochemical investigations into the regulatory role of the specific phosphorylation of myosin by the Ca^{2+}- and calmodulin-dependent enzyme myosin light chain kinase. Recent investigations have focused on demonstrating the physiological role of myosin phosphorylation in the regulation of contractility in intact smooth muscle.

593

0362-1642/85/415-0593$02.00

This review describes our current understanding of the regulation and role of myosin phosphorylation in smooth muscle contraction and relaxation. It is not historically comprehensive, and we have relied upon reviews by other authors for the citation of certain developments and perspectives. For example, Krebs & Beavo (3) have presented important criteria for establishing that an enzyme undergoes physiologically significant phosphorylation and dephosphorylation. In the context of myosin P-light chain and myosin light chain kinase phosphorylation in smooth muscle, it is worthwhile to review these criteria:

1. Demonstration in vitro that the enzyme can be phosphorylated stoichiometrically at a significant rate in a reaction(s) catalyzed by an appropriate protein kinase(s) and dephosphorylated by a phosphoprotein phosphatase(s).
2. Demonstration that functional properties of the enzyme undergo meaningful changes that correlate with the degree of phosphorylation.
3. Demonstration that the enzyme can be phosphorylated and dephosphorylated in vivo or in an intact cell system with accompaning functional changes.
4. Correlation of cellular levels of protein kinase and/or phosphoprotein phosphatase effectors and the extent of phosphorylation of the enzyme.

THE BIOCHEMICAL PROPERTIES OF MYOSIN PHOSPHORYLATION

Smooth Muscle Contractile Proteins

All smooth muscle cells contain the contractile proteins actin, myosin, and tropomyosin (4–6). The enzyme myosin is the primary protein of the thick filament in smooth muscle and is composed of two high molecular–weight subunits, or heavy chains, and two each of two types of low molecular–weight subunits, or light chains. The molecular weight of each heavy chain subunit is about 200,000 daltons, whereas the light chain subunits are 20,000 and 17,000 daltons respectively. The native hexameric form of myosin is configured as an intertwined coiled-tail region embedded in the thick filament and two globular head regions that protrude from the thick filament at regular intervals to form cross bridges. These head regions contain the actin-binding domain, the catalytic site for ATP hydrolysis, and the associated light chain subunits. According to the sliding filament theory of muscle contraction, thick (myosin) and thin (actin and tropomyosin) filaments move past one another. This process is related to the binding of cross bridges to actin and to the hydrolysis of ATP. The sliding filament theory has been developed primarily from detailed investigations of skeletal muscle, but the general organization of thin and thick filaments in smooth muscle is consistent with a similar mechanism of contraction (7–10).

Regulation by Ca^{2+}

The dominant mechanism for Ca^{2+} activation of contractile elements in vertebrate skeletal and cardiac muscle is due to a thin-filament Ca^{2+}-regulatory system, troponin-tropomyosin. The regulation of actin-myosin interactions in smooth muscle by Ca^{2+} is more complex, and different biochemical mechanisms have been proposed. These mechanisms may be differentiated into two general classes involving thick- and thin-filament regulatory processes respectively. In thick-filament regulation, Ca^{2+} binds to calmodulin and the Ca^{2+}-calmodulin complex subsequently binds to and activates myosin light chain kinase (11). Activation of this protein kinase results in the phosphorylation of the 20,000–dalton light chain subunit of myosin, the P-light chain, and the stimulation of actin-activated Mg^{2+}-ATPase activity of smooth muscle myosin (4–6). There is also evidence that phosphorylated smooth muscle myosin Mg^{2+}-ATPase activity may be further increased by Ca^{2+}, which may be related to Ca^{2+} binding directly to myosin (12–16).

Ca^{2+} may also regulate actin-myosin interaction in smooth muscle via thin-filament components. Ebashi (17) has proposed that Ca^{2+} activation is mediated by a thin-filament protein complex referred to as leiotonin. Marston (18), on the other hand, has proposed two thin filament–linked regulatory mechanisms. Isolated thin filaments, which are capable of binding Ca^{2+}, activate myosin Mg^{2+}-ATPase activity in a Ca^{2+}-dependent manner. He also found that the phosphorylation of a 21,000-dalton protein component in thin filaments is associated with an increase in the quantity of high affinity Ca^{2+} binding sites on thin filaments and a decrease in the Ca^{2+} concentration required for half-maximal activation of actin-activated myosin Mg^{2+}-ATPase activity.

In summary, the preponderance of biochemical evidence indicates that there may be more than one mechanism for Ca^{2+} regulation of smooth muscle contraction. As will be discussed below, myosin phosphorylation certainly plays a prominent role; however, it may not be the only Ca^{2+}-dependent regulatory mechanism in smooth muscle contraction. Although it is not possible to differentiate the relative importance of these other biochemical mechanisms, physiological and pharmacological investigations indicate that, in addition to the calmodulin-myosin light chain kinase system, there is probably another Ca^{2+} regulatory mechanism acting in smooth muscle contraction.

Myosin Phosphorylation and ATPase Activity

The stoichiometric phosphorylation of a single serine residue of the P-light chain of myosin is preferentially catalyzed by myosin light chain kinase, which requires two protein components for activity (4–6). One component is the ubiquitous low molecular–weight Ca^{2+}-binding protein calmodulin. The other component is the catalytic subunit of myosin light chain kinase, which has molecular weights ranging from 130,000 to 155,000 in smooth muscle cells from different animal species (19–22). The inactive enzyme exists as a monomer and is activated by the binding of one mol of calmodulin per mol of myosin light chain kinase when Ca^{2+} binds to calmodulin. The general mechanism of myosin light chain kinase activation (23) is similar to the activation scheme proposed for other calmodulin-dependent enzyme systems (24, 25):

$$4\ Ca^{2+} + \text{calmodulin} \overset{K_{Ca^{2+}}}{\rightleftharpoons} Ca^{2+}_4 \cdot \text{calmodulin} \qquad 1.$$

$$Ca^{2+}_4 \cdot \text{calmodulin} + \text{kinase} \overset{K_{CM}}{\rightleftharpoons} Ca^{2+}_4 \cdot \text{calmodulin} \cdot \text{kinase} \qquad 2.$$

It is generally accepted that at least three, if not four, Ca^{2+}-binding sites on calmodulin are occupied for the activation of the various calmodulin-dependent enzymes (24, 25). The importance of pathways for the activation and inactivation of calmodulin-activated enzymes has been emphasized in biological systems (26–28). It has been proposed that activation associated with an increase in cytoplasmic Ca^{2+} concentrations is the result of Ca^{2+} binding first to calmodulin, with subsequent binding to and activation of a calmodulin-dependent enzyme. Inactivation due to a decrease in cytoplasmic Ca^{2+} concentrations follows a different pathway, however. The rate of inactivation is about three orders of magnitude faster when Ca^{2+} first dissociates from the $Ca^{2+}_4 \cdot$ calmodulin · enzyme complex. This scheme for the activation and inactivation of myosin light chain kinase in vivo is summarized in Figure 1.

Phosphorylation of smooth muscle P-light chain by the $Ca^{2+}_4 \cdot$ calmodulin · myosin light chain kinase complex is thought to allow the activation of myosin Mg^{2+}-ATPase activity by actin, whereas dephosphorylated myosin is not activated (4–6). The quantitative relationship between the extent of P-light chain phosphorylation and actin-activated Mg^{2+}-ATPase activity has been shown not to be linear in avian gizzard smooth muscle myosin. Phosphorylation of both heads of myosin is required for the activation of myosin Mg^{2+}-ATPase activity (29-32). Although this relationship between P-light chain phosphorylation and actin-activated Mg^{2+}-ATPase activity has been demonstrated with gizzard smooth muscle myosin, it is not necessarily a universal property of myosin from all types of smooth muscle, particularly mammalian smooth muscle. Other investigators found a linear relationship between the extent of phosphorylation and actin-activated Mg^{2+}-ATPase activity of myosin purified from swine pulmonary artery (14) and bovine stomach muscle (33). Obviously, this is an important point in considering the relationship between P-light chain phosphorylation and smooth muscle contraction.

Fewer studies have been reported on the biochemical properties of myosin P-light chain phosphatases, although phosphoprotein phosphatases have been

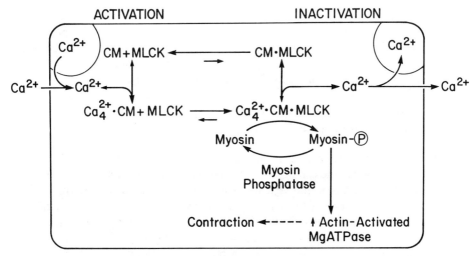

Figure 1   A general scheme for the biochemical regulation of myosin phosphorylation in smooth muscle cells. CM = calmodulin; MLCK = myosin light chain kinase; myosin-$\textcircled{P}$ = phosphory-lated myosin.

purified from smooth muscle (34, 35). A phosphatase that preferentially catalyzes the dephosphorylation of myosin has been purified from bovine aortic smooth muscle (36). Recently, a similar type of phosphatase has been purified from turkey gizzard (37). A preparation of bovine aorta containing actomyosin phosphatase activity has been demonstrated to inhibit the actin-myosin interaction as measured by the Ca^{2+}-dependent superprecipitation of aortic native actomyosin (38). These reports provide evidence of a biochemical mechanism for reversing the effect of myosin phosphorylation by myosin light chain kinase.

The biochemical investigations demonstrating specific stoichiometric phosphorylation of myosin by myosin light chain kinase, dephosphorylation by phosphoprotein phosphatase, and appropriate accompanying activation of myosin Mg^{2+}-ATPase activity satisfy criteria 1 and 2 of Krebs and Beavo mentioned above. These biochemical investigations also provide a framework for understanding the salient features of myosin phosphorylation in smooth muscle cells (Figure 1). In relaxed muscle with low cytoplasmic Ca^{2+} concentrations, little Ca^{2+} is bound to calmodulin, activation of myosin light chain kinase is minimal, and the phosphate content of P-light chain is low. During the initiation of contraction, the concentration of intracellular free Ca^{2+} increases through influx across the sarcolemma and/or through the release of Ca^{2+} from intracellular storage sites. This increase in intracellular Ca^{2+} concentration produces an increase in $Ca_4^{2+} \cdot$ calmodulin, activating myosin light chain kinase, which phosphorylates the myosin P-light chain. Phosphorylation results in an increase in myosin actin–activated Mg^{2+}-ATPase activity. Relaxation caused by the sequestration and removal of Ca^{2+} from the sarcoplasm results in the inactivation of myosin light chain kinase by dissociating Ca^{2+} from the holoenzyme complex. Dephosphorylation of myosin P-light chain by myosin phosphatase then inactivates myosin Mg^{2+}-ATPase activity.

THE REGULATION OF CONTRACTION BY Ca^{2+} AND MYOSIN PHOSPHORYLATION

The combined structural arrangement and enzymatic properties of the contractile proteins within the cell act as a chemomechanical transducer, converting the energy of hydrolysis of ATP to mechanical output. This output, determined by physical constraints on the muscle, can be expressed as force in the isometric case or force and shortening in the isotonic case. In the sliding filament theory based on extensive studies with skeletal muscle, developed force is attributed to the number of active cross bridges generating force additively, this number being regulated by the binding of Ca^{2+} to specific regulatory proteins. Shortening velocity is governed by the load against which the muscle shortens. The maximum velocity of shortening, or V_o, is interpreted as a direct reflection of cross-bridge cycling rates and appears to be determined by the isoenzymatic form of myosin in the cell. This has been demonstrated by the linear correlation between actomyosin Mg^{2+}-ATPase activity and V_o measured in skeletal muscles with widely varying speeds of shortening (39). The similar dependence of velocity on load observed in smooth muscle preparations indicates that the same basic sliding filament mechanism is shared by both muscle types (40).

The dependence of contractile force on elevated levels of calcium in the sarcoplasm surrounding the myofilaments of smooth muscle was originally demonstrated using permeabilized smooth muscle preparations that developed force as a function of calcium concentration in the presence of Mg^{2+}-ATP (41–44). Following the discovery that smooth muscle actin-activated myosin Mg^{2+}-ATPase activity increases upon phosphorylation of P-light chain by Ca^{2+}-calmodulin activated myosin light chain kinase isolated from avian gizzard muscle, more detailed studies with permeabilized or skinned smooth muscle preparations were carried out to demonstrate the significance of this reaction to contractile function. Skinned chicken gizzard preparations showed a correlation between force developed and the degree of P-light chain phosphorylation, although maximum force was produced at 0.2 mol phosphate per mol P-light chain (45). Contractions of a variety of skinned smooth muscle fibers were blocked by specific calmodulin blocking agents (46, 47), and the addition of calmodulin to these preparations enhanced developed force (48, 49). Irreversible thiophosphorylation of myosin resulted in contractions that were maintained in the absence of Ca^{2+} (50, 51). Ca^{2+}-independent contractions could also be produced by treatment with a Ca^{2+}-insensitive proteolytic fragment of myosin light chain kinase (52). These results are consistent with the notion of a Ca^{2+}- and calmodulin-regulated myosin light chain kinase system activating contraction in smooth muscle.

Stimulus-induced contractions in intact smooth muscle have also demonstrated a major role for myosin phosphorylation in the regulation of contractility; however, at the same time, studies in living cells have revealed the existence of a second Ca^{2+}-dependent regulatory event involved in contraction.

Cellular Myosin Phosphorylation and Dephosphorylation

The significant involvement of myosin phosphorylation in contractile function of intact cells has been demonstrated in studies with a variety of smooth muscle preparations in which different stimuli elicited a net increase in the phosphate content of the P-light chain (Table 1). In all cases, myosin was phosphorylated to levels above basal values during the isometric contraction. Decreases in the extent of P-light chain phosphorylation have been measured during relaxations induced by the removal of the stimulus (53–59), addition of a pharmacological antagonist (60, 61), and treatment with a relaxant agent (61–64). In bovine trachealis, the extent of both phosphorylation and force development was depressed by brief pretreatment with the β-adrenergic agonist isoproterenol (65) and the calmodulin antagonist fluphenazine (58). Thus, smooth muscle cells develop force with the phosphorylation of the contractile protein myosin.

As expected for a Ca^{2+}-dependent enzymatic process, resting values of myosin phosphorylation are generally reported to be low, averaging 0.10 mol phosphate per mol P-light chain (55, 57, 58, 66–68). A few studies have reported resting levels ranging from three to five times this value (69,70). Following protein extraction from quick-frozen tissues, the fraction of phosphorylated and non-phosphorylated P-light chain has been quantitated by determining the relative staining intensities of the two forms after separation during isoelectric focusing (53, 60, 71, 72). Erroneously high values can result from analytical overestimates, which occur if the unphosphorylated P-light chain undergoes a charge modification during electrophoresis so that it comigrates with the phosphorylated form (68). Higher resting values of myosin phosphorylation might also be attributable to differences among tissue preparations, reflecting some degree of tonic contractile activity, unphysiological stress, or possibly cell damage.

Transients in Myosin Phosphorylation

The hypothesis that P-light chain phosphorylation plays a direct role in determining isometric force by activating a certain number of cross bridges has been complicated by the observation that phosphorylation can decline in time while force is maintained (53). The correlation between P-light chain phosphoryla-

Table 1 Maximum net increase in phosphate content of myosin P-light chain in stimulated smooth muscle[a]

Tissue	Stimulus[b]	mol phosphate mol P-light chain	Stimulus duration	Animal	Reference
Carotid artery	5 µM histamine	0.59	30 seconds	pig	67
	110 mM KCl	0.37	30 seconds	pig	67
	50 µM norepinephrine	0.27	9 minutes	pig	62
	100 mM KCl	0.36	9 minutes	pig	62
Portal vein	"high" KCl	0.68	2–15 seconds	rabbit	66
Trachealis	1 µM carbachol	0.68	60 seconds	steer	65
	60 mM KCl	0.48	60 seconds	steer	65
	electrical (neural)	0.59	5 seconds	steer	59
	100 µM methacholine	0.33	30 seconds	dog	69
	10 µM carbachol	0.33	30 seconds	rabbit	55
Uterus	100 µM carbachol[c]	0.37	20 seconds	rat	63
	0.25 µM $PGF_{2\alpha}$	0.40	30 seconds	rat	64
	100 mM KCl	0.50	30 seconds	rat	68
Taenia coli	electrical[d]	0.22	5 seconds	rabbit	57

[a] Net values were calculated as the difference between the maximum reported averages for each stimulus and the average resting levels of P-light chain phosphorylation in the study.
[b] All studies were in physiological salt solutions containing 1.6–2.5 mM Ca^{2+}. Tissues were incubated at 36–37°C except those noted below.
[c] Incubated at 28°C.
[d] Incubated at 18°C.

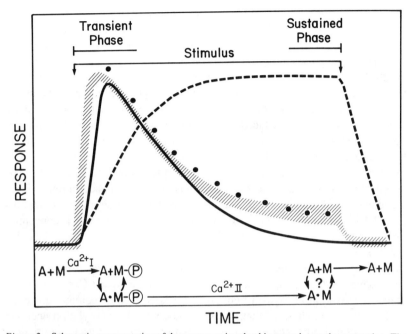

Figure 2 Schematic representative of the processes involved in smooth muscle contraction. The stimulation of resting smooth muscle results in a rapid increase in Ca^{2+}_{cell} (shaded profile), which may be transient. The first regulatory site ($Ca^{2+}I$) for initiating the cyclic interaction of myosin (M) with actin (A) is the Ca^{2+}_4 · calmodulin activation of myosin light chain kinase, which results in P-light chain phosphorylation (— and M-Ⓟ). Attached cross bridges (A•M Ⓟ or A•M) may be rapidly cycling when phosphorylated, resulting in force development (- - -) and high maximal shortening velocities (•), or non- or slowly cycling when dephosphorylated. Whether the low, but measurable, shortening velocities during the sustained phase of contraction reflect the cycling of non-phosphorylated cross bridges or the cycling of a small population of phosphorylated cross bridges is unknown. The second regulatory site ($Ca^{2+}II$) for force maintenance in the absence of myosin phosphorylation remains unidentified.

tion and isometric force has been shown to vary significantly with both contraction duration and agonist used (65, 67, 73). In the continuous presence of stimuli that maintain constant levels of isometric force, phosphorylation of the myosin P-light chain has been shown to decrease from high initial to significantly lower values in the hog carotid artery (54, 67, 74), bovine (65) and rabbit (55) trachealis, and rabbit taenia coli (57). In the carbachol-stimulated bovine trachealis, Ca^{2+}-dependent phosphorylase *a* formation, like myosin phosphorylation, has been seen to decline with time (65). Thus, the transient increase and decrease in myosin phosphorylation indicates that phosphorylation of myosin may not be the sole Ca^{2+}-dependent regulatory event in smooth muscle contraction (Figure 2).

That the phosphorylation and dephosphorylation of myosin may be related to changes in sarcoplasmic Ca^{2+} concentrations is indicated by the concomitant increase and decrease in phosphorylase a formation, which depends on Ca^{2+} and calmodulin activation of phosphorylase kinase (65, 73). Detailed studies by Murphy and co-workers (67) have confirmed the hypothesis that transients in cell $[Ca^{2+}]$ can account for the phosphorylation transients and have indirectly ruled out or relegated to a minor role three other possible causes: (a) reduced substrate (ATP depletion), (b) altered access of activated myosin to the kinase or phosphatase, and (c) reduced kinase activity secondary to its phosphorylation by cAMP-dependent protein kinase. Agonist-stimulated transients in luminescence by aequorin-loaded vascular cells have indicated that sarcoplasmic Ca^{2+} concentration may indeed vary during maintained force (75). The dependence of isometric force on sarcoplasmic Ca^{2+} concentration is illustrated in the KCl-depolarized hog carotid artery where, after myosin is dephosphorylated to near basal levels, the lowering of extracellular $CaCl_2$ concentration results in a decrease in contractile force (76). It has been hypothesized that the transient increase in myosin phosphorylation is explained by a transient rise in cell Ca^{2+} concentration and that a second regulatory site, responsible for Ca^{2+}-dependent force maintenance, necessarily has a greater Ca^{2+} sensitivity than the activation of myosin light chain kinase by $Ca_4^{2+} \cdot$ calmodulin (67).

It should be emphasized that myosin light chain phosphorylation need not always decline from high to very low values during smooth muscle contraction. The magnitude and rate of phosphorylation measured in tissues varies for both experimental and biological reasons. The time course of transients is affected by experimental temperature. Tissue thickness greatly influences agonist diffusion times. Analysis of tissues frozen soon after stimulation by adding agonist to the bathing medium reflects values in only an outer few activated cells. The true time course of cellular transients may be masked as levels of myosin phosphorylation in cells at different states of activation are averaged. This has been demonstrated by comparing rates of P-light chain phosphorylation seen with transmural electrical stimulation of the cholinergic nerves in the bovine trachealis, where activation is more synchronous than that produced by the muscarinic agonist carbachol. With neural stimulation, myosin phosphorylation reaches maximum values at five seconds, as opposed to 60 seconds in the carbachol-stimulated muscle (59, 65).

The time course of P-light chain phosphorylation also is strongly influenced by the type of smooth muscle under investigation. The activation properties of both cells and tissues are known to vary substantially depending on membrane electrical properties, the relative content of sarcoplasmic reticulum, tissue conductance and cell coupling, receptor populations and distribution, the content of non-muscle cells (mast cells, autonomic nerves, endothelial cells), and species and anatomical location (77). Any of these factors can have a significant effect on calcium distribution and handling during stimulation.

Within an individual muscle preparation, myosin phosphorylation may or may not decline to basal levels depending on stimulus conditions. P-light chain phosphorylation in the bovine trachealis has been observed during a contraction in 1 μM carbachol to decline from a maximum of 0.75 mol phosphate per mol P-light chain at one minute to resting values after two hours of maintained isometric force (Figure 3). Stimulation with 60 mM KCl, on the other hand, leads to a decline from 0.59 to only 0.40 mol phosphate per mol P-light chain after two hours of maintained force (73). Myosin phosphorylation in hog carotid artery depolarized in 110 mM KCl returns to basal levels from a maximum of 0.45 mol phosphate per mol P-light chain after 15 minutes in solutions containing 1.6 mM $CaCl_2$. In the presence of 7.5 mM $CaCl_2$, phosphate content falls from 0.65 to 0.40 mol phosphate per mol P-light chain after 15 minutes and remains unchanged for 30 minutes (67). Steady-state maintenance of P-light chain phosphorylation during contraction is presumably related to specific agonist effects on Ca^{2+} turnover and to maintaining sarcoplasmic Ca^{2+} concentrations above the threshold for myosin light chain kinase activation.

Transients in Mechanical Behavior and Energy Consumption

A more mechanistic description of the involvement of myosin phosphorylation in contractile regulation was proposed after the discovery in arterial muscle that, in parallel with phosphorylation, isotonic shortening velocity against light loads increases during the early phase of contraction and then declines while

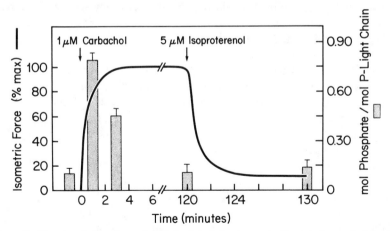

Figure 3 Phosphorylation of myosin P-light chain in bovine trachealis smooth muscle. Muscle strips were contracted by the addition of 1 μM carbachol; after two hours, 5 μM isoproterenol was added. The extent of myosin P-light chain phosphorylation was the same at both 120 and 130 minutes as that in control muscles [adapted from (22)].

force rises to a maintained maximum (74). Levels of myosin phosphorylation during maintained contractions correlate directly with V_o (cross-bridge cycling rate), and not necessarily with absolute levels of stress (number of activated cross bridges) (54). The temporal correlation between myosin phosphorylation and isotonic shortening velocity has since been observed in carbachol-stimulated rabbit trachealis (55) and neurally stimulated bovine trachealis (59). These observations have led to the hypothesis that the Ca^{2+}-dependent phosphorylation of myosin initiates rapid cycling of cross bridges, resulting in the development of isometric force, and that in the presence of a sarcoplasmic Ca^{2+} concentration sufficient to maintain force the dephosphorylation of myosin results in an attached non- or slowly cycling cross bridge (latch bridge). A second Ca^{2+}-dependent mechanism with a greater sensitivity to Ca^{2+} would operate in force maintenance when myosin is dephosphorylated. The dependence of V_o on levels of light chain phosphorylation has been interpreted to be the result of an increase in internal load due to the formation of latch bridges (76). However, a direct modulation of cross-bridge cycling rates by interacting processes activating the myosin molecules has not been ruled out (see above). Maximum velocity of shortening has been observed to be dependent on Ca^{2+} and calmodulin concentrations in skinned preparations (78–80) and on extracellular Ca^{2+} concentration in intact preparations of smooth muscle (67, 80a). While the primary Ca^{2+}-dependent regulatory event appears to be phosphorylation of the myosin P-light chain, there is evidence in intact taenia coli muscle to suggest that Ca^{2+} may have the potential to alter cross-bridge cycling rates while the level of myosin phosphorylation remains constant (80a).

Although force can be maintained in the absence of phosphorylation, these two Ca^{2+}-dependent mechanisms do not appear to be totally independent. Levels of steady-state force have been correlated to initial maximal values of P-light chain phosphorylation (73), and it has been proposed that myosin phosphorylation must precede the latch state. Studies of skinned carotid arteries have demonstrated that, while no difference in Ca^{2+} sensitivity for myosin phosphorylation and force is apparent in the development of contractions, a subsequent reduction in Ca^{2+} concentration results in a proportionally greater dephosphorylation of myosin than reduction in contractile force (81). Thus, myosin phosphorylation may be required for expression of the second Ca^{2+}-dependent mechanism involved in force maintenance during the latch state.

Mechanical (82, 83) and energetic (57) evidence also suggests the existence of a Ca^{2+}-dependent cross-bridge attachment in relaxed or relaxing smooth muscle. Following the removal of a stimulus, P-light chain phosphorylation falls rapidly to resting levels, while force declines at a slower rate (53–57, 59). The Ca^{2+} dependence on force maintenance by dephosphorylated cross bridges during relaxation has been inferred from the acceleration of relaxation by agents believed or known to lower intracellular Ca^{2+} concentration (84).

The decline in cross-bridge cycling rates during stimulation is reflected in measurements of energy consumption in contracting smooth muscle (57, 80a, 85, 86). Such studies emphasize the physiological importance of the latch state, which provides a hypothetical mechanism whereby tonic force can be maintained more efficiently by reducing the ATP consumption associated with high cross-bridge cycling rates and, to a lesser degree, by reducing phosphate turnover in the P-light chain of myosin.

The studies reviewed here fulfill the third criterion of Krebs & Beavo (3) mentioned above, which requires that concomitant functional changes in intact cells be associated with changes in enzyme phosphorylation and dephosphorylation. A simplified scheme representing processes involved with the initiation and maintenance of contractile force in smooth muscle is shown in Figure 2.

Correlation of Cellular Kinase Contents and Activities with Myosin Phosphorylation in Vivo

According to Krebs & Beavo's fourth criterion above (3), the amounts and catalytic properties of the kinase and phosphatase enzymes in the cells should be sufficient to account for the rates and extent of enzyme phosphorylation and its attendant functional alterations. Myosin light chain kinase concentration in tracheal smooth muscle homogenates has been estimated to be 0.36 μM. Assuming the maximal rate of P-light chain phosphorylation by tracheal myosin light chain kinase at 37°C to be 30 μmol phosphate incorporated per liter of intracellular water per second (87) and the rate constant for dephosphorylation to be 0.26 second^{-1} (59), maximal activation of cellular kinase will result in the incorporation of 0.65 mol phosphate per mol P-light chain after two seconds (59). The calculated maximum rate is slightly faster than that measured in the neurally stimulated tracheal smooth muscle (59) and an order of magnitude faster than measured in carbachol-stimulated trachealis (65), demonstrating that maximal rates of enzyme activation and subsequent myosin phosphorylation are not seen in tissues stimulated by externally applied agonists. The time course of P-light chain phosphorylation in the neurally stimulated smooth muscle precedes that of isometric force and coincides with the maximum velocity of shortening.

THE REGULATION OF SMOOTH MUSCLE CONTRACTION-RELAXATION BY CYCLIC AMP

Catecholamines, neurotransmitters, and many peptide hormones increase cyclic AMP formation in smooth muscle tissues by stimulating specific membrane receptors. In particular, cyclic AMP formation has been tightly linked to β-adrenergic receptors in a variety of cells and tissues, and it has been proposed that smooth muscle relaxation via stimulation of β-adrenergic receptors is mediated by cyclic AMP (88–91). In general, there is a correlation between elevated cyclic AMP content and β-adrenergic induced smooth muscle relaxation or inhibition of contraction. Isoproterenol, a β-adrenergic agonist, inhibits the rate and extent of both tension development and P-light chain phosphorylation in smooth muscle (65). However, these correlations cannot be interpreted as convincing evidence of a role for cyclic AMP in mediating smooth muscle relaxation until the precise biochemical mechanism(s) for the relaxation response has been defined. All known effects of cyclic AMP in mammalian biological systems are thought to be due to cyclic AMP activation of cyclic AMP–dependent protein kinase (3). Therefore, it is logical to propose that the relaxation of smooth muscle by β–adrenergic receptor stimulation may be mediated through the cyclic AMP activation of cyclic AMP–dependent protein kinase as well as the phosphorylation of a key protein(s) involved in the contractile process.

Decreased Sarcoplasmic Ca^{2+} Concentrations

Ca^{2+} plays a central role in eliciting contractions in smooth muscle. Therefore, investigations of mechanisms by which β-adrenergic receptor stimulation may mediate smooth muscle relaxation via cyclic AMP formation have focused on processes involved in excitation-contraction coupling. It has been proposed that cyclic AMP formation may lead to a decrease in Ca^{2+} availability to contractile proteins (88, 91). It is obvious in considering Equations 1 and 2 and Figure 1 that a decrease in Ca^{2+} concentrations in smooth muscle sarcoplasm inhibits myosin P-light chain phosphorylation by decreasing the fractional activation of myosin light chain kinase. The primary mechanisms by which β–adrenergic receptor stimulation may decrease sarcoplasmic Ca^{2+} concentrations include: (a) increased Ca^{2+} sequestration into intracellular storage sites (92–95); (b) decreased Ca^{2+} influx into smooth muscle cells (96); (c) increased Ca^{2+} efflux from smooth muscle cells (97, 98). Regarding the last mechanism, Scheid et al (99) have shown that isoproterenol activates Na^+-K^+ pumping in isolated smooth muscle cells from the toad *Bufo marinus*. These investigators also have shown that membrane fragments from these smooth muscle cells contain Na^+-K^+–dependent ATPase activity stimulated upon incubation with cyclic AMP–dependent protein kinase. These data, as well as the recent demonstration of β-adrenergic stimulation of K^+ influx and Ca^{2+} efflux in smooth muscle cells (98, 100), indicate that relaxation may be mediated in part by increasing Na^+-K^+ pump activity, with a concomitant decrease in contractility via increased Ca^{2+} extrusion by the Na^+-Ca^{2+} exchange mechanism.

Thus, published evidence indicates that β-adrenergic stimulation may decrease sarcoplasmic Ca^{2+} concentrations through three primary mechanisms involved in excitation-contraction coupling. Due to the extensive physiological and pharmacological diversity of smooth muscle cells, it seems likely that the relative importance of these mechanisms may vary from one type of smooth muscle to another. Additional investigations will be required to elucidate the biochemical mechanisms (presumably due to protein phosphorylation) involved in regulating sarcoplasmic Ca^{2+} concentrations in smooth muscle cells (25).

Myosin Light Chain Kinase Phosphorylation

In 1978, Adelstein et al (101) showed that purified turkey gizzard smooth muscle myosin light chain kinase is phosphorylated by the catalytic subunit of cyclic AMP-dependent protein kinase, which results in a decrease in the rate of P-light chain phosphorylation. Silver and DiSalvo subsequently showed that the addition of cyclic AMP-dependent protein kinase to a crude preparation of bovine aortic actomyosin markedly decreases the Ca^{2+}-dependent phosphorylation of myosin P-light chain (102). Concomitant with the inhibition of myosin P-light chain phosphorylation is a decrease in actin-activated Mg^{2+}-ATPase activity. Based upon these biochemical observations, the intriguing hypothesis was proposed that cyclic AMP may cause smooth muscle relaxation by inhibiting myosin P-light chain phosphorylation via phosphorylation of myosin light chain kinase by cyclic AMP–dependent protein kinase. This hypothesis has been extended by additional investigations on the biochemical properties of this phosphorylation reaction, and recent pharmacological and physiological studies have focused on the properties of myosin light chain kinase phosphorylation in skinned fibers and living smooth muscle cells.

Below we review the criteria of Krebs & Beavo (3) as outlined in the introduction in relation to some recent observations on the phosphorylation of myosin light chain kinase by cyclic AMP–dependent protein kinase.

STOICHIOMETRIC PHOSPHORYLATION   Two sites have been phosphorylated in purified turkey gizzard smooth muscle myosin light chain kinase by cyclic AMP–dependent protein kinase (103). In the absence of calmodulin, both sites are phosphorylated, which results in an increase in the concentration of $Ca^{2+}_4 \cdot$ calmodulin necessary for 50% activation of myosin light chain kinase activity (K_{CM}; see Equation 2). On the other hand, when calmodulin is bound to myosin light chain kinase, only one site is phosphorylated and this is associated with no change in myosin light chain kinase activity. Analogous studies have also been performed on the dephosphorylation of myosin light chain kinase by a phosphatase purified from turkey gizzard smooth muscle (34). The phosphatase dephosphorylates both sites in myosin light chain kinase in the absence of bound calmodulin. If calmodulin is bound to the diphosphorylated myosin light chain kinase, only one site is readily dephosphorylated, and it coincides with the site that is not phosphorylated by cyclic AMP-dependent protein kinase when calmodulin is bound to myosin light chain kinase.

In general, similar observations have been made on the phosphorylation properties of myosin light chain kinases purified from smooth muscle from bovine stomach (20), porcine myometrium (21), bovine aorta (104), and bovine carotid artery (105). Although myosin light chain kinases purified from bovine cardiac muscle (106) and rabbit skeletal muscle (107) are phosphorylated by cyclic AMP–dependent protein kinase with one mol of phosphate incorporated per mol of myosin light chain kinase, there are no changes in the calmodulin activation properties.

Thus, in terms of Krebs & Beavo's first criterion, it has been shown that two sites in gizzard smooth muscle myosin light chain kinase are stoichiometrically phosphorylated by cyclic AMP–dependent protein kinase. However, the effects of calmodulin on phosphorylation and dephosphorylation reactions require complex consideration. During smooth muscle contraction, calmodulin is bound to myosin light chain kinase (Figure 1). Under these conditions, one would expect a net incorporation of one mol of phosphate per mol of myosin light chain kinase because of inhibition at the other site phosphorylated by cyclic AMP-dependent protein kinase. The dephosphorylation of this site by phosphatase activity is not inhibited by calmodulin. If there were a net incorporation of only 1 mol phosphate per mol myosin light chain kinase in response to an increase in cyclic AMP formation, the calmodulin activation properties would not change.

Activation of myosin light chain kinase by the binding of calmodulin during smooth muscle contraction would also greatly impede the relaxation response due to the slow rate of dissociation of $Ca^{2+}_4 \cdot$ calmodulin from myosin light chain kinase. The calculated $t_{1/2}$ for $Ca^{2+}_4 \cdot$ calmodulin dissociation is 30–60 minutes. In this regard, it is interesting that previous investigations on skinned fibers from gizzard (108) and tracheal smooth muscle (109) have shown that previously contracted fibers are slowly relaxed over a period of one hour by the addition of the cyclic AMP–dependent protein kinase catalytic subunit.

RATE OF PHOSPHORYLATION   At 1 μM myosin light chain kinase, the initial rate of phosphorylation of the turkey gizzard enzyme in the absence of bound calmodulin is 0.2 μmol per minute per mg of cyclic AMP–dependent protein kinase catalytic subunit (103, 107). Purified bovine stomach and tracheal smooth muscle myosin light chain kinase are phosphorylated at initial rates of 0.04 and 0.14 μmol ^{32}P incorporated per minute per mg of cyclic AMP–dependent protein kinase catalytic subunit respectively at 1 μM myosin light chain kinase (20, 110). These concentrations of myosin light chain kinase are close to values thought to exist in smooth muscle (4, 19). Although the values for the kinetic parameters K_m and V_{max} for phosphorylation of smooth muscle myosin light chain kinases are not available, the published rates of phosphorylation may be compared to other physiological protein substrates phosphorylated by cyclic AMP–dependent protein kinase. These rates of phosphorylation of myosin light chain kinase are considerably slower than the rates of phosphorylation of phosphorylase kinase (111), pyruvate kinase (112), and glycogen synthase (113). The maximal rates of phosphorylation of these protein substrates range between 18–45 μmol ^{32}P incorporated per minute per mg of cyclic AMP–dependent protein kinase catalytic subunit.

A simple comparison of rates of phosphorylation of purified protein substrates for cyclic AMP–dependent kinase could be misleading in evaluating the importance of a particular phosphorylation reaction in relation to a physiological event (3). It is important to consider the relative amounts of the protein substrate, as well as cyclic AMP–dependent protein kinase, in relation to the physiological event affected. Tissues contain approximately 0.3 μM cyclic AMP–dependent protein kinase in smooth muscle, and the calculated rate of phosphorylation of myosin light chain kinase at 1 μM shows that at least 30 seconds may be required to phosphorylate the two sites in the enzyme in the absence of bound calmodulin, assuming instantaneous maximal activation of cyclic AMP–dependent protein kinase. During contraction, the rate of phosphorylation is considerably slower due to calmodulin binding to myosin light chain kinase.

THE BIOCHEMICAL EFFECT OF PHOSPHORYLATION Conti & Adelstein (103) originally found that phosphorylation of two sites in myosin light chain kinase from turkey gizzard smooth muscle by cyclic AMP–dependent protein kinase results in a 10–20 fold increase in the concentration of $Ca^{2+}_4 \cdot$ calmodulin necessary for 50% activation of myosin light chain kinase activity, i.e. a 10–20 fold increase in the K_{CM} value in Equation 2. This effect on the K_{CM} value is reversed if myosin light chain kinase is dephosphorylated by a phosphoprotein phosphatase purified from turkey gizzard smooth muscle. When calmodulin is bound to myosin light chain kinase, only one site is phosphorylated and there is no change in the calmodulin activation properties. It is not clear at this time whether phosphorylation of both sites is required for the change in the calmodulin activation properties or whether a single site may be phosphorylated with a concomitant increase in K_{CM}. Miller et al (22) found that phosphorylation of purified bovine tracheal smooth muscle myosin light chain kinase by cyclic AMP–dependent protein kinase to 2 mol phosphate per mol myosin light chain kinase results in a twelvefold increase in K_{CM}. Similar types of results have been obtained with myosin light chain kinase purified from bovine stomach smooth muscle (20), porcine myometrium (21), bovine aorta (104), and bovine carotid artery (105). Thus, myosin light chain kinase purified from a variety of smooth muscles from different animals is phosphorylated in the presence of cyclic AMP–dependent protein kinase, and phosphorylation in the absence of

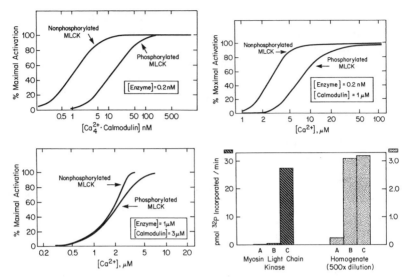

Figure 4 The activation properties of nonphosphorylated and diphosphorylated myosin light chain kinase from smooth muscle. *Upper left:* the effect of $Ca_4^{2+} \cdot$ calmodulin on kinase activities at 0.2 nM myosin light chain kinase; *upper right:* the effect of Ca^{2+} on kinase activities at 0.2 nM myosin light chain kinase and 1 μM calmodulin; *lower left:* the effect of Ca^{2+} on kinase activities at 1 μM myosin light chain kinase and 3 μM calmodulin; *lower right:* the effect of EGTA (A), 200 μM Ca^{2+} (B), or 100 nM calmodulin and 200 μM Ca^{2+} (C) on myosin light chain kinase activity of the purified enzyme (left) and in a homogenate of tracheal smooth muscle (right). Assays were performed according to conditions described in (23).

bound calmodulin results in an increase in the concentration of $Ca_4^{2+} \cdot$ calmodulin required for activation (Figure 4, upper left).

In general, the K_{CM} values change from 1 nM to 10 nM $Ca_4^{2+} \cdot$ calmodulin upon diphosphorylation. These concentrations of calmodulin are considerably lower than the total calmodulin content in smooth muscle, which has been estimated to be 3–6 μM calmodulin (4, 6, 24). However, the prediction may be made from Equations 1 and 2 that a change in the K_{CM} value for myosin light chain kinase would result in a change in the concentration of Ca^{2+} required for activation of myosin light chain kinase in the presence of a high concentration of calmodulin (Figure 4, upper right). At 1 μM calmodulin and low Ca^{2+} concentrations, there is insufficient $Ca_4^{2+} \cdot$ calmodulin for the activation of either the nonphosphorylated or the phosphorylated myosin light chain kinase. As the Ca^{2+} concentration is increased, the concentration of $Ca_4^{2+} \cdot$ calmodulin is increased due to the occupation of the four divalent binding sites on calmodulin with Ca^{2+} (Equation 1). Because diphosphorylated myosin light chain kinase requires a higher concentration of $Ca_4^{2+} \cdot$ calmodulin for activation, Ca^{2+} concentrations required for activation will be greater. Thus, in a biological setting the high concentration of calmodulin per se does not preclude the possibility that phosphorylation of myosin light chain kinase may be important in the regulation of myosin light chain kinase activity. The primary effect of diphosphorylation of the enzyme would be to increase the concentration of Ca^{2+} required for half-maximal activation in the presence of high concentrations of calmodulin.

However, there is another element that should be considered before these properties are extrapolated to living smooth muscle cells. Measurements of calmodulin or Ca^{2+} activation of myosin light chain kinase (Figure 4, upper left and right) are usually done at concentrations of enzyme that are well below K_{CM}, i.e. approximately 0.2–0.5 nM. The content of myosin light chain kinase in smooth muscle is approximately 0.5–1 μM (4, 19, 20). Thus, concentrations of myosin light chain kinase and calmodulin are both three orders of magnitude greater than K_{CM}, a factor that would have a significant effect upon activation properties (Figure 4, lower left; D. K. Blumenthal, J. T. Stull, unpublished observations). The high concentration of myosin light chain kinase acts as a buffer, so that $Ca^{2+}_4 \cdot$ calmodulin formed at low concentrations (nM range) would be bound to myosin light chain kinase. A change in K_{CM} from 1 to 10 nM would result in no significant change in the Ca^{2+} concentrations required for half-maximal activation at high enzyme and calmodulin concentrations (Figure 4, lower left). One way of resolving this dilemma is to invoke competition for $Ca^{2+}_4 \cdot$ calmodulin binding to other calmodulin binding proteins, so that the amount of $Ca^{2+}_4 \cdot$ calmodulin is not sufficient for full activation of myosin light chain kinase. We have explored this possibility by determining whether calmodulin activation of myosin light chain kinase is limiting in tracheal smooth muscle (Figure 4, lower right). As expected, purified myosin light chain kinase is not activated when Ca^{2+} is added to the reaction mixture and requires calmodulin in addition to Ca^{2+}. Myosin light chain kinase activity in a homogenate prepared from tracheal smooth muscle, on the other hand, is fully activated by the addition of Ca^{2+} and the addition of calmodulin produces no further activation. These results indicate that there is sufficient calmodulin in tracheal smooth muscle to activate fully myosin light chain kinase, and that there are not sufficient amounts of other calmodulin binding proteins to compete effectively with myosin light chain kinase for $Ca^{2+}_4 \cdot$ calmodulin.

The effect of cyclic AMP–dependent protein kinase on the calcium sensitivity of actin-myosin interactions has been investigated in a more intact protein system involving skinned bundles of different types of smooth muscles. Kerrick & Hoar (108) were the first to show that the addition of the catalytic subunit of cyclic AMP–dependent protein kinase inhibits Ca^{2+}-activated tension of skinned gizzard smooth muscle fibers. Qualitatively similar results have been obtained with skinned fibers from guinea pig taenia coli (114), hog carotid artery (115), and guinea pig trachealis (109). In most of these studies, the catalytic subunit of cyclic AMP–dependent protein kinase was preincubated with skinned fibers in the presence of a low Ca^{2+} concentration that did not elicit contraction. Under these conditions, the extent of steady-state contractile force is inhibited with increasing Ca^{2+} concentrations, in a manner similar to the effect of phosphorylation on Ca^{2+} activation of myosin light chain kinase (Figure 4, upper right). Kerrick & Hoar (108) found that the addition of 5 μM calmodulin in the presence of Ca^{2+} reverses the inhibitory effect or prevents relaxation with the subsequent addition of the catalytic subunit. Similar observations have been made by Sparrow et al (109) and Rüegg & Paul (115). Meisheri & Rüegg (116) found cyclic AMP itself relaxes skinned guinea pig taenia coli. At physiological concentrations of calmodulin (5 μM), cyclic AMP–induced relaxation is completely inhibited at low Ca^{2+} concentrations. These investigators proposed that the decrease in sarcoplasmic free Ca^{2+} concentrations by cyclic AMP may be the important determinant for the inhibition of contraction and that a direct inhibitory effect of cyclic AMP on actomyosin interaction (phosphorylation of myosin light chain kinase) plays a secondary role.

PHOSPHORYLATION IN VIVO WITH ACCOMPANYING FUNCTIONAL CHANGES   Although no measurements of myosin light chain kinase phosphorylation in vivo have been reported in which the calmodulin binding properties are also analyzed, the potential physiological role for this phosphorylation reaction has been assessed indirectly. Nishikori et al (64) have measured myosin light chain kinase activity from the uteri of estrogen-primed rats stimulated to contract with prostaglandin $F_{2\alpha}$ and then exposed to relaxin. The stimulation of cyclic AMP formation and the relaxation of uteri by relaxin decreases the extent of phosphorylation of myosin light chain and decreases myosin light chain kinase activity. However, these investigators uncovered some unusual features of myosin light chain kinase. About half of the total kinase activity was Ca^{2+}-independent, and it is this activity that primarily decreases in extracts prepared from relaxin-treated uterine smooth muscle. The Ca^{2+}-independent kinase activity may represent partially proteolyzed myosin light chain kinase or another protein kinase. The Ca^{2+} activation properties of the Ca^{2+} and calmodulin-dependent kinase activity (64) are not typical of smooth muscle myosin light chain kinase in that the curves of kinase activity do not show any positive cooperativity (6). The amount of myosin light chain kinase activity extracted from the washed myofibrillar pellets prepared from the uteri is lower by several orders of magnitude than values normally obtained (19, 20). We have found (J. R. Miller, J. T. Stull, unpublished observations) that homogenization of quick-frozen mammalian smooth muscle results in the supernatant fraction rather than the pellet containing most of the myosin light chain kinase activity. Thus, most of the uterine myosin light chain kinase activity may not have been measured. Because of these problems, it is difficult to reach a definitive conclusion about changes in the enzymatic properties of uterine smooth muscle myosin light chain kinase in response to relaxin.

Miller et al (22) have developed a simple assay for assessing changes in calmodulin activation properties that measures the ratio of myosin light chain kinase activities in the presence of 4 μM–100 μM Ca^{2+} at 1 μM calmodulin. This activity ratio in tracheal muscle strips incubated under control conditions is 0.80, a value identical to non-phosphorylated myosin light chain kinase (Figure 4, upper right). When purified myosin light chain kinase is phosphorylated at both sites by cyclic AMP–dependent protein kinase, there is a decrease in the activity ratio to 0.24, corresponding to a twelve-fold increase in K_{CM}. However, the ratio of myosin light chain kinase activity is unchanged when tracheal smooth muscle is incubated with the β-adrenergic agonist isoproterenol at a concentration sufficient to relax the muscle. These results indicate that there are no changes in the calmodulin activation properties of myosin light chain kinase in tracheal smooth muscle upon β-adrenergic stimulation. Thus, phosphorylation of both sites in myosin light chain kinase with the concomitant increase in K_{CM} may not occur in smooth muscle cells.

As pointed out previously, phosphorylation of smooth muscle myosin P-light chain can be a transient event in relation to force development. It has been found that after prolonged incubation with carbachol the extent of phosphorylation of myosin P-light chain decreases to control values after two hours while force is maintained, and the addition of isoproterenol at this time results in relaxation (Figure 3). Thus, β-adrenergic receptor stimulation may relax tracheal smooth muscle in the absence of the significant phosphorylation of myosin P-light chain. A similar experimental approach has recently been made with hog carotid artery (84). Under conditions where force is maintained and myosin P-light chain phosphorylation is at basal levels, forskolin-stimulated cyclic AMP formation relaxes the muscles with no detectable change in the extent of myosin phosphorylation. Under similar conditions adenosine, 3-isobutyl-1-methylxanthine, sodium nitroprusside, and 8-bromo-cyclic GMP also relax the muscle. Thus, these experiments show that dephosphorylation of myosin is not necessary for relaxation and in particular that agents that increase cyclic AMP formation also relax vascular smooth muscle. Jones et al (117) have measured changes in ion fluxes in relation to relaxation by forskolin contractions produced by norepinephrine, angiotensin II, and KCl depolarization in rat aorta. These authors conclude that cyclic AMP–dependent regulation of membrane ion fluxes represents a primary mechanism for relaxation and that the phosphorylation of myosin light chain kinase apparently functions in a secondary capacity. These pharmacological studies in isolated smooth muscle strips indicate that cyclic AMP–dependent effects on sarcoplasmic Ca^{2+} concentrations may be the most important process in mediating smooth muscle relaxation.

CORRELATION OF CYCLIC AMP CONTENT WITH THE EXTENT OF PHOS- PHORYLATION IN VIVO   De Lanerolle et al (61) measured the extent of radioactive phosphate incorporated into myosin light chain kinase of tracheal smooth muscle and found that the estimated phosphate incorporation under control conditions is 1.1 mol phosphate per mol myosin light chain kinase. Stimulation of cyclic AMP formation with forskolin in the absence or presence of methacholine increases the net phosphate incorporated into myosin light chain kinase by 0.6–0.8 mol phosphate per mol myosin light chain kinase respectively. When forskolin is added in the presence of methacholine, the tracheal smooth muscle relaxes. Under control conditions with low cyclic AMP levels (61) and low phosphorylation of phosphorylase (22, 65), cyclic AMP–dependent protein kinase is probably not activated. Hence, the phosphate incorporated into myosin light chain kinase under these conditions is probably not catalyzed by cyclic AMP–dependent protein kinase. Nonspecific phosphorylation in vivo is a feature common to regulated enzymes (3). During smooth muscle contraction and calmodulin activation of myosin light chain kinase, a net incorporation of 1 mol phosphate per mol myosin light chain kinase in the site that does not result in an increase in K_{CM} would be expected, and these data on the phosphorylation of myosin light chain kinase in intact tracheal smooth muscle are consistent with this notion. There have been no measurements of the calmodulin activation properties of tracheal smooth muscle myosin light chain kinase from control and forskolin-treated strips. Nor have there been any measurements of the sites phosphorylated by established peptide mapping procedures (110). Thus, no investigations with smooth muscles have yet correlated the extent of cyclic AMP formation with the phosphorylation of the two sites phosphorylated in myosin light chain kinase by cyclic AMP–dependent protein kinase.

CONCLUDING REMARKS

The Ca^{2+}-dependent phosphorylation of myosin P-light chain is an important, if not obligatory, regulatory step in the initiation of smooth muscle contraction. While myosin phosphorylation in itself may be sufficient to maintain isometric tension, it is evident that a second, as yet unidentified, Ca^{2+}-dependent regulatory mechanism is capable of operating in the maintenance of contractile force after the dephosphorylation of myosin. The identification and characterization of this second site presents an important area for future investigation.

The phosphorylation of purified smooth muscle myosin light chain kinases by cyclic AMP–dependent protein kinase results in a change in the enzymatic properties of the enzyme, with an increase in the $Ca_4^{2+} \cdot$ calmodulin concentrations required for activity. This basic observation has been used as a hypothesis for considering an important role for cyclic AMP in mediating smooth muscle relaxation via the phosphorylation of myosin light chain kinase. However, an examination of this intriguing hypothesis in relation to the specific criteria set forth by Krebs & Beavo (3) for establishing the physiological significance of a protein phosphorylation reaction reveals unresolved problems, indicating that it may not be a primary event in mediating smooth muscle relaxation associated with cyclic AMP formation. Observations with living smooth muscles indicate that a decrease in sarcoplasmic Ca^{2+} concentration may be the primary biochemical event that mediates smooth muscle relaxation upon β-adrenergic receptor stimulation.

ACKNOWLEDGMENTS

We are grateful to Ms. Nancy Bryant for her assistance in the preparation of this manuscript and to the National Institutes of Health for research support (HL23990, HL26043, HL06296, and HL32607).

Literature Cited

1. Frearson, N., Focant, B. W. W., Perry, S. V. 1976. Phosphorylation of a light chain component of myosin from smooth muscle. *FEBS Lett.* 63:27–32

2. Sobieszek, A. 1977. Vertebrate smooth muscle myosin. Enzymatic and structural properties. In *The Biochemistry of Smooth Muscle*, ed. N. L. Stephens, pp. 413–43. Baltimore: Univ. Park

3. Krebs, E. G., Beavo, J. A. 1979. Phosphorylation-dephosphorylation of enzymes. *Ann. Rev. Biochem.* 48:923–59

4. Adelstein, R. S., Eisenberg, E. 1980. Regulation and kinetics of the actin-myosin-ATP interaction. *Ann. Rev. Biochem.* 49:921–56

5. Hartshorne, D. J., Gorecka, A. 1980. Biochemistry of the contractile proteins of smooth muscle. In *Handbook of Physiology. The Cardiovascular System. Vol. 2: Vascular Smooth Muscle*, ed. D. F. Bohr, A. P. Somlyo, H. V. Sparks Jr., pp. 93–120. Bethesda: Am. Physiol. Soc.

6. Stull, J. T. 1980. Phosphorylation of contractile proteins in relation to muscle function. *Adv. Cyclic Nucleotide Res.* 13:39–93

7. Somlyo, A. V. 1980. Ultrastructure of vascular smooth muscle. See Ref. 5, pp. 33–67

8. Bagby, R. M. 1983. Organization of contractile/cytoskeletal elements. In *Bio-

chemistry of Smooth Muscle*, ed. N. L. Stephens, 1:1–84. Boca Raton: CRC

9. Small, J. V., Sobieszek, A. 1983. Contractile and structural proteins of smooth muscle. See Ref. 8, 1:85–140

10. Gabella, G. 1984. Structural apparatus for force transmission in smooth muscles. *Physiol. Rev.* 64:455–77

11. Dabrowska, R., Aromatorio, D., Sherry, J. M. F., Hartshorne, D. J. 1977. Composition of the myosin light chain kinase from chicken gizzard. *Biochem. Biophys. Res. Commun.* 78:1263–72

12. Chacko, S., Conti, M. A., Adelstein, R. S. 1977. Effect of phosphorylation of smooth muscle myosin on actin activation and Ca^{2+} regulation. *Proc. Natl. Acad. Sci. USA* 74:129–33

13. Rees, D. D., Frederiksen, D. W. 1981. Calcium regulation of porcine aortic myosin. *J. Biol. Chem.* 256:357–64

14. Chacko, S., Rosenfeld, A. 1982. Regulation of actin-activated ATP hydrolysis by arterial myosin. *Proc. Natl. Acad. Sci. USA* 79: 292–96

15. Nag, S., Seidel, J. C. 1983. Dependence on Ca^{2+} and tropomyosin of the actin-activated ATPase activity of phosphorylated gizzard myosin in the presence of low concentrations of Mg^{2+}. *J. Biol. Chem.* 258:6444–49

16. Kaminski, E. A., Chacko, S. 1984. Effects of Ca^{2+} and Mg^{2+} on the actin-

activated ATP hydrolysis by phosphorylated heavy meromyosin from arterial smooth muscle. *J. Biol. Chem.* 259: 9104–8

17. Ebashi, S. 1983. Regulation of contractility. In *Muscle and Nonmuscle Motility,* ed. A. Stracher, 1:217–32. New York: Academic

18. Marston, S. B. 1982. The regulation of smooth muscle contractile proteins. *Prog. Biophys. Mol. Biol.* 41:1–41

19. Adelstein, R. A., Klee, C. B. 1981. Purification and characterization of smooth muscle myosin light chain kinase. *J. Biol. Chem.* 256:7501–9

20. Walsh, M. P., Hinkins, S., Flink, I. L., Hartshorne, D. J. 1982. Bovine stomach myosin light chain kinase: Purification, characterization, and comparison with the turkey gizzard enzyme. *Biochemistry* 21:6890–96

21. Higashi, K., Fukunaga, K., Matsui, K., Maeyama, M., Miyamoto, E. 1983. Purification and characterization of myosin light-chain kinase from porcine myometrium and its phosphorylation and modulation by cyclic AMP–dependent protein kinase. *Biochim. Biophys. Acta* 747:232–40

22. Miller, J. R., Silver, P. J., Stull, J. T. 1983. The role of myosin light chain kinase phosphorylation in β-adrenergic relaxation of tracheal smooth muscle. *Mol. Pharmacol.* 24:235–42

23. Blumenthal, D. K., Stull, J. T. 1980. Activation of skeletal muscle myosin light chain kinase by Ca^{2+} and calmodulin. *Biochemistry* 19:5608–14

24. Klee, C. B., Crouch, T. H., Richman, P. G. 1980. Calmodulin. *Ann. Rev. Biochem.* 49:489–515

25. Rasmussen, H., Barrett, P. Q. 1984. Calcium messenger system: An integrated view. *Physiol. Rev.* 64:938–84

26. Cox, J. A., Malnoe, A., Stein, E. A. 1981. Regulation of brain cyclic nucleotide phosphodiesterase by calmodulin. A quantitative analysis. *J. Biol. Chem.* 256:3218–22

27. Huang, C. Y., Chau, V., Chock, P. B., Wang, J. H., Sharma, R. K. 1981. Mechanism of activation of cyclic nucleotide phosphodiesterase: Requirement of the binding of four Ca^{2+} to calmodulin for activation. *Proc. Natl. Acad. Sci. USA* 78:871–74

28. Chau, V., Huang, C. Y., Chock, P. B., Wang, J. H., Sharma, R. 1982. Kinetic studies of the activation of cyclic nucleotide phosphodiesterase by Ca^{++} and calmodulin. In *Calmodulin and Intracellular Ca^{++} Receptors,* ed. S.

Kakiuchi, H. Hidaka, A. R. Means, pp. 199–217. New York: Plenum

29. Ikebe, M., Ogihara, S., Tonomura, Y. 1982. Nonlinear dependence of actin-activated Mg^{2+}-ATPase activity on the extent of phosphorylation of gizzard myosin and H-meromyosin. *J. Biochem.* 91:1809–12

30. Persechini, A., Hartshorne, D. J. 1981. Phosphorylation of smooth muscle myosin: Evidence for cooperativity between the myosin heads. *Science* 213: 1383–85

31. Persechini, A., Hartshorne, D. J. 1983. Ordered phosphorylation of the two 20,000 molecular weight light chains of smooth muscle myosin. *Biochemistry* 22:470–76

32. Sellers, J. R., Chock, P. B., Adelstein, R. S. 1983. The apparently negatively cooperative phosphorylation of smooth muscle myosin at low ionic strength is related to its filamentous state. *J. Biol. Chem.* 258:14181–88

33. Chacko, S. 1981. Effects of phosphorylation, calcium ion, and tropomyosin on actin-activated adenosine 5'-triphosphate activity of mammalian smooth muscle myosin. *Biochemistry* 20:702–7

34. Pato, M. D., Adelstein, R. S. 1983. Purification and characterization of a multisubunit phosphatase from turkey gizzard smooth muscle. The effect of calmodulin binding to myosin light chain kinase on dephosphorylation. *J. Biol. Chem.* 258:7047–54

35. Pato, M. D., Adelstein, R. S. 1983. Characterization of a Mg^{2+}-dependent phosphatase from turkey gizzard smooth muscle. *J. Biol. Chem.* 258:7055–58

36. Werth, D. K., Haeberle, J. R., Hathaway, D. R. 1982. Purification of a myosin phosphatase from bovine aortic smooth muscle. *J. Biol. Chem.* 257: 7306–9

37. Pato, M. D., Kerc, E. 1984. Purification and characterization of smooth muscle phosphatase-IV from turkey gizzard. *Biophys. J.* 45:354 (Abstr.)

38. DiSalvo, J., Gifford, D., Bialojan, C., Rüegg, J. C. 1983. An aortic spontaneously active phosphatase dephosphorylates myosin and inhibits actin-myosin interaction. *Biochem. Biophys. Res. Commun.* 111:906–11

39. Bárány, M. 1967. ATPase activity of myosin correlated with speed of muscle shortening. *J. Gen. Physiol.* 50:197–218

40. Murphy, R. A. 1980. Mechanics of vascular smooth muscle. See Ref. 5, pp. 325–51

41. Filo, R. S., Bohr, D. F., Rüegg, J. C. 1965. Glycerinated skeletal and smooth muscle: calcium and magnesium dependence. *Science* 147:1581–83
42. Endo, M., Kitazawa, T., Yagi, S., Lino, M., Kakata, Y. 1977. Some properties of chemically skinned smooth muscle fibers. In *Excitation-Contraction Coupling in Smooth Muscle*, ed. R. Casteels, T. Godfraind, J. C. Rüegg, pp. 199–209. Amsterdam: Elsevier/North Holland Biomed.
43. Gordon, A. R. 1978. Contraction of detergent-treated smooth muscle. *Proc. Natl. Acad. Sci. USA* 75:3527–30
44. Saida, K., Nonomura, Y. 1978. Characteristics of Ca^{2+}- and Mg^{2+}-induced tension development in chemically skinned smooth muscle fibers. *J. Gen. Physiol.* 72:1–14
45. Kerrick, W. G. L., Hoar, P. E., Cassidy, P. S. 1980. Calcium-activated tension: The role of myosin light chain phosphorylation. *Fed. Proc.* 39:1558–63
46. Kerrick, W. G. L., Hoar, P. E., Cassidy, P. S., Bolles, L., Malencik, D. A. 1981. Calcium-regulatory mechanisms: Functional clarification using skinned fibers. *J. Gen. Physiol.* 77:177–90
47. Kreye, V. A. W., Rüegg, J. C., Hofmann, F. 1983. Effect of calcium-antagonist and calmodulin-antagonist drugs on calmodulin-dependent contractions of chemically skinned vascular smooth muscle from rabbit renal arteries. *Naunyn-Schmiedeberg's Arch. Pharmacol.* 323:85–89
48. Cassidy, P., Kerrick, W. G. L., Hoar, P. E., Malencik, D. A. 1981. Exogenous calmodulin increases Ca^{2+} sensitivity of isometric tension, activation and myosin phosphorylation in skinned smooth muscle. *Pflügers Arch.* 392:115–20
49. Sparrow, M. P., Mrwa, U., Hoffman, F., Rüegg, J. C. 1981. Calmodulin is essential for smooth muscle contraction. *FEBS Lett.* 125:141–45
50. Hoar, P. E., Kerrick, W. G. L., Cassidy, P. S. 1979. Chicken gizzard: Relation between calcium activated phosphorylation and contraction. *Science* 204:503–6
51. Peterson, J. W. III. 1982. Simple model of smooth muscle myosin phosphorylation and dephosphorylation as rate-limiting mechanism. *Biophys. J.* 37:453–59
52. Walsh, M. P., Bridenbaugh, R., Hartshorne, D. J., Kerrick, W. G. L. 1982. Phosphorylation-dependent activated tension in skinned gizzard muscle fibers in the absence of Ca^{2+}. *J. Biol. Chem.* 257:5987–90
53. Driska, S. P., Aksoy, M. O., Murphy, R. A. 1981. Myosin light chain phosphorylation associated with contraction in arterial smooth muscle. *Am. J. Physiol.* 240:C222–33
54. Aksoy, M. O., Murphy, R. A., Kamm, K. E. 1982. Role of Ca^{2+} and myosin light chain phosphorylation in regulation of smooth muscle. *Am. J. Physiol.* 242:C109–16
55. Gerthoffer, W. T., Murphy, R. A. 1983. Myosin phosphorylation and regulation of the cross-bridge cycle in tracheal smooth muscle. *Am. J. Physiol.* 244:C182–87
56. Gerthoffer, W. T., Murphy, R. A. 1983. Ca^{2+}, myosin phosphorylation, and relaxation of arterial smooth muscle. *Am. J. Physiol.* 245:C271–77
57. Butler, T. M., Siegman, M. J., Mooers, S. U. 1983. Chemical energy usage during shortening and work production in mammalian smooth muscle. *Am. J. Physiol.* 244:C234–42
58. Silver, P., Stull, J. T. 1983. Effects of the calmodulin antagonist, fluphenazine, on phosphorylation of myosin and phosphorylase in intact smooth muscle. *Mol. Pharmacol.* 23:665–70
59. Kamm, K. E., Stull, J. T. 1985. Myosin phosphorylation, force and V_o in neurally stimulated tracheal smooth muscle. *Am. J. Physiol.* In press
60. de Lanerolle, P., Stull, J. T. 1980. Myosin phosphorylation during contraction and relaxation of tracheal smooth muscle. *J. Biol. Chem.* 255:9993–10000
61. de Lanerolle, P., Nishikawa, M., Yost, D. A., Adelstein, R. S. 1984. Increased phosphorylation of myosin light chain kinase after an increase in cyclic AMP in intact smooth muscle. *Science* 223:1415–17
62. Barron, J. R., Bárány, M., Bárány, K., Storti, R. V. 1980. Reversible phosphorylation and dephosphorylation of the 20,000 dalton light chain of myosin during the contraction-relaxation-contraction cycle of arterial smooth muscle. *J. Biol. Chem.* 255:6238–44
63. Janis, R. A., Bárány, K., Bárány, M., Sarmiento, G. 1981. Association between myosin light chain phosphorylation and contraction of rat uterine smooth muscle. *Mol. Pharmacol.* 1:3–11
64. Nishikori, K., Weisbrodt, N. W., Sherwood, O. D., Sanborn, B. M. 1983. Effects of relaxin on rat uterine myosin light chain kinase activity and myosin light chain phosphorylation. *J. Biol. Chem.* 258:2468–74
65. Silver, P. J., Stull, J. T. 1982. Regula-

tion of myosin light chain and phosphorylase phosphorylation in tracheal smooth muscle. *J. Biol. Chem.* 257:6145–50

66. Somlyo, A. V., Butler, T. M., Bond, M., Somlyo, A. P. 1981. Myosin filaments have nonphosphorylated light chains in relaxed smooth muscle. *Nature* 294:567–69

67. Aksoy, M. O., Mras, S., Kamm, K. E., Murphy, R. A. 1983. Ca^{++}, cAMP, and changes in myosin phosphorylation during contraction of smooth muscle. *Am. J. Physiol.* 245:C255–70

68. Haeberle, J. R., Hott, J. W., Hathaway, D. R. 1984. Pseudophosphorylation of the smooth muscle 20,000 dalton myosin light chain: An artifact due to protein modification. *Biochim. Biophys. Acta.* 790:78–86

69. de Lanerolle, P., Condit, J. R. Jr., Tanenbaum, M., Adelstein, R. S. 1982. Myosin phosphorylation, agonist concentration and contraction of tracheal smooth muscle. *Nature* 298:871–72

70. Ledvora, R. F., Bárány, K., Van der Meulen, D. L., Barron, J. T., Bárány, M., 1983. Stretch-induced phosphorylation of the 20,000-dalton light chain of myosin in arterial smooth muscle. *J. Biol. Chem.* 258:14080–83

71. Silver, P. J., Stull, J. T. 1982. Quantitation of myosin light chain phosphorylation in small tissue samples. *J. Biol. Chem.* 257:6137–44

72. Bárány, K., Sayers, S. T., DiSalvo, J., Bárány, M. 1983. Two-dimensional electrophoretic analysis of myosin light chain phosphorylation in the heart. *Electrophoresis* 4:138–42

73. Silver, P. J., Stull, J. T. 1984. Differential regulation of myosin light chain and phosphorylase phosphorylation by K^+ depolarization and carbamylcholine in tracheal smooth muscle. *Mol. Pharmacol.* 25:267–74

74. Dillon, P. F., Aksoy, M. O., Driska, S. P., Murphy, R. A. 1981. Myosin phosphorylation and the cross-bridge cycle in arterial smooth muscle. *Science* 211:495–97

75. Morgan, J. P., Morgan, K. G. 1982. Vascular smooth muscle: The first recorded Ca^{2+} transients. *Pflügers Arch.* 395:75–77

76. Murphy, R. A., Aksoy, M. O., Dillon, P. F., Gerthoffer, W. T., Kamm, K. E. 1983. The role of myosin light chain phosphorylation in regulation of the cross-bridge cycle. *Fed. Proc.* 42:51–56

77. Bolton, T. B. 1979. Mechanisms of action of transmitters and other substances

on smooth muscle. *Physiol. Rev.* 59:606–718

78. Arner, A. 1982. Mechanical characteristics of chemically skinned guinea-pig taenia coli. *Pflügers Arch.* 395:277–84

79. Arner, A. 1983. Force-velocity relation in chemically skinned rat portal vein: Effects of Ca^{2+} and Mg^{2+}. *Pflügers Arch.* 397:6–12

80. Paul, R. J., Doerman, G., Zeugner, C., Rüegg, J. C. 1983. The dependence of unloaded shortening velocity on Ca^{++}, calmodulin, and duration of contraction in "chemically skinned" smooth muscle. *Circ. Res.* 53:342–51

80a. Siegman, M. J., Butler, T. M., Mooers, S. U., Michalek, A. 1984. Ca^{2+} can affect V_{max} without changes in myosin light chain phosphorylation in smooth muscle. *Pflügers Arch.* 401:385–90

81. Chatterjee, M., Murphy, R. A. 1983. Calcium-dependent stress maintenance without myosin phosphorylation in skinned smooth muscle. *Science* 221:464–66

82. Siegman, M. J., Butler, T. M., Mooers, S. U., Davies, R. E. 1976. Crossbridge attachment, resistance to stretch, and viscoelasticity in resting mammalian smooth muscle. *Science* 191:383–85

83. Meiss, R. A. 1982. Transient responses and continuous behavior of active smooth muscle during controlled stretches. *Am. J. Physiol.* 242:C146–58

84. Gerthoffer, W. T., Trevethick, M. A., Murphy, R. A. 1984. Myosin phosphorylation and cyclic adenosine 3',5'-monophosphate in relaxation of arterial smooth muscle by vasodilators. *Circ. Res.* 54:83–89

85. Arner, A., Hellstrand, P. 1983. Activation of contraction and ATPase activity in intact and chemically skinned smooth muscle of rat portal vein: Dependence on Ca^{++} and muscle length. *Circ. Res.* 53:695–702

86. Krisanda, J. M., Paul, R. J. 1984. Energetics of isometric contraction in porcine carotid artery. *Am. J. Physiol.* 246:C510–79

87. Stull, J. T., Blumenthal, D. K., Miller, J. R., DiSalvo, J. 1982. Regulation of myosin phosphorylation. *J. Mol. Cell Cardiol.* 14:105–10

88. Kramer, G. L., Hardman, J. G. 1980. Cyclic nucleotides and blood vessel contraction. See Ref. 5, pp. 179–99

89. Kuriyama, H., Ito, Y., Suzuki, H., Kitamura, K., Itoh, T. 1982. Factors modifying contraction-relaxation cycle in vascular smooth muscle. *Am. J. Physiol.* 243:H641–62

90. Krall, J. F., Fortier, M., Korenman, S.

G. 1983. Smooth muscle cyclic nucleotide biochemistry. See Ref. 8, 3:89–128

91. Kroeger, E. A. 1983. Roles of cyclic nucleotides in modulating smooth muscle function. See Ref. 8, 3:129–39

92. Casteels, R., Raeymaekers, L. 1979. The action of acetylcholine and catecholamines on an intracellular calcium store in the smooth muscle cells of the guinea-pig taenia coli. *J. Physiol.* 294:51–68

93. Mueller, E., van Breeman, C. 1979. Role of intracellular Ca^{2+} sequestration in β-adrenergic relaxation of a smooth muscle. *Nature* 281:682–83

94. Van Eldere, J., Raeymaekers, L., Casteels, R. 1982. Effect of isoprenaline on intracellular Ca uptake and on Ca influx in arterial smooth muscle. *Pflügers Arch.* 395:81–83

95. Itoh, T., Izumi, H., Kuriyama, H. 1982. Mechanisms of relaxation induced by activation of β-adrenoreceptors in smooth muscle cells of the guinea-pig mesenteric artery. *J. Physiol.* 326:475–93

96. Meisheri, K. D., van Breemen, C. 1982. Effects of β-adrenergic stimulation on calcium movements in rabbit aortic smooth muscle: Relationship with cyclic AMP. *J. Physiol.* 331:429–41

97. Bulbring, E., den Hertog, A. 1980. The action of isoprenaline on the smooth muscle of the guinea-pig taenia coli. *J. Physiol.* 305:277–96

98. Scheid, C. R., Fay, F. S. 1984. β-Adrenergic effects on transmembrane ^{45}Ca fluxes in isolated smooth muscle cells. *Am. J. Physiol.* 246:C431–38

99. Scheid, C. R., Honeyman, T. W., Fay, F. S. 1979. Mechanism of β-adrenergic relaxation of smooth muscle. *Nature* 277:32–36

100. Scheid, C. R., Fay, F. S. 1984. β-Adrenergic stimulation of ^{42}K influx in isolated smooth muscle cells. *Am. J. Physiol.* 246:C415–21

101. Adelstein, R. S., Conti, M. A., Hathaway, D. R. 1978. Phosphorylation of smooth muscle myosin light chain kinase by the catalytic subunit of adenosine 3':5' - monophosphate - dependent protein kinase. *J. Biol. Chem.* 253:8347–50

102. Silver, P. J., DiSalvo, J. 1979. Adenosine 3':5'-monophosphate-mediated inhibition of myosin light chain phosphorylation in bovine aortic actomyosin. *J. Biol. Chem.* 254:9951–54

103. Conti, M. A., Adelstein, R. S. 1981. The relationship between calmodulin binding and phosphorylation of smooth muscle myosin kinase by the catalytic subunit of 3':5' cAMP-dependent protein kinase. *J. Biol. Chem.* 256:3178–81

104. Vallet, B., Molla, A., Demaille, J. G. 1981. Cyclic adenosine 3',5'-monophosphate-dependent regulation of purified bovine aortic calcium/calmodulin-dependent myosin light chain kinase. *Biochim. Biophys. Acta* 674:256–64

105. Bhalla, R. C., Sharma, R. V., Gupta, R. C. 1982. Isolation of two myosin light-chain kinases from bovine carotid artery and their regulation by phosphorylation mediated by cyclic AMP-dependent protein kinase. *Biochem. J.* 203:583–92

106. Wolf, H., Hofmann, F. 1980. Purification of myosin light chain kinase from bovine cardiac muscle. *Proc. Natl. Acad. Sci. USA* 77:5852–55

107. Edelman, A. M., Krebs, E. G. 1982. Phosphorylation of skeletal muscle myosin light chain kinase by the catalytic subunit of cAMP-dependent protein kinase. *FEBS Lett.* 138:293–98

108. Kerrick, W. G. L., Hoar, P. E. 1981. Inhibition of smooth muscle tension by cyclic AMP-dependent protein kinase. *Nature* 292:253–55

109. Sparrow, M. P., Pfitzer, G., Gagelmann, M., Rüegg, J. C. 1984. Effect of calmodulin, Ca^{2+}, and cAMP protein kinase on skinned tracheal smooth muscle. *Am. J. Physiol.* 246:C308–14

110. Nishikawa, M., de Lanerolle, P., Lincoln, T. M., Adelstein, R. S. 1984. Phosphorylation of mammalian myosin light chain kinases by the catalytic subunit of cyclic AMP-dependent protein kinase and by cyclic GMP-dependent protein kinase. *J. Biol. Chem.* 259:8429–36

111. Yeaman, S. J., Cohen, P., Watson, D. C., Dixon, G. H. 1977. The substrate specificity of adenosine 3':5'-cyclic monophosphate-dependent protein kinase of rabbit skeletal muscle. *Biochem. J.* 162:411–21

112. Pilkis, S. J., El-Maghrabi, M. R., Coven, B., Claus, T. H., Tager, H. S., et al. 1980. Phosphorylation of rat hepatic fructose-1,6-bisphosphatase and pyruvate kinase. *J. Biol. Chem.* 255:2770–75

113. Proud, C. G., Rylatt, D. B., Yeaman, S. J., Cohen, P. 1977. Amino acid sequences at the two sites on glycogen synthetase phosphorylated by cyclic AMP-dependent protein kinase and their dephosphorylation by protein phosphatase-III. *FEBS Lett.* 80:435–42

114. Rüegg, J. C., Sparrow, M. P., Mrwa, U. 1981. Cyclic-AMP mediated relaxation of chemically skinned fibres of smooth muscle. *Pflügers Arch.* 390:198–201

115. Rüegg, J. C., Paul, R. J. 1982. Vascular smooth muscle. Calmodulin and cyclic AMP-dependent protein kinase alter calcium sensitivity in porcine carotid skinned fibers. *Circ. Res.* 50:394–99

116. Meisheri, K. D., Rüegg, J. C. 1983. Dependence of cyclic-AMP induced relaxation on Ca^{2+} and calmodulin in skinned smooth muscle of guinea pig *Taenia coli*. *Pflügers Arch.* 399:315–20

117. Jones, A. W., Bylund, D. B., Forte, L. R. 1984. cAMP-dependent reduction in membrane fluxes during relaxation of arterial smooth muscle. *Am. J. Physiol.* 246:H306–11

Ann. Rev. Pharmacol. Toxicol. 1985. 25:621–41

ALTERATIONS IN THE RELEASE OF NOREPINEPHRINE AT THE VASCULAR NEUROEFFECTOR JUNCTION IN HYPERTENSION

Thomas C. Westfall and Michael J. Meldrum

Department of Pharmacology, St. Louis University School of Medicine, St. Louis, Missouri 63104

INTRODUCTION

The mechanism(s) for the development of elevated blood pressure in human essential hypertension has defied precise understanding despite numerous studies. This is probably because hypertension is a multifactorial disease involving many alterations in the nervous and endocrine systems as well as alterations in vascular smooth muscle function (1–3). In an effort to obtain more information on the pathophysiology of essential hypertension, investigators have developed a large number of experimental models. The hope is that knowledge obtained about the pathophysiological mechanisms of these various experimental hypertensive models will provide clues to understanding human hypertension. Experimental hypertension has been induced by a number of procedures, including acute and chronic renal interventions, endocrine manipulations such as deoxycorticosterone (DOCA)-salt treatment, genetic inbreeding (the spontaneously hypertensive rat, or SHR, and the Dahl–salt sensitive hypertensive rat), and neurogenic manipulations.

Although other mechanisms play a role, a tremendous body of information suggests an increase in sympathetic nerve activity in the development and possibly the maintenance of hypertension in several of these models as well as

621

0362-1642/85/415-0621$02.00

in essential hypertension itself. In this review, emphasis will be placed on models where increased sympathetic nerve activity has been implicated (SHR, renal hypertension, DOCA-salt, Dahl-salt, and others). The reader is referred to several of the many recent and comprehensive reviews that discuss the evidence for increased sympathetic nerve activity in various models of hypertension (4–10).

An increase in peripheral sympathetic nerve activity may be due to alterations in either the afferent or the efferent limb of the nervous system, as well as at one or more sites within the central nervous system. Numerous studies have implicated a centrally mediated increase in sympathetic nerve activity as being of primary importance in the development and/or maintenance of hypertension in such models as the SHR (11, 12–15, 16–24), which is thought by many to be an excellent model of essential hypertension (25). Despite this fact, peripheral nerve activity may be altered independently of what occurs centrally. Such changes could take place at the vascular neuroeffector junction with the participation of either the pre- or the postsynaptic system. Alterations at the presynaptic nerve terminals could either increase or decrease the influence of impulses arriving from the central vasomotor centers. Zimmerman (26) discusses the difficulties encountered when evaluating the relative importance of peripheral or central factors in the development and maintenance of hypertension and how interpretations are tempered by imprecise methodology.

The purpose of this review is to discuss the evidence for and against the idea that alterations or dysfunction of the sympathetic nervous system at the level of the presynaptic nerve terminal of the vascular neuroeffector complex in hypertensive animals results in changes in transmitter release.

ADRENERGIC NEUROTRANSMITTER DYNAMICS IN PRESYNAPTIC NERVE TERMINALS

The events that take place in presynaptic noradrenergic nerve varicosities have been thoroughly studied and have been themselves the subject of numerous reviews (7, 8, 27–29). Only a brief summary will be presented here.

The adrenergic neurotransmitter norepinephrine is synthesized by three enzymatically controlled steps after the uptake of tyrosine into the adrenergic varicosity. Tyrosine is subsequently converted to dihydroxyphenylalanine (dopa), dopamine, and finally norepinephrine by the enzymes tyrosine-3-monooxygenase, aromatic L-amino acid decarboxylase, and dopamine-3-monooxygenase respectively. The conversion of dopamine to norepinephrine takes place in the storage vesicles, where the transmitter is stored in a complex with protein, ATP, and various ions. Upon the arrival of an action potential and depolarization of the terminal varicosity, norepinephrine is released together with other soluble contents, including dopamine ß-hydroxylase, ATP, and chromogranins, into the extracellular space. Norepinephrine migrates to the vascular effector cell, where it interacts with α_1 and/or α_2-adrenoceptors to cause vasoconstriction. In some cases it interacts with β_2-adrenoceptors to cause vasodilation. Norepinephrine's action is terminated by a specific carrier-mediated uptake system (uptake 1) across the neuronal membrane. This is an active transport process requiring Na^+ as well as energy. Following the recapture of norepinephrine inside the adrenergic varicosity, the amine is further transported into the storage vesicles for reuse or is metabolized by monoamine oxidase located on the outer membrane of the mitochondria. A second way norepinephrine is inactivated is via the extraneuronal enzyme, catechol O-methyltransferase, following uptake into smooth muscle cells (uptake 2). The synthesis, storage, release, receptor activation, and inactivation of norepinephrine are obviously subject to various control mechanisms that must operate in concert for the smooth operation of the adrenergic neurons. Much information on the regulation of these processes is available.

It is now well established that neural and hormonal substances can influence the quantitative release of norepinephrine per nerve impulse by an action on receptors located on the adrenergic varicosities and thereby influence the concentration of transmitter at the neuroeffector junction. Substances reported to decrease adrenergic neurotransmission include α_2-adrenoceptor agonists (including norepinephrine itself), purines such as ATP and adenosine, prostaglandins (PG) of the E series, acetylcholine (ACh) via muscarinic receptors, dopamine (DA), histamine, serotonin (5-HT), morphine, and opioid peptides. Substances facilitating adrenergic neurotransmission include ß-adrenergic agonists, ACh via nicotinic receptors, angiotensin (ANG), and possibly PG of the F series, and thromboxanes. In addition to influencing adrenergic neurotransmission, they may also contribute to the regulation of vascular tone by acting directly on vascular smooth muscle and/or influencing the activity of other vasoactive substances. Several extensive reviews have appeared that discuss this aspect of the control of adrenergic neuronal function in greater detail (30–37, 27, 38–41, 42). Modulation by these substances is thought to have important physiological functions and may play important pathophysiological roles as well.

EVIDENCE FOR INCREASED NORADRENERGIC TRANSMISSION IN THE BLOOD VESSELS OF HYPERTENSIVE ANIMALS

Numerous studies suggest that there is an increase in norepinephrine release from blood vessels in experimental hypertensive animals. It has been demonstrated that sympathetic nerve stimulation results in an enhancement of vaso-constriction with or without a parallel increase in the response to exogenously administered norepinephrine. This has been demonstrated in young SHR (43, 44, 11), rabbits made hypertensive by partial constriction of the abdominal aorta above the kidneys (45), the Dahl–salt sensitive genetic model of hyper-tension (46), one clip–one kidney or two-kidney renal hypertension in the dog (47, 48), and one-clip–one kidney hypertension in the rat (49). Such a situation is consistent with the increased release of norepinephrine from adrenergic nerve terminals. Studies suggesting an increase in the reactivity of blood vessels to nerve stimulation remain inconclusive and controversial, since several investi-gators have failed to observe similar increases in some of those models of hypertension (50–52).

Although there are many problems with using plasma catecholamines as an index of sympathetic nerve activity or as a marker for neurotransmitter release (see below), researchers generally agree that there is an increase in plasma catecholamines and in dopamine ß-hydroxylase in young SHR (53–56) as well as in other models of hypertension (26, 48). The interpretation of these data is more complicated, since an increase in plasma catecholamines, especially norepinephrine, could represent increased release from nerve terminals, de-creased uptake, or decreased clearance from the plasma. Plasma norepineph-rine concentrations therefore represent the net overflow of the transmitter from adrenergic nerve endings and may or may not be proportional to the amount that reaches postsynaptic receptors, thereby resulting in physiological effects. In contrast to studies in young SHR, results obtained in adult SHR are quite controversial. The majority of studies have failed to observe differences in plasma catecholamines in adult SHR compared to normotensive controls (57–61), while a few studies have reported higher values in SHR (62). Of consider-able interest is the report that the O-methylated metabolite normetanephrine is significantly higher in five– and six–month old SHR compared to Wistar-Kyoto (WKY) rats, a normotensive strain developed along with the SHR. Since normetanephrine is mainly an extraneuronal metabolite of norepinephrine, the possibility exists that its plasma concentration reflects the amount of neuro-transmitter that reaches effector cells and is consistent with an enhanced sympathetic function in adult SHR (63).

Several studies have directly demonstrated an increase in nerve traffic in peripheral sympathetic nerves of SHR or DOCA-salt hypertensive rats com-pared to normotensive controls (64–66, 12–15). Stress also results in a greater increase in peripheral sympathetic nerve activity in SHR compared to nor-motensive controls (57–61, 67–69, 44–51). Peripheral sympathectomy has been shown to markedly attenuate hypertension in the SHR (70, 71) as well as in other hypertensive models (16).

DIRECT EVIDENCE FOR THE INCREASED RELEASE OF NOREPINEPHRINE FROM THE BLOOD VESSELS OF HYPERTENSIVE ANIMALS

Although all of the studies mentioned above suggest an increase in peripheral sympathetic nerve activity in hypertensive animals over normotensive controls, they do not differentiate between the effect being mediated primarily by the increased activation of central vasomotor centers and that due to increased activity at the vascular neuroeffector junction. As already mentioned, several studies suggest that the increase in peripheral sympathetic activity in pre-, young, and established hypertensive animals is secondary to alterations in the central nervous system, with increased impulse traffic from central vasomotor systems over pre- and postganglionic sympathetic fibers (17–24).

On the other hand, several studies have directly demonstrated an increase in the release of norepinephrine from isolated blood vessels (72–76), isolated perfused organs (77–80), and isolated perfused vascular beds of SHR (81–83) compared to normotensive controls (Table 1). Such increases have been observed when both ^{3}H-norepinephrine and endogenous norepinephrine are used as markers for transmitter release (72–83). Moreover, a greater release from the blood vessels of hypertensive animals has been seen following various types of stimulation, including field stimulation, nerve stimulation, depolarization with high potassium, and the application of veratradine. It appears that the greatest release of norepinephrine occurs in pre- or young SHR animals, suggesting that the increased release of norepinephrine may participate in the development of hypertension. A greater release of norepinephrine has also been observed from the blood vessels of older SHR (28 weeks), although this has not been reported by all investigators (84). The fact that increased release of norepinephrine is seen in isolated blood vessels of hypertensive animals suggests that such alterations can take place at the level of the noradrenergic nerve terminal.

Although there have only been a few studies of other hypertensive models, results to date suggest that the enhanced release of norepinephrine from isolated blood vessels is not a property common to all types of hypertension. For instance, no difference in the field stimulation–induced release of ^{3}H-norepinephrine or endogenous norepinephrine was seen from the portal vein or caudal artery of either DOCA-salt or one-kidney, one-clip renal hypertensive rats (74, 85). The hyperresponsiveness of the mesentric vasculature to periarterial nerve stimulation in DOCA-salt hypertensive rats appears to be due to increased sensitivity of the vascular smooth muscle rather than to facilitation of transmitter release (86). Similarly, adrenergic neurotransmission is not altered in the mesenteric artery of rats with chronic neurogenic hypertension (87).

Table 1 Alterations in the release of norepinephrine from the vascular neuroeffector junction of experimental hypertensive animals

Type of hypertension (animal)	Age	Blood vessel	Observation	References
Genetic (SHR)	6 weeks	Perfused kidney	Periarterial nerve stimulation; ^{3}H release SHR>WKY	77
Genetic (SHR)	18 weeks	Perfused mesentery	Periarterial nerve stimulation; ^{3}H release SHR>WKY	81, 82
Genetic (SHR)	6, 10, 28 weeks	Isolated caudal artery	Potassium depolarization; endogenous norepinephrine SHR>WKY at all ages	72, 74
Genetic (SHR)	7–9 weeks	Isolated caudal artery	Field stimulation ^{3}H release; SHR>WKY	76
Genetic (SHR)	14–16 weeks	Perfused mesentery	Periarterial nerve stimulation; ^{3}H release SHR>WKY	83
Genetic (SHR)	6 months	Perfused kidney	Periarterial nerve stimulation; ^{3}H or endogenous norepinephrine release WKY>SHR	84
Genetic (SHR)	14–21 weeks	Perfused kidney	Periarterial nerve stimulation; ^{3}H release SHR>WKY	78, 79
Genetic (SHR)	6, 10, 28 weeks	Portal vein	Field stimulation; ^{3}H release SHR>WKY at 10 and 28 weeks	73–75
Genetic (SHR)	6, 10, 28 weeks	Caudal artery	Field stimulation; endogenous norepinephrine release SHR>WKY at all ages	74, 85
Renovascular (one clip-one kidney)		Caudal artery and portal vein	Similar increase in release of endogenous norepinephrine or ^{3}H-norepinephrine to field stimulation	85
DOCA-salt (rat)		Caudal artery and portal vein	Similar increase in release of endogenous norepinephrine or ^{3}H-norepinephrine to field stimulation	85
Neurogenic (baroreceptor deafferentation rat)		Mesenteric artery	Similar increase in release of ^{3}H-norepinephrine to field stimulation	87

Since there is evidence of increased sympathetic nerve activity in these hypertensive models as there is in young SHR, yet no evidence of enhanced release from isolated blood vessels, we suggest that in the former models increased sympathetic nerve traffic is primarily mediated by an increase in central nervous system activity, while in SHR, on the other hand, both a central and a peripheral mechanism may be operational.

PRESYNAPTIC MODULATION OF NOREPINEPHRINE RELEASE FROM THE BLOOD VESSELS OF HYPERTENSIVE ANIMALS

As mentioned above, it is now well accepted that a variety of endogenous substances can modify the evoked release of norepinephrine from the adrenergic neuroeffector junction. An examination of whether there are alterations in the activity of these release modulatory substances in hypertension has recently been undertaken as a possible explanation for the increased release of norepinephrine from the blood vessels of hypertensive animals (Table 2). The general hypothesis on which these experiments are based is that a decrease in the activity of presynaptic inhibitory receptors results in an enhancement of adrenergic neurotransmission. On the other hand, a similar enhancement would be seen if there was an increase in the activity of presynaptic facilitatory receptors.

Angiotensin is one of the substances that has been shown to enhance the evoked release of norepinephrine from adrenergic nerve terminals (88, 89). Evidence for an increased activity of presynaptic angiotensin receptors in blood vessels of SHR has been obtained in several laboratories (73–75, 81, 90). Kawasaki and co-workers (90) observed that angiotensin enhances the pressor response of the mesenteric vascular bed to periarterial nerve stimulation to a greater extent in SHR than it does in WKY. In addition, the angiotensin response to periarterial nerve stimulation is potentiated in the presence of cocaine. These results suggest that the presynaptic facilitatory modulation of adrenergic vascular neurotransmission mediated by angiotensin receptors is enhanced in the perfused mesenteric vascular bed of SHR.

Similar results were obtained by Eikenburg and co-workers using a similar preparation (81). These investigators observed that sub-pressor concentrations of angiotensin potentiate the responses to nerve stimulation in SHR to a greater extent than they do in WKY. A direct demonstration that angiotensin causes a greater enhancement of the field stimulation–induced release of norepinephrine has been obtained in the isolated superfused portal vein. In these studies, angiotensin was observed to enhance the field stimulation–induced release of ^{3}H-norepinephrine from vessels obtained from SHR to a greater extent than those of normotensive controls (73–75). Enhancement of the facilitatory

Table 2 The role of presynaptic receptors on adrenergic neurotransmission in the blood vessels of hypertensive animals

Receptor type	Type of hypertension	Blood vessel or vascular bed	Observation	References
Angiotensin	Genetic (SHR)	Caudal artery	Greater enhancement by angiotensin of endogenous norepinephrine release to field stimulation in 10 and 28 weeks SHR>WKY	74, 85
Angiotensin	Genetic (SHR)	Portal vein	Greater enhancement by angiotensin of ^{3}H-norepinephrine release to field stimulation in 10- and 28-week SHR>WKY	73–75
Angiotensin	Genetic (SHR)	Perfused mesentery	Greater enhancement by angiotensin of pressor response to periarterial nerve stimulation in 18-week SHR>WKY	81
Angiotensin	Genetic (SHR)	Perfused mesentery	Potentiation by angiotensin of the pressor response to nerve stimulation in 15–16 week SHR>WKY	90
β-Adrenoceptor	Genetic (SHR)	Portal vein	Similar enhancement by β-agonist of ^{3}H-norepinephrine release to field stimulation in 10- and 28-week SHR and WKY	73, 85
β-Adrenoceptor	Genetic (SHR)	Perfused kidney	Similar enhancement by β-agonist of ^{3}H-norepinephrine release and reactivity to field stimulation in 14-week SHR and WKY	79
β-Adrenoceptor	Genetic (SHR)	Perfused mesentery	Greater enhancement by β-agonist of the response and ^{3}H-norepinephrine release to perivascular nerve stimulation in 14–16 week SHR>WKY	83
α_2 Adrenoceptor	Genetic (SHR)	Caudal artery	Decreased enhancement by yohimbine of endogenous norepinephrine release to field stimulation or high K$^+$ in 28-week SHR versus WKY. Similar response in 6- and 10-week SHR and WKY	72–74

Receptor	Model	Preparation	Description	Ref.
α_2 Adrenoceptor	Genetic (SHR)	Portal vein	Decreased enhancement by yohimbine of ^{3}H-norepinephrine release to field stimulation of 28-week SHR versus WKY. Similar response in 6- and in 10-week SHR and WKY	74, 75
α_2 Adrenoceptor	One clip-one kidney; DOCA-salt	Caudal artery and portal vein	Similar enhancement by yohimbine of endogenous norepinephrine or ^{3}H-norepinephrine release to field stimulation in hypertensive or sham controls	74, 85
α_2 Adrenoceptor	Neurogenic baroreceptor	Mesenteric artery	Similar enhancement by phentolamine of ^{3}H-norepinephrine release to field stimulation	87
α_2 Adrenoceptor	Genetic (SHR)	Perfused mesentery	Similar enhancement by α-antagonist on response and ^{3}H-norepinephrine release to periarterial nerve stimulation in 18-week SHR and WKY	79, 101
α_2 Adrenoceptor	Genetic (SHR)	Perfused kidney	Increased inhibition by α-agonist on response and ^{3}H-norepinephrine release to periarterial	78
Purine (adenosine, ATP)	Genetic (SHR)	Perfused mesentery	Decreased inhibitory response and ^{3}H-norepinephrine release by adenosine to perivascular nerve stimulation in 5-week and 15–18 week SHR compared to WKY	107, 108
Purine (adenosine)	Renal artery	Perfused mesentery	Similar inhibitory response and ^{3}H-norepinephrine release by adenosine	80
Serotonin	Genetic (SHR)	Perfused mesentery	Decreased inhibitory response by serotonin to periarterial nerve stimulation in 15–18 week SHR compared to WKY	110

effect of angiotensin was apparent in SHR at 10 weeks of age, as it was in older animals (28 weeks of age).

Although the enhancement of norepinephrine release by angiotensin may be very important in contributing to elevated blood pressure in young SHR as well as in older animals, other mechanisms must be involved in the initial increase in transmitter release, since such an increase has been observed in animals at six weeks of age. Additional evidence for the involvement of angiotensin in hypertension development in SHR comes from studies showing that the responses to nerve stimulation, but not to norepinephrine, in SHR are decreased by captopril, a converting enzyme inhibitor. These studies further suggest a presynaptic rather than a postsynaptic effect for angiotensin in SHR (91).

In addition to angiotensin, it has been shown that activation of presynaptic ß-adrenoceptors also leads to an enhancement in the evoked release of norepinephrine from a variety of neuroeffector junctions (92–95). Whether or not there are alterations in the activity of presynaptic ß-adrenoceptors in the blood vessels of SHR or other hypertensive animals is currently unclear. Two studies have reported that the functional activity of presynaptic ß-adrenoceptors is similar in blood vessels of normotensive and hypertensive animals (75, 79). In the isolated portal vein, the effect of isoproterenol or terbutaline to enhance the field stimulation–induced release of ^{3}H-norepinephrine is similar in vessels obtained from SHR and from age-matched WKY (75). Another study reported that presynaptic ß-adrenoceptor function is similar in the isolated kidney of 14–week old SHR and WKY (79). In contrast to these two studies, it has been reported that ß-adrenoceptor agonists produce an enhancement of the response of the isolated mesenteric vascular bed from SHR compared to WKY (83). These investigators concluded that this enhancement is due to the facilitated release of neurotransmitter from adrenergic nerves mediated by presynaptic $ß_2$-adrenoceptors. The results of these studies cannot be directly compared because the studies were carried out in different preparations (i.e. an isolated blood vessel versus a perfused vascular bed). In addition, in the two studies reporting no enhancement of neurotransmission by ß-adrenoceptor agonist, transmission was evaluated by monitoring transmitter release (75, 79), while in the study reporting enhancement, changes in perfusion pressure to periarterial nerve stimulation were monitored (83). It is possible that alterations in presynaptic ß-adrenoceptor activity take place at the level of the small resistance vessels and arteries but not in larger vessels or in veins. Since the vasculature exhibits such heterogeneity, there is need for great caution when extrapolating data from one vascular preparation to another. In view of the lack of changes in prejunctional $ß_2$-adrenoceptor activity in at least two vascular preparations (portal vein and perfused kidney) in contrast to evidence for a change in the mesenteric bed, specific changes may take place at some neuroeffector junctions but not others. Clearly, additional studies are necessary to unravel the pathophysiological significance of these observations.

Even in the absence of alterations in presynaptic ß-adrenoceptor activity (i.e. increased activity), these receptors may still be implicated in hypertension. Several investigators have proposed that circulating epinephrine facilitates the release of norepinephrine by stimulating presynaptic ß-adrenoceptors. This is supported by several lines of evidence. First, presynaptic β_2-adrenoceptors have been demonstrated in human omental blood vessels (94). Second, an increase in circulating epinephrine (96, 97) has been observed in some types of hypertension. Third, the implantation of rats with a slow-release preparation of epinephrine can raise blood pressure. Moreover, it has been shown that following such implants there is an increase in the epinephrine content of tissue such as the atria (98, 99), suggesting the uptake of epinephrine into sympathetic nerve terminals. Sympathetic nerve stimulation of the atria could then lead to the release of epinephrine as a co-transmitter, which could then activate presynaptic ß-adrenoceptors, leading to the enhanced release of norepinephrine. Finally, bilateral demedullectomy has been shown to attenuate the pressor response to sympathetic nerve stimulation (100).

Several studies have been carried out to examine whether or not there are changes in presynaptic inhibitory receptor function in blood vessels of hypertensive animals. The selective prejunctional α_2-adrenoceptor antagonist yohimbine has been used to evaluate whether or not changes in the presynaptic α_2-adrenoceptors could help explain the increased field stimulation–induced release of norepinephrine from the isolated portal vein or caudal artery of SHR (72–75). Yohimbine was seen to produce the same degree of enhancement in the evoked release of ^{3}H-norepinephrine and endogenous norepinephrine from SHR (at six and ten weeks of age), one clip-one kidney renal hypertensive rats or DOCA-salt hypertensive rats compared to their respective sham controls. However, the effect of yohimbine to enhance the overflow of norepinephrine was greatly attenuated when examined in 28–week old SHR. The attenuation of the yohimbine effect was observed regardless of the way transmitter release was produced (field stimulation, potassium depolarization) and in both the caudal artery and the portal vein. These results are consistent with a decreased functional activity of presynaptic α_2-adrenoceptors in mature SHR.

The results obtained in the portal vein and caudal artery of six- and ten–week old SHR are consistent with the studies carried out in the mesenteric vascular bed in young SHR (81, 101), which suggests that presynaptic α_2–adrenoceptor mediated inhibition is similar in SHR and age-matched WKY at these ages. These investigators did not examine presynaptic α_2-adrenoceptor function in older animals, so it is not known whether the results obtained in the caudal artery and portal vein in 28–week old SHR represent only an age-related change or a difference in the response of different blood vessels.

In contrast to the results showing no difference in inhibitory presynaptic α_2-adrenoceptor function in the cadual artery, portal vein, or perfused mesenteric bed of young SHR (72–75, 81, 101) and a decreased α_2-adrenoceptor function in the caudal artery and portal vein of mature SHR (28–week old) (72–75), there is evidence for an increased α_2-adrenoceptor function in the perfused kidney of 14–week old SHR (79). It is not known whether this increased α_2-adrenoceptor activity in the kidney changes with age or whether it represents a tissue difference. Interestingly, there appears to be an increase in the binding of α_2-adrenoceptor ligands in the kidney membranes obtained from SHR compared to WKY (102–4). These results are consistent with an increase in α_2-adrenoceptors in the kidney. It is likely, however, that the vast majority of these receptors are located postsynaptically rather than presynaptically.

Adrenergic neurotransmission has been shown to be decreased by purine compounds such as adenosine and ATP (105, 106) presumably acting on purinergic receptors located on adrenergic nerve terminals. It has been observed that both ATP and adenosine inhibit the neurogenic vasoconstriction of the perfused mesenteric vascular bed to perivascular nerve stimulation in a dose-dependent manner in WKY (107). The effect of adenosine was approximately eight times greater than that of ATP. In the same preparation, isolated from 17- to 21–week old SHR, the inhibitory effects of both adenosine and ATP were significantly smaller than in WKY. In another series of experiments, adenosine was observed to decrease the efflux of ^{3}H-norepinephrine due to sympathetic nerve stimulation of the same preparation (108). The inhibition was smaller in both prehypertensive (five weeks old) and hypertensive (15–18 weeks) SHR compared with age-matched WKY. A decrease in the adenosine effect was not seen in Wistar rats rendered hypertensive by left renal artery occlusion. These results suggest that presynaptic inhibition of vascular adrenergic neurotransmission by purine compounds is reduced in SHR and that this diminished response to purines is genetically inherent to SHR. Studies carried out in the perfused kidney are at variance with the observations in the mesenteric bed (80). In the latter studies, it was observed that adenosine is equally effective in causing an inhibition of the stimulation-induced release of norepinephrine in both WKY and SHR.

Serotonin has also been shown to modulate norepinephrine release in blood vessels and other adrenergic neuroeffector junctions (109), producing both inhibition and enhancement of adrenergic transmission most likely by acting on different receptors. In the perfused mesenteric vascular bed, serotonin has been shown to augment the nerve stimulation–induced pressor response (110). In the WKY such potentiation to nerve stimulation was less than to exogenously administered norepinephrine, which is most likely due to inhibition of the nerve stimulation–induced release of norepinephrine from adrenergic nerve terminals. In SHR, unlike WKY, there was little difference between the potentiating effects of serotonin on nerve stimulation and norepinephrine-induced vasocon-striction. These results suggest that presynaptic inhibitory modulation by serotonin is diminished in the mesenteric vasculature from SHR.

ALTERATIONS IN THE SYNTHESIS STORAGE AND UPTAKE OF NOREPINEPHRINE IN PRESYNAPTIC NERVE TERMINALS IN HYPERTENSION

In addition to alterations in the release of norepinephrine and its modulation by presynaptic receptors, a large body of evidence shows changes in the synthesis, storage, and uptake of norepinephrine in adrenergic nerve varicosities in hypertensive animals and man. A discussion of this aspect of the adrenergic nerve terminal is beyond the scope of this review, and the reader is referred to several recent reviews that discuss this aspect of the pathophysiology of hypertension (7, 8, 26, 27). Because of the connection among the uptake, release, and presynaptic modulation of transmitter release, a brief summary of alterations in the uptake of norepinephrine is provided.

The principal mechanism for removing or inactivating norepinephrine from the neuroeffector junction following its release from adrenergic nerve terminals is the specific neuronal uptake process. Alterations in the uptake process can have profound biological responses, with an increase in uptake resulting in a decrease in the physiological response of the effector cell. Decreases in uptake result in an enhancement of the biological response. Several studies have examined the uptake of catecholamines in hypertensive animals, but many are controversial because of conflicting results. Most investigators report a decrease in the uptake of norepinephrine into myocardial tissue of a variety of hypertensive animals, including several strains of SHR (111–14), DOCA-salt hypertensives (115, 116), animals made hypertensive with 10% NaCl (117), adrenal regeneration hypertensives (117), and animals made hypertensive with a figure eight knot around the kidney (117). Decreased norepinephrine uptake has also been reported for the kidney of 14–week old SHR (118), the spleen of SHR (119), and the mesenteric arteries of perinephretic hypertensive dogs (120). A decreased uptake of norepinephrine into the vasculature of human essential hypertensive patients has also been reported (121).

On the other hand, a number of studies have provided evidence that there is an increase in the uptake of norepinephrine into the arteries of hypertensive animals. An increased uptake of norepinephrine has been indirectly implicated because there is a greater shift to the left of the response to sympathetic nerve stimulation or the administration of norepinephrine in SHR compared to WKY following cocaine treatment or sympathetic denervation (122). In addition, several reports indicate an increased accumulation (possibly due to increased uptake) of norepinephrine in the mesenteric and caudal artery of the SHR as well as in the ear artery of rabbits made hypertensive by placing a ligature on the abdominal aorta proximal to the kidney (45, 123–26). In the latter study, it is of interest that an increase in norepinephrine uptake and levels was seen in vessels where the blood pressure was elevated, but not in arteries below the ligature, where the pressure was normal, or in the heart or veins. A lack of increased uptake of norepinephrine into veins has been consistently seen (75).

INCREASED CATECHOLAMINE RELEASE IN ESSENTIAL HYPERTENSION IN MAN

A simple and accurate way of evaluating increased sympathetic and sympathoadrenal activity in humans is currently not available. The most common approach has been to measure plasma catecholamines. The introduction of sensitive, specific techniques for measuring plasma catecholamines (127, 128) has produced an explosion in studies attempting to relate alterations in plasma catecholamines with disease states such as hypertension (129). Increases in catecholamines do occur in many situations where there is an increase in sympathetic nerve activity. However, great caution must be used when attempting to relate plasma catecholamines to increased sympathetic nerve activity or to a specific disease such as hypertension. Such caution has been the subject of numerous reviews and editorials (e.g. 10, 130–38). Most authorities have identified at least three major problems with the use of plasma catecholamines as an index of neurogenic function. First, the assays themselves are difficult and tedious and the concentrations of catecholamines very low in most situations. Second, a large number of environmental factors contribute to the wide variation in plasma catecholamines. These include age, stress, drugs, and electrolytes, to name but a few. Third, the catecholamines found in the peripheral circulation are only a small part of the amount released from the postganglionic sympathetic nerve varicosities and the adrenal medulla. The amount of catecholamine, especially norepinephrine, that enters the circulation depends not only on the level of sympathetic nerve activity (nerve impulse frequency), but on the amount of catecholamine release per nerve impulse (subject to local regulation by release modulatory autocoids and endocoids), the extent of reuptake into nerve varicosities, the proportion metabolized in the tissues before reaching the circulation, the uptake into non-neural tissue, the binding to postjunctional receptors, the site of sampling, the rate of blood flow through the tissue, and other factors.

Recent techniques have approached the problem kinetically, utilizing the intravenous administration of high specific activity–labeled norepinephrine to reach steady-state plasma concentrations and to determine plasma norepinephrine concentration and specific activity under steady-state conditions (136, 139, 140). Such techniques allow a more accurate measurement of the rate of entry of norepinephrine into the plasma as well as the clearance of norepinephrine from the plasma. Such approaches should have some advantages over the classical techniques.

As mentioned above, as long as the various factors are kept in mind or controlled for, measurement of plasma catecholamines has provided an index of sympathetic nerve activity for comparison within individuals or among large groups. Although this approach is still extremely controversial, comparing all of the more than 90 studies appears to indicate higher catecholamine levels in hypertensives. Multiple papers and reviews have summarized the results of these many studies (130, 141–149). About 40% report a statistically significant increase in plasma catecholamines over normotensive controls. The most consistent and dramatic differences were seen among young hypertensive patients. It seems that in subpopulations of patients increased catecholamine levels are positively correlated with the disease. The occurrence of elevated norepinephrine in the young, established hypertensive patient is consistent with a pathophysiological role for increased sympathetic neural activity in this subgroup. Whether or not enhanced sympathetic nerve activity is primarily mediated by the central nervous system or the peripheral nervous system in essential hypertension remains to be established. Likewise, whether the enhanced release of catecholamines is involved in the development or maintenance of this hypertension or both is unknown.

CONCLUSION

Available evidence suggests that there is an increase in sympathetic nerve activity in the development and maintenance of many forms of experimental hypertension in animals and in human essential hypertension. In many cases, other mechanisms may also be present. Increased sympathetic nerve activity is due in part to increased activity in central vasomotor centers. In addition, alterations at the level of the adrenergic nerve terminals may also be present. There is an increase in the stimulation-induced release of norepinephrine from isolated blood vessels, isolated perfused organs, and isolated perfused vascular beds of the spontaneously hypertensive rat, considered by many a good model of essential hypertension. These effects appear to take place in addition to increased central nervous system activity. The increased release of norepinephrine may contribute to the development and/or maintenance of hypertension. Some evidence suggests that there are alterations in presynaptic receptors at the vascular neuroeffector junction. The activity of angiotensin receptors and of ß-adrenoceptors may increase and the activity of adenosine receptors may decrease. Alterations in these presynaptic receptors could contribute to the increased release of norepinephrine that has been observed. In chronic hypertensive SHR, a decrease in presynaptic α_2-adrenoceptors may take place. Because of the potential importance of these mechanisms, additional studies are clearly needed to further define the pathophysiological importance of these systems.

ACKNOWLEDGMENTS

The authors' research has been supported by grants from the Department of Health and Human Services, National Institutes of Health, NS 16215, HL 26319 and the Alcohol, Drug Abuse, and Mental Health Agency, DA-02668.

Literature Cited

1. Folkow, B. 1982. Physiological aspects of primary hypertension. *Physiol. Rev.* 62:347–504
2. Beyer, K. H., Peuler, J. 1982. Hypertension: Perspectives. *Pharmacol. Rev.* 34: 287–313
3. Khosla, M. C., Page, I. H., Bumpus, F. M. 1979. Interrelations between various blood pressure regulator systems and the mosaic theory of hypertension. *Biochem. Pharmacol.* 28:2867–82
4. Birkenhager, W. H., DeLeeuw, P. W. 1980. Pathophysiological mechanisms in essential hypertension. *Pharmacol. Ther.* 8:297–319
5. Abboud, F. M. 1982. The sympathetic system in hypertension. *Hypertension* 4(Suppl. 2):208–25
6. Chalmers, J. P. 1978. Nervous system and hypertension. *Clin. Sci.* 55:45s–56s
7. Vanhoutte, P. M., Webb, R. C., Collis, M. G. 1980. Pre- and post-junctional adrenergic mechanisms and hypertension. *Clin. Sci.* 59(Suppl. 6):211s–23s
8. Vanhoutte, P. M. 1980. The adrenergic neuroeffector interaction in the normotensive and hypertensive blood vessel wall. *J. Cardiovasc. Pharmacol.* 2(Suppl. 3):S253–67
9. Weber, M. A., Drayer, J. I. 1982. The sympathetic nervous system in primary hypertension. *Miner. Electrolyte Metab.* 7:57–66
10. Fitzgerald, G. A. 1979. Neurogenic aspects of essential hypertension in man. *Ir. J. Med. Sci.* 148:280–89
11. Bunag, R. D., Takeda, K. 1979. Sympathetic hyperresponsiveness to hypothalamic stimulation in young hypertensive rats. *Am. J. Physiol.* 237:R39–44
12. Okamoto, K., Nosaka, S., Yamori, Y., Matsumoto, M. 1967. Participation of neural factor in the pathogenesis of hypertension in the spontaneously hypertensive rat. *Jpn. Heart J.* 8:168–80
13. Iriuchijima, J. 1973. Sympathetic discharge rate in spontaneously hypertensive rats. *Jpn. Heart J.* 14:350–56
14. Takeda, K., Bunag, R. D. 1980. Augmented sympathetic nerve activity and pressor responsiveness in DOCA hypertensive rats. *Hypertension* 2:97–101
15. Judy, W. V., Watanabe, A. M., Murphy, W. R., Aprison, B. S., Yu, P. L. 1979. Sympathetic nerve activity and blood pressure in normotensive backcross rats genetically related to the spontaneously hypertensive rat. *Hypertension* 1:598–604
16. Provoost, A. P., DeJong, W. 1978. Differential development of renal, DOCA-salt and spontaneous hypertension in the rat after neonatal sympathectomy. *Clin. Exp. Hyperten.* 1:177–89
17. Haeusler, G. 1981. Central mechanism in blood pressure regulation and hypertension. *Int. J. Obesity* 5(Suppl. 1):45–50
18. Nakamura, K., Nakamura, K. 1978. Activation of central noradrenergic and adrenergic neurons in young and adult spontaneously hypertensive rats. *Jpn. Heart J.* 635–36
19. Eide, I., Myers, M. R., DeQuattro, V., Kolloch, R., Eide, K., Whigham, H. 1980. Increased hypothalamic noradrenergic activity in one kidney, one-clip neurovascular hypertensive rats. *J. Cardiovasc. Pharmacol.* 2:833–41
20. Kubo, T., Hashimoto, M. 1978. Effect of intraventricular and intraspinal 6-hydroxydopamine on blood pressure of spontaneously hypertensive rats. *Arch. Int. Pharmacol.* 232:166–76
21. Saavedra, J. M., Grobecker, H., Axelrod, J. 1978. Changes in central catecholaminergic neurons in spontaneously (genetic) hypertensive rats. *Circ. Res.* 42:529–34
22. Renaud, B., Fourniere, S., Denoroy, L., Vincent, M., Pujol, J. F., et al. 1978. Early increase in phenylethanolamine N-

methyltransferase activity in a new strain of spontaneously hypertensive rats. *Brain Res.* 159:149–59

23. Petty, M. A., Reid, J. L. 1979. Catecholamine synthesizing enzymes in brain stem and hypothalamus during the development of renovascular hypertension. *Brain Res.* 163:277–88

24. Matsuguchi, H., Sharabi, F. M., O'Connor, G., Mark, A., Schmid, P. G. 1982. Central mechanisms in DOCA-salt hypertensive rats. *Clin. Exp. Hyperten. A* 4:1303–21

25. Trippodo, N. C., Frohlich, E. D. 1981. Similarities of genetic (spontaneous) hypertension in man and rat. *Circ. Res.* 48:309–19

26. Zimmerman, B. G. 1983. Peripherial neurogenic factors in acute and chronic alterations of arterial pressure. *Circ. Res.* 53:121–30

27. Vanhoutte, P. M., Verbeuren, T. J., Webb, R. C. 1981. Local modulation of adrenergic neuroeffector interaction in the blood vessel wall. *Physiol. Rev.* 61:151–247

28. Weiner, N., Cloutier, G., Bjur, R., Pfeffer, R. I. 1972. Modification of norepinephrine synthesis in intact tissue by drugs and during short term adrenergic nerve stimulation. *Pharmacol. Rev.* 24:203–21

29. Weinshilboum, R. M. 1979. Serum dopamine ß-hydroxylase. *Pharmacol. Rev.* 30:133–66

30. Gillespie, J. 1980. Presynaptic receptors in the autonomic nervous system. *Handb. Exp. Pharmacol.* 54:169–205

31. Langer, S. Z. 1977. Presynaptic receptors and their role in the regulation of transmitter release. *Br. J. Pharmacol.* 60:481–97

32. Langer, S. Z. 1980. Presynaptic regulation of the release of catecholamines. *Pharmacol. Rev.* 32:337–62

33. Langer, S. Z., Starke, K., Dubocovich, M., eds. 1979. *Presynaptic Receptors.* New York: Pergamon

34. Patel, S., Patel, U., Vithalani, D., Verma, S. C. 1981. Regulation of catecholamine release by presynaptic receptor system. *Gen. Pharmacol.* 12:405–22

35. Paton, D. M., ed. 1979. *The Release of Catecholamines from Adrenergic Neurons,* pp. 1–393. Oxford: Pergamon

36. Starke, K. 1977. Regulation of noradrenaline release by presynaptic receptor systems. *Rev. Physiol. Biochem. Pharmacol.* 77:1–124

37. Starke, K. 1981. Presynaptic receptors. *Ann. Rev. Pharmacol. Toxicol.* 21:7–30

38. Vizi, E. S. 1979. Presynaptic modulation of neurochemical transmission. *Prog. Neurobiol.* 12:181–290

39. Westfall, T. C. 1977. Local regulation of adrenergic neurotransmission. *Physiol. Rev.* 57:659–728

40. Westfall, T. C. 1980. Neuroeffector mechanisms. *Ann. Rev. Physiol.* 42:383–97

41. Westfall, T. C. 1984. Evidence that noradrenergic transmitter release is regulated by presynaptic receptors. *Fed. Proc.* 43:1352–57

42. Lokhandwala, M. F., Eikenburg, D. C. 1983. Presynaptic receptors and alterations in noradrenaline release in spontaneously hypertensive rats. *Life Sci.* 33:1527–42

43. Collis, M. G., Vanhoutte, P. M. 1978. Neuronal and vascular reactivity in isolated perfused kidneys during the development of spontaneous hypertension. *Clin. Sci.* 55:233s–35s

44. Collis, M. G., DeMey, C., Vanhoutte, P. M. 1980. Renal vascular reactivity in the young spontaneously hypertensive rat. *Hypertension* 2:45–52

45. Bevan, R. D., Purdy, R. E., Su, C., Bevan, J. A. 1975. Evidence for an increase in adrenergic nerve function in blood vessels from hypertensive rabbits. *Circ. Res.* 37:503–8

46. Takeshita, A., Mark, A. L. 1978. Neurogenic contributions to hindquarters vasoconstriction during high sodium intake in Dahl strain of genetically hypertensive rat. *Circ. Res.* 43:I86–I91

47. Brody, M. J., Dorr, L. D., Shaffer, R. A. 1970. Reflex vasodilation and sympathetic transmission in the renal hypertensive dog. *Am. J. Physiol.* 219:1746–50

48. Zimmerman, B. G., Rolewicz, T. F., Dunham, E. W., Gisslen, J. L. 1969. Transmitter release and vascular responses in skin and muscle of hypertensive dogs. *Am. J. Physiol.* 217:798–804

49. Dargie, H. J., Franklin, S. S., Reid, J. L. 1976. The sympathetic nervous system and neurovascular hypertension in the rat. *Br. J. Pharmacol.* 56:365P

50. Touw, K. B., Haywood, J. R., Shaffer, R. A., Brody, M. J. 1980. Contribution of the sympathetic nervous system to vascular resistance in conscious young and adult spontaneously hypertensive rats. *Hypertension* 2:409–18

51. Lais, L. T., Shaffer, R. A., Brody, M. J. 1974. Neurogenic and humoral factors controlling vascular resistance in the spontaneously hypertensive rat. *Circ. Res.* 35:764–74

52. Hamed, A. T., Lokhandwala, M. F. 1982. Impairment of neurally mediated

vasoconstriction in DOCA-salt hypertensive dogs. *Clin. Exp. Hyperten. A* 4:867–81

53. Palermo, A., Constantini, C., Mara, G., Libretti, A. 1981. Role of the sympathetic nervous system in spontaneous hypertension: Changes in central adrenoceptors and plasma catecholamine levels. *Clin. Sci.* 61:195s–98s (Suppl. 7)

54. Affara, S., Denoroy, L., Renaud, B., Vincent, M., Sassard, J. 1980. Serum dopamine-ß-hydroxylase activity in a new strain of spontaneously hypertensive rat. *Experientia* 36:1207–8

55. Nagatsu, T., Kato, T., Numata, Y., Ikuta, K., Umezawa, H., et al. 1974. Serum dopamine ß-hydroxylase activity in developing hypertensive rats. *Nature* 251:630–31

56. Pak, C. H. 1981. Plasma adrenaline and noradrenaline concentrations of the spontaneously hypertensive rat. *Jpn. Heart J.* 22:987–95

57. Picotti, G. B., Carruba, M. O., Ravazzani, G., Bondiolotti, G. P., DaPrada, M. 1982. Plasma catecholamine concentrations in normotensive rats of different strains and in spontaneously hypertensive rats under basal conditions and during cold exposure. *Life Sci.* 31:2137–43

58. Chiueh, C. C., Kopin, I. J. 1978. Hyperresponsivity of spontaneously hypertensive rat to indirect measurement of blood pressure. *Am. J. Physiol.* 234:H690–95

59. Kvetnansky, R., McCarty, R., Thoa, N. B., Lake, C. R., Kopin, I. J. 1979. Sympatho-adrenal responses of spontaneously hypertensive rats to immobilization stress. *Am. J. Physiol.* 236:H457–62

60. McCarty, R., Chiueh, C. C., Kopin, I. J. 1978. Spontaneously hypertensive rats: adrenergic hyperresponsivity to anticipation of electric shock. *Behav. Biol.* 22:405–10

61. McCarty, R., Kopin, I. J. 1978. Alterations in plasma catecholamines and behavior during acute stress in spontaneously hypertensive and Wistar Kyoto normotensive rats. *Life Sci.* 22:997–1005

62. Pak, C. H. 1981. Plasma adrenaline and noradrenaline concentrations of the spontaneously hypertensive rat. *Jpn. Heart J.* 22:987–95

63. Vlachakis, N. D., Alexander, N., Maronde, R. F. 1980. Increased plasma normetanephrine in spontaneously hypertensive rats. *Clin. Exp. Hyperten.* 2:309–19

64. Thoren, P., Ricksten, S. E. 1979. Recordings of renal and splanchnic sympathetic nervous activity in normotensive

and spontaneously hypertensive rats. *Clin. Sci.* 57(Suppl. 5):197s–99s

65. Judy, W. V., Watanabe, A. M., Henry, D. P., Besch, H. R. Jr., Murphy, W. R., Hockel, G. M. 1976. Sympathetic nerve activity. Role in regulation of blood pressure in the spontaneously hypertensive rat. *Circ. Res.* 38(Suppl. 2):21–29

66. Judy, W. V., Watanabe, A. M., Henry, D. P., Besch, H. R., Aprison, B. S. 1978. Effect of L-dopa on sympathetic nerve activity and blood pressure in the spontaneously hypertensive rat. *Circ. Res.* 43:24–28

67. Yamaguchi, I., Kopin, I. J. 1980. Blood pressure, plasma catecholamines and sympathetic outflow in pithed SHR and WKY rats. *Am. J. Physiol.* 238:H365–72

68. Fujita, K., Teradaira, R., Inoue, T., Takahashi, H., Beppu, H., et al. 1982. Stress induced changes in *in vivo* and *in vitro* dopamine ß-hydroxylase activity in spontaneously hypertensive rats. *Biochem. Med.* 28:340–46

69. Hallback, M., Folkow, B. 1974. Cardiovascular responses to acute mental stress in spontaneously hypertensive rats. *Acta Physiol. Scand.* 90:684–98

70. Folkow, B., Hallback, M., Lundgren, Y., Weiss, L. 1972. The effects of "immunosympathectomy" on blood pressure and vascular reactivity in normal and spontaneously hypertensive rats. *Acta Physiol. Scand.* 84:512–23

71. Yamori, Y., Yamabe, H., DeJong, W., Lovenberg, W., Sjoersdsma, A. 1972. Effect of tissue norepinephrine depletion by 6-hydroxydopamine in spontaneously hypertensive rats. *Eur. J. Pharmacol.* 17:135–40

72. Galloway, M. P., Westfall, T. C. 1982. The release of endogenous norepinephrine from the coccygeal artery of spontaneously hypertensive and Wistar-Kyoto rats. *Circ. Res.* 51:225–32

73. Westfall, T. C., Galloway, M. P., Meldrum, M. J., Sax, R. D., Earnhardt, J. T., et al. 1983. Role of nerve impulse traffic and hypertension on prejunctional adrenoceptor function. In *Vascular Neuroeffector Mechanisms: 4th Int. Symp.*, ed. J. A. Bevan, pp. 117–24. New York: Raven

74. Westfall, T. C., Meldrum, M. J., Badino, L., Xue, C.-S. 1984. Noradrenergic transmission in blood vessels: Influence of hypertension and dietary sodium. In *Catecholamines: Basic and Peripheral Mechanisms*, ed. E. Usdin, pp. 319–26. New York: Liss

75. Westfall, T. C., Meldrum, M. J., Badino, L., Earnhardt, J. T. 1984. Noadren-

ergic transmission in the isolated portal vein of the spontaneously hypertensive rat. *Hypertension* 6:267–74

76. Zsoter, T. T., Wolchinsky, C., Lawrin, M., Sirko, S. 1982. Norepinephrine release in arteries of spontaneously hypertensive rats. *Clin. Exp. Hyperten. A* 4:431–44

77. Collis, M. G., DeMey, C., Vanhoutte, P. M. 1979. Enhanced release of noradrenaline in the kidney of the young spontaneously hypertensive rat. *Clin. Sci.* 57:233s–34s (Suppl. 5)

78. Ekas, R. D., Steenberg, M. L., Lokhandwala, M. F. 1982. Increased presynaptic α-adrenoceptor mediated regulation of noradrenaline release in the isolated perfused kidney of spontaneously hypertensive rats. *Clin. Sci.* 63:309s–11s (Suppl. 8)

79. Ekas, R. D., Steenberg, M. L., Woods, M. D., Lokhandwala, M. F. 1983. Presynaptic α- and ß-adrenoceptor stimulation and norepinephrine release in the spontaneously hypertensive rat. *Hypertension* 5:198–204

80. Ekas, R. D., Steenberg, M. L., Lokhandwala, M. F. 1983. Increased norepinephrine release during sympathetic nerve stimulation and its inhibition by adenosine in the isolated perfused kidney of spontaneously hypertensive rats. *Clin. Exp. Hyperten. A* 5:41–48

81. Eikenberg, D. C., Ekas, R. D., Lokhandwala, M. F. 1981. Presynaptic modulation of norepinephrine release by α-adrenoceptors and angiotensin II receptors in spontaneously hypertensive rats. In *Central Nervous System Mechanisms in Hypertension,* ed. J. P. Buckley, C. M. Ferraro, pp. 215–28. New York: Raven

82. Ekas, R. D., Lokhandwala, M. F. 1981. Sympathetic nerve function and vascular reactivity in spontaneously hypertensive rats. *Am. J. Physiol.* 241:R379–84

83. Kawasaki, I., Cline, W. H. Jr., Su, C. 1982. Enhanced presynaptic beta adrenoceptor mediated modulation of vascular adrenergic neurotransmission in spontaneously hypertensive rats. *J. Pharmacol. Exp. Ther.* 223:721–28

84. Vanhoutte, P. M., Browning, D., Coen, E., Verbeuren, T. J., Zonnekeyn, L., et al., 1982. Decreased release of norepinephrine in the isolated kidney of the adult spontaneously hypertensive rat. *Hypertension* 4:251–56

85. Westfall, T. C., Xue, C.-S., Carpentier, S., Meldrum, M. 1985. Modulation of noradrenaline release by presynaptic adrenoceptors in experimental hyperten-

sion. In *Pharmacology of Adrenoceptors,* ed. E. Szabadi. In press

86. Ekas, R. D., Lokhandwala, M. F. 1980. Sympathetic nerve function and vascular reactivity in DOCA-salt hypertensive rats. *Am. J. Physiol.* 239:R303–8

87. Granata, A. R., Enero, M. A., Krieger, E. M., Langer, S. Z. 1983. Norepinephrine release and vascular response elicited by nerve stimulation in rats with chronic neurogenic hypertension. *J. Pharmacol. Exp. Ther.* 227:187–93

88. Zimmerman, B. G., Whitmore, L. 1967. Effect of angiotensin and phenoxybenzamine on the release of norepinephrine in vessels during sympathetic nerve stimulation. *Int. J. Neuropharmacol.* 6:27–38

89. Zimmerman, B. G. 1978. Actions of angiotensin on adrenergic nerve endings. *Fed. Proc.* 37:199–202

90. Kawasaki, H., Cline, W. H. Jr., Su, C. 1982. Enhanced angiotensin mediated facilitation of adrenergic neurotransmission in spontaneously hypertensive rats. *J. Pharamacol. Exp. Ther.* 221:112–16

91. Antonaccio, M. J., Kerwin, L. 1980. Evidence for prejunctional inhibition of norepinephrine release by captopril in spontaneously hypertensive rats. *Eur. J. Pharmacol.* 68:209–12

92. Adler-Grascinsky, E., Langer, S. Z. 1975. Possible role of a ß-adrenoceptor in the regulation of noradrenaline release by nerve stimulation through a positive feed back mechanism. *Br. J. Pharmacol.* 53:43–50

93. Dahlof, C. 1981. Studies on ß-adrenoceptor mediated facilitation of sympathetic neurotransmission. *Acta Physiol. Scand.* 500:1–147 (Suppl.)

94. Stjarne, L., Brundin, J. 1976. ß₂-adrenoceptors facilitating noradrenaline secretion from human vasoconstrictor nerves. *Acta Physiol. Scand.* 97:88–93

95. Westfall, T. C., Peach, M. J., Tittermary, V. 1979. Enhancement of the electrically induced release of norepinephrine from the rat portal vein: Mediation by ß₂-adrenoceptors. *Eur. J. Pharmacol.* 58:67–74

96. deChamplain, J., Farley, L., Cousineau, D., Van Ameringen, M. R. 1976. Circulating catecholamine levels in human and experimental hypertension. *Circ. Res.* 38:109–14

97. Franco-Morselli, R., Baudoum-Legros, M., Guicheney, M., Meyer, P. 1968. Plasma catecholamines in essential human hypertension and in DOCA-salt hypertension in the rat. In *Circulating Catecholamines and Blood Pressure,* ed.

W. H. Birkenhager, H. E. Falks, pp. 27–38. Utrecht: Bunge

98. Majewski, H., Tung, L.-H., Rand, M. J. 1982. Adrenaline activation of prejunctional ß-adrenoceptors and hypertension. *J. Cardiovasc. Pharmacol.* 4:99–106

99. Majewski, H., Tung, L.-H., Rand, M. J. 1981. Adrenaline-induced hypertension in rats. *J. Cardiovasc. Pharmacol.* 3:179–85

100. Borkowski, K. R., Quinn, P. 1983. The effect of bilateral adrenal demedullation on vascular reactivity and blood pressure in spontaneously hypertensive rats. *Br. J. Pharmacol.* 80:429–37

101. Su, C., Kamikawa, Y., Kubo, T., Cline, W. H. Jr. 1982. Inhibitory modulation of vascular adrenergic neurotransmission in the SHR. *Proc. Springfield Blood Vessel Symp.*, ed. C. Su, pp. 33–37. Springfield: Southern Ill. Univ. Press

102. Sanchez, A., Pettinger, W. A. 1981. Dietary sodium regulation of blood pressure and renal alpha 1- and 2-receptors in WKY and SHR rats. *Life Sci.* 29:2795–802

103. Pettinger, W. A., Sanchez, A., Saavedra, J., Haywood, J. R., Gandler, T., et al. 1982. Altered renal alpha 2-adrenergic receptor regulation in genetically hypertensive rats. *Hypertension* 4(Suppl. 2):188–92

104. Graham, R. M., Pettinger, W. A., Sagalowsky, A., Brabson, J., Gandler, T. 1982. Renal alpha-adrenergic receptor abnormality in the spontaneously hypertensive rat. *Hypertension* 4:881–87

105. Su, C. 1978. Purinergic inhibition of adrenergic transmission in rabbit blood vessels. *J. Pharmacol. Exp. Ther.* 204:351–61

106. Moylan, R. D., Westfall, T. C. 1979. Effect of adenosine on adrenergic neurotransmission in the superfused rat portal vein. *Blood Vessels* 16:302–10

107. Kamikawa, Y., Cline, W. H. Jr., Su, C. 1980. Diminished purinergic modulating of the vascular adrenergic neurotransmission in the spontaneously hypertensive rat. *Eur. J. Pharmacol.* 66:347–53

108. Kubo, T., Su, C. 1983. Effects of adenosine on ^{3}H-norepinephrine release from perfused mesenteric arteries of SHR and renal hypertensive rats. *Eur. J. Pharmacol.* 87:349–52

109. McGrath, M. A. 1977. 5-Hydroxytryptamine and neurotransmitter release in canine blood vessels: Inhibition by low and augmentation by high concentrations. *Circ. Res.* 41:428–35

110. Kubo, T., Su, C. 1983. Effects of serotonin and some other neurohumoral agents on adrenergic neurotransmission in spontaneously hypertensive rat vasculature. *Clin. Exp. Hyperten. A* 5:1501–10

111. Salt, P. J., Iversen, L. L. 1973. Catecholamine uptake sites in the rat heart after 6-hydroxydopamine treatment and in a genetically hypertensive strain. *Naunyn Schmiedebergs Arch. Phamacol.* 279:381–86

112. Bell, C., Kushinsky, R. 1978. Involvement of uptake₁, uptake₂ in terminating the cardiovascular activity of noradrenaline in normotensive and genetically hypertensive rats. *J. Physiol.* 283:41–51

113. Rho, J. H., Newman, B., Alexander, N. 1981. Altered in vitro uptake of norepinephrine by cardiovascular tissues of spontaneously hypertensive rats. Part 2. Portal-mesenteric veins and atria. *Hypertension* 3:710–17

114. Howe, P. R. C., Provis, J. C., West, M. J., Chalmers, J. P. 1979. Changes in cardiac norepinephrine in spontaneously hypertensive and stroke-prone rats. *J. Cardiovasc. Pharmacol.* 1:115–22

115. deChamplain, J. 1972. Hypertension and the sympathetic nervous system. In *Perspectives in Neuropharmacology*, ed. S. H. Snyder, pp. 215–65. Oxford: Oxford Univ. Press

116. deChamplain, J., Krakoff, L. S., Axelrod, J. 1966. A reduction in the accumulation of ^{3}H-norepinephrine in experimental hypertension. *Life Sci.* 5:2283–91

117. LeLorier, J., Hedtke, J. L., Shideman, F. E. 1976. Uptake of and response to norepinephrine by certain tissues of hypertensive rats. *Am. J. Physiol.* 230:1545–49

118. Yamori, Y. 1972. Organ difference of catecholamine metabolism in spontaneously hypertensive rats. In *Spontaneous Hypertension*, ed. K. Okamoto, pp. 59–61. Tokyo: Igaku Shoin

119. Stickney, J. L. 1981. Accumulation of norepinephrine by tissue slices from spontaneously hypertensive rats. *Clin. Exp. Hyperten.* 3:141–58

120. Garrett, J., Castro-Tavares, J., Branco, D. 1981. Uptake and metabolism of noradrenaline by blood vessels of perinephrectic hypertensive dogs. *Blood Vessels* 18:100–9

121. Esler, M., Jackman, G., Bobik, A., Leonard, P., Kelleher, D., et al. 1981. Norepinephrine kinetics in essential hypertension. Defective neuronal uptake in some patients. *Hypertension* 3:149–56

122. Mulvany, M. J., Aalkjaer, C., Christensen, J. 1979. Effect of age on noradrenaline sensitivity of mesenteric resistance vessels in spontaneously hypertensive and Wistar-Kyoto rats. *Clin. Sci.* 57:43s–45s

123. Zsoter, T. T., Sirko, S., Wolchinsky, C., Kadar, D., Endrenyi, L. 1981. Adrenergic activity in arteries of spontaneously hypertensive rats. *Can. J. Physiol. Pharmacol.* 59:1104–7

124. Whall, C. W., Myers, M. M., Halpern, W. 1980. Norepinephrine sensitivity, tension development and neuronal uptake in resistance arteries from spontaneously hypertensive and normotensive rats. *Blood Vessels* 17:1–15

125. Rho, J. H., Newman, B., Alexander, N. 1981. Altered in vitro uptake of norepinephrine by cardiovascular tissues of spontaneously hypertensive rats. Part 1. Mesenteric artery. *Hypertension* 3:704–9

126. Webb, R. C., Vanhoutte, P. M. 1981. Cocaine and contractile responses of vascular smooth muscle from spontaneously hypertensive rats. *Arch. Int. Pharmacol.* 253:241–56

127. Durrett, L. R., Milano, A. J., Ziegler, M. G. 1984. Radioenzymatic assay of catecholamines. In *Norepinephrine*, ed. M. G. Ziegler, C. R. Lake, 2:27–37. Baltimore: Williams & Wilkins

128. Shoup, R. E., Kissinger, P. T., Goldstein, D. S. 1984. Rapid liquid chromatographic methods for assay of norepinephrine, epinephrine, and dopamine in biological fluids and tissues. See Ref. 127, 2:38–46

129. Goldstein, D. S. 1983. Plasma catecholamines and essential hypertension—An analytical review. *Hypertension* 5:86–99

130. Goldstein, D. S. 1981. Plasma norepinephrine in essential hypertension—A study of studies. *Hypertension* 3:48–52

131. Goldstein, D. S. 1981. Plasma norepinephrine as an indicator of sympathetic neural activity in clinical cardiology. *Am. J. Cardiol.* 48:1147–54

132. Bravo, E. 1981. Plasma catecholamines in clinical medicine. *Cardiovas. Ther.* 12:187–96

133. Folkow, B., DiBona, G. F., Hjemdahl, P., Toren, P. H., Wallin, B. G. 1983. Measurements of plasma norepinephrine concentrations in human primary hypertension—A word of caution on their applicability for assessing neurogenic contributions. *Hypertension* 5:399–403

134. Birkenhager, W. H., DeLeeuw, P. W. 1979. Pathophysiological mechanisms in essential hypertension. *Pharmacol. Ther.* 8:297–319

135. Weber, M. A., Drayer, J. I. M. 1982. The sympathetic nervous system in primary hypertension. *Miner. Electrolyte Metab.* 7:57–66

136. Esler, M. 1982. Assessment of sympathetic nervous function in humans from noradrenaline plasma kinetics. *Clin. Sci.* 62:247–54

137. Lake, C. R., Chernow, B., Feuerstein, G., Goldstein, D. S., Ziegler, M. G. 1984. The sympathetic nervous system in man: Its evaluation and the measurement of plasma NE. See Ref. 127, 2:1–26

138. Saar, N., Jackson, R., Bachmann, A., Gordon, R. 1980. Effect of sampling site and conditions on plasma levels of noradrenaline, adrenaline and dopamine. *Prog. Biochem. Pharmacol.* 17:90–97

139. Esler, M., Jackman, G., Bobik, A., Kelleher, D., Jennings, G., et al. 1979. Determination of norepinephrine apparent release rate and clearance in humans. *Life Sci.* 25:1461–70

140. Esler, M., Jackman, G., Leonard, P., Bobik, A., Skews, H., et al. 1980. Determination of noradrenaline uptake, spillover to plasma and plasma concentration in patients with essential hypertension. *Clin. Sci.* 59:311s–13s

141. Distler, A., Philipp, T. 1980. Role of sympathetic nervous system in essential hypertension. In *Contributions to Nephrology*, ed. E. Ritz, S. G. Massry, A. Heidland, K. Schaefer, 23:150–57. Basel: Karger

142. deChamplain, J., Cousineau, D., LaPointe, L. 1978. The role of the sympathetic system in the maintenance of human hypertension. *Clin. Invest. Med.* 1:123–28

143. Dustan, H. P. 1982. Physiologic regulation of arterial pressure: An overview. *Hypertension* 4:62–67

144. deChamplain, J., Van Ameringen, M. R., Cousineau, D., Marc-Aurele, J. 1977. The role of the sympathetic system in experimental and human hypertension. *Postgrad. Med. J.* 53 (Suppl.3):15–30

145. Kopin, I. J., Goldstein, D. S., Feuerstein, G. Z. 1981. Position paper: The sympathetic nervous system and hypertension. In *Hypertension Research*, ed. J. H. Laragh, F. R. Buhler, D. W. Selbin. New York: Springer-Verlag

146. Christensen, N. J. 1982. Catecholamines and essential hypertension. *Scand. J. Clin. Lab. Invest.* 42:211–15

147. Christensen, N. J. 1979. The role of catecholamines in clinical medicine. *Acta Med. Scand.* 624:9–18 (Suppl.)

148. Goldstein, D. S., Ziegler, M. G., Lake, C. R. 1984. Plasma norepinephrine in essential hypertension. See Ref. 127, 2:389–400

149. Stevo, J., Ibsen, H., Colfer, H. T. 1984. Hemodynamic and pharmacologic correlates of plasma norepinephrine in hypertension. See Ref. 127, 2:401–9

Ann. Rev. Pharmacol. Toxicol. 1985. 25:643–66

THE MECHANISMS OF ACRYLAMIDE AXONOPATHY

Matthew S. Miller and Peter S. Spencer

Institute of Neurotoxicology and Departments of Neuroscience and Pathology, Albert Einstein College of Medicine, Bronx, New York 10461

INTRODUCTION

Degeneration of the distal axons of long and large-diameter peripheral nerve fibers is perhaps the most common of all toxic peripheral nerve disorders. Degeneration commonly spreads centrally along affected nerve tracts in a dying-back fashion (1). Axonal disorders of this type are grouped under the term *central-peripheral distal axonopathy* to emphasize the contemporaneous onset of distal retrograde axonal degeneration in long nerve-fiber tracts in both the central nervous system (CNS) and the peripheral nervous system (PNS) (2). Axonopathy refers exclusively to the primary degeneration of axons, although associated changes may occur in corresponding neuronal perikarya. Schwann cells and oligodendrocytes enveloping affected axons in the PNS and CNS, respectively, commonly undergo secondary changes, including mitosis and loss of myelin maintenance, while fibroblasts and astrocytes become involved later in the degenerative process.

Distal axonopathy can result from a single or, more commonly, repeated exposure to a variety of chemically unrelated agents, or it can occur with apparent spontaneity in a number of abnormal nutritional or metabolic states (3). Although the biochemical mechanisms underlying axonal degeneration are unknown, some progress has been made in recent years in understanding the biochemical events that precede and accompany axon degeneration in certain toxic neuropathies, notably those associated with repeated exposure to acrylamide or aliphatic γ-diketones. Multidisciplinary investigation of these neuropathies in laboratory animals and organotypic tissue cultures has revealed several previously unknown basic mechanisms that may be involved in the maintenance of the axon and the initiation and regulation of the degenerative

643

0362-1642/85/415-0643$02.00

process. This review focuses on the mechanisms underlying the degeneration of the axon in acrylamide neuropathy, a subject previously reviewed by Spencer & Schaumburg (4) and Le Quesne & Tilson (5, 6). Readers interested in equally important developments in understanding γ-diketone axonopathy are referred to other review articles (7, 8).

MAINTENANCE OF THE AXON

Anatomic Considerations

An understanding of the basic processes by which normal axonal integrity is maintained is essential to any consideration of toxic/metabolic perturbations that precipitate axonal degeneration. The axon is a unique cellular process that communicates electrically encoded information over long distances. No cell other than the neuron projects cellular processes over distances comparable to that of the axon. Bipolar sensory neurons, for example, their neuronal perikarya located in lumbar spinal ganglia, project a peripheral axon that may extend the entire length of a limb to terminate in the toe while simultaneously projecting a central axon to the brain stem. In the adult human, therefore, primary sensory neurons maintain axons exceeding five feet in length.

While the mammalian axon has the metabolic machinery to synthesize proteins and lipids and to modify them post-translationally by phosphorylation and other mechanisms (9), axoplasm has a negligible capacity for lipid and protein synthesis (9, 10). Some metabolic support may be provided by Schwann cells or oligodendrocytes, but in mammals this is insufficient to maintain the axon after disconnection from its neuronal perikaryon. The axon, therefore, is largely dependent on the neuronal perikaryon for its supply of metabolic requirements (11–13). This has necessitated the development of bidirectional intraneuronal transport mechanisms to shuttle materials and information between the perikaryon, the axon, and the nerve terminal.

Axonal Transport

Axoplasmic transport may be divided into at least three anterograde and two retrograde transport systems (14, 15).

ANTEROGRADE AXONAL TRANSPORT   Materials synthesized in the neuronal perikaryon are moved distally along the axon at various velocities: at least two slow and one fast anterograde transport systems have been recognized. Slow anterograde axoplasmic transport systems supply constituents that maintain the bulk of the axonal cytoskeleton and glycolytic function. Slow component a (SCa) transports neurofilament triplet proteins and tubulin at a rate of approximately 0.1–2 mm a day; slow component b (SCb) transports a variety of structural proteins, including actin, at a rate of 2–4 mm a day (15). Several, perhaps all, glycolytic enzymes are transported in SCb (13). Thus, in a typical human nerve terminating in the foot, up to eight months may elapse before a glycolytic enzyme synthesized in the neuronal perikaryon arrives in the terminal axon.

Fast anterograde axoplasmic transport moves materials distally along the axon at rates of approximately 400 mm a day. This system is primarily involved in transporting membrane-associated proteins and glycoproteins for maintenance of axolemma, the axon surface membrane (16–18). Also transported by the fast anterograde axoplasmic transport system are peptides involved in neurotransmission, such as dopamine-β-hydroxylase, some forms of acetylcholinesterase, and substance P (19–21), as well as the classical neurotransmitters acetylcholine and norepinephrine (14). Fast anterograde axoplasmic transport therefore appears to be involved in the movement of substances required for the maintenance of axon membranes and for neurotransmission.

RETROGRADE AXONAL TRANSPORT   This transport system is the least understood component of neuronal transport. The system probably functions to communicate information on the state of the axon to the neuronal perikaryon, as well as to allow the return of certain axoplasmic constituents for reprocessing in the perikaryon (22–27).

The retrograde system translocates a variety of substances from the periphery to the soma at a rate of approximately 150–250 mm a day [reviewed in (14)]. Substances transported by the retrograde system include acetylcholinesterase, adrenergic granules, lysosomes, and fucosyl glycoproteins (28–30). In addition, a variety of endogenous or foreign substances is taken up nonspecifically by axon terminals and may utilize the retrograde transport system: these include serum albumin and horseradish peroxidase (31, 32). Nerve Growth Factor, a protein thought to act as a trophic substance in some neurons (33–35), and tetanus toxin (31, 36) interact with membrane-binding sites located on the distal terminals of neurons, undergo pinocytosis, and retrograde axon transport. The transport of Nerve Growth Factor appears to be limited to sensory and adrenergic neurons, while tetanus toxin is transported without apparent neuronal specificity (34).

A slow retrograde axoplasmic transport system also has been described (37). Transport occurs at a rate of approximately 3–6 mm a day and a single protein, thought to be albumin, is involved.

THE GRADIENT HYPOTHESIS   Proteins are probably utilized and/or degraded while undergoing anterograde axonal transport. In theory, this creates a gradient of material in which the concentration of anterogradely transported materials is greater in proximal than in distal portions of axons. Gradients of this nature have been reported in peripheral nerves for phosphoprotein, acetylcholinesterase, choline acetylase, and non-specific carboxyesterases (38). Thus, little or no surplus of axonally transported proteins may be available in distal aspects of long axons. This may render distal axons vulnerable to toxins that diminish the activity or availability of enzymes or other important proteins delivered to axoplasm by axonal transport.

ACRYLAMIDE NEUROPATHY

Introduction

Changes in axonal transport or the availability of essential materials may be essential elements of the mechanism underlying the distal retrograde axonal degeneration found in humans and animals repeatedly exposed by a systemic route to acrylamide ($CH_2 = CHCONH_2$). Although the critical biochemical events leading to axonopathy remain to be determined, acrylamide is known to react spontaneously with hydroxyl-, amino-, and sulfhydryl-containing compounds (39–44).

Neuropathy in Humans

As early as the 1950s, researchers realized that industrial workers exposed to monomeric acrylamide are at risk for peripheral neuropathy, a disorder characterized by a stocking-and-glove distribution of sensory, motor, and autonomic deficits and accompanied by excessive tiredness and ataxia (45, 46). Subjects present with cold, blue hands and commonly report unsteadiness, muscle weakness, paresthesia, and numbness in the hands and/or feet. Tendon reflexes disappear, probably in association with degenerative changes in muscle-spindle afferents (47, 48). Position sense in distal joints is commonly, but not always, lost (46). Vibration sense is lost distally, but temperature, pressure, and other objective sensory modalities remain intact (45). Recovery from mild forms of acrylamide neuropathy is usually complete, normally occurring within a few months (45, 46, 49). However, severely affected patients may never totally recover, experiencing residual ataxia, distal weakness, and sensory disturbances (50).

Experimental Neuropathy

Repeated exposure to acrylamide has been shown to produce neuropathy in cats (51–53), rats (53–56), mice (57–59), guinea pigs, rabbits, monkeys (53, 60), chickens, and goldfish (61). As with humans, laboratory animals also develop ataxia and weakness most apparent in the hind limbs.

The Disposition of Acrylamide

Numerous studies have attempted to elucidate the mechanism underlying the neurotoxic property of acrylamide. Kuperman (51) found the effects of acrylamide in the cat to be independent of route of administration or duration of intoxication, the appearance of hindlimb weakness first occurring when an apparent cumulative dose threshold had been exceeded. He believed that either acrylamide or a metabolite accumulated at the target site or the substance impaired a slowly resolving process. Functional impairment would result when a critical threshold was surpassed. While recent studies have challenged the linearity of the relationship between a cumulative dose of acrylamide and the onset of neuropathy, there is little doubt that acrylamide has cumulative effects. Thus, studies addressing the disposition of acrylamide have become essential to understanding the basis of acrylamide-induced neuropathy.

Following administration, acrylamide is rapidly distributed to all tissues, metabolized, and excreted (61–63). The distribution and elimination kinetics for acrylamide are influenced only slightly by the route of administration. Using a single dose of 2,3-^{14}C-acrylamide, Miller et al (63) demonstrated equivalent concentrations of radiolabel in all tissues except erythrocytes. Neural tissue accumulated less than 1% of the dose of acrylamide. Tissue radiolabel content decayed in a bi-exponential fashion ($t_{1/2}$ approximately equal to 5 hours). Only erythrocytes demonstrated significant retention of radiolabel (63, 64). The elimination constants for parent acrylamide ($t_{1/2}$ approximately equal to 2 hours) are faster than those for total radioactivity in all tissues. Thus, acrylamide itself is not selectively retained or concentrated in neural tissues following single (63) or repeated dosing (65). A small percentage of radiolabel persists in all tissues for several weeks ($t_{1/2}$ approximately equal to 8 days). Tissue-associated radiolabel has been reported to be protein-bound, but the possibility that metabolic fragments of acrylamide are incorporated into protein via normal protein synthetic mechanisms has not been excluded. This notion gains support from the observation that $^{14}CO_2$ is expired by laboratory animals treated with ^{14}C-acrylamide (44).

The major route of biotransformation of acrylamide is conjugation with the tripeptide glutathione (62, 63, 66). This route appears detoxifying, since depletion of tissue non-protein sulfhydryl content increases the neurotoxic potency of acrylamide (67). Acrylamide enzymatically and non-enzymatically reacts with glutathione (61–63, 67, 68) and is eventually excreted in urine as N-acetyl-S-(3-amino-3-oxypropyl)-cysteine (63, 66). Thus, it appears that neuropathy is mediated by a direct action of parent acrylamide and that conjugation of acrylamide with glutathione is a detoxification process. Acrylamide is capable of inhibiting the enzyme activity of glutathione-S-transferase both in vitro and in vivo (67–72). This suggests that acrylamide may inhibit its own detoxification along the glutathione conjugation pathway, although this has yet to be demonstrated directly.

In addition to conjugation with glutathione, acrylamide appears to undergo biotransformation mediated by the microsomal cytochrome P-450 system.

Kaplan et al (73) reported that free acrylamide disappears faster in liver homogenates prepared from animals whose microsomal cytochrome P-450 levels have been elevated by pretreatment with phenobarbitol. Further study revealed that pretreatment of rats with microsomal-inducing agents (phenobarbitol or dithiothreitol) may delay the onset of acrylamide-induced neuropathy (73, 74). However, this finding has not been confirmed by other investigators (61, 62, 65).

Structural Analogs of Acrylamide

Several structural analogs of acrylamide have been evaluated for neurotoxic potential in an attempt to determine which portion of the acrylamide molecule is involved in the induction of neuropathy (44, 61, 62, 74). Acrylamide analogs that produce neuropathy include N-isopropylacrylamide, N-methylacrylamide, methacrylamide, N-hydroxymethylacrylamide, and N,N-diethylacrylamide (74). None of these compounds demonstrates greater neurotoxic potency than acrylamide. Positive analogs (except methacrylamide) differ from acrylamide in the substitution of the amide group, although other amide-substituted analogs, such as methylene(bis)acrylamide and N,N-pentamethylene acrylamide, appear unable to produce neuropathy in laboratory animals. Reduction of the double bond of acrylamide, or deletion of the nitrogen atom, eliminates the potential of the compound to induce neuropathy. Thus, it appears that the acrylyl moiety (CH_2CHCO-) of acrylamide is essential for neurotoxic potential, while amide substitution can profoundly modify neurotoxic potential.

Acrylamide's high affinity for sulfhydryl nucleophiles has been considered a potential means by which the substance could inactivate critical axonal proteins (44, 75–82). However, no clear relationship exists between in vitro sulfhydryl reactivity and the potential to produce neuropathy, since N,N'-diethylacrylamide and N-methylacrylamide, compounds much less reactive with sulfhydryl groups than acrylamide (44), prove to be neurotoxic (61, 62). Thus, while it is possible that reaction with sulfhydryl-dependent proteins may be involved in the pathogenesis of acrylamide neuropathy, it appears that reaction with sulfhydryl moieties is not the sole mechanism by which acrylamide produces this disorder.

Effects on Axon Structure

Fullerton & Barnes (54) were the first to demonstrate the involvement of peripheral nerves in acrylamide neurotoxicity. By comparing the size distribution of myelinated fibers in nerves from acrylamide-treated and untreated rats, they were able to demonstrate a reduction in the number of large-diameter fibers in cross sections of hindlimb nerves from treated animals that revealed various stages of nerve-fiber degeneration (Figure 1). Spencer & Schaumburg

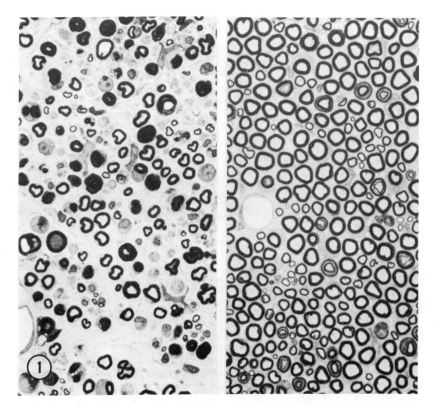

Figure 1 Left: Degeneration of myelinated fibers in the tibial nerve of a rat treated with 0.35% acrylamide in diet for 28 days. Right: Normal tibial nerve from an age-matched control rat. One-micrometer epoxy cross-sections stained with toluidine blue × 500.

(2) demonstrated the spatial-temporal evolution of retrograde degeneration in rats treated with acrylamide and showed that long nerve fibers both in peripheral nerves and in ascending tracts of the spinal cord are also involved in the dying-back process (Figure 2).

Prineas (83) first reported the ultrastructural features of axonal degeneration. Initial abnormalities include the presence of abnormally large numbers of intermediate filaments, mitochondria, and other organelles. Some of the latter appear to be sequestered and selectively removed by invaginations of adaxonal cytoplasm of the Schwann cell or oligodendrocyte (84). Shortly before the axon breaks down, there is a loss of neurotubules and neurofilaments and dissolution of the axolemma.

Schaumburg and associates (48) demonstrated that the earliest detectable morphological change produced by acrylamide in the cat occurs in the Pacinian corpuscles of the toe pads. Reduction of the generator potential of the corpuscle

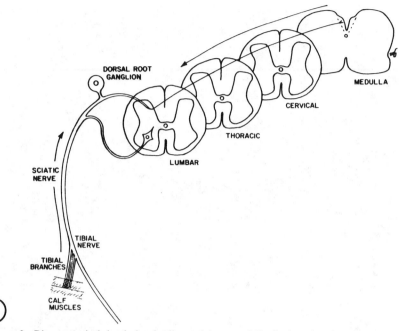

Figure 2 Diagrammatical sketch showing the spatial-temporal distribution of myelinated nerve-fiber degeneration in animals treated with acrylamide. Changes first appear in tibial branches supplying the calf musculature and in the termination of the gracile tract in the medulla oblongata. Arrows depict the temporal progression of degeneration along affected nerve-fiber pathways.

axon precedes the first structural damage produced by acrylamide, namely, loss of filopod axon processes containing microfilaments (4, 85). Sequential degeneration of adjacent primary annulospiral endings of muscle spindles, secondary muscle spindle endings, and motor nerve terminals then occurs. Degeneration is associated with accumulations of vesicles and neurofilaments in the preterminal region of the axon. This suggests that distal axonopathies, such as acrylamide neuropathy, involve a biochemical lesion that may lead to alterations in axoplasmic transport (83, 86).

Effects on Axonal Transport

Numerous studies have examined the effects of acrylamide on anterograde axonal transport in experimental animals at times when functional signs of neuropathy are evident and distal axons are undergoing degeneration (86–90). The studies of Sidenius & Jakobsen (91), Sumner and colleagues (92), and Griffin & Price (93) revealed either no change or slight decreases (10–15%) in the rate of fast anterograde axonal transport, with no detectable change in slow anterograde transport in association with acrylamide-induced neuropathy.

However, studies by Weir et al (88) and Souyri et al (89) suggest that fast anterograde transport of protein is altered by acrylamide. Furthermore, analysis of acetylcholinesterase transport in acrylamide-intoxicated chickens revealed a 60% reduction in the rapidly transported A12 form of acetylcholinesterase, while slowly transported forms (G1 and G2) were unaffected by acrylamide (94).

Caution is appropriate in the interpretation of these studies. First, it is unclear whether the reported abnormalities are associated with the cause or the effect of ultrastructural abnormalities induced by acrylamide. A second possibility is that changes in transport may occur because acrylamide impairs protein synthesis (95, 96), a property shared by acrylamide analogs that lack the ability to induce neuropathy in laboratory animals. The third important consideration is that measured changes in anterograde transport in proximal axons may differ from those occurring in distal axons.

Examination of the effect of acrylamide on bidirectional fast anterograde axoplasmic transport of radiolabeled protein revealed a large deficit in retrograde fast transport in animals that displayed ataxia and hindlimb weakness (97). Subsequent studies by Sidenius & Jakobsen (91) showed that retrograde transport is dramatically affected in acrylamide-intoxicated animals (98). The defect is characterized by a reduction in the quantity of material undergoing retrograde transport. Additionally, evaluation of retrograde axonal transport after varying doses of acrylamide revealed that alterations in retrograde transport *preceded* the development of functional signs of neuropathy (98–100). By contrast, N,N'-methylene(bis)acrylamide and N-hydroxymethylacrylamide, two acrylamide analogs that do not produce neuropathy in the doses employed, fail to affect retrograde axonal transport of protein, thereby suggesting a specific association between axonopathy and defects in retrograde transport. More recently, it has been demonstrated that acrylamide administration inhibits retrograde axonal transport but not neuronal uptake of horseradish peroxidase (HRP)(101), and that *single* doses of acrylamide produce marked deficits in the rate of retrograde axonal transport of radiolabeled Nerve Growth Factor (99) and tetanus toxin (100).

The actions of single doses of acrylamide on retrograde axonal transport have been investigated in an attempt to distinguish between the effects on axonal transport that result from the direct action of acrylamide and those that occur secondarily to axonal changes induced by repeated acrylamide dosing. Single doses of acrylamide, similar to those used for repeat-dosing studies, reduce the rate of retrograde axonal transport in a dose-dependent manner (Figure 3). Retrograde transport in sensory neurons appears more vulnerable to the actions of acrylamide than motor neurons. These data correlate well with previous electrophysiologic (47) and morphologic (48) studies demonstrating the increased susceptibility of sensory axons to acrylamide. The extent to which

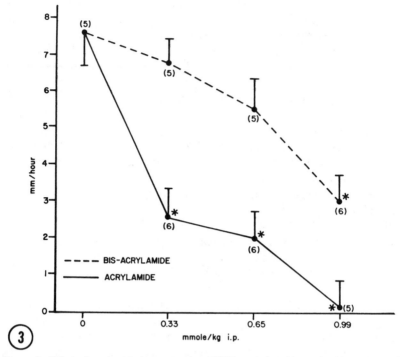

Figure 3 Effect of acrylamide (————) and N,N'-methylene-bis-acrylamide (— — — —) on rate of retrograde transport of ^{125}I-tetanus toxin. Values are mean ± SEM. Number of animals per group is in parenthesis. *p less than 0.05 versus saline-injected control value by analysis of variance and Scheffe's test. Reprinted from (100) with permission.

retrograde axonal transport is affected by acrylamide increases with repeated acrylamide administration and precedes the appearance of ataxia and weakness (Figure 4).

A recent study has examined the effects of single doses of acrylamide on slow anterograde axoplasmic transport (102). Data revealed a modest, non-specific defect in slow anterograde axonal transport of all proteins visible on fluorographs. However, the possibility that acrylamide-induced alterations in protein synthesis are responsible for the apparent slow transport defect cannot as yet be excluded.

In summary, profound changes in axonal transport are produced by single doses of acrylamide that, if repeated over the course of a few weeks, precipitate functional signs of neuropathy. These transport defects precede by many days the onset of functional or morphologic signs of axonal compromise. Further investigation is required to determine how these early changes in axonal

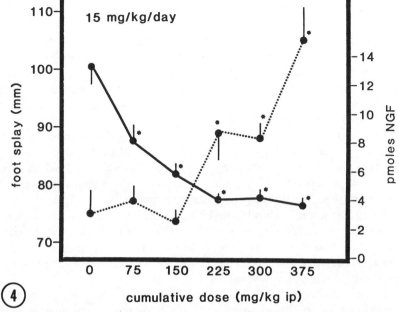

Figure 4   Effect of repeated administration of acrylamide (15 mg/kg/day, intraperitoneally) on the retrograde axonal transport of nerve growth factor (NGF)(——————) and hindlimb footsplay (— — — — —). Retrograde axonal transport was assessed by determining the quantity of ^{125}I-NGF transport to dorsal root ganglia following peripheral injection. *p less than 0.05 versus time 0 value by analysis of variance and Scheffe's test. Reprinted from (99) with permission.

transport are related to the primary biochemical lesion(s) and the subsequent axonal demise.

The Significance of Retrograde Transport Defects

Retrograde axonal transport may be instrumental in the initiation of regenerative and repair processes following neuronal injury (22). Several studies (22–27) have supported the concept that changes in retrograde transport may be one mechanism by which perikaryal responses to peripheral axon lesions are initiated. Bisby & Bulgar (22) observed that perikaryal proteins labeled with ^{3}H-leucine are transported by fast anterograde axoplasmic transport to the distal ends of both sensory and motor neurons. The direction of transport is then reversed and the radioactivity is transported in a retrograde fashion. Axonal injury by ligation causes materials transported by the fast anterograde axoplasmic transport system to turn around proximal to the ligation. These findings have led to the hypothesis that materials returning from the peripheral process via the retrograde transport system may serve to inform the soma of the integrity of the peripheral process and may be intimately involved in the initiation of the regenerative process. Recent experiments by Singer et al (27) have demonstrated that both metabolic and morphologic changes in the peri- karya following nerve transection may be delayed by administration of colchi- cine to the nerve trunk, a compound known to effect bidirectional axonal transport blockade (103–108). These data suggest that it may be the appearance of a signal, rather than the lack of one, that is responsible for initiating perikaryal responses to axon damage.

The observation that single doses of acrylamide slow retrograde transport (99, 100) has led to the hypothesis that distal axonopathy may be the result of a failure to inform the soma of the need to repair nonspecific axonal lesions. This hypothesis is supported by previous studies (109, 110) demonstrating that acrylamide significantly slows regenerative terminal sprouting, possibly as a result of interactions with sulfhydryl groups (78, 79), while fast anterograde transport of protein remains normal (110). Further support for this hypothesis is found in the studies of Cavanagh & Gysbers (111) in which the administration of acrylamide was found to potentiate retrograde degeneration of nerve fibers in the proximal stump of a severed nerve.

Taken in concert, these data suggest that acrylamide may prevent the neuronal perikaryon from responding normally to axonal transection. Several studies have suggested that repair-specific proteins are synthesized in neuronal perikarya supporting regenerating axons (11, 12, 112–116). Many of these growth-associated proteins (GAPs) are found only in regenerating axons, suggesting that they appear as a consequence of qualitative alterations in gene expression and that the synthesis of these proteins is probably dependent on transcription of new mRNA species (117–120). Whether acrylamide adminis- tration prevents the synthesis of GAPs is currently unknown. However, recent studies demonstrate that single and repeated doses of acrylamide inhibit the induction of perikaryal ornithine decarboxylase (ODC, EC 4.1.1.17) activity and the rate of total RNA synthesis in response to axon damage (121), possibly by blocking the retrograde axonal transport of putative repair-initiating fac- tor(s) (100). ODC is the rate-limiting enzyme in polyamine synthesis (122) and represents an extremely sensitive means by which perikaryal responses to peripheral nerve damage may be quantified. Polyamines are required for a variety of hyperplastic and hypertrophic cellular processes, including axonal differentiation, maturation, and regeneration (123–128). ODC has a half-life of approximately 11–15 minutes (129) and thus must be continually synthesized. Synthesis of ODC appears to be regulated predominately at the level of transcription because actinomycin D readily blocks its induction in neuronal perikarya. Although a recent study has demonstrated that induction of ODC activity may not be a prerequisite for regeneration of goldfish optic nerve (130, 131), it is apparent that ODC activity is a useful marker of alterations in

DNA-dependent transcription associated with cell proliferation, growth, or regeneration. That acrylamide inhibits the induction of ODC activity and RNA synthesis following nerve transsection supports the hypothesis that acrylamide attenuates perikaryal responses to axon damage.

Changes in Neuronal Perikarya

In addition to a possible action of acrylamide on retrograde transport–mediated perikaryal repair responses, it appears likely that acrylamide may have a direct action on the perikaryon itself. Morphologic evaluation of lumbar spinal ganglia following acrylamide administration has revealed cytoplasmic reorganization with nuclear and Nissl changes resembling chromatolysis (132–136). Chromatolysis is a poorly understood stereotypic morphologic reorganization of the perikaryon following axon transsection or injury. The intensity of the chromatolytic response increases with more proximal axon lesions and is rarely associated with distal toxic neuropathies [(83; reviewed in 137)]. Although the significance of the chromatolytic-like response in spinal ganglia following acrylamide administration is unclear, it suggests that the actions of acrylamide may in some way mimic axon transsection, possibly as a result of retrograde axonal transport blockade. It has also been suggested that acrylamide might produce distal axonopathy by disturbing the metabolic integrity of neuronal perikarya (132–135), although the observation that characteristic pathological changes appear in axons locally exposed to acrylamide (and other agents that induce axonopathy) has been taken as evidence that acrylamide is a direct axonal toxin (138).

The Mechanism of Altered Axonal Transport

ACTIONS ON TUBULIN   Bidirectional fast axonal transport is blocked by agents that bind to tubulin (103–108). Colchicine specifically binds to tubulin, resulting in the disassembly of labile microtubules, including those present in axoplasm. Similar effects are produced by the *Vinca* alkaloids, vinblastine, vincristine, and vindesine (an amide derivative), a more potent class of tubulin-binding agents. Ultrastructural studies demonstrate a rapid loss or numerical reduction of axonal microtubules following local application of tubulin-binding agents to peripheral nerves. In addition to microtubules, it has been suggested that smooth endoplasmic reticulum and neurofilaments may be important structural components of the axonal transport mechanism. No evidence for the morphologic alteration of any of the putative structural components of axonal transport, microtubules, neurofilaments, or smooth endoplasmic reticulum, is apparent in the sciatic nerve of animals treated with single doses of acrylamide that decrease rates of retrograde axonal transport (M. S. Miller, P. S. Spencer, unpublished data). Thus, it appears that acrylamide initially alters axonal transport through a biochemical lesion without obvious disruption of structural axoplasmic components.

A recent study, however, has demonstrated profound decreases in the binding of ^{3}H-colchicine to tubulin in sciatic nerve and spinal cord, but not in cerebellum or brain, following prolonged exposure to acrylamide (139). While these data might suggest that acrylamide alters existing tubulin or decreases tissue tubulin content, the time-course for the depletion of ^{3}H-colchicine binding by acrylamide appears to parallel the appearance of degenerating axons in peripheral nerves and spinal cord. Thus, it appears likely that alterations in ^{3}H-colchicine binding reflect decreases in tubulin content associated with axonal degeneration rather than specific alterations in tubulin itself. However, a direct action of acrylamide on tubulin and microtubules cannot be excluded at this time.

ACTIONS ON HIGH-ENERGY PHOSPHATE PRODUCTION   Maintenance of bidirectional fast axonal transport is clearly dependent on the constant availability of adequate supplies of high-energy phosphate [reviewed in (137)]. Transport is impaired by the specific inhibition of the metabolic steps in glycolysis, the Kreb's cycle, electron transfer chain, or terminal phosphorylation. Inhibition of axonal transport occurs when high-energy phosphate (ATP and creatine phosphate) declines to approximately half of levels found in normal mammalian nerves (140). The actual critical threshold value of axonal high-energy phosphate required to maintain fast axoplasmic transport is unknown because it is technically impossible to distinguish levels of high-energy phosphate compounds in the axon from those in Schwann cells or oligodendrocytes.

Since the enzymes involved in the production of high-energy phosphate compounds (enzymes of glycolysis and oxidative phosphorylation) undergo axonal transport, it is possible that small decrements in axonal energy production could result in dramatic deficits in the distal axon. The transport of enzymes involved in energy transformation from the neuron perikayon to the distal axon may be slowed by locally diminished high-energy phosphate supplies. Were this to occur, the failure to transport required enzymes would further compromise high-energy phosphate production, which would in turn further inhibit axonal transport. This cascade of events would result in a proximal-to-distal gradient in energy transformation, with levels in distal axons perhaps falling below those required to maintain axonal transport and, therefore, maintenance of axonal integrity more distally. Thus, a potential mechanism by which acrylamide may alter axoplasmic transport involves interference with enzymatic processes associated with the production, storage, or utilization of high-energy phosphate compounds.

Effects on Glycolytic Enzymes

Acrylamide is known to be highly reactive with cellular sulfhydryl groups (39–44) and reacts spontaneously with the non-protein sulfhydryl compound glutathione (61–63). It has been suggested that alterations in the activity of sulfhydryl-dependent glycolytic enzymes may be the critical biochemical lesion underlying acrylamide-induced distal axonopathy (76, 77, 141). Unlike other cell types, neurons with long axons would be slow to replace glycolytic enzymes irreversibly inhibited by reaction with acrylamide due to the large anatomic separation between perikaryal sites of protein synthesis and distal axoplasm. When added to purified enzyme or rat brain homogenate, acrylamide inhibits the activity of phosphofructokinase (PFK), enolase, neuron-specific enolase (NSE), and glyceraldehyde-3-phosphate dehydrogenase (GAPDH), but not lactic acid dehydrogenase (76, 77, 80–82, 142). The inhibition of glycolytic enzyme activity by acrylamide is irreversible and may be attenuated by preincubation with the sulfhydryl-protecting compound dithiothreitol. Thus, inhibition of glycolytic enzyme activity by acrylamide appears to be the result of a covalent interaction with critical enzyme sulfhydryl moieties. While inhibition of PFK and GAPDH activity by acrylamide is irreversible, the effect of acrylamide on enolase is reversed by dialysis (76, 77). This suggests that the covalent interaction of acrylamide with enolase sulfhydryl moieties is not the mechanism by which acrylamide inhibits enolase activity in peripheral nerve. Following the repeated administration of acrylamide to laboratory animals, the enzyme activities of GAPDH and NSE in peripheral nerve are reduced by approximately 35% (82). The activity of LDH or the rate-limiting glycolytic enzyme PFK remain unchanged (77). These findings raise the possibility that acrylamide alters axonal glycolysis and energy production, although it is presently impossible to determine whether changes in enzyme activity are occurring within the axon and/or the Schwann cell compartment.

Although the activity of GAPDH and NSE is diminished by acrylamide, neither enzyme is normally thought to be a rate-limiting step in glycolysis (143). Thus, the inhibition of glycolytic enzyme activity is in itself weak evidence for an alteration in glycolytic flux. Currently, no data exist to indicate that the diminished activity of glycolytic enzymes in peripheral nerve is reflected as a decrease in glycolytic flux. Furthermore, it is unclear whether these changes in enzyme activity precede or accompany the degeneration of axons in acrylamide-treated animals.

Protection Experiments

Attempts to evaluate the hypothesis that acrylamide inhibits axonal energy transformation have been frustrated by an inability to distinguish enzyme activities within the different cellular compartments of peripheral nerves. While it is possible selectively to remove the bulk of the connective tissue (epineurium and perineurium) surrounding nerve fibers, the remaining intrafascicular tissue contains endothelial cells, pericytes, fibroblasts, and a large number of Schwann cells intimately associated with axons. When intrafascicular tissue is homogenized, the anatomic separation between the axonal glycolytic enzyme and the non-axonal enzyme is lost. This allows any excess enzyme in non-axonal cells to obscure potential decreases in glycolytic flux that may be occurring specifically within the axonal compartment. Thus, indirect means of evaluating the hypothesis have been attempted.

One recent approach has been to investigate the effects on peripheral nerves of the repeated systemic administration of iodoacetic acid, a known inhibitor of glycolysis (M. S. Miller, P. S. Spencer, unpublished data). Measurement of glycolytic enzyme activity in the peripheral nerve demonstrated a greater degree of inhibition than that produced by doses of acrylamide high enough to precipitate nerve degeneration, yet no neuropathy resulted in the animals treated with iodoacetic acid. These data suggest that altered peripheral nerve glycolytic enzyme activity is not the sole mechanism by which acrylamide produces distal axonopathy. In addition, studies by Hashimoto and Aldridge (44) demonstrated no changes in pyruvate or lactate concentrations in brain exposed to acrylamide in vitro or in vivo.

Another indirect approach to examining the role of energy transformation in the genesis of acrylamide neuropathy has been to supplement animals with pyruvate during the period of intoxication in an attempt to circumvent the putative blockade in glycolytic function produced by acrylamide. Early studies using small numbers of animals found that administration of sodium pyruvate delayed the onset of acrylamide neuropathy (144, 145). This finding was only partially confirmed by Sterman et al (146). More recently, Dairman et al (145) have reported the results of a series of studies using a large number of animals that were subjected to detailed functional, morphological, and biochemical analyses of CNS and PNS tissues. These studies demonstrated conclusively that the administration of pyruvate, either the sodium salt or the free acid, delays the appearance of axonal degeneration and functional neuropathy. While these results are consistent with a potential role for altered glycolysis in the etiology of neuropathy, the mechanism underlying protection is unknown. The failure of exogenous pyruvate administration to prevent the development of neuropathy suggests that either the dose of pyruvate employed was submaximal or that altered glycolysis is not the sole pathologic mechanism underlying the development of this disorder.

A similar protective effect has been reported in animals supplemented with pyridoxine (vitamin B_6) (147). Pyridoxine is a cofactor required by many enzymatic reactions, including a number of amino-acid (aspartate, glutamate) transaminase reactions that supply pyruvate, oxaloacetate, 2-keto-glutarate, and succinate to the tricarboxylic acid cycle, as well as enzymes regulating the metabolism of glycogen to glucose (148).

The mechanisms underlying pyruvate- and pyridoxine-induced retardation of acrylamide neuropathy are unknown. The development of acrylamide axonopathy can be delayed by several non-specific methods, including the modulation of non-protein sulfhydryl content and altered pharmacokinetics. Therefore, it is critical that the means by which exogenously administered compounds delay or prevent acrylamide axonopathy be confirmed prior to interpretation.

SUMMARY

The neurotoxic property of acrylamide has been studied for more than 30 years. Recognition that the underlying lesion involves distal retrograde degeneration of long and large-diameter axons demonstrated that acrylamide neuropathy belongs to the class of central-peripheral distal axonopathies. This is a relatively common response of the nervous system found in a large number of unrelated toxic-metabolic states. The ready availability of pure acrylamide and the ability to reproduce a reliable model of acrylamide neuropathy in laboratory animals encouraged many investigators to focus on this disorder as a paradigm with which to study the cellular and biochemical mechanisms underlying distal axonopathies.

The discovery that abnormalities of energy-dependent axonal transport are associated with nerve fiber degeneration led investigators to explore the possibility that energy flux in axons is perturbed by the action of acrylamide. This hypothesis has proved as yet untestable by direct means, due to an inability to separate glial contributions to energy production from those of the axon. Indirect means of addressing this hypothesis have, however, yielded data suggestive of a role for altered glycolysis in the etiology of acrylamide axonopathy. However, it is becoming apparent that, if diminished glycolytic flux is involved in the etiology of axonopathy, it is unlikely to be the sole pathologic mechanism and may in fact represent only one facet of a complex series of biochemical events underlying axonopathy.

A recent hypothesis has suggested that alterations in axon-perikaryal interactions may underlie acrylamide-induced axonopathy. Evidence exists to indicate that alterations in the retrograde axonal transport of axon-derived maintenance- or repair-initiating factors may prevent or attenuate the perikaryal responses necessary to repair and maintain the distal axon in the presence of acrylamide. Thus, acrylamide-induced axonopathy may be the result of at least two biochemical lesions: (a) A relatively non-specific axonal lesion that may be the inhibition of glycolytic enzyme activity or some other axon lesion resulting from the interaction of acrylamide with sulfhydryl, amino, and/or hydroxyl moieties associated with axonal constituents. (*b*) Inhibition of perikaryal-mediated axon repair and maintenance mechanisms that could occur as a result of alterations in retrograde axonal transport of one or more lesion-associated factors or as a result of a direct action of acrylamide on the perikaryon. A third hypothesis suggests that a direct action of acrylamide on the neuronal perikaryon alone may result in a generalized, non-specific metabolic lesion that stresses the neuron to a point where the distal end can no longer be maintained.

Regardless of the actual mechanism of acrylamide-induced axonopathy, recent investigations by several laboratories have provided new and exciting insights into the possible mechanism of distal axonopathy, the means by which axon-perikaryal communication occurs, and the manner in which the perikaryon responds to axon damage. In addition to the obvious significance that understanding mechanisms of toxin-induced peripheral nerve degeneration has to the toxicologist, toxic neuropathy may be a means by which the basic mechanisms underlying comparable human neurodegenerative disorders may profitably be studied.

ACKNOWLEDGEMENTS

These studies were supported by federal grants from NIH NINCDS NS19611, NIOSH OH 00851, and OH 00535.

Literature Cited

1. Cavanagh, J. B. 1964. The significance of the "dying-back" process in experimental and human neurological disease. *Int. Rev. Exp. Pathol.* 3:219–67
2. Spencer, P. S., Schaumburg, H. H. 1977. Ultrastructural studies of the dying-back process. IV. Differential vulnerabilities of PNS and CNS fibers in experimental central-peripheral distal axonopathies. *J. Neuropathol. Exp. Neurol.* 36:300–20
3. Spencer, P. S., Miller, M. S., Ross, S. M., Schwab, B., Sabri, M. I. 1985. Biochemical mechanisms underlying primary degeneration of axons. In *Handbook of Neurochemistry*, ed. A. Lajtha. 9:31–66. New York: Plenum
4. Spencer, P. S., Schaumburg, H. H. 1974. A review of acrylamide neurotoxicity. II. Experimental animal neurotoxicity and pathologic mechanisms. *Can. J. Neurol. Sci.* 1:152–64
5. Le Quesne, P. M. 1980. Acrylamide. In *Experimental and Clinical Neurotoxicology*, ed. P. S. Spencer, H. H. Schaumburg, pp. 309–25. Baltimore, MD: Williams & Wilkins

6. Tilson, H. A. 1981. The neurotoxicity of acrylamide: an overview. *Neurobehav. Toxicol. Teratol.* 3:437–44
7. Spencer, P. S., Schaumburg, H. H., Sabri, M. I., Veronesi, B. 1980. The enlarging view of hexacarbon neurotoxicity. *CRC Crit. Rev. Toxicol.* 3:279–356
8. Couri, D., Milks, M. 1982. Toxicity and metabolism of the neurotoxic hexacarbons *n*-hexane, 2-hexanone, and 2,5-hexanedione. *Ann. Rev. Pharmacol. Toxicol.* 22:145–66
9. Ochs, S., Sabri, M. I., Ranish, N. 1970. Somal site of synthesis of fast transported material in mammalian nerve fibers. *J. Neurobiol.* 1:329–44
10. Singer, M., Salpeter, M. M. 1966. Transport of tritium-labelled I-histidine through the Schwann and myelin sheaths into the axon of peripheral nerves. *Nature* 210:1225–1227
11. Skene, J. H. P., Willard, M. 1981. Axonally transported proteins associated with axon growth in rabbit central and peripheral nervous systems. *J. Cell Biol.* 89:96–103
12. Skene, J. H. P., Willard, M. 1981.

Changes in axonally transported proteins during axon regeneration in toad retinal ganglion cells. *J. Cell Biol.* 89:86–95

13. Brady, S. T., Lasek, R. J. 1981. Nerve-specific enolase and creatinine phosphokinase in axonal transport: Soluble proteins and the axoplasmic matrix. *Cell* 23:515–23

14. Schwartz, J. H. 1979. Axonal transport: Components, mechanisms and specificity. *Ann. Rev. Neurosci.* 2:467–504

15. Black, M. M., Lasek, R. J. 1979. Axonal transport of actin: Slow component b is the principal source of actin for the axon. *Brain Res.* 171:401–13

16. Goldberg, D. J., Sherbany, A. A., Schwartz, J. H. 1978. Kinetic properties of normal and perturbed axonal transport of serotonin in a single identified axon. *J. Physiol.* 281:559–79

17. Ochs, S. 1975. Retention and redistribution of proteins in mammalian nerve fibers by axoplasmic transport. *J. Physiol.* 253:459–75

18. Gross, G. W., Beidler, L. M. 1975. A quantitative analysis of isotope concentration profiles and rapid transport velocities in the C-fibers of the garfish olfactory nerve. *J. Neurobiol.* 6:213–32

19. Brimijoin, S. 1975. Stop-flow: A new technique for measuring axonal transport of dopamine-B-hydroxylase. *J. Neurobiol.* 6:379–94

20. Brimijoin, S., Lundberg, J. M., Brodin, E., Hokfelt, T., Nilsson, G. 1980. Axonal transport of substance P in the vagus and sciatic nerves of the guinea pig. *Brain Res.* 191:443–57

21. Hanson, M. 1978. A new method to study fast axonal transport *in vivo*. *Brain Res.* 153:121

22. Bisby, M. A., Bulgar, V. T. 1977. Reversal of axonal transport at a nerve crush. *J. Neurochem.* 29:313–20

23. Grafstein, B. 1975. The nerve cell response to axotomy. *Exp. Neurol.* 48:32–51

24. Cragg, B. C. 1970. What is the signal for chromatolysis? *Brain Res.* 23:1–21

25. Kristensson, K., Sjostrand, J. 1972. Retrograde transport of protein tracer in rabbit hypoglossal nerve regeneration. *Brain Res.* 45:175–81

26. Pilar, G., Landmesser, L. J. 1972. Axotomy mimicked by local colchicine application. *Science* 177:1116–18

27. Singer, P. A., Mehler, S., Fernandez, H. L. 1982. Blockade of retrograde axonal transport delays the onset of metabolic and morphologic changes induced by axotomy. *J. Neurosci.* 2:1299–306

28. Droz, B., Rambourg, A., Koenig, H. L.

1975. The smooth endoplasmic reticulum: Structure and role in the renewal of axonal membranes and synaptic vesicles by fast axonal transport. *Brain Res.* 93:1–13

29. Holtzman, E., Teichberg, S., Abrahams, S. J., Citkoitz, E., Kawai, N., Peterson, E. R. 1973. Notes on synaptic vesicles and related structures, endoplasmic reticulum, lysosomes and peroxisomes in nervous tissue and adrenal medulla. *J. Histochem. Cytochem.* 21:349–85

30. Sahenk, Z., Mendell, J. R. 1978. Abnormal retrograde axoplasmic transport in the pathogenesis of experimental dying-back neuropathy of BOTZ. *Neurology* 28:357

31. Price, D. L., Griffin, J., Young, A., Peck, K., Stocks, A. 1975. Tetanus toxin: Direct evidence for retrograde intraaxonal transport. *Science* 188:945–47

32. Bunt, A. H., Haschke, R. H., Lund, R. D., Calins, D. F. 1976. Factors affecting retrograde axonal transport of horseradish peroxidase in the visual system. *Brain Res.* 102:152–55

33. Hendry, I. A., Stach, R., Herrup, K. 1974. Characteristics of the retrograde axonal transport system for nerve growth factor in the sympathetic nervous system. *Brain Res.* 82:117–28

34. Stoeckel, K., Schwab, M., Thoenen, H. 1975. Comparison between the retrograde axonal transport of nerve growth factor and tetanus toxin in motor, sensory and adrenergic neurons. *Brain Res.* 99:1–16

35. Miller, M. S., Buck, S. H., Sipes, I. G., Yamamura, H. I., Burks, T. F. 1982. Regulations of substance P by nerve growth factor: disruption by capsaicin. *Brain Res.* 250:193–96

36. Stoeckel, K., Schwab, M., Thoenen, H. 1977. Role of gangliosides in the uptake and retrograde axonal transport of cholera and tetanus toxin as compared to nerve growth factor and wheat germ agglutinin. *Brain Res.* 132:273–85

37. Fink, D. J., Gainer, H. 1980. Retrograde axonal transport of endogenous proteins in sciatic nerve demonstrated by covalent labelling in vivo. *Science* 208:303

38. Porcellati, G. 1969. Peripheral nerve. See Ref. 3, 11:393–422

39. Bikales, N. M., Kolodny, E. R. 1963. Acrylamide. In *Encyclopedia of Chemical Technology*, ed. A. Standen, pp. 274–84. New York: Interscience. 2nd ed.

40. Bikales, N. M. 1970. Acrylamide and related amides. In *High Polymers, Vinyl and Diene Monomers*, ed. E. C. Leonard, pp. 81–104. New York: Wiley

41. Cavins, J. F., Friedman, M. 1967. Specific modification of protein sulfhydryl groups with alpha,beta-unsaturated compounds. *Fed. Proc.* 26:822

42. Cavins, J. F., Friedman, M. 1967. New amino acids derived from reaction of E-amino groups in protein with alpha,beta-unsaturated compounds. *Biochemistry* 6: 3766–70

43. Druckery, H., Consbruch, U., Schmahl, D. 1953. Effects of monomeric acrylamide on proteins. *Z. Naturforsch.* 86: 145–50

44. Hashimoto, K., Aldridge, W. N. 1970. Biochemical studies on acrylamide, a neurotoxic agent. *Biochem. Pharmacol.* 19:2591–604

45. Auld, R. B., Bedwell, S. F. 1967. Peripheral neuropathy with sympathetic overactivity from industrial contact with acrylamide. *Can. Med. Assoc. J.* 96: 652

46. Garland, T. O., Patterson, M. H. 1967. Six cases of acrylamide poisoning. *Br. Med. J.* 4:134–38

47. Sumner, A. J., Asbury, A. K. 1975. Physiological studies of the dying-back phenomenon. Muscle stretch afferents in acrylamide neuropathy. *Brain* 98:91–100

48. Schaumburg, H. H., Wisniewski, H. M., Spencer, P. S. 1974. Ultrastructural studies of the dying-back process: I. Peripheral nerve terminal and axon degeneration in systemic acrylamide intoxication. *J. Neuropathol. Exp. Neurol.* 33:260–84

49. Kesson, C. M., Baird, A. W., Lawson, D. H. 1977. Acrylamide poisoning. *Postgrad. Med. J.* 53:16–17

50. Fullerton, P. M. 1969. Electrophysiological and histological observations on peripheral nerves in acrylamide poisoning in man. *J. Neurol. Neurosurg. Psych.* 32:186–92

51. Kuperman, A. S. 1958. Effects of acrylamide on the central nervous system of the cat. *J. Pharmacol. Exp. Ther.* 123:180–92

52. Leswing, R. J., Ribelin, W. E. 1969. Physiologic and pathologic changes in acrylamide neuropathy. *Arch. Environ. Health* 18:22–29

53. McCollister, D. D., Oyen, F., Rowe, V. K. 1964. Toxicology of acrylamide. *Toxicol. Appl. Pharmacol.* 6:172–81

54. Fullerton, P. M., Barnes, J. M. 1966. Peripheral neuropathy in rats produced by acrylamide. *Br. J. Indust. Med.* 23:210–21

55. Suzuki, K., Pfaff, L. D. 1973. Acrylamide neuropathy in rats—An electron microscopic study of degeneration and regeneration. *Acta Neuropath.* 24:197–213

56. Tilson, H. A., Cabe, P. A., Spencer, P. S. 1979. Acrylamide behavioral toxicity in rats: A correlated neurobehavioral and pathological study. *Neurotoxicology* 1: 89–104

57. Bradley, W. G., Asbury, A. K. 1970. Radioautographic studies of Schwann cell behavior. I. Acrylamide neuropathy in the mouse. *J. Neuropathol. Exp. Neurol.* 29:500–6

58. Evans, H., Teal, J. J. 1981. Appetitive behaviors as models of the neurotoxicity of acrylamide. *Fed. Proc.* 40:677

59. Gilbert, S. G., Maurissen, J. P. 1982. Assessment of the effects of acrylamide, methylmercury, and 2,5-hexanedione on motor functions in mice. *J. Toxicol. Environ. Health* 10:31–41

60. Hopkins, A. P. 1970. The effect of acrylamide on the peripheral nervous system of the baboon. *J. Neurosurg. Psychiatr.* 33:805–16

61. Edwards, P. M. 1975. Neurotoxicity of acrylamide and its analogues and effects of these analogues and other agents on acrylamide neuropathy. *Br. J. Ind. Med.* 32:31–38

62. Edwards, P. M. 1975. The distribution and metabolism of acrylamide and its neurotoxic analogues in rats. *Biochem. Pharmacol.* 24:1277–82

63. Miller, M. J., Carter, D. E., Sipes, I. G. 1982. The pharmacokinetics of acrylamide in Fisher 344 rats. *Toxicol. Appl. Pharmacol.* 63:36–44

64. Pastoor, T., Richardson, R. J. 1981. Blood dynamics of acrylamide in rats. *Toxicologist* 1:53

65. Rylander-Yueh, L. A., Carter, D. E. 1982. Tissue disposition of acrylamide in multiply-dosed 5-week vs. 11-week male Holtzman rats. *Toxicologist* 2:1–50

66. Pastoor, T., Heydens, W., Richardson, R. J. 1980. Time and dose-related excretion of acrylamide metabolites in the urine of Fisher 344 rats. In *Mechanisms of Toxicity and Hazard Evaluation Developments in Toxicology and Environmental Science, Vol. 8*, ed. B. Holmstedt, R. Lauwerys, M. Mercier, M. Roberfraid. New York: Elsevier-North Holland

67. Dixit, R., Seth, P. K., Mukhtar, H. 1980. Brain glutathione-S-transferase catalyzed conjugation of acrylamide: A novel mechanism for detoxification of neurotoxin. *Biochem. Int.* 1:547–52

68. Dixit, R., Husain, R., Mukhtar, H., Seth, P. K. 1981. Acrylamide induced inhibition of hepatic glutathione-S-

transferase activity in rats. *Toxicol. Letts.* 7:207–10

69. Dixit, R., Husain, R., Seth, P. K., Mukhtar, H. 1980. Effect of diethylmaleate on acrylamide induced neuropathy in rats. *Toxicol. Letts.* 6:417–21

70. Dixit, R., Mukhtar, H., Seth, P. K., Krishna, C. R. 1980. Binding of acrylamide with glutathione-S-transferases. *Chem. Biol. Interact.* 32:353–59

71. Mukhtar, H., Dixit, R., Seth, P. K. 1981. Reduction in cutaneous and hepatic glutathione contents, glutathione-S-transferase and aryl hydrocarbon hydroylase activities following topical application of acrylamide to mouse. *Toxicol. Letts.* 9:153–56

72. Das, M., Mukhtar, H., Seth, P. K. 1982. Effect of acrylamide on brain and hepatic mixed-function oxidase and glutathione-S-transferase in rats. *Toxicol. Appl. Pharmacol.* 66:420–26

73. Kaplan, M. L., Murphy, S. D., Gilles, F. H. 1973. Modification of acrylamide neuropathy in rats by selected factors. *Toxicol. Appl. Pharmacol.* 24:564–79

74. Hashimoto, K., Sakamoto, J., Tannii, H. 1981. Neurotoxicity of acrylamide and related compounds and their effects on male gonads in mice. *Arch. Toxicol.* 47:179–89

75. Howland, R. D. 1981. The etiology of acrylamide neuropathy: Enolase, phosphofructokinase, and glyceraldehyde-3-phosphate dehydrogenase activity in peripheral nerve, spinal cord, brain and skeletal muscle of acrylamide-intoxicated cats. *Toxicol. Appl. Pharmacol.* 60:324–33

76. Howland, R. D., Vyas, I. L., Lowndes, H. E. 1980. The etiology of acrylamide neuropathy: Possible involvement of neuron specific enolase. *Brain Res.* 190:529–35

77. Howland, R. D., Vyas, I. L., Lowndes, H. E., Argentieri, T. M. 1980. The etiology of toxic peripheral neuropathies: In vitro effects of acrylamide and 2,5-hexanedione on brain enolase and other glycolytic enzymes. *Brain Res.* 202:131–42

78. Kemplay, S., Cavanagh, J. B. 1984. Effects of acrylamide and other sulfhydryl compounds in vivo and in vitro on staining of motor nerve terminals by the zinc iodide-osmium technique. *Muscle Nerve* 7:94–100

79. Kemplay, S., Cavanagh, J. B. 1984. Effects of acrylamide and some other sulfhydryl reagents on spontaneous and pathologically induced terminal sprout-ing from motor end-plates. *Muscle Nerve* 7:101–9

80. Sabri, M. I., Spencer, P. S. 1980. Inhibition of glyceraldehyde-3-phosphate and other glycolytic enzymes by acrylamide. *Neurosci. Letts. Suppl.* 5:455

81. Sabri, M. I., Moore, C. L., Spencer, P. S. 1979. Studies on the biochemical basis of distal axonopathies I. Inhibition of glycolysis by neurotoxic hexacarbon compounds. *J. Neurochem.* 32:683–89

82. Sabri, M. I. 1983. Mechanism of action of acrylamide on the nervous system. *Biol. Mem.* 8:16–27

83. Prineas, J. 1969. The pathogenesis of dying-back polyneuropathies. II. An ultrastructural study of experimental acrylamide intoxication in the cat. *J. Neuropathol. Exp. Neurol.* 28:598–621

84. Spencer, P. S., Thomas, P. K. 1974. Ultrastructural studies of the dying-back process. II. The sequestration and removal by Schwann cells and oligodendrocytes of organelles from normal and diseased axons. *J. Neurocytol.* 3:763–83

85. Hanna, R. B., Spencer, P. S., Pappas, G. D. 1976. Structural differences in membranes in the pacinian corpuscle. A freeze-fracture study. *Neurosci. Abstr.* 2:404

86. Pleasure, D. E., Mishner, K. C., Engel, W. K. 1969. Axonal transport of proteins in experimental neuropathies. *Science* 166:524–25

87. Bradley, W. G., Williams, M. H. 1973. Axoplasmic flow in axonal neuropathies. *Brain* 96:235–46

88. Weir, R. L., Glaubiger, G., Chase, T. N. 1978. Inhibition of fast axoplasmic transport by acrylamide. *Environ. Res.* 17:251–55

89. Souyri, F., Chretien, M., Droz, B. 1981. Retention of proteins conveyed with fast axonal transport in acrylamide-induced neuropathy. I. Light radioautographic study: Focal retention of fast transported proteins in preterminal axons. *Brain Res.* 205:1–13

90. Chretien, M., Patey, G., Souyri, F., Droz, B. 1981. Acrylamide induced neuropathy and impairment of axonal transport of proteins. II. Abnormal accumulations of smooth endoplasmic reticulum at sites of focal retention of fast transported proteins. Electron microscope radioautographic study. *Brain Res.* 205:15–28

91. Sidenius, P., Jakobsen, J. 1983. Anterograde axonal transport in rats during intoxication with acrylamide. *J. Neurochem.* 40:697–704

92. Sumner, A., Pleasure, D., Ciesielka, K. 1976. Slowing of fast axoplasmic transport in acrylamide neuropathy. *J. Neuropathol. Exp. Neurol.* 35:319 (Abstr.)

93. Griffin, J. W., Price, D. L. 1976. Axonal transport in motor neuron pathology. In *Recent Research Trends,* ed. J. Andrews, R. Johnson, M. Brazier, p. 33–67. New York: Academic

94. Couraud, J. Y., Di Giamberardino, J., Chretien, M., Souyri, F., Fardeau, M. 1982. Acrylamide neuropathy and changes in the axonal transport and muscular content of the molecular forms of acetylcholinesterase. *Muscle Nerve* 5:302–12

95. Schotman, P., Gipon, L., Jennekens, F. G. I., Gispen, W. H. 1978. Polyneuropathies and CNS protein metabolism III. Changes in protein synthesis rate induced by acrylamide intoxication. *J. Neuropathol. Exp. Neurol.* 37:820–37

96. Hashimoto, K., Ando, K. 1973. Alteration of amino acid incorporation into proteins of the nervous system in vitro after administration of acrylamide to rats. *Biochem. Pharmacol.* 22:1057–66

97. Sahenk, Z., Mendell, J. R. 1981. Acrylamide and hexanedione neuropathies: Abnormal bidirectional transport rate in distal axons. *Brain Res.* 219:397–405

98. Jakobsen, J., Sidenius, P. 1983. Early and dose-dependent decrease of retrograde axonal transport in acrylamide-intoxicated rats. *J. Neurochem.* 40:447–54

99. Miller, M. S., Miller, M. J., Burks, T. F., Sipes, I. G. 1983. Altered retrograde axonal transport of nerve growth factor after single and repeated doses of acrylamide in the rat. *Toxicol. Appl. Pharmacol.* 69:96–101

100. Miller, M. S., Spencer, P. S. 1984. Single doses of acrylamide reduce retrograde transport velocity. *J. Neurochem.* 43(5):1401–8

101. Kemplay, S., Cavanagh, J. B. 1983. Effects of acrylamide and botulinum toxin on horseradish peroxidase labelling of trigeminal motor neurons in the rat. *J. Anat.* 137:477–82

102. Gold, B. G., Griffin, J. W., Price, D. L. 1983. Slow axonal transport following single high-dose acrylamide administration. *Soc. Neurosci. Abstr.* 9:669

103. Kreutzberg, G. W. 1968. Histochemical demonstration of a colchicine-induced blockage of enzyme transport in axons of peripheral nerves. *Proc. 3rd Int. Congr. Histochem. Cytochem.,* pp. 133–34. New York: Springer-Verlag

104. Kreutzberg, G. W. 1969. Neuronal dynamics and axonal flow. IV. Blockage of intra-axonal enzyme transport by colchicine. *Proc. Natl. Acad. Sci. USA* 62:722–28

105. Karlsson, J. O., Hanson, H. A., Sjostrand, J. 1971. Effect of colchicine on axonal transport and morphology of retinal ganglion cells. *Z. Zellforsch. Mikrosk. Anat.* 115:265–83

106. Karlsson, J. O., Sjostrand, J. 1969. The effect of colchicine on the axonal transport of protein in the optic nerve and tract of the rabbit. *Brain Res.* 13:617–19

107. Hanson, M., Edstrom, A. 1978. Mitosis inhibitors and axonal transport. *Int. Rev. Cytol.* 7:373–402

108. Samson, F. E. 1976. Pharmacology of drugs that affect intracellular movement. *Ann. Rev. Pharmacol. Toxicol.* 16:143–59

109. Morgan-Hughes, J. A., Sinclair, S., Durston, J. H. J. 1974. The pattern of peripheral nerve regeneration induced by crush in rats with severe acrylamide neuropathy. *Brain* 97:235–50

110. Griffin, J. W., Price, D. L., Drachman, D. B. 1977. Impaired axonal regeneration in acrylamide intoxication. *J. Neurobiol.* 8:355–70

111. Cavanagh, J. B., Gysbers, M. F. 1980. "Dying-back" above a nerve ligature produced by acrylamide. *Acta Neuropathol.* 51:169–77

112. Benowitz, L. I., Sashoua, V. E., Yoon, M. G. 1981. Rapidly transported proteins in the regenerating optic nerve of goldfish. *J. Neurosci.* 1:300–7

113. Bisby, M. A. 1980. Changes in the composition of labeled protein transported in motor axons during their regeneration. *J. Neurobiol.* 11:435–45

114. Giulian, D., Des Ruisseaux, H., Cowburn, D. 1980. Biosynthesis and intraaxonal transport of proteins during neuronal regeneration. *J. Biol. Chem.* 255:6494–501

115. Perry, G. W., Wilson, D. L. 1981. Protein synthesis and axonal transport during nerve regeneration. *J. Neurochem.* 37:1203–17

116. Perry, G. W., Krayanek, S. R., Wilson, D. L. 1983. Protein synthesis and rapid axonal transport during regrowth of dorsal root axons. *J. Neurochem.* 40:1590–98

117. Gunning, P. W., Kaye, P. L., Austin, L. 1977. In vivo RNA synthesis within the rat nodose ganglia. *J. Neurochem.* 28:1237–40

118. Gunning, P. W., Kaye, P. L., Austin, L. 1977. In vivo synthesis of rapidly labelled RNA within the rat nodose gan-

glia following vagotomy. *J. Neurochem.* 28:1245–48

119. Kaye, P. L., Gunning, P. W., Austin, L. 1977. In vivo synthesis of stable RNA within the rat nodose ganglia following vagotomy. *J. Neurochem.* 28:1241–43

120. Langford, C. J., Scheffer, J. W., Jeffrey, P. L., Austin, L. 1980. The in vitro synthesis of RNA within the rat nodose ganglion following vagotomy. *J. Neurochem.* 34:531–39

121. Miller, M. S., Spencer, P. S. Inhibition by acrylamide of increased ornithine decarboxylase activity and RNA synthesis in dorsal root ganglion following sciatic nerve transsection. *J. Neurochem.* Submitted for publication

122. Russell, D. H., Snyder, S. H. 1968. Amine synthesis in rapidly growing tissues: Ornithine decarboxylase in rat liver. *Endocrinology* 86:1414–19

123. Russell, D. H. 1980. Ornithine decarboxylase as a biological and pharmacological tool. *Pharmacology* 20:117–29

124. Slotkin, T. A. 1979. Ornithine decarboxylase as a tool in developmental neurobiology. *Life Sci.* 24:1623–30

125. Slotkin, T. A., Seidler, F. J., Whitmore, W. L., Weigel, S. J., Slepetis, R. J., et al. 1983. Critical periods for the role of ornithine decarboxylase and the polyamines in growth and development of the rat: Effects of exposure to alpha-difluoromethylornithine during discrete prenatal or postnatal intervals. *Int. J. Devl. Neurosci.* 1:113–127

126. Slotkin, T. A., Whitmore, W. L., Lerea, L., Slepetis, R. J., Weigel, S. J., et al. 1983. Role of ornithine decarboxylase and the polyamines in nervous system development: Short-term postnatal administration of alpha-difluoromethylornithine, an irreversible inhibitor of ornithine decarboxylase. *Int. J. Dev. Neurosci.* 1:7–16

127. Ingoglia, N. A., Sturman, J. A., Eisner, R. A. 1977. Axonal transport of putrescine, spermine, and spermidine in normal and regenerating goldfish optic nerves. *Brain Res.* 130:433–45

128. Rochel, S., Margolis, F. L. 1980. The response of ornithine decarboxylase during neuronal degeneration and regeneration in olfactory epithelium. *J. Neurochem.* 35:850–60

129. Russell, D. H. 1973. Polyamines in growth—Normal and neoplastic. In *Polyamines in Normal and Neoplastic Growth,* ed. D. H. Russell, pp. 1–13. New York: Raven

130. Kohsaka, S., Heacock, A. M., Klinger, P. D., Porta, R., Agranoff, B. W. 1982. Dissociation of enhanced ornithine decarboxylase activity and optic nerve regeneration in goldfish. *Dev. Brain Res.* 4:149–56

131. Kohsaka, S., Schwartz, M., Agranoff, B. W. 1981. Increased activity of ornithine decarboxylase in goldfish following optic nerve crush. *Dev. Brain Res.* 1:391–401

132. Sterman, A. B. 1982. Cell body remodeling during dying-back axonopathy: DRG changes during advanced disease. *J. Neuropathol. Exp. Neurol.* 41:400–11

133. Sterman, A. B. 1982. Acrylamide induces early morphologic reorganization of the neuronal cell body. *Neurology* 32:1023–26

134. Sterman, A. B. 1983. Altered sensory ganglia in acrylamide neuropathy: Quantitative evidence of neuronal reorganization. *J. Neuropathol. Exp. Neurol.* 42:166–76

135. Cavanagh, J. B. 1982. The pathokinetics of acrylamide intoxication: A reassessment of the problem. *Neuropathol. Appl. Neurobiol.* 8:315–36

136. Cavanagh, J. B., Gysbers, M. F. 1983. Ultrastructural features of the purkinje cell damage caused by acrylamide in the rat: a new phenomenon in cellular neuropathology. *J. Neurocytol.* 12:413–37

137. Ochs, S. 1982. In *Axoplasmic Transport and its Relation to Other Nerve Functions,* pp. 148–77. New York: Wiley

138. Griffin, J. W., Hoffman, P. N., Price, D. L. 1982. Axoplasmic transport in B,B'-Iminodipropionitrile neuropathy. In *Axoplasmic Transport in Physiology and Pathology,* ed. D. G. Weiss, A. Gorio, pp. 109–18. Berlin: Springer-Verlag

139. Tanii, H., Hashimoto, K. 1983. Neurotoxicity of acrylamide and related compounds in rats: Effects on rotorod performance, morphology of nerves and neurotubulin. *Arch. Toxicol.* 54:203–13

140. Sabri, M. I., Ochs, S. 1971. Inhibition of glyceraldehyde-3-phosphate dehydrogenase in mammalian nerve by iodoacetate. *J. Neurochem.* 13:1509–14

141. Spencer, P. S., Sabri, M. I., Schaumburg, H. H., Moore, C. L. 1978. Does a defect of energy metabolism in the nerve fiber underlie axonal degeneration in polyneuropathies? *Ann. Neurol.* 5:501–7

142. Spencer, P. S., Sabri, M. I., Politis, M. 1980. Methyl-*n*-butyl ketone, carbon disulfide, and acrylamide: Putative mechanism of neurotoxic damage. In *Advances in Neurotoxicology,* ed. L. Manzo, pp. 173–80. New York: Pergamon

143. Lehninger, A. L. 1975. *Biochemistry.* New York: Worth. 2nd ed.

144. Sabri, M. I., Dairman, W., Juhasz, L., Bischoff, M. C., Spencer, P. S. 1981. Is acrylamide neurotoxicity pyruvate sensitive? *Trans. Am. Soc. Neurochem.* 12:155

145. Dairman, W., Sabri, M. I., Bischoff, M., Juhasz, L., Ng, T., Spencer, P. S. 1984. Dietary pyruvate suppresses acrylamide neuropathy in male rats. *Ann. Neurol.* Submitted for publication

146. Sterman, A. B., Panasci, D. J., Persons, W. 1983. Does pyruvate prevent acrylamide neurotoxicity? Implications for disease pathogenesis. *Exp. Neurol.* 82:148–58

147. Loeb, A. L., Anderson, R. J. 1981. Antagonism of acrylamide neurotoxicity by supplementation with vitamin B_6. *Neurotoxicology* 2:625–33

148. Metzler, D. E. 1977. *Biochemistry. The Chemical Reactions of Living Cells.* New York: Academic

Ann. Rev. Pharmacol. Toxicol. 1985. 25:667–89

PHARMACOKINETIC PITFALLS IN THE ESTIMATION OF THE BREAST MILK/PLASMA RATIO FOR DRUGS

John T. Wilson, R. Don Brown, James L. Hinson, and John W. Dailey

Departments of Pharmacology and Therapeutics and Pediatrics, Louisiana State University School of Medicine in Shreveport, Shreveport, Louisiana 71130-3932

INTRODUCTION

We hold these truths to be self-evident. The concentration of a drug in milk is time dependent. Concurrence does not necessarily exist between milk and plasma drug concentration profiles. Presumed concurrence undermines the study design and weakens the reliability of data. A pharmacokinetic model is a requisite foundation for studies of drugs in breast milk. A test of the model applicable to each drug allows the most accurate estimates of the milk-to-plasma (M/P) ratio. Pragmatic utilization of study data is often a function of a valid M/P ratio as it impacts on an assessment of dose and safety for the nursing infant.

The milk-to-plasma (M/P) ratio of drug concentration is often used to estimate the dose of maternal drug delivered via breast milk to the infant. An accurate ratio applicable to different dose strengths and chronicity of dosing is very useful when the concentration of drug in a mother's plasma, but not in her milk, is known. An inaccurate ratio, or one that cannot be used under the desired clinical circumstances, produces erroneous estimates of the amount of drug in milk.

Pitfalls exist in the estimation of the M/P ratio. The most common one is an implicit assumption that milk and plasma drug concentrations parallel each other throughout dosing, i.e. that a concurrence exists between the milk and plasma drug concentration profiles. This review emphasizes this and other potential problems by developing pharmacokinetic models, simulating illustrations, and citing studies reported for a few drugs.

667

0362-1642/85/415-0667$02.00

A focused review cannot appropriately consider all aspects of this important subject. Additional information is available from recent reviews of a selective or comprehensive nature on the following topics: pharmacokinetics (1–5), general aspects (6–22), and safety evaluations (23–24). We hope that the reader who reviews work in this field will question study design as it impacts on the accuracy of the reported M/P ratio and consequently on the estimation of drug dose in milk received by the nursing infant.

BACKGROUND

The Use of the M/P Ratio

The M/P ratio is used essentially to estimate the dose of a drug in milk as a function of the maternal plasma drug concentration. The M/P ratio adjusts for the factors that can change this concentration in either fluid. For example, an increase in dose or the use of multiple doses is expected to produce a higher concentration of drug in plasma, and hence in milk, than a lower or single dose. The ratio between milk and plasma concentrations expresses these changes without the need for a nomogram of maternal drug dose versus concentration of drug in milk. The usefulness of a nomogram is limited by the multiple influences on maternal drug disposition. The M/P ratio captures the net result of maternal drug dosing and disposition, i.e. the resultant plasma concentration, and the transfer of drug into milk. However, the M/P ratio is not necessarily constant under all conditions and at all times after dosing of a particular drug. The ratio may be affected by factors that alter either the delivery of blood to the breast or the bidirectional transfer of drug between plasma and milk. Some of these factors include pharmacokinetic characteristics of the drug itself (e.g. deep-compartment distribution behavior), physiochemical properties of the drug (pKa) and pH of the milk, the period of lactation, the maturity of the milk, the frequency of suckling, and maternal illness. These may perturb the expected concurrence of the milk and plasma drug concentration profiles and hence destabilize a M/P ratio determined under dissimilar conditions.

Utilizing the M/P ratio for the estimation of infant drug dose via breast milk is shown by the equations in Table 1 (3). An interdose plasma average is often used for the M/P ratio. Use of this equation presupposes a concurrence of milk and plasma profile during the dosing interval. It also presupposes that the M/P ratio for a single dose is the same as that for multiple dose administration under steady state conditions.

Prerequisites for an Estimate of Drug Concentration in Breast Milk

As emphasized previously (4), three components are needed for a comprehensive study of drug dosing via breast milk: maternal pharmacokinetics, mam-

Table 1 Drug dose given to infant via breast milk[a]

General calculation

$C_{avg} \times M/P \times$ milk volume (ml/kg/d) = dose (mg/kg/d)

Worse case analysis

$C_{max} \times M/P \times$ milk volume (ml/kg/d) = dose (mg/kg/d)

C_{avg} and C_{max} are respective averages and maximum drug concentrations in plasma at time of feeding. M/P is the milk to plasma ratio of drug concentration and is assumed to be invariate with regard to time after dosing.

Milk volume average is 150 ml/kg/d.

[a]Taken from (3).

Table 2 Interrelation of factors in mother and infant as they affect drug dose in milk and safety to infant

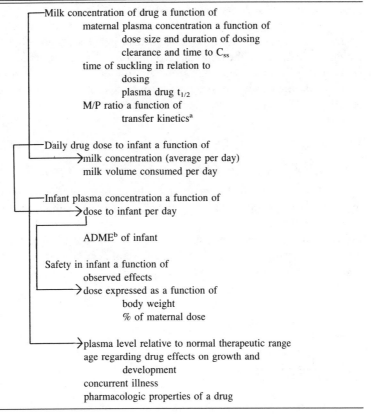

— Milk concentration of drug a function of
    maternal plasma concentration a function of
        dose size and duration of dosing
        clearance and time to C_{ss}
    time of suckling in relation to
        dosing
        plasma drug $t_{1/2}$
    M/P ratio a function of
        transfer kinetics[a]

— Daily drug dose to infant a function of
    → milk concentration (average per day)
    milk volume consumed per day

— Infant plasma concentration a function of
    → dose to infant per day

    ADME[b] of infant

Safety in infant a function of
    observed effects
    → dose expressed as a function of
        body weight
        % of maternal dose

    → plasma level relative to normal therapeutic range
    age regarding drug effects on growth and
        development
    concurrent illness
    pharmacologic properties of a drug

[a] Transfer kinetics is broadly defined as all those events that determine the concentration of drug in milk at a certain time.

[b] ADME is absorption, distribution, metabolism, and excretion of a drug.

mary pharmacokinetics, and infant pharmacokinetics. The first two components interact to determine the time course profile of the M/P ratio. Resultant infant plasma concentrations (as well as the estimated dose in milk) are used to assess safety in addition to the intrinsic pharmacologic properties of a drug. This review addresses maternal and mammary pharmacokinetics as determinants of the M/P ratio and hence the amount of drug in breast milk.

The cascade of events starts with the excretion of drug in breast milk and ends with assessment of safety for the nursing infant (Table 2). Milk is seldom analyzed for drug concentration, so estimates are usually derived from maternal plasma levels and a reported value for the M/P ratio. An error in the estimation of drug concentration in milk can confound an evaluation of safety unless plasma drug concentrations are analyzed in the infant. Such analyses should be done at the time of predicted steady state conditions in the infant; otherwise drug concentrations will be underestimated. When only the calculated dose in milk is used as a guide, an accurate M/P ratio is crucial.

Use of a single-point-in-time M/P ratio or an average ratio calculated with single-dose area-under-the-curve (AUC) data is not sufficient for all drugs. Neither ratio attests to the importance of the time-dependent variation of drug concentration in milk. This time dependency presents pitfalls in determining an accurate M/P ratio as well as estimates of drug dose in milk at the time of infant suckling.

PITFALLS IN THE ESTIMATION OF THE M/P RATIO

Applicable Models and Simulated Profiles of the M/P Ratio

The M/P ratio is a function of the model that best describes maternal drug distribution and elimination. Drug profiles have been simulated for several models in order to show model-dependent effects on the M/P ratio as well as to illustrate the pharmacokinetic nature of pitfalls in estimation of the ratio.

A one-compartment open model, inclusive of central, peripheral, and milk compartments, is shown below:

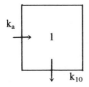

For this and subsequent models oral dosing is used and the absorption rate constant is k_a. The overall elimination rate constant is k_{10}. Simulations of each model utilize equations designed to elicit the amount of drug in a compartment. Conversion to drug concentration units requires information about the apparent drug distribution volume of each compartment. This has not been assessed for each model nor is it important for the purpose of this review. The M/P ratios reported for the simulations illustrate the effects of particular combinations of pharmacokinetic rate constants on the amounts of drug rather than on drug concentrations. The resultant trend of M/P ratios for drug amounts should correspond closely to the trend of M/P ratios for drug concentrations in these models. However, the value of the M/P ratio for drug concentrations may not be the same as that for the M/P ratio for drug amount unless the apparent volumes of distribution for the two compartments are the same. For this and other models we have assumed that infant suckling does not occur or has no effect on the simulated profile[1].

A simulated drug concentration and derived M/P ratio profile for the one-compartment open model is shown in Figure 1. The M/P ratio essentially does not change in relation to time after single or multiple doses. The value of the M/P ratio for this and other simulations is determined solely by the pharmaco-kinetic parameters, without regard to drug-partitioning characteristics among fluids of different pH. It is quite likely that the distribution rate constants incorporate (or are largely a function of) the ion-partitioning characteristics of a drug. Observation of a similarity between the predicted and observed ultrafil-trate M/P ratio may require determining the M/P ratio under post-distribution conditions. This is apparent from a review of the following simulations, which emphasize the relative time dependency rather than absolute M/P ratio.

A two-compartment open model, including the peripheral and milk compart-ments, is shown as:

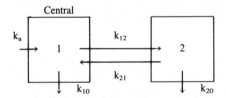

Corresponding simulations of drug amount in plasma and milk are shown in Figure 2. Note that the time dependency of the M/P ratio derived after a single dose is a function of the value of the distribution rate constants. A linear relationship has been found for the asymptotic value of the M/P ratio and the slope of the initial phase of the ratio obtained after a single dose. This relationship prevails in a two-compartment open model when the hybrid α rate constant is unchanged even though the k_{12}/k_{21} ratio changes. However, the rate constants for β and k_a confound the relationship. Given these restrictions on the

[1]For example, k_{20} in the succeeding two-compartment model has not been incorporated into our simulations.

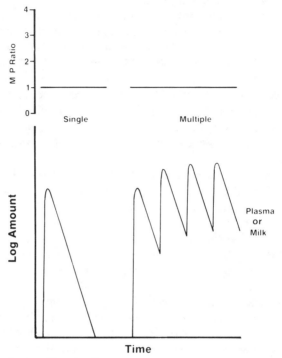

Figure 1 Simulated profiles of milk and plasma drug amounts and derived M/P ratios for a one-compartment open model after single and multiple doses. Oral dosing and a one-compartment open model are assumed. Suckling did not occur. Pharmacokinetic parameters used for the simulation are: $k_a = 5.35$, $\beta = 0.4$ hour-1. The dosing interval is three hours.

relationship, it is apparent that a higher M/P ratio, as observed with weakly basic drugs, is probably associated with a greater degree of change in the M/P ratio during early post-dose periods. A concentration-time profile must be described for such drugs in order to derive an accurate M/P ratio.

Figure 3 shows simulations of the drug amount and M/P ratio profiles for a two-compartment open model after multiple doses. It is apparent that the M/P ratio for single or multiple doses is a function of the time at which it is determined after dosing. This time dependency is exaggerated for drugs with rate constants similar to those used for Figure 2B and 2D, as shown by parts A and B of Figure 3. The deep-compartment behavior of a drug in milk, as shown by the simulation in Figure 4, produces a more marked change in the M/P ratio as dosing continues. In this example, the M/P ratio increases as a function of dose number. This is expected for filling a deep compartment. Accurate determination of the M/P ratio requires information about the drug-

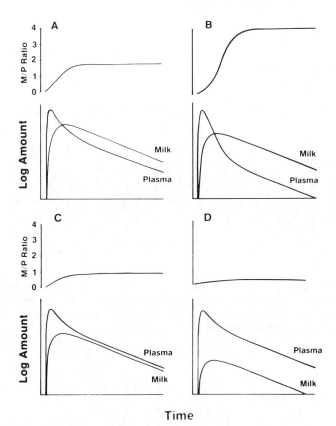

Time

Figure 2 Simulated profiles of milk and plasma drug amounts and derived M/P ratios for a two-compartment open model after a single dose. Oral dosing and a two-compartment open model are assumed. Suckling did not occur. Equations for this model as described in (25, 26) were used. Pharmacokinetic parameters for each part of this figure are:

	A	B	C	D
	(hour^{-1})			
k_a	4.0	4.0	4.0	4.0
k_{el}	0.2	0.2	0.2	0.2
α	1.5	1.5	0.56	0.272
k_{10}	0.53	1.0	0.37	0.25
k_{12}	0.60	0.4	0.087	0.0047
k_{21}	0.56	0.3	0.30	0.22

concentration time-course profile in each fluid after a dose as well as the number of doses preceding the profile.

The three-compartment open model can exist in several forms, two of which are shown below:

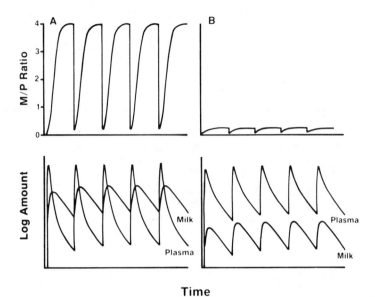

Figure 3 Simulated profiles of milk and plasma drug amounts and derived M/P ratios for a two-compartment open model after multiple doses. Pharmacokinetic parameters shown for Figure 2B and 2D were used for parts A and B of this figure respectively. A dosing interval of eight hours was used and plasma steady-state conditions are shown.

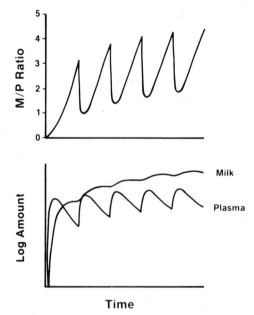

Figure 4 Simulated profiles of milk and plasma drug amounts for a two-compartment open model: dose number and interval dependency of the M/P ratio. The parameters are: $k_a = 0.7$, $k_{el} = 0.0318$, $\alpha = 0.5$, $k_{10} = 0.1987$, $k_{12} = 0.2531$, $k_{21} = 0.08$ hour^{-1}. The dosing interval was every eight hours and dosing continued to attainment of plasma steady-state conditions.

Mamillary

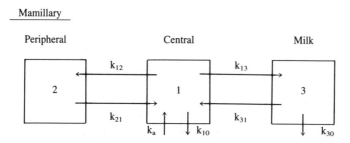

Simulations for this model are likely to be similar to those for the two-compartment open model. Note that compartment #3 (milk) can be either deep or shallow and may not necessarily have the same characteristics as compartment #2. An example of milk as a deep compartment in this model is shown by the simulation in Figure 5. An enhanced M/P ratio occurs with each successive dose and depends on both dose number and interdose interval.

Sequential

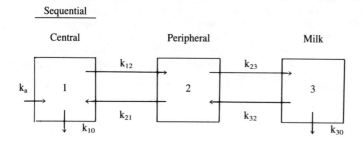

In this model, milk compartment #3 contains a drug amount limited by that of compartment #2. This model was suggested previously, as was the mamillary model above (2). Either model allows the depth (and capacity) of the milk compartment to be estimated in a manner that distinguishes it from other compartments. This is advantageous since breast blood flow and milk production may alter the characteristics of the milk compartment irrespective of other compartments during various periods of lactation. It is not appropriate to assume that the characteristics of a peripheral compartment as determined by an analysis of plasma drug disposition are also applicable to the milk compartment. An analysis of drug concentration in both plasma and milk at various post-dose intervals may allow each compartment to be distinguished so that a model that best fits the data can be selected. Simulations of profiles for the sequential three-compartment open model are shown in Figure 6. The M/P ratio is a function of transfer kinetics operative for all three compartments and this

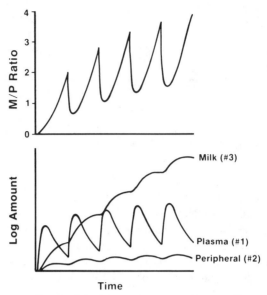

Time

Figure 5 Simulated profiles of milk and plasma drug amounts for a mamillary three-compartment open model: dose number and interval dependency of the M/P ratio. The compartment corresponding to each fluid is numbered. The following pharmacokinetic parameters were used for this simulation: $k_a = 0.7$, $\alpha = 0.52$, $\beta = 0.184$, $\gamma = 0.026$, $k_{10} = 0.2$, $k_{12} = 0.08$, $k_{21} = 0.25$, $k_{13} = 0.15$, $k_{31} = 0.05$ hour^{-1}. The dosing interval was every eight hours to the point of steady state. Milk is the third compartment and suckling did not occur (i.e. $k_{30} = 0$). The following differential equations were used to prepare the simulation:

1. $dXa/dt = -k_aX_a$
2. $dX_1/dt = k_aX_a - (k_{10} + k_{12} + k_{13})X_1 + k_{21}X_2 + k_{31}X_3$
3. $dX_2/dt = k_{12}X_1 - k_{21}X_2$
4. $dX_3/dt = k_{13}X_1 - (k_{30} + k_{31})X_3$

X_i is the amount of drug in compartment i, and k_{ij} represents the transfer rate constant between two compartments. Since suckling is assumed not to occur, k_{30} can be set to zero. The solution was obtained by using input and disposition functions as described by Benet (27). Taking the Laplace transform of each equation yields a system of linear equations solvable by matrix algebra. Inverse transformation of the resulting solutions is accomplished using the general partial fraction theorem, as shown by Benet & Turi (28). For each compartment, the equation that relates the amount of drug in the compartment versus time contains the expected four exponential terms and this was used to construct the simulations. Programs using these solutions were executed by the Cromemco model Z-2D and Tektronix 4054 computers. Computation of α, β, and γ was accomplished by Bairstow's method for extracting polynomial roots.

produces a time dependency in the M/P ratio after a single dose. A dose-number dependency can also occur in this model (Figure 7). Caveats expressed about this finding in relation to the two-compartment and the mamillary three-compartment models are pertinent here also.

A four-compartment open model can contain features of the mamillary and sequential forms of the three-compartment open model:

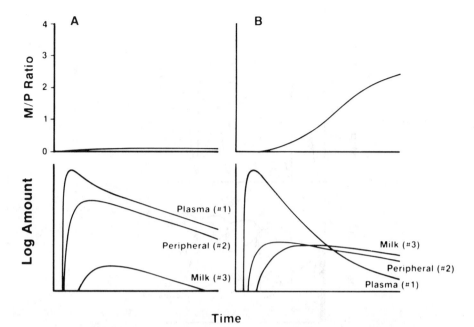

Time

Figure 6   Simulated profiles of milk and plasma drug amounts and derived M/P ratios for a sequential three-compartment open model after a single dose. See legend of Figure 5 for the development of mathematical solutions for this model needed to prepare the simulations. Pharmacokinetic parameters are:

	A	B
	(hour^{-1})	
k_a	3.87	3.87
α	1.75	1.72
β	1.02	0.73
γ	0.20	0.10
k_{10}	0.36	0.63
k_{12}	0.50	0.10
k_{21}	0.93	0.27
k_{23}	0.11	0.80
k_{32}	1.06	0.75

The simulation described by a sequential three-compartment open model was developed by use of differential equations where milk was the third compartment:

1. $dX_a/dt = -k_a X_a$
2. $dX_1/dt = k_a X_a - (k_{10} + k_{12})X_1 + k_{21}X_2$
3. $dX_2/dt = k_{12}X_1 - (k_{21} + k_{23})X_2 + k_{32}X_3$
4. $dX_3/dt = k_{23}X_2 - (k_{30} + k_{32})X_3$

X_i is the amount of drug in compartment i, and k_{ij} represents the transfer rate constants between two compartments. Since suckling is assumed not to occur, k_{30} can be set to zero.

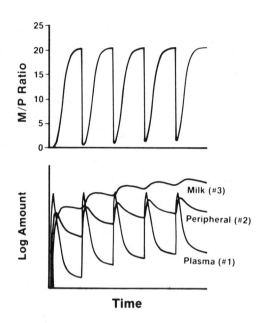

Figure 7 Simulated profiles of milk and plasma drug amounts for a sequential three-compartment open model: dose number and interval dependency of the M/P ratio. A dosing interval of twelve hours and the following pharmacokinetic parameters were used: $k_a = 2.5$, $\alpha = 1.45$, $\beta = 0.7595$, $\gamma = 0.02297$, $k_{10} = 0.63$, $k_{12} = 0.6$, $k_{21} = 0.2$, $k_{23} = 0.6$, $k_{32} = 0.2$ hour^{-1}. See legend of Figure 5 for development of mathematical solutions for this model needed to prepare the simulations. Suckling did not occur (i.e. $k_{30} = 0$). A further exaggeration of the M/P ratio dose number dependency pattern is seen when $k_a = 1.5$, $\alpha = 1.174$, $\beta = 0.3726$, $\gamma = 0.0132$, $k_{10} = 0.9$, $k_{12} = 0.25$, $k_{21} = 0.08$, $k_{23} = 0.25$, and $k_{32} = 0.08$ hour^{-1}.

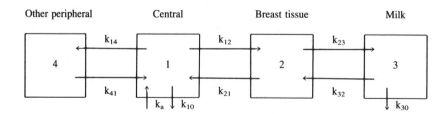

This model allows breast tissue (as a specific peripheral compartment #2) to be distinguished from other peripheral compartments, including milk (#3). Physiological changes in lactation are expected to make compartment #2 discernable. This model allows a study of drug-transfer mechanisms from the central

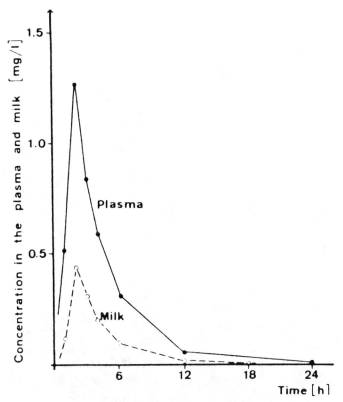

Figure 8 Praziquantel concentrations (mg/l) in breast milk and plasma at various time intervals after a single oral dose of about 50 mg/kg. The arithmetic mean of data from five women studied by Putter et al (29) is shown.

to the milk compartment. Mathematical solutions for this model are being developed.

Reported Profiles of Milk and Plasma Drug Concentrations

Reported examples of milk and plasma drug concentrations illustrate the time dependent nature of the M/P ratio as predicted from the simulations illustrated above. This ratio has been calculated for several reported drug studies in order to emphasize presence or absence of a concurrent profile for drug in plasma and milk. A concurrent profile is one in which the M/P ratio remains relatively flat following single or multiple drug doses. This has been found for several drugs after a single-dose administration to lactating women. The concentration profiles for a single dose of praziquantel (Figure 8) (29) are typical. The M/P ratio at any time after dosing is generally applicable to any other time, and a reliable average dose in milk can be estimated from an M/P ratio calculated from

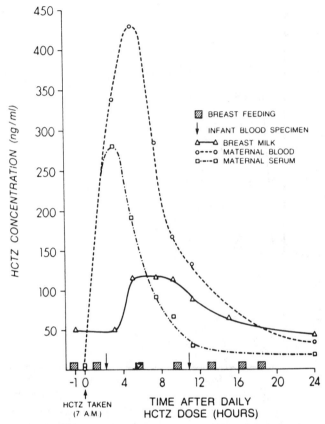

Figure 9 Hydrochlorothiazide concentrations in breast milk, blood and serum over a 24-hour dosing interval. The two indicated blood specimens from the baby showed no detectable hydrochlorothiazide. Interdose data were obtained from a woman studied by Miller et al (30).

concentration or AUC data. Concurrent profiles found for single doses should be tested under steady-state conditions for lack of change in the observed M/P ratio.

A perturbed concurrence between milk and plasma drug concentrations is found for several drugs. The concentration of drug in milk and the timing of breast feeding to deliver the lowest amount of drug are affected accordingly. Previous reports show pitfalls in the M/P ratio caused by a lack of concurrent drug concentration profiles. A notable example is that of hydrochlorothiazide concentration in milk and plasma (Figure 9) (30). Nadolol milk and plasma concentrations show a marked difference with chronic dosing and after the drug is discontinued (Figure 10) (31). A similar single versus chronic dose discrepancy has been found for cimetidine such that the drug appears to accumulate in milk more than in plasma after multiple doses (32).

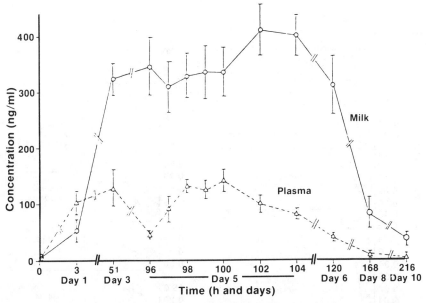

Figure 10   Nadolol concentrations in breast milk and serum. The mean data from twelve subjects were obtained by Devlin et al (31). The drug was given once per day orally for five days.

The M/P ratios derived from reported milk and plasma drug concentration profiles are shown in Figures 11 and 12. The data are arbitrarily grouped for M/P ratios less than 0.2 and 0.2 to approximately one (Figure 11) and the same as or greater than one (Figure 12). Several observations of practical importance emerge from an analysis of M/P ratios for a wide variety of drugs. First, most drugs show a variable M/P ratio during the early periods following a dose. The variability appears to be less for drugs with an M/P ratio less than one. This is consistent with the relationship found between the initial slope and the asymptotic phase of the M/P ratio in profiles simulated for a two-compartment open model after a single dose. Second, a discrepancy in the single versus multiple dose M/P ratio has been found for nadolol and propranolol as seen in Figure 12 and as reported for cimetidine (32). This discrepancy is apparent with pharmacokinetic parameters used in our multiple dose simulations wherein a dose number dependency has been observed. Some drugs, notably those with an M/P ratio greater than one, may have milk distribution characteristics that enhance this discrepancy in single versus multiple dose M/P ratios. These are the drugs that may produce the highest concentrations in milk after multiple doses and hence may pose a risk to the infant. Overall, the derived M/P ratios in Figures 11 and 12 must be defined according to the post-dose interval and presumably also in relation to the single or multiple dose conditions. The third point of emphasis is that only eleven of the studies have data for more than one

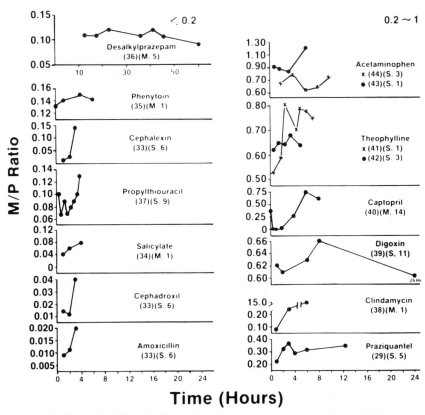

Time (Hours)

Figure 11   Reported profiles of milk and plasma drug concentrations for a calculated M/P ratio of less than one. The milk and plasma (serum or blood) concentration data depicted in tables or graphs of the cited reference (first parenthetical number) was used to calculate the M/P ratio for each drug shown. Midpoint estimations and extrapolations by sight were used in some cases so that milk and plasma concentrations could be paired. The parenthetical material corresponds to data from a single (S) dose or after the administration of multiple (M) doses by the oral route. The number of patients is also shown. The metabolite of prazepam, desalkylprazepam, is shown because the parent drug was not detected in milk or plasma after three days of administration (36).

subject. It is difficult to apply a single subject–derived M/P ratio to the general population. Studies of appropriate design and in a sufficient number of lactating women are needed so that proposed models can be validated and generally applicable drug dose-in-milk calculations can be made.

Milk Volume and Its Constituent Effects on the M/P Ratio

Our previous review (2) emphasized the effects of milk volume, pH, fat, and water on the total amount of drug excreted in breast milk. Less well appreciated (and apparently not well studied) is the role of these factors on the M/P ratio.

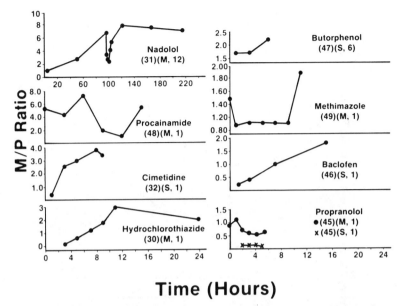

Time (Hours)

Figure 12   Reported profiles of milk and drug concentrations for a calculated M/P ratio of greater than one. See legend of Figure 11.

For example, a weakly acidic and very fat-soluble drug may show a change in M/P ratio as a function of pH and fat content of milk, as predicted in Figure 13. These predicted effects are of practical importance, since milk pH and fat increase as a function of feeding time (fore versus hind milk) (50–51). A combined effect of milk fat and pH on the M/P ratio is probably reflected in the overall drug distribution rate constants as previously discussed. The possible contribution of these effects is seen in the relationship shown in Figure 13.

The quantity of drug in the milk compartment and the value of the M/P ratio are probably a function of both volume of milk and protein content as well as fat and pH. Each could give milk deep-compartment characteristics. In one study (44), the breast milk protein binding of acetaminophen was 13% that of plasma. This factor is quite likely reflected in the pharmacokinetic rate constants for a particular model.

Drug Metabolism Effects on the M/P Ratio

While major attention is given to maternal drug disposition as it affects the M/P ratio, conceivable effects arise from in situ drug metabolism by breast tissue. This could limit the entry of drug to milk or selectively enhance drug metabolite excretion in milk. This is another phenomenon that could be incorporated by rate constants that fit a pharmacokinetic model. The inhibition of drug binding to milk protein via metabolite competition for binding sites is also possible. The

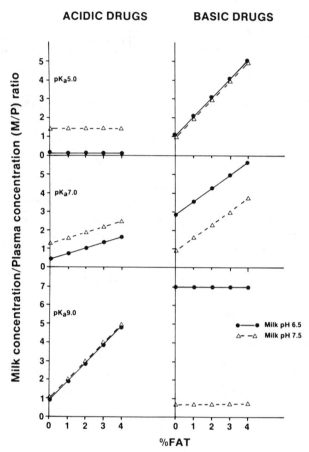

Figure 13 Predicted change in the M/P ratio with increasing milk fat content. For these predictions, it was assumed that breast milk volume is much less than plasma volume, so that changes in M/P ratio do not cause plasma concentration to change. It was also assumed that the drugs were 100 times more soluble in fat than in water and that milk behaves as a simple two-phase system at the point of equilibrium with plasma. Acidic and basic drugs of various pK_a are shown.

excretion of drug metabolites, either formed in situ or elsewhere, in breast milk should be examined with an approach not unlike that used for the parent drug. Metabolites in breast milk have been shown for the following drugs: disopyramide (52), procainamide (48), salicylazosulfapyridine (53, 54), isoniazid (55), and prazepam (36). Metabolites of antipyrine (56) and acetaminophen (43) have not been found in breast milk. An extensive analysis (57) has revealed multiple drug metabolites in breast milk after the administration of a combination drug product containing aspirin, caffeine, phenacetin, and codeine (Table 3). The M/P ratio of these drugs does not necessarily correspond

Table 3 M/P ratios of parent drug and metabolites[a]

Time (hours)	Phenacetin	Acetaminophen	Codeine	Morphine	Salicylate	Caffeine
			(M/P concentration ratio)			
0.5	0.54	0.40	1.35	0.23	0.01	0.31
1.0	0.84	0.38	2.55	0.99	0.02	0.57
1.5						
2.0	0.88	0.65	2.52	1.56	0.03	0.86
3.0	0.55					
4.0	0.55	0.77	1.92	2.0	0.04	0.86
7.0	1.02	1.25	2.14	3.48	0.09	0.92
12.0	0.37	1.63	1.67	5.07	0.31	0.85
			(AUC_M/AUC_P)			
	0.67	0.81	2.16	2.46	0.05	0.82

[a] Adapted from Findlay et al (57) and from data they supplied to us for their subject #1. Single-dose administration of a compound analgesic preparation containing aspirin, phenacetin, caffeine, and codeine was studied in one subject. Concentration values were used to calculate M/P ratios at times shown. Area under the curve (AUC) estimates were used to derive the average AUC ratios.

to the value- or time-dependent profile of their respective metabolites. The dose of drug metabolites in breast milk is important if such metabolites are pharmacologically active and/or require excretion by immature systems in the nursing infant.

Maternal Disease Effects on the M/P Ratio

Breast feeding women who take medicines presumably do so for the treatment of an illness. The effect of illness per se on either the M/P ratio or amount of drug excreted in milk has not been systematically studied. Diseases known to affect the amount of free drug in plasma may change the amount of drug in milk and possibly the M/P ratio.

Drug Interaction Effects on the M/P Ratio

Not unlike disease effects, the influence of drug-drug interactions on the M/P ratio has not been well studied. Competing for milk binding sites or transfer mechanisms are loci for potential drug interactions, with resultant changes in the M/P ratio as well as total drug excreted in milk. This includes the coexistence of metabolites as well as parent drug in milk.

Interindividual Differences in the M/P Ratio

Each drug or biological factor discussed above may interact to give a distinct value to the M/P ratio in an individual at a certain period of lactation. The collective contribution has not been assessed in a controlled manner. That interindividual variation in the M/P ratio probably exists is shown by the wide range of percent of maternal dose in milk values for antipyrine (0.56–2.38%) (56). Other drugs with reported interindividual variation in either breast milk drug concentrations or the M/P ratio are atenolol and propranolol (58), methyldopa (59), lormetazepam (60), phenytoin, (35), valproic acid (61, 62), and dyphylline (63). These few existing population studies highlight the weakness of an M/P ratio derived from a single case report.

CONCLUSIONS

This review of pharmacokinetic pitfalls in the M/P ratio serves as a guideline for the design of studies that formulate an M/P ratio applicable to drugs used by lactating women. Errors implicit in an uncritical interpretation of existing data are highlighted by an appreciation of these pitfalls. The M/P ratio is a very important factor in the equation used to calculate dose of drug in milk delivered to the nursing infant. It is this factor that corrects for dose strength, duration of dosing, and maternal variations in drug disposition. A systematic study of probable influences on the M/P ratio should yield a valid parameter for the assessment of infant dose and for the safety of breast feeding by mothers who require drug therapy during lactation.

ACKNOWLEDGEMENTS

The authors appreciate the skilled secretarial assistance of Mrs. Carole Webb. We thank Dr. John W. A. Findlay and his coworkers for sharing their original data with us.

Literature Cited

1. Wilson, J. T., Brown, R. D., Cherek, D., Dailey, J. W., Hilman, B., et al. 1980. Drug excretion in breast milk: Principles, pharmacokinetics and projected consequences. *Clin. Pharmacokinet.* 5:1–66
2. Wilson, J. T. 1981. *Drugs in Breast Milk.* Australia: ADIS Press. 110 pp.
3. Wilson, J. T. 1983. Determinants and consequences of drug excretion in breast milk. *Drug Metab. Rev.* 14:619–52
4. Wilson, J. T. 1983. Contamination of human milk by drugs and chemicals. *Nutr. Health* 2:191–201
5. Wilson, J. T. 1984. Chemical contaminants of cow's milk and human milk. In *Health Hazards of Milk,* ed. D. L. J. Freed, pp. 12–26. London: Bailliere Tindall
6. Platzker, A. C. D., Lew, C. D., Stewart, D. 1980. Drug "administration" via breast milk, *Hosp. Pract.* 15:111–22
7. Buchanan, N. 1981. Commentary: Drugs in pediatric practice. I. Principles of drug therapy in pediatric practice. II. The problems of drug therapy in pregnancy. III. Drugs and breast feeding: A practical approach, *Aust. Paediatr. J.* 17:219–23
8. Savage, R. L. 1977. Drugs and breast milk, *J. Hum. Nutr.* 31:459–64
9. O'Brien, T. E. 1974. Excretion of drugs in human milk. *Am. J. Hosp. Pharm.* 31:844–54
10. Chaplin, S., Sanders, G. L., Smith, J. M. 1982. Drug excretion in human breast milk. *Adverse Drug React. Acute Poisoning Rev.* 1:255–87
11. Reisner, S. H., Eisenberg, N. H., Stahl, B., Hauser, G. J. 1983. Maternal medications and breast-feeding. *Dev. Pharmacol. Ther.* 6:285–304
12. George, D. I., O'Toole, T. J. 1983. A review of drug transfer to the infant by breast-feeding: Concerns for the dentist. *J. Am. Dent. Assoc.* 106:204–8
13. Berlin, C. M. 1981. Pharmacologic considerations of drug use in the lactating mother. *Obstet. Gynecol.* 58:17S–23S
14. Giacoia, G. P., Catz, C. S. 1979. Drugs and pollutants in breast milk. *Clin. Perinatol.* 6:181–96
15. Kochenour, N. K., Emery, M. G. 1981. Drugs in lactating women. *Obstet. Gynecol. Ann.* 10:107–26
16. Anderson, P. O. 1977. Drugs and breast feeding, *Drug Intell. Clin. Pharm.* 11:208–23
17. Hervada, A. R., Feit, E., Sagraves, R. 1978. Drugs in breast milk. *Perinatal Care* 2:19–25
18. Welch, R. M., Findlay, J. W. A. 1981. Excretion of drugs in human breast milk. *Drug Metab. Rev.* 12:261–77
19. Arena, J. M. 1980. Drugs and chemicals excreted in breast milk. *Pediatr. Ann.* 9:452–57
20. Berlin, C. M. 1980. The excretion of drugs in human milk. In *Drug and Chemical Risks to the Fetus and Newborn,* ed. R. J. Schwarz, S. J. Yaffe, pp. 115–27. New York: Liss. 166 pp.
21. Sannerstedt, R., Berglund, F., Flodh, H., Hedstrand, A. G. 1980. Medication during pregnancy and breast-feeding—A new Swedish system for classifying drugs. *Int. J. Clin. Pharmacol. Ther. Toxicol.* 18:45–49
22. White, G. J., White, M. K. 1980. Breast-feeding and drugs in human milk. *Vet. Hum. Toxicol.* 22:1–44
23. Committee on Drugs. 1983. The transfer of drugs and other chemicals into human breast milk. *Pediatrics* 72:375–83
24. Bowes, W. A. 1980. The effect of medications on the lactating mother and her infant. *Clin. Obstet. Gynecol.* 23:1073–80
25. Wagner, J. G. 1975. Linear compartment models. In *Fundamentals of Clinical Pharmacokinetics,* ed. J. G. Wagner, pp. 102–6. Hamilton, Ill.: Drug Intell. Publ. 461 pp.
26. Gibaldi, M., Perrier, D. 1975. Multicompartment models. In *Pharmacokinetics,* ed. J. Swarbuik, pp. 48–86. New York: Dekker. 329 pp.
27. Benet, L. Z. 1972. General treatment of

linear mammillary models with elimination from any compartment as used in pharmacokinetics. *J. Pharm. Sci.* 61: 536–41

28. Benet, L. Z., Turi, J. S. 1971. Use of general partial fraction theorem for obtaining inverse laplace transforms in pharmacokinetic analysis. *J. Pharm. Sci.* 60:1953–54

29. Putter, J., Held, F. 1979. Quantitative studies on the occurrence of praziquantel in milk and plasma of lactating women. *Eur. J. Drug Metab. Pharmacokinet.* 4:193–98

30. Miller, M. E., Cohn, R. D., Burghart, P. H. 1982. Hydrochlorothiazide disposition in a mother and her breast fed infant. *J. Pediatrics.* (5) 101:789–91

31. Devlin, R. G., Duchin, K. L., Fleiss, P. M. 1981. Nadolol in human serum and breast milk. *Br. J. Clin. Pharmacol.* 12:393–96

32. Somogyi, A., Gugler, R. 1979. Cimetidine excretion into breast milk. *Br. J. Clin. Pharmacol.* 7:627–28

33. Kafetzis, D. A., Siafas, C. A., Georgakopoulos, P. A., Papadatos, C. J. 1981. Passage of cephalosporins and amoxicillin into the breast milk. *Acta Paediatr. Scand.* 70:285–88

34. Bailey, D. N., Weibert, R. T., Naylor, A. J. 1982. A study of salicylate and caffeine excretion in the breast milk of two nursing mothers. *J. Anal. Toxicol.* 6:64–68

35. Steen, B., Rane, A., Lonnerholm, G., Falk, O., Elwin, C-E., Sjoqvist, F. 1982. Phenytoin excretion in human breast milk and plasma levels in nursed infants, *Ther. Drug Monit.* 4:331–34

36. Brodie, R. R., Chasseaud, L. F., Taylor, T. 1981. Concentrations of N-descyclopropylmethylprazepam in whole-blood, plasma, and milk after administration of prazepam to humans. *Biopharm. Drug Dispos.* 2:59–68

37. Kampmann, J. P., Johansen, K., Hansen, J. M., Helweg, J. 1980. Propylthiouracil in human milk. *Lancet* 1:736–38

38. Steen, B., Rane, A. 1982. Clindamycin passage into human milk. *Br. J. Clin. Pharmacol.* 13:661–64

39. Reinhardt, D., Richter, O., Genz, T., Potthoff, S. 1982. Kinetics of the translactal passage of digoxin from breast feeding mothers to their infants. *Eur. J. Pediatr.* 138:49–52

40. Devlin, R. G., Fleiss, P. M. 1981. Captopril in human blood and breast milk. *J. Clin. Pharmacol.* 21:110–13

41. Yurchak, A. M., Jusko, W. J. 1976. Theophylline secretion into breast milk. *Pediatrics* 57:518–20

42. Stec, G. P., Greenberger, P., Tsuen, I. R., Henthorn, T., Morita, Y., et al. 1980. Kinetics of theophylline transfer to breast milk. *Clin. Pharmacol. Ther.* 28(3):404–8

43. Berlin, C. M., Yaffe, S. J., Ragni, M. 1980. Disposition of acetaminophen in milk, saliva, and plasma of lactating women. *Pediatr. Pharmacol.* 1:135–41

44. Bitzen, P. O., Gustafsson, B., Jostell, K. G., Melander, A., Wahlin-Boll, E. 1981. Excretion of paracetamol in human breast milk. *Eur. J. Clin. Pharmacol.* 20:123–25

45. Bauer, J. H., Pape, B., Zajicek, J., Groshong, T. 1979. Propranolol in human plasma and breast milk. *Am. J. Cardiol.* 43:860–62

46. Eriksson, G., Swahn, C.-G. 1981. Concentrations of baclofen in serum and breast milk from a lactating woman, *Scand. J. Clin. Lab. Invest.* 41:185–87

47. Pittman, K. A., Smyth, R. D., Losada, M., Zighelboim, I., Maduska, A. L., Sunshine, A. 1980. Human perinatal distribution of butorphanol. *Am. J. Obstet. Gynecol.* 138(7):797–800

48. Pittard, W. B. III, Glazier, H. 1983. Procainamide excretion in human milk. *J. Pediatrics* 102(4):631–33

49. Tegler, L., Lindstrom, B. 1980. Antithyroid drugs in milk. *Lancet* 2:591

50. Neville, M. C., Allen, J. C., Watters, C. 1983. The mechanism of milk secretion. In *Lactation,* ed. M. C. Neville, M. R. Neifert, pp. 49–102. New York/London: Plenum. 466 pp.

51. Hall, B. 1975. Changing composition of human milk and early development of appetite control. *Lancet* 1:779–82

52. Barnett, D. B., Hudson, S. A., McBurney, A. 1982. Disopyramide and its N-monodesalkyl metabolite in breast milk. *Br. J. Clin. Pharmacol.* 14:310–12

53. Berlin, C. M., Yaffe, S. J. 1980. Disposition of salicylazosulfapyridine (azulfidine) and metabolites in human breast milk. *Dev. Pharmacol. Ther.* 1:31–39

54. Azad Khan, A. K., Truelove, S. C. 1979. Placental and mammary transfer of sulphasalazine. *Br. Med. J.* 2:1553

55. Berlin, C. M., Lee, C. 1979. Isoniazin and acetylisoniazid disposition in human milk, saliva and plasma. *Fed. Proc.* 38:426

56. Berlin, C. M. 1978. Antipyrine appearance and decay in human breast milk and saliva. *Pharmacologist* 20:219

57. Findlay, J. W. A., DeAngelis, R. L.,

Kearney, M. F., Welch, R. M., Findlay, J. M. 1981. Analgesic drugs in breast milk and plasma. *Clin. Pharmacol. Ther.* 29:625–33

58. Thorley, K. J., McAinsh J. 1983. Levels of the beta-blockers atenolol and propranolol in the breast milk of women treated for hypertension in pregnancy. *Biopharm. Drug Dispos.* 4:299–301

59. Hoskins, A., Holliday, S. B. 1982. Determination of α-methyldopa and methyldopate in human breast milk and plasma by ion-exchange chromatography using electrochemical detection. *J. Chromatog.* 230:162–67

60. Humpel, M., Stoppelli, I., Milia, S., Rainer, E. 1982. Pharmacokinetics and biotransformation of the new benzo-

diazepine, lormetazepam, in man. *Eur. J. Clin. Pharmacol.* 21:421–25

61. von Unruh, G. E., Froescher, W., Hoffmann, F., Niesen, M. 1984. Valproic acid in breast milk: How much is really there? *Ther. Drug Monit.* 8:301–5

62. Nau, H., Rating, D., Koch, S., Hauser, I., Helge, H. 1981. Valproic acid and its metabolites: Placental transfer, neonatal pharmacokinetics, transfer via mother's milk and clinical status in neonates of epileptic mothers. *J. Pharmacol. Exp. Ther.* 219:768–77

63. Jarboe, C. H., Cook, L. N., Malesic, I., Fleischaker, J. 1981. Dyphylline elimination kinetics in lactating women: Blood to milk transfer. *J. Clin. Pharmacol.* 21:405–10

Ann. Rev. Pharmacol. Toxicol. 1985. 25:691–714

THE PHARMACOLOGY OF ALDOSE REDUCTASE INHIBITORS[1]

Peter F. Kador, W. Gerald Robison, Jr., and Jin H. Kinoshita

National Eye Institute, National Institutes of Health, Bethesda, Maryland 20205

INTRODUCTION

Despite the advent of life-prolonging insulin for the treatment of diabetes, the appearance and progression of many of the disabling complications associated with this disease cannot be prevented through the administration of insulin. Clinically, the onset and rate of progression of diabetic complications, including cataract, corneal epitheliopathy, microangiopathy, nephropathy, neuropathy, and retinopathy, appear to be dependent upon both the duration and the severity of the diabetes. Moreover, many of the cells in tissues displaying diabetic complications are capable of insulin-independent glucose transport so that the intracellular glucose levels in these cells can mirror blood glucose concentrations, with increased blood glucose levels leading to increased levels of intracellular glucose (1).

The intracellular glucose in turn is utilized primarily for energy production, although it can also be used for special reactions such as the synthesis of polysaccharides, collagen, mucin, or for the glycosylation of proteins. Utilization for glycolysis, however, requires that glucose first be phosphorylated to glucose-6-phosphate by the enzyme hexokinase. Alternatively, glucose can be converted to fructose, which can then undergo glycolysis following phosphorylation by fructokinase. This conversion of glucose to fructose proceeds in two steps through the intermediate sorbitol in what is commonly called the sorbitol or polyol pathway. In the first step of this pathway, aldose reductase (alditol: $NADP^+$ oxidoreductase, EC 1.1.1.21) utilizes NADPH to reduce the aldehyde form of glucose to its corresponding sugar alcohol, sorbitol. In the second step, sorbitol dehydrogenase (1-iditol dehydrogenase, ED 1.1.1.14) utilizes NAD^+ to oxidize sorbitol to fructose.

---

[1]The US Government has the right to retain a nonexclusive royalty-free license in and to any copyright covering this paper.

691

$$\text{glucose} + \text{NADPH} \xrightarrow{\text{aldose reductase}} \text{sorbitol} + \text{NADP}^+$$

$$\text{sorbitol} + \text{NAD}^+ \xrightarrow{\text{sorbitol dehydrogenase}} \text{fructose} + \text{NADH}$$

The sorbitol pathway was first observed in 1956 in the seminal vesicles, where it appears to have a physiological function in the production of fructose for sperm (2). Since then, its presence has been observed in a variety of tissues, including those that display diabetes-associated pathology. In these tissues, aldose reductase can compete directly with hexokinase for the utilization of glucose. The affinity of aldose reductase for glucose, however, is much less than that of hexokinase, so that under normal physiological conditions available glucose is rapidly phosphorylated by hexokinase rather than being reduced to sorbitol by aldose reductase. It is only under nonphysiological conditions, such as in diabetes where the elevated levels of glucose can saturate hexokinase, that a physiologically significant level of sorbitol is produced. Moreover, under these conditions sorbitol can be produced more rapidly than it is converted to fructose, resulting in an accumulation of sorbitol. This accumulation is enhanced by the polar nature of the sugar alcohol, since its polarity prevents facile membrane penetration and subsequent removal through diffusion. The intracellular accumulation of a polar sugar alcohol can thus produce an hyperosmotic effect, which results in an infusion of fluid to counteract the osmotic gradient produced. This fluid influx has been observed to lead to membrane permeability changes and the onset of cellular pathology (3).

In addition to reducing glucose, aldose reductase possesses broad substrate specificity, with the ability to reduce a variety of aromatic and aliphatic aldehydes, including the aldoses galactose, xylose, and arabinose (4–8). Moreover, the enzyme displays a greater affinity for galactose than for glucose, so that the increased levels of galactose are more readily reduced to dulcitol (galactitol) than glucose to sorbitol. The dulcitol is not further oxidized by sorbitol dehydrogenase, so that the intracellular levels of this polar sugar alcohol remain elevated.

$$\text{galactose} + \text{NADPH} \xrightarrow{\text{aldose reductase}} \text{dulcitol} + \text{NADP}^+$$

$$\text{dulcitol} + \text{NAD}^+ \xrightarrow{\text{sorbitol dehydrogenase}} \text{NR}$$

The increased intracellular levels of galactose can result in a more rapid and greater hyperosmotic effect than that from glucose. Tissues accumulating dulcitol develop cellular pathology similar to that observed in diabetic tissues. Therefore, through the use of galactosemic and diabetic animal studies, evidence linking the aldose reductase–initiated accumulation of sugar alcohols with the pathogenesis of diabetic complications is rapidly increasing. These observations suggest that the inhibition of aldose reductase represents a novel, potentially direct pharmacological approach toward the treatment of certain diabetic complications—an approach distinct from the improved control of blood sugar levels. This novel approach has evolved from studies on the mechanisms of diabetic cataract formation.

ALDOSE REDUCTASE IN DIABETIC CATARACTS

Diabetic cataracts have been extensively studied since the 1930s, when it was demonstrated that cataracts could easily be produced in rats either by the removal of the pancreas or through the destruction of pancreatic beta cells by the injection of alloxan or streptozotocin. Despite intensive research, however, it has taken over 50 years to elucidate the mechanism of cataract formation in diabetic animals. The solution to the question of diabetic cataract formation had its beginning in 1959, when van Heyningen found the presence of sorbitol in the lenses of diabetic rats, indicating that the enzyme aldose reductase was functioning in the lens (9). Prior to van Heyningen's finding, it was thought that the sorbitol pathway primarily functioned in certain reproductive tissues; however, this finding spurred others to uncover aldose reductase in other tissues, especially those tissues affected by diabetes.

The lenticular accumulation of sorbitol, which was known to poorly penetrate biological membranes, immediately became suspect as the cause of osmotic changes observed in histopathological studies of diabetic lenses (10). These studies had revealed that the earliest visible change was the appearance of swollen lens fibers caused by an increase in lens hydration. The swollen lens fibers eventually ruptured, with liquifaction of the fibers resulting in vacuole formation. Thus, sorbitol formation within the lens cells created a hypertonicity that was corrected by an influx of water to maintain isotonicity with the environment. This, as events were to prove later, is the initiating step in the development of the diabetic cataract.

The argument for polyol-initiated osmotic changes was strengthened by the identification of dulcitol in the lenses of galactosemic rats and by studies that indicated that excess galactose feeding of rats could induce cataracts histologically similar to diabetic cataracts. Moreover, from the more favorable substrate affinity of galactose and the lack of metabolism of dulcitol by sorbitol dehydrogenase, one could predict that the lens polyol level should be higher and the onset of cataract earlier than in the diabetic rat. This was indeed the case with polyol levels of 72 mmol per Kg of lens found in the 50% galactose–fed rats, at least twice the level found in diabetic lenses (11). The cataracts also appear earlier in the galactosemic rats, with the dense nuclear cataract occurring after three weeks of the galactosemic state compared to two months for the diabetic rat (11). Thus, the galactose model is much more convenient to study the details of aldose reductase–initiated cataract formation. Moreover, if aldose reductase is involved in the development of other diabetic complications, then they should be reproducible in the galactosemic state as well.

Osmotic Hypothesis

The sequence of events leading to the formation of diabetic cataract is summarized in Figure 1 (3). Although the K_m for glucose is high, so that at ambient levels of glucose very little sorbitol is formed, the availability of high glucose levels in diabetes in a sense activates aldose reductase to produce substantial amounts of sorbitol, some of which is converted to fructose. The increase in osmolality caused by the accumulation of sorbitol and fructose draws water into the lens fibers, causing them to swell. The swelling has adverse effects as it increases the permeability to substances normally retained in the lens at concentrations higher than the surrounding intraocular fluids. Thus, concentrations of K^+, amino acids, glutathione, inositol, and ATP begin to decrease, and Na^+ and Cl^- ions slowly begin to build up. As the process continues, a secondary osmotic change results from the electrolyte changes of increased Na^+ and Cl^- ions; eventually the increases in these electrolytes become the predominant factor in lens swelling. The lens membranes become freely permeable to all substances other than the larger proteins. In this later stage, swelling is explained by the Donnan principle. It is accompanied by the appearance of the dense nuclear cataract.

Protein synthesis also ceases, even in the early stages of these sugar cataracts (12). Normally, there is continual growth of the lens, due to new fibers being laid down from the elongation of epithelial cells at the lens equator. Concomitant with this growth is the synthesis of new lens proteins. However, in these cataracts growth of the lens is retarded as protein synthesis is decreased. Apparently the potassium-sodium ratio governs the degrees of protein synthesis. In the lens the normally high K^+/Na^+ environment is conducive to protein synthesis. However, in these sugar cataracts, where the intracellular concentration of K^+ is lowered and Na^+ is increased, protein synthesis is depressed. If the cation concentrations are returned to near normal, as in the reversal of galactose cataract, protein synthesis also returns to normal (12). The control of lens protein synthesis by electrolytes appears to be a general phenomenon, since other osmotic cataracts have shown defects in protein synthesis similar to those found in sugar cataracts (13, 14).

The fact that all the secondary changes shown in Figure 1 are related to the osmotic event has been verified by in vitro lens culture studies. By this technique, lenses can be maintained in a control medium with normal glucose concentrations while their contralateral lenses are placed in a medium containing high levels of glucose, simulating the hyperglycemic state (15–17). The lenses in the control medium remain clear and transparent while the lenses exposed to high sugar gain water, become cloudy and develop vacuoles at the

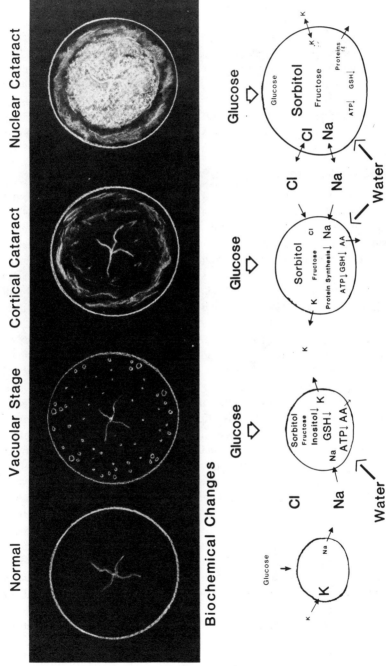

Figure 1 Summary of changes occurring in the rat lens during sugar cataract formation. K indicates potassium; Na, sodium; Cl, chloride; GSH, reduced glutathione; AA, amino acids; ATP, adenosine-5'-triphosphate.

equator region, just as do the lenses in diabetic animals. By this approach, a quantitative relationship showing that sorbitol accumulation is paralleled by an increase in lens hydration was clearly established, and biochemical changes related to the osmotic effect were observed. These biochemical changes can be prevented by preventing the lens swelling from occurring despite the accumulation of polyol by adding an amount of sorbitol to the medium equivalent to that formed in the lens. Under these conditions, normal lens volume was maintained despite the accumulation of sorbitol, and the biochemical parameters remained normal so that no changes in the levels of electrolytes, amino acids, glutathione, or inositol could be observed.

Aldose Reductase Inhibitors

Although biochemical and in vitro culture studies indicated that the aldose reductase–initiated accumulation of polyols induces lens swelling, which in turn results in other changes leading to cataract formation, the most convincing evidence for aldose reductase's role in diabetic cataracts has emerged from studies with aldose reductase inhibitors (3). These studies, which indicate that inhibition of aldose reductase can successfully prevent the onset of cataract, have led to the development of a variety of structurally diverse inhibitors. Through their use, evidence for the involvement of aldose reductase in other serious diabetic complications has evolved (18).

Initial studies in the late 1960s indicated that long-chain fatty acids could inhibit aldose reductase in lens homogenates (7). This led to the development of tetramethylene glutaric acid (TMG), the first inhibitor to reveal that the cataractous process could be altered by modifying the activity of aldose reductase (3, 19). Lens culture studies in which the lens was incubated in a high-galactose medium revealed that TMG is effective in blocking dulcitol synthesis and accumulation, that it minimizes increases in lens hydration, and that it prevents the appearance of vacuoles. Its inability to penetrate membranes, however, made the compound ineffective in vivo. The first in vivo active inhibitor was N-(3-nitro-2-pyridyl)-3-trifluoromethyl-aniline (AY-20,263) (3). Significant solubility problems were encountered with this compound, which was administered by intraocular injection as a dimethylsulfoxide solution. This was shortly followed by the development of the water-soluble inhibitor alrestatin (3-dioxo-1-H-benz[de]isoquinoline-2(3H)-acetic acid, AY-22,284) (20). This compound, when administered orally to galactosemic rats, delays the appearance of the nuclear opacity. Since alrestatin, the development of a number of more potent organic acids as aldose reductase inhibitors has been pursued. From these studies several compounds, including 3-(4-bromo-2-fluorobenzyl-4-oxo-3H-phthalazine-1-ylacetic acid (ICI 128,436), N-[(5-(trifluoromethyl)-6-methoxy-1-naphthalenyl)thioxomethyl]-N-methylglycine (tolrestat, AY 22,773) and (E)-5-[(E)-2-methyl-3-phenylpropenylidene] rhodanine-3-acetic acid (ONO 2235) have evolved as clinical trial candidates (21–23). By the mid-1970s a number of flavonoids were observed to have aldose reductase–inhibitory activity (24). These included quercetin [2-(3',4'-dihydroxyphenyl)-3,5,7-trihydroxy-4-oxo-4H-chromen] and its 3-rhamnoside quercitrin. Solubility problems were also encountered in the evaluation of certain flavonoids; however, replacement of the aromatic 2-phenyl substituents with a nonaromatic carboxyl group increased the water solubility of these inhibitors (25). Moreover, this indicated that the 4-oxo-4H-chromen ring system of flavonoids appeared to be necessary for inhibitory activity. Because of the structural similarities of the 2-chromone carboxylic acid with the antiallergy agonist disodium cromoglycate, examination of a variety of other classes of antiallergy agonists have been pursued. These led to the observation that many antiallergy compounds that contained the chromone ring system or analogs of this system, including quinolones, coumarins, chalcones, fluorenones, xanthones, 11-oxo-11H-pyrido[2,1b]quinazoline-8-carboxylic acids, 1,6-dihydro-6-oxo-2-phenylpyrimidine-5-carboxylic acids, and oxazolidines, could also inhibit aldose reductase (26). The chroman ring has also been combined with a hydantoin ring to form the potent inhibitor sorbinil (S-6-fluoro-spirochroman-4-4'-imidazolidine-2',5'-dione,CP45,634) (27). This compound was the first in vivo effective oral inhibitor that could prevent the entire cataractogenic process when administered to either galactosemic or diabetic rats (28). Moreover, through its use relationships between aldose reductase and a variety of other diabetic complications has been uncovered, so that today sorbinil may be considered a benchmark by which the potency and effectiveness of other aldose reductase inhibitors are measured. Sorbinil in turn has led to the development of several other spirohydantoins and related thiazolidine-2,4-dione and oxazolidine-2,4-dione analogs (29–32).

Although aldose reductase inhibitors appear to be diverse, certain similarities can be seen among them. Both kinetic and competition studies with purified enzyme reveal that the inhibitors interact with aldose reductase at a common site independent of either the substrate or the nucleotide cofactor fold. This site appears to be stereospecific and contains a nucleophilic residue that can reversibly interact with the inhibitors (33, 34). The steric requirements of this site may vary with enzymes from different tissues and species. Through the use of computer modeling and molecular orbital calculations, steric and electronic similarities among the inhibitors have also become apparent (33). By superimposing specific aromatic residues common to most inhibitors, a common molecular conglomerate can be formed that consists of a generally planar structure with two aromatic (hydrophobic) regions and a common carbonyl region susceptible to reversible nucleophilic attack. From this conglomerate, a schematic inhibitor site model has been postulated. Inhibitor attachment to this site results from a combination of hydrophobic bonding and a reversible charge-transfer reaction between the nucleophilic residue and the reactive carbonyl moiety. Thus, the inhibitory potency of a compound would be expected to increase either by the addition of selective lipophilic substituents that could through enhanced hydrophobic bonding increase its affinity for the inhibitor site or by the addition of groups that could more readily undergo nucleophilic attack (e.g. thiocarbonyl versus carbonyl). In addition, hydrogen bonding sites located near the two lipophilic regions can also help to orient the inhibitor onto this site. For this orientation several selective hydroxyl groups appear to be required that correspond to regions encompassed by the 7-position on the 4-oxo-4H-chromen ring and the 2-(4'-hydroxyphenyl) position. From this model the pharmacophor requirements for an aldose reductase inhibitor have been defined.

For the in vitro analyses of these inhibitors, aldose reductase from a variety of different sources and species have been employed, including bovine, rabbit, rat, dog, and human lens, human placenta, and the Engelbreth-Holm-Swarm (EHS) tumor cell line (35–40). Although kinetic studies indicate that aldose reductases from different species and tissues display similar substrate affinities, differences in the susceptibility to inhibition of aldose reductases from various sources have been observed through the use of these structurally diverse inhibitors. These studies reveal no specific trends; human placental aldose reductase is generally less susceptible to inhibition, and increasing certain steric bulk on the inhibitors makes the human placental enzyme less susceptible to inhibition than enzyme from other sources. The inhibitory susceptibility of isolated aldose reductase can also change with enzyme purification; highly purified enzyme often is less susceptible to inhibition (41). These studies suggest that no universally potent inhibitor currently exists.

A number of in vivo studies on the effect of aldose reductase inhibitors on the progression of diabetic or galactosemic rats have also been reported (Table 1). These studies, which employed various routes of administration, conclude that the ability of the inhibitor to delay or prevent the onset of cataract formation is proportional to the inhibitory potency of the drug. Their potency can also be gauged by their effectiveness in offsetting the effects produced by diets containing increasing amounts of galactose, with effectiveness against a 50% galactose diet considered the acid test for inhibitory potency.

From the studies illustrated in Table 1, it is very evident that the cataractous process can be prevented if an aldose reductase inhibitor potent enough to completely block polyol formation is administered at the onset of hyperglycemia or hypergalactosemia. However, can an aldose reductase inhibitor reverse the cataractous process once the process gets underway? This question was addressed in galactosemic rat studies, where it was shown that, when rats are fed a diet of 50% galactose, the cataractous process can be reversed only when galactose is withdrawn from the diet six days after its inception (42).

Table 1 In vivo effects of aldose reductase inhibitors on rat sugar cataracts

Inhibitor		Cataract type	Dose	Effect	Reference
Structure	Name				
	AY 20,263	Galactose (50% diet)	Intravitreal injection 0.8 mg in 10 μl DMSO	Eighteen-day delay of nuclear opacity	3
	AY 22,284 Alrestatin	Galactose (30% diet)	0.96 g/kg/day oral	80% delay of cataract after 29 days	20
		Galactose (50% diet)	10% topical 2×/day	Seven-day delay of nuclear opacity	98
	Quercetin	Galactose (50% diet)	Oral, 2.5% of diet	After 12 days lens fiber integrity and growth preserved	99
	Gossypin	Galactose (30% diet)	15 mg/kg oral	60% delay of cataract after 28 days	100

Structure	Compound	Condition	Dose	Result	Ref
	3-Vicianosyl quercetin	Galactose (20% diet)	100 mg/kg/day ip 4 days after start of diet	28% decrease at nine days of ophthalmoscopic ring opacities	101
	—	Galactose (20% diet)	100 mg/kg/day ip 4 days after start of diet	38% decrease at nine days of ophthalmoscopic ring opacities	101
	RS 7535	Galactose (35% diet)	2% topical 2×/day	30% delay of bilateral cataract after 29 days	102
	CP 45,634 Sorbinil	Diabetic	60 mg/kg/day oral	No lens change after six months	103
		Galactose (50% diet)	60 mg/kg/day oral	No lens change after eight months	28
	M 79175	Galactose (30% diet)	1 mg/kg po/day	No opacity after 33 days	29
	AI 1567	Galactose (30% diet)	4 mg/kg/day oral	No opacity after 32 days	30

Structure	Compound	Condition	Dose	Result	Ref.
	ICI 105,552	Diabetic	50 mg/kg/day intubation	170 day delay for 50% of lenses with greater than punctate opacities	104
	ICI 128,436	Diabetic	25 mg/kg/day oral	No lens change after 74 days	21
	ONO 2235	Diabetic	50 mg/kg/day oral	Significant decrease in lens sorbitol after five months	77
	AY 27,773 Tolrestat	Galactose (50% diet)	56 mg/kg/day oral	No opacities after nine months	See footnote a below

[a] D. Dvornik, personal communication

After six days on the galactose diet, reversal of the cataractous process is not possible, with the vacuolar stage continuing to the dense nuclear cataract even though the rats are on a normal diet. A similar point of no return has been observed with sorbinil, which can reverse the appearance of cataract in the galactose-fed rats as long as it is administered prior to the sixth day of galactose feeding. The reversal of the cataract with sorbinil has been accomplished despite the continuation of the galactose diet. However, when sorbinil is applied after the sixth day the cataractous process continues, leading to opacification of the lens.

Human Diabetic Cataracts

The appearance of true diabetic cataracts seems to occur only rarely in young diabetics. In older individuals, however, diabetes hastens cataracts. Evidence for this clinical impression was provided by an epidemiological study that clearly demonstrated that diabetics between 55 and 64 years of age have a three-fold greater risk of developing cataracts than nondiabetics (43). Diabetes, therefore, appears to be one of many factors that contribute to cataract formation.

In the human lens, aldose reductase activity is not as substantial as in the rat lens. As a result, some have claimed that aldose reductase may not be active enough to accumulate sorbitol to levels sufficient for an osmotic effect (44). Analysis of cataracts extracted from diabetic patients, however, reveals that the amount of sorbitol and fructose recovered parallels the level of HbA1C, with the levels of polyol and fructose as high as 19 mmol per Kg per lens (45, 46). If these products of the sorbitol pathway are confined to the regions of the lens where aldose reductase is found, polyol may have an osmotic effect.

OTHER OCULAR DIABETIC COMPLICATIONS

Cornea

Diabetic corneal effects were unknown prior to the advent of vitrectomy, a surgical procedure used to remove blood or tissues obscuring the path of light onto the retina from the vitreous. Following insertion of the vitrectomy instrument into the eye, the corneal epithelium of diabetics often becomes cloudy, obscuring the vision of the surgeon who must view the surgical procedures through the patient's cornea. Consequently, the epithelium must be removed to permit surgery. Under normal circumstances, stripping the corneal epithelium does not present a problem because reepithelialization occurs rapidly. In diabetic patients, however, it was found that a delay in epithelial regeneration and persistent epithelial defects were serious post-surgical complications.

A similar delay in the reepithelialization of denuded corneas has been reproduced in diabetic and galactosemic rats (11, 47, 48). Moreover, the reepithelialized corneas of both diabetic and galactosemic rats appeared hazy and edematous, while the corneas stripped of their epithelium were characterized by a swelling of the stroma and marked invasion of polymorphonuclear leucocytes. Treatment with a number of aldose reductase inhibitors completely abolished the delay in the rate of reepithelialization and resulted in resurfaced corneas that were clear and transparent (11, 48). Histologically, the epithelia of the inhibitor–treated corneas also appeared healthier, multilayered, and thicker than those of untreated diabetic or galactosemic corneas, with leucocytes appearing less prominently in the treated ones.

Clinically, the aldose reductase inhibitor sorbinil has been employed in an interesting case of corneal keratopathy involving a 24-year-old female diabetic whose diabetes was poorly controlled (49). Following laser treatment for retinopathy, spontaneous bilateral corneal erosion developed. Since conventional treatment was ineffective, a single case protocol calling for the use of sorbinil eye drops was drafted and a single masked study was arranged in which one eye was treated with sorbinil while the other was given placebo eye drops. The sorbinil-treated eye slowly responded and the inflammatory signs and epithelial defects disappeared, while the placebo-treated eye worsened and eventually perforated, requiring an emergency corneal transplant. The keratoplast appeared successful until a few days after the operation, when the cornea developed the characteristic diabetic defects. At this point this eye was also treated with sorbinil. It responded favorably, and after a year both eyes appear stable.

The presence of aldose reductase in the corneal and conjunctival epithelium has been demonstrated by the immunoperoxidase method, which shows aldose reductase to be particularly rich in the basal layer of cells (50). Moreover, the fact that the delay of reepithelialization can be reproduced in the galactosemic as well as the diabetic rats strongly suggests the involvement of aldose reductase in diabetic corneal epitheliopathy. These observations, combined with the fact that aldose reductase inhibitors produce beneficial effects, indicate that aldose reductase is involved in diabetic abnormalities of the epithelium when the cornea is stressed in vitrectomy or when it is compelled to regenerate the epithelial layer.

Retina

Diabetic retinopathy, one of the leading causes of blindness, increases in prevalence with the duration of diabetes. Among the characteristics of early nonproliferative retinopathy are vascular changes of the retinal capillary bed, with the formation of microaneurysms, exudates, and small intraretinal hemorrhages. The hallmark of early retinopathy is the selective loss of retinal capillary pericytes (mural cells) versus endothelial cells; however, electroretinogram (ERG) pattern changes, color vision shifts, and capillary basement membrane thickening also have been observed (51).

Currently, only secondary evidence links aldose reductase with diabetic retinopathy. Histochemically, this enzyme has been localized in all human retinal regions displaying diabetic pathology. These include the pericytes of retinal capillaries, the Mueller cells, ganglion cells, and selective cone cells (50, 52, 53).

The first evidence suggesting the pathological involvement of aldose reductase in diabetic retinopathy, especially pericyte loss, evolved from studies with isolated monkey retinal capillary cells (54). Endothelial cells cultured in high glucose medium remained viable, while pericytes cultured in high glucose showed a threefold increase in sorbitol and cellular degeneration. However, rapid progress in this area has been hampered by the lack of a convenient, short-term animal model capable of displaying human-like retinal pathology, especially the selective loss of pericytes.

In streptozotocin diabetic rats, increased sorbitol levels have been detected in the retina and these increased levels have been reduced by the administration of the aldose reductase inhibitor 1-(3,4-dichlorobenzyl)-3-methyl-1,2-dihydro-2-oxoquinol-4-ylacetic acid (ICI 105552) (55). Retinal capillary basement membrane thickening, which has been observed to occur in both diabetic and galactosemic rats (see below), can also be controlled by the administration of aldose reductase inhibitors (56, 57). Through histochemistry, aldose reductase has been localized in the Mueller cells, ganglion cells, and pericytes of rat retinas (58, 59). The formation of pericyte ghosts as observed in human retinopathy, however, has not been equivocably demonstrated in either diabetic or galactosemic rats (57).

Long-term studies with alloxan diabetic dogs indicate that these animals are unique in developing retinopathy with a selective loss of pericytes demonstrable after 60 months of diabetes (60). Recently, an identical retinopathy, which includes the presence of retinal capillary aneurysms, hemorrhages, exudates, pericyte ghosts, and capillary basement membrane thickening, has been demonstrated to occur in dogs after 32 months of 30% galactose feeding (61). Increased polyol levels have also been detected in isolated canine retinal vessels cultured with high levels of either glucose or galactose (62). This formation of polyols was reduced by the addition of the aldose reductase inhibitor sorbinil to the culture medium. Upon histochemical examination of isolated canine retinal capillaries with antibodies prepared against purified dog lens aldose reductase, the presence of aldose reductase could only be detected in the pericytes (37).

These canine studies clearly suggest the involvement of aldose reductase in the pathogenesis of diabetic retinopathy. Confirmation, however, must wait until current long-term galactose-feeding studies with aldose reductase inhibitors are complete.

DIABETIC NEUROPATHY

A majority of all diabetics are afflicted to some degree with neuropathy. Diabetic neuropathy may express itself in many ways, ranging from subtle changes in nerve conduction velocity and axoplasmic flow to complete loss of various neurons and a myriad of clinical manifestations, which can include some of the most disabling complications of long-term diabetes mellitus (63). The role of aldose reductase in the pathogenesis of this diabetic complication has been established through basic laboratory and animal studies as well as through clinical trials. Aldose reductase has been localized to the Schwann cells of the myelin sheath, and the accumulation of sorbitol in these cells may result in osmotic swelling similar to that observed in the lens (64, 65). In vitro incubation of rat sciatic nerves in high glucose medium has been demonstrated to result in the accumulation of sorbitol, and this accumulation can be prevented by the administration of a variety of aldose reductase inhibitors, including alrestatin, sulindac, and sorbinil (65, 66). In streptozotocin diabetic rats, nerve sorbitol levels have been observed to increase within three days following induction of diabetes (67). This increase in the nerve sorbitol concentration was accompanied by significant decreases in the motor nerve conduction velocities of the sciatic nerves, whether the duration of diabetes was two, five, or nine months (68). The accumulation of sorbitol was therefore associated with impairments of nerve conduction velocities, which are among the earliest and most easily quantifiable signs of diabetic neuropathy. Treatment for four weeks with the potent aldose reductase inhibitor sorbinil reduced the sorbitol concentration in the sciatic nerve and increased motor nerve conduction to normal levels, even though high blood glucose persisted.

Similar neurological changes have been observed in galactosemic animals, with nerve swelling in a galactosemic model similar to that reported in streptozotocin-induced diabetic rats (69). The swollen sciatic nerves of galactosemic rats have been shown to contain increased polyol (dulcitol) concentrations and increased water content, concomitant with decreased nerve conduction velocity. These changes can be reversed either by removal of the rats from the galactose diet or by the administration of aldose reductase inhibitors, suggesting that the water content and nerve conduction velocity are related to the polyol pathway. In rats fed a 50% galactose diet for forty-four weeks, the sciatic nerves are decidedly swollen compared to those of rats on a normal, control diet (35% increase in diameter) (70). Nerve swelling has not been found in rats receiving the galactose diet containing the inhibitor sorbinil.

In addition to nerve conduction velocity, the axonal transport of choline acetyltranferase has been demonstrated to decrease in either diabetic or galactosemic rats (71). This decreased axonal transport, another early sign of diabetic neuropathy, can be reversed through the use of aldose reductase inhibitors. Impaired orthograde axonal transport of choline acetyltransferase has been demonstrated by ligature of the sciatic nerve in diabetic rats and has been reversed by treatment with ICI 105,552.

Several clinical trials with aldose reductase inhibitors have been reported. Early trials with alrestatin on long-term diabetics suggested qualitatively that treatment could improve peripheral nerve function and the relief of pain (72, 73). Recent reports suggest that within a few days of treatment with the more potent inhibitor sorbinil, several patients with severely painful diabetic neuropathy experienced decreased pain, improved sensory perception, increased muscle strength, and normalization of nerve conduction velocities (74, 75).

In an effort to quantitate the effects of the aldose reductase inhibitor sorbinil on neuropathy, a multicenter, randomized, doubly masked crossover trial was undertaken (76). Following a six-week baseline study, patients chosen for good blood glucose control were randomized as to treatment received. Half received 250 mg sorbinil per day for nine weeks while the other half received placebo for nine weeks; then the treatments were reversed for a second nine-week period. Finally, all patients received placebo treatment for another three weeks to allow a masked assessment of drug washout for each patient. In order to evaluate the effect of the drug, nerve conduction velocities of peroneal motor nerve, median motor nerve, and median sensory nerve were measured at three-week intervals throughout the twenty-seven-week study. As expected, during their placebo treatment, whether this was received first or last, all patients exhibited decreased nerve conduction velocities in all three nerves. During treatment with sorbinil, however, the nerve conduction velocities of all three nerves rose significantly. Conduction decreased again during the three-week sorbinil washout.

The apparent initially positive clinical results of sorbinil further strengthen the link between the polyol pathway and the neuropathy of diabetes mellitus. Successful utilization of several unrelated inhibitors of aldose reductase has demonstrated the improbability of nonspecific inhibition of the polyol pathway. Moreover, the possibility that the hydantoin entity common to many of the aldose reductase inhibitors might affect mainly the central nervous system, having only indirect effects on the polyol pathway, has been eliminated by work with several hydantoin-free compounds such as the 1-(3,4-dichlorobenzyl)-3-methyl-1,2-dihydro-2-oxoquinol-4-ylacetic acid (ICI

105552) and (E)-5-[(E)-2-methyl-3-phenylpropenylidene]rhodanine-3-acetic
acid (ONO 2235) (71, 77).

DIABETIC ANGIOPATHY

Capillary Basement Membrane Thickening

A striking morphological change occurring consistently in all tissues of diabetics and animal models of diabetes is the frank thickening of capillary basement
membranes (78). These so-called membranes are thin, extracellular matrices
consisting of a unique type IV collagen bound to varying degrees with several
proteoglycans, glycoproteins, and an amyloid (79). They form enveloping
sheaths that surround the capillary and separate the pericytes and endothelial
cells of the capillary wall from adjacent tissues. Pathophysiologically, capillary
basement membrane thickening has been considered the fundamental structural
lesion of the small blood vessels in diabetic patients and the ultrastructural
hallmark of diabetic microangiopathy (78, 80). It is believed to be involved in
several diabetic complications, including both diabetic retinopathy and nephropathy, since the basement membranes of both retinal capillaries and kidney
glomerular capillaries thicken progressively in diabetics (80, 81). Failure of
glomerular filtration is accompanied by massive accumulations of basement
membrane material surrounding the endothelial cells and pericytes (masangial
cells) of the capillaries, leaving little surface area for filtration to occur.
Basement membrane thickness in capillaries of muscle biopsies has been
utilized as a sign of microangiopathy in asymptomatic diabetic patients (82).

An understanding of the pathogenesis of capillary basement membrane
thickening in diabetics has been complicated because factors other than abnormal carbohydrate metabolism can contribute to basement membrane thickening
(78). These include hypertension and aging. Moreover, many of the results
obtained have been controversial due to the measurement methodologies employed (78, 83). However, a possible breakthrough in the study of basement
membrane thickening has come from studies using precise, reproducible computer planimetry techniques that indicate that galactosemic animals can form
thickened capillary basement membranes that appear to be ultrastructurally
similar to those of diabetics (56). Basement membranes from galactosemic and
diabetic rats and dogs contain fibrous collagen with banding patterns, clear
vacuoles, and areas of irregular thicknesses and multilaminar composition, all
of which are seen seldom in controls (56, 57, 61).

In rats fed from weaning a diet containing 50% galactose, a 57% thickening
of capillary basement membranes in the outer plexiform layer of the retina was
observed after 28 weeks, and a twofold thickening after 44 weeks, compared to
controls fed a normal diet (56). This thickening was prevented in another

galactose-fed group by the concomitant daily administration of .04% sorbinil mixed into the diet (56). Similar results were obtained with the structurally unrelated aldose reductase inhibitor tolrestat at both .03% and .04% levels in the diet. Rats fed a 30% galactose diet also developed significant thickening of retinal capillary basement membranes after 15 to 21 months that was more pronounced in hypertensive than in normotensive rats (57). This thickening was also prevented by sorbinil. Significant retinal capillary basement membrane thickening has also been reported in rats two months after the induction of diabetes with streptozotocin (84). This thickening was prevented by treatment with the inhibitor dl-spiro-(2-fluorofluoren-9'4'-imidazolidine)-2'5'-dione (AL 1567).

It is known that basement membrane thickening can result from high serum hexose levels, and the prevention of thickening by these diverse aldose reductase inhibitors suggests that aldose reductase may play a role in the biochemical mechanism leading to the excessive formation of basement membranes. This possibility is currently being investigated in the Engelbreth-Holm-Swarm (EHS) tumor, a tissue that produces relatively large quantities of basement membrane (85). When grown in galactosemic mice, these tumor cells can accumulate dulcitol (40). Moreover, enzyme studies indicate the presence of an apparent aldose reductase in this tumor tissue that can be inhibited by a variety of aldose reductase inhibitors.

The observation that diabetes-like basement membrane thickening occurs in galactosemic animals, combined with the fact that aldose reductase inhibitors can prevent this thickening in either galactosemic or diabetic animals, strongly suggests that aldose reductase may regulate basement membrane thickening, although the mechanism remains unknown. While the regulation of blood sugar levels has been known to mediate basement membrane thickness, the prevention of thickening by inhibition of aldose reductase represents a novel approach toward the regulation of basement membrane thickness, an approach independent of blood sugar control.

Erythrocytes and Platelets

Among the factors contributing to diabetic angiopathy are altered blood flow characteristics, including enhanced erythrocyte aggregation, increased plasma viscosity, increased resistance to blood flow, and increased platelet aggregation (1). Human erythrocyte sorbitol levels in insulin-dependent diabetics have been clearly demonstrated to be above those of nondiabetics after an eight-hour fast (86). Statistically significant correlations have also been observed between the levels of red cell sorbitol and erythrocyte deformability measured as a filtration index. In diabetics this factor is substantially diminished (87). In vitro culture of intact human erythrocytes in high glucose medium also results in the increased intracellular accumulation of sorbitol, and this accumulation of sorbitol can be inhibited by either tetramethylene glutaric acid or sorbinil (86). Moreover, the sorbitol levels in red blood cells of diabetic rats have been shown to be directly related to nerve sorbitol levels (88). Both red blood cells and nerves appear to be equally susceptible to inhibition by the aldose reductase inhibitor sorbinil. These results clearly demonstrate the presence of aldose reductase in the red blood cell. Although no beneficial effect has been reported to result from the inhibition of red blood cell aldose reductase, measuring its levels has become a convenient method for monitoring the plasma levels of aldose reductase inhibitor in clinical trials (88).

Sorbitol is also present in the platelets of diabetics. The accumulation of sorbitol has been demonstrated in human platelets incubated in high glucose medium, and this accumulation can be inhibited with the aldose reductase inhibitor alrestatin (89). However, no correlation between platelet aggregation and sorbitol accumulation has been reported. Therefore, it has been concluded that the sorbitol accumulation in platelets is not responsible for the abnormal platelet formation or morphology observed in diabetes.

DIABETIC NEPHROPATHY

Loss of renal function associated with diabetic nephropathy leads to death in about half of all insulin-dependent diabetics. Diabetic changes of the kidney generally involve alterations of the glomerular capillaries and associated arterioles, which lead to changes in filtration, proteinuria, and eventually impaired renal failure. Clinically, the earliest feature of diabetic nephropathy is symptomless proteinuria (1, 80).

Currently, little evidence implicating aldose reductase in the pathogenesis of diabetic nephropathy exists. The renal presence of aldose reductase has been demonstrated in the interstitial cells, Henle's loop, and collecting tubules of the dog; in Henle's loop, collecting tubules, and glomerular podocytes of the rat; and in the glomeruli of the human (59, 90, 91). The polyol pathway has also been observed to be present in cultured monkey kidney epithelial cells, which accumulate sorbitol upon culture in a high glucose medium (92). Moreover, the addition of either of the aldose reductase inhibitors tetramethylene glutaric acid, 1-(3,4-dichlorobenzyl)-3-methyl-1,2-dihydro-2-oxoquinol-4-ylacetic acid (ICI 105552), 7-0-(β-hydroxyethyl)quercetin, or 5,7,3',4,'-tetra-0-(β-hydroxyrutin) to the culture medium results in the decreased formation of sorbitol (93).

However, some implications of a potential role for aldose reductase in nephropathy have recently emerged. Consistently higher kidney wet weights have been observed in rats fed a 50% galactose diet for 25 days, than in those fed a normal diet, despite the fact that the body weights of the galactosemic rats were 55% lower (94). Differences in the wet to dry weight ratios suggest that the apparent hypertrophy involved both increased fluid content and renal mass. Furthermore, this apparent hypertrophy has been prevented by concomitant treatment of the galactose-fed rats with the aldose reductase inhibitor sorbinil. Increased levels of sorbitol have also been observed in isolated glomeruli from streptozotocin diabetic rats, and the level of sorbitol in the glomeruli from similar rats treated with sorbinil has also been reduced (95). Unique protein pattern changes in the urine of these diabetic rats can also be detected with the prolonged onset of diabetes (96). These changes, suggestive of proteinuria, were diminished by sorbinil treatment.

These preliminary observations, suggesting potential beneficial effects of the aldose reductase inhibitor sorbinil for the treatment of nephropathy, should stimulate further work in establishing the relationships between aldose reductase and the pathogenesis of diabetic nephropathy.

CONCLUSION

Work on the role of aldose reductase in diabetic complications has progressed from initial studies limited to cataracts to current studies of virtually all tissues that display diabetic pathology. For these studies, recently developed potent aldose reductase inhibitors used on appropriate diabetic and galactosemic animal models have provided powerful tools for elucidating the relationship between aldose reductase and diabetic complications. Inhibition of aldose reductase has been demonstrated to prevent the onset of cataract, to reverse problems in the reepithelialization of denuded corneas, to reverse decreases in both nerve conduction velocity and axonal transport, and to prevent retinal capillary basement membrane thickening. Evidence for the involvement of aldose reductase in retinopathy and possibly nephropathy is also mounting. Results suggest that in order to be effective, aldose reductase inhibitors must be used at the onset or during very early stages of diabetes. Moreover, while the physiological role of this enzyme remains unknown, no significant adverse effects have been reported from long-term aldose reductase inhibition in rats or dogs. These studies have provided the basis for several clinical trials that will eventually determine the effect of aldose reductase inhibition on diabetic man.

The aldose reductase–initiated intracellular accumulation of polyols has been shown to result in an hyperosmotic effect on either the lens or nerve. However, the possibility that aldose reductase has adverse effects other than osmotic changes must also be considered. Recent nuclear magnetic resonance (NMR) studies have revealed that the flux of glucose through the sorbitol pathway appears to be more substantial than indicated by the levels of polyols observed (97). If this is the case, then the amount of NADPH utilized may be substantial and it may be diverted from reactions in which it is normally used. This deflection of the cofactor to the aldose reductase reaction can result in adverse metabolic consequences. Another interesting observation in all tissues displaying diabetic complications in which aldose reductase is thought to be involved is the inverse relationship between the levels of sorbitol and myo-inositol. As the sorbitol levels increase in these tissues, the inositol levels decrease. Inositol loss in the lens appears to be due to leakage; however, other possibilities may also exist. Except for experimental diabetic cataracts, the exact mechanism by which aldose reductase is involved in the diabetic complication needs to be clarified.

Until then, we propose that certain guidelines be established in linking aldose reductase to diabetic complications: (a) aldose reductase should be present in the tissue in question; (b) the complication should occur in the galactosemic as well as in the diabetic state; (c) the complication should occur earlier and be more severe in galactosemia than in diabetes; (d) aldose reductase inhibitor should prevent or delay the appearance of the complication; and (e) more than one aldose reductase inhibitor should be effective.

Literature Cited

1. Dvornik, D. 1978. Chronic complications of diabetes. *Ann. Rep. Med. Chem.* 13:159–66
2. Hers, H. G. 1956. Le mecanisme de la transformation de glucose en fructose par les vesicules seminals. *Biochim. Biophys. Acta* 22:202–3
3. Kinoshita, J. H. 1974. Mechanism initiating cataract formation. Proctor Lecture. *Invest. Ophthalmol.* 13:713–24
4. Kinoshita, J. H. 1965. Cataracts in galactosemia. The Jonas Friedenwald Memorial Lecture. *Invest. Ophthalmol.* 4:786–99
5. Obazawa, H., Merola, L. O., Kinoshita, J. H. 1974. Effects of xylose on the isolated lens. *Invest. Ophthalmol.* 13:204–9
6. Keller, H. W., Koch, H. R., Ohrloff, C. 1977. Experimental arabinose cataracts in young rats. *Ophthal. Res.* 9:205–12
7. Hayman, S., Kinoshita, J. H. 1965. Isolation and properties of lens aldose reductase. *J. Biol. Chem.* 240:877–82
8. Herrmann, R. K., Kador, P. F., Kinoshita, J. H. 1983. Rat lens aldose reductase: Rapid purification and comparison with human placental aldose reductase. *Exp. Eye Res.* 37:467–74
9. van Heyningen, R. 1959. Formation of polyols by the lens of the rat with "sugar" cataract. *Nature* 184:194–95
10. Friedenwald, J. S., Rytel, D. 1955. Contributions to the histopathology of cataract. *Arch. Ophth.* 53:825–33
11. Kinoshita, J. H., Fukushi, S., Kador, P., Merola, L. O. 1979. Aldose reductase in diabetic complications of the eye. *Metabolism* 28:462–69
12. Kador, P., Zigler, J. S., Kinoshita, J. H. 1979. Alteration of lens protein synthesis in galactosemic rats. *Invest. Ophthalmol. Vis. Sci.* 18:696–702
13. Piatigorsky, J., Fukui, H. N., Kinoshita, J. H. 1978. Differential metabolism and leakage of protein in an inherited cataract and a normal lens cultured with ouabain. *Nature* 274:558–62
14. Piatigorsky, J., Kador, P. F., Kinoshita, J. H. 1980. Differential synthesis of protein in the hereditary Philly mouse cataract. *Exp. Eye Res.* 30:69–78
15. Chylack, L. T., Kinoshita, J. H. 1969. Biochemical evaluation of a cataract induced in high glucose medium. *Invest. Ophthalmol.* 8:401–12
16. Kinoshita, J. H., Barber, W. G., Merola, L. O., Tung, B. 1969. Changes in the levels of free amino acids and myoinositol in the galactose-exposed lens. *Invest. Ophthalmol.* 8:625–36
17. Kinoshita, J. H., Merola, L. O., Hayman, S. 1965. Osmotic effects on the amino acid concentrating mechanism in the rabbit lens. *J. Biol. Chem.* 240:310–15
18. Kador, P. F., Kinoshita, J. H. 1984. Diabetic galactosemic cataracts. *Ciba Found. Symp. Human Cataract Formation* 106:110–23
19. Jedziniak, J. A., Kinoshita, J. H. 1971. Activators and inhibitors of aldose reductase. *Invest. Ophthalmol.* 10:357–66
20. Dvornik, D., Simard-Duquesne, N., Kraml, M., Sestanj, K., Gabbay, K. H., et al. 1973. Inhibition of aldose reductase in vivo. *Science* 182:1146–47

21. Stribling, D., Mirrless, D. J., Harrison, H. E., Earl, D. C. N. 1984. Properties of ICI 128,436: A novel aldose reductase inhibitor and its effects on diabetic complications in the rat. *Metabolism*. In press

22. Sestanj, K., Bellini, F., Fung, S., Abraham, N., Treasurywala, A., et al. 1984. N - [(5 - (trifluoromethyl) - 6 - methoxy - 1 - naphthalenyl)thioxomethyl] - N - methylglycine (Tolrestat), a potent, orally active aldose reductase inhibitor. *J. Med. Chem.* 27:255–56

23. Terashima, H., Hama, K., Yamamoto, R., Tsuboshima, M., Kikkawa, R., et al. 1984. Effects of a new aldose reductase inhibitor on various tissues in vitro. *J. Pharmacol. Exp. Ther.* 229:226–30

24. Varma, S. D., Kinoshita, J. H. 1976. Inhibition of lens aldose reductase by flavonoids. *Biochem. Pharmacol.* 25:2505–13

25. Kador, P. F., Sharpless, N. E. 1978. Structure-activity studies of aldose reductase inhibitors containing the 4-oxo-4H-chromen ring system. *Biophys. Chem.* 8:81–85

26. Kador, P. F., Sharpless, N. E., Goosey, J. D. 1982. Aldose reductase inhibition by anti-allergy drugs. *Prog. Clin. Biol. Res.* 114:243–59

27. Peterson, M. J., Sarges, R., Aldinger, C. G., MacDonald, D. P. 1979. CP-45634: A novel aldose reductase inhibitor that inhibits polyol formation pathway activity in diabetic and galactosemic rats. *Metabolism* 28:456–61

28. Fukushi, S., Merola, L. O., Kinoshita, J. H. 1980. Altering the course of cataracts in diabetic rats. *Invest. Ophthalmol. Vis. Sci.* 19:313–15

29. Ono, H., Nozawa, Y., Hayano, S. 1980. Effects of M79175, an aldose reductase inhibitor, on experimental sugar cataracts. *Nippon Ganka Gakki Zasshi* 86:1343–50

30. York, B. M. 1983. *European Patent Application 0 092 385*

31. Sohda, T., Mizuno, K., Imamiya, E., Tawada, H., Meguro, K., et al. 1982. *Chem. Pharm. Bull.* 30:3601–16

32. Schnur, R. C., Sarges, R., Peterson, M. J. 1982. Spiro oxazolidinedione aldose reductase inhibitors. *J. Med. Chem.* 25:1451–54

33. Kador, P. F., Sharpless, N. E. 1983. Pharmacophor requirements of the aldose reductase inhibitor site. *Mol. Pharmacol.* 24:521–31

34. Kador, P. F., Goosey, J. D., Sharpless, N. E., Kolish, J., Miller, D. D. 1981. Stereospecific inhibition of aldose reductase. *Eur. J. Med. Chem.* 16:293–98

35. Okuda, J., Miwa, I., Inakagi, K., Horie, T., Nakayama, M. 1982. Inhibition of aldose reductases from rat and bovine lenses by flavonoids. *Biochem. Pharmacol.* 31:3807–22

36. Tanimoto, T., Fukuda, H., Kawamura, J. 1984. Characterization of aldose reductases la and lb from rabbit lens. *Chem. Pharm. Bull.* 32:1025–31

37. Kador, P. F., Millen, J., Akagi, Y., Kinoshita, J. H. 1984. Dog lens aldose reductase: Purification and comparison with the rat lens enzyme. *Invest. Ophthalmol. Vis. Sci.* 25:47 (Suppl.)

38. Kador, P. F., Merola, L. O., Kinoshita, J. H. 1979. Differences in the susceptibility of various aldose reductases to inhibition. *Doc. Ophthalmol. Proc. Ser.* 18:117–24

39. Kador, P. F., Kinoshita, J. H., Tung, W. H., Chylack, L. T. 1980. Differences in the susceptibility of aldose reductase to inhibition. II. *Invest. Ophthalmol. Visual Sci.* 19:980–82

40. Millen, J., Kador, P. F., Kinoshita, J. H., Vogeli, G. 1984. Aldose reductase and basement membrane production. *Invest. Ophthalmol. Vis. Sci.* 25:154 (Suppl.)

41. Kador, P. F., Shiono, T., Kinoshita, J. H. 1983. Studies with purified aldose reductase. *Invest. Ophthalmol. Vis. Sci.* 24:267 (Suppl)

42. Hu, T. S., Datiles, M., Kinoshita, J. H. 1983. Reversal of galactose cataract with sorbinil in rats. *Invest. Ophthalmol. Vis. Sci.* 24:640–44

43. Ederer, F., Hiller, R., Taylor, H. R. 1981. Senile lens changes and diabetes in two population studies. *Am. J. Ophthalmol.* 91:381–95

44. Jedziniak, J. A., Chylack, L. T. Jr., Cheng, H. M., Gillis, M. K., Kalustian, A. A., et al. 1981. The sorbitol pathway in the human lens: Aldose reductase and polyol dehydrogenase. *Invest. Ophthalmol. Vis. Sci.* 20:314–26

45. Lerner, B. C., Varma, S. D., Richards, R. D. 1984. Polyol pathway metabolites in human cataracts. *Arch. Opthalmol.* 102:917–20

46. Varma, S. D., Schocket, S. S., Richards, R. D. 1979. Implications of aldose reductase in cataracts of human diabetes. *Invest. Ophthalmol. Vis. Sci.* 18:237–41

47. Fukushi, S., Merola, L. O., Tanaka, M., Datiles, M., Kinoshita, J. H. 1980. Reepithelialization of denuded corneas in diabetic rats. *Exp. Eye Res.* 31:611–21

48. Datiles, M. B., Kador, P. F., Fukui, H. N., Hu, T. S., Kinoshita, J. H. 1983. Corneal re-epithelialization in galactosemic rats. *Invest. Ophthalmol. Vis. Sci.* 24:563–69

49. Cobo, L. M. 1984. Aldose reductase and

diabetic keratopathy. In *Aldose Reductase and Complications of Diabetes,* mod. D. G. Cogan, *Ann. Intern. Med.* 101:82–91

50. Akagi, Y., Yajima, Y., Kador, P. F., Kuwabara, T., Kinoshita, J. H. 1984. Localization of aldose reductase in the human eye. *Diabetes* 33:562–66

51. Kuwabara, T., Cogan, D. G. 1963. Retinal vascular patterns VI. Mural cells of the retinal capillaries. *Arch. Ophthalmol.* 69:492–502

52. Akagi, Y., Kador, P. F., Kuwabara, T., Kinoshita, J. H. 1983. Aldose reductase in human retinal mural cells. *Invest. Ophthalmol. Vis. Sci.* 24:1516–19

53. Jahn, C. E., Schindler, E., Holbach, L., Kador, P. F. 1984. Immunohistologische lokalisation der aldose reductase in menschlichen auge durch monoclonale antikoerper. *Fortschr. Ophthalmol.* In press

54. Buzney, S. M., Frank, R. N., Varma, S. D., Tanishima, T., Gabbay, K. H. 1977. Aldose reductase in retinal mural cells. *Invest. Ophthalmol. Vis. Sci.* 16:392–96

55. Poulsom, R., Heath, H. 1983. Inhibition of aldose reductase in five tissues of the streptozotocin-diabetic rat. *Biochem. Pharmacol.* 32:1495–99

56. Robison, W. G. Jr., Kador, P. F., Kinoshita, J. H. 1983. Retinal capillaries: Basement membrane thickening by galactosemia prevented with aldose reductase inhibitor. *Science* 221:1177–79

57. Frank, R. N., Kern, R. J., Kennedy, A., Frank, K. W. 1983. Galactose-induced retinal capillary basement membrane thickening: Prevention by sorbinil. *Invest. Ophthalmol. Vis. Sci.* 24:1519–24

58. Akagi, Y., Kador, P., Kuwabara, T., Kinoshita, J. 1983. Aldose reductase localization in retinal mural cells. *Invest. Ophthalmol. Vis. Sci.* 24:257 (Suppl.)

59. Ludvigson, M. A., Sorenson, R. L. 1980. Immunohistochemical localization of aldose reductase II. Rat eye and kidney. *Diabetes* 29:450–59

60. Engerman, R., Bloodworth, J. M. B. Jr., Nelson, S. 1977. Relationship of microvascular disease in diabetes to metabolic control. *Diabetes* 26:760–69

61. Engerman, R. L., Kern, T. S. 1984. Experimental galactosemia produces diabetic-like retinopathy. *Diabetes* 33:97–100

62. Kern, T. S., Engerman, R. L. 1984. Hexitol production by canine retinal microvessels. *Invest. Ophthalmol. Vis. Sci.* 25:159 (Suppl)

63. Ellenberg, M. 1983. Diabetic neuropathy. In *Diabetes Mellitus, Theory and Practice,* ed. M. Ellenberg, H. Rifkin, pp. 777–801. New York: Med. Exam.

64. Ludvigson, M. A., Sorenson, R. L. 1980. Immunohistochemical localization of aldose reductase. I. Enzyme purification and antibody preparation—localization in peripheral nerve, artery, and testes. *Diabetes* 29:438–49

65. Gabbay, K. H. 1973. The polyol pathway and the complications of diabetes. *N. Engl. J. Med.* 288:831–36

66. Jacobson, M., Sharma, Y. R., Cotlier, E., Hollander, J. D. 1983. Diabetic complications in lens and nerve and their prevention by sulindac or sorbinil: Two novel aldose reductase inhibitors. *Invest. Ophthalmol. Vis. Sci.* 24:1426–29

67. Ward, J. D. 1973. The polyol pathway in the neuropathy of early diseases. In *Advances in Metabolic Disorders, Supplement 2,* pp. 425–29. New York: Academic

68. Yue, D. K., Hanwell, M. A., Satchell, P. M., Turtle, J. R. 1982. The effect of aldose reductase inhibition on motor nerve conduction velocity in diabetic rats. *Diabetes* 31:789–94

69. Gabbay, K. H. 1973. Role of sorbitol pathway in neuropathy. See Ref. 67, pp. 417–24

70. Robison, W. G. Jr., 1984. Aldose reductase and diabetic neuropathy. See Ref. 49, pp. 85–87

71. Tomlinson, D. R., Holmes, P. R., Mayer, J. H. 1982. Reversal, by treatment with an aldose reductase inhibitor, of impaired axonal transport and motor nerve conduction velocity in experimental diabetes mellitus. *Neurosci. Lett.* 31:189–93

72. Gabbay, K. H., Spack, N., Loo, S., Hirsch, H. J., Ackil, A. A. 1979. Aldose reductase inhibition: Studies with alrestatin. *Metabolism* 28:471–76 (Suppl. 1)

73. Fagius, J., Jameson, S. 1981. Effects of aldose reductase inhibitor treatment in diabetic polyneuropathy—A clinical and neurophysiological study. *J. Neurol. Neurosurg. Psych.* 44:991–1001

74. Young, R. J., Ewing, D. J., Clarke, B. F. 1983. A controlled trial of sorbinil, an aldose reductase inhibitor, in chronic painful diabetic neuropathy. *Diabetes* 32:938–42

75. Jaspan, J., Herold, K., Maselli, R., Bartkus, C. 1983. Treatment of severely painful diabetic neuropathy with an aldose reductase inhibitor: Relief of pain and improved somatic and autonomic nerve function. *Lancet* 2:758–62

76. Judzewitsch, R., Jaspan, J. B., Polonsky, K. S., Weinberg, C. R., Halter, J. B., et al. 1983. Aldose reductase inhibition improves motor nerve conduction

velocity in diabetic patients. *N. Engl. J. Med.* 308:119–25

77. Hotta, N., Kakuta, H., Kimura, M., Fukasawa, H., Koh, N., et al. 1983. Experimental and clinical trial of aldose reductase inhibitor in diabetic neuropathy. *Diabetes* 32:98A (Suppl. 1)

78. Williamson, J. R., Kilo, C. 1977. Current status of capillary basement membrane disease in diabetes mellitus. *Diabetes* 26:65–75

79. Lubec, G. 1984. Definition of glomerular basement membrane. *Renal Physiol.* 7:1–2

80. Osterby, R. 1983. Basement membrane morphology in diabetes mellitus. See Ref. 63, pp. 323–41

81. Ashton, N. 1974. Vascular basement membrane changes in diabetic retinopathy. *Br. J. Ophthalmol.* 58:344–66

82. Camerini-Davalos, R. A., Velasco, C., Glasser, M., Bloodworth, J. M. B. Jr. 1983. Drug-induced reversal of early diabetic microangiopathy. *N. Eng. J. Med.* 309:1551–56

83. Siperstein, M. D., Unger, R. H., Madison, L. L. 1968. Studies of muscle capillary basement membranes in normal subjects, diabetic, and prediabetic patients. *J. Clin. Invest.* 47:1973–99

84. Chandler, M. L., Shannon, W. A., DeSantis, L. 1984. Prevention of retinal capillary basement membrane thickening in diabetic rats by aldose reductase inhibitors. *Invest. Ophthalmol. Vis. Sci.* 25:159 (Suppl.)

85. Rohrbach, D. H., Wagner, C. W., Star, V. L., Martin, G. R., Brown, K. S., et al. 1983. Reduced synthesis of basement membrane heparan sulfate proteoglycan in streptozotocin-induced diabetic mice. *J. Biol. Chem.* 258:11672–77

86. Malone, J. I., Knox, G., Benford, S., Tedesco, T. A. 1980. Red cell sorbitol: An indicator of diabetic control. *Diabetes* 29:861–64

87. Carandente, O., Colombo, R., Girardi, A. M., Margonto, A., Pozza, G. 1982. Role of red cell sorbitol as determinant of reduced erythrocyte filtrability in insulin-dependent diabetics. *Acta Diabetol. Lat.* 19:359–68

88. Malone, J. I., Leavengood, H., Peterson, M. J., O'Brien, M. M., Page, M. G., et al. 1984. Red blood cell sorbitol as an indicator of polyol pathway activity: Inhibition of sorbinil in insulin-dependent diabetic subjects. *Diabetes* 33:45–49

89. Bidot-Lopez, P., Robertson, S., O'Mallay, B. C. 1979. Sorbitol accumulation in human diabetic and in normal platelets

incubated in glucose. *Clin. Res.* 27:363A

90. Kern, T. S., Engerman, R. L. 1982. Immunohistochemical distribution of aldose reductase. *Histochem. J.* 14:507–15

91. Corder, C. N., Braughler, J. M., Culp, P. A. 1979. Quantitative histochemistry of the sorbitol pathway in glomeruli and small arteries of human diabetic kidney. *Folia Histochem. Cytochem.* 17:137–46

92. Hutton, J. C., Williams, J. F., Schofield, P. H., Hollows, F. C. 1974. Polyol metabolism in monkey kidney epithelial cell cultures. *Eur. J. Biochem.* 49:347–53

93. Boot-Hanford, R., Heath, H. 1981. The effects of aldose reductase inhibitors on the metabolism of cultured monkey kidney epithelial cells. *Biochem. Pharmacol.* 30:3065–69

94. Beyer-Mears, A., Cruz, E., Dillon, P., Tanis, D., Roche, M. 1983. Diabetic renal hypertrophy diminished by aldose reductase inhibitor. *Fed. Proc.* 42:505

95. Beyer-Mears, A., Ku, L., Cohen, M. P. 1984. Glomerular polyol accumulation in diabetes and its prevention with sorbinil. *Diabetes* 33:89A (Suppl.)

96. Varagiannis, E., Beyer-Mears, A., Cruz, E. 1984. Diminished proteinuria by an aldose reductase inhibitor. *Diabetes* 33:43A (Suppl.)

97. Gonzalez, R. G., Barnett, P., Aguayo, J., Cheng, H. M., Chylack, L. T. Jr. 1984. Direct measurement of polyol pathway activity in the ocular lens. *Diabetes* 33:196–99

98. Varma, S. D., Kinoshita, J. H. 1976. Topical treatment of galactose cataracts. *Doc. Opthalmol. Proc.* 8:305–9

99. Beyer-Mears, A., Farnsworth, P. N. 1979. Diminished sugar cataractogenesis by quercetin. *Exp. Eye Res.* 28:709–16

100. Parmar, N. S., Ghosh, M. N. 1979. Effects of gossypin, a flavonoid, on the formation of galactose-induced cataract in rats. *Exp. Eye Res.* 29:229–32

101. Fauran, F., Feniou, C., Mosser, J., Thibault, A., Andre, C., Prat, G. 1980. Benzopyran glycosides acetals and ketals. US Patent 4,211,772

102. Waterbury, D. L. 1980. Xanthone carboxylic acids for preventing diabetic complications. US Patent 4,232,040

103. Datiles, M., Fukui, H., Kinoshita, J. H. 1982. Galactose cataract prevention with sorbinil, an aldose reductase inhibitor: A light microscopic study. *Invest. Opthalmol. Vis. Sci.* 22:174–79

104. Poulsom, R., Boot-Handford, R. P., Heath, H. 1983. Some affects of aldose reductase inhibition upon the eyes of long-term streptozotocin diabetic rats. *Cur. Eye Res.* 2:351–54

Ann. Rev. Pharmacol. Toxicol. 1985. 25:715–44

THE REGULATION OF HEPATIC GLUTATHIONE[1]

Neil Kaplowitz, Tak Yee Aw, and Murad Ookhtens

Liver Research Laboratory, Medical and Research Services, Wadsworth Veterans Administration Hospital, and University of California School of Medicine, Los Angeles, California 90073

INTRODUCTION

Glutathione (GSH) is a peptide composed of glutamate, cysteine, and glycine that exists in thiol-reduced (GSH) and disulfide-oxidized (GSSG) forms. GSH has been the subject of intense interest in the past decade and numerous symposia and reviews have been written about its function and regulation since 1980 (1–7). We propose to review some of the recent exciting developments in this field, with a particular focus on the regulation of hepatic GSH. We will not exhaustively review the literature and therefore apologize for inadvertent or intentional omissions. We hope to bring a personal and different perspective to this subject.

A few words about the functions of GSH will focus on the importance of elucidating the physiology and biochemistry of the regulation of this vital substance. GSH is a fairly ubiquitous substance in aerobic life forms and tissues and generally exists in millimolar concentrations. The liver is among the organs with the highest content of GSH. The heterogeneity of GSH content in tissues has been observed. Thus, periportal hepatocytes may contain approximately twice the centrilobular concentration, enterocytes at the villus tip have a higher content than the crypts, and proximal tubular cells of kidney have more GSH than other parts of the nephron (8–10).

GSH plays a critical role in detoxification reactions. It is a specific substrate for GSH peroxidase (11) and GSH S-transferases (12), and it participates in microsomal peroxidase and radical scavenging reactions (13, 14). In this regard, probably the key function of GSH is reducing hydrogen peroxide (H_2O_2), a reaction catalyzed by GSH peroxidase. H_2O_2 production is a by-product of oxygen-requiring metabolism. It has been estimated that approximately 5% of hepatic mitochondrial O_2 consumption generates H_2O_2. GSH peroxidase seems to be more important in reducing H_2O_2 than catalase, which is restricted by peroxisomal compartmentation (15). Therefore, GSH plays a critical role in the defense against oxygen toxicity by breaking the chain of reactions leading from superoxide anion to the very active membrane peroxidizing hydroxyl radical through intermediate H_2O_2. Undoubtedly, the status and efficiency of this reaction, coupled with other endogenous mechanisms for scavenging oxygen radicals, are important in modulating the aging process.

The GSH S–transferase catalyzed reactions represent another important function of GSH. The detoxification of electrophilic metabolites of xenobiotics is exemplified by the role of GSH in protecting the liver against acetaminophen-quinoneimine and the detoxification of polycyclic hydrocarbon epoxides. Thus, GSH-dependent detoxification may play a vital role in preventing cellular injury and cancer. Recently, endogenous substrates for these reactions have been identified. Thus, it has been recognized that GSH is involved in prostaglandin and leukotriene biosynthesis (16).

GSH exists in the reduced and disulfide forms. The relationship between these two forms has an important effect on the oxidation-reduction state of protein thiols. Thus, it has been suggested that the oxidation-reduction status of GSH may act as a third messenger in either enhancing or diminishing the activities of a variety of biological processes, such as enzyme catalysis, protein synthesis, and receptor binding (17).

It has become apparent that GSH is a substance with a broad range of vital functions that include detoxification reactions catalyzed by enzymes such as GSH peroxidase and GSH S-transferases, for which GSH is the only significant endogenous substrate, and the modulation of cellular thiol-disulfide status. This review focuses on hepatic GSH. The liver, having the greatest content of GSH, is the major organ involved in the elimination and detoxification of xenobiotics, and it also seems to play a central role in the interorgan relationships of GSH. As is discussed below, GSH is synthesized from precursor amino acids in virtually all cells. However, the liver is unique in two major aspects of GSH regulation: it has the ability to convert methionine to cysteine, and it efficiently exports GSH mainly into plasma at a rate that accounts for nearly all of its hepatic biosynthesis.

HEPATIC GSH SYNTHESIS

The maintenance of hepatocellular GSH is a dynamic process. Its steady-state cellular concentration is achieved by a balance between the rate of synthesis, catalyzed by γ-glutamylcysteine synthetase and GSH synthetase or GSSG reductase, the rate of utilization through redox (GSH peroxidase) and alkylat-

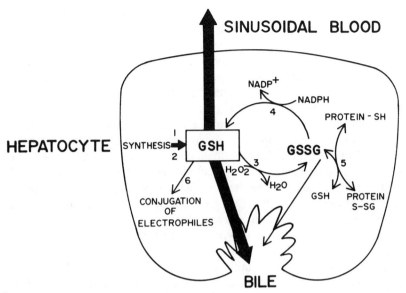

Figure 1   The regulation of hepatic glutathione. Reaction 1: γ-glutamylcysteine synthetase; reaction 2: GSH synthetase; reaction 3: GSH peroxidase; reaction 4: GSSG reductace; reaction 5: thioltransferase; reaction 6: GSH S-transferase. This model does not show the mitochondrial pool, which seems to have the same enzymes and distinct GSH regulation. [Reprinted with permission (2).]

ing (GSH S-transferase) reactions, and the rate of GSH export from hepatocytes (Figure 1).

Enzymes of GSH Biosynthesis

The enzymes of GSH synthesis were first described and characterized over 30 years ago by Bloch and coworkers (18, 19). The synthesis of GSH from its constituent amino acids, L-glutamate, L-cysteine, and L-glycine, involves two ATP-requiring enzymatic steps. The first, which is rate-limiting in GSH synthesis, is the formation of γ-glutamylcysteine from L-glutamate and L-cysteine. γ-Glutamylcysteine synthetase, the enzyme that catalyzes this reaction, is specific to the γ-glutamyl moiety and is regulated by (*a*) feedback competitive inhibition of the γ-glutamate binding site by GSH (K_i = 2.3 mM) (20, 21) and (*b*) the availability of its precursor, cysteine (22–24). The K_m of γ-glutamylcysteine synthetase for its two substrates, cysteine and glutamate, are 0.35 mM and 2 mM (21). Recent studies of this enzyme have concentrated on the purification, identification, and characterization of the nature of its active site (25, 26). Purification of the enzyme from rat liver has not been reported, but the purified γ-glutamylcysteine synthetase from rat kidney has a M_r of 100,000 daltons, with heavy (M_r = 74,000) and light (M_r = 24,000) subunits (27). Seelig & Meister (25) have demonstrated the presence of one disulfide bond and two free sulfhydryl groups in the kidney enzyme, only one of which is involved in the active site. Other recent studies have shown that γ-glutamylcysteine synthetase is inhibited by several analogs of methionine sulfoximine, such as propionine and buthionine sulfoximine (28, 29). The potency of inhibition is in the increasing order: methionine, propionine, and buthionine (28, 29). It is suggested that the S-alkyl moiety of sulfoximine binds to the enzyme at a site that normally accepts L-cysteine (28), and that the mechanism of inhibition appears to involve the phosphorylation of the sulfoximine by ATP [the formation of sulfoximine phosphate (30)]. Chung & Maines (31) further demonstrated that γ-glutamylcysteine synthetase is inducible by treating rats with sodium selenite via a mechanism that involves new protein synthesis. Conversely, Hill & Burk have demonstrated that selenium deficiency induces the activity of this enzyme (32).

The second enzyme in the biosynthetic pathway is GSH synthetase, which catalyzes the formation of a peptide bond between γ-glutamylcysteine and L-glycine in a reaction that utilizes 1 mole of ATP. The regulation of this enzyme has received less attention than has γ-glutamylcysteine synthetase, but some very early studies in hog and pigeon liver suggested that ADP may play a regulatory role (19, 33). Purification of GSH synthetase from rat kidney has been achieved. It has been shown to have a M_r of 118,000, with two identical subunits (34). Studies of the substrate binding sites on the enzyme have demonstrated that the enzyme binds glycine and cysteine but not glutamate very specifically. The L-glutamyl moiety may be replaced by its D-isomer and several other substituted glutamyl compounds (34). Purification of the enzyme from rat liver has not been reported. In contrast to γ-glutamylcysteine synthetase, GSH synthetase is not subject to feedback inhibition by GSH.

The Availability of Precursors

As alluded to earlier, hepatic GSH synthesis is largely limited by the availability of its precursor, L-cysteine (22–24). The free cysteine pool in the liver (0.2–0.5 mM) is at least an order of magnitude lower than that of GSH (5 mM), but it is approximately the same as the K_m of γ-glutamylcysteine synthetase for cysteine (21). Under physiological conditions, cysteine is derived mainly from the diet or from protein breakdown. Cystine, which is the predominant form in plasma, is poorly taken up by hepatocytes (35, 36) and is therefore not a ready, direct source of cellular GSH. Alternatively, cysteine may be derived from dietary methionine, which can serve as a major source of cellular cysteine via the transsulfuration pathway in the liver (24, 35–37). Experimentally, the supply of precursors for hepatic GSH synthesis is normally achieved by exposing hepatocytes to either cysteine or methionine (22–24, 35–39). Recently, a derivative of cysteine, L-2-oxo-thiazolidine-4-carboxylate, has been synthesized (40). Within the hepatocytes, the thiazolidine is converted to free cysteine by the action of 5-oxo-L-prolinase (41). Cysteine is often difficult to handle because of its rapid autoxidation rate, and the thiazolidine, which is more stable, is a useful alternate source of cellular cysteine. When administered to mice, cellular GSH concentration is maintained in the face of the GSH depletors diethylmaleate and acetaminophen (42). Furthermore, the oxothiazolidine protects the liver against acetaminophen toxicity (40, 42). However, it remains to be shown whether this compound is as effective in promoting hepatic GSH synthesis in other animal models, such as the rat.

Recent studies have demonstrated that GSH levels can be increased by supplying amino acid precursors for its hepatic synthesis and by supplying it directly to hepatocytes as esters (43). Puri & Meister have shown (43) that the treatment of mice with GSH esters causes a substantial elevation in cellular GSH in the liver and kidney. They suggest that, in contrast to GSH, the monomethyl and monoethyl esters of GSH are taken up by the hepatocytes, which are then hydrolyzed to release free GSH within the cell. By this means, hepatocellular GSH concentrations twofold above the basal level have been obtained two hours after the administration of the thiol esters to mice (43). They further demonstrated that the esters maintain the hepatic GSH level in the presence of acetaminophen, a depletor of cellular GSH. One other interesting approach to raising hepatic GSH has been employed by Wendel & Jaeschke in which GSH is delivered directly to cells via carrier liposomes (44–46). These researchers noted that GSH delivered in this manner to mice via intravenous injection in the tail vein is able to maintain hepatic GSH concentrations in the face of increased utilization by acetaminophen (44, 46). This technique therefore offers a useful approach to the study of hepatoprotection by GSH against drug-induced toxicity, since GSH itself is not taken up by the liver to any appreciable extent. GSH administered free or in vesicles similarly increases liver GSH. Free GSH given intravenously would be expected to break down in the kidney with cysteine, thereby becoming available to the liver. However, vesicle GSH exerts greater hepatoprotection. It remains to be determined whether these two forms of GSH affect different cell types in the liver or distribute differentially in the hepatic acinus. This experimental model has a further potential, namely, the delivery of enzymes and other substances that do not generally traverse cell membranes.

The Cystathionine Pathway

The liver's ability to utilize methionine effectively for GSH synthesis is relatively unique. This is because of the presence of an efficient transsulfuration pathway in the liver that is absent or insignificant in other GSH-synthesizing systems, either in normal (47, 48) or in transformed tissues (36, 48, 49). First described by du Vigneaud & Binkley (50, 51), the cystathionine pathway, as it is generally called, has been studied and characterized in the liver principally through the efforts of Reed and coworkers using the isolated hepatocyte model (24, 35, 37). Methionine is sequentially converted to cysteine via several enzymatic steps, the first of which involves the activation of methionine to S-adenosylmethionine. Subsequent demethylation and the removal of the adenosyl moiety yields homocysteine. Homocysteine condenses with serine to form cystathionine in a reaction catalyzed by cystathionine synthetase. Cleavage of cystathionine releases free cysteine. Cystathionase, the enzyme that catalyzes this cleavage, is strongly inhibited by propargylglycine, a potent irreversible inhibitor of methionine-dependent GSH synthesis (24, 52). Experimentally, the use of propargylglycine has been instrumental in demonstrating the significance of the pathway in hepatic GSH synthesis (24, 37). Data accumulated from several laboratories (22, 24, 35–39) have verified the importance of the cystathionine pathway as a major supplier of cysteine for hepatic GSH synthesis in isolated hepatocytes. However, its quantitative contribution to in vivo GSH synthesis in the liver remains to be established. Currently, little is known about the regulatory controls for this pathway. Dietary methionine appears to play an important role. Some studies have shown a correlation between changes in the hepatic levels of enzymes in the pathway and dietary levels of methionine in the rat (53). Other evidence suggests that regulation of the cellular homocysteine pool may be an important control factor (54). It is not clear if cysteine itself exerts a regulatory effect on its own synthesis.

The GSH Redox Cycle

Reduced GSH and its oxidized form, GSSG, is the major thiol redox system of the cell. Therefore, the redox state of this couple is of major importance for cellular function. Cellular GSH redox status is maintained by the proper distribution of GSH among all its major chemical forms: GSH, GSSG, and mixed disulfides. Oxidation-reduction and thiol-disulfide exchange reactions from normal metabolism or toxicological perturbations can cause the redistribution of some or all of these forms. GSH status in the liver is maintained mainly in the reduced state (GSH:GSSG 250), which is achieved by the efficient GSH peroxidase and reductase system coupled to the $NADP^+/NADPH$ redox pair. The oxidation of GSH to GSSG normally occurs through the reduction by GSH of the endogenous H_2O_2 catalyzed by GSH peroxidase. At the expense of cellular NADPH, GSSG is effectively reduced back to GSH by NADPH:GSSG reductase, thus maintaining thiol balance. As a result, GSSG reductase has a great capacity to protect cells against oxygen toxicity from endogenous active oxygen species (i.e. H_2O_2 and $O_2^{\cdot}$). This enzyme has recently been shown to be inducible in rat liver by dietary selenium, in parallel with γ-glutamylcysteine synthetase (31). Hydroperoxide metabolism and its relation to cellular GSH status has been extensively pursued, and the reader is referred to the review by Chance et al for a detailed discussion of the topic (55). The hepatoprotective role of GSSG reductase and its importance in maintaining cellular thiol redox balance has been verified in studies using 1,3-bis(2-chloro-ethyl)-1-nitrosourea (BCNU), a potent inhibitor of the enzyme (56). The hepatoprotective role of GSSG reductase against adriamycin-mediated toxicity in rats has recently been demonstrated by Wallace (57) and by Babson et al (58). In support of this, Meredith & Reed showed that the inhibition of the reductase by BCNU potentiates the injurious effect of adriamycin in rats, presumably by enhancing lipid peroxidation due to the depletion of cytosolic and especially mitochondrial GSH (59).

During oxidative stress, excessively high intracellular GSSG accumulates that renders cells more oxidized. This can have deleterious effects on cell integrity and metabolic processes. An example of this phenomenon is the regulation of Ca^{2+} homeostasis in the hepatocyte, an area that has received considerable attention and is still being actively pursued. Reduced GSH is implicated as playing a critical role in protecting microsomal Ca^{2+} sequestration and plasma membrane Ca^{2+} release, presumably by preventing the oxidation of thiol groups critical for Ca^{2+} ATPase activity (60–63). The protective effect of other thiols, such as dithiothreitol, supports this suggestion (63). Recently, increasing attention has also been given to the significance of protein mixed disulfides and the potential biological regulatory role of membrane and enzyme protein thiols (64). Mixed disulfides are formed in a reaction catalyzed by thiol transferase:

$$protein{-}SH + GSSG \rightleftharpoons protein{-}SSG + GSH$$

A hepatic thiol transferase from rat cytosol has been isolated (65). Brigelius et al (66) have recently demonstrated a linear relationship between cellular GSSG concentration and GSH protein mixed disulfide. By raising intracellular GSSG with either paraquat, t-butylhydroperoxide, or nitrofurantoin, they observed a parallel quantitative increase in protein mixed disulfide (GSSG:mixed disulfide ratio = 1:1). Furthermore, they also found that, concomitant with increased GSSG formation elicited by paraquat, the $NADPH/NADP^+$ ratio decreases from 5:1 to 2:3 (67). They expressed uncertainty about the form of thiol that exists as mixed disulfide, however, and have noted that the thiol released from mixed disulfide mainly is not GSH. The increase in protein mixed disulfides may suggest changes in regulatory functions such as in enzymes of the pentose phosphate pathway.

One final consideration about the GSH redox cycle is the supply of NADPH. The steady-state production of NADPH depends on the presence of glucose and its flux through the pentose phosphate pathway, mitochondrial production, and shuttles. Therefore, changes in shunt activity are expected to affect NADPH supply and consequent GSH/GSSG status. Pentose phosphate shunt activity may be controlled by substrate supply (glucose) or enzyme function (the inhibition of glucose-6-phosphate dehydrogenase by NADPH is alleviated by GSSG). Recently, Brigelius and colleagues have suggested that this pathway in the liver may be stimulated by the redox cycling compound paraquat (67). Increased consumption of NADPH by paraquat (67) via redox cycling can cause cellular NADPH concentration to fall 50% below that required to sustain normal metabolism. Other researchers have suggested further that the toxicity of paraquat may be at least partly due to its modulation of the redox state of the pyridine nucleotides. Earlier studies by Thurman et al have shown that mitochondrial production of NADPH supports NADPH-dependent P450-catalyzed reactions under conditions of decreased pentose phosphate shunt activity (68, 69). Whether mitochondrial production similarly plays a significant role in the maintenance of cellular GSH redox status remains to be established.

HEPATIC GSH TRANSPORT

The liver releases glutathione in both oxidized and reduced forms. Hepatocytes are polar cells with functionally and anatomically distinct plasma membrane domains. The canalicular domain differs in several respects from the sinusoidal domain in terms of the release of GSH and GSSG.

Sinusoidal GSH Transport

The perfused liver model and in vivo studies have been utilized to characterize GSH release. GSH is released into the perfusate at a rate of 12–18 nmol per minute $^{-1}$ per gram^{-1} (70–75). Virtually no GSSG is found in the perfusate under basal conditions. In vivo, the concentration of plasma GSH leaving the liver is much greater than that entering the liver (73, 76, 77) and estimates of efflux rates are comparable to the data in the isolated organ. The rate of efflux of GSH in vitro and in vivo into plasma approximates the turnover rate of hepatic GSH (15–20% per hour^{-1}) and therefore quantitatively is the major component of intracellular degradation. This has recently been verified by turnover studies in vivo that demonstrated that GSH release quantitatively accounts for nearly all of the turnover of hepatic GSH (77).

The release of GSH from the sinusoidal side of the liver has been well documented in the perfused liver and in vivo. In the perfused liver, our laboratory has studied the kinetics of efflux in relation to hepatic GSH concentrations (74, 75). We have observed a saturable export of GSH so that, when hepatic concentrations are raised by phenobarbital, 3-methylcholanthrene, or cobaltous chloride, the efflux rate remains nearly constant (Figure 2). Depletion of hepatic GSH below fasting is associated with a fall in efflux rate. The

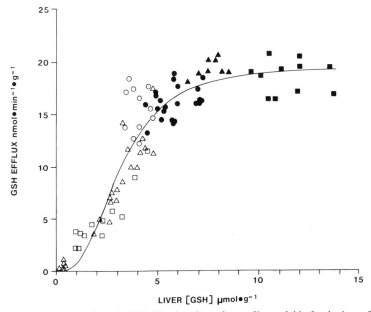

Figure 2   The kinetics of hepatic GSH efflux into the perfusate of hemoglobin-free in situ perfused rat liver. Each data point represents the mean efflux of GSH from a single liver perfused over a one-hour interval. Symbols defining conditions and treatments: fed (●), 48-hour fasted (○), diethylmaleate (△), buthionine sulfoximine (□), 3-methylcholanthrene (▲), and CoCl₂ (■). The curve represents the best (least-squares) fit obtained using the Hill model. The kinetic parameters defined by the fit are: V_{max} = 20 nmol per minute^{-1} per gram^{-1}, k_m = 3.2 μmol. per gram^{-1}, and n ≈ 3. [Reprinted with permission (75).]

apparent K_m for GSH efflux is about 3 μmol per gram. Thus, under normal circumstances (such as the fasting or fed state) GSH export is zero order and the rate is near maximum. This strongly suggests that the release of GSH into plasma is by carrier-mediated transport. Further support for a carrier-mediated process for sinusoidal GSH efflux comes from studies in isolated hepatocytes, which have demonstrated that methionine selectively inhibits GSH efflux (Figure 3), suggesting that methionine shares the same carrier (78). No other amino acids inhibit GSH efflux, and the methionine effect occurs in the presence or absence of sodium as well as in the presence or absence of the inhibition of γ-glutamyl-transferase or cystathionase. This observation requires further characterization regarding mechanism but suggests that GSH efflux is a mediated event rather than a diffusional one. Moreover, methionine maintains hepatic GSH by inhibiting efflux as well as by serving as a cysteine precursor. In GSH-repleted states, cellular GSH is conserved almost exclusively by the inhibition of efflux, whereas in depleted states GSH synthesis is stimulated by methionine; efflux is already suppressed in relation to lower

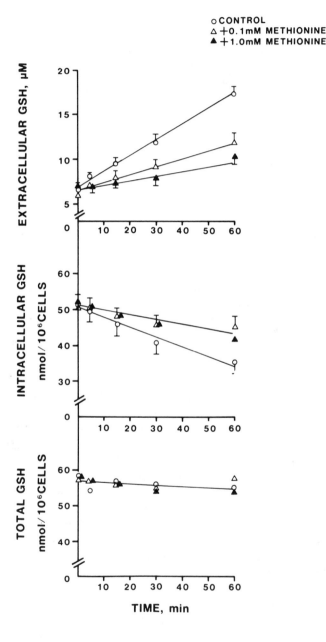

Figure 3   Inhibition of GSH efflux by methionine. Incubations (10^6 hepatocytes per ml) were carried out in the absence (0) or presence of 0.1 mM ($\triangle$) or 1.0 mM ($\blacktriangle$) methionine. At indicated times, samples were removed and cells were separated from media by centrifugation. Extracellular and intracellular GSH were measured. Data are mean ± SE for six separate cell preparations. Top: accumulation of extracellular GSH with time; center: intracellular GSH remaining with time; bottom: total GSH with time. [Reprinted with permission (79).]

cellular GSH. Interestingly, GSH is not taken up by the intact liver (79), an observation that is not surprising, considering that its entry into hepatocytes would be against a substantial electrochemical gradient.

Recently, Inoue et al have characterized GSH transport in sinusoidal-enriched membrane vesicles (80). Transport was studied in right-side out vesicles and the uptake of GSH determined. Saturable GSH transport into an osmotically active space was observed, with two kinetically distinct components of transport: one having $K_m = 0.3$ mM and the other having $K_m = 3.3$ mM. Only the latter is inhibited by glutathione conjugates. Remarkably, both transporters are probably saturated at physiological hepatic GSH, and the kinetics of the high-K_m transporter seem to correspond to those we have observed in the intact organ.

Canalicular GSH Transport

The efflux of GSH into bile, initially studied in the perfused liver, is almost exclusively GSSG. However, this work is complicated by two factors: (a) GSH rapidly autoxidizes in bile, and (b) GSH efflux into bile precipitously declines in the perfused liver model. Eberle et al recognized the autoxidation of GSH in bile (81). When inhibited, about two-thirds of the GSH in bile is in the reduced form. The concentration of GSH in bile is 1–2 mM, a lower value than that in the liver (~6 μmol per gram). However, a significant proportion of GSH in bile may be degraded by γ-glutamyl transferase in biliary epithelial brush border. When this enzyme is inhibited, the concentration of GSH in bile approaches that in liver (3). The release of GSH into bile seems to be directly proportional to hepatic GSH levels in vivo, with no evidence of saturation (73, 82). However, controversy exists regarding the relationship between GSH efflux into bile and bile flow. One group has suggested that choleresis induced by the infusion of various cholephilic substances increases GSH output (82), whereas others have found that choleresis from taurocholate (73) and dehydrocholate (83) lowers GSH concentration in bile without affecting output. The lack of saturability of GSH output into bile and possible flow dependence favor the view that GSH efflux into bile is a passive diffusional process. However, organic anions such as sulfobromophthalein (BSP) (83) inhibit GSH efflux into bile and phenobarbital induces GSH efflux into bile (73), an effect that can be dissociated from the transient choleresis from a single dose of phenobarbital. These data might support the carrier-mediated transport of GSH into bile. However, they must be interpreted cautiously; BSP may exert nonspecific toxicity and phenobarbital's effect may be indirect, e.g. may be a change in the permeability of the membrane to the passive movement of GSH. Nevertheless, sufficient data exist to warrant the hypothesis that GSH efflux into bile is carrier mediated. The recent work of Inoue et al using isolated canalicular membrane vesicles has characterized a GSH transport process (84). This carrier has a low

K_m for GSH (0.1 mM), which suggests that it is operating at capacity (saturated) even when liver GSH is severely depleted (1 mM). Therefore, it is difficult to relate the characteristics of this carrier to the concentration-dependent efflux of GSH into bile in vivo.

Canalicular GSSG Transport

GSSG is formed under basal conditions and its concentration in liver (15–20 nmol per gram) is near the equilibrium concentration relative to GSH for NADPH:GSSG reductase (85). Normally, GSSG appears in bile in concentrations 10–20-fold greater than in liver (81, 82, 85). Increasing the dead space of bile collections does not seem to affect this concentration (81), suggesting that minimal autoxidation of GSH occurs during bile transit. Thus, GSSG appears to be exported into bile in a concentrative fashion. Increased GSSG production is associated with increased GSSG appearance in bile in direct relation to the hepatic concentration (82, 85). At levels of up to 200 μM GSSG in intact liver, this process is not saturated (85). Using canalicular membrane vesicles oriented right side out, a saturable GSSG uptake process has been observed with K_m equalling 0.4 mM (86). Thus, high enough concentrations may not have been achieved in the in vivo studies to demonstrate saturability.

An active transport of GSSG from inverted red cell plasma membrane preparations has been observed (87–90). This transport process has two distinct kinetic components: a low K_m (0.1 mM) that is not inhibited by thiol reagents or glutathione-chlorodinitrobenzene conjugate (GSH–DNP), and a high K_m (7 mM) transport that is inhibited by thiol reagents and GSH–DNP. This transport is unique in having a direct ATP requirement ($K_{mATP} = 0.6$–1.2 mM). The studies using canalicular membranes identified a single kinetic component and were performed with right-side out vesicles and thus could not assess the requirement for ATP.

It seems very clear at this point that sinusoidal GSH release is a carrier-mediated process despite the fact that GSH moves down a steep electrochemical gradient. The physiological explanation for GSSG release into bile may be quite similar to that of red cell transport. However, more work is required to characterize the energetics of this process. The predominant mechanism for GSH release into bile remains the least clear. Although a transport system for GSH has been observed in canalicular-membrane vesicles, the explanation for the bulk of GSH release into bile is uncertain. Controversy exists about its relation to bile flow. The efflux of GSH into bile does not appear to be saturable in vivo. The explanation for its stimulation by phenobarbital and its inhibition by BSP but not BSP–GSH requires more work.

The Competition for Transport

An area that requires more work is the nature of the interaction of the transport of GSH, GSSG, and GSH conjugates. Evidence from the sinusoidal membrane preparation indicates that GSSG and GSH–DNP inhibit GSH transport by the high-K_m system and vice versa (80). However, the nature of the inhibition has not been established. In the canalicular preparation, GSH transport has been inhibited by probenecid, GSSG, and GSH–DNP, suggesting a common carrier (84, 86, 91). However, in vivo studies have strongly suggested that GSH and GSSG are exported into bile by distinct mechanisms (73, 82, 85, 92, 93). Thus, GSH–DNP has been shown to inhibit only GSSG export into bile (92). Interestingly, only the export of stimulated GSSG is inhibited, whereas basal GSSG export seems to be unaffected (92). Some investigators have noted the inhibition of GSSG export by BSP–GSH (82) in vivo, whereas others have not observed this phenomenon in vivo (73, 83) or in the canalicular preparation (91). Moreover, increased GSSG production and biliary release through the oxidation of substrates for flavin monooxygenase has not affected GSH release into bile (93). Thus, we are currently faced with some uncertainty about the relationship between the canalicular excretion of GSH and of GSSG. It seems likely that the GSSG transport system makes only a negligible contribution to GSH efflux into bile and that the true physiological mechanism of GSH efflux into bile must be considered unsettled. The transport of GSH conjugates into bile probably interacts with the GSSG transport system, although not all GSH conjugates interact and, even in the case of those that do, alternative transport systems may also exist. The sinusoidal efflux of GSH seems to be preferential; it requires unphysiologically high concentrations of GSSG or GSH–DNP to inhibit GSH transport in the sinusoidal vesicle preparation. Thus, considering the abundance of GSH in hepatocytes relative to GSSG or conjugates that may form, the sinusoidal membrane seems to transport GSH preferentially. In contrast, as noted above, the canalicular membrane seems to transport GSH and GSSG independently, at least according to what appears in bile. GSH conjugates may interact with the GSSG carrier and other organic anion transport mechanisms; possibly they overlap.

GSH and Metals

The relationship between GSH export and trace metals and elements is intriguing. Selenium deficiency seems to induce compensatory changes in hepatic GSH metabolism such as increased γ-glutamylcysteine synthetase and markedly increases hepatic GSH release into plasma (72). The physiological explanation for this increase is uncertain but may reflect the induction or loss of inhibition of a sinusoidal GSH transport carrier. The biliary export of GSH has been coupled with that of heavy metals (mercury, copper, zinc) found in bile predominantly in a GSH-chelated form. Young rats exhibit both low-bile GSH export and diminished metal excretion (94). Factors that increase or decrease bile excretion affect metal excretion in parallel (83). It is uncertain whether GSH in bile simply serves as a sink to chelate metals and minimize "free" metals or whether metals and GSH are actually transported by a common or independent carrier.

Mention should be made of the relationship between GSH transport and membrane potential. Since GSH is negatively charged in cells and the internal milieu is negatively charged (-30 mV for hepatocytes), perturbations of membrane potential are likely to have an influence on GSH efflux. This has been assessed so far in right–side out canalicular membrane vesicles in which an inside-positive potassium diffusion potential increases GSH and GSH–DNP transport (84, 91). Thus, one might expect that differences in hepatic lobular O_2 concentration, ATP content, or sodium-coupled transport (uptake) of bile acids and amino acids lead to variations in hepatocyte membrane potential that influence the rate of GSH efflux. Such physiological perturbations may have important influences on hepatic and extrahepatic GSH content and turnover.

It should be noted that the efflux of GSH and GSSG seems to occur as a general phenomenon with tissues other than liver. Lymphoid cells (95), fibroblasts (96), and kidney (97) export GSH, whereas GSSG export has been recently characterized in heart (98). The heart has a small, slowly turning over GSH pool, very low GSSG reductase content, and a low-K_m (~30 μM) saturable GSSG export system with very limited capacity. As a consequence, the heart's content of GSSG can change profoundly in response to oxidant stress.

The Functions of Plasma GSH

Systemic plasma contains a significant level of glutathione (10–20 μM), mainly in the GSH form, but that autoxidizes or is destroyed very quickly in vitro, leading to artifactual levels (99). The liver is the major source of plasma GSH (77). It has been suggested that plasma GSH reflects liver content (100). Since the clearance of plasma GSH is very rapid (77, 101), the plasma level reflects mainly hepatic GSH output. Although one can demonstrate a relationship between severe GSH depletion and decreased GSH efflux, many other factors may influence hepatic GSH transport and the peripheral utilization of plasma GSH, making it difficult to use plasma levels as a reliable index of liver GSH content. For example, GSH output in the fasted and fed states are not significantly different in the perfused liver (74, 75), whereas in selenium deficiency enhanced output has been observed and methionine may inhibit hepatic GSH efflux (79). Recently, increased hepatic GSH output into plasma has been described in vivo during fasting, as has the increased clearance of plasma GSH (73). Thus, to directly relate plasma to liver GSH concentration is an oversimplification.

The kidney removes a large proportion of plasma GSH, with estimates indicating that two-thirds of plasma GSH clearance is renal (76, 102, 103). Interestingly, 80% of the GSH in plasma that enters the kidney is removed.

However, only 30% is filtered by the glomeruli. Thus, there appears to be a polarity of tubular epithelium for the handling of GSH. The portion that enters the tubular lumen is hydrolyzed by γ-glutamyltransferase and cysteinylglycine dipeptidase. The γ-glutamate may be transferred to acceptor amino acids and to peptides such as cystine. The γ-glutamyl amino acids are taken up intact (97, 102, 104). In the case of γ-glutamylcystine formed from transpeptidation, after transport into tubular epithelial cells intracellular thiol-disulfide exchange liberates cysteine and γ-glutamylcysteine for GSH synthesis (104). The cysteine is a substrate for γ-glutamylcysteine synthetase, which is autoregulated by cellular GSH concentration. The γ-glutamylcysteine bypasses autoregulation and can drive the GSH concentration to supranormal levels (104). It is unclear to what extent γ-glutamyl amino acid transport occurs in tissues other than kidney, and whether this transport is localized to any particular domain of the tubular cell is uncertain.

GSH interacting with the blood pole of the renal tubular epithelia is rapidly oxidized by a thiol oxidase in the plasma membrane (76, 102). Recently, GSH has been shown to be transported by a sodium-coupled, saturable carrier-mediated process into osmotically sensitive vesicles prepared from renal baso-lateral membrane (Figure 4) (105). Whether GSSG is similarly taken up and what the tissue and membrane-domain localization of this process is remain to be determined. Since γ-glutamyltransferase is also found in the basolateral domain of kidney epithelia (106), the quantitative contribution of sodium-coupled GSH transport to renal plasma GSH clearance is uncertain. The preliminary work of L. Lash & D. Jones suggests a similar transport process in the basolateral membrane of the intestinal epithelium (Lash, Jones, personal communication). Recent work suggests that plasma GSH is taken up by lung, but it is uncertain whether this is direct transport or transport mediated by enzymatic hydrolysis initiated by γ-glutamyltransferase (106).

Thus, an hypothesis is emerging that describes the liver as a GSH source for many extrahepatic tissues (Figure 5). The liver exports GSH into plasma at near-maximum rates in both fasting and fed rats, thereby providing a constant source of GSH for plasma. Since the liver is relatively unique in its ability to convert methionine to cysteine, which is rapidly incorporated into GSH, one can hypothesize that the hepatic release of GSH is a mechanism for stabilizing and carrying cysteine (derived by hepatic synthesis) to other tissues at fairly constant rates somewhat independently of the dietary supply of cysteine. Plasma or bile GSH can thus support extrahepatic GSH levels in two ways: (*a*) GSH or GSSG can be hydrolyzed, particularly by brush border γ-glutamyltransferase in kidney and intestine, providing these tissues with cysteine that can be utilized for GSH synthesis or that returns to the liver; (*b*) plasma GSH may be directly taken up by certain epithelia. The relative contribution of these two pathways in vivo requires more study.

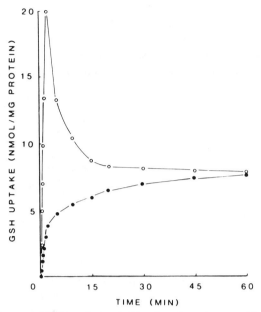

Figure 4   Time course of GSH uptake in renal basolateral membrane vesicles. Incubations of membrane vesicles with glycine-2-^{3}H GSH (1 mM) were performed with 250 mM sucrose (●) or 100 mM NaSCN and 50 mM sucrose (○). Points are mean of three studies. Sodium-dependent GSH uptake is seen, with characteristic overshoot demonstrating transient concentrative uptake energized by a sodium gradient. [Reprinted with permission (105).]

The physiological significance of the oxidation of plasma GSH by thiol oxidase remains uncertain. In addition, the functional role of extracellular GSH and GSSG in maintaining the thiol-disulfide redox status of plasma proteins and membrane proteins is intriguing.

The export of GSH by hepatocytes has been linked directly to the availability of cysteine (35, 36). In contrast to many tissues that preferentially transport cystine as opposed to cysteine, the liver seems to function in a converse fashion. Since the bulk of circulating cysteine is in the disulfide form, it has been suggested that GSH exported from liver interacts with cystine through a thiol-disulfide exchange to liberate cysteine for hepatic uptake. This process has been documented in suspensions of freshly isolated hepatocytes and provides a one-for-one exchange of exported GSH for cysteine uptake. Thus, an additional proposed function of GSH export from liver is to provide cysteine. The mixed disulfide of GSH and cysteine would undergo further exchange to GSSG. Both GSSG and the mixed disulfide would then be available for extrahepatic utilization. It remains to be established whether this process of GSH interaction with cystine is physiologically important.

INTERORGAN GSH HOMEOSTASIS

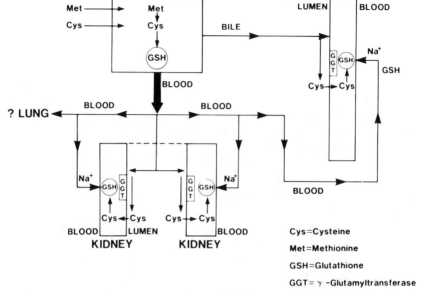

Figure 5 Model proposed to explain interorgan GSH homeostasis. The liver plays a central role, synthesizing GSH from precursor cysteine or methionine; GSH is exported into blood and bile. Luminal renal or intestinal GSH is hydrolyzed by γ-glutamyltransferase. Potential basolateral transport of GSH is shown in the kidney and intestine. The alternative contribution of γ-glutamyltransferase exposed to plasma GSH is not shown in the diagram but may be important. Also not shown is the recycling of cysteine from sites of extrahepatic breakdown of GSH back to the liver.

TURNOVER OF HEPATIC GSH

Under normal steady-state conditions, the hepatic pool of GSH is depleted at the same rate as it is repleted, so that homeostasis is maintained. This dynamic equilibrium is therefore maintained (or perturbed) by a continuous turnover (synthesis-degradation) of hepatic GSH. The degradation of hepatic GSH is achieved in several ways. As we have discussed, the foremost and major component, accounting for about 90–95% of the rate of hepatic GSH depletion, has been found to be the efflux of GSH across sinusoidal and canalicular membranes. The sinusoidal efflux comprises about 80–85% of the total efflux. Another 5–10% of the rate of hepatic GSH degradation may be accounted for by consumption by conjugation reactions, oxidation to GSSG, or enzymatic breakdown. The principal enzyme that hydrolyzes GSH is γ-glutamyltransferase. This enzyme is externally oriented and is present in relatively small concentrations in rat liver (107, 108). Therefore, the hepatic enzyme makes a negligible direct contribution to hepatocyte GSH turnover.

Heretofore, numerous studies have been conducted to estimate the rate of hepatic GSH turnover (109–120). The main aspects of these studies and the estimated half-lives ($t_{1/2}$) of turnover have been compiled in Table 1. As can be seen, a wide variety of labeled tracers (different amino acids and even GSH) have been administered through different routes and the $t_{1/2}$ of turnover has been estimated by different approaches.

In studies conducted between 1941 and 1951, incorporation of the labeled precursor amino acids into liver GSH commonly was used, along with some assumptions, to calculate the replacement or turnover rate. The wide variability among the estimates of the $t_{1/2}$ of GSH turnover in these studies may be due in part to a near-complete lack of precursor radioactivity data.

In studies conducted between 1955 and 1974, improved quantitative methods were used to study hepatic GSH turnover. In most cases, longer-term data were obtained to estimate more reliably the rate of decay of the specific activity of the GSH pool. Also, complete precursor-product data at times were analyzed by compartmental models (115). These studies generally resulted in shorter estimated half-lives than the earlier ones. This outcome was due in part to the fact that these studies: (*a*) avoided the underestimation of the turnover rate due to lack of information about the kinetics of turnover of precursor pools (especially when the tracer dose was introduced by stomach tube, resulting in slow incorporation); (*b*) provided a closer correlation of the slope of the decline of the product (GSH) pool to the fractional rate of turnover when the label of the precursor pool diminished more rapidly [more likely the case in the intravenous (iv) injections].

Higashi et al (116) extended the observation of the specific activity of the hepatic GSH pool to 72 hours following the administration of radiolabeled amino acids. However, in their study, the tracers were given orally to rats and measurements were begun 15 hours later. Although the label in plasma and liver protein pools showed slow components of turnover, no accounting was made for their possible contribution to the hepatic GSH radioactivity data. The researchers analyzed the biexponential decline of labeled GSH to define $t_{1/2}$'s of the two phases at 1.7 and 28.5 hours (Table 1). They suggested that these results might indicate the existence of two pools of hepatic GSH, a labile pool that turns over rapidly, and a more stable, slow pool that is about 50% of the total hepatic GSH. Recently, Lauterburg & Mitchell (118) have proposed that this slower component probably represents the delayed and slow (rate-limiting) recycling of the label from the protein pool. The results of the recent experiments by Meredith & Reed (119), however, suggest that the recycling of labeled cysteine (presumably reabsorbed following breakdown of circulating

Table 1 Past studies of hepatic glutathione turnover measured in vivo on the intact organ

Species	Tracer	Route of administration	Method used to estimate GSH turnover $t_{1/2}$	$t_{1/2}$ of hepatic GSH turnover (h)	Year	Reference
rat	[15N] glycine	stomach tube	incorporation of label	8	1941	109
rabbit	[15N] glycine	stomach tube	incorporation of label	18	1941	109
rat	DL-[15N] glutamate	stomach tube	incorporation of label	2–4	1942	110
rabbit	DL-[15N] glutamate	stomach tube	incorporation of label	2–4	1942	110
rat	DL-[35S] cysteine	stomach tube	incorporation of label	3[a]	1951	111
rabbit	[14C] glycine	iv[b]	precursor-product	8	1955	112
rat	[14C] glycine	ip[c]	slope of decline of sp. act.	4	1956	113
rat	[14C] glycine	iv tail	precursor-product	1.7	1957	114
mouse	L-[14C] glutamate	ip	two-compartment model for precursor-product	2.4	1974	115
rat	L-[35S] cysteine and L-[3H] cystine	oral	slope of decline of sp. act.	1.7, 28.5	1977	116
rat	L-[u-14C] cysteine or L-[u-14C] glutamate or [2-3H] glycine or L-[2-3H] glycine-glutathione	iv	slope of decline of sp. act.	6 weeks old: 1.3 / 24 weeks old: 5.8	1980	117
rat	[35S] cysteine or L-[G-3H] glutamate	iv	slope of decline of sp. act. and two-compartment model	fed 3.7 / 48-h-fasted-refed: 2.8 / 48-h-fasted: 1.6	1981	118
rat	[35S] methionine	ip prelabeled cell	slope of decline of sp. act. / slope of decline of sp. act. cytosol: mitochondria	2 / 2, 30	1982	119

[a] time of maximum incorporation
[b] Intravenously
[c] Intraperitoneally

GSH by renal γ-glutamyltranspeptidase) is the most likely cause of a slow component of the magnitude reported by Higashi et al. Thus, in tracer experiments conducted in vivo, the effect of extrahepatic events in the measurement of hepatic turnover rates cannot be discounted.

Meredith & Reed (119) also have studied the turnover of hepatic GSH in both isolated hepatocytes and in vivo. The cellular studies were done by prelabeling the hepatocytes for two hours with [^{35}S]-methionine and studying the subsequent decline of specific activity of GSH for three hours after the cells were washed and resuspended. Both cytosolic and mitochondrial turnovers were studied after rapid isolation techniques using digitonin. The cystolic pool showed a turnover $t_{1/2}$ of approximately 2.1 hours and the turnover $t_{1/2}$ of the mitochondrial pool was estimated to be approximately 30 hours. Thus, it has been found that the mitochondrial pool functions as a metabolically isolated pool from the cytosol. It appears to synthesize its own GSH with no substantial transport of GSH between the two pools. Agents such as diethyl maleate and bis-1,3-(2-chloroethyl)-1-nitrosurea have been found to deplete the cytosolic pool selectively, leaving the mitochondrial pool intact. Meredith & Reed (119) conducted their in vivo turnover studies by intraperitoneal (ip) injection of [^{35}S]-methionine into rats fasted for twelve hours that had been supplemented with 11 mmol per kilogram of unlabeled methionine four hours prior to the injection of the label. At the time of supplementation, half of the rats were also given (ip) 0.5 mmol per kilogram of AT-125, a potent inhibitor of γ-glutamyltransferase. The specific activity of hepatic GSH was measured at different times up to 13 hours. The control group (those not receiving AT-125) showed the typical biphasic decline in GSH specific activity, with the short $t_{1/2}$ (≥ 2 hours) followed by a long one (~ 36 hours). The group receiving AT-125 had a somewhat faster initial decline $t_{1/2}$ (~ 2 hours) followed by a slower one (~ 38.5 hours). Dramatic difference in the two sets of data was observed; the control group's slower phase of decline had much higher specific activity (Figure 6). This difference has been interpreted to be the result of extensive recycling of the label from the vascular pool as a result of the breakdown of labeled GSH, probably by renal γ-glutamyltransferase, and reabsorption of the labeled amino acids. The slow phase of decline of radioactivity in the AT-125 injected group has been interpreted to be the mitochondrial pool's radioactivity, since it corresponds to very low specific activities. It is worth noting that the hepatic GSH pool size of this group, unlike that of the controls, was not at steady-state throughout the turnover study; it appeared to remain constant for two to three hours; thereafter, it declined to less than half the zero-time value at eight hours and seemed to be rebounding afterward, although it remained at half the zero-time value. It is difficult to account for the effect of this non-steady state on the outcome and interpretation of the specific activity data. Moreover, the near-plateau of hepatic GSH specific activity in the control group (Figure 6) demonstrates the very large component of recycling of precursor from the extrahepatic site of breakdown to the liver. The quantitative importance of this recycling observed beyond two hours suggests to us that it cannot be viewed as negligible in the first few hours of turnover, when hepatic GSH specific activity is falling, particularly when very few data points are obtained. Thus, Meredith & Reed's data suggest to us a very large and continual reutilization of precursor through interorgan-related reactions. Therefore, we feel that in the performance of in vivo turnover studies, ignoring the reutilization of labeled precursor by determining specific activity only at early time points may markedly underestimate the true hepatic GSH turnover rates.

The turnover studies of Lauterburg et al use a technique, referred to as the acetaminophen probe, developed in their laboratory (117, 118). The basic premise of this technique is that administered small doses of acetaminophen are cleared by the liver and a small fraction is activated by cytochrome P450 to a metabolite conjugated with GSH without stimulating GSH turnover. Then the GSH conjugate is rapidly excreted into bile after conjugation with hepatic GSH. Thus, the specific activity of the GSH in the adduct reflects the specific

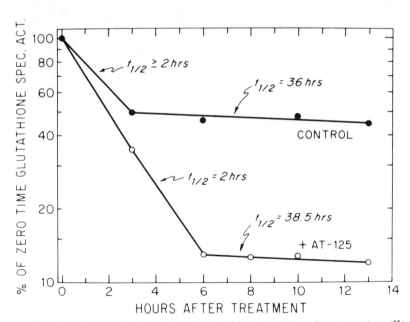

Figure 6   The effect of AT-125 on the turnover of liver glutathione. Rats were given [^{35}S] methionine four hours prior to the administration of AT-125 and unlabeled methionine. The high relative constant specific activity of hepatic GSH after three hours in controls reflects the large interorgan recycling of label. The slow turnover of GSH in rats treated with AT-125 probably represents the hepatic mitochondrial pool. [Reprinted with permission (119).]

activity of the hepatic GSH pool (provided, of course, that the latter is a single, homogeneous, well-mixed pool). This technique then allows serial and nondestructive sampling of the hepatic GSH pool for turnover studies. The researchers label the hepatic GSH pool with an intravenous injection of radioactive cysteine, glycine, glutamic acid, or GSH in different groups of rats. Then the turnover of hepatic GSH is studied for several hours by the periodic administration of the acetaminophen probe. The specific activity-time data from studies using different tracer precursors apparently all have similar features. Using the slope of the declining phase of the specific activity data (117), they have calculated a rate constant of 0.12 hours $^{-1}$, corresponding to a $t_{1/2}$ of 5.8 hours in 24-week-old rats. The rate constant is 0.52 hour^{-1}, the equivalent to a $t_{1/2}$ of 1.3 hours in six-week-old rats, indicating a much faster fractional turnover in younger animals. The acute depletion of GSH by diethylmaleate causes a doubling of the fractional turnover rate in all age groups. In subsequent studies (118), Lauterburg et al used the same technique and found that the fractional turnover of hepatic GSH in the rat is increased by fasting. It rises from 0.19 hour^{-1} ($t_{1/2}$ = 3.6 hours) in the livers of rats on regular diets to 0.25 hour^{-1} ($t_{1/2}$ = 2.8 hours) in the livers of rats refed for 4 hours after a 48-hour fast to 0.43 hour^{-1} ($t_{1/2}$ = 1.6 hours) in 48-hour-fasted livers. Using their measured hepatic GSH values of 4.7, 4.8, and 3.6 μmol per gram liver for the above three groups respectively and assuming quasi-steady state conditions for the hepatic GSH pool sizes, the corresponding turnover flux can be calculated to be 14.3, 18.3, and 25.0 nmol per minute per gram. Thus, it is apparent that precursor availability in fasting is sufficient to support a large increase in GSH synthesis. Nevertheless, hepatic GSH content falls with fasting, which might indicate a relative decrease in the availability of precursor to support GSH synthesis and maintain the fed steady state. However, other possible explanations for this occurrence need to be examined.

The phenomenon of the increased turnover of hepatic GSH caused by fasting was observed in some earlier studies (120), but no apparent mechanism was proposed for it. Lauterburg & Mitchell initially proposed that this increased turnover perhaps is due to the increased consumption of GSH because γ-glutamyl transpeptidase is elevated by fasting and by the conversion of GSH to mixed disulfides, which increase with fasting from 32 to 54% of total liver GSH (118). However, the induction of hepatic γ-glutamyltransferase would not influence hepatic GSH turnover unless either a redistribution of enzyme in hepatocytes occurs, making intracellular GSH accessible to the enzyme, or a bilio-hepatic cycle exists for the recovery of cysteine liberated in the canalicular or bile duct lumen (unlikely possibilities that require study). In addition, turnover studies have been performed after a prolonged fast, at which time maximal protein-mixed disulfide has already formed. Therefore, a dynamically expanding pool of mixed disulfide is not present to influence the turnover rate.

It is worth noting that our studies with perfused rat livers have shown that a 30% fall in hepatic GSH content, induced by a 48-hour fast, is not accompanied by a concurrent fall in the sinusoidal GSH efflux (74, 75). Thus, the fractional rate of sinusoidal efflux is higher by 40% in fasted livers compared to those of the fed. This alone can account for about 30–40% of the increased hepatic GSH turnover observed in fasting. However, recent in vivo studies by Lauterburg et al offer an explanation for the marked increase in GSH turnover with fasting (77). These researchers have observed an actual increase in sinusoidal GSH output from the fasted liver into blood that can account for nearly all of the increased turnover. Since we have not observed an increment in GSH efflux in the hemoglobin-free perfused liver, we conclude that fasting in some way perturbs GSH transport characteristics in vivo. The mechanism for this effect needs to be defined. Although increased plasma clearance of GSH accompanied by lower steady-state plasma GSH concentration has been observed with fasting, it is uncertain whether this serves as a signal to the liver for increased GSH transport by establishing a more favorable concentration gradient for hepatic GSH export. However, in the perfused liver we have not observed any effect of adding GSH (up to 40 μM) to the perfusate entering the liver on hepatic GSH efflux. Thus, more work is required to elucidate the mechanism for increased GSH efflux during fasting.

Other critical issues must be examined before a clear picture of the turnover of hepatic GSH is obtained. The most important of these issues are:

1. Homogeneity of the hepatic GSH pool. Lauterburg & Mitchell have proposed that the hepatic GSH pool behaves as a kinetically homogeneous pool (118). They have made simultaneous determinations of the specific activities of hepatic GSH and the GSH-acetaminophen adduct excreted into bile. These measurements show that at different times, following the administration of the labeled precursor, the two specific activities mentioned are identical. However, Meredith & Reed have shown (119) that there is an inhomogeneity caused by the compartmentation and apparent metabolic isolation of the mitochondrial GSH pool from the cytosolic one. Since the mitochondrial pool comprises about 10% of the total hepatic GSH pool and turns over much more slowly than the cytosolic one, it can easily be masked within the experimental error of most intact organ or cell turnover studies. Thus, special provisions are required (e.g. selective depletion of the cytosolic pool) to conduct studies in which both the cytosolic and the mitochondrial turnover of GSH are revealed.

2. Precursor-product relationships. In many of the turnover studies conducted heretofore, precursor-product relationships have not been determined. Obviously, when the tracer amino acids are introduced by stomach tube, the absorption and appearance of the label in the hepatic precursor amino acid, and thus the GSH pool, are not instantaneous. In fact, there is evidence that even an intraperitoneally injected precursor amino acid (L-[^{14}C]glutamate) itself may

turn over with a $t_{1/2}$ as slow as approximately 10 minutes in the liver (115). It is also possible that tracer amino acid injected intravenously and cleared rapidly from the circulation ($t_{1/2}\sim$ a few minutes) may not insure an impulse-like labeling of the precursor pool in the liver. Therefore, the $t_{1/2}$ of the declining phase of hepatic GSH specific activity rarely correlates with the turnover rate of hepatic GSH pool. It generally causes an overestimation of the turnover $t_{1/2}$ or an underestimation of the fractional rate of turnover. In fact, under circumstances in which the precursor pool's fractional turnover rate is rate-limiting compared to the product pool, the slope of the declining phase of the specific activity of the product pool reflects more closely the fractional turnover of the precursor pool. In addition, if the precursor pool turns over much more rapidly than the product pool, the time at which the maximum specific activity of the product pool is attained (t_{max}) is very short. It is only under the latter conditions that the decline (semi-log scale) of the product pool's specific activity equals the fractional rate of turnover of the product pool.

In many instances, when early samples have been obtained, the t_{max} of GSH has been found to be delayed as much as one hour following intravenous injection of labeled amino acids (117). This implies that the $t_{1/2}$ of the precursor pool is not shorter than twenty minutes; otherwise t_{max} would be reached sooner than in one hour's time (e.g. if the precursor amino acid pool has a $t_{1/2}$ of approximately three minutes and the GSH pools $t_{1/2}$ is approximately two hours, then a t_{max} of approximately fifteen minutes can be expected after an impulse labeling of the precursor pool). In simulations of two-compartment (precursor-product) models for GSH turnover in which the precursor pool's turnover is very rapid, t_{max} is predicted to be less than twelve minutes (118).

The possible ways in which the t_{max} is delayed are:

1. The passage and subsequent dilution of the label in synthetic intermediate pools. However, the sizes of these pools need to be sufficiently large to cause the necessary delay. This possibility is probably remote, but it needs to be ruled out unequivocally.
2. The kinetic inhomogeneity of the hepatic GSH pool (beyond the relatively small inhomogeneity caused by the mitochondrial GSH pool). This type of inhomogeneity requires that the GSH pool from which the acetaminophen-conjugate forms becomes labeled later than other pools (113). Lauterburg & Mitchell have presented data that seem to overrule these types of inhomogeneities (118).
3. Delayed precursor pool turnover due to recycling; this is the most likely possibility. As noted above, Meredith & Reed have presented data (119) showing that when the extrahepatic γ-glutamyl cycle is blocked by AT-125 in vivo, liver GSH specific activity declines somewhat faster ($t_{1/2}$ = two hours) than that of the controls ($t_{1/2} \geqslant$ two hours). In the control group, a

very slowly declining ($t_{1/2}$~ 36 hours) component with very high specific activity (half of zero-time) has been observed. This has been interpreted as the recycling of the label from the vascular amino acid pool after the labeled GSH is degraded by renal γ-glutamyltransferase. This observed response requires that no tissue other than the liver can take up any of the cysteine generated by the breakdown of circulating labeled GSH. Therefore, the liver and kidney must act virtually as a closed system. In addition, the size of the pool from which the label is recycled must be about half the size of the liver GSH pool. Thus, a major pitfall in in vivo studies of hepatic GSH turnover is the major quantitative contribution of the interorgan recycling of the labeled precursor. Most work on hepatic GSH turnover has not accounted for this component by determining the precursor pool specific activity and turnover. Substantial inaccuracy may result from such omissions.

CONCLUSION

A picture is emerging of the complex interorgan regulation of cysteine and GSH metabolism. The liver appears to play a critical role in this process by exporting nearly all the GSH produced in hepatic cytosol at a rapid rate, mainly into plasma. The liver is also unique in its ability to generate cysteine from methionine. In this way, the capacity of the liver to synthesize GSH is not limited by the availability of dietary cysteine. Thus, the liver has the ability to maintain or increase GSH export in the face of limited dietary precursors. This may serve a critical role in supplying extrahepatic tissues with GSH or its component amino acids. The interorgan cycle seems to be completed by a quantitatively important reutilization of these amino acids in the liver for GSH synthesis. Key steps in the cycle are the cystathionine pathway in the liver, carrier-mediated GSH transport (efflux) in the liver, and mechanisms for tissue utilization of plasma GSH. A great deal more needs to be learned about the regulation of these events and their interactions.

Literature Cited

1. McIntyre, T. M., Curthoys, N. P. 1980. The interorgan metabolism of glutathione. *Int. J. Biochem.* 12:545–51
2. Kaplowitz, N. 1981. The importance and regulation of hepatic glutathione. *Yale J. Biol. Med.* 54:497–502
3. Meister, A., Anderson, M. E. 1983. Glutathione. *Ann. Rev. Biochem.* 52:711–60
4. Meister, A. 1983. Selective modification of glutathione metabolism *Science* 220: 473–77
5. Orrenius, S., Ormstad, K., Thor, H., Jewell, S. A. 1983. Turnover and func-

tions of glutathione studied with isolated hepatic and renal cells. *Fed. Proc.* 42:3177–88
6. Meister, A. 1984. New developments in glutathione metabolism and their potential application in therapy. *Hepatology* 4:739–42
7. Larsson, A., Orrenius, S., Holmgren, A., Mannervik, B., eds. 1983. *Functions of Glutathione: Biochemical, Physiological, Toxicological, and Clinical Aspects.* New York: Raven. 393 pp.
8. Smith, M. T., Loveridge, N., Wills, E.

D., Chayen, J. 1979. The distribution of glutathione in the rat liver lobule. *Biochem. J.* 182:103–8

9. Cornell, J. S., Meister, A. 1976. Glutathione and γ-glutamyl cycle enzymes in crypt and villus tip cells of rat jejunal mucosa. *Proc. Natl. Acad. Sci. USA* 73:420–22

10. Brehe, J. E., Chan, A. W., Alvey, T. R., Burch, H. B. 1976. Effect of methionine sulfoximine on glutathione and amino acid levels in the nephron. *Am. J. Physiol.* 23:1536–40

11. Stadtman, T. C. 1980 Selenium-dependent enzymes. *Ann. Rev. Biochem.* 49:93–110

12. Kaplowitz, N. 1980. Physiologic significance of the glutathione S-transferases. *Am. J. Physiol.* 239:439–44

13. Reddy, C. C., Tu, C.-P. D., Burgess, J. R., Ho, C.-Y., Scholz, R. W., Massaro, E. J. 1981. Evidence for the occurrence of selenium-independent glutathione peroxidase activity in rat liver microsomes. *Biochem. Biophys. Res. Commun.* 101:970–78

14. Burk, R. F. 1983. Glutathione-dependent protection by rat liver microsomal protein against lipid peroxidation. *Biochem. Biophys. Acta* 757:21–28

15. Jones, D. P. 1982. Intracellular catalase function: Analysis of the catalytic activity by product formation in isolated liver cells. *Arch. Biochem. Biophys.* 214:806–14

16. Grundfest, C. C., Chang, J., Newcombe, D. 1982. Arcolein: A potent modulator of lung macrophage arachidonic acid metabolism. *Biochim. Biophys. Acta* 713:149–59

17. Gilbert, H. F. 1982. Biological disulfides: The third messenger? *J. Biol. Chem.* 257:12086–91

18. Snoke, J. E., Bloch, K. 1952. Formation and utilization of γ-glutamylcysteine in glutathione synthesis. *J. Biol. Chem.* 199:407–14

19. Snoke, J. E., Yanan, S., Bloch, K. 1953. Synthesis of glutathione from γ-glutamylcysteine. *J. Biol. Chem.* 201:573–86

20. Davis, J. S., Balinsky, J. B., Harrington, J. S., Shepherd, J. B. 1973. Assay, purification, properties and mechanism of action of γ-glutamylcysteine synthetase from the liver of the rat and *Xenopus laevis. Biochem. J.* 133:667–78

21. Richman, P. G., Meister, A. 1975. Regulation of γ-glutamylcysteine synthetase by non-allosteric feedback inhibition by glutathione. *J. Biol. Chem.* 250:1422–26

22. Thor, H., Moldéus, P., Hermanson, R.,

Högberg, J., Reed, D. J., Orrenius, S. 1978. Metabolic activation and hepatotoxicity: Toxicity of bromobenzene in hepatocytes isolated from phenobarbital and diethylmaleate-treated rats. *Arch. Biochem. Biophys.* 188:122–29

23. Vinã, J., Reginald, H., Krebs, H. A. 1978. Maintenance of glutathione content in isolated hepatocytes. *Biochem. J.* 170:627–30

24. Beatty, P. W., Reed, D. J. 1980. Involvement of the cystathionine pathway in the biosynthesis of glutathione by isolated rat hepatocytes. *Arch. Biochem. Biophys.* 204:80–87

25. Seelig, G. F., Meister, A. 1984. γ-Glutamylcysteine synthetase. Interactions of an essential sulfhydryl group. *J. Biol. Chem.* 259:3534–38

26. Seelig, G. F., Meister, A. 1982. Cystamine-sepharose. A probe for the active site of γ-glutamylcysteine synthetase. *J. Biol. Chem.* 257:5092–96

27. Sekura, R., Meister, A. 1977. γ-Glutamylcysteine synthetase. Further purification, "half of the sites" reactivity, subunits, and specificity. *J. Biol. Chem.* 252:2599–605

28. Griffith, O. W., Meister, A. 1979. Potent and specific inhibition of glutathione synthesis by buthionine sulfoximine (S-n-butyl homocysteine sulfoximine). *J. Biol. Chem.* 254:7558–60

29. Griffith, O. W., Anderson, M. E., Meister, A. 1979. Inhibition of glutathione biosynthesis by propionine sulfoximine (S-n-propyl homocysteine sulfoximine), a selective inhibition of γ-glutamylcysteine synthetase *J. Biol. Chem.* 254:1205–10

30. Griffith, O. W. 1982. Mechanism of action, metabolism, and toxicity of buthionine sulfoximine and its higher homologs, potent inhibitors of glutathione synthesis. *J. Biol. Chem.* 257:13704–12

31. Chung, A., Maines, M. D. 1981. Effect of selenium on glutathione metabolism. Induction of γ-glutamylcysteine synthetase and glutathione reductase in the rat liver. *Biochem. Pharmacol.* 30:3217–23

32. Hill, K. E., Burk, R. F. 1982. Effect of selenium deficiency and vitamin E deficiency on glutathione metabolism in isolated rat hepatocytes. *J. Biol. Chem.* 257:10668–72

33. Yanari, S., Snoke, J. E., Bloch, K. 1953. Energy sources in glutathione biosynthesis. *J. Biol. Chem.* 201:561–71

34. Oppenheimer, L., Wellner, V. P., Griffith, O. W., Meister, A. 1979. Glutathione synthetase. Purification from rat

kidney and mapping of the substrate binding sites. *J. Biol. Chem.* 254:5184–90

35. Reed, D. J., Orrenius, S. 1977. The role of methionine in glutathione biosynthesis by isolated hepatocytes. *Biochem. Biophys. Res. Commun.* 77:1257–64

36. Reed, D. J., Brodie, A. E., Meredith, M. J. 1983. Cellular heterogeneity in the status and functions of cysteine and glutathione. See Ref. 7, pp. 39–49

37. Reed, D. J., Beatty, P. W. 1980. Biosynthesis and regulation of glutathione: toxicological implications. In *Review of Biochemical Toxicology*, ed. E. Hodgson, J. R. Bend, R. N. Philpot, pp. 213–41. New York: Elsevier North Holland

38. Beatty, P., Reed, D. J. 1981. Influence of cysteine upon the glutathione states of isolated rat hepatocytes. *Biochem. Pharmacol.* 30:1227–30

39. Hill, K. E., Burk, R. F. 1983. Effect of methionine and cysteine in glutathione synthesis by selenium-deficient isolated rat hepatocytes. See Ref. 7, pp. 117–24

40. Williamson, J. M., Meister, A. 1981. Stimulation of hepatic glutathione formation by administration of L-2-oxo thiazolidine-4-carboxylate, a 5-oxo-L-prolinase substrate. *Proc. Natl. Acad. Sci. USA* 78:936–39

41. Williamson, J. M., Meister, A. 1982. New substrates of 5-oxo-L-prolinase. *J. Biol. Chem.* 257:12039–42

42. Williamson, J. M., Boettcher, B., Meister, A. 1982. Intracellular cysteine delivery system that protects against toxicity by promoting glutathione synthesis. *Proc. Natl. Acad. Sci. USA* 79:6246–49

43. Puri, R. N., Meister, A. 1983. Transport of glutathione, as γ-glutamylcysteinylglycyl ester, into liver and kidney. *Proc. Natl. Acad. Sci. USA* 80:5258–60

44. Wendel, A., Jaeschke, H., Glager, M. 1982. Drug-induced lipid peroxidation in mice. 2. Protection against paracetamol-induced liver necrosis by intravenous liposomally-entrapped glutathione. *Biochem. Pharmacol.* 31:3601–5

45. Wendel, A., Jaeschke, H. 1982. Drug-induced lipid peroxidation in mice. 3. Glutathione content of liver, kidney and spleen after intravenous administration of free and liposomally-entrapped glutathione. *Biochem. Pharmacol.* 31: 3607–11

46. Wendel, A., Jaeschke, H. 1983. Differential hepatoprotection against paracetamol-induced liver necrosis in mice by

free and liposomally-entrapped glutathione. See Ref. 7, pp. 139–47

47. Moldéus, P., Ormstad, K., Reed, D. J. 1981. Turnover of cellular glutathione in isolated rat kidney cells. *Eur. J. Biochem.* 116:13–16

48. Brodie, A. E., Potter, J., Reed, D. J. 1982. Unique characteristics of rat spleen lymphocyte, L1210 lymphoma and HeLa cell in glutathione biosynthesis from sulfur-containing amino acids. *Eur. J. Biochem.* 123:159–64

49. Brodie, A. E., Potter, J., Ellis, W. W., Evenson, M. D., Reed, D. J. 1981. Glutathione biosynthesis in murine L5178 Y lymphoma cells. *Arch. Biochem. Biophys.* 210:437–44

50. Binkley, F., du Vigneaud, V. 1942. The formation of cysteine from homocysteine and serine by liver tissue of rats. *J. Biol. Chem.* 144:507

51. Binkley, F. 1951. Synthesis of cystathionine by preparations from rat liver. *J. Biol. Chem.* 191:531–34

52. Abeles, R., Walsh, C. 1973. Acetylenic enzyme in activators. Inactivation of cystathionase, *in vitro* and *in vivo* by propargylglycine. *J. Am. Chem. Soc.* 95:6124

53. Finkelstein, J. D., Mudd, S. H. 1967. Transsulfuration in mammals. The methionine sparing effect of cystine. *J. Biol. Chem.* 242:873–80

54. Finkelstein, J. D., Kyle, W. E., Harris, B. J. 1971. Methionine metabolism in mammals: Regulation of homocysteine methyl-transferase in rat tissue. *Arch. Biochem. Biophys.* 146:84–92

55. Chance, B., Sies, H., Boveris, A. 1979. Hydroperoxide metabolism in mammalian organs. *Physiol. Rev.* 59:527–605

56. Babson, J. R., Reed, D. J. 1978. Inactivation of glutathione reductase by 2-chloroethyl nitrosourea-derived isocyanates. *Biochem. Biophys. Res. Commun.* 83:754–62

57. Wallace, K. B. 1983. Hepatic redox homeostasis following acute adriamycin intoxication in rats. *Biochem. Pharmacol.* 32:2577–82

58. Babson, J. R., Abell, N. S., Reed, D. J. 1981. Protective role of the glutathione redox cycle against adriamycin-mediated toxicity in isolated hepatocytes. *Biochem. Pharmacol.* 30:2299–304

59. Meredith, M. J., Reed, D. J. 1983. Depletion *in vitro* of mitochondrial glutathione in rat hepatocytes and enhancement of lipid peroxidation by adriamycin and 1,3-Bis (2-chloroethyl)-1-nitrosourea (BCNU). *Biochem. Pharmacol.* 32:1383–88

60. Bellomo, G., Jewell, S. A., Thor, H.,

Orrenius, S. 1982. Regulation of intracellular calcium compartmentation: Studies with isolated hepatocytes and t-butyl hydroperoxide. *Proc. Natl. Acad. Sci. USA* 79:6842–46

61. Bellomo, G., Mirabelli, F., Richelmi, P., Orrenius, S. 1983. Critical role of sulfhydryl group(s) in ATP-dependent Ca^{2+} sequestration by the plasma membrane fraction from rat liver. *FEBS Lett.* 163:136–39

62. Jewell, S. A., Bellomo, G., Thor, H., Orrenius, S., Smith, M. T. 1982. Changes in the surface structure of isolated hepatocytes during drug metabolism are caused by alterations in intracellular thiol and Ca^{2+} homeostasis. *Science* 217:1257–59

63. Jones, D. P., Thor, H., Smith, M. T., Jewell, S. A., Orrenius, S. 1983. Inhibition of ATP-dependent microsomal Ca^{2+} sequestration during oxidative stress and its prevention by glutathione. *J. Biol. Chem.* 258:6390–93

64. Mannervik, B., Axelsson, K. 1980. Role of cytoplasmic thioltransferase in cellular regulation by thiol-disulfide interchange. *Biochem. J.* 190:125–30

65. Axelsson, K., Eriksson, S., Mannervik, B. 1978. Purification and characterization of cytoplasmic thioltransferase (glutathione:disulfide oxidoreductase) from rat liver. *Biochemistry* 17:2978–84

66. Brigelius, R., Muckel, C., Akerboom, T. P. M., Sies, H. 1983. Identification and quantitation of glutathione in hepatic protein mixed disulfides and its relationship to glutathione disulfide. *Biochem. Pharmacol.* 32:2529–34

67. Brigelius, R., Lenzen, R., Sies, H. 1982. Increase in hepatic mixed disulfide and glutathione disulfide levels elicited by paraquat. *Biochem. Pharmacol.* 31: 1637–41

68. Thurman, R. G., Lurquin, M., Evans, R., Kauffman, F. C. 1977. Role of reducing equivalents generated in mitochondria in hepatic mixed-function oxidations. In *Microsomes and Drug Oxidations,* ed. V. Ullrich, p. 315. Oxford: Pergamon

69. Reinke, L. A., Kauffman, F. C., Belinsky, S. A., Thurman, R. G. 1980. Interactions between ethanol metabolism and mixed-function oxidation in perfused rat liver: Inhibition of p-nitroanisole 0-demethylation. *J. Pharm. Exp. Ther.* 213:70–78

70. Bartoli, G. M., Sies, H. 1978. Reduced and oxidized glutathione efflux from liver. *FEBS Lett.* 86:89–91

71. Sies, H., Bartoli, G. M., Burk, R. F.,

Waydhas, C. 1978. Glutathione efflux from perfused rat liver after phenobarbital treatment, during drug oxidations, and in selenium deficiency. *Eur. J. Biochem.* 89:113–18

72. Hill, K. E., Burk, R. F. 1982. Effect of selenium deficiency and vitamin E deficiency on glutathion metabolism in isolated rat hepatocytes. *J. Biol. Chem.* 257:10668–72

73. Kaplowitz, N., Eberle, D. E., Petrini, J., Touloukian, J., Corvasce, M. C., Kuhlenkamp, F. 1983. Factors influencing the efflux of hepatic glutathione into bile in rats. *J. Pharm. Exp. Ther.* 224:141–47

74. Ookhtens, M., Hobdy, K., Kaplowitz, N. 1983. Sinusoidal efflux of hepatic glutathione: Evidence for a carrier-mediated process. *Hepatology* 3:325

75. Ookhtens, M., Hobdy, K., Corvasce, M. C., Aw, T. Y., Kaplowitz, N. 1985. Sinusoidal efflux of glutathione in the perfused rat liver: evidence for a carrier-mediated process. *J. Clin. Invest.* In press.

76. Anderson, M. E., Bridges, R. J., Meister, A. 1980. *Biochem. Biophys. Res. Commun.* 96:848–53

77. Lauterburg, B. H., Adams, J. D., Mitchell, J. R. 1984. Hepatic glutathione homeostasis in the rat: Efflux accounts for glutathione turnover. *Hepatology* 4:586–90

78. Aw, T. Y., Ookhtens, M., Kaplowitz, N. 1984. Inhibition of glutathione efflux from isolated rat hepatocytes by methionine. *J. Biol. Chem.* 259:9355–58

79. Hahn, R., Wendel, A., Flohe, L. 1978. The fate of extracellular glutathione in the rat. *Biochim. Biophys. Acta* 539:324–37

80. Inoue, M., Kinne, R., Tran, T., Arias, I. M. 1984. Glutathione transport across hepatocyte plasma membranes: Analysis using isolated rat-liver sinusoidal vesicles. *Eur. J. Biochem.* 138:491–95

81. Eberle, D., Clarke, R., Kaplowitz, N. 1981. Rapid oxidation *in vitro* of endogenous and exogenous glutathione in bile of rats. *J. Biol. Chem.* 256:2115–17

82. Lauterburg, B. H., Smith, C. V., Hughes, H., Mitchell, J. R. 1984. Biliary excretion of glutathione and glutathione disulfide in the rat. Regulation and response to oxidative stress. *J. Clin. Invest.* 73:124–33

83. Ballatori, N., Clarkson, T. W. 1983. Biliary transport of glutathione and methylmercury. *Am. J. Physiol.* 244: 6435–41

84. Inoue, M., Kinne, R., Tran, T., Arias, I.

M. 1983. The mechanism of biliary secretion of reduced glutathione: Analysis of transport process in isolated rat-liver canalicular membrane vesicles. *Eur. J. Biochem.* 134:467–71

85. Akerboom, T. P. M., Bilzer, M., Sies, H. 1982. The relationship of biliary glutathione disulfide efflux and intracellular glutathione disulfide content in perfused rat liver. *J. Biol. Chem.* 257:4248–52

86. Akerboom, T., Inoue, M., Sies, H., Kinne, K., Arias, I. M. 1984. Biliary transport of glutatione disulfide studies with isolated rat liver canalicular-membrane vesicles. *Eur. J. Biochem.* 141:211–15

87. Kondo, T., Dale, G. L., Beutler, E. 1980. Glutathione transport by inside-out vesicles from human erythrocytes. *Proc. Natl. Acad. Sci. USA* 77:6359–62

88. Board, P. G. Transport of glutathione S-conjugate from human erythrocytes. *FEBS Lett.* 124:163–65

89. Kondo, T., Dale, G. L., Beutler, E. 1981. Studies on glutathione transport utilizing inside-out vesicles prepared from human erythrocytes. *Biochim. Biophys. Acta* 645:132–36

90. Kondo, T., Murao, M., Taniguchi, N. 1982. Glutathione S-conjugate transport using inside-out vesicles from human erythrocytes. *Eur. J. Biochem.* 125:551–54

91. Inoue, M., Akerboom, T. P. M., Sies, H., Kinne, R., Thao, T., Arias, I. M. 1984. Biliary transport of glutathione S-conjugate by rat liver canalicular membrane vesicles. *J. Biol. Chem.* 259:4998–5002

92. Akerboom, T. P. M., Bilzer, M., Sies, H. 1982. Competition between transport of glutathione disulfide (GSSG) and glutathione S-conjugates from perfused rat liver into bile. *FEBS Lett.* 140:73–76

93. Krieter, P. A., Ziegler, D. M., Hill, K. E., Burk, R. F. 1984. *Mol. Pharmacol.* 26:122–27

94. Ballatori, N., Clarkson, T. W. 1982. Developmental changes in the biliary excretion of methylmercury and glutathione. *Science* 216:61–62

95. Griffith, O. W., Novogrodsky, A., Meister, A. 1979. Translocation of glutathione from lymphoid cells that have markedly different γ-glutamyl-transpeptidase activities. *Proc. Natl. Acad. Sci. USA* 76:2249–52

96. Bannai, S., Tsukeda, H. 1979. The export of glutathione from human diploid cells in culture. *J. Biol. Chem.* 254:3444–50

97. Griffith, O. W., Meister, A. 1979. Translocation of intracellular glutathione to membrane-bound γ-glutamyltranspeptidase as a discrete step in the γ-glutamylcycle: Glutathionuria after inhibition of transpeptidase. *Proc. Natl. Acad. Sci. USA* 76:268–72

98. Ishikawa, T., Sies, H. 1984. Cardiac transport of glutathione disulfide and S-conjugate studies with isolated perfused rat heart during hydroperoxide metabolism. *J. Biol. Chem.* 259:3838–43

99. Anderson, M. E., Meister, A. 1980. Dynamic state of glutathione in blood plasma. *J. Biol. Chem.* 255:9530–33

100. Adams, J. D., Lauterburg, B. H., Mitchell, J. R. 1983. Plasma glutathione and glutathione disulfide in the rat: Regulation and response to oxidative stress. *J. Pharmacol. Exp. Ther.* 227:749–54

101. Wendel, A., Akryt, P. 1980. The level and half-life of glutathione in human plasma. *FEBS Lett.* 120:209–11

102. Jones, D. P., Moldéus, P., Stead, H., Ormstad, K., Jornvall, H., Orrenius, S. 1979. Metabolism of glutathione and glutathione conjugate by isolated kidney cells. *J. Biol. Chem.* 254:2787–92

103. Ormstad, K., Lastbom, T., Orrenius, S. 1980. Translocation of amino acids and glutathione studied with the perfused kidney and isolated renal cells. *FEBS Lett.* 112:55–59

104. Anderson, M. E., Meister, A. 1983. Transport and direct utilization of γ-glutamylcysteine for glutathione biosynthesis. *Proc. Natl. Acad. Sci.* 80:707–11

105. Lash, L. H., Jones, D. P. 1983. Transport of glutathione by renal basal-lateral membrane vesicles. *Biochem. Biophys. Res. Commun.* 112:55–60

106. Dawson, J. R., Vahakangas, K., Jernstrom, B., Moldéus, P. 1984. Glutathione conjugation by isolated lung cells and the isolated, perfused lung. Effect of extracellular glutathione. *Eur. J. Biochem.* 138:439–43

107. Horuichi, S., Inoue, M., Morino, Y. 1978. Glutamyl transpeptidase: Sidedness of its active site on renal brush-border membrane. *Eur. J. Biochem.* 87:429–37

108. Tsao, B., Curthoys, N. P. 1980. The absolute asymmetry of orientation of γ-glutamyltranspeptidase and aminopeptidase on the external surface of the rat renal brush border membrane. *J. Biol. Chem.* 255:7708–11

109. Waelsch, H., Rittenberg, D. 1941. Glutathione. 1. The metabolism of glutathione studied with isotopic glycine. *J. Biol. Chem.* 139:761–74

110. Waelsch, H., Rittenberg, D. 1942. Glu-

tathione. 2. The metabolism of glutathione studied with isotopic ammonia and glutamic acid. *J. Biol. Chem.* 144:53–58

111. Anderson, E. L., Mosher, W. A. 1951. Incorporation of S^{35} from DL-cystine into glutathione and protein in the rat. *J. Biol. Chem.* 188:717–22

112. Henriques, O. B., Henriques, S. B., Neuberger, A. 1955. Quantitative aspects of glycine metabolism in the rabbit. *Biochem. J.* 60:409–24

113. Douglas, G. W., Mortensen, R. A. 1956. The rate of metabolism of brain and liver glutathione in the rat studied with C^{14}-glycine. *J. Biol. Chem.* 222:581–85

114. Henriques, S. B., Henriques, O. B., Mandelbaum, F. R. 1957. Incorporation of glycine into glutathione and fibrinogen of rats under adrenaline treatment. *Biochem. J.* 66:222–27

115. Sekura, R., Meister, A. 1974. Glutathione turnover in the kidney; considerations relating to the γ-glutamyl cycle and the transport of amino acids. *Proc.* *Natl. Acad. Sci. USA* 71:2969–72

116. Higashi, T., Tateishi, N., Naruse, A., Sakamoto, Y. 1977. A novel physiological role of liver glutathione as a reservoir of L-cysteine. *J. Biochem.* 82:117–24

117. Lauterburg, B. H., Vaishnav, Y., Stillwell, W. G., Mitchell, J. R. 1980. The effect of age and glutathione depletion on hepatic glutathione turnover *in vivo* determined by acetaminophen probe analysis. *J. Pharmacol. Exp. Ther.* 213:54–58

118. Lauterburg, B. H., Mitchell, J. R. 1981. Regulation of hepatic glutathione turnover in rats *in vivo* and evidence for kinetic homogeneity of the hepatic glutathione pool. *J. Clin. Inv.* 67:1415–24

119. Meredith, M. J., Reed, D. J. 1982. Status of the mitochondrial pool of glutathione in the isolated hepatocyte. *J. Biol. Chem.* 257:3747–53

120. Tateishi, N., Higashi, T., Shinya, S., Naruse, A., Sakamoto, Y. 1974. Studies of the regulation of glutathione in rat liver. *J. Biochem.* 75:93–103

Ann. Rev. Pharmacol. Toxicol. 1985. 25:745–67

THE MECHANISTIC TOXICOLOGY OF FORMALDEHYDE AND ITS IMPLICATIONS FOR QUANTITATIVE RISK ESTIMATION

Thomas B. Starr and James E. Gibson

Chemical Industry Institute of Toxicology, P. O. Box 12137, Research Triangle Park, North Carolina 27709

INTRODUCTION

In 1980 the Chemical Industry Institute of Toxicology (CIIT) issued preliminary results from a chronic toxicity and carcinogenicity study of inhaled formaldehyde in rats and mice. These results, which pertained to 18 months of formaldehyde exposure, indicated that formaldehyde is carcinogenic in rats (1). A final report published in 1983 (2) confirmed the preliminary findings. Specifically, inhalation exposure to formaldehyde concentrations of 5.6 or 14.3 ppm, six hours per day, five days per week, for 24 months caused squamous cell carcinomas in the nasal cavities of approximately 50% of the rats in the high-exposure group and 1% of the rats in the low-exposure group (5.6 ppm). Mice also proved susceptible to formaldehyde's carcinogenicity, but tumors were observed only at the highest exposure concentration (14.3 ppm) and with an incidence of 1%.

Because formaldehyde is a major building-block chemical used in a multitude of industrial processes and consumer products, these findings have provoked widespread concern about the possible effects of formaldehyde exposure on human health (3, 4). In 1983, for example, the estimated US production of

745

0362-1642/85/415-0745$02.00

formaldehyde as a 37% solution was 5.7 billion pounds (5). Formaldehyde's major end uses include adhesives (60%) and plastics (15%), with the main derivatives being urea-formaldehyde resins, phenol-formaldehyde resins, polyacetal, and butanediol. Formaldehyde-derived resins are used primarily in manufacturing particleboard, plywood, insulation, appliances, and automobiles, and residual formaldehyde vapors are known to off-gas from some of these products. The potential for both occupational and environmental exposures to this chemical is thus considerable.

In order to assess adequately the cancer risk from low-level formaldehyde exposures, critical issues of mechanism must be considered in addition to the basic finding that formaldehyde is carcinogenic in rats and mice. Two important mechanistic factors are the physiologic responses to sensory irritation produced by formaldehyde exposure and the effects of such exposure on the mucociliary clearance apparatus of the nasal cavity. These factors control the local rate of delivery of airborne formaldehyde to underlying target tissues. Also critical are the cellular proliferation response to formaldehyde-induced cytotoxicity and the disposition of delivered formaldehyde within target cells via metabolism and macromolecular binding. All four of these mechanistic aspects of formaldehyde toxicology are directly relevant to both the low-dose and interspecies risk extrapolation problems because they determine the form of the functional relationship between the concentration of formaldehyde in ambient air and the amount of formaldehyde that ultimately reaches and interacts with the genetic material of target cells. When such mechanistic information is incorporated properly into quantitative dose-response models, more accurate and scientifically defensible estimates of low-dose cancer risk should result.

Following a brief summary of the major findings of the CIIT chronic inhalation bioassay, this review focuses on results from selected mechanistic studies that appear to be directly applicable to the problem of assessing carcinogenic risk from exposure to gaseous formaldehyde. The concluding section illustrates how the data regarding biological defense mechanisms can be incorporated into the quantitative risk assessment process.

A SUMMARY OF THE CIIT CHRONIC FORMALDEHYDE INHALATION BIOASSAY FINDINGS

The Chemical Industry Institute of Toxicology commissioned the Battelle Memorial Institute, Columbus Laboratory, in Columbus, Ohio, to undertake a 24-month toxicity and carcinogenicity study of inhaled formaldehyde in male and female B6C3F1 mice and Fischer-344 rats. One hundred-twenty animals of each sex and species began inhalation exposure to formaldehyde at target concentrations of 0, 2, 6, and 15 ppm six hours per day, five days per week.

The mean formaldehyde concentrations in the test chambers over the 24-month exposure period were: 2.0 ± 0.6, 5.6 ± 1.2, and 14.3 ± 2.8 ppm. Interim necropsies of randomly selected animals were completed at 6, 12, 18, and 24 months after exposure commenced. Some female mice and male and female rats were followed for an additional three-to-six months after completion of the planned 24-month exposures.

The major toxicological finding from this study was the induction of squamous cell carcinomas in the nasal cavities of 103 rats in the 14.3-ppm group, two rats in the 5.6-ppm group, and two male mice in the 14.3-ppm group (Table 1). Two nasal carcinomas, one carcinosarcoma, one undifferentiated carcinoma, and one undifferentiated sarcoma were also observed in rats in the 14.3-ppm exposure group. In addition, an exposure-related induction of squamous metaplasia was found in the respiratory epithelium of the anterior nasal passages of rats in all formaldehyde-exposed groups (2). In mice, however, the irritant-induced effects were essentially limited to the group exposed to 15 ppm and no effects were observed at lower concentrations. The animals from the low and intermediate exposure groups that were allowed to recover after 24 months of formaldehyde exposure showed an apparent regression of metaplasia in all affected sites of the nasal cavity (2).

A number of polypoid adenomas were also observed in the nasal cavities of exposed and control rats (Table 1). Although the incidence of these benign lesions in the exposed animals was not significantly elevated over that in controls in an adjusted pairwise analysis, an adjusted trend test indicated that formaldehyde exposure increases the frequency of this lesion (2). However, the observed incidence of adenomas did not increase as a function of airborne formaldehyde concentration. Adenomas were found in 3.4, 2.6, and 2.2% of the animals exposed to 2.0, 5.6, and 14.3 ppm formaldehyde respectively. This compares to an incidence of 0.4% (one case) in control animals. An independent review of these findings (Pathology Working Group, unpublished observations) yielded a consensus among participating pathologists regarding the benign nature of the observed polypoid adenomas. Moreover, these reviewers concluded that "there was no morphological evidence that these lesions progressed to squamous cell carcinomas." The squamous cell carcinomas and polypoid adenomas were thought to be readily separable lesions that should not be combined solely for statistical and risk estimation purposes.

PHYSIOLOGIC RESPONSES TO SENSORY IRRITATION

The respiratory tract membranes contain a wide variety of sensory nerve endings that can respond to chemical and/or physical stimuli. One group of these nerve endings, located in the nasal mucosa, is associated with the maxillary and ophthalmic divisions of the trigeminal nerve. Stimulation of

Table 1 Summary of neoplastic lesions in the nasal cavity of Fischer-344 rats exposed to formaldehyde gas[a]

Exposure group	0 ppm		2.0 ppm		5.6 ppm		14.3 ppm	
Sex	M	F	M	F	M	F	M	F
Diagnosis								
Number of nasal cavities evaluated	118	114	118	118	119	116	117	115
Squamous cell carcinoma	0	0	0	0	1	1	51	52
Nasal carcinoma	0	0	0	0	0	0	1[b]	1
Undifferentiated carcinoma/sarcoma	0	0	0	0	0	0	2[b]	0
Carcinosarcoma	0	0	0	0	0	0	1	0
Polypoid adenoma	1	0	4	4	6	0	4	1
Osteochondroma	1	0	0	0	0	0	0	0

[a] Adapted from (16).
[b] One rat in this group also had a squamous cell carcinoma.

these nerve endings by airborne chemical irritants such as formaldehyde evokes a painful burning sensation, a desire to withdraw from the contaminated atmosphere, and a decrease in the rate of respiration (6). Collectively, these responses to sensory irritation have been termed the common chemical sense, separating them from more specialized chemical senses such as olfaction and gustation (7). All substances that excite the common chemical sense are potentially noxious and lung damaging, and the reflex responses to sensory irritation comprise an important respiratory tract defense mechanism that serves to minimize the inhalation of noxious agents and warn of their presence through the perception of pain (6, 8, 9).

Decreases in respiratory rate during inhalation exposure can be used to quantitate the sensory irritation potential of chemicals (6). For formaldehyde, this property is well established in laboratory animals (10–12). Experimental results indicate that mice are far more sensitive to formaldehyde exposure than rats. For example, the formaldehyde concentration required to elicit a 50% decrease in respiratory rate (RD_{50}) in naive animals is 3.13 ppm for Swiss-Webster mice (10) and 4.9 ppm for B6C3F1 mice (12) but is 31.7 ppm for Fischer-344 rats (12). Chang and colleagues have shown that associated changes in tidal volume do not compensate entirely for the decreased respiratory rate in both rats and mice (12). As a result, minute volumes (the product of respiratory rate and tidal volume) for naive animals of these species decrease during exposure to sufficiently high formaldehyde concentrations.

Significant differences between rats and mice in the magnitude of their response to sensory irritation have also been observed following pretreatment with four six-hour-per-day exposures to 2, 6, and 15 ppm formaldehyde (12). While respiration was depressed in a concentration-dependent manner in both species, the amplitude of the response was always greater in mice. This can be interpreted as a shift in the concentration-response curves for mice relative to those for rats to lower concentration ranges, with RD_{50} values ranging from 2–6 ppm in the mice compared to 23–32 ppm in rats. Minute volumes at the RD_{50} values are also decreased by approximately 50%. However, it is notable that rats pretreated to 15 ppm did have some degree of tidal volume compensation, as evidenced by a decrease of only 37.5% in minute volume following pretreatment to 15 ppm formaldehyde (12). These results suggest that the B6C3F1 mouse respiratory tract may be better protected against chronic exposure to high airborne formaldehyde concentrations than is the respiratory tract of the Fischer-344 rat.

Testing this hypothesis of differential protective capability in these two species has been possible because the formaldehyde toxicity induced by chronic inhalation exposure appears to be limited to the nasal cavity (1, 2). The localization of toxicity is due in large part to the high-water solubility of formaldehyde and the fact that rodents are obligatory nose breathers. Assuming that all inhaled formaldehyde is deposited in the nasal cavity, a theoretical deposition rate on the mucosal surface can be obtained by dividing the amount of formaldehyde inhaled per unit time by the nasal cavity surface area. For a ten-minute exposure to 15 ppm formaldehyde, this deposition rate for rats is twofold larger than that for mice (13, 14). Although the disparity between these species in the calculated deposition rate is consistent with the parallel disparity in nasal tumor incidence following chronic exposure (2), additional studies were required to determine whether or not this difference in delivered dose is maintained during chronic exposure conditions.

The persistence of this effect has been evaluated in rats and mice pretreated to 6 and 15 ppm formaldehyde six hours per day for four days (15). On the fifth day, minute volume was measured during a six-hour exposure to 6 and 15 ppm. During exposure to 15 ppm formaldehyde, the time-weighted average deposition rate for mice continued to be approximately half that for rats, while at 6 ppm both species appeared to receive similar delivered doses.

The species difference predicted at 15 ppm was also assessed by comparative autoradiography, histopathology, and cell turnover studies (15). Whole-body autoradiographic studies of rats and mice exposed to [^{14}C]formaldehyde revealed that radioactivity was heavily deposited in the anterior nasal cavity, with much less deposition in olfactory regions. This anterior-posterior gradient is consistent with the high-water solubility and chemical reactivity of formaldehyde. In addition, whole-body autoradiography qualitatively confirmed the difference in delivered dose in rats compared with mice identically exposed to 15 ppm formaldehyde (15). Histopathologic examination of the nasal cavities of rats and mice after one and five days of exposure to 15 ppm formaldehyde demonstrated that rats had more severe lesions than mice. Cell turnover studies of nasal respiratory epithelium have also revealed much higher cell proliferation in rats compared with that observed in mice (15). When comparing the responses of different species to the same airborne concentration of formaldehyde, it is therefore essential to adjust for the interspecies differences in pulmonary ventilation and nasal cavity surface area.

The effects of exposure on pulmonary ventilation must also be considered when comparing the responses of a single species to different airborne concentrations of a sensory irritant. This is particularly important when estimating the shape of the dose-response curve for risk assessment purposes. For example, rats exposed to 15 ppm formaldehyde for six hours inhale only twice the amount of formaldehyde per unit time as do rats similarly exposed to 6 ppm (16). This mildly nonlinear relationship between the inhalation rate for rats and the concentration of formaldehyde in ambient air is due to the larger depression of minute volume induced in rats by exposure to 15 ppm formaldehyde relative to that induced by exposure to 6 ppm (16). Thus, the precipitously steep rise in squamous cell carcinoma incidence from 1% among rats chronically exposed to

5.6 ppm formaldehyde to nearly 50% among rats similarly exposed to 14.3 ppm (Table 1) actually appears even steeper, i.e. more severely nonlinear, when the amount of formaldehyde inhaled per unit time, rather than ambient air concentration, is used as the measure of exposure.

THE EFFECTS OF EXPOSURE ON MUCOCILIARY FUNCTION

Many factors are expected to influence the distribution of lesions induced by irritant materials in the nasal passages (17). These include species-specific anatomy and physiology, nasal cavity airflow dynamics, mucociliary flow rate and direction, as well as exposure level and tissue-specific susceptibility. The amount of airborne formaldehyde that reaches the surface of the nasal epithelium is clearly dependent on its ambient air concentration and the rate at which inspired air passes through the nose. Furthermore, airflow patterns within the nose modulate the amount of gas reaching specific areas, while the nature and movement of the surface secretions are likely to affect absorption of formaldehyde and its subsequent fate.

As noted previously, chronic exposure to high concentrations of formaldehyde induced squamous cell carcinomas in the nasal passages of rats, and exposure was also weakly associated with an increased incidence of polypoid adenomas (2). Because detailed mapping of the locations of these neoplasms within the nasal passages was not attempted during the original chronic inhalation study (1, 2), the histologic sections of this bioassay were reexamined to determine the locations and apparent site of origin of the observed tumors (17a).

The majority of the squamous cell carcinomas occurred in two main locations. The first region is lateral to the nasoturbinate, extending from the ventral margin of this turbinate to the lateral wall just dorsal to the maxilloturbinate, at a level measured along the long axis of the nose just posterior to the incisor tooth. The second region is comprised of the ventral and middle nasal septum approximately at the level of the incisive papilla. In contrast, polypoid adenomas occurred just posterior to the vestibule, on the naso- and maxilloturbinates and the adjacent lateral wall. These three regions of the nose are lined with respiratory epithelium, which is protected by the nasal mucociliary apparatus (18). Because of the potential importance of the mucociliary apparatus in modulating the delivery of formaldehyde to target cells in the nasal passages, studies of the effects of formaldehyde on the mucociliary apparatus have also been undertaken. The current state of knowledge about this system and the results of some initial studies are summarized below.

The nasal mucociliary apparatus of the rat provides a continuous layer of watery mucus that covers the respiratory epithelium (19, 20). Formaldehyde would be expected to dissolve readily in this layer and thus be removed from the inspired airstream. It has been demonstrated that almost 100% of inspired gaseous formaldehyde is removed in the upper airways in dogs (21), but the retention efficiency of the rat nose for formaldehyde has yet to be established directly. The approximate thickness of the mucus (20), its flow patterns (20, 22), and its flow rate (20) have been determined in the rat nose. The layer of nasal mucus flows continuously over the surface of the nasal mucosa and is cleared eventually toward the nasopharynx (20, 22), where it is swallowed with any entrapped or dissolved materials. Recent studies have demonstrated that the nasal and tracheal mucociliary clearance mechanisms in the guinea pig can respond to formaldehyde exposure with an increased rate of clearance (23). If mucus clearance does result in the removal of formaldehyde from the nose, then increased clearance rates in response to exposure would be expected to increase the efficiency of this potentially protective mechanism.

However, exposure to sufficiently high formaldehyde concentrations is also known to have inhibitory effects upon mucociliary function. The mucociliary apparatus consists of several main components that have been reviewed in detail elsewhere (18). Each component may be influenced adversely by exposure to formaldehyde. Cilia, which are microscopic, hair-like processes of the epithelial cells, drive the mucus over the surface by their coordinated beating. Formaldehyde has been found to be ciliastatic in several species (19), and it causes slowing of mucus flow in the anterior nasal passages of humans during inhalation exposure (24). Studies with a frog palate preparation indicate that formaldehyde induces slowing of mucus flow before it inhibits ciliary activity, probably as a result of biochemical reactions with constituents of the mucus blanket (25). Nasal mucus consists principally of water (~95%), mucus glycoproteins (0.5–1%), free proteins and salts, and other materials in much smaller amounts (25a). Formaldehyde reacts readily with proteins (25b) and with polysaccharides at room temperature (25c). Similar reactions may be responsible for the slowing of mucus flow in humans.

At high concentrations, formaldehyde has been found to induce both mucostasis and ciliastasis in rats following in vivo inhalation exposure (19). Studies with rats using a rapid postmortem assessment of nasal mucociliary function following inhalation exposures to formaldehyde revealed a clear concentration-response relationship for the inhibition of nasal mucociliary function, with 0.5 ppm being a no-observed-effect concentration (26). This concentration-response relationship closely parallels that for formaldehyde-induced lesions observed in the chronic inhalation study (2). It therefore has been postulated that localized disruption of mucociliary function accounts in part for the subsequent appearance of epithelial lesions in the affected locations (16).

The areas of inhibition of mucociliary function and acute cytotoxicity in the nasal epithelium (20) include the regions in which squamous cell carcinomas occurred. However, acute changes also appeared consistently on the medial aspect of the maxilloturbinate at 6 and 15 ppm (20, 26). The latter region was rarely a site of squamous cell carcinoma development, indicating possible regional differences in the susceptibility of the rat nasal epithelium to the carcinogenic effects of formaldehyde.

In the chronic inhalation study (2), the polypoid adenomas occurred in the anterior nasal passages, a region lined by sparsely ciliated respiratory epithelium with generally very slow mucus flow rates (20). Mucus in this region is derived from mucus streams that originate in more dorsal or more posterior regions of the nose. Mucus flow results in the translocation of materials deposited on the surface and may thus influence the final site at which the nasal epithelium is exposed to inspired materials. Formaldehyde absorbed more posteriorly might be carried forward toward the point at which the polypoid adenomas occurred. Macklin has proposed that mucus flow patterns in the lower respiratory tract account for the distribution of air-pollutant-induced cancer in the trachea and bronchi of humans (27), and similar reasoning may be applicable to the distribution of formaldehyde-induced lesions in the rat nasal cavity.

Mucus flow may thus play an important role in determining the distribution and frequency of neoplasia in the nasal passages of rats exposed to formaldehyde by modulating delivery of this chemical to the nasal epithelium in specific regions of the nose. However, anatomic or physiologic characteristics of the rat nose may also render this species either hyper- or hyposensitive to formaldehyde-induced nasal cancer. Thus, comparative studies in rats and humans of nasal air flow, mucus flow, other physiologic characteristics, and their effects on the delivered dose will provide additional information valuable for risk-assessment purposes.

THE CELL PROLIFERATION RESPONSE TO TISSUE INJURY

Cell proliferation is a critical factor in chemical carcinogenesis. Numerous studies with a broad range of chemicals have demonstrated that cell replication is required for the initiation and promotion of chemical carcinogenesis. When promutagenic DNA adducts are present during de novo DNA synthesis, the likelihood of inserting a wrong nucleotide greatly increases, and such events, if unrepaired before replication, result in permanent mutations. Cell proliferation is also responsible for expanding the clonal population of initiated cells to a cancerous mass. Furthermore, in the case of formaldehyde-induced neoplasia, cell replication is thought to be important in the initial binding of the chemical to DNA, since formaldehyde is known to bind only to single-stranded DNA (28, 29). The number of single-stranded sites is much greater in replicating

DNA than in non-replicating DNA. Thus, the likelihood of formaldehyde binding to DNA, errant DNA synthesis, and expansion of initiated cell populations to neoplasia are all related to cell proliferation.

Morphologic changes in the nasal respiratory mucosa of Fischer-344 rats have been observed following a single six-hour exposure to 15 ppm formaldehyde gas. These changes consisted of acute degeneration and swelling, with the formation of dense bodies and vacuoles within epithelial cells (15, 30). Three to five similar exposures (one per day) produced ulceration of the respiratory epithelium in a high proportion of the animals. After nine days of exposure, restorative hyperplasia and metaplasia were observed. Rats exposed to 6 ppm exhibited milder degenerative changes but prominent hyperplasia of the respiratory epithelium. In contrast, no morphologic changes were evident by light microscopy in rats exposed to 0.5 or 2 ppm formaldehyde.

In order to better understand these cytotoxic and restorative responses to different concentrations and durations of formaldehyde exposure, a series of investigations was undertaken to identify and elucidate the effects of formaldehyde exposure on cell replication in the respiratory epithelium of rodent nasal passages. Initial studies (31) have demonstrated that marked increases in cell proliferation were present in the second level of the nasal passages, the same region that had the acute pathology and that developed most of the squamous cell carcinomas in the CIIT bioassay (2). Rats exposed to 6 or 15 ppm formaldehyde for three six-hour-per-day exposures had ten to twenty fold increases in [^{3}H]thymidine labeling. No increase over controls was detected in rats exposed to 0.5 or 2 ppm nor in mice exposed to 0.5, 2, or 6 ppm formaldehyde. Mice exposed to 15 ppm formaldehyde showed a tenfold increase in de novo DNA synthesis. Subsequent studies have shown that administration of [^{3}H]thymidine at 18 rather than two hours after the last exposure is a more sensitive method for evaluating the effects of formaldehyde on cell proliferation (31). Rats exposed to 15 ppm formaldehyde for a single six-hour period already showed a greater than tenfold increase in cell proliferation relative to controls. By five days of exposure, this increase exceeded twentyfold. Similar increases have been demonstrated in mice.

It is important to know how much of this response is due to the duration of exposure and how much is due to formaldehyde concentration, since markedly different results were evident in the histopathology of rats exposed for six months to 15 ppm formaldehyde, six hours per day, five days per week, (450 ppm-hours per week) (1, 2, 32) compared to that of rats exposed to 3 ppm, 22 hours per day, seven days per week (462 ppm-hours per week) (33). Animals on the latter exposure regimen exhibited much less toxicity. To evaluate this discrepancy, rats and mice were exposed to 12 ppm formaldehyde for three hours per day, 6 ppm for six hours per day, or 3 ppm for twelve hours per day (31). Exposures were conducted for three and ten days, with [^{3}H]thymidine

Table 2   Effects of formaldehyde concentration versus cumulative exposure on cell turnover in Fischer-344 rats[a]

| | Percent labeled cells[b] | | |
| | Level 1 | Level 2 | |
Exposure	3 days	3 days	10 days
Control	3.00 ± 1.56	0.54 ± 0.03	0.26 ± 0.02
3 ppm × 12 hours	16.99 ± 1.50	1.73 ± 0.63	0.49 ± 0.19
6 ppm × 6 hours	15.46 ± 10.01	3.07 ± 1.09	0.53 ± 0.20
12 ppm × 3 hours	16.49 ± 2.02	9.00 ± 0.88	1.73 ± 0.65

[a] Adapted from (31).
[b] Mean ± standard error.

administered 18 hours after the last exposure. Sections from the most anterior and the second level of respiratory mucosa were prepared for autoradiography and the labeling index was determined. Table 2 shows that the most anterior level of the respiratory epithelium (level 1) had a similar fivefold increase in cell proliferation in all three concentration-time groups. This is in marked contrast to the adjacent, more posterior section (level 2), where a distinct relationship between concentration and cell turnover is evident. In this section, the marked increase in proliferation is also a somewhat transient event, since its magnitude decreased with time.

These concentration-time data are consistent with the recent data on the effects of formaldehyde on the mucociliary clearance apparatus (20, 26). The lack of a concentration effect in the anterior section reflects the fact that this region has minimal mucociliary clearance. In contrast, the adjacent more posterior section normally has a continuous flow of mucus over its surface. As the concentration of formaldehyde increases, larger areas of the mucus blanket become immobilized, effectively removing this protective mechanism (26). The efficacy of mucociliary clearance is thus likely to be greatest at low concentrations of formaldehyde.

In ongoing experiments following a protocol similar to that employed by Swenberg et al (31) except that the pulse of [^{3}H]thymidine was administered 18 hours after the last exposure, slight increases in cell proliferation were evident in rats exposed to 0.5 and 2 ppm formaldehyde in one six-hour exposure, but not after three or nine such exposures (33a). In contrast, much higher labeling indices were observed in 6-ppm exposed rats after one and three days. These data show a distinct nonlinear dependence of the labeling indices on formaldehyde concentration. A threefold increase in formaldehyde concentration from 2 to 6 ppm resulted in an eightfold increase in cell proliferation after one day of exposure and nearly a 25-fold increase after three days of exposure.

These data are consistent with nonlinear data on the covalent binding of formaldehyde to respiratory mucosal DNA (34) and carcinogenesis (16).

THE BIOCHEMICAL DISPOSITION OF INHALED FORMALDEHYDE

Formaldehyde is known to react with DNA in cultured mammalian cells in vitro, forming DNA-protein cross-links (35, 36), and this reaction may be a critical factor in the transformational (37), mutagenic (38), and carcinogenic (2) actions of formaldehyde. It is therefore important to determine whether inhaled formaldehyde can react with DNA in vivo and, if this reaction occurs, to quantify the amount of formaldehyde that reacts with DNA in target tissues as a function of its airborne concentration.

Evidence that inhaled formaldehyde reacts with respiratory mucosal DNA has been obtained by Casanova-Schmitz & Heck (39). These researchers observed that exposure of Fischer-344 rats to formaldehyde concentrations equal to or greater than 6 ppm resulted in a statistically significant decrease in the amount of DNA that could be extracted from proteins in homogenates of the respiratory mucosa. The extraction of the solubilized tissue homogenates was carried out using a strongly denaturing aqueous-immiscible organic solvent mixture. When the tissue was extracted in this manner, the DNA separated into two fractions (39). The aqueous (AQ) phase contained DNA that by all spectrophotometric and chromatographic criteria appeared to be pure, double-stranded DNA. An interfacial (IF) layer also contained DNA, but this DNA appeared to be cross-linked to proteins, since the DNA could not be released without digestion of the interface using proteinase K. Importantly, the quantity of IF DNA was dependent on the airborne formaldehyde concentration to which the rats had been exposed, increasing as the concentration increased. The investigators therefore concluded that formaldehyde does react with respiratory mucosal DNA following in vivo inhalation exposures, and that this reaction might well play a critical role in the development of nasal cancer during chronic formaldehyde inhalation exposures.

The inability to extract DNA from proteins does not, however, constitute proof of the formation of DNA-protein cross-links. Additional evidence is required to ensure the validity of this conclusion. To obtain such evidence, and to determine, if possible, the amount of formaldehyde that becomes covalently bound, additional experiments have been performed to investigate the mechanisms of labeling of respiratory mucosal DNA following inhalation exposure of rats to [^{14}C]- and [^{3}H]formaldehyde (34). The labeling of macromolecules (DNA, RNA, and protein) in the respiratory mucosa has been studied in rats that were pre-exposed for six hours to unlabeled formaldehyde on the day preceding exposure to the labeled compound. Pre-exposure was undertaken to stimulate cell turnover in the respiratory mucosa, a physiological response to toxic injury that appears to play an important role in the induction of nasal cancer by formaldehyde (30). The pre-exposure to unlabeled formaldehyde and the exposure to [^{14}C]- and [^{3}H]formaldehyde were both carried out at the same airborne concentrations. The specific activities of IF and AQ DNA obtained from the respiratory mucosa following in vivo exposure to 0.3, 2, 6, 10, and 15 ppm of [^{14}C]- or [^{3}H]formaldehyde were determined. The [^{14}C]-specific activity of the total DNA rose to a peak at 6 ppm and then decreased at higher concentrations. In addition, the ^{14}C-specific activity of the AQ DNA fraction was found to be significantly greater than that of the IF DNA fraction at 6 ppm, but no significant difference between the specific activities of IF and AQ DNA was found at other concentrations.

Based on several arguments advanced by Casanova-Schmitz et al (34), it was concluded that the major route of DNA labeling in the respiratory mucosa is metabolic incorporation. The maximum in the specific activity of the DNA at 6 ppm therefore implies that the metabolic incorporation of [^{14}C]formaldehyde into respiratory mucosal DNA is maximal at this concentration. This result is consistent with the observation that the incorporation of [^{3}H]thymidine into respiratory mucosal DNA after exposure to formaldehyde at 6 ppm is higher than after exposure to 15 ppm (31). The smaller amount of metabolic incorporation of ^{14}C into DNA that occurs at 10 and 15 ppm relative to that at 6 ppm is probably due to the cytotoxic effects of formaldehyde at these high concentrations.

The finding that the ^{14}C-specific activity of respiratory mucosal AQ DNA is significantly higher than that of IF DNA at 6 ppm is an extremely important one. This result implies that the AQ DNA incorporates a significantly larger amount of ^{14}C than the IF DNA at 6 ppm. In addition, this result implies that the two DNA fractions must differ structurally, for otherwise they could not have been separated by solvent extraction into portions with differing specific activities. However, no difference between the specific activities of AQ and IF DNA has been found at either 0.3 or 2 ppm, demonstrating that the structural difference noted above is not an inherent property of respiratory mucosal DNA but must have been induced in the DNA by exposure to formaldehyde at 6 ppm. A plausible explanation for this structural difference is that formaldehyde exposure at 6 ppm results in the formation of DNA-protein cross-links in the IF DNA fraction.

It may at first seem contradictory that the specific activity of IF DNA is lower than that of AQ DNA at 6 ppm since the IF DNA is presumed to contain covalently bound formaldehyde. However, this result is consistent with DNA-protein cross-linking because the major route of DNA labeling is metabolic incorporation. The formation of cross-links decreases the rate of incorporation of [^{14}C]formaldehyde metabolites into DNA by preventing the dissociation of proteins from DNA necessary for de novo DNA synthesis to occur. An inhibition of DNA synthesis by formaldehyde has been shown to occur in yeast under conditions in which DNA-protein cross-links were induced (40).

The most direct evidence for the formation of covalently bound formaldehyde in DNA and proteins in the respiratory mucosa has been provided by determinations of the $^3H/^{14}C$ ratios in respiratory mucosal macromolecules following exposure of rats to [^{14}C]- and [^3H]formaldehyde (34). The $^3H/^{14}C$ ratios in the IF DNA and proteins increased with increasing formaldehyde concentrations, but no increases in the $^3H/^{14}C$ ratios of the AQ DNA and RNA have been observed. As discussed in detail by Casanova-Schmitz et al (34), increased $^3H/^{14}C$ ratios in macromolecules with increasing formaldehyde concentrations provide evidence of the covalent binding of formaldehyde. Thus, only the IF DNA and proteins contain measurable quantities of covalently bound formaldehyde.

The differences between the $^3H/^{14}C$ ratios in IF and AQ DNA are statistically significant at formaldehyde concentrations equal to or greater than 2 ppm. These differences therefore indicate that at these concentrations the mechanisms of labeling of IF and AQ DNA are significantly different: AQ DNA is labeled primarily or exclusively by metabolic incorporation, whereas IF DNA is labeled by both metabolic incorporation and covalent binding. Strong support for the conclusion that the difference between the $^3H/^{14}C$ ratios in the two DNA fractions is due to DNA-protein cross-linking is provided by the strong correlation between the difference in the $^3H/^{14}C$ ratios in IF and AQ DNA fractions and the percent interfacial DNA that was obtained in each experiment (34). It should be noted that, although a significant difference between the $^3H/^{14}C$ ratios of IF and AQ DNA has been detected at 2 ppm and above, the percentage of interfacial DNA is significantly increased relative to the level in control rats only at concentrations equal to or greater than 6 ppm (39). This indicates that the isotope ratio method is a more sensitive technique for the detection of DNA-protein cross-links than is the measurement of DNA extractability.

Casanova-Schmitz et al (34) also have shown that the $^3H/^{14}C$ ratio of a macromolecule following exposure to formaldehyde labeled with both isotopes is quantitatively related to the fraction of the total ^{14}C that is due to covalent binding, f_b, as follows:

$$f_b = \frac{(^3H/^{14}C)_o - (^3H/^{14}C)_m}{(^3H/^{14}C)_b - (^3H/^{14}C)_m} .$$

The terms in this equation include: $(^3H/^{14}C)_o$ = the observed $^3H/^{14}C$ ratio of macromolecule; $(^3H/^{14}C)_m$ = $^3H/^{14}C$ ratio characteristic of metabolic incorporation of ^3H and ^{14}C (derived from [^3H]- and [^{14}C]formaldehyde) into the macromolecule; $(^3H/^{14}C)_b$ = $^3H/^{14}C$ ratio characteristic of covalent binding of

Table 3 Absolute and relative concentrations of covalently bound [^{14}C]formaldehyde in respiratory mucosal DNA of Fischer-344 rats[a]

Airborne formaldehyde concentration (ppm)	Absolute concentration of covalently bound [^{14}C]formaldehyde (nmol/mg DNA)	Relative concentration of covalently bound [^{14}C]formaldehyde[b] (nmol/mg DNA/ppm)
0.3	0.002 ± 0.003[c]	0.007
2.0	0.022 ± 0.006	0.011
6.0	0.233 ± 0.023	0.039
10.0	0.406 ± 0.099	0.041
15.0	0.631 ± 0.064	0.042

[a] Adapted from (41).

[b] Absolute amount of covalent binding in nmol/mg DNA divided by airborne formaldehyde concentration.

[c] Mean $\pm$ standard error as determined by Casanova-Schmitz et al (34).

[^{3}H]- and [^{14}C]formaldehyde to the macromolecule under the reaction conditions. The values of these isotope ratios can be determined by methods described in Casanova-Schmitz et al (34). Hence, the fraction of covalently bound [^{14}C]formaldehyde can be calculated. Knowing the total ^{14}C concentration in the macromolecule permits determination of the concentration of covalently bound formaldehyde. The results of calculating the concentrations of covalently bound formaldehyde in respiratory mucosal DNA at 0.3, 2, 6, 10, and 15 ppm of inhaled formaldehyde are summarized in Table 3.

These data show that the concentration-response profile for covalent binding of [^{14}C]formaldehyde to DNA is sigmoidal, increasing gradually between 0.3 and 2 ppm, steeply between 2 and 6 ppm, and less steeply at the higher concentrations. The observed concentration of covalently bound formaldehyde at 2 ppm is significantly lower than the value predicted by linear extrapolation from the concentration measured at 6 ppm to the origin. In contrast to the results obtained with respiratory mucosal DNA, covalent binding of [^{14}C]formaldehyde to respiratory mucosal proteins depends in an apparently linear manner on the formaldehyde concentration throughout the concentration range (34).

The explanation for nonlinearity in the binding of formaldehyde to respiratory mucosal DNA is presently unknown. However, at least two mechanisms may account for the nonlinear behavior. First, the physiological and biochemical defense mechanisms such as mucociliary clearance, metabolism, and DNA repair could be inactivated or become less efficient with increasing formaldehyde concentrations, resulting in a disproportionate increase in the concentration of DNA-protein cross-links. Second, the marked increase in cell turnover caused by formaldehyde exposure at 6 ppm relative to that at 2 ppm

(31) could increase the availability of sites in DNA for reaction with formaldehyde. As noted above, we know that formaldehyde binds to single-stranded regions of DNA but not to double-stranded regions (28, 29).

Also important is the fact that the relative disposition of formaldehyde in respiratory mucosal tissues is concentration dependent. Casanova-Schmitz et al (34) have shown that the percentage of total ^{14}C in respiratory mucosal DNA and proteins due to covalent binding increases with concentration. If the disposition of formaldehyde in the respiratory mucosa were governed by purely linear kinetics, then the percentage of the total ^{14}C due to covalent binding would be constant, i.e. independent of the airborne concentration. Nonlinear kinetics must therefore be involved.

THE IMPLICATIONS FOR QUANTITATIVE RISK ESTIMATION

Nearly four years have elapsed since the first report that the chronic inhalation of gaseous formaldehyde induces nasal cancer in Fischer-344 rats (1). During that time, research into the mechanisms of formaldehyde toxicity has yielded a great deal of additional information directly relevant to concerns about the potential adverse effects of formaldehyde exposure on human health. As reviewed above, this research has focused on the biological defenses that protect organisms from toxicity at low-level formaldehyde exposures. It has also elucidated the mechanisms by which high-level formaldehyde exposures impair these defenses and thereby enhance nonlinearly the probability of irreversible toxic effects.

Nevertheless, low-dose risk estimates that result from the typical approach to quantitative risk assessment, namely, a linearized multistage model analysis of bioassay tumor incidence versus administered dose, do not utilize this additional mechanistic information. Indeed, such risk estimates would be no different had none of the research described above been undertaken. The process of quantitative risk estimation can be improved in this regard by utilizing the available mechanistic data to construct a measure of exposure that is more realistic and biologically meaningful than administered dose, as is summarized below.

The key issue in the use of mechanistic data in quantitative risk estimation concerns the form of the relationship between two distinct measures of exposure denoted by the terms *administered dose* and *delivered dose* (41). The administered dose is an external measure of exposure directly controlled in laboratory studies of toxicity. For inhalation studies, it refers to the concentration of a test chemical in the inhalation chamber air. In contrast, the delivered dose is an internal measure of exposure referring to the quantity or concentration of the biologially active form of a test chemical present in specific target tissues. This latter measure is presumed to be the direct causative variable in mechanistic descriptions of the carcinogenic process at the cellular and molecular levels (42).

The relationship between administered and delivered doses reflects the entire spectrum of biological responses to exposure, ranging from physiologic responses of the whole organism to intracellular biochemical responses in target tissues. Thus, the administered dose actually provides no more than an indirect, surrogate measure of the delivered dose, and the relationship between these two measures of exposure need not be a simple linear one. This is especially important because low-dose risk extrapolations based on the assumption of linearity are known to yield risk estimates that are either excessively conservative (too high) or anticonservative (too low) when the true administered-delivered dose relationship is nonlinear (42).

In the case of formaldehyde, the extensive mechanistically oriented studies reviewed above have identified four biological responses that appear to be important determinants of the formaldehyde dose delivered to target tissues in the rodent nasal cavity. The first of these is the minute volume depression in response to sensory irritation. In Fischer-344 rats and B6C3F1 mice it is an important factor only at formaldehyde concentrations above 6 ppm. Still, the fact that it is induced at these concentrations has three important consequences. First, the amount of formaldehyde entering the rat or mouse nasal cavity is not linearly proportional to formaldehyde concentrations in inspired air greater than 6 ppm. Second, the precipitously steep rise in squamous cell carcinoma incidence from about 1% among rats chronically exposed to 5.6 ppm formaldehyde to nearly 50% among rats similarly exposed to 14.3 ppm (Table 1) is actually steeper, i.e. more severely nonlinear, when the amount of formaldehyde inhaled per unit time is used as the measure of exposure rather than the ambient air formaldehyde concentration. Third, the marked disparity in tumor response between rats and mice identically exposed to 14.3 ppm formaldehyde (Table 1) can be reconciled by measuring exposure in terms of the rate, adjusted for the interspecies difference in nasal cavity surface area, at which formaldehyde is actually deposited in the nasal cavity.

Two other factors that must be considered are the inhibition of mucociliary clearance and the stimulation of cell proliferation that are both induced by exposure to high but not low formaldehyde concentrations. Both tend to increase disproportionately the dose delivered to target tissues at high formaldehyde concentrations, thus counterbalancing and probably overriding any reduction in delivered dose associated with minute volume depression. The inhibition of mucociliary clearance contributes to this effect by eliminating a pathway for the removal of formaldehyde from the nasal cavity before it penetrates to underlying epithelial cells. Increased cell proliferation enhances the likelihood of irreversible genotoxic events once formaldehyde reaches the target cells by increasing the number of single-stranded DNA sites at which formaldehyde may covalently bind and by decreasing the amount of time available for the repair of such lesions before they become fixed during cell replication.

Finally, studies of the disposition of formaldehyde in nasal cavity tissues have provided the first direct quantitative measurements of the amount of formaldehyde delivered to target-tissue DNA. These studies are of critical importance for several reasons. First, they have demonstrated that the delivered dose/administered dose relationship is distinctly nonlinear, as would be expected from considering the observed spectrum of effects of inhaled formaldehyde on minute volume, mucociliary clearance, and cell proliferation. Second, the studies also provide evidence that in target tissues, metabolic incorporation, a process by which delivered formaldehyde is detoxified, is less efficient at high airborne formaldehyde concentrations than it is at low concentrations. Thus, another removal pathway that protects against formaldehyde toxicity at low airborne concentrations appears to be compromised at formaldehyde concentrations greater than 2 ppm. Third, the data for the covalent binding of formaldehyde to target-tissue DNA are in a form that makes it possible to reanalyze the nasal tumor results from the chronic bioassay with the delivered formaldehyde dose rather than the airborne formaldehyde concentration as the measure of exposure. Such a reanalysis has been completed recently (41), and a brief summary of the principal results is provided below.

Tumor incidence rates nearly identical to those used by Cohn (43) were employed since his analysis of the chronic bioassay results figured prominently in the US Consumer Product Safety Commission's decision to ban the sale of urea-formaldehyde foam insulation in the United States (3). Concentrations of formaldehyde covalently bound to respiratory mucosal DNA corresponding to the airborne formaldehyde concentrations employed in the chronic bioassay were derived from those reported by Casanova-Schmitz et al (34). Four commonly used quantal response models, namely, the multistage, Weibull, logit, and probit, were used for low-dose extrapolation. Model parameters were estimated using standard maximum likelihood (ML) techniques. Both ML estimates of risk and their upper 95% confidence bounds were calculated for three airborne formaldehyde concentrations, 0.1, 0.5, and 1.0 ppm. For these concentrations, it was assumed that the delivered dose/administered dose relationship was linear and given by a straight line passing from the origin through the concentration of covalently bound formaldehyde observed at 2 ppm (34). As noted by Starr & Buck (41), this low-dose linearity assumption probably overestimates the amount of covalent binding that actually occurs at these airborne concentrations.

The maximum likelihood (ML) estimates of risk and their upper 95% confidence bounds are shown in Tables 4 and 5 respectively. It is readily

Table 4 Maximum likelihood estimates of risk based on administered dose (A) and delivered dose (D) at selected ambient air formaldehyde concentrations[a]

Airborne concentration (ppm)	Dose measure	Maximum likelihood risk estimates			
		Probit	Logit	Weibull	Multistage
0.1	A	< 1.00(−26)[b]	3.92(−11)	2.20(−10)	2.51(−7)
	D	< 1.00(−26)	7.40(−13)	6.20(−12)	4.70(−9)
0.5	A	5.16(−17)	9.85(− 8)	2.75(− 7)	3.14(−5)
	D	< 1.00(−26)	9.76(−10)	4.27(− 9)	5.88(−7)
1.0	A	2.65(−11)	2.87(− 6)	5.94(− 6)	2.51(−4)
	D	4.00(−20)	2.15(− 8)	7.13(− 8)	4.70(−6)

[a] Reprinted with permission from (41).
[b] Values in parentheses are powers of ten.

Table 5 Upper 95% confidence bounds on risk based on administered dose (A) and delivered dose (D) at selected ambient air formaldehyde concentrations[a]

Airborne concentration (ppm)	Dose measure	Upper 95% confidence bounds on risk			
		Probit	Logit	Weibull	Multistage
0.1	A	< 1.00(−26)[b]	2.84(−10)	1.57(− 9)	1.56(−4)
	D	< 1.00(−26)	6.19(−12)	5.12(−11)	6.19(−5)
0.5	A	7.69(−16)	5.13(− 7)	1.41(− 6)	8.09(−4)
	D	< 1.00(−26)	6.31(− 9)	2.73(− 8)	3.10(−4)
1.0	A	2.58(−10)	1.24(− 5)	2.54(− 5)	1.80(−3)
	D	7.09(−19)	1.22(− 7)	3.98(− 7)	6.24(−4)

[a]Reprinted with permission from (41).
[b]Values in parentheses are powers of ten.

apparent that the estimates obtained with delivered dose are unilaterally lower than the corresponding estimates obtained with administered dose. For ML estimates, the ratios of risk based on administered dose to risk based on delivered dose range from 35 (Weibull: 0.1 ppm) to more than nine orders of magnitude (probit: 0.5 ppm). The multistage ML risk estimates based on delivered dose are uniformly lower by a factor of 53. For upper 95% confidence bounds, corresponding risk reduction factors range from 2.5 (multistage: 0.1 ppm) to more than ten orders of magnitude (probit: 0.5 ppm).

These results demonstrate that the incorporation of delivered dose into low-dose extrapolation procedures leads to a unilateral reduction in estimates of cancer risk associated with exposure to low airborne formaldehyde concentrations. Because the use of this exposure measure allows much of the information already obtained from mechanistic studies of formaldehyde toxicity to enter the risk assessment process in a meaningful and relevant manner, the resulting risk estimates reflect what is known of the underlying biological reality more faithfully than do previous estimates based solely on findings from the chronic bioassay. Additional research is of course required to further refine and elaborate the delivered dose concept, especially for humans. Comparative studies of the physiologic and biochemical responses to formaldehyde exposure are especially important. In addition, predictive mechanistic models that explicitly incorporate the influences of these phenomena on the covalent binding of formaldehyde to target tissue DNA and on the promotional stages of the carcinogenic process must be constructed and validated.

Literature Cited

1. Swenberg, J. A., Kerns, W. D., Mitchell, R. E., Gralla, E. J., Pavkov, K. L. 1980. Induction of squamous cell carcinomas of the rat nasal cavity by inhalation exposure to formaldehyde vapor. *Cancer Res.* 40:3398–402

2. Kerns, W. D., Pavkov, K. L., Donofrio, D. J., Gralla, E. J., Swenberg, J. A. 1983. Carcinogenicity of formaldehyde in rats and mice after long-term inhalation exposure. *Cancer Res.* 43:4382–92

3. US Consumer Product Safety Commission. 1982. Part IV: Consumer Product Safety Commission ban of urea formaldehyde foam insulation, withdrawal of proposed labeling rule, and denial of petition to issue a standard. *Fed. Reg.* 47:14366–419

4. US Environmental Protection Agency. 1984. Formaldehyde: Determination of significant risk. *Fed. Reg.* 49(101): 21870–98

5. Greek, B. F. 1984. US farming pickup helps natural gas-based petrochemicals. *Chem. Eng. News* 62(5):10–14

6. Alarie, Y. 1973. Sensory irritation by airborne chemicals. *CRC Crit. Rev. Toxicol.* 2:299–363

7. Keele, C. A. 1962. The common chemical sense and its receptors. *Arch. Int. Pharmacodyn. Ther.* 139:547–57

8. Widdicombe, J. G. 1977. Defense mechanisms of the respiratory tract and lungs. In *Respiratory Physiology II*, ed. J. G. Widdicombe, 14:291–315. Baltimore: Univ. Park

9. Comroe, J. H. Jr. 1974. *Physiology of Respiration*, pp. 220–28. Chicago: Year Book. 2nd ed.

10. Kane, L. E., Alarie, Y. 1977. Sensory irritation of formaldehyde and acrolein during single and repeated exposures in mice. *Am. Ind. Hyg. Assoc. J.* 38:509–22

11. Kulle, T. J., Cooper, G. P. 1975. Effects of formaldehyde and ozone on the trigeminal nasal sensory system. *Arch. Environ. Health* 30:237–43

12. Chang, J. C. F., Steinhagen, W. H., Barrow, C. S. 1981. Effects of single or repeated formaldehyde exposure on mi-

nute volume of B6C3F1 mice and F-344
rats. *Toxicol. Appl. Pharmacol.* 61:451–
59
13. Gross, E. A., Swenberg, J. A., Fields,
S., Popp, J. A. 1982. Comparative morphometry of the nasal cavity in rats and
mice. *J. Anat.* 135:83–88
14. Barrow, C. S., Steinhagen, W. H.,
Chang, J. C. F. 1983. Formaldehyde sensory irritation. In *Formaldehyde Toxicity,* ed. J. E. Gibson, pp. 16–25. New
York: Hemisphere
15. Chang, J. C. F., Gross, E. A., Swenberg, J. A., Barrow, C. S. 1983. Nasal
cavity deposition, histopathology, and
cell proliferation after single or repeated
formaldehyde exposures in B6C3F1 mice
and F-344 rats. *Toxicol. Appl. Pharmacol.* 68:161–76
16. Swenberg, J. A., Barrow, C. S.,
Boreiko, C. J., Heck, H. d'A., Levine,
R. J., et al. 1983. Non-linear biological
responses to formaldehyde and their implications for carcinogenic risk assessment. *Carcinogenesis* 4:945–52
17. Walker, D. 1983. Histopathology of the
nasal cavity in laboratory animals exposed to cigarette smoke and other irritants. In *Nasal Tumors in Animals and
Man,* ed. G. Reznik, S. F. Stinson,
3:115–35. New York: CRC
17a. Jiang, X.-Z., Morgan, K. T.,
Beauchamp, R. O. Jr. 1985. Histopathology of acute and subacute nasal toxicity.
In *Toxicology of the Nasal Passages,* ed.
C. S. Barrow. New York: Hemisphere.
In press
18. Proctor, D. F. 1982. The mucociliary
system. In *The Nose, Upper Airway
Physiology and the Atmospheric Environment,* ed. D. F. Proctor, I. Anderson, pp. 245–70. Amsterdam: Elsevier
North Holland
19. Morgan, K. T., Patterson, D. L., Gross,
E. A. 1983. Formaldehyde and the nasal
mucociliary apparatus. In *Formaldehyde
Toxicology, Epidemiology, and Mechanisms,* ed. J. J. Clary, J. E. Gibson, R. S.
Waritz, pp. 193–210. New York: Dekker
20. Morgan, K. T., Jiang, X. Z., Patterson,
D. L., Gross, E. A. 1984. The nasal
mucociliary apparatus. Correlation of
structure and function in the rat. *Am. Rev.
Resp. Dis.* 130:275–81
21. Egle, J. L. 1972. Retention of inhaled
formaldehyde, propionaldehyde and
acrolein in the dog. *Arch. Environ.
Health* 25:119–24
22. Lucas, A., Douglas, L. C. 1934. Principles underlying ciliary activity in the respiratory tract. *Arch. Otolaryngol.*
20:518–41

23. Marshall, T. C., Hahn, F. F., Henderson, R. F., Silbaugh, S. A., Hobbs, C.
H. 1982. Subchronic inhalation exposure
of guinea pigs to formaldehyde. In *Inhalation Toxicology Res. Inst. Ann.
Rep., 1981–1982, LMF-102, UC-48,* pp.
423–27. Albuquerque: Lovelace Biomed. Environ. Res. Inst.
24. Anderson, I., Molhave, L. 1983. Controlled human studies with formaldehyde. See Ref. 14, pp. 154–65
25. Morgan, K. T., Patterson, D. L., Gross,
E. A. 1984. Frog palate mucociliary
apparatus: Structure, function and response to formaldehyde gas. *Fund. Appl.
Toxicol.* 4:58–68
25a. Creeth, J. M. 1978. Constituents of
mucus and their separation. *Br. Med.
Bull.* 34:17–24
25b. French, D., Edsall, J. T. 1945. The
reactions of formaldehyde with amino
acids and proteins. *Adv. Prot. Chem.*
2:277–335
25c. Kihara, Y., Kasuga, M., Tonaka, K.
1962. Reaction of aldehydes on starch.
Denpun Kogyo Gakkaishi 10:1–6
26. Morgan, K. T. 1983. Localization of
areas of inhibition of nasal mucociliary
function in rats following in vivo exposure to formaldehyde. *Am. Rev. Resp.
Dis.* 127:166 (Abstr.)
27. Macklin, C. C. 1956. Induction of bronchial cancer by local massing of carcinogen concentrate in outdrifting mucus. *J.
Thor. Surg.* 31:238–44
28. von Hippel, P. H., Wong, K.-Y. 1971.
Dynamic aspects of native DNA structure: Kinetics of the formaldehyde reaction with calf thymus DNA. *J. Mol. Biol.*
61:587–613
29. Lukashin, A. V., Vologodskii, A. V.,
Frank-Kamenetskii, M. D., Lyub-
chenko, Y. L. 1976. Fluctuational opening of the double helix as revealed by
theoretical and experimental study of
DNA interaction with formaldehyde. *J.
Mol. Biol.* 108:665–82
30. Swenberg, J. A., Gross, E. A., Martin,
J., Popp, J. A. 1983. Mechanisms of
formaldehyde toxicity. See Ref. 14, pp.
132–47
31. Swenberg, J. A., Gross, E. A., Randall,
H. W., Barrow, C. S. 1983. The effect of
formaldehyde exposure on cytotoxicity
and cell proliferation. See Ref. 19, pp.
225–36
32. Kerns, W. D., Donofrio, D. J., Pavkov,
K. L. 1983. The chronic effects of formaldehyde inhalation in rats and mice: a
preliminary report. See Ref. 14, pp. 111–
31
33. Rusch, G. M., Bolte, J. F., Rinehart, W.

E. 1983. A 26-week inhalation toxicity study with formaldehyde. See Ref. 14, pp. 98–110

33a. Swenberg, J. A., Gross, E. A., Randall, H. W. 1985. Localization and quantitations of cell proliferation following exposure to nasal irritants. See Ref. 17a

34. Casanova-Schmitz, M., Starr, T. B., Heck, H. d'A. 1984. Differentiation between metabolic incorporation and covalent binding in the labeling of macromolecules in the rat nasal mucosa and bone marrow by inhaled [^{14}C]-and [^{3}H]formaldehyde. *Toxicol. Appl. Pharmacol.* 76:26–44

35. Ross, W. E., Shipley, N. 1980. Relationship between DNA damage and survival in formaldehyde-treated mouse cells. *Mut. Res.* 79:277–83

36. Grafstrom, R. C., Fornace, A. J. Jr., Autrup, H., Lechner, J. F., Harris, C. C. 1983. Formaldehyde damage to DNA and inhibition of DNA repair in human bronchial cells. *Science* 220:216–18

37. Ragan, D. L., Boreiko, C. J. 1981. Initiation of C3H/10T1/2 cell transformation by formaldehyde. *Cancer Lett.* 13:325–31

38. Goldmacher, V. S., Thilly, W. G. 1983.

Formaldehyde is mutagenic for cultured human cells. *Mut. Res.* 116:417–22

39. Casanova-Schmitz, M., Heck, H. d'A. 1983. Effects of formaldehyde exposure on the extractability of DNA from proteins in the rat nasal mucosa. *Toxicol. Appl. Pharmacol.* 70:121–32

40. Magana-Schwenke, N., Moustacchi, E. 1980. Biochemical analysis of damage induced in yeast by formaldehyde. III. Repair of induced cross-links between DNA and proteins in the wild-type and in excision-deficient strains. *Mut. Res.* 70:29–35

41. Starr, T. B., Buck, R. D. 1984. The importance of delivered dose in estimating low-dose cancer risk from inhalation exposure to formaldehyde. *Fund. Appl. Toxicol.* 4:740–53

42. Hoel, D. G., Kaplan, N. L., Anderson, M. W. 1983. Implication of nonlinear kinetics on risk estimation in carcinogenesis. *Science* 219:1032–37

43. Cohn, M. S. 1981. *Revised Carcinogenic Risk Assessment of Urea-Formaldehyde Foam Insulation: Estimates of Cancer Risk due to Inhalation of Formaldehyde Released by UFFI.* Oct. 26. Washington, DC: US Cons. Prod. Safety Comm.

Ann. Rev. Pharmacol. Toxicol. 1985. 25:769–75

REVIEW OF REVIEWS

E. Leong Way

Department of Pharmacology, University of California, San Francisco, California
94143

NEW SERIES

Supply and demand are the cornerstone of a free economy and, although I am
an advocate of the system, I sometimes am bewildered by its economics. This
past year a number of new book series have emerged, so publishers must
believe that their ventures are likely to reap a profit. However, at the prices
some of these new publications cost, will they?

Libraries, let alone individuals, would strain to pay eight hundred dollars a
year for twelve issues of a volume (1) whose list of authors and titles offers no
greater enticements than existing series. Granted that it is produced by a
non-profit organization, what a bargain the Annual Reviews volume is and, in
contrast, what a profit some private publishers seek. Of course, some series are
being offered at prices more reasonable than eight hundred dollars, but they still
are not inexpensive.

Grahame-Smith, Hippius & Winokur tackle a highly ambitious undertaking
in their two-volume biennial critical survey of the international literature in
psychopharmacology (2). Part 1 of this work discusses the preclinical and Part
2 the clinical aspects of the topic. The first volume covers the basic pharmacology of agents used to treat the psychiatric states as well as the pharmacology of
abused drugs. In general, the discussion attempts to relate drug affinity,
binding sites, and neuroamine disposition to pathological states and drug
action. Conceding that most of the drugs in use have been discovered serendipi-
tously, the authors offer some arguments about why deeper insight into mental
illness can come only from an understanding of the basic processes involved.
However, they also have caveats. Even though excellent correlations can be
drawn between the disposition of an endogenous substance and the beneficial
effect of a drug, this does not necessarily mean that the relationship is primary.
For example, the impressive correlation between the ability of the phe-

769

0362-1642/85/415-0769$02.00

nothiazines to block the action of dopamine in the brain and their antipsychotic potency implied a disturbance in dopaminergic neuronal function that led to the dopamine hypothesis of schizophrenia. However, the possibility that drug effects are mediated at a secondary level can easily lead to erroneous conclusions. It has not been established that dopamine is a primary etiological factor in schizophrenia, and in fact such evidence is meager, if not missing. By analogy, albeit a foolish one, we can make a case for a cholinergic hypothesis based on curare's ability to prevent physical violence during a schizophrenic paranoid delusion.

Part 2 of their survey of psychopharmacological literature, edited by Hippius & Winokur, deals with the clinical aspects of psychopharmacology, but the initial chapters seem to differ little from some of those in Part 1. The meat of the volume is the chapters updating the clinical pharmacology of the conventional psychotropic drugs (neuroleptics, antidepressants, tranquilizers, stimulants, and lithium). Also considered as a cause of mental disorder are hormones, peptides, and miscellaneous agents. Pharmacologists can be educated about the clinical application of certain agents whose rationale is not clear (e.g. lithium in cluster headaches, tricylic antidepressants in chronic pain, and imipramine in enuresis). The book also contains interesting chapters on drugs for the treatment of social, sexual, and childhood disorders, and a fairly comprehensive chapter on alcoholism. Both volumes are informative and useful but, with so many authors, the editors will have quite a task updating the volumes on a biennial basis.

Parnham & Bruinvels edit a new series, *Discoveries in Pharmacology* (3), to compete with *Chronicles of Drug Discovery,* which I reviewed here two years ago (4). The first volume of the present series emphasizes psycho- and neuropharmacology. Bonta's introduction mixes story telling with smatterings of history and science; the author unabashedly admits this but writes a chapter that is fun to read. The main thesis of the presentation by Kramer & Merlin on the ancient use of psychoactive drugs is that such use was practiced widely in the Old World and was a key element in shaping North African, Asiatic, and European cultures. Microfossil evidence is cited to show that Neanderthal man, a subspecies of *Homo sapiens,* was buried with plants used locally even in modern times.

Moving into more current aspects of the subject, Bacq provides an intimate account of the controversy over the theory of the chemical transmission of nerve impulses. Sharp discussions ventilate without acrimony the arguments of the two opposing schools, led by Dale (pro) and Eccles (con). This great debate is a model of how scientific discussion can be conducted with friendly feeling and mutual respect. Bowman's style is monographic in his chronological account of the development of our knowledge of peripherally acting muscle relaxants. The chapter on the use of drugs for testing psychotic behavior is divided into several subsections, and some of the authors of these subsections played a part in the introduction of drugs for this purpose. Their discoveries, emanating largely from the clinic rather than the laboratory, were not always well received. Initially the therapeutic application of chlorpromazine, lithium, tricyclic antidepressants, and monoamine oxidase inhibitors was opposed vigorously by many experts in the field.

Sourkes & Gaulthier trace the discovery of levodopa and dopamine agonists in the treatment of Parkinson's disease. In this instance, the application of these agents resulted from information on dopamine generated in the laboratory using histochemical, metabolic, and pathological techniques. Hulzer & Lembeck's account of our developing understanding of pain makes rather dull reading because their recitation is telegraphic, but Livingston compensates in part with an account on the development of anesthesia. Garretta and I provide a history of the narcotic antagonists, pointing out that the conceptualization and development of narcotic antagonists were a significant achievement because so much practical knowledge has grown out of their discovery, prime examples being the development of potent analgetics with low-addiction potential, the isolation of opiopeptins (or endorphins), and the characterization of opiate receptors. There are also chapters on hypnotics by Koppanyi, antiepileptics by Meijer, Meinardi, & Binnie, benzodiazepines by Halfly, and neuropeptides by de Wied. In general, the *Discoveries in Pharmacology* is of greater reading interest than its older competitor. We will have to wait and see whether both volumes can survive.

CAFFEINE

Dew has edited a monograph on caffeine, important mainly for its timely analysis of the possible long-range effects of the substance (5); activist groups questioning the innocuousness of beverages containing caffeine have pressed the regulatory agencies of several countries to reevaluate the consequences to society of caffeine intake. First, one chapter covers thoroughly the bioavailability of caffeine, including its measurement in body fluids, absorption, distribution, metabolism, and excretion, followed by an interspecies comparison of these aspects of the subject. Epidemiological studies of the intake of coffee, tea, cocoa, and soft drinks provide a measure of the range of consumption, including the maximum amount of caffeine likely to be ingested. The discussion then centers on the cardiovascular, behavioral, and neuroendocrine effects of caffeine and their dose-response relationships. Finally, the teratogenic, mutagenic, carcinogenic, and genotoxic potential of caffeine is critically analyzed. The reviewers do not question that high doses of caffeine can produce serious pharmacological and toxicological effects. However, the experts overwhelmingly agreed that the amount of caffeine in the daily diet does not constitute a health hazard. Nonetheless, it would not surprise me if in a few years another isolated study reporting adverse toxic effects of high doses of caffeine will result in another inquiry.

NEW CARDIOVASCULAR AGENTS

Scriabine edits a review of thirteen cardiovascular drugs recently approved for use or under clinical investigation (6). The calcium channel blockers receive considerable attention, although under this category are various types of drugs that may act preferentially at different sites to find selective, sometimes overlapping, applications. Four antihypertensives are discussed, including an angiotensin converting–enzyme inhibitor (enalapril), a β-receptor antagonist (celiprolol), a calcium channel inhibitor (nitrendipine), and a loop diuretic (muzolimine). Under the rubric of antiarrhythmics, another calcium channel blocker (verapamil) and a prolongator of action potential duration (clofilium) are considered. Four antianginal agents are covered, including two more calcium entry inhibitors (dilitiazem and bepridil), a vascular smooth muscle relaxant (molidomine), and a new type of agent that acts to slow the heart by an effect on the pacemaker cells of the cardiac sinus node (alinidine). Prenalterol, a selective β-adrenoreceptor agonist, is listed as a cardiac stimulant, and yet another calcium entry blocker is listed as a cerebral antihypoxic agent for treating migraine (flunarizine).

RECEPTOLOGY

Kenakin provides a thorough critical analysis of the theory and methods used to classify drug and drug receptors in isolated tissues (9). The reader cannot help but be impressed by the scope and depth of his coverage as well as by his scholarly, authoritative treatment of the subject matter. Kenakin points out, for instance, that if two agonists under comparison have large differences in receptor reserve, selective desensitization or the selective irreversible inhibition of responses by an alkylating agent can yield misleading information. Thus, if one agonist has a 90% receptor reserve and another a 40% receptor reserve, then the responses to the latter agonist will be more sensitive to the removal of portions of the receptor pool either by desensitization or by alkylation. In addition, the application of theoretical considerations can be useful in the screening of new drugs. Thus, the most potent agonist may not be the most useful if its potency is related mainly to a high efficacy rather than to a high affinity, because drugs of high affinity but low efficacy are more susceptible to the efficiency of receptor coupling than are drugs of high efficacy. Moreover, the concept that a screening program can stress high selectivity presupposes the existence of a unique receptor or mechanism, but two activities in one molecule may be critical to the selectivity or overall activity of that molecule in vivo. The presentation is invaluable for the graduate student and the post-doctoral fellow.

OPIOIDS

Duggan & North provide a comprehensive review of the electrophysiology of opioids, implicating calcium in opioid action (7). The coverage includes in vitro as well as in vivo systems and an analysis of the methods used for opioid administration. Considerable evidence is cited to support the notion that calcium is more basic to the acute action of opioids than adenosine $3'-5'$-cyclic monophosphate (cAMP). Although the inhibition of adenylate cyclase has been popular as the suggested mechanism by which opioids produce their effects on neurons, electrophysiological studies do not to support this hypothesis; manipulations designed to elevate cellular cAMP by administering dibutyryl cAMP or a phosphodiesterase inhibitor (isobutylmethylxanthine) failed to alter neuronal firing in systems known to be highly sensitive to opioids.

Opioids inhibit neuronal firing in sensitive cells that contain a high density of opiate binding sites. In certain exceptional cases, when excitation is noted, the effect can be considered the result of disinhibition. The inhibition of neuronal firing after the acute administration of opioids is believed to be due to a reduction in the release of excitatory neurotransmitters that is calcium dependent. However, the mode by which calcium may be involved has not been clearly established. The mechanism the authors seem to opt for is that opioids cause cell membrane hyperpolarization that, following a period of repetitive firing, is particularly susceptible to enhancement by opiates. Other possibilities whereby transmitter release can be reduced by opioids can be attributed to hyperpolarization of nerves leading to propagation block, to a block of voltage-dependent calcium currents, or to interference with the ability of intracellular calcium currents to promote release. Based on studies in slices of the *locus caeruleus* and *substantia gelatinosa,* the researchers concluded that hyperpolarization induced by opioids results from an increase in potassium conductance that then could lead to a shunting of the calcium action potential and an inhibition of transmitter release. The mechanism for the increased potassium conductance has not been determined, but the elevation of intracellular calcium as a result of its displacement from sequestered sites has been suggested. This seems reasonable, since the binding of calcium in an enriched nerve ending preparation has been shown to be altered by opiates at the inner synaptic plasma membrane and synaptic vesicles. These findings are contained in our review summarizing the neurochemical evidence for implicating calcium in the acute and chronic actions of opiates (8).

Akil and company review the current knowledge of the biology and function of opiopeptins (endogenous opioids) (10). The various types of opiopeptins, their biosynthesis, processing, anatomy, and possible function are discussed in an attempt to provide some understanding of a rapidly moving field. To this end, the committee of six have succeeded in authoring a concise summary of the state of knowledge of the three opioid gene families, their distribution in the central nervous system (and the periphery as well), and the multiple receptors through which they interact. Their possible relevance to homeostatic function, which is related to stress, pain, and cardiovascular action, is presented in an interesting and provocative manner. The omission of their relationship with other anterior pituitary hormones is disappointing; nevertheless, this review is recommended for its readability and its expertise.

DRUG DEPENDENCE

In addition to the usual original reports on the chemistry and the basic and clinical pharmacology of substances of abuse, the proceedings of the 45th annual meeting of the Committee on Problems of Drug Dependence, edited by Harris, contains several presentations of general pharmacological interest (11). Isbell eulogizes H. Frank Fraser, who made many notable contributions to psychopharmacology, including the development of a quantitative methodology for the assessment of the behavioral effects of drugs in human subjects. He also carried out extensive studies with the opiates, nalorphine, and the barbiturates on addicts at the Addiction Research Center at the US public health hospital in Lexington. Isbell, the late Abe Wikler, and Fraser were the acknowledged giants in research on drug dependence and made the center internationally renowned.

Nathan B. Eddy award winner Eric Simon summarizes his work on the isolation of the opiate receptor. Of particular interest is his evidence for a physical separation of the κ site from the μ and δ sites. Martin, who developed the multireceptor concept for opiates, offers a steric theory of opioid agonist, antagonist, antagonist-agonist, and partial agonist action. He uses three-dimensional models to explain the diverse effects of these substances and considers a large number of reactive sites that play two roles: their occupancy initiates a pharmacological action and they orient the drug in the receptor. Kornetsky cautions that attempts to relate the endorphins (or opiopeptins) to analgesia may overlook a more general role for these endogenous substances in stress as well as a possible role for them in modulating the attentional component of perception. O'Brien discusses the role of conditioning in drug dependence and describes problems in attempts to apply extinction methodology to the treatment of drug addicts. Kadden, Pomerleau, & Meyer examine a number of clinical and experimental findings that implicate conditioned respondents as a factor in the stimulus control of problem drinking.

Peturrsson & Lader have put together a volume on dependence on tranquilizers (12). The term *tranquilizer* is restricted to the diazepams and I rather like that. I never could reconcile myself to using the terms *major tranquilizers* for antipsychotic drugs and *minor tranquilizers* for anti-anxiety agents. In recent years dependence on diazepams has become an increasingly apparent problem. Duration of intake is the most reliable measure of the likelihood of developing physical dependence, but dosage, of course, is also a major consideration. High dosage intake for four months can lead to physical dependence, and, although a withdrawal syndrome becomes apparent in only 5–10% of misusers after six months of use, the incidence increases to 25–45% after two to four years. Withdrawal signs and symptoms include severe sleep disturbance, irritability, increased tension and anxiety, perceptual hypersensitivity, panic attacks, tremors, sweating, nausea, retching, and weight loss. The direct way to handle this problem is to educate primary-care physicians to detect diazepam dependence and to treat it by graded withdrawal. Most important, however, physicians must learn not to prescribe such agents indiscriminately.

Literature Cited

1. Sartorelli, A. C., Bowman, W. C., Breckenridge, A. M. 1983. *Pharmacology and Therapeutics*. Oxford: Pergamon
2. Grahame-Smith, D. G., Hippius, H., Winokur, G., eds. 1983. *Psychopharmacology. 1. A Biennial Critical Survey of the International Literature. Part 1: Preclinical, Part 2: Clinical*. Princeton: Excerpta Medica. 482 pp; 456 pp.
3. Parnham, M. J., Bruinvels, J. 1983. *Discoveries in Pharmacology. Vol. 1: Psycho- and Neuro-Pharmacology*. New York: Elsevier. 507 pp.
4. Way, E. Leong. 1983. Review of reviews. *Ann. Rev. Pharmacol. and Toxicol.* 23:646–56
5. Dew, P. B. 1984. *Caffeine—Perspective from Recent Research*. Berlin: Springer Verlag. 260 pp.
6. Scriabine, A. 1984. *New Drugs Annual: Cardiovascular Drugs Vol. 2*. New York: Raven. 273 pp.
7. Duggan, A. W., North, R. A. 1984. Electrophysiology of opioids. *Pharmacol. Rev.* 35:219–81
8. Chapman, D., Way, E. L. 1983. Pharmacologic consequences of calcium interactions with opioid alkaloids and peptides. *Am. Chem. Soc. Symp.* Ser. 201:119–42
9. Kenakin, T. P. 1984. The classification of drugs and drug receptors in isolated tissues. *Pharmacol. Rev.* 36:165–222
10. Akil, H., Watson, S., Young, E., Lewis, M., Khachaturian, H., Walker, J. 1984. Endogenous opioids: Biology and function. *Ann. Rev. Neurosci.* 7:223–55
11. Harris, L. S., ed. 1983. Problems of drug dependence. *Proc. Ann. Meet. Comm. Probl. Drug Depend.* 45th NIDA Res. Monogr. 49. Washington, D.C.: GPO. 455 pp.
12. Peturrsson, H., Lader, M. 1984. *Dependence on Tranquilizers*. Oxford: Oxford Univ. Press. 130 pp.

SUBJECT INDEX

CUMULATIVE INDEXES

CONTRIBUTING AUTHORS, VOLUMES 21–25

A

Abou-Donia, M. B., 21:511–48
Alarie, Y., 25:325–47
Alousi, A. A., 24:275–328
Andresen, B. D., 21:575–96
Antonaccio, M. J., 22:57–87
Aposhian, H. V., 23:193–215
Archer, S., 25:485–508
Aw, T. Y., 25:714–44
Awouters, F., 23:279–301

B

Baird, A., 25:463–83
Banner, W. Jr., 24:65–83
Beckman, D. A., 24:483–500
Bend, J. R., 25:97–125
Bernstein, K. N., 24:105–20
Bianchetti, A., 25:249–73
Bianchine, J. R., 21:575–96
Bloom, F. E., 23:151–70
Böhlen, P., 25:463–83
Bolard, J., 23:303–30
Bolender, R. P., 21:549–73
Bourne, H. R., 21:251–64
Boyd, M. R., 23:217–38
Brajtburg, J., 23:303–30
Brammer, G. L., 22:643–61
Brater, D. C., 23:45–62
Brent, R. L., 24:483–500
Brezenoff, H. E., 22:341–81
Brown, R. D., 25:667–89

C

Camitta, B. M., 21:231–49
Cannon, J. G., 23:103–30
Caranasos, G. J., 25:67–95
Carr, C. J., 22:19–29
Casida, J. E., 23:413–38
Cauvin, C., 23:373–96
Chan, W. Y., 23:131–49
Chen, K. K., 21:1–6
Chenoweth, M. B., 25:33–40
Cluff, L. E., 25:67–95
Cohen, M. L., 25:307–23
Cooper, S. A., 23:617–47
Correia, M. A., 23:481–503

D

Couri, D., 22:145–66
Creese, I., 21:357–91
Critchley, J. A. J. H., 23:87–101
Cuatrecasas, P., 23:461–79

Dailey, J. W., 25:667–89
Davis, H. P., 21:323–56
Dedrick, R. L., 24:85–103
Dixon, R. L., 25:567–92
Duckles, S. P., 24:65–83
Duran, D. O., 21:575–96
Durant, N. N., 23:505–39

E

Eisen, H. J., 21:431–62
Eneanya, D. I., 21:575–96
Eneroth, P., 23:259–78
Esch, F., 25:463–83
Evans, R. H., 21:165–204

F

Fahim, M., 22:465–90
Fara, J. W., 24:199–236
Farah, A. E., 24:275–328
Farfel, Z., 21:251–64
Foreman, J. C., 21:63–81
Fridovich, I., 23:239–57
Fudenberg, H. H., 24:147–74
Furchgott, R. F., 24:175–97

G

Gammon, D. W., 23:413–38
Gibson, J. E., 25:745–67
Giuliano, R., 22:341–81
Glickman, A. H., 23:413–38
Goldberg, A. M., 25:225–47
Goldstein, D. B., 24:43–64
Guillemin, R., 25:463–83
Gustafson, E., 25:413–31
Gustafsson, J. Å., 23:259–78
Guth, P. S., 22:383–412
Guzelian, P. S., 22:89–113

H

Halpert, J., 22:321–39
Han, J. S., 22:193–220
Handwerger, S., 25:349–80
Harper, G. P., 21:205–29
Harris, R. A., 21:83–111
Henderson, E. G., 23:505–39
Herbette, L., 22:413–34
Hershey, L., 24:361–86
Hinson, J. L., 25:667–89
Hirasawa, K., 25:147–70
Hjelmeland, L. M., 21:431–62
Ho, I. K., 21:83–111
Hodgson, E., 24:19–42
Hökfelt, T., 23:259–78
Holaday, J. W., 23:541–94
Holcenberg, J. S., 21:231–49
Holohan, P. D., 23:65–85
Hondeghem, L. M., 24:387–423

I

Ignarro, L. J., 25:171–91
Inscoe, M. N., 22:297–320
Iversen, L. L., 23:1–28

J

Jacobs, S., 23:461–79
Jamasbi, R., 21:113–63
Janssen, P. A. J., 23:279–301
Johnson, E. M., 21:417–29

K

Kador, P. F., 25:691–714
Kadowitz, P. J., 25:171–91
Kamm, K. E., 25:593–620
Kaplowitz, N., 25:715–44
Katz, A. M., 22:413–34
Katzung, B. G., 24:387–423
Keats, A. S., 25:41–65
Kendrick, Z. V., 25:275–305
Kinoshita, J. H., 25:691–714
Knutson, J. C., 22:517–54
Kobayashi, G. S., 23:303–30
Kulkarni, A. P., 24:19–42

792

CHAPTER TITLES, VOLUMES 21–25

ORDER FORM

Annual Reviews Inc.

A NONPROFIT SCIENTIFIC PUBLISHER

4139 EL CAMINO WAY • PALO ALTO, CA 94306-9981 • (415) 493-4400

Orders for Annual Reviews Inc. publications may be placed through your bookstore; subscription agent; participating professional societies; or directly from Annual Reviews Inc. by mail or telephone (paid by credit card or purchase order). Prices subject to change without notice.

Individuals: Prepayment required in U.S. funds or charged to American Express, MasterCard, or Visa.
Institutional Buyers: Please include purchase order.
Students: Special rates are available to qualified students. Refer to Annual Reviews *Prospectus* or contact Annual Reviews Inc. office for information.
Professional Society Members: Members whose professional societies have a contractural arrangement with Annual Reviews may order books through their society at a special discount. Check with your society for information.

Regular orders: When ordering current or back volumes, please list the volumes you wish by volume number.
Standing orders: (New volume in the series will be sent to you automatically each year upon publication. Cancellation may be made at any time.) Please indicate volume number to begin standing order.
Prepublication orders: Volumes not yet published will be shipped in month and year indicated.
California orders: Add applicable sales tax.
Postage paid (4th class bookrate /surface mail) by Annual Reviews Inc.

ANNUAL REVIEWS SERIES		Prices Postpaid per volume USA/elsewhere	Regular Order Please send:	Standing Order Begin with:
			Vol. number	Vol. number
Annual Review of ANTHROPOLOGY				
Vols. 1-10	(1972-1981)	$20.00/$21.00		
Vol. 11	(1982)	$22.00/$25.00		
Vols. 12-13	(1983-1984)	$27.00/$30.00		
Vol. 14	(avail. Oct. 1985)	$27.00/$30.00	Vol(s). _____	Vol. _____
Annual Review of ASTRONOMY AND ASTROPHYSICS				
Vols. 1-19	(1963-1981)	$20.00/$21.00		
Vol. 20	(1982)	$22.00/$25.00		
Vols. 21-22	(1983-1984)	$44.00/$47.00		
Vol. 23	(avail. Sept. 1985)	$44.00/$47.00	Vol(s). _____	Vol. _____
Annual Review of BIOCHEMISTRY				
Vols. 29-34, 36-50	(1960-1965; 1967-1981)	$21.00/$22.00		
Vol. 51	(1982)	$23.00/$26.00		
Vols. 52-53	(1983-1984)	$29.00/$32.00		
Vol. 54	(avail. July 1985)	$29.00/$32.00	Vol(s). _____	Vol. _____
Annual Review of BIOPHYSICS				
Vols. 1-10	(1972-1981)	$20.00/$21.00		
Vol. 11	(1982)	$22.00/$25.00		
Vols. 12-13	(1983-1984)	$47.00/$50.00		
Vol. 14	(avail. June 1985)	$47.00/$50.00	Vol(s). _____	Vol. _____
Annual Review of CELL BIOLOGY				
Vol. 1	(avail. Nov. 1985)	est. $27.00/$30.00	Vol. _____	Vol. _____
Annual Review of EARTH AND PLANETARY SCIENCES				
Vols. 1-9	(1973-1981)	$20.00/$21.00		
Vol. 10	(1982)	$22.00/$25.00		
Vols. 11-12	(1983-1984)	$44.00/$47.00		
Vol. 13	(avail. May 1985)	$44.00/$47.00	Vol(s). _____	Vol. _____
Annual Review of ECOLOGY AND SYSTEMATICS				
Vols. 1-12	(1970-1981)	$20.00/$21.00		
Vol. 13	(1982)	$22.00/$25.00		
Vols. 14-15	(1983-1984)	$27.00/$30.00		
Vol. 16	(avail. Nov. 1985)	$27.00/$30.00	Vol(s). _____	Vol. _____

1

		Prices Postpaid per volume USA/elsewhere	Regular Order Please send:	Standing Order Begin with:
			Vol. number	Vol. number

Annual Review of **ENERGY**

Vols. 1-6	(1976-1981)	$20.00/$21.00		
Vol. 7	(1982)	$22.00/$25.00		
Vols. 8-9	(1983-1984)	$56.00/$59.00		
Vol. 10	(avail. Oct. 1985)	$56.00/$59.00	Vol(s)._____	Vol._____

Annual Review of **ENTOMOLOGY**

Vols. 8-16, 18-26	(1963-1971; 1973-1981)	$20.00/$21.00		
Vol. 27	(1982)	$22.00/$25.00		
Vols. 28-29	(1983-1984)	$27.00/$30.00		
Vol. 30	(avail. Jan. 1985)	$27.00/$30.00	Vol(s)._____	Vol._____

Annual Review of **FLUID MECHANICS**

Vols. 1-5, 7-13	(1969-1973; 1975-1981)	$20.00/$21.00		
Vol. 14	(1982)	$22.00/$25.00		
Vols. 15-16	(1983-1984)	$28.00/$31.00		
Vol. 17	(avail. Jan. 1985)	$28.00/$31.00	Vol(s)._____	Vol._____

Annual Review of **GENETICS**

Vols. 1-15	(1967-1981)	$20.00/$21.00		
Vol. 16	(1982)	$22.00/$25.00		
Vols. 17-18	(1983-1984)	$27.00/$30.00		
Vol. 19	(avail. Dec. 1985)	$27.00/$30.00	Vol(s)._____	Vol._____

Annual Review of **IMMUNOLOGY**

| Vols. 1-2 | (1983-1984) | $27.00/$30.00 | | |
| Vol. 3 | (avail. April 1985) | $27.00/$30.00 | Vol(s)._____ | Vol._____ |

Annual Review of **MATERIALS SCIENCE**

Vols. 1-11	(1971-1981)	$20.00/$21.00		
Vol. 12	(1982)	$22.00/$25.00		
Vols. 13-14	(1983-1984)	$64.00/$67.00		
Vol. 15	(avail. Aug. 1985)	$64.00/$67.00	Vol(s)._____	Vol._____

Annual Review of **MEDICINE: Selected Topics in the Clinical Sciences**

Vols. 1-3, 5-15	(1950-1952; 1954-1964)	$20.00/$21.00		
Vols. 17-32	(1966-1981)	$20.00/$21.00		
Vol. 33	(1982)	$22.00/$25.00		
Vols. 34-35	(1983-1984)	$27.00/$30.00		
Vol. 36	(avail. April 1985)	$27.00/$30.00	Vol(s)._____	Vol._____

Annual Review of **MICROBIOLOGY**

Vols. 17-35	(1963-1981)	$20.00/$21.00		
Vol. 36	(1982)	$22.00/$25.00		
Vols. 37-38	(1983-1984)	$27.00/$30.00		
Vol. 39	(avail. Oct. 1985)	$27.00/$30.00	Vol(s)._____	Vol._____

Annual Review of **NEUROSCIENCE**

Vols. 1-4	(1978-1981)	$20.00/$21.00		
Vol. 5	(1982)	$22.00/$25.00		
Vols. 6-7	(1983-1984)	$27.00/$30.00		
Vol. 8	(avail. March 1985)	$27.00/$30.00	Vol(s)._____	Vol._____

Annual Review of **NUCLEAR AND PARTICLE SCIENCE**

Vols. 12-31	(1962-1981)	$22.50/$23.50		
Vol. 32	(1982)	$25.00/$28.00		
Vols. 33-34	(1983-1984)	$30.00/$33.00		
Vol. 35	(avail. Dec. 1985)	$30.00/$33.00	Vol(s)._____	Vol._____

SEE ORDERING INFORMATION ON PAGE 4